Y0-AGF-128

AMERICAN HANDBOOK OF PSYCHIATRY

Volume Four

AMERICAN HANDBOOK OF PSYCHIATRY

Silvano Arieti, EDITOR-IN-CHIEF

Volume One
The Foundations of Psychiatry
EDITED BY SILVANO ARIETI

Volume Two
Child and Adolescent Psychiatry, Sociocultural and Community Psychiatry
EDITED BY GERALD CAPLAN

Volume Three
Adult Clinical Psychiatry
EDITED BY SILVANO ARIETI AND EUGENE B. BRODY

Volume Four
Organic Disorders and Psychosomatic Medicine
EDITED BY MORTON F. REISER

Volume Five
Treatment
EDITED BY DANIEL X. FREEDMAN AND JARL E. DYRUD

Volume Six
New Psychiatric Frontiers
EDITED BY DAVID A. HAMBURG AND H. KEITH H. BRODIE

AMERICAN HANDBOOK OF PSYCHIATRY

Silvano Arieti · Editor-in-Chief

VOLUME FOUR

Organic Disorders and Psychosomatic Medicine

MORTON F. REISER · *Editor*

BASIC BOOKS, INC., PUBLISHERS · NEW YORK

Library of Congress Cataloging in Publication Data
Main entry under title:

Organic disorders and psychosomatic medicine.

(American handbook of psychiatry, second edition;
vo. 4)
Includes bibliographies.
1.   Neuropsychiatry.   2.   Medicine, Psychosomatic.
I.   Reiser, Morton F., 1919–   II.   Series.
RC435.A562 vol. 4 [RC343] 616.8′9′008s [616.08]
ISBN 0-465-00150-5   75-26588

Second Edition
Copyright © 1975 by Basic Books, Inc.
Printed in the United States of America
75 76 77 78 79   10 9 8 7 6 5 4 3 2 1

CONTRIBUTORS

Hyman Bakst, M.D.
Associate Attending in Medicine, Beth-Israel Hospital, New York; Assistant Clinical Professor of Medicine, Mount Sinai School of Medicine of the City University of New York.

D. Frank Benson, M.D.
Director, Neurobehavioral Center, Boston Veterans' Administration Hospital; Professor of Neurology, Boston University School of Medicine.

Malcolm B. Bowers, Jr., M.D.
Associate Professor of Psychiatry, Yale University School of Medicine, New Haven; Chief of Psychiatry, Yale-New Haven Hospital.

Henry Brill, M.D.
Regional Director, New York State Department of Mental Hygiene, Hauppaauge, New York; Clinical Professor of Psychiatry, Downstate Medical Center at Stony Brook, New York.

Jason W. Brown, M.D.
Associate Clinical Professor of Neurology, New York University Medical Center, New York.

Hilde Bruch, M.D.
Professor of Psychiatry, Baylor College of Medicine, Houston.

Walter L. Bruetsch, M.D.
Professor Emeritus, Neurology and Neuropathology, Indiana University School of Medicine, Indianapolis; Former Director, Research Laboratories, Central State Hospital, Indianapolis.

Ewald W. Busse, M.D.
J. P. Gibbons Professor of Psychiatry, Duke University, Durham, North Carolina; Associate Provost and Director, Medical and Allied Health Education, Duke University Medical Center.

George L. Engel, M.D.
Professor of Psychiatry and Professor of Medicine, University of Rochester School of Medicine, Rochester, New York.

Armando Ferraro, M.D.
Retired; Formerly, Clinical Professor of Psychiatry, College of Physicians and Surgeons, Columbia University, New York; Formerly, Head of the Research Department of Neuropathology, New York State Psychiatric Institute, New York.

Irving Fish, M.D.
Assistant Professor of Neurology (Pediatrics) and Acting Director, Division of Pediatric Neurology, New York University Medical Center, New York.

Shervert H. Frazier, M.D.
Psychiatrist-in-Chief, McLean Hospital, Belmont, Massachusetts; Professor of Psychiatry, Harvard Medical School, Boston.

Daniel X. Freedman, M.D.
Louis Block Professor of Biological Sciences and Chairman, Department of Psychiatry, University of Chicago Pritzker School of Medicine.

Sterling D. Garrard, M.D.
Chief of the Medical Division, Walter E. Fernald State School, Waltham, Massachusetts; Director, University Affiliated Program, Eunice Kennedy Shriver Center for Mental Retardation, Waltham.

Norman Geschwind, M.D.
James Jackson Putnam Professor of Neurology, Harvard Medical School, Boston.

Gilbert H. Glaser, M.D.
Professor of Neurology and Chairman, Department of Neurology, Yale University School of Medicine, New Haven; Neurologist-in-Chief, Yale-New Haven Hospital.

Kurt Goldstein, M.D.
Deceased.

Stanley S. Heller, M.D.
Assistant Professor of Clinical Psychiatry, College of Physicians and Surgeons, Columbia University, New York; Director, Psychiatric Consultation Service, St. Luke's Hospital, New York.

Myron A. Hofer, M.D.
Associate Attending Psychiatrist, Montefiore Hospital and Medical Center, Bronx, New York; Associate Professor of Psychiatry, Albert Einstein College of Medicine, Bronx.

George A. Jervis, M.D.
Director, Institute of Basic Research in Mental Retardation, Richmond, New York; Clinical Professor of Psychiatry, College of Physicians and Surgeons, Columbia University, New York.

Ismet Karacan, M.D., Med.D.Sc.
Professor of Psychiatry, Baylor College of Medicine, Houston; Associate Chief of Staff for Research, Veterans' Administration Hospital, Houston.

Mavis A. Kaufman, M.D.
Pathologist, New York State Psychiatric Institute, New York; Associate Professor of Neuropathology, College of Physicians and Surgeons, Columbia University, New York.

Chase Patterson Kimball, M.D.
Professor of Psychiatry, Medicine, and Behavioral Science, University of Chicago Pritzker School of Medicine.

Peter H. Knapp, M.D.
Associate Chairman, Division of Psychiatry, Boston University School of Medicine.

Lawrence C. Kolb, M.D.
Professor and Chairman, Department of Psychiatry, College of Physicians and Surgeons, Columbia University, New York; Director, New York State Psychiatric Institute, New York.

Donald S. Kornfeld, M.D.
Chief, Psychiatric Consultation Service, Columbia-Presbyterian Medical Center, New York; Professor of Clinical Psychiatry, College of Physicians and Surgeons, Columbia University, New York.

Zbigniew J. Lipowski, M.D.
Professor of Psychiatry, Dartmouth Medical School, Hanover, New Hampshire; Director, Psychiatric Consultation Service, Dartmouth-Hitchcock Medical Center.

F. Patrick McKegney, M.D.
Professor, Department of Psychiatry, University of Vermont College of Medicine, Burlington; Director, Consultation-Liaison Service, University of Vermont.

John W. Mason, M.D.
Chief, Department of Neuroendocrinology, Division of Neuropsychiatry, Walter Reed Army Institute of Research, Walter Reed Army Medical Center, Washington.

Nancy K. Mello, Ph.D.
Lecturer, Harvard Medical School, Boston; Psychologist, McLean Hospital, Belmont, Massachusetts.

Jack H. Mendelson, M.D.
Professor of Psychiatry, Harvard Medical School, Boston; Director, Alcohol and Drug Abuse Research Center, McLean Hospital, Belmont, Massachusetts.

J.P. Mohr, M.D.
Assistant Neurologist, Massachusetts General Hospital, Boston; Assistant Professor of Neurology, Harvard Medical School, Boston.

Donald Oken, M.D.
Professor and Chairman, Department of Psychiatry, Upstate Medical Center, State University of New York, Syracuse.

Joseph Ransohoff, M.D.
Professor and Chairman, Department of Neurosurgery, New York University Medical Center, New York; Director, Neurosurgery, Bellevue Hospital Center, New York.

Morton F. Reiser, M.D.
Professor and Chairman, Department of Psychiatry, Yale University School of Medicine, New Haven.

Julius B. Richmond, M.D.
Professor of Child Psychiatry and Human Development, and Professor of Preventive and Social Medicine in the Faculty of Public Health and the Faculty of Medicine, Harvard Medical School, Boston; Director, Judge Baker Guidance Center, Boston.

Leon Roizin, M.D.
Chief of Psychiatric Research (Neuropathology), New York State Psychiatric Institute, New York; Professor of Neuropathology, College of Physicians and Surgeons, Columbia University, New York.

Edward J. Sachar, M.D.
Professor of Psychiatry and Neuroscience, Albert Einstein College of Medicine, Bronx, New York.

I. Herbert Scheinberg, M.D.
Professor of Medicine, Albert Einstein College of Medicine, Bronx, New York; Visiting Physician, Bronx Municipal Hospital Center.

Raul C. Schiavi, M.D.
Associate Professor of Psychiatry, Mount Sinai School of Medicine of the City University of New York; Associate Attending Psychiatrist, Mount Sinai Hospital, New York.

John J. Schwab, M.D.
Professor and Chairman, Department of Psychiatry and Behavioral Sciences, University of Louisville School of Medicine, Louisville, Kentucky.

Murray Sidman, Ph.D.
Professor of Psychology, Northeastern University, Boston; Director of Behavioral Research, Eunice Kennedy Shriver Center for Mental Retardation of the Walter E. Fernald State School, Waltham, Massachusetts.

Marvin Stein, M.D.
Professor and Chairman, Department of Psychiatry, Mount Sinai School of Medicine of the City University of New York.

Albert J. Stunkard, M.D.
Professor of Psychiatry, Stanford University School of Medicine, Stanford, California.

Kenneth Tuerk, M.D.
Assistant Professor of Neurosurgery, School of Medicine, University of California at San Francisco; Assistant Chief of Neurosurgery, San Francisco General Hospital, San Francisco.

Herbert Weiner, M.D.
Chairman, Department of Psychiatry, Montefiore Hospital and Medical Center, Bronx, New York; Professor of Psychiatry and Neuroscience, Albert Einstein College of Medicine, Bronx.

John R. Whittier, M.D.
Director of Psychiatric Research, Creedmoor Institute for Psychobiologic Studies, New York State Department of Mental Hygiene, Queens Village, New York; Assistant Clinical Professor of Psychiatry, College of Physicians and Surgeons, Columbia University, New York.

Robert L. Williams, M.D.
D. C. and Irene Ellwood Professor and Chairman of Psychiatry, Baylor College of Medicine, Houston, Texas; Chief, Psychiatry Service, Methodist Hospital Texas Medical Center, Houston, Texas.

CONTENTS

Volume Four

PART TWO: *Psychosomatic Medicine*

PART ONE

Organic Disorders

PHYSICAL ILLNESS, THE PATIENT AND HIS ENVIRONMENT: PSYCHOSOCIAL FOUNDATIONS OF MEDICINE

Zbigniew J. Lipowski

❨ Introduction

THE DOMINANT FOCUS of this Volume is is on mind-body-environment interrelationships as they determine health and disease. Whether we talk of psychosomatic medicine, of organic brain syndromes, or of psychosocial aspects of physical illness, we are looking at different facets of the same basic theme, namely the interplay between man as a psychobiological unit and his environment as it pertains to health and disease.

The present Chapter has a twofold purpose: to outline briefly the contemporary conceptions of disease, and to provide a comprehensive framework for organizing our knowledge about human experience and behavior in physical illness and disability. The writer's approach to both these topics is both *holistic* and *ecological*. The holistic viewpoint sees body and personality as two integral aspects of a larger whole: *The person*. Soma and psyche are constructs reflecting two different modes of abstraction and methodological approaches to the study of man, the biophysical and the psychological, respectively. These different approaches involve two distinct languages for description of the phenomena studied and for the formulation of relevant explanatory statements.[117] Human body and personality constitute a unit shaped by continuous interplay between man's genetic endowment and his social and physical environment. The ecological perspective stresses the ways in which environment influences man and he in turn affects it.[122,174] Mind, body, and environment are viewed as elements of a dynamically interacting system. Human health and disease are a continuum of psychobiological states determined to a varying extent by biophysical, psychological, and social variables. These states involve all levels of human organization, from the molecular to the symbolic. This view is equally valid for what, in our dualistic language, we call psychiatric and physical, or mental and organic disorders.

A traditional approach in medicine has been to distinguish sharply between etiological and reactive factors in disease. This distinction still has some practical value in the search for specific causal agents and for preventive action. Yet dichotomies like "etiological" versus "reactive," "organic" versus "mental," or "psychosomatic" versus "somatopsychic," are becoming less sharp now with the emergence of multicausal and dynamic conceptions of disease and the recognition of complex feedback mechanisms.[79] For practical purposes, however, it is still useful to talk of psychological responses to physical illness, while keeping in mind that they are an integral part of it.

To reflect contemporary trends in both medicine and psychiatry it is appropriate to introduce this Volume with a conceptual bridge between medicine and behavioral sciences, and psychiatry, which has its roots in both. We shall call this approach *psychobiological ecology* of man. To develop it, we need to cross interdisciplinary boundaries in quest of a unified knowledge of mind-body-environment transactions. This quest has emerged as one of the most important scientific challenges of our times.

The major sections of this chapter are:

1. Contemporary conceptions of health and disease in man.
2. Determinants of psychological reaction to disease.
3. Modes of psychological response to physical disease, injury, and disability.
4. Personal meanings of illness.
5. The stages of illness and related challenges.
6. Terminal illness and management of the dying patient.

The above schema is an attempt to organize a complex and fragmented field for didactic purposes. It is a formidable task, but it is worth attempting to bring together a body of observations, concepts, and hypotheses equally relevant for the psychiatrist and other health professionals, as well as for behavioral scientists concerned with matters of human health and disease.

⟨ Contemporary Conceptions of Health and Disease in Man

The concept of disease has undergone repeated changes throughout the history of medicine.[38] A *unified concept* of it has been gaining ground in the 1970s. It reflects the influence of psychosomatic and ecological thought, as well as of social pressures for both personalized and universally available medical and psychiatric care. Current emphasis on a *comprehensive* approach to the prevention of disease and management of patients favors the holistic and ecological approaches. Social trends and involvement of behavioral scientists in medicine have combined to endorse psychosomatic thought which enriched the medical model of man as a biological *organism* with a psychosocial perspective of him as a person and a member of a given social group with which he interacts. The definition of disease in a recent medical dictionary reflects a contemporary concept of it. Disease is the "sum total of the reactions, physical and mental, made by a person to a noxious agent entering his body from without or arising within . . . , an injury, a congenital or hereditary defect, a metabolic disorder, a food deficiency or a degenerative process."[137]

The above definition conceives of disease as a state having no separate existence apart from a patient, a person. This is still a controversial point. Feinstein[49] advocates a distinction between the meaning of the terms "disease" and "illness," respectively. The former refers to data described in *impersonal* terms: anatomical, chemical, microbiological, physiological, etc.; the latter designates *clinical phenomena*, such as the host's subjective sensations (i.e., symptoms), and certain objective findings (i.e., signs).

In this writer's opinion the dictionary definition of disease is preferable to Feinstein's. For one thing, his concept of disease leaves out many psychiatric disorders which are not at this time describable in "impersonal" terms and would thus constitute nondiseases. Feinstein's distinction between disease and illness has a limited application and does not do justice to the contemporary trends to define disease, at least in part, by subjective and social as well as biophysical criteria. To avoid semantic confusion we use the terms "illness" and "disease" interchangeably.

The concept of disease is intimately related to prevailing views on etiology and pathological mechanisms. We note that the dictionary definition quoted above confines the range of causal factors to the biological, physical, and chemical ones. This leaves out *psychosocial factors* as a class of potentially noxious and pathogenic agents. *Symbolic stimuli* emanating from man's environment and impinging on him as information may be no less noxious than the other etiological factors listed.[122] Information evaluated by the recipient in terms of personal threat, loss, failure, or punishment, or eliciting conflicts and frustration with their concomitant affects, may result in disturbed

homeostasis and some degree of adaptive failure. The latter involves biological, psychological, and social aspects. These facts reflect man's unique capacity to create symbols in thought and language, and respond to them at all levels of his organization. This capacity is predicated on cerebral activity which not only subserves mental activity but also mediates between man's environment and his internal milieu which it controls and on which it is also dependent. We shall elaborate these concepts further while discussing psychological stress. They are also mentioned in Chapter 2 (p. 97), in which causes and psychological effects of cerebral damage and dysfunction will be discussed.

A unified concept of disease, elaborated by Dubos,[38] Engel,[42] and Wolff,[223] takes full cognizance of man's capacity for symbolic activity, which adds a crucial dimension to his adaptation to the social and physical environments, and to maintenance of health, as well as susceptibility to disease. As Wolff[223] put it: "It is unprofitable to establish a separate category of illness to be defined psychosomatic or to separate sharply—as regards genesis—psychiatric, medical, and surgical diseases." This view has been influenced by the general system theory[212] and is rapidly replacing earlier, reductionist concepts of static, single-factor, unilinear causal sequences, be they expressed as germ theory or psychogenesis.

The characteristics of the unified approach to disease may be formulated in the following postulates, equally applicable to somatic and psychiatric disorders:

Relativity of the Concepts Health and Disease

There is no sharp boundary between health and disease, between normality and abnormality. They are relative concepts defined by changing statistical, subjective, and social criteria, as well as by abstract, utopian notions of an ideal state and varying degrees of deviation from it. For Dubos[38] health implies "a modus vivendi enabling imperfect men to achieve a rewarding and not too painful existence while they cope with an imperfect world." Disease connotes "failures or disturbances in the organism as a whole or any of its systems."[42] Thus health and disease are viewed as states constituting a continuum divided by an arbitrarily and conventionally defined boundary.

Multifactorial Etiology

No disease is caused by a single factor, although one factor may outweigh all the others in determining a given disease state. Etiologic factors include enduring predispositions or vulnerabilities of genetic and acquired origin, as well as current susceptibility, psychic and/or somatic, of the individual to noxious agents ranging from physical, chemical, and biological to symbolic, which exert a strain on his current adaptive capacities. These causal factors vary in their respective relevance from case to case, and evaluation of their relative contribution to a patient's malfunction and discomfort constitutes the process of comprehensive diagnosis.[201]

Ecologic Viewpoint

The study of every disease must include the person, his body, and his human and non-human environment as essential components of the total system. This involves the employment of methodologies, explanatory concepts, and terminologies derived from physical, biological, and behavioral sciences. For reasons of research strategy these different components are broken down and studied in isolation from those belonging to the other levels. But the determinants of health and disease in an individual always involve complex interactions between him and his total environment.*

Disease as Dynamic State

It is customary to distinguish etiological and reactive aspects of disease as if they represented two different categories of phenomena. This is largely an artifact, although it has some heuristic value. The whole constellation of factors listed under *Multifactorial Etiology* above

* See references 38, 64, 74, 75, 122, 174, and 201.

continues to influence the course of any disease. There is dynamic interplay among these factors and numerous feedback loops having a beneficial or deleterious effect on the disease as a process and on its outcome. This is particularly true of the currently prevalent chronic diseases, in many of which the point of onset cannot be identified. In them it is quite arbitrary to distinguish between causal and reactive factors.

Psychosocial Stress

When the meaning of any information input, internal or external, is construed by the subject in terms of threat of, or actual loss or injury to his psychic and/or physical integrity, we talk of *psychological stress*. This theoretical construct has been plagued by ambiguity, despite numerous attempts at its clear formulation.[43,111,113] The most lucid and comprehensive discussion of psychological stress has been given by Lazarus,[111,112] that of social stress, by Levine and Scotch.[113] Semantic confusion, however, should not obscure the mass of accumulated evidence, clinical and experimental, that events and situations in an individual's life affect his health. When such events are interpreted by the subject in terms of meanings mentioned above and result in disturbances of his psychological and/or somatic homeostasis straining his current adaptive and coping capacities, we can apply the term psychological stress. It is a general concept encompassing disturbing stimuli (stressors), their cognitive assessment, and the resulting emotional, physiological, and coping responses.[111]

Psychological stress need not have pathological consequences unless it is sustained, or of such a magnitude for a given person at a given time that it results in a breakdown of adaptive mechanisms, somatic, psychological, or both. Such a breakdown has been expressed in the concept of *general susceptibility* to disease.[75,204] Whether the latter occurs and what form it takes is determined by a variety of factors, enduring and current, residing within the individual (host) and in his social and physical environment. Recent psychosomatic research has used a three-pronged approach to the investigation of the chain of events leading from a social stimulus to disease.[119,123] The first approach emphasizes epidemiological methods, and focuses on temporal relationships between specific *life changes*, or demanding *life situations*, e.g. family or occupational, in groups of individuals and their morbidity.[75,171] The second approach takes as its starting point an individual's *psychological state*, the realm of thought and feeling, in response to life events and situations which are disturbing to him.[178] The third approach aims at identifying *physiological mechanisms and pathways* mediating between symbolic stimuli, a disturbed psychic state, and evidence of pathology and/or dysfunction in a given organ or tissue.[74,119]

Engel [43] distinguishes three broad classes of psychologically stressful events: *loss* or threat of loss of psychic objects, i.e. people, possessions, ideals, etc., having ego-sustaining value for the person; actual or threatened *injury* to the body; and *frustration of drives*. This list is not exhaustive. One could add to it the disorienting rate of social change; value, choice, and decision conflicts; wants, created by the existing economic system, coupled with aroused expectations and inability to meet them; status inconsistency,[36,215] and a host of other social situations and events which cannot be reduced to Engel's three main categories.[122] It must be emphasized, however, that despite observed similarities of people's responses to external events, the ultimately decisive factor is the *individual's* evaluation of his perceptions, and his personal interpretation of them.

Bodily injury or illness, or threat of either, constitute one of the major sources of psychological stress. This view links etiological factors with reactive ones. Thus, psychosocial factors may not only contribute to disease onset, but illness itself includes psychosocial responses which may increase or reduce the initial psychological stress and thus influence the course and outcome of the illness.*

* See references 20, 36, 40, 64, 74, 75, 82, 92, 94, 111, 121, 126, 171, 193, 204, 210, 211, 215, 216, 224, and 226.

(Determinants of Psychological Reaction to Disease

The multiple determinants of every patient's psychological reaction to his physical illness, injury, defect, and/or disability may be assigned to the following classes:

1. Intrapersonal factors, which include biological variables, such as age, sex, and constitution; and psychological, i.e., personality in all its aspects, past experience with illness in oneself and others, etc. Both these classes of variables inherent in the person include his enduring psychobiological predispositions and states as well as those obtaining at the onset of illness and throughout its duration.

2. Interpersonal factors, i.e., nature of patient's relationships with other people, especially family and health professionals, both before and during his illness.

3. Pathology-related factors, i.e., spatio-temporal characteristics of disease or injury and the subjective meaning they have for the patient in relation to his past history, knowledge, values, and current adaptive capacity.

4. Sociocultural and economic factors, i.e., values and attitudes toward illness as such and specific diseases prevalent in the patient's social milieu; beliefs about medical care delivery and its practitioners; economic consequences of illness for patient; etc.

5. Nonhuman environmental factors, i.e., physical aspects of environment in which patient lives during his illness.

The varying influence of the above factors determines the unique quality of the experience and behavior of every patient in any given episode of illness. No single set of generalizations can fully account for the individual nuances of response to illness. Yet generalizations are practically useful to allow grouping of patients showing common features and as a basis for the clinical approach to every individual. Each of the five classes of determinants must be taken into account for a *comprehensive* diagnosis and management.

Intrapersonal Factors

These are the *psychobiological characteristics* of the patient and his premorbid life history as experienced by him. Those aspects of his past experience are relevant which influence the meaning for him and his attitude toward his particular illness or disability and its consequences.

The psychological impact of any illness differs depending on its timing in a person's life cycle. The experience of being sick and the psychological resources to cope with disability are different in a child, adolescent, or an old person. Thus *age* is an important variable.

Illness, disability, or injury in *childhood**deserve special attention. They may interfere with the child's maturation and optimal psychological development.[22] The quality of the illness experience, influenced by the behavior of the important adults toward the sick child, may determine his reactions to illness in later life, such as excessive fear of, sense of weakness and shame in relation to, or, on the contrary, eager acceptance and even simulation of illness as a psychologically rewarding state. A child has a limited repertoire of cognitive and other coping strategies available to him, and his usual defense is regression. Yet, as Langford[109] points out, such regression is "strategic withdrawal for regrouping of strengths" rather than a pathological development. Most children cope with illness surprisingly well and may come out of it with increased maturity and vigor. To achieve this favorable outcome, however, the child needs the understanding and support of those taking care of him, particularly if the illness is severe, prolonged, and requiring hospitalization.[169,208]

Physical illness during *adolescence*[130] imposes an additional stress at a time when the tasks of gaining independence from the parents and developing a stable body and self-image provide a formidable challenge. Some adolescents tend to fear the passivity and de-

* See references 32, 105, 109, 138, 169, and 208.

pendence imposed by the illness and may readily interpret it as a punishment for sexual and aggressive feelings and activities. Others may welcome it. Physical illness during adolescence is particularly likely to engender intense conflicts and anxiety. They may be manifested directly or take the form of lack of cooperation with health professionals, and denial of and attempted flight from illness. Examples of this are provided by juvenile diabetics[181] and adolescents suffering from malignant neoplasms.[152]

Illness, even relatively mild, in a *middle-aged* person who has enjoyed good health, may trigger off thoughts of approaching old age, infirmity, and death. Such associations may evoke an emotional response more intense than the nature of the illness would warrant. This intensity may be further enhanced if the illness occurs close to the age at which a parent or other significant person died.[129]

Old age frequently adds an important variable influencing the response to illness: some degree of brain damage and consequent proneness to cerebral decompensation. The latter often complicates physical illness and hospitalization in persons over 65 years.[114,124] Cognitive disorganization impairs rational evaluation of the illness and environment, and adds a source of psychological stress and disorganizing anxiety. There is also the grave hazard of extension of the irreversible brain damage.

Thus, the psychological impact of illness or disability varies with the developmental phases of the human life cycle. A congenital deformity or functional handicap will help shape a person's body image and influence the direction of growth of his personality. Acquired at any stage from birth on an injury or illness carries a potential for psychological growth as well as for crippling maladjustment. Anything that disturbs functions of the body affects the psyche and vice versa.

The patient's sex influences reaction to diseases which impair bodily attributes or functions valued for their enhancement of the sex role. Injury or deformity which mars esthetic quality of the body is likely to have more serious emotional significance for a woman than a man. He is more likely to be affected by any chronic illness which enforces dependence on others and interferes with capacity for work, a source of gratification in its own right. In either sex, disease affecting sexual function or secondary sex characteristics may undermine his or her sexual role and identity, and intensify related unconscious conflicts. Unconscious symbolic meaning of the affected body part may have a sexual connotation, and injury to it, the nose for example,[11] may be unconsciously interpreted as castration with consequent anxiety or depression.[177]

The patient's *personality style* influences the meaning and experience of illness, as many authors have emphasized.[8,85,86] Myocardial infarction, for example, evokes different responses in an obsessional, schizoid, paranoid, hysterical, or impulsive[33] personality type. Personality attributes comprise the individual's *cognitive and perceptual style*, such as field dependence or independence;[222] his unconscious *conflicts*, characteristic *ego defenses*, and *coping styles* with psychological stress of any type; *ego strength, intelligence, values,* and *knowledge; body image* and *self-concept*; and other relatively enduring qualities which all play a major part in determining the total psychological response to disease. These factors influence behavior to all facets and at all stages of illness, and hence their assessment should be part of a comprehensive diagnosis as a basis for an individually tailored management plan for every patient. The clinical relevance of these variables will be discussed in more concrete terms in the subsequent sections.

Apart from enduring personality characteristics, the patient's *psychobiological state* at the onset and during the course of his illness must also be taken into account. His level of consciousness and his cognitive and perceptual capacity, will influence his ability to appraise his illness, diagnostic procedures, etc. His ability to cope with the illness also depends on his current mood, state of unconscious and conscious conflicts, and stability of life situation. It has been observed that the greater are the magnitude of *life change* and the related conflicts, adaptive demands, and

affective arousal, the more likely is an illness to occur[171] and be severe.[226] This suggests that psychosocial stress plays a dual part in that it both enhances susceptibility to illness and impairs the host's capacity to cope with it physiologically and psychologically. Since illness itself changes the quality of subjective experience, producing unpleasant mood and disturbing perceptions and thoughts, a vicious circle results. Increasing psychophysiological arousal and distress may readily ensue and add to the initial psychological stress.*

Interpersonal Factors

The quality of the individual's interpersonal relationships before and after the onset of his illness exerts a profound effect on his experience and coping capacity. When illness comes on, as it often does, in a setting of interpersonal, say marital, conflict, or of loss of a close person, or work-related stress, its impact tends to be greater, its course more stormy and the recovery protracted or absent. Findings of higher than average morbidity and mortality rates among the recently bereaved, for example[139,160,172] may reflect both increased susceptibility to disease and reduced ability and/or willingness to cope with it. Loss of an important relationship, whether actual, anticipated or even imagined, is said to be a common trigger for the so-called *giving up–given up complex*.[179] That psychological state, consisting of negative appraisals of self and environment, and concomitant affects of helplessness or hopelessness, has been observed to be a *common antecedent* of many illnesses. It appears that the more intense those affects are, the greater the tendency to give up the struggle for survival, psychologically and biologically.[178]

Increasing attention has been given lately to the crucial importance of *family relationships* in influencing the course and outcome of illness. These factors will be discussed in more detail later. It suffices to stress at this point that viewing the patient apart from his social

---

* See references 9, 42, 82, 83, 102, 143, and 193.

context results in an incomplete picture of illness and its deficient management.[132]

Relationships between the patient and the health professionals with whom he comes into contact invariably influence, for better or worse, the course and outcome of his illness. Other relevant relationships include those with employers, friends, neighbors, etc., who constitute the patient's social milieu. All these factors will be considered in some detail in the later sections.

Pathology–Related Factors

The nature and characteristics of the pathological process or injury are a class of biological variables pertaining to the integrity of the body and its functions. These factors acquire psychological significance as they, and/or their consequences, give rise to perceptions, thoughts, feelings, communications, and actions. There is some indication that subliminal interoceptive stimuli may influence conscious psychic processes and dream contents and thus provide clues to a still covert pathological process.[187] It would be valuable for preventive medicine if such clues could be reliably identified, but this is not yet feasible.

Variables, such as the site and extent of the lesion, rate of onset and progression, the kind and degree of functional derangement, as well as duration of the pathological process, all influence the patient's emotional response. Specific organs and physiological functions have different psychological significance and symbolic value for each person, related to his unique life experience, body image, and personality. These values may have little relevance to the issue of survival. Injury to the face or an abdominal scar may have greater subjective significance than impairment of organs essential for survival. The particular experiential history of the patient, his conscious and unconscious conflicts and beliefs, sociocultural influences, and other factors, determine what significance and value he attaches to the given body part or function. The extent to which the disease process changes one's *somatic sensory input and body image* also influences how one responds to disease or

injury. Last but not least, *impairment of cerebral function* by disease, its nature, and the degree of its reversibility or compensability, is important.*

An organ or biological function has especial subjective significance[118] for a person when it:

1. constitutes a source of pleasure, pride, self-esteem, and effective coping with the environment;
2. helps maintain satisfying relationships with others;
3. helps alleviate intrapsychic conflicts and thus protects against experience of painful affects;
4. enhances sense of personal identity, self-concept, and stability of his body image;
5. helps maintain social roles and occupational capacity;
6. has unconscious symbolic meaning which imparts to it a vital value in his psychic economy.

Any disease, injury, or disability which jeopardizes or destroys such personal values has an intense subjective meaning for and emotional effects on the patient.

Sociocultural and Economic Factors

This is the domain of *values, beliefs,* and *attitudes* related to matters of health and disease. They are generally shared by members of a given social group and class, and affect every patient's emotional response to illness, as well as his illness behavior.[146,206] These factors have been studied extensively by medical sociologists.†

Everyone holds views about the significance, etiology, likely effects, and prognosis of the more prevalent diseases. Such beliefs influence the meaning of his illness for the patient and what he does or fails to do about it. His behavior also expresses his image of the health professionals and medical institutions. If this image is largely unfavorable, the pa-

* See references 11, 23, 32, 52, 78, 124, 125, 129, 177, 183, 186, 194, 202, 210, 216, and 218.
† See references 84, 98, 146, 147, 161, and 206.

tient tends to avoid seeking medical help and resorts to folk medicine and self-medication. Members of the lower socioeconomic groups tend to be wary of doctors and hospitals, less likely to evaluate symptoms as indicative of disease, and more likely to trust their own understanding of health.[135,200] Poor people from city slums or rural areas have often different medical values and customs from those of health professionals and other members of the higher socioeconomic groups. These factors, combined with the cost of medical care, contribute to the medically deprived position of the poor.[200]

Attitudes in a patient's social milieu toward being sick, as well as derogatory and fearful views of certain diseases, influence his willingness to accept the sick role,[146,200] and reveal his symptoms to others. Some diseases carry a *stigma*[99] and to suffer from one of them may evoke shame, guilt, self-devaluation, and social withdrawal. Such responses add to the other stresses of illness, and promote attempts at its concealment. Venereal diseases, epilepsy, leprosy, or tuberculosis are often stigmatized because of their negative moral connotation, fears of contagiousness, and/or frightening outward manifestations. Cancer is so dreaded at all levels of American society that about 60 percent of adults queried in a large poll stated that they would conceal it from others.[63] Many people believe that cancer is contagious and fear contracting it from or transferring it to members of their family. Such fears are particularly strong in patients suffering from an illness believed to be contagious who harbor conflicts over hostile impulses and feel guilty about them. If such an illness intensifies the patient's hostility, he may have unconscious wishes to infect others and suffer intense guilt as a consequence.

Knowledge of scientific medicine varies with socioeconomic grouping[135] and is usually lowest in those with a low level of education and income. Yet irrational beliefs about medical matters are not confined to any class. Nor does possession of medical knowledge automatically ensure rational behavior in illness, as any physician who has treated his colleagues can testify.

Nonhuman Environmental Factors

Psychological effects of the physical environment in which the sick person lives, be it home or hospital, are an important, although neglected subject. Various hospital environments affect the patients. Esthetic qualities of the surroundings, quantity and quality of the sensory input, and appearance of diagnostic and therapeutic implements may influence the patient's mood and at times arouse anxiety or facilitate cognitive disorganization on account of their novelty, unfamiliarity, monotony, etc.[104]

The above list of determinants of psychological reactions to disease is not meant to be exhaustive. Their outline underscores the large number and diversity of variables which influence the experience and behavior of the sick.

(Modes of Psychological Response to Disease

We will describe patients' responses to disease, in both their *subjective* and *observable* aspects. Three such overlapping aspects will be distinguished:

1. The intrapsychic (experiential), which refers to what the patient perceives, thinks, and feels, that is to perceptual, affective, and cognitive components of his subjective response to his illness;
2. The behavioral, that is, how the patient communicates with others and acts in regard to his illness;
3. The social, which concerns his interactions with others, particularly his family and the health professionals.

The Intrapsychic (Experiential) Aspect

Disease and the suffering it causes are universal components of the human condition. Stripped of its abstract, scientific connotations, "disease" and "illness" are labels for an essentially personal experience, one known only through introspection. It may be communicated to others and has to be received with empathy to result in meaningful information. Such procedure is often dismissed as unscientific and the data as anecdotal. Yet this is not a valid reason to leave out of account what matters the most to every patient, to every one of us, personally. The subjective aspects of illness may be described and studied in two distinct ways: as a *total experience*, by obtaining introspective reports; and *atomistically* by applying scientific psychological terminology and observation methods, and breaking down the patient's experience as an integrated whole into its *perceptual, cognitive*, and *emotional* components. The former method will be briefly discussed first.

An illness colors to some extent the sick person's experience of his body, self, and environment, his values and goals. Novelists, like Proust or Chechov, writers of diaries, and some existentialists,[207] have written sensitive accounts of how the sick feel. Of particular interest are autobiographical descriptions of specific illness experiences written by physicians.[168] While every episode of illness is a unique experience, certain common trends may be discerned. Narrowing of interests, egocentricity, increased attention and responsiveness to bodily perceptions and functions, irritability, increased sense of insecurity and longing for human support and closeness, are commonly reported inner changes.[6] There is often an unpleasant change in the general body feeling, or coenesthesis, experienced as malaise or the feeling of sickness, usually associated with an active pathology. Negative emotional experiences are not invariably reported, however. Some sufferers from chronic illness or disability experience an increased awareness of esthetic and intellectual values and enhanced intensity of spiritual life in general.[168]

PERCEPTUAL, COGNITIVE, AND AFFECTIVE COMPONENTS OF RESPONSE

Perception of all the sensory input relevant to one's illness depends on the *attributes of the perceiving individual*, the *characteristics of perception* itself, and *the situation* in which the patient finds himself. The quality, intensity, and spatiotemporal features of the perception are important. A sudden attack of vertigo, bleeding, severe pain, or marked shortness of breath are more likely to force an appraisal of what is happening with greater urgency than a painless lump or transient bowel dysfunction. Yet already at this stage the characteristics of the perceiving individual come into play.

One such characteristic is the *perceptual style*, whether conceptualized as *perceptual reactance*, that is, augmentation or reduction of what is being perceived;[166] as *repression-sensitization*;[18] or some other hypothesized continuum of perceptual reactivity. Habitual augmenters tend to perceive somatic sensations, such as pain, more keenly and appraise them more readily in terms of threat or harm than the reducers. The latter find it easier to ignore and deny the significance of their symptoms. Sensitizers are liable to report greater frequency and/or severity of symptoms, and higher total numbers of complaints and visits to physicians, than repressors. These observations seem to represent differences in perception concerning illness and corresponding responses to it.[18]

Individuals differ with regard to their responsiveness to somesthetic stimuli. Some may mislabel their interoceptive cues. These individual differences reflect early learning of both somatic responses and their symbolic, linguistic equivalents. The latter are influenced by sociocultural and ethnic factors.[228]

Cognition refers to thinking, concept formation, and problem-solving. *Cognitive aspects* of the psychological response reflect an individual's *cognitive style*. Two such styles pertain to illness experience: *vigilant focusing on and need to explain* illness-related perceptions and events; and *minimization*, that is, a habitual tendency to play down the significance of any perceived bodily changes, etc.[120]

Cognitive evaluation of illness is partly conscious and partly unconscious. Unconscious cognition involves primary process thinking, that is one characterized by distortions of facts according to the person's wishes, conflicts, fears, repressed memories and fantasies, etc.

Different organs and bodily functions have unconscious symbolic meanings derived from early childhood experiences and never influenced by factual knowledge. Thus, perception of abdominal distension due to a malignancy may arouse unconscious fantasies of pregnancy, for example. Much has been written about unconscious sexual symbols of the nose, neck, eyes, or teeth. Any body orifice may symbolically represent a female genital. Illness may be interpreted, consciously or not, as just or unjust punishment for repudiated wishes or actions which had aroused feelings of guilt; as enemy; challenge; weakness; irreparable damage; or as value.[120] Such subjective views of illness or injury influence the patient's conscious attitude, feelings, and overt behavior.[120,177]

An almost universal cognitive response to illness is an attempt to *explain its origin*. Two most common modes of explanation are to *blame* oneself or another person or nonhuman agent for having caused the disease.[5] Such beliefs about etiology may vary from rational and scientifically sound ones to irrational and delusional.[135] In any case, to "explain" the origins and mechanisms of the illness may offer a comforting illusion of mastery over it and help reduce ambiguity, uncertainty and anxiety. Yet this is not always so. Sometimes the evolved explanation may result in a sense of guilt, grievance, and anguish.[120]

The emotional responses to illness vary in quality, intensity, and duration. They both reflect and influence the personal meaning of illness, the nature and degree of symptoms and disability, and the degree of support the patient gets from his environment. *Anxiety, grief, depression, shame, guilt, anger*—these are the affects most often elicited. Less common are *apathy, indifference, elation, or euphoria*. Whether one judges a patient's affective response as normal or not depends on its *appropriateness*, that is, degree of correspondence to the severity of the pain, losses, and suffering. Such judgment is obviously value-laden and the borderline between normal and abnormal responses is an arbitrary one. Practically more important is the degree to which the affective response impairs a pa-

tient's capacity for recovery and/or adjustment. Pathological emotional responses which are components of identifiable psychiatric syndromes, neurotic or psychotic, are discussed in detail in a paper devoted to the psychopathology related to physical illness.[125]

The Behavioral Aspect

The *communications* and *actions* of the patient in relation to his illness comprise the behavioral aspect of his total psychological response. Mechanic[147] introduced the concept "illness behavior" to designate "the ways in which given symptoms may be differentially perceived, evaluated, and acted (or not acted) upon by different kinds of persons." Yet perception and evaluation of symptoms do not logically belong to behavior as usually defined in psychology, but communications and actions do. Illness behavior should be confined to the latter.

COMMUNICATIVE BEHAVIOR

What the patient communicates regarding his symptoms or distress, when he does it, to whom and how, is important for delivery of medical care and a satisfactory doctor–patient relationship. Communication is a two-way process, modified by the manner in which messages are responded to by the recipients. In the case of illness, the patient's communications influence and are influenced by the responses of his doctors, family members, or other concerned persons. This aspect of illness behavior has attracted considerable attention in the 1970s because of its relevance to the diagnostic decision and the patient's compliance with medical recommendations.*

Only selected examples of studies in this area are mentioned here. Zola[230,231] emphasizes the influence of *sociocultural factors* on the manner in which patients communicate their symptoms to the doctor. He found that Irish and Italian patients attending outpatient clinics of a general hospital presented their complaints differently. The Irish tended to understate their difficulties, to refer their com-

---

* See references 1, 39, 149, 196, 213, 228, 230, and 231.

plaints mostly to the eyes, ears, nose, and throat, and to deny that they felt pain. Italians, on the contrary, dramatized their complaints, referred symptoms to many parts of the body, and claimed that their distress interfered with their social relationships. More Italians were labelled as "psychiatric problems" by the doctors, suggesting that the way in which symptoms are communicated tends to influence diagnostic reasoning. Zola observes that the doctor "can block or reject the patient's communication by his very reaction, or lack of reaction, to the patient's concerns" and thus obtain inaccurate and misleading information. Similar conclusion was reached by Duff and Hollingshead[39] from their study of medical inpatients.

Zborowski[228] studied responses to *pain* manifested verbally and nonverbally by patients of Old American, Jewish, Irish, and Italian origin. Patients of Jewish and Italian origin tended to be more emotional while experiencing and communicating pain than the Anglo-Saxons (Old Americans). They also tended to emphasize their perception of pain and its severity. The Old Americans and Irish tended to play down pain, report it unemotionally, and describe it typically as stabbing and sharp. The Irish were vague and confused in their description of perceptions and feelings about pain. Italians related more often than others that their pain was constant rather than intermittent. They and the Jewish patients made no effort to conceal their pain, and manifested it by crying, moaning, etc., suggesting their desire to communicate their suffering both verbally and nonverbally.

Patients often communicate selectively what they believe the doctors are interested in, namely somatic complaints. This expectation may make the patient express his psychological distress in terms of somatic complaints and metaphors. Such skewed communication readily leads to diagnostic errors, and unnecessary and costly investigations of nonexistent organic disease. Another source of diagnostic error is provided by patients who complain in terms of psychological distress and withhold information about their somatic symptoms.[175] Others habitually express their disturbed feel-

ings in *somatic* terms.[173] Such somatizing patients predominate in the lower economic classes and the rural areas.[29,133]

Special problems are presented by patients suffering from disorders of communication, for example aphasia, or those who communicate in an idiosyncratic idiom, as many schizophrenics do, or overdramatize their symptoms as an expression of hysterical personality. Such patients may fail to make themselves understood or believed with possible errors in diagnosis.

COPING BEHAVIOR

The *actions* taken by the patient in relation to his illness are an aspect of his overall *coping behavior*.[28] The concept of coping designates "instrumental behavior and problem-solving capacities of persons in meeting life demands and goals."[146] A narrower definition confines it specifically to strategies of dealing with psychological stress.[111] Physical illness and disability are a category of psychological stress with one crucial characteristic: the primary source of stressors lies within the person's body boundaries. Coping in this context may be defined as cognitive and psychomotor activities which a sick person employs to preserve his bodily and psychic integrity, to recover reversibly impaired function, and compensate to the attainable limit for residual irreversible impairment.[120]

One may distinguish behavioral coping *styles* and *strategies*.[120] The former refer to *enduring dispositions* to act in a certain manner in response to threat or loss involving one's body. Strategies refer to the *actual techniques* which the patient employs in dealing with a particular illness or disability. They are a resultant of both his coping style and current situational constraints. The latter include the particular form of disability suffered from, say paraplegia or aphasia, as well as the whole constellation of intrapersonal and environmental factors accompanying a given illness episode. Behavioral coping styles may be classified as *tackling*, *capitulating*, and *avoiding*.[120]

Tackling means a tendency to adopt an active attitude toward challenges and tasks imposed by illness or disability. In its extreme form, it is manifested by a tendency to "fight" illness at any cost. The patient acts as if the disease was an enemy to be combated and may engage in behavior inimical to his health, for example by continuing strenuous physical activity in the presence of coronary artery disease or rheumatoid arthritis. Adaptive manifestations of this style include rationally modulated activities aimed at early recovery, or compensation for residual disability. Timely seeking of medical advice, compliance with therapeutic regimens, active information-seeking, searching for substitute skills and gratifications to replace the lost ones—these are desirable coping strategies reflecting the tackling style.

Capitulating refers to one's habitual way of dealing with threats and losses by adopting a passive stance and either withdrawal from or dependent clinging to others. Patients displaying this style create problems for physicians because of their inadequate cooperation, or excessive demands for support, reassurance and care-taking, respectively. This way of coping should not be confused with adaptive passivity during the acute stage of any serious illness.

Avoiding pertains to active attempts to get away from the exigencies and challenges of the illness. It is characteristically displayed by individuals for whom acceptance of illness, hospitalization, treatment, etc., signifies a severe threat to their self-concept as independent or invulnerable, or, on the contrary, excessively vulnerable. Its intrapsychic concomitant is usually either a marked degree of denial of illness or of manifest anxiety.

Coping behavior in patients has been studied in particular detail in relation to such conditions as chronic illness and disability,[6,32,60,225] severe burns,[70] acute poliomyelitis,[208] diabetes,[105] and other illnesses. It is a clinically useful universal concept as it allows the physician to identify a given patient's dispositions and actual techniques for dealing with his illness, and intervene to encourage adaptive ones. Excellent examples of such intervention are given by Hackett and Weisman[67,68] who describe psychiatric techniques of managing psychological disturbances related to surgery.

The Social Aspect

The social aspect of the patient's response to illness refers to his interactions with concerned others, especially his family and health professionals. This aspect has been studied extensively by sociologists, who have proposed relevant explanatory hypotheses and introduced organizing theoretical constructs. The most influential of the latter has been that of the sick role, developed by Parsons.[161] As Kasl and Cobb[91] put it, "Parsons observed with great insight that when one becomes ill, one does not simply drop one's customary roles—the role of parent, spouse, or provider; one actually adopts a new role which supersedes the others." Parsons called this the *sick role*. This concept is reviewed here as it is pertinent to the patient's interactions with his social environment.

The concept of any role involves two kinds of expectations: That the individual will adopt certain attitudes and follow certain actions; and that others should behave toward him according to explicit and implicit rules. The sick role implies the following expectations: 1. Exemption from the responsibilities and obligations of the premorbid social roles (for example, as wage earner) in relation to the nature and severity of illness; 2. Obligation to seek the health and comply with advice of competent persons; and 3. Surrender of the sick role as soon as possible. It is thus expected that playing the sick role has a time limit and the patient should do his best to achieve functional recovery. This is in accordance with the prevailing values and norms of the American society, which extol self-reliance, individual initiative, efficiency, and achievement. The sick role is a deviant one, but distinguished from other deviant roles by the fact that the sick person is not held responsible for his condition.

The sick role is a heuristically fertile concept, which provides a *sociological* framework for the study of illness as an indispensable complement to the biological and psychological approaches. The concept has been criticised on theoretical and practical grounds. The main criticisms are that it is inadequate for the study of minor as well as of incurable and stigmatized diseases; and that it is not applicable to illness behavior not involving contact with physicians. It is also not applicable to the characteristics of other cultures.[206] These criticisms do not detract from the originality and methodological value of Parsons' contribution.

The patient may take one of several courses of action with regard to acceptance of the sick role: (1) He may accept it realistically, as society expects him to do, and surrender it upon recovery; (2) He may attempt to reject or avoid it, even if this is harmful to him; (3) He may adopt it readily and refuse to give it up despite the doctor's opinion that he is fit to do so; and (4) He may strive to avoid it, then give in to and cling to it. All these patterns of sick role behavior are encountered in clinical practice and influence the course, duration, and outcome of any illness or injury. They are determined by the interplay between the patient, his illness, and his social environment. A person who views dependence, helplessness, and physical incapacity as threatening or degrading has difficulty in accepting the sick role and engaging in rational illness behavior. Interaction between the patient and members of *his family* on the one hand, and the *health professionals* on the other, influences his sick role behavior and will now be discussed.

THE PATIENT AND HIS FAMILY

The relationship between illness and family dynamics may be approached from several overlapping points of view: (1) The influence of family interaction, say marital conflict, on the development of illness or injury;[24,30,148,151] (2) The role of the family in the learning of particular modes of illness behavior. For example, children may adopt through identification and imitation specific attitudes toward the sick role as well as predisposition to evaluate given symptoms or types of disability as threatening, shameful, etc. Children rewarded for being ill may acquire a tendency to view illness as a potential source of gratification;[188]

(3) The impact of illness in a given family member on the stability of the family as a whole; (4) The interactions between the sick member and other members of the family as they affect the patient and his spouse, children, parents or siblings; and (5) The influence of the family dynamics on the timing of seeking medical consultation and hospitalization.[16,17]

All these aspects of the relationship between illness and family interactions have been studied and there is growing appreciation of their importance for medicine.[132] Only selected observations and theoretical formulations may be touched upon here.

An influential set of theoretical formulations in this area has been contributed by Parsons and Fox.[162] They pointed out that the modern American family by virtue of its small size and relative isolation is exceptionally vulnerable to the impact of illness of one of its members. The illness in the mother is disturbing because of her unifying and emotionally supporting role within the family. Her illness may deprive husband and children of her customary support, while imposing additional stresses and demands on her. Illness of the father, as the main provider and status-bearer, undermines the social and economic position of the family as a whole, and by attracting mother's concerns deprives the children of her support. Illness of a child could increase marital strain and enhance sibling rivalry, for example. The intrafamily dynamics could be further disturbed if the sick member used his illness as a strategy aimed at escape and relief from obligations and demands within and outside the family. The adjustment to illness and disability involves learning by the patient how to be sick and by the family how to respond to his sickness. Both these tasks are demanding and may evoke disruptive emotional responses.

Many studies have focussed on the impact of severe illness in a child on family dynamics.* Friedman et al.[57] made a detailed analysis of parents' reactions and coping strategies in response to neoplastic disease, mostly leukemia, in a child. The common sequence of

---

* See references 30, 57, 138, 169, and 208.

parental reactions began with a feeling of shock when diagnosis was disclosed, followed by a tendency to self-blame and guilt for imaginary errors of omission and neglect with regard to early manifestations of disease. Such guilt feelings tended to be transient and gave way to seeking of information about the illness and its etiology as an attempt at mastery of an uncontrollable situation. The coping behavior of the parents included defense mechanisms of isolation of affect, intellectualization, and, less often, denial. Poor operation of such defenses was associated with manifest anxiety and depression which hampered a parent's ability to care for the sick child. Hope in the parents was common and gradually gave way to anticipatory grief, manifested by somatic symptoms, apathy, and preoccupation with thoughts about the ill child.

As part of this study[57] an attempt was made to assess the degree of psychological stress in the parents by determining urinary 17-hydroxycorticosteroid levels and relate them to the observed coping behavior and affects. It was found that the excretion rates were relatively stable and the investigators concluded that the more any defense mechanism protected the individual from the impact of the chronic stress of a child's illness, the lower and less fluctuating would be the associated 17-OHCS levels. Such levels were among the lowest in parents who displayed marked denial mechanisms.[58]

This study[58] stands out as one of the most thorough of its kind and is using a psychophysiological approach. It shows that a person's coping strategies have *both psychological and physiological* aspects and consequences for him.

The impact of specific diseases and disabilities in *adults* on the family interaction has been less extensively studied. A few representative examples will be cited to emphasize the diversity of the related problems which await further research.

Disability in *husbands and fathers* has been studied from the point of view of the patients. The latter reported the main changes in their family relationships in the following order: (1) greater responsibilities for the wives in the management of the home; (2) reduction of social and recreational activities; (3) more duties for the children around the house; (4) incurred debts; (5) changed plans for a larger family; (6) necessity of wife's employment; (7) increased marital discord; (8) changed plans for children's education; and (9) changed living accomodation. The disabled head of the family perceived significant shifts in the respective roles of the family members, with his own role being undermined in the process. There was also evidence of marital friction and decline in social and economic status of the family.[140] Shifts of roles within the family may create conflicts when the husband eventually recovers and claims his previous dominant role and its prerogatives. This writer has observed psychological decompensation in several wives as a result of such repeated role reversal.

The impact of chronic illness upon the *spouse* was studied in a sample of men and women belonging mostly to the lower class.[100] The healthy spouses reported new or increased symptoms, such as nervousness or fatigue. There were indications of increased interpersonal conflict (role tension) expressed by irritability and readiness to feel depressed in both partners. Greater symptomatic distress of the patient caused more emotional tension in the spouse, and vice versa.

An interesting relationship has been observed among physical disability, and need and marriage satisfaction in couples in which the *wife* was severely disabled.[50] "Severe disability" was defined as a physical impairment interfering with homemaking activities. Some of the women were bedridden and unable to move. The physical condition of the disabled woman was not a reliable predictor of need or marriage satisfaction in either partner. Greater mobility of the wife did not invariably result in greater need or marriage satisfaction. There was no simple relationship between the wife's level of functional mobility and the husband's need satisfaction. Severe disability provided the patient with a less ambiguous role and thus less conflict and demand for efforts to improve her ability to meet obligations. The disabled woman's sexual satisfaction was positively correlated with her marriage satisfaction. Physical condition of disabled persons had little effect on marital sexual activity. Similar observations have been made in paraplegics and quadriplegics.[66]

In general, the following conclusions may be drawn from the available studies: (1) Evaluation of any patient is incomplete without a detailed inquiry into his family interactions and the ways and degree in which they are affected by the patient's illness and, in turn, affect him;[132] (2) The quality of *communications* between the patient and his family members should be assessed in a marital couple or family interview. There is often skewed communication, and in cases of fatal illness a conspiracy of silence, which imposes a strain on all concerned; (3) In the case of a married patient it is essential to inquire into the effect of the disabling illness on the respective *roles* of the couple, their sexual adjustment, and the related marital tensions. The sense of sexual identity of either partner may be undermined as a result of illness and reactivate related intrapsychic conflicts. This may occur if the wife is forced to play a more active role both as breadwinner and sexual partner (for example, husband's paraplegia or painful back may preclude his taking an active role during sexual intercourse). The reverse situation and role shift may occur if the husband of a disabled woman has to assume housekeeping and other functions conflicting with his self-concept as a male; (4) The response of a "healthy" family member may aid and abet the *maintenance of the sick role*. Or, on the contrary, a hostile response toward the ill member may prompt him to attempt to give up the sick role prematurely. When the former interaction is at play, the healthy member, be it parent or spouse, may derive gratification from playing a supporting and nurturing role. He or she may then interfere with treatment of the patient, foster his dependence, and decompensate psychologically if the patient recovers; (5) Chronic or fatal illness and disability often tend to accentuate *ambivalence* in the relationship between the sick member and the one most concerned with

his care. Negative aspects of the ambivalence are then a source of guilt and provoke renewed attempts at compensation with resulting increased resentment leading to more guilt, etc. Such a vicious circle is commonly observed, increases psychological stress for both partners, and predisposes to pathological forms of grief when the sick member dies; (6) Illness *does not always disorganize* a family, but at times helps it to rally together and consolidate itself.

THE PATIENT AND HEALTH PROFESSIONALS: THE DOCTOR–PATIENT RELATIONSHIP

The importance of the *doctor–patient relationship* for the course and outcome of the illness has long been recognized and there is extensive literature[10,108,146] on the subject. Only some salient theoretical models and studies are mentioned here.

Henderson[73] proposed an early model of doctor–patient interaction. He defined it concisely: "A physician and a patient taken together make up a social system. They do so because they are two and because they have relations of mutual dependence." Parsons[161] has carried a *sociological* analysis of the doctor–patient system further. He points out that the role of the physician "centers on his responsibility for the welfare of the patient in the sense of facilitating his recovery from illness to the best of the physician's ability." A doctor's judgment confers on a sick person the status of a "patient." This is a prerogative of the physician's social role.

The *social role* of the physician is only one aspect of the doctor–patient relationship. The analysis of the latter should include three basic elements: (1) The individual predispositions of the physician, including his unconscious motivations and responses;[227] (2) His internalized standards of professional behavior; and (3) The specific stimulus complex provided by the patient.[10]

Szasz and Hollender[203] describe three types of doctor–patient relationship: *activity–passivity*, in which the patient is helpless and passive and the physician treats him in a manner similar to that of the parent of a helpless infant;

guidance–cooperation, implying that the patient is capable of following directions and exercising judgment. He is, however, expected to comply with the physician as a competent guide. This model has its prototype in the relationship of the parent and his child (or adolescent); *mutual participation,* a model most appropriate for the management of chronic illness in which the patient is largely responsible for his care and consults the doctor only occasionally. The physician helps the patient to help himself. This is a relationship between two adults.

While each of the above models is appropriate for certain types or stages of illness as well as in relation to the patient's age, intelligence and cognitive clarity, the actual relationship may be inappropriate for the given patient and situation. Thus a comprehending adult may be treated as if he were a child. Such a relationship may be initiated by either doctor or patient, but willing cooperation of both is needed for the inappropriate relationship to become established and flourish. How can this happen? The answer lies in the fact that neither doctors nor patients are just rational adults and that both are influenced by unconscious motives related to dependent, sexual and/or power needs. The degree to which such elements enter into the doctor–patient relationship influences its quality and therapeutic efficacy. We speak of *transference* and *countertransference* in this relationship to mean distortion of the mutual perceptions of the doctor and patient, respectively, and consequently of their relationship, by the significant past relationships of each of them. Such influence is usually unconscious and may result in intense feelings of attraction, suspicion, hostility, competition, regressive dependence, etc., which tend to impair the professional relationship. Transference and countertransference do not mean conscious feelings of liking, trust, sympathy, or antipathy which are universal aspects of human relationships. They refer only to *distortion* of present relationships in terms of the past, usually childhood ones.

A common aspect of the doctor–patient relationship is *ambivalence,* which may be mutual. The doctor lends himself to contradictory feelings by virtue of his role itself. He is in some respects an authority, a judge and bearer of good or bad news related to the patient's future, to matters of suffering and death. The doctor may feel attracted to a patient, or repulsed and exploited by his demands, lack of progress, irrational behavior, or ingratitude. A physician's knowledge and therapeutic efficacy are limited, giving rise to doubts, sense of failure and other self-devaluating feelings which for some are hard to bear. The hallmarks of the patient's situation are *uncertainty* and, if treatment is undertaken, *dependence* on the doctor's judgment, competence, and information he chooses to transmit. This unique type of social relationship may arouse mutual mixed feelings in both partners. Whether such feelings remain within manageable bounds, or acquire disturbing intensity, depends both on the personality of the patient and the doctor's maturity, attitude, and conduct. A measure of self-awareness can certainly help the physician to avoid countertransference reactions burdensome for him and antitherapeutic for the patient.

One of the crucial aspects of the doctor–patient relationship is the quality of their mutual *communications,* verbal and nonverbal.[72] This subject was discussed in an earlier section dealing with the patients' communicative behavior (see p. 20). The other side of the dialogue is what the doctor communicates to the patient, how he does it, where and when. Studies relevant to this topic lead to the following conclusions: Information given by physician to patient affects the quality and course of treatment. The patient's compliance with medical advice is closely related to the degree of his satisfaction with having his need for information met. Insufficient, contradictory, or confusing information results in the patient's dissatisfaction and noncompliance.[34] The patient's postoperative course is improved by providing information before surgery. The degree of the information about illness transmitted by the physician to the patient depends on characteristics (personality, ethnic, cultural) of the physician and patient, and on the situation in which the information is communicated. If the doctor succeeds in giving accurate information in a manner understandable and emotionally acceptable to the patient and his family, he has a better chance of obtaining a meaningful history and cooperation.[213]

The quality of the doctor–patient relationship influences—for better or worse—the patient's response to his illness and its course and outcome. To some extent the same holds true for other health professionals, especially nurses involved in his care during hospitalization.[110]

(Personal Meanings of Illness

The central unifying concept in a discussion of psychological response to disease, injury, or disability is that of the *personal meaning* which illness in all its aspects has for the patient. It refers to the subjective significance of all the information input, internal and external, which the patient receives and appraises in the light of his values, beliefs, memories, conflicts, etc. The meaning is a product of the interplay between the patient, his illness and environment. It links conceptually the determinants and modes of the psychological response to disease. Symptoms, diagnostic label, lesion, functional impairment, doctors' statements, and other facets of the total illness experience are appraised by the patient, consciously and unconsciously. This process of evaluation, resulting in meaning, continues unabated throughout the course of every illness. It is a dynamic process reflecting continuity of the information inputs. One could talk of many changing meanings, but it is helpful to identify a dominant personal meaning of the illness or disability as a whole.[183]

What his illness means to a patient is influence by the determinants listed earlier (see p. 7), as well as by the quality of the emotional response elicited in and results of actions taken by him. The evolved meaning modifies and is in turn modified by the patient's emotions and perceptions. The dynamic interplay among these factors and the related feedback

effects contribute to the complexity of this subject and the difficulty in explaining it clearly. Some clinical examples may illustrate it.

To understand why a patient feels and acts in a particular manner it is necessary to gain insight into what his particular illness or disability means to him. For example, people who value their *physical* appearance highly are prone to psychological breakdown as a result of mutilation or disfigurement.[136] Impairment of *intellectual* or *perceptual* functions by disease of the brain, or sensory organs or pathways, will disrupt the main adaptive coping mechanisms and source of pride and security in any individual for whom intellectual achievement or perceptual clarity are indispensable conditions for self-esteem, pleasure, a sense of competence, and economic security. A man whose major source of gratification is *sexual* prowess and ability to procreate is likely to be disturbed by impotence due to spinal injury, diabetes, or prostatectomy, for example. Mastectomy, hysterectomy, or masculinization induced by hormones in a woman may have similar emotional effects, as well as revive latent intrapsychic conflicts over her sexual identity and role. Persons who attach particular importance to personal *cleanliness* as part of an obsessional personality style are liable to feel dirty and devalued after construction of a colostomy.[37] Urinary or fecal incontinence may have similar effects.[158] Some paraplegic patients seen by the writer were more disturbed by loss of sphincter control than by paralysis.

Such examples may be multiplied. In each of them the specific personal meaning of the disease, dysfunction, etc., for the particular individual is a crucial factor in determining his emotional and behavioral responses. The latter are also influenced by the attitudes of the patient's environment to both his illness and behavior. In general, there is no organ or physiological function whose disturbance, damage, or loss could not disturb a given individual's sense of security and personal worth because of its personal value-laden meaning for him. The psychological impact of illness or disability depends in part on the individual's vulnerability related to his personality and past experience.

Categories of Meaning

It is helpful for clinical assessment of patients to distinguish four broad categories of subjective meaning of illness, injury, disability, and its consequences for the patient:[118] 1. threat 2. loss 3. gain or relief 4. insignificance.

Threat implies anticipation of harm to one's physical and/or psychic integrity whose occurrence would cause suffering. Such anticipation may follow perception of any bodily change if this is interpreted by the person as signifying danger to him. At times, no threat is perceived until the patient is told by a doctor that an illness is present. Tendency to interpret somatic perceptions as threatening varies widely and appears to be an enduring personality trait acquired through earlier learning. Some people respond with alarm to any novel somatic perception or even one, say palpitations, which they may have been told repeatedly to disregard as harmless. Others equally consistently minimize and ignore even obvious and painful bodily changes.

Anticipation of danger, whether realistic or not, characteristically evokes *anxiety* or *fear*.[51,189] To avoid semantic confusion, the term anxiety is used exclusively in this discussion. This affect is accompanied by individually varied patterns of physiological arousal which may give rise to somatic perceptions, such as palpitations, sweating, shortness of breath, etc. These may, in turn, be interpreted as danger signals and result in augmentation of anxiety—an example of a positive feedback. Anxiety tends to increase vigilance to threat and to set off cognitive and behavioral activities aimed at avoidance, tackling, or minimization of the anticipated danger, and thus reduction of the unpleasant experience of the anxiety state itself. The coping strategies employed by people to reduce or eliminate anxiety include the unconsciously operating ego mechanisms of defense as well as deliberate actions, such as intake of drugs or alcohol, compulsive overwork or sexual activity. Thus

threat and anxiety have both physiological and behavioral consequences which may be adaptive or harmful. Excessive physiological arousal may complicate and exacerbate an existent pathological process, and precipitate cardiac decompensation or fatal arrhythmia in a patient with heart disease, for example. Coping with anxiety may harm the individual, if he engages in actions inimical to his health. Excessive intensity of the aroused anxiety may lead to delay or, on the contrary, undue haste in seeking medical help. A moderate degree of anxiety results in optimal adjustment to illness and its consequences.[82]

Loss in this context means not only actual damage to the person's bodily integrity, that is loss of body parts and functions, but also *symbolic losses* resulting from disease or disability. Such losses refer to deprivation of personally significant needs and values. The latter are related chiefly to *self-esteem, security, and gratification of needs*. Any illness or disability may result in partial or total loss of gratification derived from eating; from physical, sexual, or intellectual activities; esthetic qualities of physical appearance, and so forth. These various activities and attributes lost evoke an emotional response *in proportion to their subjective value and importance to the individual*.

The common emotional response to real or anticipated loss, whether concrete or symbolic, takes the form of *grief*. This may merge imperceptibly into a depressive syndrome. Less often, reaction to loss may take the form of any psychiatric disorder, neurotic or psychotic, or antisocial behavior, or somatic illness. Grief is a normal affective reaction to any type of loss, including that of a bodily part or function. Its intensity and duration are roughly proportional to the subjective importance of the loss. Grief is considered by many authors as a necessary step in the work of mourning which results in eventual acceptance and adjustment to what is irreparably lost.[83,180,225] The desirability of grieving is often taken for granted in the literature, especially that inspired by psychoanalytic theory. Lack of grief in the face of loss is usually assigned to the working of the mechanism of *denial*, which is also invoked when a person shows no anxiety in response to threat. Yet absence of anxiety may be a sign of good adjustment and is not always presumptive evidence of the operation of denial.[185] Lack of grief may mean that the given event was not perceived by the patient as a loss. More systematic research is needed in this area to validate the prevailing hypotheses and caution is indicated in accepting them as universally valid facts.[144]

Gain or *relief* refer to a personal significance of illness, conscious or unconscious, as a source of psychological, social and/or economic advantage for the patient. From the psychological viewpoint, any illness or disability may facilitate resolution, gratification, or avoidance of intrapsychic conflicts over disavowed impulses: aggressive, sexual, dependent or powerseeking. Illness may provide a legitimate reason for avoidance of conflictual situations and actions. An epileptic, for example, may avoid contacts with the opposite sex on the grounds that he might develop a seizure in the presence of his partner, or that he is unfit to be married, have children, etc. Another patient may justify outbursts of anger or avoidance of competitive situations by invoking his particular illness or disability. Open expression of dependent needs and demands for their gratification may be legitimized in the patient's view by the special status conferred on him by his disease or disability. Thus illness may provide rationalization for either avoidance of or indulgence in behavior which the patient could not otherwise face or engage in without conflict. In other cases, a painful or otherwise disabling illness may satisfy a psychological, usually unconscious, need for suffering as atonement for unacceptable impulses or fantasies. When such psychic factors are present, the patient may have a vested interest in maintaining his illness and react adversely to its improvement.[78] The patient's manifest attitude to his illness may be entirely at variance with his unconscious view of it and its psychological advantages. He may deplore in good faith that he is ill and clamor for relief and cure, while his nonverbal behavior may express the opposite attitude of which he is unaware and which he may explicitly deny.

From the *social* viewpoint, illness may provide a patient with a strategy used to avoid social demands and responsibilities, and secure attention, support, and compliance of others, especially his family members. Some patients derive a sense of identity, pride, and satisfaction from being ill, particularly if the illness is unusual and attracts attention and curiosity of others, including doctors. A patient with a rare disease may attract much medical attention, be repeatedly displayed and discussed by physicians, and puzzle them. He may learn to enjoy the exhibitionistic aspects of such interest and the perplexity of the doctors. For some individuals this may be the only claim to distinction. They are not likely to give up these advantages readily.

One may propose this generalization: A patient's overall response to illness and disability, and his motivation to get well, are related to the subjectively experienced losses and/or gains derived from the illness.

Insignificance refers to a relative absence of personal meaning of one's illness or symptoms. Early symptoms of a neoplasm, for example, may be ignored by the patient if they do not signify a threat to him. This may be a result of incorrect appraisal due to lack of medical knowledge, but may also stem from indifference to symptoms in someone who is withdrawn, depressed, apathetic, or who believes himself invulnerable.

Illness experience and behavior change as illness progresses and full recovery, a downward course, or some degree of permanent disability follow. The view of illness as a *process* involving a *time dimension* may be clarified if we describe it as comprising a series of *phases* or *stages*.[199] As the patient moves from one stage to the next, he faces novel tasks which impose demands upon him.

(Stages of Illness

The terms "acute" and "chronic" are commonly used in medical and psychiatric practice and connote rate of onset, duration, and reversibility of disease. These terms are ambiguous. It is difficult to identify clearly any group of individuals as the chronically ill, or the acutely ill, or those with disabilities. Within most diagnostic categories there are patients who are more disabled than ill, more acutely ill than chronically ill, and so on. The term "chronic illness", as commonly used, is synonymous with disability.[183]

We will attempt to give a meaningful presentation here of a patient's progress, the changing tasks, stresses, and pitfalls he has to face on the road to recovery, or when chronic illness, disability, or fatal disease preclude return to full health. Not every patient goes through all the stages. His illness may become arrested at any of them. An acute phase may never occur. There are only three possible outcomes: recovery, chronicity, or death. The following stages will be described:

1. symptom perception,
2. decision making,
3. medical contact,
4. acute illness,
5. convalescence or rehabilitation,
6. chronic illness or disability.

The Symptom-Perception Stage

Psychological characteristics of this phase of any illness are: *perception* of change within one's body boundaries and its *evaluation*.

Traditionally, a *symptom* has been defined as a manifestation of disease apparent to the patient himself; a *sign* denotes a manifestation of disease that only the physician perceives. This distinction is misleading. Engel[41] proposes that "the presence of a complaint must be regarded as presumptive evidence of disease." A symptom is a phenomenon belonging to the realm of subjective perception which may or may not be observable by others, or communicated to them as a complaint. A *sign* connotes an *inference* made by a qualified observer that what the patient reports and/or the observer notices directly, or discovers by means of special techniques, indicates the presence of a particular disease. Such an inference may be made not only by a doctor, but at times also by a lay observer, and may

be at variance with what the patient perceives, reports, or even explicitly denies.

A person's interpretation of the significance of his symptoms determines his affective responses and subsequent action or lack of it. Symptoms are perceived and evaluated differentially by different individuals and in different social situations. Such differences reflect both culturally and socially learned responses, and the subject's personality.[146]

Sociocultural differences result in different patterns of response to symptoms of illness. For instance, upper-class persons are more likely than lower-class members to see themselves as ill when they experience particular symptoms.[103] Ethnic factors were discussed before in relation to studies by Zola and Zborowski. As symptoms become more severe, continuous, unfamiliar, and unpredictable in their course, however, the sociocultural and ethnic factors become less important.[146] Pain, the commonest symptom, is likely to motivate a search for a medical consultation.[41,149,194,202]

A different approach to the perception and evaluation of symptoms uses the concept of *body image* as a basis for explanatory hypotheses and research methodology.[177] Every individual has a unique concept of his body as a psychological object. Alterations of body perception which occur in illness are responded to cognitively and emotionally in a manner and intensity which are partly dependent on the subject's body concept. Sensations arising from areas assigned high significance in the person's body gestalt are more likely to be registered and interpreted.[23] The vast literature on the body image has recently been reviewed by Fisher,[52] and the concept itself critically analyzed by Shontz.[184] The reader is referred to these sources as well as to Chapter 33 of this Volume.

A *psychodynamic* approach to somatic symptoms is represented by a study by Silverman.[186] He claims that the development of physical symptoms, regardless of whether they are due to organic disease, is related to "an insufficiency of the psychological systems for handling the stimulus influx mobilized by stress." This study represents an attempt to explore an important dimension of somatic symptoms, namely their *unconscious symbolic meaning and determinants*. This area of investigation still suffers from the lack of reliable methods of validating the proposed links between observation records on the one hand, and inferences made from them, on the other. In general, the more the meaning of perceived symptoms is influenced by unconscious needs, fantasies, and conflicts, the more irrational, idiosyncratic, and unpredictable is the patient's overt response. Panic, massive denial, and disregard of the likely significance of symptoms, their delusional misinterpretations, marked delay or, on the contrary, undue haste in seeking medical help—these are familiar examples of responses to symptoms which are more influenced by unconscious factors than by rational reasoning and knowledge.

Experiential factors related to previous illness episodes in oneself, or in a person close to the patient, tend to influence the meaning of symptoms and affective response to them. One who lost a close relative by cancer or heart disease may become sensitized to and fearful of any associatively linked symptom in himself. This may be an expression of identification with or guilt toward the deceased individual.

Physicians commonly speak of "organic" or "functional" symptoms. This distinction is meaningless since every illness has both physiological and psychic components and the crucial question is *how much both of them* contribute to the patient's clinical picture.[116] It may help the clinician to assess such a relative contribution if he has a clear grasp of complaints which indicate *psychic distress* regardless of whether a physical illness is present. The following classification may serve as a guide to complaints or symptoms pertaining to the body, but indicative of psychological distress or disorder. Such symptoms are variously referred to as "psychogenic," "psychophysiological," "psychosomatic," or "somatization reactions"—all vague and misused terms.

1. Physiological correlates of *affective arousal*,[9] such as anxiety or anger, or somatic manifestations of an *affective disorder*, mainly depressive or anxiety syndromes, e.g., pain, palpitations, diarrhea, hyperventilation syndrome, polyuria, etc.[193] Of course, none of these symptoms is pathognomonic of a psychiatric disorder.

2. Somatic expression and communication of ideational, often conflict-related, mental contents, which originate at the symbolic level of organization and attempt to imitate a physical illness to meet the patient's psychosocial needs. These are the *conversion symptoms*.[44]

3. Secondary symbolic elaborations, manifested as conversion symptoms, of perceived somatic changes of any etiology, e.g., hysterical fits coexisting with epilepsy.[127]

4. Excessive preoccupation with bodily sensations, functions and appearance, often accompanied by increased sensitivity to normally subliminal somesthetic sensations. This is *hypochondriasis*.*

5. Nosophobia, that is morbid fear of disease, such as cancer, venereal or heart disease, etc.[116]

6. Somatic delusions, that is, *false convictions* of bodily change, disfigurement or disease, e.g., of changing one's sexual characteristics or having parasites, expressive of unconscious fantasies and signifying schizophrenic or depressive *psychosis*, or occurring transiently in *delirium*.

7. Communication of psychological distress in *bodily metaphors*, e.g. "my heart is heavy," "my head is empty."

8. Psychogenic *body image disturbances*, that is, subjective sense of change in color, shape, weight, size, position, etc., of the body and/or its parts. Such symptoms occur in association with schizophrenia, depression, severe anxiety states, and the depersonalization syndrome.[52,177]

9. Somatic symptoms representing *residues* of earlier responses to stress,[195] or memories of somatic symptoms experienced during a forgotten childhood illness and reexperienced through associative links with a current psychosocial stress.

The above symptoms may be present alone or coexist with and mask those of a physical illness, just as the latter may be present as a disorder of mood or higher mental func-

---

* See references 96, 97, 128, 167, and 177.

tions.[116] At any given time, symptoms may be manifestations of primarily organic pathology, the affective response to it and the associated physiological arousal, and of the symbolic meaning of the other symptoms. A patient may experience combinations of symptoms having different mechanisms and diagnostic significance.[143]

The Decision-Making Stage

A patient's response to his symptoms has a bearing on his *decision to seek medical help*.[17,134,197,232] Studies of medical care in the United States and England show that in a population of 1000 adults over sixteen years of age, in an average month 750 experience an episode of illness, but only 250 of these consult a doctor.[213] In certain population groups, such as the aged, nine out of ten illness episodes are not treated by a physician.[232] At least three sets of factors influence the patient's decision to seek medical help: (1) his objective clinical disorder and symptoms, as well as his perception, knowledge, beliefs, and attitudes about having a particular disorder; (2) his attitudes and expectations of the doctor and medical services; and (3) his definitions of "health," "sickness," and need for medical care.[197] These factors vary in the population and reflect individual, ethnic, and sociocultural variables discussed earlier.

Many people seek medical consultation during periods of *life stress*.[17,90,91,197] Psychophysiological reactions evoked by such stress are a source of discomfort and may also prompt attention to symptoms which were previously ignored. Life stress may foster the adoption of the sick role regardless of presence or absence of a physiological change or dysfunction.[3] The onset of a psychiatric disorder in response to psychosocial stress may bring the patient to a doctor, but be expressed in terms of the somatic complaints listed earlier.

The patient's decision-making process is practically important for two reasons: (1) It has a bearing on *preventive medicine* and *timely* utilization of medical facilities; and (2) It is related to *overuse* of medical care. The former problem has been studied to identify

psychosocial causes of *delay* in seeking medical help for serious conditions, mostly cancer and heart disease.*

Delay may be computed from the date of first appearance of symptoms or from the time a symptom is recognized by the patient as requiring medical attention.[91] It is this latter, "avoidable," delay which has attracted particular attention. Many different factors have been suggested as influencing delay: 1. *age*, older patients being more likely to delay; 2. *ethnic factors*; 3. *lower socioeconomic status*; 4. *site of symptoms*, those noticeable by others may lead to greater delay;[63] 5. *personality variables*.

Most studies identify two sets of relevant factors: *excessive anxiety* related to the appraisal of symptoms as highly threatening; and ignorance, minimization, and/or denial of the significance of symptoms accompanied by *low anxiety*.† Denial and extreme anxiety may not, however, be the only relevant factors. *Severe depression* related to a life crisis may make some patients relatively indifferent to somatic symptoms, or be accompanied by self-destructive or masochistic tendencies with resulting inaction. A *schizophrenic* may be indifferent to pain of a myocardial infarction, for example.

Excessive use of medical facilities has been less often studied than delay, even though undue tendency to respond to subjective discomfort by seeking medical help contributes to the cost of medical care. Such behavior may be a manifestation of hypochondriasis.[96,97,128,167] Some patients suffering from *anxiety neurosis* may displace their anxiety from inner conflicts onto somatic concerns and fear of disease. A doctor may reinforce such fears by telling the patient that he has a "weak heart" or "tired blood," for example. Many patients come to medical clinics or doctors' offices because they need sympathetic advice about *psychosocial problems*. If the doctor ignores this need, the patient may continue to return to him and present ever new somatic symptoms until a doctor opens up a discussion of the patient's real concerns, or attaches a medi-

---

* See references 19, 27, 61, 63, 67, 71, 90, and 91.
† See references 19, 27, 61, 63, 67, and 71.

cal label to his complaints. In the latter case the patient may "organize" his illness and enter a long-term "patient career."[3,145] Such patients are likely to become chronic attenders of clinics, etc., and are often called "crocks" by the exasperated doctors.[128] Early inquiry into the reasons underlying the patient's complaints and the timing of his visits may lead to a talk about his psychosocial problems, usually family or job related. This may satisfy the patient's need and prevent repeated and fruitless attendance.[3,159,196,197]

The Medical Contact Stage

Once a person has decided to consult a doctor, a new element enters the picture: *patient–doctor interaction*.[14] This aspect of illness has been discussed earlier and only a few additional comments need be added.

Both the patient and physician bring certain expectations into their encounter. They are partly related to their respective *social roles* which consist of conventionally defined attitudes, rights, and duties assigned to each participant. Patients tend to evaluate the physician by nonprofessional criteria which are influenced by their cultural background and conceptions of what constitutes a *good doctor*. Surveys indicate that people single out competence, interest in patients, and a sympathetic and concerned manner, as the chief qualities of a good doctor.[146] The success of a visit to a physician, judged by the patient's satisfaction and willingness to comply with the doctor's advice, depends to a large extent on whether the patient's expectations are met.

For the doctor, the purpose of a consultation is to arrive at a diagnosis. "The satisfaction felt by the physician when he is able to assign a name, hopefully the correct one, to the patient's illness is matched only by the layman's relief when he hears that he is suffering from aplastic anemia and not leukemia."[45] This wry comment reflects a deplorable aspect of current medical practice. To diagnose means more than attach a medical label. It also includes an assessment of the patient's

personality and current level of psychological functioning; his family, occupational, social, and economic situation; and his attitude toward his illness and symptoms. To achieve a *comprehensive* diagnosis the doctor observes the patient's appearance and verbal and nonverbal behavior, takes an extensive history, and performs a manual and instrumental examination. These aspects of a medical consultation cannot be discussed in detail here. The reader is referred to selected references.*

The doctor's diagnostic reasoning process and the decision reached are influenced by his interaction and communication with the patient. These, in turn, are affected by the doctor's personality and whether he is *physical-minded* or *psychological-minded*, respectively. The former is typically less reflective, introspective, and interested in abstract psychological ideas than the latter.[214] These personality characteristics determine if the doctor pays attention and tries to deal with his patients' psychosocial concerns.

Whatever the result of the doctor's diagnostic reasoning may be, he has to convey his opinion and advice to the patient. The manner in which he does it influences the patient's affective response and his cooperation or lack of it.[34,62,72] The doctor should state his findings and opinions clearly, bearing in mind the kind of person he is dealing with. The patient's ability to comprehend and his need for information and likely reaction to it have to be assessed. An intelligent, obsessional patient needs more information to allay his anxiety than one whose intellectual capacity and need for understanding are less. Medical jargon, ambiguous statements, or vague innuendoes may increase the patient's anxiety and open the way to misinterpretations.[62] A patient who habitually minimizes and denies the significance of danger must be recognized and given an unambiguous statement of what the physician thinks and recommends. Disclosure of diagnosis of a serious and potentially fatal illness will be discussed later (see p. 50). When no evidence of organic disease is found,

---

* See references 14, 45, 46, 49, 108, and 154.

the patient should be told so and asked about other possible reasons for his symptoms. To tell him that his complaints are "imaginary" or "functional" and he is really well, only serves to antagonize him and belies his subjective perception of ill health. The doctor should state that while there is no evidence of organic illness, there must be a reason for the patient's discomfort, possibly related to his life situation. In this way an inquiry into the latter and possible preparation for a psychiatric consultation may be broached.[123]

The Acute Illness Stage

An acute illness implies relatively sudden onset and brief duration. A mild, commonplace acute illness is usually self-limited and may not even bring a patient to the doctor. If the illness is serious, however, it drastically interrupts a person's way of life and readily arouses fears of death, incapacity, dependence on others, and personal losses discussed earlier. Pain, if present, adds to the other stresses. The patient often responds with shock, disbelief, and sometimes attempts at escape from the threatening situation.[102] Thus a patient with an acute myocardial infarction may attempt to continue his activities and dismiss his symptoms as "indigestion" or some other harmless condition.[210] He may display unconcern and even bravado which mask his anxiety and may be mistaken for courage. An acutely ill patient needs the doctor's emotional support and reassuring firmness.

The characteristics of this phase, or type, of illness are: adoption of some degree of *dependence* on others; *confinement* at home or a hospital; and *uncertainty* about the outcome. The latter may be full recovery, death, or some degree of irreversible damage and thus chronicity. An acute illness may be a transient or terminal phase of a chronic one. Since the other aspects of illness have been discussed before, we will focus on one common feature of acute illness: *hospitalization* and the hospital as a *social milieu* with which the patient interacts.

RESPONSE TO HOSPITALIZATION

Admission to a medical ward is for many a novel and anxiety-provoking experience, for some a welcome respite. As an inpatient one becomes a member of a specific social milieu in which the chief roles are played by the health professionals. A person accustomed to privacy and independence has to surrender them, and his freedom of action is curtailed by the authority of doctors and nurses. He is subjected to often irksome rules. Members of the clinical team decide what is wrong with him, what investigations and therapies he is to undergo, what restrictions to observe, and what behavior is acceptable or not. The physical environment itself is for many unfamiliar and often frightening. The patient brings to this situation his habitual attitudes toward and modes of coping with novelty, dependence, passive submission, authority figures, and uncertainty—hallmarks of his condition as a hospitalized patient. Most people manage to adjust to this situation, some enjoy it, some find it distressing.[35,116,123] The patient engages in interactions with other patients and ward personnel, and the more *anxious* and/or angry he is, the more likely is he to fall into conflict with some member of the ward community. He is then liable to be branded a "management problem" or a "difficult patient," and referred for a psychiatric consultation.[115]

The mere event of admission to a medical ward may be a source of stress. Corticosteroid and catecholamine responses, respectively, were studied in two groups of normal adults admitted to a hospital research ward. Urinary 17-hydroxycorticosteroids, epinephrine, and norepinephrine values were higher on the day of admission than later in hospitalization. This suggests that hospital admission involves elements of novelty, threat, and unpredictability which are associated with stress and psychophysiological arousal.[142,205]

Ward rounds[93] and laboratory procedures may be emotionally stressful.[89] Yet predictions of what may disturb a given patient are not easy. This is illustrated by a study of women awaiting breast biopsy for suspected cancer.[92] Despite the obvious uncertainty and unpredictability of this situation for the patients, the majority of them did not show manifest breakdown of psychological defenses. This was reflected in the normal range of hydrocortisone production rates. Thus it is incorrect to assume a priori that what to an observer may appear as "stress" actually evokes emotional *distress* in a given individual or group. The distress depends on how a potentially threatening situation is individually perceived, interpreted, and defended against. Some patients react with excessive emotions to hospitalization, investigations, surgery, etc.

It is largely up to the doctors and nurses to ensure that a medical ward should have a therapeutic effect. To prevent psychological crises in the ward milieu it is important to ensure maintenance of *communication* between patients and staff.[115] This helps prevent interpersonal conflicts related to fears, mutual distrust, and distorted perceptions among members of the ward community. Some physicians and nurses readily provoke in many of their patients unduly dependent, hostile, anxious, or seductive responses which interfere with professional relationships. Such complications are avoidable and may call for a clarifying and mediating intervention of a psychiatric consultant.[115]

Understanding of the patient's personality and some degree of psychological self-awareness on the part of the staff facilitate therapeutic and preventive actions. The latter, called by some "adaptive intervention" or "therapeutic manipulation," involve *personality diagnosis, suggestion,* and *clarification.*[8,86] The use of such methods need not be confined to psychiatric consultants. Properly trained nurses may apply some of these techniques, for example in *group therapy* sessions for the inpatients in a general hospital. Such intervention may help them adjust to hospitalization, illness, investigative and therapeutic procedures, etc.[110]

There is a growing trend to create a *therapeutic social milieu* in the general hospital.[83] This involves attention by the staff to the patients' emotional needs and their fears and uncertainties, which are often either unexpressed

spontaneously or acted out in behavior disruptive of ward routine.

The Convalescent or Rehabilitation Stage

Physiological recovery from illness should lead to surrender of the sick role. This applies to all acute and fully reversible illness as well as that which leaves physically nondisabling residual damage. When convalescence and/or rehabilitation is indicated, the patient should cooperate. Yet psychosocial factors may interfere with these goals and prolong disability beyond the physiological recovery and despite the doctor's judgment that the patient is well. A physical illness or injury may be followed by some degree of disability due to psychosocial factors, that is, by *psychological invalidism*. Intrapsychic as well as socioeconomic factors may contribute.[31,80,176]

INTRAPSYCHIC FACTORS

Ruesch[176] studied a sample of patients with *delayed recovery*. He frequently found conflicts over dependency and aggression in men, and conflicts related to self-love and the feminine role in women. The men tended to be dependent and passive, the women dominant, aggressive, and overprotective. The sick role provided these patients with a *primary gain*, that is reduction of intensity of intrapsychic conflicts and related unpleasant affects. When physical illness or injury occurred in a setting of *psychological stress* or *interpersonal conflict*, recovery was delayed. Psychologically traumatic implications of disease or therapeutic procedures had the same effect.[176]

Other studies of patients with delayed recovery from a variety of infections, or cardiovascular and other diseases generally concur with Ruesch's findings. Severe psychological trauma in their early lives, proneness to depression, and a disturbed life situation and depression before or after illness, characterizes many patients who have prolonged convalescence.[80] Slow recovery from infectious mononucleosis was correlated with lower scores of ego-strength.[80] Protracted convalescence in women who underwent radical mastectomy

could be predicted by
relation between the ...
that of the delayed ...
sample of patients ...
cardial infarction ...
meaning of the h ...
determinant of ...
themselves to ...
able.[101,126]

Thus endu ...
the concurre ...
and/or inte ...
covery. The ...
ary gains a ...
to psychological, ...
vantages which a patien ...
illness. One should make ...
ever, between conscious ...
lection to illness on the ...
tence of somatic sympton ...
arousal on the other. In the ...
tional and *attitudinal* factors ...
role; in the second case, the ...
illness merges with a *psycho...* ...,
as anxiety, depressive, conversion, or hypochondriacal neurosis, and related perception
of symptoms.[125,210] This distinction is important for treatment. If the patient suffers from
an anxiety state, for example, psychotherapy
and use of psychotropic drugs may help accelerate his recovery.

Social and Economic Factors

The doctor–patient relationship plays a
part in delayed recovery and rehabilitation.
The amount and quality of *information* which
the physician transmits to the patient is important.[39] This is well illustrated by the effects of
the extent of medical information given to patients suffering from a first coronary occlusion.
The nature and adequacy of information
given to such patients is associated with the
frequency and timing of return to work. Anxiety and depression are common in these patients and related to the inability of doctors to
confront and answer patients' questions about
the meaning and implications of their illness.[141,155] Treating patients' symptoms related to psychological distress as if they were
manifestations of continuing physical illness is

member may reinforce the patient's secondary
gains from being sick by meeting his dependent needs to a much greater extent than
when he was well. Anxiety in the spouse may
increase that of the patient. If there is convergence between the latter's motivation, conscious or unconscious, to remain ill and a
gratifying family response to his persisting
complaints, prolonged psychogenic disability
may ensue.

Social security disability programs, workmen's compensation insurance, compensation
and medical malpractice suits, and other *economic* incentives may contribute to the patient's secondary gains and invalidism.[217]

The Chronic-Illness Stage

Chronic illness implies a significant degree
of *irreversibility* of the pathological process or
damage to the body and the related *disability*.
It is an ill-defined category[183] and includes
such diverse conditions as congenital defects,
acquired injuries and illnesses leaving residual

* See references 12, 101, 141, 155, and 221.

damage, and incurable diseases with a progressive or remitting course. It is difficult and misleading to generalize about such diverse pathological conditions. Their importance lies in the fact that chronic illnesses are the leading cause of morbidity in advanced societies.[36] The literature on the psychological aspects of specific types of chronic illness and disability is extensive.*

To discuss meaningfully psychological responses to chronic illness or disability, one has to classify categories according to several criteria:

1. Time of onset. It is important if the given defect, disease, or disability was present at or acquired after birth. If the latter, then at what point in the person's life cycle did it appear? We do not deal here with congenital defects or deformities, since they must be considered part of the individual's somatic endowment and not a stage of an illness.

2. Rate of onset: acute or gradual. The latter allows the patient more time to develop coping mechanisms and is usually less traumatic psychologically than the former.

3. Presence or absence of progression. If the disability results from an accident, for example, and a *stable* condition ensues, the patient is dealing with some form and degree of permanent disability, loss of function, or disfigurement, to which he has to adjust. If the pathological condition is potentially *progressive*, this adds an element of *uncertainty* about the future. Many people find uncertainty more distressing than a serious but definite loss. Sufferers from many chronic illnesses, such as multiple sclerosis, find it hard to plan for the future which for them is unpredictable.[127] A terminal illness adds the challenge of facing early death.

4. Degree of reversibility of and/or compensability for the impaired function. These factors determine realistic planning for rehabilitation and adjustment, and the setting of goals toward which the patient may strive and whose achievement may be a source of pride and enhanced self-esteem.[53]

* See references 6, 32, 60, 144, and 225.

We will describe some of the more commonly observed *response patterns* to *severe disability* and *fatal illness*, especially *cancer*, respectively. Much of what was discussed in relation to the other stages of illness is equally relevant to the present stage and will not be repeated.

Chodoff[25,26] offers a classification and description of *patterns of psychological adjustment* to chronic illness and disability. It will be used as a general framework and basis for discussion. The proposed three major response patterns are:

1. *Insightful acceptance,* characterized by a lack of bitterness and hostility, and of a sense of personal devaluation. The patient copes adaptively, cooperates with rehabilitation plans, tries to learn substitute skills, and find new sources of gratification. This is the most desirable response both for the patient and those concerned with his care.

2. *The denial pattern,* characterized by negation of objective facts of illness, for example of paralysis; of significance of disability, such as the need to be cared for or to avoid certain activities; and of one's emotional response to illness, like anxiety, depression, or anger. Denial may be applied to one or all of the above aspects of illness and vary in extent. It may be explicitly or implicitly expressed. As such it is neither necessarily pathological nor maladaptive. Some degree of it may help maintain optimal psychic adaptation. Denial is pathological only if it concerns obvious facts and/or prevents the patient from behaving in a manner respecting his limitations and requirements of treatment.

3. *The regressive pattern* is characterized by exaggerated *dependence* and *passivity*, often with thinly veiled anger and hostility. A regressed patient plays up his disability and demands maximum attention and care from his environment. He exaggerates his helplessness and suffering and uses his illness as a strategy to manipulate others by playing on their sympathy or feelings of guilt. This pattern is most often observed in hysterical personalities who are typically overly dependent and dramatize their feelings, as well as in

some people who overemphasize their physical prowess and independence.

Such classifications are deficient in several respects. They are static and obscure clinical observations that the chronically ill and disabled go through various *phases* of psychological response. Patients may experience shock, denial, grief, anger, apathy, and euphoria, that is, display a wide spectrum of emotional reactions and defensive strategies before settling in one or another response pattern. In practice one must consider the changing, *dynamic* aspects of every patient's illness behavior.[183] General classifications tend to ignore inherent personality *assets* which are present to some extent in *every patient* and must be used to the best advantage in his rehabilitation. If a patient is just labelled as a "denier" or "regressed," this may lead to therapeutic nihilism and failure to tap whatever usable personality resources he may possess. Even small gains in a sense of self-esteem and meaningful existence in the severely disabled are a worthwhile goal of rehabilitation efforts.[183] Categorizing patients in terms of their ego mechanisms of defence gives no indication of what specific affects they are defending against. Is it anxiety, grief, shame, guilt, envy, resentment, or hopelessness? Identification of the specific affective response in the individual patient may offer important clues for therapeutic intervention, be it individual or group psychotherapy, behavior therapy, or use of psychotropic drugs.

In conclusion, generalizations or labels should not obviate the need for repeated evaluation of each patient's psychological assets and liabilities as a basis for an *individually tailored* and periodically reassessed management approach.*

The same holds for every patient regardless of the nature of his disease or disability. Patients suffering from *cancer* provide another important example.[76] There is a vast literature on psychological aspects of cancer, with 126 citations in English between 1970–1973 alone.[170] There too we see attempts to classify psychological response patterns which cancer patients evolve.[182] Such descriptive categories may serve only as guidelines in evaluating a given patient's most dominant concerns and emotional reaction at a given time. Few patients display an invariable response pattern throughout their illness and its treatment. One must be sensitive to shifts in the psychological responses and encourage the most adaptive ones. Problems of communicating diagnosis of cancer,[95,106,152,156] patterns of communication,[1] and psychological aspects of the management of cancer[59,163] cannot be discussed here. The question whether psychological factors influence prognosis of cancer patients has attracted attention. In one study, those with a most favorable outcome had a high proportion of individuals who had strong *hostile* drives without loss of emotional control.[192] Others report that cancer patients who were *aware* of the nature of their illness lived longer than those who were not, while those who suffered from concomitant *depression* tended to die sooner than those not depressed.[2]

Conclusion

The same general determinants of psychological responses operate at all stages and in all types of physical illness. A multifactorial scheme for the clinical evaluation and study of such responses has been proposed in this Chapter. This general model is applicable to any disease or injury, acute or chronic, mild or severe. The relative weight of the different factors obviously varies from patient to patient, but they all contribute to illness experience and behavior. Assessment of these factors is a necessary part of comprehensive diagnosis as a basis for efficient clinical management of all patients.

(Terminal Illness and Its Management

Terminal illness connotes impending death. Finality replaces uncertainty about the future.

---

* See references 26, 53, 59, 60, 81, 144, and 225.

It is the last phase of the human life cycle evoking intense psychological responses in patients, their families, and the health professionals. Its specific problems justify a separate discussion.

The scientific study of attitudes toward death and the experience of dying has a short history. Few systematic studies had been published until about twenty years ago. By 1964, a bibliography on death and bereavement listed 321 entries of which about one-third had been published after 1960.[87] A more recent annotated bibliography on death and dying deals with the more important works which had appeared up to 1969.[88] This upsurge of scientific interest in death and dying continues and is one of the most remarkable developments in contemporary culture. We now have a body of factual knowledge which allows formulation of guidelines for the management of the dying. We first discuss briefly some salient observations and then principles of management.

One should first distinguish different foci of studies related to death and dying: (1) of psychological and cultural *attitudes* toward death in the general population; (2) of the *fear* of death, one's own or of others; (3) of the *concept of death* in various populations, such as children; (4) of *thanatophobia*; (5) of the attitudes, experiences and communications of the *moribund patient*; and (6) of the actual *experience of dying*.

Only the last two types of studies can be considered here. The reader is referred to several recent books which together offer comprehensive coverage of the whole subject.*

Weisman and Kastenbaum[220] have written a lucid account of a study of the terminal phase of life. Their method, "the psychological autopsy," was an interdisciplinary conference that attempted to reconstruct the preterminal and terminal phases of life of a recently deceased patient and evaluate the role of psychosocial factors in his death. Their patient sample consisted of eighty elderly men and women, inmates of a hospital for the aged.

* See references 13, 48, 107, 165, 220, and 219.

The authors emphasize that dying is a *natural event* in the life cycle. There is a distinct *preterminal period* that may be regarded as a developmental phase serving as preparation for and adaptation to impending death. The dying process must not be viewed as a "mental health problem." Four attitudes toward death could be distinguished: 1. *acceptance*; 2. *apathy*; 3. *apprehension*; and 4. *anticipation*, i.e. acceptance plus an explicit wish for death. Acceptance was more often the attitude of well-adjusted patients, while death anxiety was associated with moderately severe organic and psychiatric deterioration.[219,220]

Those findings were obtained retrospectively and from a restricted patient population. It would be erroneous to generalize from them. Thus, observations of terminal cancer patients revealed that nearly all of them were deeply concerned about dying, depressed, and frightened.[163] Kübler-Ross, in her valuable book *On Death and Dying*,[107] reports on a study of over 200 terminal patients. She describes five major stages in the psychological response to the awareness of dying: (1) *Denial and isolation*. This initial phase was present in both those who were told that they would die and those who came to this conclusion independently. A characteristic verbal response was: "No, not me, it cannot be true." Denial was at least partially used by almost all patients during the first stage of terminal illness, and intermittently later on. It was, for a time, a healthy way of dealing with an uncomfortable and inexorable situation. Denial sustained to the end did not bring distress. Most patients, however, gradually gave up denying the reality of their situation and displayed other responses; (2) *Anger*. When denial could no longer be maintained, it was often replaced by feelings of anger, rage, envy, and resentment. The typical question at this stage was: "Why me?" The patients readily projected their anger and blame on family and staff. They were aggrieved by and found fault with everything. Such hostile behavior was aggravated by angry responses of family and the ward staff; (3) *Bargaining*. This stage was characterized by patients' attempts to avert their fate by being amiable and cooperative as if this could be rewarded by postponement or warding off death; (4) *Depression*. When progression of his disease was unmistakable, the patient reacted with a sense of loss and grief. *Reactive grief or depression* was related to the losses of body parts through surgery and the symbolic losses of self-esteem, etc., accompanied by feelings of guilt or shame. *Preparatory depression*, on the contrary, signified anticipation of the ultimate loss of life itself. This second type of depression was a necessary stage in coming to terms with the impending loss of all the love objects; and (5) *Acceptance*. This stage required time to be achieved and help in working through the preceding stages. The patient was neither depressed nor angry, but almost devoid of feeling and increasingly detached. He tended to be silent and wished to be left alone. *Hope* usually persisted through all the stages. If a patient gave up hoping, it was usually a sign of imminent death.

Death has different *meanings* for different individuals: the personified destroyer; relief from pain; reunion with one's family; loss of control; punishment; loneliness. *Attitudes* toward death can vary in the same individual, ranging from fear, defiance, and denial, to uneasy resignation and calm acceptance.[48] For some, the approach of death may become a stimulus to psychological growth and creativity.[229]

Descriptions of the subjective *experience of dying* have been obtained from patients resuscitated after cardiac arrest. They related a pleasant feeling as though they were entering a peaceful sleep. None of them recalled any fear or other unpleasant feeling while losing consciousness. It seems that "biologic death" is not an unpleasant experience.[15]

Psychological complications tend to occur if the dying person suffers from unresolved feelings of *guilt*; a sense of *unfulfillment* or wasted opportunities; and a marked susceptibility to *separation anxiety*. These are conditions in which psychiatric consultation, sometimes supplemented by talks with a clergyman may help alleviate the patient's anguish. The incidence of "psychopathological" reactions in terminal patients is unknown. Some patients are delirious or comatose in the final stages of life.

The Management of the Dying Patient

The doctor's personal attitude toward his own death influences his views on how the dying patient should be managed. Death is an ultimate challenge to the physician's knowledge and skill and a disturbing reminder of their limitations. Some doctors experience their failure to save the patient as a personal defeat and humiliation. They may respond with feelings of guilt, shame, and resentment. To cope with his own emotions, the doctor may simply avoid the patient, or become awkward and detached in his contacts with him. The doctor's withdrawal tends to increase the patient's sense of helplessness and loneliness. Often the patient, his family, and the doctor attempt to maintain the denial of the impending dissolution and an awkward game of mutual deception and avoidance of facing the facts takes the place of open communication. How can this common and regrettable situation be avoided? We may offer some general clinical guidelines.

1. The issue to be faced and settled by all concerned is that of *communication of diagnosis* and its consequences. The perennially controversial question is: "To tell or not to tell?" It is remarkable that extensive polls conducted among physicians and laymen, respectively, reveal almost diametrically opposite views on this issue. Eighty to ninety percent of healthy subjects, as well as cancer patients, questioned responded that they wished to be told that they had cancer or another fatal illness.[21,95] However, 40 percent of dying patients, who were asked if they wanted to be told *when* they would die, answered in the negative.[21] And how about the doctors? Of 219 physicians questioned by Oken,[156] ninety percent said that they did not disclose diagnosis of cancer as a usual policy. In a general poll of 5000 American doctors, twenty-two percent said that they never told

patients that they had cancer.[156] Yet doctors usually affirm that they would personally want to be told if critically ill.

Whether or not the patient is told that he has cancer, or another fatal illness, he sooner or later guesses the truth from the nonverbal cues. How should this problem be handled? The question is *not* whether to tell, but *who should do it, how and when.* Communication should be the responsibility of someone close to the patient and his family. Time must be allowed for the facts to sink in and for questions to arise. The patient should not be told that there is no more that can be done for him. The way the news is broken should depend on the patient's personality, intelligence, religion, and the indirect clues he provides about how he is likely to deal with the disclosure. Some should not be told until a strong relationship with a staff member has developed. Clearly, a general rule of thumb has no place here.[106]

2. The management involves sustained and supportive *communication* after the disclosure of diagnosis.

3. Some patients benefit from psychological intervention and counseling. The latter should have the following aims: *Encouragement of competent behavior,* that is, helping the patient maintain his remaining competence and capacity for achievement; *preservation of rewarding relationships* with the family and friends; *maintenance of a dignified self-image* by providing environment, activities, and relationships enhancing the patient's sense of his own worth; *attainment of an acceptable death* by helping the patient resolve his intrapsychic conflicts and emphasizing his achievements and autonomy.[219]

4. Communication with and support of the patient's *family.*

In summary, management of the dying patient is one of the most important and demanding tasks for all health professionals involved in his care. Adequate communication with the patient, sustained contact and emotional support *to the very end* are mandatory. These tasks belong to the health professionals in attendance, and *not* primarily to the psychiatrist. His role should be confined to consulting and therapeutic intervention in selected cases only. The management of the dying must be adapted to their individual needs and capacities. The physician must also at times face the decision when to withhold treatment and distinguish between prolongation of life and prolonging dying.[13]

Conclusion

There is a major increase of interest in the psychological aspects of death and the process of dying. This area of study is far from finished and its results are still inconclusive. It imposes serious emotional demands upon the investigator, who can hardly remain detached and separate research from therapy. There are many modes of dying. The patient's age, sex, personality, circumstances of his terminal illness, his religious beliefs, the degree of support he receives from his environment, his state of consciousness, and amount of physical pain are all significant factors.

⟮ Bibliography

1. ABRAMS, R. D. "The Patient with Cancer—His Changing Pattern of Communication," *N. Engl. J. Med.,* 274 (1966), 317–322.
2. ACHTE, K. and J. L. VAUKHONEN. *Cancer and Psyche. Part 1: Psychic Factors in Cancer.* Helsinki: Monograph from the Psychiatric Clinic of the Helsinki University Central Hospital, 1970.
3. BALINT, M. *The Doctor, His Patient and the Illness.* London: Pitman, 1957.
4. BARD, M. "The Use of Dependence for Predicting Psychogenic Invalidism following Radical Mastectomy," *J. Nerv. Ment. Dis.,* 122 (1955), 152–160.
5. BARD, M. and R. B. DYK. "The Psychodynamic Significance of Beliefs Regarding the Cause of Serious Illness," *Psychoanal. Rev.* 43 (1956), 146–162.
6. BARKER, R. G., B. A. WRIGHT, L. MEYERSON et al. *Adjustment to Physical Handicap and Illness.* New York: Social Science Research Council, 1953.
7. BELLAK, L., ed. *Psychology of Physical Illness.* New York: Grune & Stratton, 1952.
8. BIBRING, G. L. "Psychiatry and Medical

Practice in a General Hospital," *N. Engl. J. Med.*, 254 (1956), 366–372.

9. BLACK, P., ed. *Physiological Correlates of Emotion.* New York: Academic, 1970.

10. BLOOM, S. W. *The Doctor and His Patient.* New York: Russell Sage Foundation, 1963.

11. BOOK, H. E. "Sexual Implications of the Nose," *Compr. Psychiatry*, 12 (1971), 450–455.

12. BREWERTON, D. A. and J. W. DANIEL. "Factors Influencing Return to Work," *Br. Med. J.*, 4 (1971), 277–281.

13. BRIM, O. G., JR., H. E. FREEMAN, S. LEVINE et al., eds. *The Dying Patient.* New York: Russell Sage Foundation, 1970.

14. BROWNE, K. and P. FREELING. *The Doctor–Patient Relationship.* Edinburgh: E. & S. Livingstone, 1967.

15. BURCH, G. E., N. P. DE PASQUALE, and J. H. PHILLIPS. "What Death Is Like," *Am. Heart J.*, 76 (1968), 438–439.

16. BURSTEN, B. "Family Dynamics, the Sick Role, and Medical Hospital Admissions," *Family Process*, 4 (1965), 206–216.

17. ———. "Psychosocial Stress and Medical Consultation," *Psychosomatics*, 6 (1965), 100–106.

18. BYRNE, D., M. A. STEINBERG, and M. S. SCHWARTZ. "Relationship Between Repression-Sensitization and Physical Illness," *J. Abnorm. Psychol.*, 73 (1968), 154–155.

19. CAMERON, A. and J. HINTON. "Delay in Seeking Treatment for Mammary Tumors," *Cancer*, 21 (1968), 1121–1126.

20. CANTER, A., J. B. IMBODEN, and L. E. CLUFF. "The Frequency of Physical Illness as a Function of Prior Psychological Vulnerability and Contemporary Stress," *Psychosom. Med.*, 28 (1966), 344–350.

21. CAPPON, D. "Attitudes of and Towards the Dying," *Can. Med. Assoc. J.*, 87 (1962), 693–700.

22. CAREY, W. B. "Psychologic Sequelae of Early Infancy Health Crises," *Clin. Pediatr.*, 8 (1969), 459–463.

23. CASSELL, W. A. "Individual Differences in Somatic Perception," in Advances in Psychosomatic Medicine, Vol. 8, Z. J. Lipowski, ed., *Psychosocial Aspects of Physical Illness*, pp. 86–104. Basel: Karger, 1972.

24. CHESTER, R. "Health and Marriage Breakdown: Experience of a Sample of Divorced Women," *B. J. Prev. Soc. Med.*, 25 (1971), 231–235.

25. CHODOFF, P. "Adjustment to Disability. Some Observations on Patients with Multiple Sclerosis," *J. Chronic Dis.*, 9 (1959), 653–670.

26. ———. "Understanding and Management of the Chronically Ill Patient. Part 1. Who Are the Chronically Ill?" *Am. Practitioner*, 13 (1962), 136–144.

27. COBB, B., R. L. CLARK, JR., C. McGUIRE et al. "Patient Responsible Delay in Cancer Treatment; Social Psychological Study," *Cancer*, 7 (1954), 920–926.

28. COELHO, G. V., D. A. HAMBURG, R. MOOS et al., eds. *Coping and Adaptation. A Behavioral Sciences Bibliography.* Chevy Chase, Md.: National Institute of Mental Health, 1970.

29. CRANDELL, D. L. and B. P. DOHRENWEND. "Some Relations Among Psychiatric Symptoms, Organic Illness, and Social Class," *A. J. Psychiatry*, 123 (1967), 1527–1537.

30. CRAWFORD, C. O., ed. *Health and the Family.* New York: Macmillan, 1971.

31. CROOG, S. H., S. LEVINE, and Z. LURIE. "The Heart Patient and the Recovery Process," *Soc. Sci. Med.*, 2 (1968), 111–164.

32. CRUICKSHANK, W. M., ed. *Psychology of Exceptional Children and Youth.* 3rd ed., Englewood Cliffs, N.J.: Prentice-Hall, 1971.

33. DAVIS, H. K. and R. L. ZAPALAC. "The Immature Personality with a Physical Illness," *South. Med. J.*, 61 (1968), 985–989.

34. DAVIS, M. S. "Variation in Patients' Compliance with Doctors' Orders: Medical Practice and Doctor–Patient Interaction," *Psychiatry Med.*, 2 (1971), 31–54.

35. DEWOLFE, A. S., R. P. BARRELL, and J. W. CUMMINGS. "Patient Variables in Emotional Response to Hospitalization for Physical Illness," *J. Consult. Psychol.*, 30 (1968), 68–72.

36. DODGE, D. L. and W. T. MARTIN. *Social Stress and Chronic Illness.* Notre Dame, Ind.: University of Notre Dame Press, 1970.

37. DRUSS, R. G., J. F. O'CONNOR, J. F. PRUDDEN et al. "Psychologic Response to Colectomy," *Arch. Gen. Psychiatry*, 18 (1968), 53–59.

38. DUBOS, R. *Man, Medicine, and Environment.* New York: Praeger, 1968.

39. DUFF, R. S. and A. B. HOLLINGSHEAD. *Sickness and Society.* New York: Harper & Row, 1968.

40. ELIOT, R. S., ed. *Stress and the Heart*. Mount Kisco, N.Y.: Futura, 1974.

41. ENGEL G. L. "'Psychogenic' Pain and the Pain-Prone Patient," *Am. J. Med.*, 26 (1959), 899–918.

42. ———. "A Unified Concept of Health and Disease," *Perspect. Biol. Med.*, 3 (1960), 459–485.

43. ———. *Psychological Development in Health and Disease*. Philadelphia: Saunders, 1962.

44. ———. "Conversion Symptoms," in C. M. MacBryde and R. S. Blacklow, eds., *Signs and Symptoms*, pp. 650–668, 5th ed., Philadelphia: Lippincott, 1970.

45. ENGLE, R. L., JR. and B. J. DAVIS. "Medical Diagnosis: Present, Past, and Future," *Arch. Intern. Med.*, 112 (1963), 512–519.

46. FAUCETT, R. L. "Psychiatric Interview as Tool of Medical Diagnosis," *JAMA*, 162 (1956), 537.

47. FEIFEL, H. *The Meaning of Death*. New York: McGraw-Hill, 1959.

48. ———. "Attitudes toward Death: A Psychological Perspective," *J. Cons. Clin. Psychol.*, 33 (1969), 292–295.

49. FEINSTEIN, A. R. *Clinical Judgment*. Baltimore: Williams & Wilkins, 1967.

50. FINK, S. L., J. K. SKIPPER, JR., and P. HALLENBECK. "Physical Disability and Problems in Marriage," *J. Marriage Family*, 30 (1968), 64–73.

51. FISCHER, W. F. *Theories of Anxiety*. New York: Harper & Row, 1970.

52. FISHER, S. *Body Experience in Fantasy and Behavior*. New York: Appleton-Century-Crofts, 1970.

53. FOGEL, M. L. and R. H. ROSILLO. "Correlation of Psychological Variables and Progress in Physical Rehabilitation. II. Motivation, Attitudes, and Flexibility of Goals," *Dis. Nerv. Syst.*, 30 (1969), 593–600.

54. FOX, R. C. *Experiment Perilous: Physicians and Patients Facing the Unknown*. Glencoe, Ill.: Free Press, 1959.

55. ———. "Medical Evolution" in J. J. Loubser et al., eds., *Explorations in Social Science Theory*, pp. 1–52. New York: Free Press, 1973.

56. FREIDSON, E. *Profession of Medicine*. New York: Dodd-Mead, 1970.

57. FRIEDMAN, S. B., P. CHODOFF, J. W. MASON et al. "Behavioral Observations on Parents Anticipating the Death of a Child," *Pediatrics*, 32 (1963), 610–625.

58. FRIEDMAN, S. B., J. W. MASON, and D. HAMBURG. "Urinary 17-Hydroxysteroid Levels in Parents of Children with Neoplastic Disease: A Study of Chronic Psychological Stress," *Psychosom. Med.*, 25 (1963), 364–376.

59. GARNER, H. H. *Psychosomatic Management of the Patient with Malignancy*. Springfield, Ill.: Charles C. Thomas, 1966.

60. GARRETT, J. F. and E. S. LEVINE, eds. *Psychological Practices with the Physically Disabled*. New York: Columbia University Press, 1962.

61. GOLD, M. A. "Causes of Patient's Delay in Diseases of the Breast," *Cancer*, 17 (1964), 564–577.

62. GOLDEN, J. S. and G. D. JOHNSTON. "Problems of Distortion in Doctor–Patient Communications," *Psychiatry Med.*, 1 (1970), 127–149.

63. GOLDSEN, R. K. "Patient Delay in Seeking Cancer Diagnosis: Behavioral Aspects," *J. Chronic Dis.*, 16 (1963), 427–436.

64. GORDON, G., O. W. ANDERSON, H. P. BREHM et al. *Disease, the Individual, and Society*. New Haven, Conn.: College & University Press, 1968.

65. GUSSOW, Z. "Behavioral Research in Chronic Disease: A Study of Leprosy," *J. Chronic Dis.*, 17 (1964), 179–189.

66. GUTTMAN, L. "The Married Life of Paraplegics and Tetraplegics," *Paraplegia*, 2 (1964), 182–188.

67. HACKETT, T. P. and N. H. CASSEM. "Factors Contributing to Delay in Responding to the Signs and Symptoms of Acute Myocardial Infarction," *Am. J. Cardiol.*, 24 (1969), 651–658.

68. HACKETT, T. P. and A. D. WEISMAN. "Psychiatric Management of Operative Syndromes: 1. The Therapeutic Consultation and the Effect of Noninterpretive Intervention," *Psychosom. Med.*, 22 (1960), 267.

69. ———. "Psychiatric Management of Operative Syndromes: II. Psychodynamic Factors in Formulation and Management," *Psychosom. Med.*, 22 (1960), 356.

70. HAMBURG, D. A., B. HAMBURG, and S. DE GOZA. "Adaptive Problems and Mechanisms in Severely Burned Patients," *Psychiatry*, 16 (1953), 11–20.

71. HAMMERSCHLAG, C. A., S. FISHER, J. DE COSSE et al. "Breast Symptoms and Patient Delay: Psychological Variables Involved," *Cancer*, 17 (1964), 1480–1485.

72. HARPER, A. C. "Towards a Job Description for Comprehensive Health Care—a Framework for Education and Management," *Soc. Sci. Med.*, 7 (1973), 291–303.

73. HENDERSON, L. J. "The Patient and Physician as a Social System," *N. Engl. J. Med.*, 212 (1935), 819–823.

74. HINKLE, L. E., JR. "Relating Biochemical, Physiological, and Psychological Disorders to the Social Environment," *Arch. Environ. Health*, 16 (1968), 77–82.

75. HINKLE, L. E., JR., W. N. CHRISTENSON, F. D. KANE et al. "An Investigation of the Relation between Life Experience, Personality Characteristics, and General Susceptibility to Illness," *Psychosom. Med.*, 20 (1958), 278.

76. HOLLAND, J. "Psychologic Aspects of Cancer," in J. F. Holland and E. Frei, eds., *Cancer Medicine*. Philadelphia: Lea & Febiger, 1973.

77. HONEYMAN, M. S., H. RAPPAPORT, M. REZNIKOFF et al. "Psychological Impact of Heart Disease in the Family of the Patient," *Psychosomatics*, 9 (1968), 34–37.

78. HOROWITZ, M. J. *Psychosocial Function in Epilepsy*. Springfield, Ill.: Charles C. Thomas, 1970.

79. HUGHES, G. M., ed. *Homeostasis and Feedback Mechanisms*. New York: Academic, 1964.

80. IMBODEN, J. B. "Psychosocial Determinants of Recovery," in Advances in Psychosomatic Medicine, Vol. 8, Z. J. Lipowski, ed., *Psychosocial Aspects of Physical Illness*, pp. 142–155. Basel: Karger, 1972.

81. JACO, E. G., ed. *Patients, Physicians, and Illness*. Glencoe, Ill.: Free Press, 1958.

82. JANIS, I. L. *Psychological Stress*. New York: Wiley, 1958.

83. JANIS, I. L. and H. LEVENTHAL. "Psychological Aspects of Physical Illness and Hospital Care," in B. Wolman, ed., *Handbook of Clinical Psychology*, pp. 1360–1377. New York: McGraw-Hill, 1965.

84. JENKINS, D. C. and S. J. ZYZANSKI. "Dimensions of Belief and Feeling Concerning Three Diseases, Poliomyelitis, Cancer, and Mental Illness: A Factor Analytic Study," *Behav. Sci.*, 13 (1968), 372–381.

85. KAHANA, R. J. "Studies in Medical Psychology: A Brief Survey," *Psychiatry Med.*, 3 (1972), 1–22.

86. KAHANA, R. J. and G. L. BIBRING. "Personality Types in Medical Management," in E. N. Zinberg, ed., *Psychiatry and Medical Practice in a General Hospital*, pp. 108–123. New York: International Universities Press, 1964.

87. KALISH, R. A. "Death and Bereavement: An Annotated Social Science Bibliography Through 1964," *SK&F Psychiatr. Rept.*, March–April, 1965.

88. ——. "Death and Dying. A Briefly Annotated Bibliography," in O. G. Brim, H. E. Freeman, S. Levine et al., eds., *The Dying Patient*. New York: Russell Sage Foundation, 1970.

89. KAPLAN, S. M. "Laboratory Procedures as an Emotional Stress," *JAMA*, 161 (1956), 677–681.

90. KASL, S. V. and S. COBB. "Health Behavior, Illness Behavior and Sick-role Behavior. 1. Health and Illness Behavior," *Arch Environ. Health*, 12 (1966), 246–266.

91. ——. "Health Behavior, Illness Behavior and Sick-role Behavior. 2. Sick-role Behavior," *Arch. Environ. Health*, 12 (1966), 531–541.

92. KATZ, J. L., H. WEINER, T. F. GALLAGHER et al. "Stress, Distress, and Ego Defenses," *Arch. Gen. Psychiatry*, 23 (1970), 131–142.

93. KAUFMAN, R. M., A. N. FRANZBLAU, and D. KAIRYS. "The Emotional Impact of Ward Rounds," *J. Mount Sinai Hosp.*, 23 (1956), 782–803.

94. KELLNER, R. "Psychiatric Ill Health Following Physical Illness," *Br. J. Psychiatry*, 112 (1966), 71–73.

95. KELLY, W. D., and S. R. FRIESEN. "Do Cancer Patients Want To Be Told?" *Surgery*, 27 (1950), 822–826.

96. KENYON, F. E. "Hypochondriasis: A Clinical Study," *Br. J. Psychiatry*, 110 (1964), 467.

97. ——. "Hypochondriasis: A Survey of Some Historical, Clinical, and Social Aspects," *Br. J. Med. Psychol.*, 38 (1965), 117.

98. KING, S. H. *Perceptions of Illness and Medical Practice*. New York: Russell Sage Foundation, 1962.

99. KLECK, R. "Physical Stigma and Nonverbal Cues Emitted in Face-to-Face Interaction," *Hum. Rel.*, 21 (1968), 19–28.

100. KLEIN, R. F., A. DEAN, and M. D. BOGDONOFF. "The Impact of Illness Upon the Spouse," *J. Chronic Dis.*, 20 (1967), 241–248.

101. KLEIN, R. F., A. DEAN, M. L. WILLSON et al. "The Physician and Postmyocardial Infarction Invalidism," *JAMA*, 194 (1965), 123–128.

102. KOLLAR, E. J. "Psychology of the Acutely Sick and Injured," *Int. Psychiatry Clin.*, 3 (1966), 83–91.

103. KOOS, E. L. *The Health of Regionville*. New York: Columbia University Press, 1954.

104. KORNFELD, D. S. "The Hospital Environment: Its Impact on the Patient," in Advances in Psychosomatic Medicine, Vol. 8, Z. J. Lipowski, ed., *Psychosocial Aspects of Physical Illness*, pp. 252–270. Basel: Karger, 1972.

105. KOSKI, M. L. "The Coping Processes in Childhood Diabetes," *Acta Paediatr. Scand.*, Suppl. 198 (1969).

106. KRANT, M. J. "The Organized Care of the Dying Patient," *Hosp. Practice*, 7 (1972), 101–108.

107. KÜBLER-ROSS, E. *On Death and Dying*. London: Macmillan, 1969.

108. LAIN-ENTRALGO, P. *Doctor and Patient*. London: Weidenfeld & Nicolson, 1969.

109. LANGFORD, W. S. "The Child in the Pediatric Hospital: Adaptation to Illness and Hospitalization," *Am. J. Orthopsychiatry*, 31 (1961), 667–684.

110. LANGLOIS, P. and V. TERAMOTO. "Helping Patients Cope with Hospitalization," *Nurs. Outlook*, 19 (1971), 334–336.

111. LAZARUS, R. S. *Psychological Stress and the Coping Process*. New York: McGraw-Hill, 1966.

112. LAZARUS, R. S. "Psychological stress and coping in adaptation and illness," *Psychiatry Med.* (in press).

113. LEVINE, S. and N. A. SCOTCH, eds. *Social Stress*. Chicago: Aldine, 1970.

114. LIPOWSKI, Z. J. "Delirium, Clouding of Consciousness and Confusion," *J. Nerv. Ment. Dis.*, 145 (1967), 227–255.

115. ———. "Review of Consultation Psychiatry and Psychosomatic Medicine. 1. General Principles," *Psychosom. Med.*, 29 (1967), 153–171.

116. ———. "Review of Consultation Psychiatry and Psychosomatic Medicine. 2. Clinical Aspects," *Psychosom. Med.*, 29 (1967), 201–224.

117. ———. "Review of Consultation Psychiatry and Psychosomatic Medicine. 3. Theoretical Issues," *Psychosom. Med.*, 30 (1968), 395–422.

118. ———. "Psychosocial Aspects of Disease," *Ann. Intern. Med.*, 71 (1969), 1197–1206.

119. ———. "New Perspective in Psychosomatic Medicine," *Can. Psychiatr. Assoc. J.*, 15 (1970), 515–525.

120. ———. "Physical Illness, the Individual and the Coping Processes," *Psychiatry Med.* 1 (1970), 91–102.

121. LIPOWSKI, Z. J., ed. *Psychosocial Aspects of Physical Illness*, Vol. 8 of Advances in Psychosomatic Medicine. Basel: Karger, 1972.

122. ———. "Psychosomatic Medicine in a Changing Society: Some Current Trends in Theory and Research," *Compr. Psychiatry*, 14 (1973), 203–215.

123. ———. "Consultation-Liaison Psychiatry: An Overview," *Am. J. Psychiatry*, 131 (1974), 623–630.

124. ———. "Organic Brain Syndromes: An Overview and Classification," in F. D. Benson and D. Blumer, eds., *Psychiatric Aspects of Neurologic Disorders*. New York: Grune & Stratton, forthcoming.

125. ———. "Psychiatry of Somatic Diseases: Epidemiology, Pathogenesis, Classification," *Compr. Psychiatry*, in press.

126. ———. "Psychophysiological Cardiovascular Disorders," in A. M. Freedman, H. I. Kaplan, and B. Sadock, eds., *Comprehensive Textbook of Psychiatry*, 2nd ed. Baltimore: Williams & Wilkins, forthcoming.

127. LIPOWSKI, Z. J. and R. Z. KIRIAKOS. "Borderlands Between Neurology and Psychiatry: Observations in a Neurological Hospital," *Psychiatry Med.*, 3 (1972), 131–147.

128. LIPSITT, D. R. "Medical and Psychological Characteristics of 'Crocks,'" *Psychiatry Med.*, 1 (1970), 15–25.

129. LITTLE, C. J. "The Athlete's Neurosis—A Deprivation Crisis," *Acta Psychiatr. Scand.*, 45 (1969), 187–197.

130. LITTLE, S. "Psychology of Physical Illness in Adolescents," *Pediatr. Clin. North Am.*, 7 (1960), 85–96.

131. LIVSEY, C. G. "Family Therapy: Role of the Practicing Physician," in E. T. Lisansky, and B. R. Shochet, eds., *Psychiatry in Medical Practice*, pp. 806–820. New York: Harper & Row, 1969.

132. ———. "Physical Illness and Family Dynamics," in Advances in Psychosomatic Medicine, Vol. 8, Z. J. Lipowski, ed., *Psychosocial Aspects of Physical Illness*, pp. 237–251. Basel: Karger, 1972.

133. Lowy, F. "Patients Who Somatize," Paper presented at 52nd Annu. Meet. of the Ontario Psychiatr. Assoc., Toronto, Ont.: January 29, 1972.

134. Ludwig, E. G. and G. Gibson. "Self Perception of Sickness and the Seeking of Medical Care," *J. Health Soc. Behav.*, 10 (1969), 125–133.

135. Mabry, J. H. "Lay Concepts of Etiology," *J. Chronic Dis.*, 17 (1964), 371–386.

136. MacGregor, F. C. *Transformation and Identity.* New York: Quadrangle, 1974.

137. MacNalty, A. S., ed. *The British Medical Dictionary.* Philadelphia: Lippincott, 1963.

138. Maddison, D. and B. Raphael. "Social and Psychological Consequences of Chronic Disease in Childhood," *Med. J. Aust.*, 2 (1971), 1265–1270.

139. Maddison, D. and A. Viola. "The Health of Widows in the Year Following Bereavement," *J. Psychosom. Res.*, 12 (1968), 297–306.

140. Marra, J. and F. Novis. "Family Problems in Rehabilitation Counseling," *Personnel Guidance J.*, 38 (1959), 40–42.

141. Martin, H. L. "The Significance of Discussion with Patients about Their Diagnosis and its Implications," *Br. J. Med. Psychol.*, 40 (1967), 233.

142. Mason, J. W., E. J. Sachar, J. Fishman et al. "Corticosteroid Responses to Hospital Admission," *Arch. Gen. Psychiatry*, 13 (1965), 1–8.

143. Matarazzo, R. G., J. D. Matarazzo, and G. Saslow. "The Relationship between Medical and Psychiatric Symptoms," *J. Abnorm. Soc. Psychol.*, 62 (1961), 55–61.

144. McDaniel, J. W. *Physical Disability and Human Behavior.* New York: Pergamon, 1969.

145. McKinlay, J. B. "The Concept of 'Patient Career' as a Heuristic Device for Making Medical Sociology Relevant to Medical Students," *Soc. Sci. Med.*, 5 (1971), 441–460.

146. Mechanic, D. *Medical Sociology.* New York: Free Press, 1968.

147. ———. "The Concept of Illness Behavior," *J. Chronic Dis.*, 15 (1962), 189–194.

148. Meissner, W. W. "Family Dynamics and Psychosomatic Processes," *Family Process*, 5 (1966), 142–161.

149. Melzack, R. and W. S. Torgerson. "On the Language of Pain," *Anesthesiology*, 34 (1971), 50–59.

150. Mering, O. von, and L. Kasdan. *Anthropology and the Behavioral and Health Sciences.* Pittsburgh: University of Pittsburgh Press, 1970.

151. Meyer, R. J. and R. J. Haggerty. "Streptococcal Infections in Families," *Pediatrics*, 29 (1962), 539–549.

152. Moore, D. C., C. P. Holton, and G. W. Marten. "Psychologic Problems in the Management of Adolescents with Malignancy. Experiences with 182 Patients," *Clin. Pediatr.*, (1969), 464–473.

153. Moos, R. H. and G. F. Solomon. "Personality Correlates of the Degree of Functional Incapacity of Patients with Physical Disease," *J. Chronic Dis.*, 18 (1965), 1019–1038.

154. Morgan, W. L., Jr. and G. L. Engel. *The Clinical Approach to the Patient.* Philadelphia: Saunders, 1969.

155. Nagle, R., R. Gangola, and I. Picton-Robinson. "Factors Influencing Return to Work after Myocardial Infarction," *Lancet*, 2 (1971), 454–456.

156. Oken, D. "What to Tell Cancer Patients," *JAMA*, 175 (1961), 1120–1128.

157. Olsen, E. H. "The Impact of Serious Illness on the Family System," *Postgrad. Med.*, 47 (1970), 169–174.

158. Orbach, C. E., M. Bard, and A. M. Sutherland. "Fear and Defensive Adaptations to the Loss of Anal Sphincter Control," *Psychoanal. Rev.*, 44 (1957), 121–175.

159. Palmer, R. S. "Psychiatry and Internal Medicine," *N. Engl. J. Med.*, 263 (1960), 14–18.

160. Parkes, C. M. *Bereavement.* New York: International Universities Press, 1972.

161. Parsons, T. *The Social System.* Glencoe, Ill.: Free Press, 1951.

162. Parsons, T. and R. Fox. "Illness, Therapy, and the Modern Urban American Family," *J. Soc. Issues*, 8 (1952), 31–44.

163. Payne, E. C., Jr. and M. J. Krant. "The Psychosocial Aspects of Advanced Cancer," *JAMA*, 210 (1969), 1238–1242.

164. Pearsall, M. *Medical Behavioral Science: A Selected Bibliography of Cultural Anthropology, Social Psychology, and Sociology in Medicine.* Lexington, Ky.: University of Kentucky Press, 1963.

165. Pearson, L., ed. *Death and Dying.* Cleveland: Press of Case Western Reserve University, 1969.

166. PETRIE, A. *Individuality in Pain and Suffering*. Chicago: University of Chicago Press, 1967.

167. PILOWSKY, I. "Primary and Secondary Hypochondriasis," *Acta Psychiatr. Scand.*, 46 (1970), 273–285.

168. PINNER, M. and B. F. MILLER, eds. *When Doctors Are Patients*. New York: Norton, 1952.

169. PRUGH, D. G., E. M. STAUB, H. H. SANDS et al. "A Study of the Emotional Reactions of Children and Families to Hospitalization and Illness," *Am. J. Orthopsychiatry*, 23 (1953), 70–106.

170. *Psychological Aspects of Cancer, January 1970–March 1973*. Washington, D.C.: U.S. Department of Health, Education and Welfare, 1973.

171. RAHE, R. H. "Subjects' Recent Life Changes and Their Near-future Illness Susceptibility," in Advances in Psychosomatic Medicine, Vol. 8, Z. J. Lipowski, ed., *Psychosocial Aspects of Physical Illness*, pp. 2–19. Basel: Karger, 1972.

172. REES, D. W. and S. G. LUTKINS. "Mortality of Bereavement," *Br. Med. J.*, 4 (1967), 13–16.

173. RICKELS, K., R. W. DOWNING, and M. H. DOWNING. "Personality Differences between Somatically and Psychologically Oriented Neurotic Patients," *J. Nerv. Ment. Dis.*, 142 (1966), 10–18.

174. ROGERS, E. S. *Human Ecology and Health*. New York: Macmillan, 1960.

175. ROSNER, B. L. "The Use of Valid Psychological Complaints to Screen, Minimize or Deny Serious Somatic Illness," *J. Nerv. Ment. Dis.*, 143 (1966), 234.

176. RUESCH, J. *Chronic Disease and Psychological Invalidism*. Berkeley: University of California Press, 1951.

177. SCHILDER, P. *The Image and Appearance of the Human Body*. New York: International Universities Press, 1950.

178. SCHMALE, A. H., JR. "Giving Up as a Final Common Pathway to Changes in Health," in Advances in Psychosomatic Medicine, Vol. 8, Z. J. Lipowski, ed., *Psychosocial Aspects of Physical Illness*, pp. 20–40. Basel: Karger, 1972.

179. SCHMALE, A. H., JR. and G. L. ENGEL. "The Giving up—Given up Complex Illustrated on Film," *Arch. Gen. Psychiatry*, 17 (1967), 135–145.

180. SCHOENBERG, B., A. C. CARR, D. PERETZ et al. *Loss and Grief: Psychological Management in Medical Practice*. New York: Columbia University Press, 1970.

181. SEIDMAN, F. and C. SWIFT. "Psychologic Aspects of Juvenile Diabetes Mellitus," in H. S. Traisman, ed., *Management of Juvenile Diabetes*, pp. 162–170. St. Louis, Mo.: Mosby, 1971.

182. SENESCU, R. A. "The Development of Emotional Complications in the Patient with Cancer," *J. Chronic Dis.*, 16 (1963), 813–832.

183. SHONTZ, F. C. "Severe Chronic Illness", in J. F. Garrett and E. S. Levine, eds., *Psychological Practices with the Physically Disabled*. New York: Columbia University Press, 1962.

184. ———. *Perceptual and Cognitive Aspects of Body Experience*. New York: Academic, 1969.

185. ———. "Physical Disability and Personality: Theory and Recent Research," *Psycholog. Aspects Disability*, 17 (1970), 51–69.

186. SILVERMAN, S. *Psychological Aspects of Physical Symptoms*. New York: Appleton-Century-Crofts, 1968.

187. ———. *Psychological Cues in Forecasting Physical Illness*. New York: Appleton-Century-Crofts, 1970.

188. SPERLING, M. "Transference Neurosis in Patients with Psychosomatic Disorders," *Psychoanal. Q.*, 36 (1967), 342–355.

189. SPIELBERGER, C. D., ed. *Anxiety: Current Trends in Theory and Research*. New York: Academic, 1972.

190. STALLONES, R. A. "Community Health," *Science*, 175 (1972), 839.

191. STARKEY, P. D. "Sick-role Retention as a Factor in Nonrehabilitation," *J. Couns. Psychol.*, 15 (1967), 75–79.

192. STAVRAKY, K. M., C. W. BUCK, S. J. LOTT et al. "Psychological Factors in the Outcome of Human Cancer," *J. Psychosom. Res.*, 12 (1968), 251–259.

193. STERN, R. M. and D. J. HIGGINS. "Perceived Somatic Reactions to Stress: Sex, Age and Familial Occurrence," *J. Psychosom. Res.*, 13 (1969), 77–82.

194. STERNBACH, R. H. *Pain: A Psychophysiological Analysis*. New York: Academic, 1968.

195. STEVENSON, I. "Single Physical Symptoms as Residues of an Earlier Response to Stress," *Ann. Intern. Med.*, 70 (1969), 1231–1237.

196. STOECKLE, J. D. and G. E. DAVIDSON. "Communicating Aggrieved Feelings in the Patient's Initial Visit to a Medical Clinic," *J. Health Human Behav.*, 4 (1963), 199–206.

197. STOECKLE, J. D., I. K. ZOLA, and G. E. DAVIDSON. "On Going to See the Doctor, the Contributions of the Patient to the Decision to Seek Medical Aid," *J. Chronic Dis.*, 16 (1963), 975–989.

198. STRAUS, R. "Behavioral Science in the Medical Curriculum," *Ann. N.Y. Acad. Sci.*, 128 (1965), 599–606.

199. SUCHMAN, E. A. "Stages of Illness and Medical Care," *J. Health Human Behav.*, 6 (1965), 114–128.

200. ———. "Health Attitudes and Behavior," *Arch. Environ. Health*, 20 (1970), 105–110.

201. SUSSER, M. *Causal Thinking in the Health Sciences*. New York: Oxford University Press, 1973.

202. SZASZ, T. S. *Pain and Pleasure*. New York: Basic Books, 1957.

203. SZASZ, T. S. and M. H. HOLLENDER. "A Contribution to the Philosophy of Medicine: The Basic Models of the Doctor–Patient Relationship," *Am. Med. Assoc. Arch. Intern. Med.*, 97 (1956), 585.

204. THURLOW, J. H. "Illness in Relation to Life Situation and Sick-role Tendency," *J. Psychosom. Res.*, 15 (1971), 73–88.

205. TOLSON, W. W., J. W. MASON, E. J. SACHAR et al. "Urinary Catecholamine Responses Association with Hospital Admission in Normal Human Subjects," *J. Psychosom. Res.*, 8 (1965), 365–372.

206. TWADDLE, A. C. "The Concepts of the Sick Role and Illness Behavior," in Advances in Psychosomatic Medicine, Vol. 8, Z. J. Lipowski, ed. *Psychosocial Aspects of Physical Illness*, pp. 162–179. Basel: Karger, 1972.

207. VAN DEN BERG, J. H. *The Psychology of the Sickbed*. Pittsburgh: Duquesne University Press, 1966.

208. VERNON, D. T. A., J. M. FOLLEY, R. R. SIPOWICZ et al. *The Psychological Responses of Children to Hospitalization and Illness*. Springfield, Ill.: Charles C. Thomas, 1965.

209. VERWOERDT, A. *Communication with the Fatally Ill*. Springfield, Ill.: Charles C. Thomas, 1966.

210. ———. "Psychopathological Responses to the Stress of Physical Illness," in Advances in Psychosomatic Medicine, Vol. 8, Z. J. Lipowski, ed., *Psychosocial Aspects of Physical Illness*, pp. 119–141. Basel: Karger, 1972.

211. VISOTSKY, H. M., D. A. HAMBURG, M. A. Goss et al. "Coping Behavior under Extreme Stress," *Arch. Gen. Psychiatry*, 5 (1961), 423–448.

212. VON BERTALANFFY, L. *General System Theory*. New York: Brazillier, 1968.

213. WAITZKIN, H. and J. D. STOECKLE. "The Communication of Information about Illness," in Advances in Psychosomatic Medicine, Vol. 8, Z. J. Lipowski, ed., *Psychosocial Aspects of Phyical Illness*, pp. 180–215. Basel: Karger, 1972.

214. WALTON, H. J. "Effect of the Doctor's Personality on His Style of Practice," *J. R. Coll. Gen. Pract.*, 16 (1968), 113–126.

215. WAN, T. "Status Stress and Morbidity: A Sociological Investigation of Selected Categories of Work-Limiting Chronic Conditions," *J. Chronic Dis.*, 24 (1971), 453–468.

216. WARM, J. S. and E. A. ALLUISI. "Behavioral Reactions to Infection: Review of the Psychological Literature," *Percept. Mot. Skills*, 24 (1967), 755–783.

217. WEINSTEIN, M. R. "The Illness Process," *JAMA*, 204 (1968), 209–213.

218. WEINSTEIN, S., R. VETTER, and E. SERSEN. "Physiological and Experiential Concomitants of the Phantom," quoted in J. W. McDaniel, *Physical Disability and Human Behavior*, p. 32. New York: Pergamon, 1969.

219. WEISMAN, A. D. *On Dying and Denying*. New York: Behavioral Publ., 1972.

220. WEISMAN, A. D. and R. KASTENBAUM. "The Psychological Autopsy," *Community Ment. Health J.*, Monogr. 4 (1968).

221. WISHNIE, H. A., T. P. HACKETT, and N. H. CASSEM. "Psychological Hazards of Convalescence Following Myocardial Infarction," *JAMA*, 215 (1971), 1292–1296.

222. WITKIN, H. A., R. B. DYK, H. F. PATERSON et al. *Psychological Differentiation*. New York: Wiley, 1962.

223. WOLFF, H. G. "A Concept of Disease in Man," *Psychosom. Med.*, 24 (1962), 25–30.

224. ———. *Stress and Disease*. 2nd ed. rev., S. Wolf and H. Goodell, eds., Springfield, Ill.: Charles C. Thomas, 1968.

225. WRIGHT, B. *Physical Disability: A Psychological Approach*. New York: Harper & Row, 1960.

226. WYLER, A. R., M. MASUDA, and T. H. HOLMES. "Magnitude of Life Events and Seriousness of Illness," *Psychosom. Med.*, 33 (1971), 115.

227. ZABARENKO, R. N., L. ZABARENKO, and R. A. PITTENGER. "The Psychodynamics of Physicianhood," *Psychiatry*, 33 (1970), 102–118.

228. ZBOROWSKI, M. *People in Pain*. San Francisco: Jossey-Bass, 1969.

229. ZINKER, J. C. and S. L. FINK. "The Possibility of Psychological Growth in a Dying Person," *J. Gen. Psychol.*, 77 (1966), 185–199.

230. ZOLA, I. K. "Problems of Communication, Diagnosis, and Patient Care: The Interplay of Patient, Physician and Clinic Organization," *J. Med. Educ.*, 38 (1963), 829.

231. ———. "Culture and Symptoms: An Analysis of Patients' Presenting Complaints," *Am. Sociol. Rev.*, 31 (1966), 615–630.

232. ———. "Studying the Decision to See a Doctor," in Advances in Psychosomatic Medicine, Vol. 8, Z. J. Lipowski, ed., *Psychosocial Aspects of Physical Illness*, pp. 216–236. Basel: Karger, 1972.

CHAPTER 2

DELIRIUM AND
RELATED PROBLEMS

Stanley S. Heller and Donald S. Kornfeld

THE GOLDEN BOUGH[22], by Sir James Frazier, began as a study of the rule of succession to the priesthood at Ariccia in the Alban Hills of Italy. However, to understand this, Frazier was required to continually examine larger questions, until he ended with twelve volumes and a comprehensive theory of primitive religion. At one time, an article about delirium might have been simple; all that would have been required was to catalogue the myriad syndromes that affect the brain, as though the severity of the central nervous system insult explained all. But the story turns out to be a good deal more complicated than that. The investigation of the multitude of factors actually responsible for delirium production has raised general and profound questions concerning the nature of brain function, the mechanisms of sleep and dreams, the importance of man's environment, the interaction of mind and body, and the mode of action of licit and illicit drugs. Delirium is the psychosomatic syndrome par excellence, a final pathway of often coexistent physical and psychological disturbance. Yet, as recently as 1967, Lipowski[50] lamented that delirium was the "Cinderella of English-language psychiatry: taken for granted, ignored and not considered worthy of study." New developments in brain physiology, the advent of Rapid Eye Movement technology (REM) allowing new insight into sleep and dreaming, research into sensory deprivation and overstimulation, the model psychoses of hallucinogenic drugs, the development of medical–surgical techniques causing delirium, e.g., open-heart surgery, or preventing it, e.g., renal dialysis, have all combined to cause considerably more interest in this increasingly complex subject. Ten years ago it was simpler; intensive care units (ICU) could be built without windows since patients would be unconscious or semiconscious and not need them. It is now recognized that of all the facilities of a general hospital, the ICU and recovery rooms need windows the most.

There used to be a saying that to understand syphilis was to understand all of medicine. To understand delirium fully requires us to understand fully the patient's world: physical, environmental, social, and intrapsychic. The concept of multidetermination is as applicable to delirium as to symptom or dream formation. We will begin by looking at the syndrome in general terms, and then turn to the specific situations in the general hospital where delirium is most likely to occur.

(History

Delirium is such a ubiquitous phenomenon that it was well known to the ancient world. The Greeks and Romans clearly identified an acute reversible brain syndrome distinguishable from chronic mental illness, and called it "phrenitis" or "phrensy."[29] Fever was a common cause, and Hippocrates noted visual hallucinations and picking at bed sheets. Plato and Aristotle noted the similarity of dreams to the visions of the mentally ill.[16] Celsus saw the relationship between mind and body, realizing that delirium was caused by debilitating systemic illness, and was a serious prognostic sign auguring death. Delirium tremens was described by Aretaeus and Galen and in the fifth century by Cassius Felix.

The Talmud, compiled in the first five hundred years A.D., describes a reversible syndrome of "Kordiakos," attributed to drinking new wine from a vat.[29] When convulsions were described, light wine was prescribed for therapy, and this might very well also have been related to delirium tremens.

Delirium was of course known to poets and writers before it attracted the attention of modern scientists. As has been noted,[31,44] Shakespeare eloquently describes Falstaff's final illness in Henry V. "For often I saw him fumble with the sheets and play with flowers and smile upon his fingers' ends, I knew there was but one way, for his nose was sharp as a pen, and a'babbled of green fields." (II,iii). He also recognized the role of psychological stress, "The king has kill'd his heart." (II,i).

In the modern era, Thomas Willis's conceptualization has been summarized by Li-powski.[50] Wilson realized that delirium could be produced by infection, intoxication, malnutrition, and visceral disorders. Postsurgical delirium was described by Pare in the sixteenth century, and investigated by Dupuytren in 1819.[57] The nineteenth century witnessed great interest in the phenomenon of hallucinations, as schizophrenia was delineated, and the effect of hashish studied.

Freud's contribution to the theory of delirium has not received sufficient notice. In the Interpretation of Dreams,[24] he pointed out that the content of deliria is partly related to the individual's experience; "even the deliria of confusional states may have a meaning . . . they are unintelligible to us owing to the gaps in them." In the essay on Leonardo da Vinci,[25] he pointed out the similar mechanisms of dreaming and hallucinations; "a phantasy . . . must have some meaning in the same way as any other psychical creation: a dream, a vision or a delirium." In this connection he quotes Radestock:[63] "Both in patients suffering from fever and in dreamers, memories arise from the remote past, both sleeping and sick men recollect things which waking and healthy men seem to have forgotten." Freud also saw the working of the mental apparatus, and that even in delirious states the unconscious never overcomes the resistance of consciousness "so that the secret of the childhood experiences is not betrayed even in the most confused delirium."[23]

As Lipowski[50] has noted, the German psychiatrist Bonhoeffer classified deliria, noting that specific etiologies could produce many types of delirium reactions. Nonetheless there remained great terminological confusion, partly relieved by the authoritative work of Engel and Romano.[15] Delirium was conceptualized as a syndrome of cerebral insufficiency, that could be monitored by following the slowing of the electroencephalogram (EEG). Hyperactivity, hallucinations, or agitation were not necessary for the diagnosis. Delirium was defined as any acute, reversible syndrome of cerebral insufficiency. Lipowski[50] has introduced the concept of delirium as a psychosomatic condition, in which both physical and psychological factors interact causally. Psychological factors, such as sensory input, sleep deprivation, the stress, setting and care of the medical illness, all were seen as possible precipitating or intensifying factors in delirium etiology.

(Classification

A number of related terms are used with different meaning to different people. *Delirium*, which dynamically and historically should include all acute brain syndromes, is used by many people to refer only to agitated hallucinating patients. *Confusion, metabolic encephalopathy, acute brain syndrome*, and *psychosis associated with organic brain syndrome* are, conversely, sometimes applied only to the apathetic confused patient. The issue is further complicated by the suggestion that the terms hyper- and hypoactive delirium be used to make that distinction.[3] However, this overlooks the shifting and protean nature of the symptoms of delirium in any given patient. These distinctions are quantitative, not qualitative. Delirium represents a broad syndrome of disturbances in sensation, perception, memory, thought, and judgment. It can run the gamut from a slight reduction in alertness to coma, and indeed patients may pass through this sequence in both directions, as their disease waxes and wanes.

In its mildest form it resembles alcohol intoxication, or hypnagogic or hypnopompic phenomena, particularly in a strange place. It begins with a mild clouding of perceptions, with a subjective lack of focus, blurring or haziness. It is only with an effort that thought processes can be channeled into logical and coherent patterns. Memory, especially for recent events, becomes impaired. Speech and thinking become slowed, and the right answer is obtained with delay. Perplexity, uncertainty, and vagueness are communicated as the patient looks around searching for an answer. With partial preservation of cerebral functioning, there may be moments of insight into the perceptual, thought, and memory disturbances. Symbolic and abstract thinking dwin-

dle. Time disturbance appears with inability to give the day of the week, hour of the day, or date. Place disorientation may occur, with the hospital identified as home or as a branch of the hospital close to home. Grasp, retention, and the capacity for attention are impaired. Patients become distracted and fail to distinguish the relevant from the irrelevant. Conversation becomes limited, with a tendency to short monosyllabic phrases. Thought becomes disordered and fragmented with perseveration, and an ultimate poverty of ideas. Drowsiness follows in many patients, while others are restless and unable to sleep. Affect can be shallow or, in more labile forms, irritation and agitation appear, with hypersensitivity to light and noise. Headache may be present.

In the fully developed syndrome, the clouded sensorium and disorientation proceed, and thinking may be so disconnected as to produce incoherent speech. No matter how great the effort, reading becomes impossible, and so may conversation. Progressive loss of motor control appears with drooling, food spilling, poor food intake and hygiene, and unkemptness. Ultimately, incontinence of urine and feces occur. This may occur initially in dreams with ensuing shame, but in the end even the social excretory conventions may be lost. Lack of contact with the environment may be extreme, with total time and place disorientation and misidentification of family members. Motor signs such as tremor, slurred speech, seizures, increased autonomic activity appear, with fever, sweating, injected conjunctivae, flushed countenance, rapid pulse, pilomotor responses, and diarrhea. Patients may sleep only during the day when sensory cues are sufficient to reorient and lessen anxiety, but night combines anxiety with reduced sensory input, preventing sleep.

The fully developed syndrome is not merely the worsening of the mild form but contains novel elements of the greatest scientific interest. It is the appearance of hallucinations, initially reported as dreams, that raise major questions. As Lipowski has noted, there is difficulty in estimating their frequency, with a range of 39–73 percent.[50] Visual hallucinations are generally the most prominent, although the auditory modality is frequently involved, and authors have commonly observed proprioceptive hallucinations in postcardiotomy and tank respirator patients. Hallucinations are less marked in the aged and in chronic disease. Lipowksi has raised three critical questions with regard to the hallucinations: Why do they occur at all? Why are they largely visual? How are they shaped by the ego's conflicts?

West[74] has provided a framework for answering these questions. His analogy conveys the reciprocal relationship between reality and illusion . . . "a man in his study standing at a closed glass window opposite the fireplace, looking out at his garden in the sunset. He is absorbed by the view of the outside world. He does not visualize the interior of the room in which he stands. As it becomes darker outside, however, images of the objects in the room behind him can be seen reflected dimly in the window glass. For a time he may see either the garden (if he gazes into the distance) or the reflection of the room's interior (if he focuses on the glass a few inches from his face). Night falls, but the fire still burns brightly in the fireplace and illuminates the room. The watcher now sees in the glass a vivid reflection of the interior of the room behind him, which appears to be outside the window. This illusion becomes dimmer as the fire dies down, and finally, when it is dark both outside and within, nothing more is seen. If the fire flares up from time to time, the visions in the glass reappear." For West, "perceptual release" explains both the hallucinations of the delirious and the sleeper's dream. For both to occur, there must be a decrease in strength of the inhibiting forces controlling release of recorded precepts, along with sufficient preservation of arousal to permit the discharge of perception-bearing circuits. With relative sensory deprivation during sleep, as well as in sensory restriction experiments, and perhaps in delirium, residual awareness no longer competes with current awareness, and the perceptual traces are released and reexperienced, sometimes in rearranged form. This would also explain the effect of sensory overload which "jams the circuits." In sleep, environmental awareness diminishes, yet the cortex is functioning sufficiently to allow for discharge of memory, altered by the censorship of the weakened sleeping ego. Optimal conditions for hallucinations (or hallucinogens) would be disturbed sensory input while maintaining or enhancing arousal. Similarly, subhallucinogenic drug doses in the presence of sleep deprivation may also produce hallucinations.

By inference, it would appear that delirious hallucinations are primarily visual, for the same reason that dreams are. It is likely there is a greater amount of visual memory, of unusual intensity. It seems less likely that nonspecific visual stimuli, produced within the visual pathway's anatomy provides the raw material, awaiting only secondary elaboration.

The visual hallucinations themselves vary widely in duration, vividness, complexity, and relationship to other modalities. Particularly vivid, intense hallucinations are seen in withdrawal syndromes, and we have also seen them in postcardiotomy delirium.

(Course

The course of delirium is characterized by fluctuation and variation, often in the presence of apparently constant organic findings. In many instances, this may be due to variations in emotional and environmental factors, although unrecognized physiological changes in brain metabolism may also occur.

Symptoms may last from moments to weeks, but rarely longer than a month. Postcardiotomy delirium generally lasts several days. In the series by Morse et al. on postoperative delirium[56–58] over half of the patients recovered within a week, and three-quarters eventually recovered completely. Termination can also be by death or by passing into a chronic dementia. Together with Frank,[21] we have shown the absence of permanent organic deficits in patients with the postcardiotomy syndrome. Obviously the likelihood of persistent organic deficiencies are dependent on the nature of the physical factors contributing to the delirium.

During the acute phase, with the savage physical assault on brain function, various release phenomena appear. Unchecked id or sadistic superego are no longer counterbalanced. Lack of inhibition, or depression and paranoia can emerge. Once again, the more acute the syndrome, the more disruptive it is to the defensive apparatus, and more primitive defenses appear. Given overwhelming catastrophe there is a great tendency to blame the self or others. In *Risk*,[52] the author hallucinates that the surgeon has operated on her to "get a brilliant article." A frequent delusion is that the staff is out to kill the patient, which is also a projection of the rage felt for being forced to endure pain and suffering.

Obviously, the premorbid personality determines the quality of release phenomena. Obsessive–compulsive personalities with emphasis on performance may be hit hard by their inability to meet self-set standards, and be terrified by weakly opposed aggressive and sexual impulses. Soiling may produce extreme humiliation. Active personalities may react with outward blame and heightened vigilance. For each patient, the unique blend of premorbid personality, organic insult and clinical setting will shape the content and even appearance of delirium.

⟮ Examination of the Delirious Patient

The skilled interviewer can often detect reduction in the level of cognition during a routine history. Woven into such an interview can be questions about dates of onset, admission, length of time in the hospital, vital statistics etc., so that considerable information can be gained without exposing the patient to a humiliating quiz in which he knows few of the answers. The exposure of deficits may hinder further cooperation and foster antagonistic attitudes. Arithmetic calculations are often used in less obvious cases. The use of serial sevens and repetition of digits backward has been

scored by Katz et al.[39] It has value in obtaining sequential state measures, but fails in deliria characterized by relatively clear cognition, but with perceptual aberrations or place disorientation. In severe cases, the month and year may provide an easily obtainable barometer. In answering questions, the delirious patient may not only make errors, but may respond slowly, utilize concrete aids, like his fingers, or try to conceal his deficit by attacking the question.

⟮ Differential Diagnosis

Delirium must be suspected in any behavioral or emotional problem in a patient who is seriously ill or exposed to sensory or movement restriction. Dementia or chronic organic brain syndrome is usually ruled out by a history of long-standing intellectual deficit, along with a relative absence of agitation, affect, and hallucinations. However, dementia may only be diagnosed when the underlying acute precipitant is treated and cognitive deficits persist. Quite common is the worsening of a mild dementia by an acute organic illness or stress to create a delirium, just as the added insult of sodium amytal may precipitate severe confusion in a mildly organic patient.

At the other extreme, delirium must be distinguished from purely functional illness. The EEG can often answer such a dilemma. Intravenous sodium amytal, judiciously given, can also be helpful in the differential diagnosis since the patient with delirium will get worse. In a patient with a functional disorder, this etiology will become more apparent. This test should be given with great care in situations where the patient's physical condition can be compromised by its use. Most difficult is the clinical differentiation between retarded delirium and retarded depression. The depressed patient may complain of memory loss related to his lack of interest, difficulty in concentrating, and need for self-abuse. However, the mental status should reveal the absence of confusion. The hallucinating schizophrenic tends to be younger and have primarily auditory hallucinations. Once again, the sensorium will be clear. Dissociative patients tend to not know who they are, a great rarity in delirium. They generally also have a model for their symptoms, a history of previous hysterical symptomatology, and are in a stressful situation to which the delirium-like symptom is a compromise solution.

❲ Incidence

As Reding and Daniel[64] have pointed out, delirium is frequently missed because of inadequate mental status examination, failure to notice nurses' notes, difficulties in distinguishing between normal aging and pathology, and insufficient use of the EEG. They also cite an overemphasis on psychodynamics. There is no doubt that nonpsychiatrists often miss the diagnosis. Stated most baldly by Hoaken,[33] "On surgical wards . . . the last thing of interest . . . is the patient's general behavior and mental state." In view of these problems of diagnosis, the true incidence of delirium can only be estimated. Select groups, such as cardiac surgery patients, have a high incidence, and the presence of large numbers of such patients can skew a sample. Nonetheless, Skoog[69] reported a 15 percent incidence in patients admitted to a Swedish hospital. As in certain other studies, women had a greater susceptibility. Foreigners were particularly vulnerable probably because of lack of social and linguistic contact. In 1938, Cobb and McDermott[9] made the same observation of a high incidence in foreigners, some of whom lacked obvious physical explanations. Even then, they suggested loneliness and strangeness as possibly causal factors. Lipowski,[50] in reviewing the German literature, cites the estimate of Bleuler et al.[7] that 30 percent of the 20–70 year old population will, within their lifetime, sustain an episode of delirium, and that 5–10 percent of medical patients in a general hospital suffer from it. The rate is clearly higher for patients over sixty years, where it may approach 50 percent.[88] One estimate[50] is that one-sixth of psychiatric consultations in the general hospital are requested for organic brain syndrome.

❲ Brain Pathophysiology

Although toxic factors are not the whole story of delirium, consistent brain pathophysiological problems have been demonstrated in metabolic encephalopathies. The brain's problems in oxidative metabolism can be replicated at altitudes over 12,000 ft. and at blood sugar levels below 60 mg. percent.[15] Posner[62] has summarized the pertinent neurophysiology. For reasons that are not well understood, cerebral oxygen uptake declines in proportion to the severity of the metabolic brain disease. The normal brain receives 55 ml. of blood per minute, about 15 percent of the resting cardiac output. If the flow falls, more oxygen and glucose are initially extracted. But if the oxygen tension of cerebral tissues falls below 4 mm. Hg, unconsciousness is inevitable. There is no cerebral storage of oxygen and within only six seconds of deprivation, coma occurs. A four-minute interruption of oxygen supply almost always causes irreversible damage, and after fifteen minutes virtually all nerve cells are dead. The brain is less demanding for glucose, its only physiological substrate. One hundred g. of brain utilizes 5.5 mg. glucose per minute, 85 percent of which reacts with oxygen. There is a reserve of 2 g. of glucose to allow 90 minutes of metabolism without irreversible damage.

In addition, the brain requires enzymes and cofactors (vitamins and electrolytes) to function. It is believed that metabolic derangements such as vitamin deficiency, electrolyte imbalance, and exogenous and endogenous poisons operate by inhibition of the cofactors. Nonetheless, the precise mechanism of uremic and hepatic coma, two of the most common metabolic poisonings, are not even known. Although diminished oxygen uptake is a biochemical common denominator, there is no proven anatomic one. Moreover, there is even disagreement as to which area of the brain is most vulnerable to metabolic insult. The traditional view was that the most primitive neural structures were best preserved, and the most recent phylogenetic acquisitions least protected. In this sequence, the cortex is affected initially, then subcortical structures. Pathological studies of anoxia and hypoglycemia support this view, as do animal studies where cortical electrical activity disappears first. A more recent theory holds that the brain stem reticular formation is most vulnerable and that cortical neurons stop functioning when no longer stimulated from below. In some animal studies, electrical transmission through the reticular formation ceases while the cortical neurons are still able to receive other afferent input. Clinically, it would seem that the cortex is first attacked as decline in cortical function preceded alteration of consciousness. Posner[62] concludes that regional issues such as energy needs, blood supply, etc., may determine the point of maximum vulnerability.

❨ Electroencephalographic Findings

The normal EEG has an 8–13 cycle per second (cps) base frequency. The degree of slowing from this baseline parallels the degree of dysfunction. In metabolic disease bilateral synchronous bursts of 1–3 cps are superimposed on a 5–7 cps background. This slowing is an extremely consistent finding, and monitoring it allows for an accurate reading of the clinical state. Slowing parallels worsening and acceleration improvement. Change is more important than absolute values; an initially high-frequency alpha may fall into a normal range with delirium. The EEG is not specific to any single etiology, but is affected by the intensity and duration of the metabolic problem. Recent advances in computer technology have allowed the study of evoked responses. Anticholinergic drug-induced delirium has been associated with abolition of visual response after rhythm, resembling those of sleep.[67] Itil[35] found anticholinergic hallucinogens to produce EEG's with a marked increase of slow waves with superimposed high-

frequency fast activity. Fast beta waves were related to an increase in hallucinations. Studies of the EEG during REM sleep may shed further light on the electrical manifestations of image formation.

Of great theoretical significance is the discovery that sensory restriction can produce EEG changes. This material has been summarized by Schultz.[66] Heron[32] was able to show progressive slowing of the EEG and dysynchronization of the alpha rhythm persisting for hours after a sensory restriction experiment. There were noticeable EEG changes during hallucinatory periods. Zubek et al.[80] found less alpha activity during hallucinations, as well as an excess of theta activity especially over the temporal lobes. Later[79] he demonstrated a mean decrease in occipital lobe frequency, albeit a highly variable one. This variability may be related to differential susceptibility to sensory restriction. Moreover, Zubek and Wilgosh[81] showed occipital lobe slowing following immobilization in a coffin-like box without sensory restriction. In this connection, it was also shown[78] that the EEG slowing due to sensory restriction could be diminished if exercise was permitted. Immobilization alone could also produce intellectual and perceptual impairments.

❨ Metabolic Disturbances in Delirium

All diseases that can disturb the brain's homeostasis can produce delirium. There is little specificity to any etiologic agent. Specificity would have to be associated with a selective rather than general effect on the brain. Sedative or alcohol withdrawal syndromes which produce extreme agitation and florid hallucinations may be such an instance. The intensity is also related to their acute onset, while chronic debilitating illness leads to a quieter syndrome. It should be borne in mind that organic factors often coexist with one another in producing delirium, and that their effect is modified by psychological and environmental factors. An outline of the protean types of disorders that can contribute to delirium is given in the following list.

Organic Causal Factors in Delirium

I. Intrinsic central nervous system (CNS) disease
  A. Tumor
    (1) Primary
    (2) Secondary
  B. Infections
    (1) Encephalitis
    (2) Abscess
    (3) Meningitis
    (4) Neurosyphilis
    (5) Fungal and protozoan
  C. Epilepsy
  D. Ischemic
    (1) Diffuse or multifocal blood vessel obstruction
    (2) Large-vessel disease
      a. Thrombosis
      b. Embolism
    (3) Intravascular coagulation
      a. Collagen disease
      b. SBE (subacute bacterial endocarditis)
  E. Hypertensive encephalopathy
  F. CNS bleeding
    (1) Subarachnoid
    (2) Subdural hematoma
    (3) Bleeding diathesis
      a. Purpura
      b. Clotting disturbance
      c. Leukemia
  G. Degenerative
    (1) Senile
    (2) Presenile
    (3) Metabolic errors
    (4) Demyelinating

II. Non-CNS vascular disorders
  A. Hypoxia due to pulmonary disease
  B. Hypoxia due to cardiac disease
    (1) Congestive heart failure
    (2) Arrhythmia including cardiac arrest and Stokes-Adams
    (3) Shock as with myocardial infarction
    (4) Valvular disease as with aortic stenosis
  C. Reduced peripheral resistance
  D. Disorders of blood volume and viscosity
    (1) Polycythemia
    (2) Cryo- and macroglobulimemia
  E. Anemias and hemoglobinopathies
    (1) Pernicious anemia
    (2) Carbon monoxide
    (3) Methemoglobinemia

III. Non-CNS organic disease
  A. Liver
  B. Kidney
  C. Lung

IV. Endocrine hypo- or hyperfunction
  A. Thyroid-myxedema, thyrotoxicosis
  B. Parathyroid: hypo- and hyperfunction
  C. Adrenal: Addison's and Cushing's, pheochromocytoma
  D. Pancreas: diabetes, hypoglycemia
  E. Pituitary hypofunction

V. Ionic or Acid–base Imbalance
  A. Water intoxication or dehydration
  B. Hyper- and hyponatremia
  C. Hyper- and hypokalemia
  D. Hyper- and hypocalcemia
  E. Hyper- and hypomagnesomia
  F. Acidosis, metabolic or respiratory

VI. Infections
  A. Acute, such as: pneumonia, typhoid, malaria, acute rheumatic fever
  B. Chronic

VII. Environment
  A. Low-oxygen hypoxia
  B. Starvation hypoglycemia
  C. Vitamin deficiencies: thiamin, niacin, pyridoxine, B_{12}, folic acid
  D. Heat and electricity
  E. Radiation

VIII. Exogenous Poisons
  A. Medications
    (1) Sedatives, barbiturates, and other hypnotics
    (2) Minor tranquilizers: diazepam, chlordiazepoxide
    (3) Phenothiazines
    (4) Opiates
    (5) Anticholinergics
    (6) Tricyclic antidepressants

(7) Alcohol
(8) Anticonvulsants
(9) Digitalis
(10) Quinidine
(11) Salicylates
(12) L-Dopa
(13) Penicillin
(14) Steroids

B. Poisons
(1) Methyl alcohol
(2) Ethylene glycol
(3) Organic solvents
(4) Heavy metals
(5) Organophosphorus insecticides

IX. Withdrawal syndromes
A. Alcohol
B. Sedatives and hypnotics

In tropical countries, special emphasis must be placed on trypanosomiasis and malaria as causes of delirium. They may produce either gross or localized disturbances in the sensorium or seemingly functional syndromes. Trypanosomiasis, with its insidious course, may particularly lead to loss of interest in work, avoidance of friends, and cyclothymia, before proceeding to confusion, lethargy, and somnolence. Falciparum malaria infections produce a more acute syndrome. Parasitized red cells with greater adhesiveness and reduced deformability block central nervous system capillaries, until the lumens are obliterated by vast numbers of parasites (Figure 2–1).[5] Characteristic changes can then be seen in anoxic neurons (Figure 2–2). Later changes, with peripheral hemorrhage, including necrosis, demyelination, and gliosis are shown in Figure 2–3). There is a danger, however, that an erroneous causal connection is made when malarial parasites are found in the blood of a delirious patient. Other causes of delirium must be excluded.

It should be underscored that failure to recognize and treat the physical causes of acute delirium may result in permanent brain damage. Unrecognized, and hence untreated myxedema and pernicious anemia are particularly tragic examples of this. The diagnosis of pernicious anemia may be especially difficult

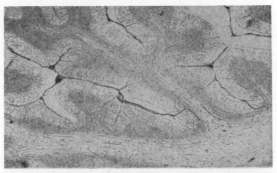

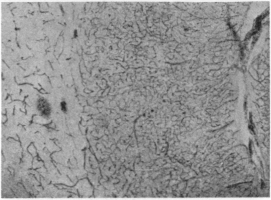

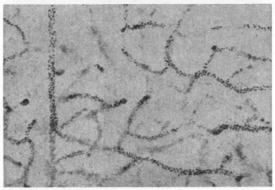

Figure 2–1. (top) Case of cerebral malaria due to *Plasmodium falciparum*. Photomicrographs from unstained frozen sections, 120 to 200 microns thick. The malarial pigment, which is contained in the vessels, outlines the vascular pattern. Cerebellar angioarchitecture (low magnification). (center) Section from a cerebral area (low magnification), showing the difference in the vascular pattern in the cortex (right part of the picture) and in the white matter (left part). In the white matter it is possible to recognize a small hemorrhagic area, represented by a group of extravasated dots of pigment. (bottom) Section from a cortical area (medium magnification), revealing that the coloration is due to the granules of malarial pigment contained in the capillaries. (Courtesy of Dr. Silvano Arieti and the Archives of Neurology and Psychiatry.)

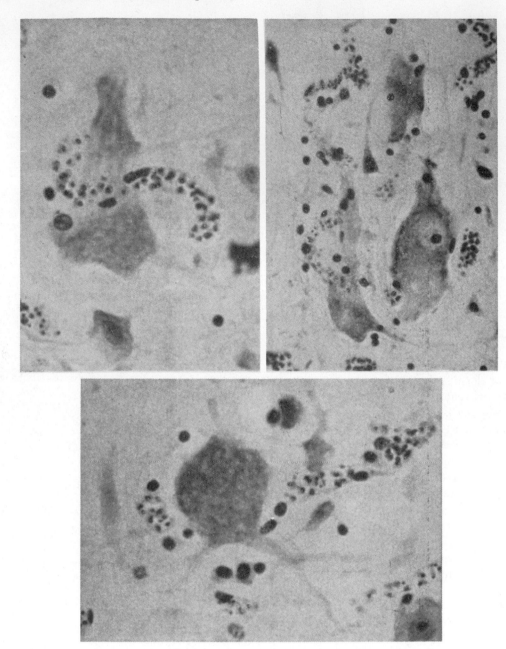

Figure 2–2. (upper left) Case of cerebral malaria due to *Plasmodium falciparum*. Betz's cell, surrounded by a capillary loaded with parasites. Notice the dissolution of tigroid substance in the cytoplasm of the nerve cell. (upper right) Betz's cells, showing retrograde (axonal) degeneration. The nucleus is displaced, and the tigroid substance is dissolved in the center of the cell but preserved at the periphery. Notice, also, the large number of parasites in the neighboring capillaries. (bottom) Ganglion cell of the motor area, showing acute swelling. Nissl stain, high magnification. (Courtesy of Dr. Silvano Arieti and the Archives of Neurology and Psychiatry.)

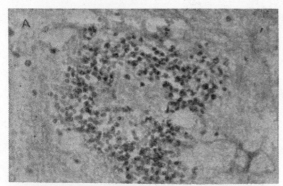

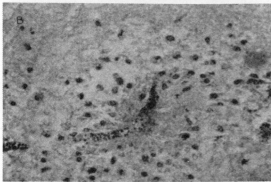

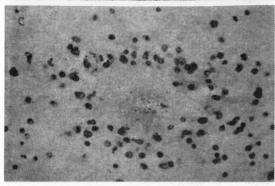

Figure 2-3. (top) Case of cerebral malaria due to *Plasmodium falciparum*. Formation of a pseudo-granuloma. In a small subcortical hemorrhage, the red cells have almost completely disappeared from the center of the area (only a few are left in radial positions) but are still numerous at the periphery. Mallory stain, medium magnification. (center) The red cells have disappeared from the peripheral area also. This area appears edematous and of loose consistency and shows proliferation of glial cells. Note also a central capillary loaded with parasites. Giemsa stain, medium magnification. (bottom) The Pseudogranuloma is now almost formed. At the center one sees in cross section a capillary loaded with parasites. A necrotic central area is surrounded by a peripheral cuffing consisting predominantly of glial cells. Nissl stain, medium magnification. (Courtesy of Dr. Silvano Arieti and the Archives of Neurology and Psychiatry.)

when folic acid treatment prevents the characteristic hematological picture from emerging, also emphasizing the lack of correlation between the anemia itself and cerebral symptoms. The latter may be produced by endarteritis leading to anoxia (Figure 2-4) and accompanied by demyelination (Figure 2-5).[17]

(Roads to Hallucinations and Cognitive Dysfunction

The general hospital provides natural experiments in which the following conditions, that can cause delirium, are combined.

Causes of Perceptual and Cognitive Impairment

    I. Organic insult
    II. Sensory monotony
    III. Sensory overload
    IV. Sleep and dream deprivation
    V. Immobilization
    VI. Overwhelming anxiety

Sensory deprivation is believed to be responsible for the hallucinations of sailors, explorers, and perhaps even religious figures. Numerous studies have demonstrated the frequent development of hallucinations, impairment of time sense, and impaired perceptual-motor performance following sensory monotony. It is most effective when combined with immobilization, as in total-immersion experiments. Similarly, sensory bombardment[26] via immersion in a geodesic dome with psychedelic light and sound can also produce cognitive impairment, particularly in field-dependent subjects.

Subjects deprived of sleeping and dreaming also develop cognitive dysfunction, at times with hallucinations. Hallucinations of a purely functional nature arise when massive anxiety requires the use of primitive mechanisms of denial and projection. In this regard, Arieti's concept of the expectant attitude is relevant. The paranoid listens to the environment expecting to hear his own critical self-appraisal.

As we shall see, there are situations in the general hospital highly conducive to delirium production. Each of them will be examined in turn. However, virtually all patients are subjected to some of the etiologic factors. A physical disease is invariably present. Patients are separated from their familiar environment, family, and even their clothes, and placed in single rooms fostering monotony, or in busy wards leading to overstimulation. Hearing aids or glasses are misplaced or removed for

fear of loss. The same may also be true of television sets and radios. Physical symptoms or the strange environment may interfere with sleep. Sedatives that can cloud consciousness are prescribed for sleep or tranquilization and given in larger doses if not initially successful. Anxiety is rampant and suspiciousness regarding medical care is always possible. Margolis,[53] has focused on the violations of patient's privacy in the ICU. Processions of doctors, nurses, aides, volunteers, equipment mechanics, floor scrubbers, relatives, and friends may

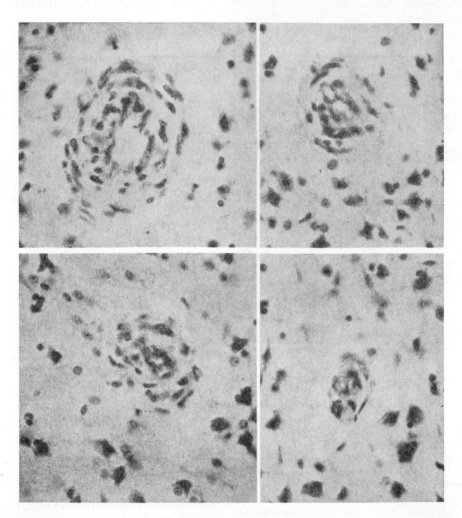

Figure 2–4. (upper left) Progressive stages of endoarteritis in brain of patient suffering from psychosis accompanying pernicious anemia. Vascular walls moderately thickened. (lower left) More advanced stage. Vascular lumen conspicuously reduced. (upper right) The lumen of the vessel is considerably narrowed. Recanalization has already taken place. (lower right) Cortical capillary, the lumen of which is completely occluded. Nissl stain. (Courtesy of Drs. Armando Ferraro, Silvano Arieti, and W. H. English and the *Journal of Neuropathology and Experimental Neurology.*)

troop through. They see the patient at his worst, his weakness exposed.

In the laboratory, subdelirium levels of one factor combined with subdelirium levels of another can produce delirium. Safer[65] duplicated West's finding with anticholinergic hallucinogens and sleep deprivation. Half of a hallucinogenic dose of scopolamine plus one

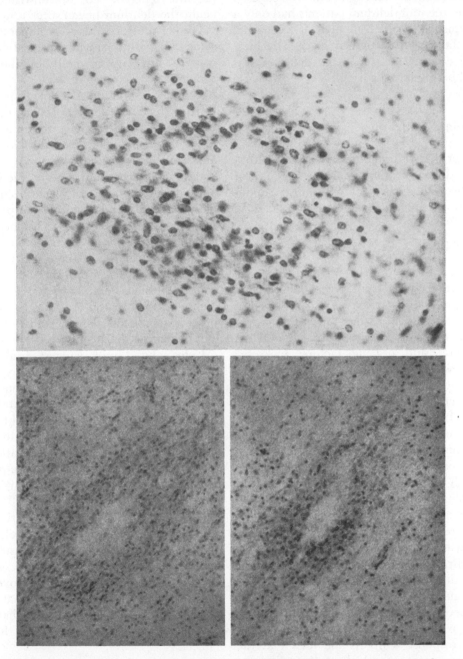

Figure 2–5. (top) Case of psychosis accompanying pernicious anemia. Nissl stain. Typical Lichtheim's plaque consisting of a central degenerated area surrounded by a crown of glial nuclei. (lower left) Plaque showing two acellular areas. (lower right) Plaque showing an elongated acellular area which probably follows the course of a vessel. (Courtesy of Drs. Armando Ferraro, Silvano Arieti, and W. H. English and the *Journal of Neuropathology and Experimental Neurology*.)

sleepless night was equivalent to a full hallucinogenic dose.

In 1936, while investigating the delirium associated with a course of five to ten hyperthermia treatments, Ebaugh et al.[13] discovered that 43 percent of delirium patients had only a single episode, 80 percent of which occurred during the first induction of fever. The inescapable conclusion is that the delirium was fostered by the initial anxiety.

◖ Special Syndromes

A number of syndromes are associated with a high incidence of delirium. Since they are of great theoretical, as well as clinical significance, they will be examined in detail.

Eye Surgery

With the former practice of patching both eyes after cataract surgery, sudden visual deprivation was imposed. This produced a delirium referred to as the "black patch psychosis" which illustrates the interaction of environmental and organic factors. Jackson[36] has reviewed the extensive literature in this area over the last eighty years.

Cataract patients tend to be old and already suffering from some chronic brain impairment. Retinal detachment patients are younger, but have a more acute illness and greater restriction of postoperative movement. Both groups have high levels of anxiety about the possibility of blindness. Colman[11] in 1894, first reported postoperative hallucinations. In 1900, Posey[61] reported twenty-four cases of delirium in elderly patients with patched eyes. "The delirium began with mental restlessness and rapidly progressed to hallucinations and ideas of persecution. Delirium developed during the second day for eight patients; the third day for six; and the fourth day for two." This delayed response supports the idea that the restriction operates gradually to contribute to the delirium. Moreover, the eye surgery, done under local anesthesia, does not provide a fresh organic insult to the brain. In 1913 Parker[60] reviewed the charts of a large series of cataract extractions. Patients were described as "restless, maniacal, suspicious, uncontrollable, and disoriented; getting out of bed; talking incoherently and removing their patches" (maybe not so unwisely!). Once again the delirium began after a latent interval from one to six days postoperatively, the same range as in most postsurgical delirium. A report in 1917 by Brownell[8] described the syndrome as lasting a day or two.

Our understanding of etiology is enhanced by the dramatic discovery that, despite the covering of both eyes, the delirium was more apt to begin and/or worsen at night. Weisman and Hackett[73] eloquently wrote ". . . night . . . is the time when a hush falls on the ward, and auditory cues, which may have been responsible for alerting and orienting the patient during the day are replaced by silence with an occasional whispered conversation and the soft sporadic sounds of the night. Under these circumstances . . . misinterpretations may become delusions and anxiety may become panic." Added to this is the mystique of the night symbolizing danger and vulnerability, and increasing the anxiety.

Coles and Linn[10] suggest trial patching prior to surgery if it is absolutely required. Delirium could be predicted when the EEG was abnormal and the sodium amytal test positive. In high-risk patients, surgical techniques may have to be modified, keeping in mind the patient's likelihood of noncooperation. Early mobilization and stimulation of the patient, as might be obtained in a two- to four-bed room, were recommended. Ziskind et al[77] reported the highest delirium incidence in the non-English speaking, the deaf, alcoholics, or those with obvious brain damage. Jackson[36] noted the great variability in insight, and that patches were most frequently removed by patients at night. It seems clear that bilateral patching should be avoided and that removal of patches may have dramatic therapeutic effects.

Respirator Delirium

The phenomena of respirator-induced delirium was described by Holland and Coles[34] in 1955 following an outbreak of poliomyelitis. Forty percent of bulbar polio patients developed delirium beginning from one to ten days after entering the respirator. Hallucinations and delusions were of a pleasurable nature, frequently involving motion and travel. The emotional stress was enormous. Patients feared that they would be unable to summon help, since they could not close their tracheotomies should there be a power failure or the plug be pulled accidentally. They faced the prospect of possibly permanent paralysis or even death. As time in the tank progressed, patients became depressed, finally showing hostility and anxiety with weaning from the respirator. Disorientation and confusion were also noticed.

Mendelsohn and Foley[54] provide an explanation of this syndrome. The hallucinations occurred in a quasi-twilight state. They disappeared when the patients' limbs were manipulated or when someone spoke to them about their real surroundings. They could not see their bodies, their vision was restricted, hearing was impaired due to the repetitious motor sound, and mobility was restricted by the paralysis and tank confinement.

Extending their clinical observations, seventeen normal control subjects were put in the respirator. Only five could remain in it longer than thirty-six hours. Eight sustained hallucinations and all were unable to concentrate or judge time. Four had to terminate abruptly due to severe anxiety. Moreover, the subjects were not febrile, and they knew they could get out, walk, and breathe at any time.

Mendelsohn et al.[55] structurally analyzed the hallucinations. In general, hallucinations are wish-fulfilling or defensive. The latter tend to be auditory, the former multisensory. They are facilitated by great anxiety and need in schizophrenia, or in the nonschizophrenic subjected to enormous stress. The polio patients' hallucinations had both wish-fulfilling and defensive characteristics. Movement motifs were enhanced by the vibration of the pump motor. Hallucinations were extremely colorful, three dimensional, and generally pleasant. They served the wish of being able to move again, yet reality intruded to the extent that tank-type structures followed them along as they anticipated their future lives.

The tank-respirator syndrome is now observed in patients with chronic lung disease, such as kyphoscoliosis. It is also seen in neurological diseases, especially if they combine paralysis with decreased sensation. Intermittent removal from the tank, if possible, is recommended.

Cardiac Surgery

In 1964, Blachly,[6] Egerton[14] and Kornfeld et al.[47] described a syndrome occurring in the open heart recovery room (OHRR), three to five days postoperatively. Logically, it was named postcardiotomy delirium. It often began with illusions based on sounds created by the machinery in the room, and with frequent proprioceptive distortions such as a rocking or floating sensation. Patients would become briefly, or persistently, disoriented. Delusions were common, sometimes with a frank paranoid flavor. One patient thought a record player had been placed under her bed to torture her. She also hallucinated the voices of absent family members. Like most patients, she improved after transfer from the OHRR. Thirty-eight percent of Kornfeld patients were adjudged delirious by chart review, and fully seventy percent of those followed throughout the surgical experience had delirium symptoms. Kornfeld confirmed Blachly's finding that degree of preoperative illness predisposed to delirium. Also confirmed was Blachly's finding of a higher incidence in double-valve replacement cases, and an association between prolonged cardiopulmonary bypass time and delirium.

Kornfeld reasoned that the lucid interval of several days postoperatively suggested that postoperative factors played a role in delirium causation. Similarities were noted between the OHRR experience and sleep and sensory deprivation studies. It was postulated that the intense anxiety the cardiac surgery patient experienced might also play a part.

A number of recommendations were made to lessen delirium incidence and severity. Uninterrupted sleep was to be encouraged. Individual rooms were suggested to minimize patients waking each other or witnessing anxiety-provoking emergencies. Less obtrusive monitoring equipment was advocated to minimize sensory monotony and anxiety. Increased mobility with early removal of wires and tubes was recommended. The monotonous noise of oxygen, cooling, and air-conditioning apparatus was to be minimized. Television sets, radios, clocks, and calendars were to be supplied to increase stimuli and provide reality cueing.

A more detailed longitudinal study reported in 1970[30] of 142 survivors showed a decrease in delirium incidence since the early report. Now only 24 percent experienced the delirium after a lucid interval, while 9 percent had evidence of an organic mental syndrome upon awakening from anesthesia. These latter patients were hypoactive and tended to lack florid symptomatology. They tended to have severe organic illnesses.

The lucid interval delirium group was intensively studied. Organic factors clearly played a role, since advanced age, and severity of pre- and postoperative illness, and time on the cardio-pulmonary bypass were all correlated significantly with delirium.

An effort was made in the 1970s to understand the reduced incidence. Decreased bypass time appeared to play a role, as within each operative category reduction in incidence paralleled the varying reduction in bypass time. It was also postulated that the adopted suggestions with regard to sleep and environment, and the less panicky attitude of patients and staff might also be responsible. Other investigators confirmed the role of social-environmental factors in delirium incidence. Lazarus and Hagens[49] studied two groups undergoing open-heart surgery by the same surgeon at different hospitals. In one hospital, modifications designed to lessen anxiety, sensory monotony, and sleep deprivation halved the incidence of delirium. Layne and Yudofsky[48] reported that patients who did not express preoperative anxiety had double the incidence of delirium of anxiety expres-

sors. It seems clear that pre- and postoperative emotional ventilation would play a prophylactic role. This view was further confirmed when a member of our research team reviewed the charts of patients seen by the research group and a comparable group that had not been seen. The interviewed group had half the delirium incidence of the unseen group.

The present authors have undertaken a detailed study of the personality and psychological factors associated with postcardiotomy delirium. Organic factors were once again found to be significantly related. A new finding, based on statistically significant psychological test reports and suggestive psychiatric ratings, was that patients characterized by dominance, aggressivity, confidence, and an active orientation seemed more vulnerable to delirium. It was reasoned that for such individuals, the passive, immobilized patient role in the OHRR would be more stressful than it would be for more passive patients. For the active group, the OHRR experience is an exact opposite to their usual functioning and produces intense conflicts. Denying anxiety, this group would be unable to benefit from preoperative psychological ventilation which might reduce postoperative anger and paranoia.

All these factors, it should be emphasized, complement rather than conflict with organic risk factors. Other investigators have presented new evidence confirming the importance of organic factors. Tufo[70] has shown that operative hypotension is associated with postoperative organicity. Kimball[41] has emphasized the significance of previous central nervous system insult. Willner et al.[75] have found organically based disturbance of analogy reasoning predictive of delirium.

Our work has shown a high incidence of delirium, approaching 40 percent, in patients undergoing saphenous vein coronary artery bypass surgery. This is believed to be related to relatively lengthy bypass times and possibly the active-dominant character of the sample. These patients often manifest the time urgency and aggressivity characteristically associated with early onset of coronary disease.

General Surgery

The most straightforward study suggesting that psychological factors play a role in general surgical delirium comes from two small hospitals in El Dorado, Arkansas.[76] The two hospitals have the same bed capacity and medical staff, and accept random admissions. One of the ICUs is windowless, the other has windows. Controlled factors were age, type of procedure, and postoperative temperature. There were no differences between the two groups. Yet the windowless ICU had a 40 percent delirium incidence as compared with 18 percent in the windowed unit. Although it can be argued that there is an unidentified causal difference, it would seem that a room without windows during the critical immediate postoperative period is deleterious.

Comprehensive information concerning general surgical delirium is found in the work of Morse et al.[56–58] Probably related to the excellent medical and surgical care at the Mayo Clinic, the overall operative delirium rate was only 0.5 percent. Sixty delirious patients, equally divided between retarded and hyperactive forms were compared with a control group, matched for type of operation, age, and sex. Twenty-two percent of the delirium group had open-heart surgery, 18 percent hip or other fractures, 12 percent spinal fusion, 10 percent colectomy; the remainder had miscellaneous surgery. Delirium occurred from the third to the seventh day postoperatively. Delusions were found in two-thirds of the cases. As would be expected, 55 percent of the delirium patients were over sixty. Age over sixty and duration over one week were bad prognostic signs for recovery.

Abundant support was obtained for the general theory that organic, social-environmental, and emotional factors combine to cause delirium. To be sure, organic physical factors were extremely important. All parameters studied were more likely to be abnormal in the delirium group, and the following significantly so: abnormal EKG (electrocardiogram), albuminuria, alkalosis, anemia, azotemia, hypochloremia, hypokalemia, hyponatremia, and leukocytosis. The delirium group had significantly more cardiac failure, cardiovascular disease, infection, drug or alcohol intoxication or withdrawal, history of organic brain syndrome, preoperative disorientation, operative procedure longer than four hours, emergency operation, postoperative complications, and use of more than five drugs postoperatively. It should be noted, however, that the abnormalities were not confined to the delirium group.

Yet nonorganic factors also correlated significantly with delirium. Morbid preoperative expectation was associated with a 33 percent delirium incidence as compared with 3 percent not showing pessimism. Sensory distortion, caused by visual disorders or partial deafness, was also much more common in the delirium group, as was a history of more than two previous operations. Denial of preoperative fear was associated with a lower incidence of delirium.

Other, purely psychiatric factors were also significantly correlated with delirium: a history of alcoholism or depression, a family history of psychosis, functional GI (gastrointestinal) disturbance, insomnia, paranoid personality or psychosis, history of previous postoperative psychosis, history of psychiatric treatment, or retirement problems. Patients of the highest social class seemed less susceptible to delirium. Clinical vignettes also supported the psychobiological thesis. In one case, delirium cleared when a misplaced hearing aid was found; in another, it worsened with a son's departure.

Renal Disease

With the development of hemodialysis and transplantation surgery, there has been a renewal of interest in the previously largely academic question of neuropsychological disorders in end-stage renal failure.[71] Untreated, the mental changes show gradual onset and hence tend to less dramatic manifestations. The usual sequence of events for chronic delirium is followed. Difficulty in concentration and memory change appear associated initially with normal or minimally changed EEG's. This may long precede the development of azotemia. Prodromal symptoms are followed by irritability, labile affect, manifest disorientation and confusion, with delusions and hallucinations. With the neurotoxic crumbling of the personality, dietary indiscretions increase, creating a vicious cycle. Periods of lucidity decline and torpor is common as myoclonus and fasciculations, asterixis and convulsions develop. Lassitude passes into stupor and then coma, usually with heightened muscle tone. Any improvement occurs in reverse order to the loss.

EEG changes parallel the clinical disorder, with slowing usually accompanying BUN (blood urea nitrogen) levels over 60 mg. percent. Initially there is slight slowing with a tendency to disorganization of alpha activity, followed by progressive slowing and disorganization with paroxysms of greater slowness, leading to diffuse slowing and spiking. Tyler[71] claims that the EEG is similar, but not identical to those of hepatic decompensation. Kiley and Hines[40] noted that wave frequency becomes slower before obvious electrolyte changes. Some photic driving, as in a drug withdrawal syndrome, is seen particularly during recovery phases, raising the provocative question of a withdrawal syndrome to an unidentified toxin. Of course, no single electrolyte correlates with EEG abnormalities, but rapid shifts in electrolytes cause worsening of the EEG and the clinical state. Klinger[43] reports photogenic abnormal occipital sharp waves and Lossky-Nekhorocheff et al.[51] showed disappearance of the alpha rhythm and disturbance of the arresting reaction. Complete records of abnormal slow waves preceded imminent death. Eighty percent of irrational confused patients had abnormally slow frequencies, and if 40 percent of the record is abnormally slow, psychological testing would show cognitive impairment. It should be noted that frequently coexisting diseases, such as anemia and hypertension, can also affect the EEG. Yet the EEG can be used as an indicator for dialysis when there is slowing to less than 6 cps.

But is the treatment any better than the disease? The life of a dialysis patient is dominated by conflicts about the value of staying alive. In the series by Foster, Cohn et al.[20] almost 50 percent of the dialysis patients made suicidal threats. Interestingly, three of the four patients who made attempts succumbed to their disease. Survival was related to physical factors, such as low mean BUN, but also to Catholicism, the presence of parents, and indifference to the fate of other dialysis patients.

Abram[1,2] has greatly expanded our knowledge of the inner life of the chronic dialysis patient. He classifies the uremic syndrome into the following categories: asthenic, restless, hallucinating, schizophreniform, depressed, manic, and paranoid. The asthenic category predominates. In a series of thirty-eight patients, psychological testing revealed evidence of organicity in all, with poor visual-motor coordination, and difficulty in nonverbal abstraction and attention. Few patients had acute hyperactive episodes, and when they did occur it was usually during the first episode of uremia, as in the hyperthermia study, again suggesting multifactorial causation.

The initial adjustment to dialysis is euphoria as toxic apathy clears. Anxiety appears at about the third to fifth dialyses, followed by depression as the problems of the treatment become undeniable. Conflicts about dependency and independence emerge and psychotherapy is frequently indicated. From the third to the twelfth month the issue of whether life is worth living becomes paramount. Viederman[72] has well described these problems. The patient has surrendered his autonomy, his clothes are removed, privacy is denied, intake and elimination become subject to the orders of others. There is no dietary freedom. Pain and exposure are experienced two or three times a week for five to eight hours a day tied to a machine. The dialysis bath comes to symbolize the womb and birth, and a love–hate relationship develops with the machine. It becomes the frustrating bad mother, breaking down frequently with ruptured coils and causing weakness, cramps, and hypotension. Such experiences resonate with early maternal encounters. The content of a delirium will clearly reflect this. One of Viederman's patients had the delusion she had been cured by God, and no longer needed dialysis. Another had the somatic delusion of bodily disintegration with holes in the skin.

According to Abram, life with the machine preoccupies the patient. He becomes a compulsive gambler knowing the only roulette wheel in town is rigged against him, but unable to stop using it. He fantasies or threatens to cut his shunt, the weakest link, the umbilical cord to the machine. He frequently imagines himself a Frankenstein and in his drawings sees himself as increasingly resembling a dialyzer. He has become a semiartificial man, a zombie, the living dead. In fantasy or delusion, mechanical monsters with malevolent intent are after him. Even the nurses dream of the ubiquitous machine and of being dialyzed. They develop psychosomatic illnesses and there is a rapid staff turnover.

Intense relationships develop between patients and staff in this setting. Male patients seeing themselves as castrated may exhibit themselves to the nurses. Particularly where transplantation is considered, patients have great difficulty in expressing anger to the staff for fear of being labelled noncooperative and excluded from the hoped-for miracle surgery. In addition, intense conflicts are experienced concerning family members who do or do not offer their kidneys, and over assuming the identity of the donor. Therefore, both the precipitation and content of any delirious episode must be viewed in the widest possible context.

Hepatic Coma

The delirium associated with liver disease is in many ways similar to that of uremia. In both, we witness a final chapter in a long process resulting in a complex metabolic poisoning. Delirium in liver disease can be divided into two groups, that of hepatic failure, and of portal shunting to the systemic circulation.

The treatment of liver failure, despite the recent use of L-Dopa,[18] leaves much to be desired. There is no hepatic dialysis and symptoms tend to be progressive. A prodromal syndrome is followed by impending coma, often with asterixis (liver flap), and with characteristic, if not specific, EEG findings.[19] There are paroxysms of bilaterally symmetrical high-voltage delta waves $1\frac{1}{2}$–3 cps, along with relatively normal alpha waves.

Organic brain syndromes in patients with liver disease need not be hepatic coma.[46] Delirium can also be caused by anoxia from anemia following gastrointestinal bleeding; central nervous system bleeding caused by a clotting diathesis or head trauma, especially in the alcoholic; inadequately metabolized sedatives or tranquilizers; and the effects of alcohol or its withdrawal.

The differentiation between delirium tremens (DT) and hepatic coma is particularly important since sedative-replacement therapy can be lethal for the impending hepatic-coma patient.[12] The DT's patient will characteristically have abstained from alcohol one to three days before the appearance of symptoms, be more alert, aggressive, and have more vivid hallucinations. His tremor will be coarse and rhythmic. The chronic liver-disease patient, on the other hand, is hypoactive, tends not to have intense hallucinations, and has an irregular and flapping tremor.

Portal-systemic encephalopathy is the term applied to delirium caused by portal shunting, which may be congenital or surgically acquired. It can be produced with or without accompanying liver disease.[68] Clinically it is similar to impending hepatic coma, although at times there may be unique elements. It has a chronic course with recurrent episodes of stupor or coma. Patients may also manifest other neurological signs and symptoms as the illness progresses. These may become irreversible. These patients can mistakenly be thought to be taking excessive quantities of sedatives or tranquilizers. They often suffer from headaches and the analgesics taken for their relief can be inadequately metabolized, complicating the picture further. The drowsy periods may follow meals with too much nitrogen content, since these patients are particularly sensitive to nitrogenous substances. The rigorous need for a protein-free intake may create psychological problems. This syndrome has been attributed to the introduction of intestinal absorption products directly into the systemic circulation. The blood ammonium is usually raised,[68] but it does not always correlate with the neurological state.

Burn Patients

The psychiatric aspects of extensive burn patients have been largely ignored. Yet a third of the patients with significant burns[4] may develop delirium. Half of the delirium patients were hallucinating and thrashing, half were somnolent. The extensiveness of the burn and its associated metabolic derangements were obviously related to delirium causation. Premorbid psychopathology was also implicated. It would seem that sensory restriction may also play a role with limited mobility and impaired sensory input. Certainly, massive anxiety would be mobilized by the traumatic event and the threat of disfigurement and death.

Intensive Care Units

The ICU may reproduce many of the etiological factors in delirium. The patients are quite sick and vulnerable, and even if delirium is not caused, environmental factors may add to agitation, anxiety, and depression. The cardiac care unit is similar in many ways to the OHRR. There are intravenous (IV) catheters, electrocardiogram (EKG) cables, flashing EKG oscilloscopes with bell alarms (with inevitable false alarms), and an omnipresent defibrillator. A cardiac arrest brings a stampede of house officers. Parker and Hodge[59] have reported delirium in these units which they attribute to sensory monotony. On the other hand, Hackett and Cassem[27] did not find significant psychopathology. It should be noted that the units vary greatly in environment and personnel. In some converted units there is only curtain separation, while newly constructed units have cubicles and concealed monitoring equipment. The number of patients in a unit also varies. The observation of death and complications in other patients can be particularly distressing with predictable autonomic reactions, which could not come at a worse time. Even patients who deny anxiety related to another patient's death would prefer to be in private rooms.[27]

Caution should be used in applying the term ICU syndrome to delirium in this setting. These patients are severely medically ill, or they would not be there. They are also receiving complex medical regimens. Although we should be aware of environmental factors, our nonpsychiatric colleagues must be urged to explore all possible medical causes for delirium before invoking a purely environmental explanation.

Departure from ICU's can also be traumatic. It is frequently abrupt, and viewed as a rejection with ensuing cardiovascular problems related to increased catecholamine excretion.[42] Symptoms akin to traumatic neurosis can be produced which manifest themselves with delayed insomnia and nightmares. Patients frequently are discharged from the units without adequate recommendations to minimize over- and underactivity.

❨ Treatment

The multifactorial causation of delirium requires a multifactorial therapy. The role of psychic factors does not diminish in the slightest the need for correction of underlying physical abnormalities, which may be brain- and lifesaving. Delirium is a medical emergency; the brain cannot wait. Not only should specific factors related to illnesses and medications be sought, but the general physical condition of the patient, his hemoglobin level, hydration, and nutrition must all be considered. Osler's rule of 1892 still applies, "procure sleep and support the strength."[31]

The consulting psychiatrist often finds that the patient with delirium has already been inappropriately treated with a minor tranquilizer or barbiturate. Indeed, the most common recommendation is the withdrawal of barbiturates or minor tranquilizers and substitution by phenothiazines. Barbiturates and minor tranquilizers are only indicated in withdrawal syndromes, and may worsen or precipitate a delirium. On the other hand, chlorpromazine is particularly useful. It should be given 25 mgs. intramuscularly, and repeated as needed. Usually 25 mg. IM (intramuscular), or 50 to 100 mg. by mouth every four to six hours is sufficient. A standing order, to be given when the patient is awake, is generally preferable to awaiting severe symptoms. If excessive somnolence is produced, a less sedating phenothiazine, such as thioridazine or trifluoperazine, can be substituted for part or all of the dosage. The drugs have a potent antipsychotic effect, and provide "chemical restraint" which is far superior to physical. It may be necessary to assuage the undue fear internists and surgeons have of these medications causing hepatitis and hypotension. Generally the benefits far outweigh the risk. However, a greater risk is that effective symptomatic treatment may dissuade the referring physician from vigorously pursuing the etiology of the delirium once behavioral problems have diminished.

Prevention and therapy should also include minimizing sleep interruption and sensory restriction or overload. An overly sterile, monotonous, instrument-laden hospital room provides a blank screen upon which the patient can project his fantasies. Immobilization is also unnatural and should be avoided. Familiar figures from the patient's life should be available to him as much as is feasible. Stays in OHRRs or ICUs should be as brief as possible. The staff should be helped to provide a warm, trusting relationship.

Psychotherapy visits should be brief and frequent. Recognizing the precarious state of integration of these patients, efforts should be made at support and ego enhancement, rather than at exposing deficits. Efforts should be made to provide cueing, and to reduce the harsh criticisms of performance failures. The psychiatrist must convey that he understands what the patient is experiencing. Patients should be told that they have a reversible condition for which there is appropriate treatment. They can be reassured that there is a specific, usually correctable stress, and that they are not "going crazy." They should be encouraged to report unusual experiences to the staff. Encouragement can be provided as recovery begins. After recovery, patients should be given the opportunity to understand and integrate their experience.

(Bibliography

1. ABRAM, H. S. "The Psychiatrist, the Treatment of Chronic Renal Failure and the Prolongation of Life 1," *Am. J. Psychiatry*, 124 (1968), 1351–1357.

2. ———. "The Prosthetic Man," *Compr. Psychiatry*, 11 (1970), 475–481.

3. ADAMS, R. D. and M. VICTOR. "Delirium and Other Confusional States and Korsakoff's Amnestic Syndrome," in M. W. Wintrobe et al., eds., *Harrison's Textbook of Medicine*, pp. 185–193. New York: McGraw-Hill, 1970.

4. ANDREASEN, N. C., R. NOYES et al. "Management of Emotional Reactions in Seriously Burned Adults," *N. Engl. J. Med.*, 286 (1972), 65–69.

5. ARIETI, S. "Histopathologic Changes in Cerebral Malaria and Their Relation to Psychotic Sequels," *Arch. Neurol. Psychiatry*, 56 (1946), 79.

6. BLACHLY, P. H. and A. STARR. "Post-cardiotomy Delirium," *Am. J. Psychiatry*, 121 (1964), 371–375.

7. BLEULER, M., J. WILLI et al. *Akute Psychische Begleiterscheinungen koerperlicher Krankheiten*. Stuttgart: Thieme, 1966.

8. BROWNELL, M. E. "Cataract Deliriums. A Complete Report of the Cases of Cataract Delirium Occurring in the Ophthalmologic Clinic of the University of Michigan Between the Years 1904 and 1917," *J. Mich. State Med. Assoc.*, 16 (1917), 282–286.

9. COBB, S. and N. T. McDERMOTT. "Clinic of Doctors Cobb and McDermott," *Med. Clin. North Am.*, (1938), 569–576.

10. COLES, R. S. and L. LINN. "Behavior Disturbances Related to Cataract Extraction," *Eye, Ear, Nose, Throat Monthly*, 35 (1956), 111–113.

11. COLMAN, W. S. "Hallucinations in the Sane, Associated with Local Organic Disease of the Sensory Organs, etc.," *Br. Med. J.*, 1 (1894), 1015–1017.

12. DAVIDSON, E. A. and P. SOLOMON. "The Differentiation of Delirium Tremens from

Impending Hepatic Coma and DT's," *J. Ment. Sci.*, 104 (1958), 226–333.

13. EBAUGH, F. G., C. H. BARNACLE et al. "Delirious Episodes Associated with Artificial Fever: A Study of Two Hundred Cases," *Am. J. Psychiatry*, 93 (1936), 191–217.

14. EGERTON, N. and J. H. KAY. "Psychological Disturbances Associated with Open-Heart Surgery," *Br. J. Psychiatry*, 110 (1964), 433–439.

15. ENGEL, G. L. and J. ROMANO. "Delirium, a Syndrome of Cerebral Insufficiency," *J. Chronic Dis.*, 9 (1959), 260–277.

16. EVARTS, E. V. "A Neurophysiologic Theory of Hallucinations," in L. J. West, ed., *Hallucinations*, pp. 1–14. New York: Grune & Stratton, 1962.

17. FERRARO, A., S. ARIETI, and W. H. ENGLISH. "Cerebral Changes in the Course of Pernicious Anemia and Their Relationship to Psychic Symptoms," *J. Neuropathol. Exp. Neurol.*, 4 (1945), 217.

18. FISCHER, J. E. and R. J. BALDESSARINI. "False Neurotransmitters and Hepatic Failure," *Lancet*, 2 (1971), 75–79.

19. FOLEY, J. M., C. W. WATSON et al. "Significance of EEG Changes in Hepatic Coma," *Trans. Am. Neurol. Assoc.*, 75 (1950), 61.

20. FOSTER, F. G., G. L. COHN et al. "Psychobiologic Factors and Individual Survival on Clinical Renal Hemodialysis, a Two Year Follow-Up 1," *Psychosom. Med.*, 35, (1973), 64–82.

21. FRANK, K. A., S. S. HELLER et al. "Long-Term Effects of Open-Heart Surgery on Intellectual Functioning," *J. Thorac. Cardiovasc. Surgery*, 64 (1972), 811–815.

22. FRAZIER, J. G. *The Golden Bough*, abr. ed., New York: MacMillan, 1951.

23. FREUD, S. (1897) "Letter to Fliess," Number 69, in J. Strachey, ed., *Standard Edition*, Vol. 1, pp. 259–260. London: Hogarth, 1966.

24. ———. (1900) *The Interpretation of Dreams* in J. Strachey, ed., *Standard Edition*, Vol. 4. London: Hogarth, 1953.

25. ———. (1910) "Leonardo da Vinci and a Memory of His Childhood," in J. Strachey, ed., *Standard Edition*, Vol. 11, pp. 63–137. London: Hogarth, 1957.

26. GOTTSCHALK, C. A., J. L. HAER et al. "Effect of Sensory Overload on Psychological State Changes in Social Alienation, Personal Disorganization and Cognitive-Intellectual Impairment," *Arch. Gen. Psychiatry*, 27 (1972), 451–457.

27. HACKETT, T. P., N. H. CASSEM et al. "The Coronary Care Unit, an Appraisal of Its Psychological Hazards," *N. Engl. J. Med.*, 279 (1968), 1365–1370.

28. HACKETT, T. P. and A. D. WEISMAN. "Psychiatric Management of Operative Syndromes II. Psychodynamic Factors in Formulation and Management," *Psychosom. Med.*, 22 (1960), 356–372.

29. HANKOFF, L. D. "Ancient Descriptions of Organic Brain Syndrome: the 'Kordiakos' of the Talmud," *Am. J. Psychiatry*, 129 (1972), 233–236.

30. HELLER, S. S., K. A. FRANK et al. "Psychiatric Complications of Open-Heart Surgery: a Re-Examination," *N. Engl. J. Med.*, 283 (1970), 1015–1020.

31. HENRY, D. W. and A. M. MANN. "Diagnosis and Treatment of Delirium," *J. Can. Med. Assoc.*, 93 (1965), 1156–1166.

32. HERON, W. "Cognitive and Physiological Effects of Perceptual Isolation," in P. Solomon et al., eds., *Sensory Deprivation.* Cambridge, Mass.: Harvard University Press, 1961.

33. HOAKEN, P. "Discussion of R. M. Morse, and E. M. Linin, 'Anatomy of a Delirium'," *Am. J. Psychiatry*, 128 (1971), 115.

34. HOLLAND, J. C. and M. R. COLES. "Neuropsychiatric Aspects of Acute Poliomyelitis," *Am. J. Psychiatry*, 114 (1957), 54–63.

35. ITIL, T. and M. FINK. "Anticholinergic Drug-Induced Delirium, Experimental Modification, Quantitative EEG and Behavioral Correlations," *J. Nerv. Ment. Dis.*, 143 (1966), 492–507.

36. JACKSON, C. W., JR. "Clinical Sensory Deprivation: a Review of Hospitalized Eye Surgery Patients," in J. P. Zubek, ed., *Sensory Deprivation: Fifteen Years of Research*. New York: Appleton-Century-Crofts, 1969.

37. JOHNSON, M. H. "Drugs of Choice in Confusional States," *Med. Times*, 100 (1972), 92–99.

38. KAPLAN, D. "Emotional Reaction of Patients on Chronic Hemodialysis," *Psychosom. Med.*, 30 (1968), 521–533.

39. KATZ, N. M., D. P. AGLE et al. "Delirium in Surgical Patients under Intensive Care, Utility of Mental Status Examination," *Arch. Surg.*, 104 (1972), 310–313.

40. KILEY, J. and O. HINES. "Electroencephalographic Evaluation of Uremia," *Arch. Intern. Med.*, 116 (1965), 67–73.

41. KIMBALL, C. P. "The Experience of Open-Heart Surgery III: Toward a Definition and Understanding of Post-Cardiotomy Delirium," *Arch. Gen. Psychiatry*, 27 (1972), 57–63.

42. KLEIN, R. F., V. S. KLINER et al. "Transfer from a Coronary Care Unit," *Arch. Intern. Med.*, 122 (1968), 104–108.

43. KLINGER, M. "EEG Observations in Uremia," *Electroencephalogr. Clin. Neurophysiol.*, 6 (1954), 519.

44. KOLB, L. C. *Modern Clinical Psychiatry.* Philadelphia: Saunders, 1973.

45. KORNFELD, D. S. "Psychiatric Problems of an Intensive Care Unit," *Med. Clin. North Am.*, 55 (1971), 1353–1363.

46. ———. "Psychiatric Aspects of Liver Disease," in A. Linder, ed., *Emotional Factors in Gastrointestinal Disease*, pp. 166–181. Amsterdam: Excerpta Medica, 1974.

47. KORNFELD, D. S., S. ZIMBERG et al. "Psychiatric Complications of Open-Heart Surgery," *N. Engl. J. Med.*, 273 (1965), 287–292.

48. LAYNE, O. L. and S. C. YUDOFSKY. "Post-Operative Psychosis in Cardiotomy Patients," *N. Engl. J. Med.*, 284 (1971), 518–520.

49. LAZARUS, H. R. and J. H. HAGENS. "Prevention of Psychosis Following Open-Heart Surgery," *Am. J. Psychiatry*, 124 (1968), 1190–1195.

50. LIPOWSKI, Z. J. "Delirium, Clouding of Consciousness and Confusion," *J. Nerv. Ment. Dis.*, 145 (1967), 227–255.

51. LOSSKY-NEKHOROCHEFF, I., J. L. LERIQUE-KOECHLIN et al. "EEG dans les Anuries Aigues Hyperazoteniques," *Rev. Neurol.*, 100 (1959), 317.

52. MACKENZIE, R. *Risk.* New York: Viking, 1970.

53. MARGOLIS, A. J. "Post-Operative Psychosis in the Intensive Care Unit," *Comp. Psychiatry*, 8 (1967), 227–232.

54. MENDELSOHN, J. and J. FOLEY. "An Abnormality of Mental Function Affecting Patients with Poliomyelitis in a Tank-Type Respirator," *Trans. Am. Neurol. Assoc.*, 8 (1956), 134–138.

55. MENDELSOHN, J., P. SOLOMON et al. "Hallucinations in Poliomyelitis Patients During Treatment in a Respirator," *J. Nerv. Ment. Dis.*, 12 (1958), 421–428.

56. MORSE, R. M. "Post-Operative Delirium: A Syndrome of Multiple Causation," *Psychosomatics*, 11 (1970), 164–168.

57. MORSE, R. M. and E. M. LITIN. "Post-Operative Delirium: a Study of Etiologic Factors," *Am. J. Psychiatry*, 126 (1969), 388–395.

58. ———. "Anatomy of a Delirium," *Am. J. Psychiatry*, 128 (1971), 111–116.

59. PARKER, D. L. and J. R. HODGE. "Delirium in a Coronary Care Unit," *JAMA*, 20 (1967), 702–703.

60. PARKER, W. R. "Post-Cataract Extraction Delirium," *JAMA*, 61 (1913), 1174–1177.

61. POSEY, W. C. "Mental Disturbances after Operations upon the Eye," *Ophthalmol. Rev.*, 19 (1900), 235–237.

62. POSNER, J. B. "Delirium and Exogenous Metabolic Brain Disease," in P. Beeson, and W. McDermott, eds., *Cecil and Loeb Textbook of Medicine*, pp. 88–95. Philadelphia: Saunders, 1971.

63. RADESTOCK, P. *Schlaf und Traum.* Leipzig: 1879.

64. REDING, G. R. and R. S. DANIELS. "Organic Brain Syndromes in a General Hospital," *Am. J. Psychiatry*, 120 (1964), 800–801.

65. SAFER, D. J. "The Concomitant Effects of Mild Sleep Loss and an Anti-Cholinergic Drug," *Psychopharmacologia*, 17 (1970), 425–433.

66. SCHULTZ, D. P. "Physiological Effects of Sensory Restriction—Electroencephalographic Changes," in D. P. Schultz, ed., *Sensory Restriction*, pp. 35–42. New York: Academic, 1965.

67. SHAGASS, C. "Electrophysiological Studies of Psychiatric Problems," *Can. Biol. Rev.*, 31 Suppl. (1972), 77–95.

68. SHERLOCK, S., W. H. SUMMERSKILL, JR. et al. "Portal—Systemic Encephalopathy," *Lancet*, 2 (1954), 453–457.

69. SKOOG, G. "The Course of Acute Confusional States," *Acta Psychiatr. Scandinavica*, Suppl. 203 (1968), 29–32.

70. TUFO, H. M., A. M. OSTFELD et al. "Central Nervous System Dysfunction following Open-Heart Surgery," *JAMA*, 212 (1970), 1333–1340.

71. TYLER, H. R. "Neurologic Disorders in Renal Failure," *Am. J. Med.*, 44 (1968), 734–748.

72. VIEDERMAN, M. "Adaptive and Maladaptive

Regression in Hemodialysis," *Psychiatry*, 37 (1974), 68–77.

73. WEISMAN, A. D. and T. P. HACKETT. "Psychosis after Eye Surgery," *N. Engl. J. Med.*, 258 (1968), 1284–1289.

74. WEST, L. J. "A General Theory of Hallucinations and Dreams," in L. J. West, ed., *Hallucinations*, pp. 275–291. New York: Grune & Stratton, 1962.

75. WILLNER, A. E., C. J. RABINER et al. "Analogical Reasoning, Rheumatic Heart Disease and Post-Operative Outcome in Patients Scheduled for Open-Heart Surgery." Unpublished.

76. WILSON, L. M. "Intensive Care Delirium: The Effect of Outside Deprivation in a Windowless Unit," *Arch. Intern. Med.*, 130 (1972), 225–226.

77. ZISKIND, E. and H. JONES. "Observations on Mental Symptoms in Eye Patched Patients: Hypnagogic Symptoms in Sensory Deprivation," *Am. J. Psychiatry*, 116 (1960), 893–900.

78. ZUBEK, J. D. "Counteracting Effects of Physical Exercises Performed during Prolonged Perceptual Deprivation," *Science*, 142 (1963), 504–506.

79. ———. "Behavioral and EEG Changes after Fourteen Days of Perceptual Deprivation," *Psychonom. Sci.*, 1 (1964), 57–58.

80. ZUBEK, J. P., D. PUSHKAR et al. "Perceptual Changes after Prolonged Sensory Isolation (Darkness and Silence)," *Can. J. Psychol.*, 15 (1961), 83–100.

81. ZUBEK, J. P. and L. WILGOSH. "Prolonged Immobilization of the Body: Changes in Performance and in the Electroencephalogram," *Science*, 140 (1963), 306–308.

CHAPTER 3

AGING AND PSYCHIATRIC DISEASES OF LATE LIFE*

Ewald W. Busse

⟦ Terms and Definitions

AGING when applied to living organisms is used to identify changes that take place gradually and end with death. Such changes may be a decline in body efficiency, a change in structure, and a stoppage or reversal of growth. *Primary aging* refers to biological processes that are apparently inborn and inevitable detrimental changes which are time related but influenced by stress, trauma, and environment. All people, animals, plants, as well as nonliving matter become older, and all undergo identifiable changes with the passage of time. Primary aging processes are not identical in all people, and those that take place do not progress at the same rate. *Secondary aging* refers to disabilities resulting from trauma and disease. The terms *growth* and *development* usually represent biological processes which are the opposite of aging. Living things must, of course, grow older; hence both growth and aging can take place in the same living organisms at the same time.[12]

The designation *aged* is often used arbitrarily to denote or define persons who have achieved a certain chronological age within a given environment. Utilizing chronological age to place a person in a group is a great convenience for society, but the age of an individual does not reflect the individual's abilities. Furthermore, a person is considered old or aged at forty in so-called underdeveloped nations, while in an industrialized or advanced society, a person can live many more years before being considered aged.

Some scientists and scholars believe that the term *aging* is misleading and prefer to use the term *senescence* to stand for the deterioration that accompanies the passage of time. This term is, therefore, essentially the same as primary aging. *Senility,* or senile changes, refers to what has been previously described as *secondary aging.* The science of aging, called

* Additional information can be found in Vol. 6, Chap. 42, of this *Handbook.*

gerontology, includes all of its aspects—biological, psychological, and sociological. *Geriatrics* is a more restricted term applied to the biomedical aspects of gerontology.

Expectation of life, that is, the average number of years of life remaining to persons at a given age, is an estimate based upon the assumption that the death rate in a single year or over some period of time will remain completely unchanged in the future. Obviously any event that influences future death rates alters the accuracy of the estimate called "life expectancy." Life expectancy at birth in the United States between 1900 and 1902 was as follows: white males, 48.2 years; white females, 52.2 years. In 1968, the life expectancy of American white males was 67.5 years, and of white females, 74.9 years. Nonwhite males had increased to 60.1 years, and nonwhite females to 67.5 years.[7]

Negroes of all ages compose approximately 11 percent of the population of the United States. However, because of the lower life expectancy, older Negroes are underrepresented in both the total population and in the Negro population.

In 1970, 9.9 percent of the United States' citizens were 65 years of age and over. This means that every tenth American is considered to be an older American. In 1870, only 2.9 percent were 65 years and over. This shift in the age distribution of our population is particularly significant to physicians and psychiatrists. However, of equal if not greater importance to our society and to psychiatry is the growing predominance of women. This is discussed further in the section, The Older Population.

Longevity, the state of living considerably beyond the normal expectation, is said to occur in identifiable groups of humans. A group of people that have received particular public attention are the inhabitants of Abkhasia in southern Russia. News media reports based upon articles by the Soviet Russian scientist Basilevich, the American anthropologist Sula Benet, and Alexander Leaf of Harvard University indicate that a significant number of elderly individuals reach the age of 100 years or more.[4,31] Although they show age changes affecting the hair and skin, they reportedly have keen eyesight and most have their own teeth. The latter is particularly remarkable when one considers the loss of teeth in elderly Americans. The Abkhasians are reported to be extremely active people who are slender and agile and maintain physical cleanliness and neat clothing. They rarely marry before the age of 30, and virginity for the bride is an absolute requirement. Yet sex is considered good and pleasurable. Retirement is unknown and the status of the aged in the community increases with age. Abkhasians themselves attribute their longevity to their work patterns, sex, and dietary habits.

Although many individuals express the hope and belief that it is possible to extend the life span, the hope of delaying aging focuses, for most individuals, on the continuation of sexual vigor and reproductive capacity. Perhaps the best known attempt to find prolonged youth is the medieval search for the Fountain of Youth. It was taken seriously and was based upon a science-fictionlike account written in the second century. Ponce de Leon's expedition in 1512 and his exploration of Florida were actually organized and financed to specifically search for the Fountain of Youth. Rejuvenation efforts have existed for centuries in the Near and Far East. Efforts to maintain and restore youth were primarily rooted in the practice of gerocomy. *Gerocomy* is the belief and practice that men absorb virtue and youth from women, particularly young women. King David in the Old Testament believed it and practiced it accordingly. In more recent times, Mahatma Gandhi practiced a form by sleeping with his niece.[22] According to Comfort[17] this concept has some support from modern experimental studies. Aged male rats respond favorably when a young female rat is placed among them. Her presence and activities greatly improve their condition and prolong their survival.

❨ Theories of Aging

There is no unified theory of aging because of the complexity of the interaction of biological, psychological, and sociological processes. A discussion of social theories can be found in Vol. 6, Chap. 42 of this *Handbook*. A brief and oversimplified review of the biological and psychological theories of aging follows.

Biological Theories

There are three distinct biological components of the bodies of humans and higher animals. Two of the components are cellular and one is noncellular. One of the cellular components is made up of cells that are capable of reproducing themselves throughout the animal or person's life span. Skin and white blood cells are examples of such cells that have the capacity to reproduce. The second component is made up of those cells that cannot reproduce and cannot be replaced. Such cells are the neurons of the brain and of the nervous system. The third biological component is noncellular; that is, it is the material that occupies the space between the cells. It appears that aging is different in each of these components. Consequently, many so-called aging processes have been described and theories advanced. Some of these aging changes take place in at least two of the components, but at this time none is applicable to all three components of the body. One early biological explanation of aging rests on the assumption that a living organism contains a fixed supply of energy not unlike that contained within a coiled watch spring. When the spring of the watch is unwound or the energy consumed, life ends (exhaustion theory). The accumulation of harmful matter is another simple theory based upon the increasing failure of the organism to dispose of waste products.

Deliberate biological programming is another explanation of aging and death. The vital functions and the duration of the life of a cell are determined by an intracellular memory stored in a DNA (dioxyribo nucleic acid) controller gene.[43] Hayflick contends that dividing cells have a finite capacity for doing so.[27] He has demonstrated that human embryonic fibroblasts divide approximately 50 times and then die. Cells created at about age 20 years approximately double 30 times, and cells acquired at a later age show a progressive decline in their doubling capacities.[27]

Another theory that has received considerable attention in the laboratory relates to the reduction of life span of most organisms exposed to ionizing radiation. Although radiation does produce disruption of many functions, the changes and shortening of life resulting from radiation are significantly different from those associated with the aging process. However, aging and radiation effects do have some common features. For example, both are accompanied by alterations in the structure of the gene transmitting DNA molecule.

Another aging process that has received considerable laboratory attention is the cross-linkage or eversion theory. The initial research was directed towards collagen, the most abundant body protein found in the noncellular component. One strand of the polypeptide that composes collagen is gradually chemically linked with another, reducing the elasticity of the material. Some investigators have claimed that cross-linkage occurs in other proteins in the body, particularly those within cells.

Two interesting theories are the free-radical and the immunologic theory of aging. Free radicals are highly reactive molecular fragments which are ubiquitous in living substances and are produced by normal metabolic processes, as well as exposure to ionizing radiation. Initiators of free radicals include ozone, the allotropic form of oxygen, and hydrogen peroxide. However, it is not known whether ozone is produced internally in the human body. The introduction into the body of free-radical inhibitors has been carried out with mice with some success. The existence of free radicals within the body and their deleterious effects upon the central nervous system (CNS) cannot be ignored. But it has yet to be demonstrated how to reduce the deleterious effect without producing adverse side effects.[26,39]

Wolford[52] has given considerable attention to the immunologic theory of aging. He believes that the phenomenon called autoimmunity is one of several aging processes that may stem from a common "first cause" or single etiology. There is little doubt that the immunologic processes in the advanced years of life are considerably altered from that found in the young and middle-aged adult[6] and contribute to many of the disabilities that are present in late life.

It is conceivable that the autoimmune process is responsible for the loss of brain cells in humans as well as in experimental animals.[45]

Psychological Theories

Theories of aging emanating from psychologists and related behavioral sciences are almost as numerous and diversified as those coming from the biological scientists. Psychological theories of aging are often the extension of personality and developmental theories into middle and late life. Erikson is one of the few theorists who have acknowledged the state of late adulthood. He holds that at this stage of life the status of ego integrity is of fundamental importance.[21] The basic conflict is between the acceptance of one's life as useful and successful versus a sense of despair and fear of death. Such personality theories usually consider the innate human needs and forces that motivate thought and behavior, and the modification of these biologically based energies by the experience of living in a physical and social environment. In early childhood, according to the theories of the development of personality, the physiological changes of the growing child and the interaction with the mother set the stage for basic personality characteristics and determine the relationship between the existence of the individual and his environment. There is no doubt that certain often unidentified characteristics are set early in childhood. There is no escaping the fact that as humans pass through their life experience they become increasingly different rather than similar. This divergence in psychological and behavioral characteristics continues as a response to the large array of possible learning and living experiences. The increasing differences seems to continue until old age when it is possible that the very aged return to greater similarity in certain charac-

teristics, as they share similar declines in biological functioning and socioeconomic constraints.

Neugarten and his associates[34] have attempted to explore patterns of personality in middle and late life. They concluded that when 60-year olds are compared to 40-year olds, the former see the environment as more complex and dangerous. The older adult is less ready to contribute actively to society and to influence persons in his environment; he moves from an outer to an inner world orientation. In addition, older men seem to be more conscious than younger men of their own "affiliative, nurturant, and sensual prompting." Older women become more self-accepting of their own "aggressive and eccentric impulses."[34]

Much of the investigation concerned with psychological functioning in the aged is directed towards cognitive function and learning. It is evident that the decline in intellectual functioning does not affect all elderly people equally and that some elderly people preserve their intelligence late in life. This maintenance of psychological capabilities appears to be related to a number of variables including general health, educational attainment, lifelong patterns of learning, and economic conditions. Such studies give credence to a so-called cybernetic or activity theory. The proponents of this theory maintain, "To become functional early in life, neurons must be activated. To retain their position of control, they must be reactivated repeatedly. We believe that aging involves deterioration of neuronic control which proceeds more rapidly if the cybernetic control systems are not used."[42] Thus the cybernetic theory implies that previously established patterns of learning and social activity are the determinants of patterns in late life.

⟮ The Older Population

In the United States there are approximately 20,000,000 men and women aged 65 and over. The 1970 census showed that the older population (i.e., 65 years and over) increased faster in the preceding ten-year period than the remaining population,—an increase of 21.1 versus 12.5 percent. Of even greater importance to the nursing home is the increase of those aged 75 and over. This truly aged group (75+) increased by 37.1 percent.[11] At least one in every 11 persons in the United States is 65 or over. There is considerable variation from sate to state in the percentage of 65-year-olds and over. Florida ranks first with 14.5 percent.[1] In 1900, 4.1 percent of the population of the United States were in the older age group. By 1965 this figure had increased to 9.4 percent. While the percentage has doubled, the actual number of aged persons has increased six to seven-fold, i.e., from 3 to more than 20 million.

At the turn of the century the difference in the number of elderly men and women was not significant. Of particular importance to today's society is the growing predominance of women. Even though there are more boys than girls born, the longer life expectancy for females results in a gradual shift in percentages; therefore, after the age of 18 there are 105.5 females for every 100 males in the total population. In the population 65 years and over, there are 138.5 females per 100 males. This proportion increases after age 75 to 156.2 females to every 100 males. The ever-growing number of widows and single elderly women is presenting a very serious problem, as it is necessary to find avenues of social participation which are rewarding to single elderly women as opposed to married elderly men and women.[5]

Retirement

Although age 65 is often used as the date for enforced retirement and for the beginning of social security benefits, the assumption that most individuals at age 65 experience a major change in their physical health and mental efficiency is very misleading. Generally speaking, individuals between 65 and 75 are healthy and capable of living rewarding lives. From a health statistical viewpoint, age 75 is a more important date than 65 because life expec-

tancy at age 75 is about nine years and it is then the health problems increase significantly.

Persons 75 years or older are restricted in their activities because illness confines them about 12 days more per year than those age 65 to 74. The person in the older age group is in bed at least eight days more per year, and is limited in general activity as the result of chronic conditions. Of persons 75 and over, 23.7 percent are unable to carry on a major activity as opposed to 9.7 percent of those between 65 and 74 years. Individuals of 75 or over are often referred to as aged persons. This class comprises 8.1 percent of the institutionalized, as opposed to 2 percent of those between 65 to 74 years.

There is no doubt that compulsory retirement and retirement because of poor health account for many people leaving the labor force. However, considering the persons who are compelled to retire because of employer policy, there is no doubt that a significant percentage would be capable of functioning for at least five to ten years past the retirement age. Compulsory retirement plans are primarily associated with economic conditions and the condition of the labor market rather than with the individual's capability of performing in some financially rewarding capacity.

Prejudice

Elderly people are the victims of widespread prejudice and bias.[30] Discrimination takes all forms, but one of the most difficult problems is the fact that elderly people are ridiculed when they continue to strive for love and affection, seek pleasure, and wish to maintain their self-esteem. This widespread prejudice is the result of early acquired attitudes towards the aged and can be attributed to a number of factors including socioeconomic changes. Unfortunately, these prejudices are found not only in the lay public but also in professional and volunteer workers who are products of the society and therefore bring to their relationship with elderly people the predetermined attitudes and patterns which are common in society. A British scientist noting the extent of this prejudice has referred to it as *gerontophobia*. If the elderly persons are to receive the care which they need and deserve, it is important that these prejudices be eliminated, and their previous contributions and present values and needs be recognized.

Physical and Mental Health

In the older population the close relationship between physical and psychological state is particularly apparent. Chronic illnesses are prevalent and their occurrence increases steadily with age. In earlier adulthood, that is, up to 45 years of age, 45.3 percent of persons have one or more annoying chronic condition. Fortunately these produce limitations of major activity in only 7.4 percent. Between the ages of 45 and 64 chronic conditions are present in 61.3 percent and limitations of activity in 18.3 percent. After age 65 chronic disorders increase to 78.7 percent and disability to 45.1 percent. Those bedfast comprise 2.3 percent of the aged, while 6.1 percent are confined to their rooms or living quarters. Of the remaining, 86.2 percent can go out without difficulty, while 5.4 percent must exert considerable effort in order to venture out from their confined environment.[19] Obviously confined persons are in danger of isolation and have difficulty maintaining social activity, intellectual stimulation, and opportunities for learning. This undoubtedly accounts in large measure for their decline in mental capacities. The decline in intellectual and mental abilities have a clear relationship to institutionalization in approximately 80 percent of the cases studied.[29]

Need for Self-esteem

Self-esteem is a composite of innumerable self-ratings that are socially influenced, but in a large measure constructed, measured, and valued by the individual. Two components of self-esteem, which are often extremely important to the elderly person, are his measure of whether he feels his life has any value to himself and to others, and the more subtle but extremely important measure of his capacity to deal successfully with physical disease and trauma. Some individuals believe that they have resources that make it possible for them to survive any period of illness successfully. However, there are others who do not have this reserve strength and are completely at the mercy of others to take care of them during an illness. Some individuals can control this situation by economic resources, while others must be highly dependent upon being liked and respected, and being considered sufficiently worthwhile by others that they will be adequately cared for during their illness. Chronic disability plays an important role in these measures of self-esteem, since a disabled person may find it very difficult to feel that his life is meaningful and justified and, in addition, may deplete his resources so that his comfort and survival are tied to the goodwill of others.

❰ Types of Mental Problems in the Aged Population

Health and service professionals working with elderly people refer to the frequency of hypochondriacal and depressive reactions. Obviously, these professionals are working with elderly who are in need of help whether it be medical or socioeconomic. Therefore, in a cross-section of elderly people the question arises, "How often does one encounter these reactions?" One of our early studies indicated that 40 percent of elderly people were free of psychological problems and another 54 percent were functioning well enough to be classified as nonpsychotic even though they had various mental symptoms. The remaining 6 percent were psychotic but functioning at a socially acceptable level in the community and participated in our research. Although it would be convenient for discussion purposes to indicate that the psychoneurotic could clearly be separated into a distinguishable diagnostic group, this was not actually the case. Thirty-three percent of all of the subjects had mild to severe hypochondriasis. Of the approximately 11 percent classified as severely psychoneurotic, depressive features and "intense body concern," that is, hypochondriasis, were major features of the psychoneurotic reactions.[6] Of interest are the group of psychotic elderly individuals who were functioning in the community. What permits these individuals to function at a socially acceptable level? The study[6] includes a social-activity score, and this does appear to be an important dimension. The neurotic group was markedly less active in a social sense than the "normal" subjects. Thus the psychotics approached the normal level of social activity. They were able to hold in check and balance their psychotic thinking (which was detected by a psychiatric examination) by maintaining a near-normal level of social activity.

(The Use of Psychiatric Facilities

Kramer, et al. are responsible for most of the following information.[30] In 1946, state, county, and private psychiatric hospitals accounted for 42 percent of all hospital beds in the United States. About 80 percent of the mental beds were located in state and county mental hospitals. In 1969, psychiatric beds had dropped to 31 percent of all hospital beds, but 80 percent of the mental hospital beds were still in state and county hospitals. This happened despite the fact that 1400 general hospitals report routinely admitting psychiatric patients and that over 2000 outpatient psychiatric clinics were in operation. Studies of first admissions to public hospitals continue to show that certain persons are more vulnerable to mental disorders than others. These contributing factors hold regardless of age; socioeconomic group; color; urban as compared to rural resident; and marital status. Between 1946 and 1955, the number of first admissions being returned to the community increased from 50 to 63 percent. However, for those who remained in the hospital longer than one year the chances of ever returning to the community decreased rapidly with increasing length of hospitalization. Such patients are usually diagnosed as schizophrenics and they have a

high likelihood of growing old in the hospital. During this same period, the public mental hospital continued to struggle with the problem of providing medical and psychiatric care to large numbers of aged with brain syndromes associated with senile brain disease and cerebral arteriosclerosis.

It does appear that between 1950 and 1968 there was either a remarkable change in the number of mental disorders of the senium, or alternatives for prolonged hospitalization were being developed, as there was a decrease of 32.1 in the percentage of resident patients in public hospitals with mental disorders of old age. Kramer also points out that there was a sharp reduction in first admission for patients 65 years and over. Many state hospital systems adopted policies that resulted in these reductions which, in turn, led to an increased use of nursing homes and related facilities for aged patients. As a consequence, between 1962 and 1965 the rate of first admission for the age group 65 years and over dropped by 9.1 percent for males, 11.5 percent for females; and 10.5 percent for both sexes combined. Between 1965 and 1969, the corresponding decreases were 19 percent for males, 43 percent for females, and 31 percent for both sexes combined.

Between 1946 and 1968, there was a rapid growth of *outpatient psychiatric clinics*. Approximately 500 clinics were functioning in 1946. This number expanded to almost 2000 by 1968. However, these facilities have had an interesting distribution when one compares the age at termination of the patients they served. These facilities have been used to a large extent by children and adolescents under 18 years who account for about 33 percent of the patient load. Adults in the age group 18 to 44 years account for another 51 percent; patients 45 to 54 years for 10 percent; 55 to 64, 4 percent; and 65 years and over only 2 percent. On the basis of population composition alone, the aged are clearly under represented, as at that time they composed approximately 9 percent of the population. In addition, *day-care services* seemed to be playing a relatively minor role in the care of aged patients. Of the estimated 11,000 admissions (nationwide basis) to day-care programs of community mental health centers during 1969, only 2.6 percent, or 260 persons, were 65 years of age or older. Day activities of other types, such as workshops, do exist for elderly people, but they are designed for prevention rather than treatment, and serve the relatively normal aged. Although useful, there are too few to have any substantial impact upon the health and adjustment of the elderly.

Community mental health centers, as defined by the criteria necessary for Federal funding, also do not appear to be carrying a proportionate load of aged patients. As of 1969, only 4 percent of admissions were 65 years and over. Psychiatric services in general hospitals are carrying a greater load, as 13 percent of the termination from these services were 65 years and older.

In the last 20 years the number of *nursing homes* in operation have increased twentyfold and the number of beds over thirty times. Much of the recent increase has been due to the impact of Medicaid and Medicare.

Among the institutionalized elderly individuals suffering from mental illness, the distribution is approximately as follows: 51 percent are patients in state and county mental hospitals; 43 percent are in nursing homes and related facilities; 5 percent are occupants of Veterans Administration beds; and 1 percent are in private mental hospitals. However, the percentage of mentally ill aged in nursing homes is probably a minimum estimate, as Kramer and his colleagues question the accuracy of the diagnosis submitted from nursing homes. They believe that the actual number of mentally ill aged in nursing homes has surpassed the number of mentally ill aged residents in all other types of psychiatric inpatient facilities.

⟨ Depressive Episodes in the Elderly

Evidence indicates that depressive episodes increase in frequency and depth in the advanced years of life. Elderly subjects are aware of these more frequent and more annoying depressive periods, and they report that during such episodes they feel discouraged, worried, and troubled and often see no reason to continue their existence.[9] However, only a small number admit entertaining suicidal ideas, but a larger percentage state that during such depressive episodes they would welcome a painless death. During such periods, the elderly are more or less incapacitated, but they rarely seek medical help. This type of reaction must be distinguished from the much more serious psychotic depressive illness which is a common cause of hospitalization.

The observation that elderly subjects were aware that they were experiencing more frequent and more annoying depressive episodes is based upon a study made some years ago and confirmed by more recent longitudinal studies.[10] Observations indicate that there is a difference in the process leading to depressive episodes in the elderly as compared with the middle-aged or young adults. Guilt and the turning inward of unconscious impulses (interjection) that are unacceptable to the ego are common mechanisms in the depressions of young adults. This is not the case with elderly subjects. Depressive episodes can be readily linked with the loss of so-called narcissistic supplies. The older subject becomes depressed when he cannot find ways of gratifying his needs; that is, when social environmental changes or the decreased efficiency of his body prevent him from meeting his needs and reducing his tensions. He is likely to have a loss of self-esteem; hence he feels depressed.

There is clear evidence that the frequency of depressive episodes is influenced by the life situation. For example, three groups of subjects reported mood disturbances occurring at least once a month and lasting from a few hours to a few days.[13] The highest number of subjects (48 percent) reporting mood disturbances occurred in persons over the age of 60, unable to work, attending an outpatient clinic for various physical disorders, and suffering financial hardships. Depressive spells occurred in 44 percent who were retired, in good health, and in acceptable financial condition. However, only 25 percent of subjects continuing to work past the usual age of retirement reported such experiences. Most of the subjects in the three groups denied that they had experienced depressive spells of similar frequency or duration earlier in life.

To fully appreciate the factors that are important to depressive episodes in the elderly, particular attention must be given to attitudes toward chronic disease, disability, and death. When studied longitudinally, the importance of physical health as a determinant of depressive feelings becomes increasingly evident. It appears that the aged person can tolerate the loss of love objects and prestige better than a decline in health, as physical disability often disrupts mobility and results in partial isolation. Hence the opportunities for restoration of self-esteem are reduced.[10]

Important factors that contribute to depressive feelings in elderly persons are often conscious, as approximately 85 percent of elderly subjects are able to identify the specific event or stimulus that precipitated the feelings of depression. Therefore, many depressive episodes in the elderly are a realistic grief response to a loss and not primarily influenced by unconscious mechanisms. Hence the symptom is relieved when the actual loss or threat is removed or compensated for.

Simon[41] believes we need to know more about the crisis of bereavement of widowhood not only in late life, but also in the middle years. There is evidence that the death rate is increased among newly widowed persons for several years at least. Generally, there are more women than men among depressed persons in their fifties and sixties. After 65, it is about evenly divided between women and men. Simon states that the bereaved constitute a high-risk group that must be recognized and offered help.[41]

Somewhat different statistics given in the Russian literature[40] indicate that after the age of 50, women are three to four times more likely than men to develop depressions. However, when men become depressed, they are more likely to be in the age group 50 to 59, while women are more likely to be between 60 and 69 years of age. A smaller peak is reached for women who have their first depressive episode before age 45.

As to premorbid personality traits, although a variety were common, only 10 percent presented evidence of premorbid abnormalities which could be considered pronounced psychopathology.

"Organically colored" depressions were identified in 13 percent of those between the ages of 50 and 59; 8.3 percent between 60 and 69; and 28.7 percent after the age of 70. Before the age of 70, anxious-hypochondriacal and anxious-delusional syndromes associated with the depressions were the most common occurring in 31.5 and 26.7 percent, respectively.

Depression and Dementia

Depressive symptoms are not unusual in patients with organic brain disease. The majority of clinical studies indicate that depressive symptoms are more common in cerebral arteriosclerosis and cerebral vascular brain disturbances than in senile dementia. One explanation is that insight is less frequently observed in senile dementia.

Some years ago depression in the elderly was often considered "prodromal depression" or the "neuroasthenic stage" of cerebral arteriosclerosis or senile dementia. English investigators have demonstrated that elderly depressives do not subsequently develop cerebral degeneration any more than do elderly people in general.[37]

Wang[48] uses the term *brain impairment* to designate measures of loss of brain function based on a number of laboratory procedures including EEG (electroencephalogram), cerebral blood flow, cerebral metabolism, etc. The degree of dementia is determined by psychological tests and/or clinical measures of intellectual performance and emotional variations. Wang and Busse point out that there is all too often a lack of correlation between these two types of evaluations. Of particular concern are the discrepancies found in patients with a precipitous decline observed clinically, but not paralleled by evidence of rapid physiological brain changes. Careful consideration of factors, such as general physical health, economic status, social environment, and previous living habits, forces the clinician to concede that he is faced with an illness of multiple etiology.[48]

Pseudodementia

Depressed elderly patients occasionally present a clinical picture of pseudodementia.[36] According to Post, such patients appear to be severely perplexed and disoriented, and have memory defects. They may show the "syndrome of approximate answers." Two observations help to exclude the existence of true organic brain disease: (1) The history indicates a recent abrupt onset of defective memory and judgment plus depressive symptoms; (2) negativism is common; for example, the patient replies, "I don't know," rather than confabulate as do many patients with brain impairment.

To summarize, for the latter part of the life span of most Americans—particularly for those over the age of 65—life is replete with events that are losses. In addition, the elderly person often does not have the socioeconomic resources that would permit him or her to deal effectively with such losses. The large number of elderly who do maintain a reasonable emotional balance is evidence of the capacity of people to withstand stress, deprivation, pain, and discomfort.

◖ Hypochondriasis

Hypochondriasis is another common mental problem that is encountered in elderly people. Hypochondriasis is ubiquitous but particularly common in elderly people who seek help in a university clinic. It is generally accepted that hypochondriasis is not a disease entity but a syndrome consisting of an anxious preoccupation with the body or a portion of the body which the patient believes is either diseased or not functioning properly. Hypochondriasis may be part of a symptom pattern in a neurosis, a psychosis, a psychophysiological reaction or a personality disturbance. Cross-sectional and longitudinal studies have provided an opportunity to observe hypochondriacal tendencies in elderly subjects residing in the community or seeking medical help. Of elderly people in the community, 33 percent were found to have varying degrees of hypochondriacal symptoms. A much greater number showed what was called "high body concern," because in many of these cases the degree of concern was probably reality determined, that is, organic disease actually existed and the complaints were not solely of neurotic origin.

In the *psychodynamics* of hypochondriasis three major components are recognized: (1) The patient's interest may be withdrawn from other persons or objects around him and be centered upon himself, his body, and its functions; (2) the restrictions and discomforts produced by this psychic illness may be utilized by the patient as punishment and partial atonement for guilt resulting from feelings of hostility and a desire for revenge; and (3) the symptom can be caused by a shift of anxiety from some specific area of psychic conflict to a less threatening concern with bodily function. It has been our observation that although the guilt mechanism is found in young hypochondriacs, it is rarely encountered in older persons. The older person's high body concern is more likely to result from a withdrawal of his interests in other persons or objects, and/or displacement of his anxiety.

Observations indicate that the frequency of persistent hypochondriacal syndrome encountered in the patient population is not necessarily paralleled in our community subjects. Studies showed that hypochondriacal episodes were not infrequent in elderly persons who did not necessarily seek medical help. The depressive element in the hypochondriacal reaction in community subjects was easily recognized. For reasons previously mentioned, the investigators preferred to rate "high body concern." Other scales, based on specific criteria, were used to rate the subjects in a number of areas of functions and activities. The results of the entire medical (physical) examination were summarized in terms of a five-point scale representing the objective health status of the subject.

A subject's health was considered to be medically good if there were no symptoms of disease or, if the symptoms existed, the individual suffered no more than 20 percent limitation of normal functioning. Subjects with limitations of 20 percent or more were considered to be in poor health. The subject was also given an opportunity to make a self-assessment of his health. In this particular study a number of other observations were included as important. Consideration was given to the IQ as determined by performance on the WAIS (Wechsler Adult Intelligence Scale). The existence of excessive preoccupation with health in the psychiatric examination was considered, as well as a count of symptoms or complaints from the physical examination. Morale was measured in terms of a Havighurst Attitude Scale, and the level of activity was determined by an Activity Scale. Social placement factors were also included in the study. Considered were age, sex, race, change in work role, and socioeconomic status. Each subject had an opportunity by letter and personal contact to be informed of his objective health status as evaluated by the examining physicians.

The data from the original observations indicated that in 65 percent of the subjects there was congruity between self-assessment and the medical evaluation of health. Incongruity of self-assessment of health and medical evaluation occurred almost without regard of the objective health status. Of the subjects considered to be in good health, 31 percent were health pessimists, and of those in poor health, 44 percent were optimists. Thus, approximately one-third of elderly persons could not be relied upon to give an accurate self-assessment of their physical health. Subjects whose health was medically good and who had realistic self-appraisal were likely to be older (that is, age 70 or above), to occupy a higher social status, and to maintain a high level of social activity. In subjects of poor health, it appeared that the younger was more likely to be pessimistic, while the older subject used denial and maintained an optimistic view. There was also a sex difference; pessimism was more characteristic of women, in spite of the fact that the mortality rate favors the older woman. The pessimistic or hypochondriacal person was likely to have low morale, to be poorly adjusted to the environment, to report past and current periods of depression, and to express feelings of neglect.[32]

The persistent optimist uses his opportunity to pursue the busy life to the point where he is too busy to recognize the appearance of physical disease and disability. Consequently, the optimist is unlikely to have the attention of a physician until the disease has become so serious that it cannot be denied. At that point such a person often becomes seriously depressed and requires support and skillful redirection to activities consistent with the disability. The person using the mechanism of denial should not be seen as a courageous person. A courageous person realistically appraises the situation, determines the odds, accepts the challenge, and moves ahead.

(Organic Brain Syndromes

The sequence of the disease discussed (disorders caused by or associated with impairment of brain-tissue function) is essentially that found in DSM II *The Diagnostic and Statistical Manual of Mental Disorders*.[1] Under the entry of organic brain syndrome are included all those diseases which result in mental changes that can be attributed to diffuse or significant involvement of brain-tissue function. The disease should be designated as either psychotic or nonpsychotic, and the extent of the mental change whether it be mild, moderate, or severe, should be identified. Furthermore, it is important to distinguish acute from chronic brain disorders. The term *acute* is not used to indicate a sudden onset of the disease, but implies reversibility. Both "acute" and "chronic" are descriptive terms which are unrelated to etiology, as the same causative agent can produce in one individual a temporary, that is, acute, disorder, while in a second individual it may produce a chronic, that is, permanent, disability.

The diagnosis of an acute brain disorder indicates that the patient is expected to recover and that his physiological brain functioning will return to normal. Unfortunately, particularly for the elderly patient, the experience of an acute brain disorder often leaves the patient with a prolonged adverse effect upon psychological functioning. The recovered elderly person is seriously concerned that the brain disorder heralds the beginning of intellectual decline and death. The anxiety and depression associated with the recovery period from an acute organic brain reaction must be recognized and relieved. Generally speaking, an acute brain disorder that occurs in older persons is either a toxic or ischemic reaction. Recovery is dependent upon elimination of the toxic substance and restoration of the brain to normal metabolic functioning.

The criteria are limited to distinguish psychotic from nonpsychotic reactions. DSM II[1] [p.31] describes patients as psychotic "when their mental functioning is sufficiently impaired to interfere grossly with their capacity to meet the ordinary demands of life." The description of the nonpsychotic organic brain syndrome is not extensive. It is mentioned that mild brain damage often manifests itself by hyperactivity, short attention span, easy detractibility, and impulsiveness. Conversely, sometimes the patient is withdrawn, listless, perseverative, and unresponsive. It is also evident that some symptoms, particularly in older individuals, are superimposed responses to the mental changes that are the direct result of the organic brain change.

According to the accepted diagnostic nomenclature, the word "dementia" occurs in relationship to senile and presenile dementias that are considered psychoses associated with organic brain syndromes. Unfortunately, there is considerable discrepancy as to how clinicians and investigators utilize the term dementia. Webster's *Third International Dictionary* defines dementia as "A condition of deteriorated mentality, however caused; mental abnormality that is characterized by a marked decline from the individual's former intellectual level and often by emotional apathy." The 1969 edition of *A Psychiatric Glossary*[3] defines dementia as "an old term denoting madness or

insanity; now used entirely to denote organic loss of intellectual function." John G. Allee's version of Webster's definitions calls dementia "an incipient loss of reason." This broadening of the definition is the trend in medicine, as the term is being increasingly used to designate any intellectual decline or organic cause, whether it be mild, moderate, or severe. This possible conflict and confusion in the diagnostic terms should be carefully considered by a psychiatrist, as the litigation of wills, testamentary capacity, and competence frequently rest upon an accurate diagnosis and description. The nonpsychotic nature of an early senile dementia should be clearly stated.

Organic brain syndromes are likely to be accompanied by important alterations in the person's thinking and behavior. The so-called cognitive functions which include comprehension, calculation, problem-solving, learning, and judgment are impaired. Memory is spotty and orientation for time, place, and person is faulty. Emotional responses are easily elicited and are disproportionate or inappropriate to the stimulus. This basic clinical picture characteristic of an organic brain disorder may be associated with a wide variety of other symptoms. The type and severity of the symptoms are not necessarily directly proportional to the extent of the physiological disturbance, as they are often influenced by psychological patterns of long standing and the particular psychological state of the patient at the time the physiological disorder develops.

Dementia in Late Life

Several of the dementias that develop in the latter part of life appear at least in some cases to be influenced by genetic factors. The evidence for genetic transmission is strong in some dementias and less in others. Still, in other diseases, the principle of "genetic heterogeneity" appears to operate, which states that the phenotypic similarity, that is, the clinical manifestations of the disease, may be produced by genotypically different conditions.[25] Some of the differences reported in various studies of heredity may be distorted by the diagnostic criteria used.

Pratt[38] reports on more than a dozen families in which a condition developed that is identical with if not indistinguishable from Alzheimer's disease that is transmitted as a regularly manifested dominant trait. The regular transmission of dementia differs from the common form of Alzheimer's disease, for a slight though definite tendency to familial aggregation of the disorder is common. Furthermore, Pick's disease, while pathologically distinct, is clinically difficult to differentiate from Alzheimer's disease. However, Pick's disease does appear to be associated with a dominant autosomal mode of inheritance. The transmission of senile dementia appears to be either a multifactorial or a dominant mode of transmission. Close relatives of patients with senile dementia have a risk four times that of the general population of developing the disease. Studies conducted in Sweden have indicated that senile dementia is determined by a single autosomal dominant gene carried by 12 percent of the general population and reaching 40 percent manifestation at the age of 90 years. This evidence indicates that senile dementia is qualitatively distinct from ordinary senescence. It is also reasonable to assume that some specific enzyme or other biochemical defect is the first cause of senile dementia. Alzheimer's disease, the most common of the presenile dementia, was not found in excess within families of senile dementia, suggesting that it is in part determined by factors that do not operate in senile dementia. Pratt concludes that the evidence is more in keeping with a polygenic inheritance, with a shared predisposition to both Alzheimer's disease and senile dementia.[38] As to concordance rates in identical twins, senile dementia occurs in 43 percent from monozygotic and 8 percent from dizygotic twins. If Alzheimer's disease affects one of a monozygotic pair, it is highly likely that the other will develop the same manifestations of dementia.

Slow Virus and Dementia

The possibility that some of the dementias in late life can be attributed to a slow virus cannot be disregarded. In 1968, Gibbs and his co-workers reported the transmission of a disease from a patient diagnosed as having Creutzfeldt-Jakob's disease to a monkey.[23] The following year the same investigators reported successful transmission from man to monkey in six of eight patients suffering from the same disorder, which is also known as spongiform encephalopathy. Other investigators have reported the observation of viruslike particles by electron microscope in patients with spongiform encephalopathy. Familial instances of this disease have been reported, but this may be the result of the transmission of the slow-acting virus rather than the result of a genetically determined condition.

Differential Diagnosis

This discussion of differential diagnosis is primarily concerned with senile dementia and the presenile dementias known as Alzheimer's and as Pick's disease. Experienced clinicians have repeatedly found that there is no reliable criteria to distinguish senile dementia from Alzheimer's or from Pick's disease. There are clear-cut anatomical differences between Pick's and Alzheimer's disease, but most pathologists doubt that any valid histological distinction can be made between senile dementia and Alzheimer's disease. To further complicate the picture, there is in at least 20 percent of autopsy cases a coexistence of senile and arteriosclerotic brain changes. Post does not agree with the assertion that patients with Pick's disease tend to repeat words or brief phrases in a stereotyped manner and that they are less restless and hyperkinetic than those with Alzheimer's.[36]

Both Alzheimer's and Pick's disease have an early date of onset. Hence the age of the sick patient is often used as an important diagnostic criterion. Some clinicians believe that senile dementia, in contrast to Alzheimer's disease, is accompanied by other evidence of exaggerated aging affecting the entire body. Frequently there is a general wasting of muscles, shrinkage of soft tissue, loss of elasticity of the skin, thinning and graying of the hair, and easy fatigability. However, the fact that senile dementia has its onset considerably later in life could explain why these aging symptoms are also observed. Hence, they could be an aging phenomenon and not necessarily a manifestation of the disease.

ALZHEIMER'S DISEASE

This illness was described by Louis Alzheimer in 1906. Its average onset is the mid portion of the fifth decade of life. Occasionally, it begins in the fourth decade of life. It is probably the most common of the presenile dementias as it is found in 4 percent of the autopsies in a psychiatric institution. Its sex distribution is in favor of females, the ratio being three to two. The familial possibilities of this disorder have been discussed earlier (p. 79). Another clinical feature that may have importance is the recognition that in spite of the loss of memory, illogical reasoning, etc., insight is often preserved in patients with Alzheimer's disease which results in a distressing awareness of impending insanity. As the deterioration continues, speech becomes seriously disturbed and involuntary movements of arms and legs are frequently observed. The course of the disease is progressively deteriorating with invariable fatal conclusions. The duration of the disease varies from two to ten years and sometimes more. The average is usually believed to be approximately four years. No specific treatment is known for this disorder, and symptomatic environmental measures are the sole relief that can be offered.[8]

PICK'S DISEASE

Pick's disease is generally characterized as a presenile dementia, although it is doubtful that it is the result of the premature onset of an aging process. The age of onset is very similar to that of Alzheimer's disease. It most frequently appears at approximately age 54, although occasionally it occurs as early as the fortieth year of life. The recognition of this disease is attributed to A. Pick, who lived in Prague and first published his work in 1802. Pick's original purpose was to illustrate the different types of aphasic manifestations which can occur in senile brain diseases. It was really the efforts of other scientists that established Pick's disease as a distinct clinical pathological entity. It is truly a rare disease, and the female ratio is two to one. Again, the onset of aging is one of the primary distinguishing features of Pick's disease to senile dementia. Symptoms of focal cortical damage, usually frontal or temporal in origin, are sometimes of help. Pneumoencephalographic studies reveal the areas of localized atrophy. The areas of most frequent involvement and their characteristic pathological condition are described in Chapter 4.

Subtypes of senile dementia have been described by Ehrentheil.[20] The distinctions are often overlapping but include: (1) simple deterioration; (2) the depressed and agitated type; (3) the delirious and confused type; (4) the hyperactive type with motor restlessness and loquaciousness; and (5) the paranoid type.

Experience indicates that approximately 50 percent of patients follow a pattern of simple deterioration, with transient episodes of a wide variety of reactions. However, a substantial number deteriorate without any dramatic events accompanying the illness, and these people do not produce a serious disturbance in the community. Hence they are kept in a protected environment until they have reached an advanced stage of senile mental deterioration. Of the disturbing types of reactions, the paranoid are probably the most common and constitute 15 to 25 percent of the major manifestations of this disorder.

Pathophysiology of Cerebral Vascular Disease

Cerebral vascular disease is often explained on the basis of vascular insufficiency. Unfortunately, cerebral vascular insufficiency is not a phenomenon that is amenable to direct observation. We are dependent upon assuming its existence on the basis of other observations.[35] Vascular insufficiencies are believed to exist when it appears that the blood supply of the brain is inadequate to meet its metabolic needs. It may be present continuously, or occur intermittently when the blood flow falls below acceptable levels, or it could occur if the metabolic activity of the brain increased to a point that the normal supply was insufficient. There is a natural tendency for a clinician to assume that the blood pressure is the primary contributor to the presence or absence of vascular insufficiency. It must be remembered that it is the cerebral blood flow, not the blood pressure, that is the ultimate factor in determining the availability of oxygen to the brain. Cerebral blood flow, usually expressed in ml. of blood per 100 g. of brain per minute, is the result of two forces. Although blood pressure is important, it is only one of several factors that must be considered in cerebral blood flow. The first is the available pressure called the pressure head, that is, the difference between the pressure on the arterial and that on the venous side. The second factor is the cerebral vascular resistance. It is influenced by the structure of the walls of the blood vessels, by the functional tone of the vessels, the pressure on the vessels from without, that is, the intercranial pressure, and the viscosity of the blood passing through the vessels.[33] Cerebral blood flow is clearly an extremely complicated phenomenon, as it is also influenced by the metabolic demands of the brain. If the brain metabolism is decreased, cerebral blood flow is also decreased. For this reason, it is often extremely difficult to decide if a lowered cerebral blood flow may be contributing to a decrease in brain metabolism, or is its result.

The caliber of the cerebral arteries is mainly determined by chemical balance, especially by the concentration of carbon dioxide, CO_2. It is the partial CO_2 pressure in the blood which normally determines the caliber of the cerebral arteries. A rise in the CO_2 pressure of the blood produces cerebral vasodilatation. Interestingly, this takes place without simultaneous systemic vasodilatation, so that the cerebral blood flow is increased until the excess CO_2 is removed. Although many pharmacological agents aimed at improving the blood supply to the brain have been tried, most, if not all, appear to be ineffective. This is because these pharmacological agents produce systemic vasodilation which causes a fall in blood pressure which, in turn, is compensated for by brain vascular changes so that the cerebral blood flow remains unchanged. On the other hand, oxygen, doubtless, has an effect upon the cerebral circulation acting as a vasoconstrictor. The inhalation of 100 percent oxygen produces a fall in cerebral blood flow of approximately 13 percent.

Episodic disturbances commonly referred to as transient ischemic attacks are not infrequent in the older population. The majority of these episodes are probably attributable to thrombi and emboli affecting areas where restoration of collateral supply is possible. However, there is increasing evidence that prolonged, marginal cerebral blood flow can produce degenerative changes in the brain which lead to behavioral and intellectual impairment.

Hyperbaric Therapy

In 1969, the Veterans Administration Hospital in Buffalo, New York, reported that repeated exposures to hyperbaric oxygen (O_2) may have a positive effect on cognitive functioning in elderly patients for the diagnosis of chronic brain syndrome.[28] However, Goldfarb, et al. reported in 1970 that they were unable to demonstrate this effect in a series of randomly selective patients with "organic brain syndrome."[24] L. W. Thompson[44] and his colleagues at Duke University consider their results to be equivocal, but have shown some positive changes in approximately 50 percent of their subjects.

The hyperbaric treatment program used by Thompson et al.[18] consists of thirty exposures to 2.5 atm. of absolute pressure, (the duration of each exposure is 90 min.). The experimental group receives 100 percent oxygen which provides alveolar oxygen (O_2) tensions of approximately 1800 mm. Hg. The control subjects breathe normal air at 1.3 atm. of pressure which provides alveolar O_2 tension levels slightly higher than air at one atmosphere.

¶ Psychosis Associated with Other Cerebral Conditions

Cerebral Arteriosclerosis and Cerebral Vascular Disturbance

It is worthwhile again to caution the clinician to recognize that if the mental disturbance is not of psychotic proportions, the condition is classified under nonpsychotic organic brain syndrome with circulatory disturbance, not with cerebral arteriosclerosis. This can be a cause of diagnostic confusion. Furthermore, if the mental reactions result from such problems as cardiac decompensation, it is necessary to include the underlying pathology as an additional diagnosis. (See DSM II, p. 31).[2]

Dementia associated with cerebral arteriosclerosis not infrequently appears before the age of 70. The disease may appear in persons as young as 45 and can develop at any time in the late years of life. As all atherosclerotic diseases, it is more common in males than in females (three times as common in males than in females). Apparently female hormones do play a protective role, and there are some clinicians who advocate the continuation of supplemental estrogenic hormones in females for a number of reasons, including the prevention of arteriosclerotic disease. Vascular pathology is not only confined to the brain, but is usually found in other parts of the body. The duration of the illness is difficult to determine, but the average appears to be near 3.5 years.

Some clinicians indicate that more than 50 percent of cases with cerebral arteriosclerosis demonstrate their first symptomatology by suddenly developing a delirium manifested by confusion, incoherence, restlessness, and not infrequently accompanied by hallucinations. However, this delirious picture does subside and leaves the patient at a considerably reduced functioning level from which he gradually declines further. As previously noted, this gradual decline is first seen as defects of memory and then errors in judgment. Some individuals become very irritable, aggressive, and quarrelsome. In contrast with senile dementia, these patients are more likely to have some insight into the fact that they are losing some of their intellectual skills. Depression complicates the picture, and suicidal impulses may produce a serious problem for the family and physician.

¶ Changes of EEG in Late Life

Focal abnormalities of EEG, predominantly over the temporal areas of the brain, and maximally on the left, have been repeatedly observed in 30 to 40 percent of apparently healthy elderly people. This finding was first reported by Busse et al.[13] in 1955. Since that date the observation of the frequent occurrence of a left-temporal focus in old people has been reported by other investigators. A study of healthy volunteers between the ages of 20 and 60 reveals that only 3 percent of normal adults under the age of 40 years have temporal lobe EEG changes. This increases so that in the 20 years between 40 and 60, 20 percent of the subjects show temporal lobe irregularities. After age 60, the focal disturbance tends to be stabilized, as very few elderly subjects studied longitudinally have developed a focus or have shown an increase in the degree of abnormality once they have entered the latter part of their life.[16]

The exact origin of these foci as well as their significance is still not clear. The localized EEG abnormality is usually episodic in nature and is composed of high-voltage waves in the delta and theta range, occasionally accompanied by focal short waves. The disturbance is found in the waking record, is maximum in the drowsy state, and disappears in sleep.[15] In 75 to 80 percent of the cases the abnormality is at a maximum or completely confined to the left side of the brain. It is not related to handedness, and although it is evidently episodic in nature, it is unrelated to seizures. There are indications that these temporal foci commonly seen in normal senescence are associated with a localized cerebral circulatory insufficiency.

Another common characteristic of EEG changes is the progressive slowing of the dominant frequency involving the alpha frequency and the appearance of slow waves in the theta or delta range. A slight slowing of the alpha index is not pathognomonic for any particular brain disorder. However, moderate to severe slowing is characteristically found in brain disorders whether they are classified as degenerative or vascular in origin. Elderly subjects in good health are found to have a mean occipital frequency which is almost a full cycle slower than that found in healthy young adults. Furthermore, about 7 percent of the EEG's in the elderly subjects were dominated by slow waves in the theta range, that is, 6 to 8 per second.[47] Since a good correlation has been demonstrated between EEG frequency and cerebral oxygen consumption or blood flow, the slowing of the dominant frequency in the majority of elderly people may indicate a depression of cerebral metabolism.

The correlation between EEG changes with advancing age and reduced intellectual functions indicates that, in residents of old age homes and other institutions, alterations are related to measures of brain impairment. Unfortunately, this correlation is not nearly as clear in subjects remaining in the community. It is possible that those who live in the community are actually adjusting at a borderline level and may be vulnerable to disruption in functioning which would precipitate the appearance of organic brain disease. The focal disturbances in senescent EEG's have not been consistently correlated with any particular psychological function or measure. However, a review of our longitudinal studies indicates that the presence of a focus in the left anterior temporal region is closely associated with a decline in verbal abilities, while the diffuse slowing in the occipital rhythm is associated with a decline in performance abilities.[49] However, it is necessary to remember that these findings may be influenced by such factors as levels of arousal, medication, and innumerable other influences which require further study.

There appears to be a relationship between EEG frequency and blood pressure, as the correlation between these two variables in healthy elderly subjects is highly significant. Included in a study[42] were also those individuals with compensated heart disease, but who had significantly higher blood pressure than those without heart disease. In these individuals with mild and moderate hypertension, a somewhat faster EEG frequency is associated with less evidence of brain disorder than in those individuals without heart disease. All of these findings suggest that there is an impairment of cerebral vascular autoregulation in many elderly subjects, and consequently the cerebral blood flow has become more dependent upon the blood pressure. It appears that moderate elevation of blood pressure in many individuals helps to preserve the brain.[50] However, sustained severe diastolic hypertension (106+) is often associated with intellectual decline.[51]

EEG's taken of elderly subjects in their sleep reveal some very important changes. Elderly subjects require a longer period to fall asleep and their sleep is lighter. There are more frequent wakenings, and deep sleep (stage 4) virtually disappears. These changes are considerably more pronounced in persons with significant organic brain disease.

(The Nursing Home

One of the most difficult tasks is the selection of a nursing home for a chronically ill person, particularly if mentally impaired and advanced in age. If one approaches such a complex task, it is essential not only to have guidelines and standards for the services in a nursing home, but also one must evaluate the patient so that the environment and activities selected are best suited to meet his needs.[11] For this purpose it is necessary to evaluate the extent of the overt incapacities which reduce the individual's capabilities for his own daily personal care; for instance, the inability of a person to bathe and dress without assistance, and the physical and mental capacity to be responsible for mobility, either walking or through private or public conveyances.

Other changes occur in the later years which are not as easily recognized and yet are very important to the total functioning of the individual and for life satisfactions. For example, there may be a decline in a person's capacity to taste, smell, feel pain and temperature changes, to hear, and to see. The process of senescence, or so-called normal aging, brings with it a decline in the ability to hear certain high-frequency sounds and to separate from a number of sounds those which are most meaningful. It also affects the speed in which a person can adjust when moving from a dark to a lighted room or vice versa. Also, the elderly person requires greater illumination to work and to see such things as utensils and food. Such changes require that the environment be structured to meet the needs of the elderly. This environment is quite different from that which is best suited for the health and adjustment of a younger person. The age changes mentioned above appear relevant to the criteria used in selecting a nursing home.

What Is a Nursing Home?

Unfortunately, what is legally considered a nursing home may be considerably different from one locality to another. A dimension was added to the long-term health care of the elderly when the term "extended care" was introduced by Public Law 89-97 amendments to the Social Security Act of 1965. Extended care and the extended-care facility conceived under Medicare legislation are intended to be an extension of hospital care. It is meant to be an active-treatment program aimed at restoring the patient to an acceptable level of functioning within the community. The term "extended care" has been, but should not be, confused with long-term care or continuing care. This type of care involves patients who are unable to remain at home because they cannot, physically or mentally, either independently or with assistance, maintain a satisfactory adjustment. Generally speaking, such long-term facilities are classified as nursing homes, but there are states such as New York that permit one facility to offer both such services, that is, nursing-home care and extended care. Obviously, extended care is oriented towards rehabilitation, while nursing-home care is geared to maintaining life at a level as satisfactory as possible. There is a financial differentiation, particularly important as extended care can be financed by Medicare. The situation is confused, since it is often difficult to distinguish between the patient's need for extended care and for nursing-home care. In determining eligibility, one of the primary determinants is the prediction of the patient's ability to regain capacity to care for himself. Once it is determined that the patient requires chronic or long-term institutional care, the patient is probably no longer eligible for Medicare benefits, even though his health status may be such that he requires constant attention. Long-term care is often provided in proprietary nursing homes, in a few publicly sponsored chronic-disease hospitals or homes for the aged and infirm, and in state mental institutions.

In selecting a long-term care facility, the advice of a knowledgeable physician, though of value, may have limited use because of the complexity and the fluidity of long-term facilities and programs. The physician, of course, is interested in maintaining good communication with the nursing-home administrator and the skilled health personnel on the staff. He is particularly interested in ensuring that good records are kept so that he can evaluate the health status of the patient and ensure his prescribed medication and programs are accurately followed.

Administration

One of the most serious drawbacks in either a proprietary or public nursing home is usually the remoteness of the director. The owner or the director of a proprietary nursing home should be continually involved with the services, as it is as easy to make the assumption that the home is functioning very effectively because the purchasing systems, the accounting methods, etc., are efficient. It is important to make certain that the administrator does have the capacity to make judgments regarding policy changes in patient care.

Nursing Home Location

Firm guidelines cannot be developed as to the urban, rural, or semirural location of a nursing home. Regardless of where the home is located, there should be sufficient stimuli in the environment to keep the person alert and interested. An elderly person can be very lonely regardless of where the home is located. Many approaches can be utilized to maximize the stimuli from the environment. For example, in an air-conditioned nursing home, externally located pickups transmit into the dining and living areas the familiar early morning songs of birds. Such devices can be extended to a bird identification by song or bird-watching activity which can add an important dimension to living.

The nursing home cannot expect to function effectively as an isolated unit. It must have intimate and continuing relationships with community activity and resources. The administrator and personnel of the nursing home must have good working relationships with church groups and any other public or private groups or agencies that can be of value to the residents of the home. Periodic visits and projects by such organizations as Girl Scouts have proved to be of great value.

The Quality of Nursing Care

The personnel who come in day-to-day contact with the residents of a nursing home include those associated with the so-called nursing service, the food service, and other supporting service people. Employees associated with the nursing service include registered nurses, practical nurses, nursing aides, and attendants. All of these individuals offer what is called nursing care. It is not merely the administration of drugs and the applications of treatment techniques but an extremely

demanding relationship with elderly people that is necessary in order to make the older resident feel that he is understood, that his needs are appreciated, and that his health and well-being are important to those who come in contact with him. A chronically ill elderly person is particularly aware of his high dependence upon nursing personnel, as he can easily be deprived of many satisfactions if they become annoyed or angry with him. Consequently, some patients try to be modest in their requests, so that in the event they are in desperate need, nursing personnel will adequately respond to their needs. Often an older person feels that he is not being properly cared for but is afraid to express his displeasure because he may antagonize the very ones who are responsible for his care.

Recent studies in Great Britain indicate that there is a serious misconception regarding nursing by many nursing-home administrators. They seem to believe that geriatric patients require less nursing skill and fewer nurses than acute medical and surgical patients. Detailed records and observations indicate that this is not true, particularly in homes which have admitted or accumulated a large number of seriously ill people. The range of diagnoses and treatment regimes is wide, requiring great knowledge and skill, and many of the chronic illnesses are complicated by mental confusion and the burden of fecal and urinary incontinence. Dr. Robin E. Irvien and Miss B. J. Smith reported to the British Geriatric Society in London (Spring, 1970) that many geriatric units require a very high nurse–patient ratio, a ratio of one-to-one being the best.

Serious Illness

Although it is extremely important that the residents of a nursing home have the services of a physician when required, it is obvious that many of the complicated diagnostic procedures cannot possibly be carried out within a nursing home. Therefore, transportation should be readily available for the patient to be moved to the medical facility where diagnostic procedures can be carried out, or to a hospital if necessary.

Food Service

The dietician and the administrator responsible for the preparation and the serving of food to residents of nursing homes must be aware of the physiological and pathological changes that accompany old age. The decline in ability to taste and to smell are directly relevant to the dietary service. In addition, the normal changes of aging require better lighting in order to adequately see certain objects. The loss of teeth often makes it necessary for the dietician to make foods attractive and distinctive without having them appear as a pureed, undifferentiated mass.

The weak and unsteady hands of many elderly persons make it embarrassing to attempt to cut food or to properly prepare it, such as the buttering of bread and biscuits. Assistance in the preparation of food must be done in an unobtrusive, helpful manner that is not embarrassing to the patient. The plates must be deep, and some nursing homes prefer to use compartment plates. Cups and glasses must be of adequate size, but not heavy. The silverware, too, must be efficient but lightweight. The process of eating is often a social event, and therefore it is essential that the persons can sit comfortably, eat at a reasonable pace, and have an opportunity for conversation after the meal. The chairs should be comfortable and the tables large enough to permit adequate distances between the diners. It is important that the consumption of food be observed so that adequate intake is assured without forcing the elderly person as some people force children to eat all that is placed before them.

There is no doubt that there is a continuing shortage of well-trained and capable individuals in these service fields. Food service is no exception, and it is unfortunate that many nursing homes are aware of deficiencies within their food services but cannot find capable personnel, even though they are willing to pay adequately. Consequently, it is often necessary for family and friends to assist whenever possible and to make certain that food intake is pleasant and adequate.

A number of investigators have found that the addition of beer and wine to the routine of a nursing home or a chronic-care unit has proved to be extremely effective toward improving patient morale. It is known that alcohol is a sedative, but the availability and the addition of beer and wine have increased conversation and social interaction. Certainly, people who have been accustomed to such beverages throughout their life should not be denied the opportunity to enjoy them in old age. Alcoholism or excessive alcohol intake can be a problem at any age, but fortunately its consumption can be carefully controlled in most nursing homes.

Activities

Visits to randomly selected nursing homes reveal that a large number of patients appear to be withdrawn, unsociable, and virtually unreachable. Purposeful mass activity has been found to be a very useful device in breaking down this wall separating the elderly person from the world.

Physical Environment

Room arrangement, a roommate, ease of the residents' movement in their rooms and to recreational areas are all of utmost importance. The nursing home should be a "home" in the true sense, offering security, comfort, and stimulation. Residents in a nursing home should participate fully in planning and carrying out social activities and have an opportunity to make suggestions regarding not only the services rendered but the appearance and structure of the environment. Lighting is of particular importance. Night lights are necessary in many locations, as elderly people find it particularly difficult to move around in the dark and cannot move from a well-lighted room to a dark room without a lengthy delay in visual accommodation. With advancing age there appears to be a rather capricious intolerance to changes in temperature. It is important that the temperature of the building be held as constant as possible so that the variation in how an elderly person responds to the temperature can be individualized and handled by the addition of wraps or the reduction in the number of clothes. The floor of a nursing home should be level, avoiding even small steps. For example, bathroom floors should not be raised requiring an older person to step up or down. Handrails for assistance should be adjacent to commodes and bathtubs.

Nursing-Home Care Versus Hospitalization

In the 1970s, the proportion of older persons in mental hospitals has increased steadily. At any given time, at least one of three beds in a public mental hospital is occupied by a person 65 years or older. Approximately one-third to one-half of the persons in the 65 or older age group in public mental hospitals are admitted at an earlier age. However, the remaining one-half or more were admitted at age 65 or older. Eighty-three percent of first-admission older patients are diagnosed as having senile brain disease and/or arteriosclerotic brain damage. The reliability of these clinical diagnoses has been questioned and has been under study for many years. The coexistence of senile and arteriosclerotic brain disease is not unusual and is discussed in Chapter 4.

Nursing homes have become a major resource for the placement of aged patients from state mental hospitals. Questions have been raised as to whether these homes are appropriate for this type of patient. Investigators at the Boston State Hospital conducted a one-year controlled study of sixteen nursing homes housing approximately 14,000 patients. They found institutional deprivation—physical, intellectual, or spiritual—to be a common problem. Deprivation in nursing homes was found to be particularly related to: (1) lack of stimulation; (2) lack of adequate walking space inside and outside the homes; (3) lack of recreational and occupational therapy; (4) lack of space for group socialization and activities; (5) lack of a common dining room forcing patients to eat from trays in their rooms; (6) absence of volunteer workers from the community; (7) separation of patients on different floors, reducing the possibility of interaction; and (8) minimal socialization between male and female patients. This study indicated that regressive behavior can be the result of deprivation rather than organic changes. Regressive behavior is manifested by withdrawal, seclusiveness, uncooperativeness, incontinence, refusal to eat, loss of interest in personal hygiene, loss of ability to perform self-care functions, and grossly inappropriate social behavior. Some investigators believe that the nursing supervisor is the key staff member in a nursing home. The type of person, selected by the administrator and owner to be the nursing supervisor, is of great importance. At least three types of nursing supervisors can be identified. The *permissive* supervisor leads to an indifferent staff and anxious patients. The *dominant* supervisor, although running a home that is a model of efficiency and neatness, lowers the self-esteem of the staff and is likely to disregard patients' emotional needs. A *staff-centered* supervisor who shares control of responsibility and planning with the staff is much more likely to contribute to the effectiveness of the home program. A nursing supervisor who has produced the best climate for the patient is desirable, but may not be appreciated because some people prefer to have cleanliness and neatness take priority over meeting emotional needs.

⟨ Bibliography

1. AGING. "Great Variations Found in State Aging Populations Patterns," 204 (1971), 10–11.
2. AMERICAN PSYCHIATRIC ASSOCIATION. *Diagnostic and Statistical Manual of Mental Disorders* (DSM-II). Washington, D.C.: APA 1968.
3. ———. *A Psychiatric Glossary*, 3rd ed. Washington, D.C.: APA., 1969.
4. BENET, S. "Why They Live to Be 100 or Even Older in Abkhasia," *N.Y. Times Magazine*, Dec. 26, 1971.
5. BROTMAN, H. E. *Facts and Figures on Older Americans. The Older Population Revisited*, Publication 182. Washington, D.C.: U.S.

Department of Health, Education, and Welfare, Administration on Aging, 1971.

6. BUCKLEY, C. E. and F. C. DORSEY. "Serum Immunoglobulin Levels Throughout the Life-Span of Healthy Man," *Ann. Intern. Med.*, 75 (1971), 673–682.

7. BUREAU OF THE CENSUS. *Expectation of Life*, Statistical Abstract of the United States, Life Table Values No. 69, p. 53. Washington, D.C.: Bureau of the Census, 1971.

8. BUSSE, E. W. "Psychopathology," in J. Birren, ed., *Handbook of Aging and the Individual*, pp. 364–399. Chicago: University of Chicago Press, 1959.

9. ———. "Psychoneurotic Reactions and Defense Mechanisms in the Aged," in P. H. Hoch and J. Zubin, eds., *Psychopathology of Aging*, pp. 274–284. New York: Grune & Stratton, 1961.

10. ———. "The Mental Health of the Elderly," *Int. Ment. Health Res. Newsletter*, 10 (1968), 13–16.

11. ———. "The Geriatric Patient and the Nursing Home," *N.C. Med. J.*, 33 (1972), 218–222.

12. ———. "Aging," to be published in the *World Book Encyclopedia*, Chicago, 1975.

13. BUSSE, E. W., R. H. BARNES, A. J. SILVERMAN et al. "Studies in the Processes of Aging. X: The Strengths and Weaknesses of Psychic Functioning in the Aged," *Am. J. Psychiatry*, 111 (1955), 896–901.

14. BUSSE, E. W., R. H. DOVENMUEHLE, and R. G. BROWN. "Psychoneurotic Reactions of the Aged," *Geriatrics*, 15 (1960), 97–105.

15. BUSSE, E. W. and W. D. OBRIST. "Significance of Focal Electroencephalographic Changes in the Elderly," *Postgrad. Med.*, 34 (1963), 179–182.

16. ———. "Presenescent Electroencephalographic Changes in Normal Subjects," *J. Gerontol.*, 20 (1965), 315–320.

17. COMFORT, A. *Ageing: The Biology of Senescence*. London: Routledge and Kegan Paul, 1964.

18. DAVIS, G. C., L. THOMPSON, and A. HEYMAN. "Hyperbaric Treatment in Dementia." Paper presented American Academy of Neurology, Boston, April 1973.

19. DEPARTMENT OF HEALTH, EDUCATION, AND WELFARE. *Public Health Service Health Statistics*, PHS Publ. No. 580-536. Washington, D.C.: U.S. Govt. Print. Off., Oct. 1962.

20. EHRENTEIL, O. "Differential Diagnosis of Organic Dementias in Affective Disorders in Aged Persons," *Geriatrics*, 12 (1957), 426.

21. ERIKSON, E. H. *Identity and the Life Cycle*. Psychological Issues Vol. 1, No. 1. New York: International Universities Press, 1959.

22. ———. *Gandhi's Truth*, pp. 21, 403–406. New York: Norton, 1969.

23. GIBBS, C. J., D. GADJUSKE, D. ASHER et al. "Creutzfeldt-Jakob Disease: Transmission to the Chimpanzee," *Science*, 161 (1968), 388–389.

24. GOLDFARB, A. I., N. HOCHSTADT, and J. H. JACOBSON. "Hyperbaric O_2 Treatment of Organic Mental Syndrome in Aged Persons," *Gerontologist*, 10 (1970), 30.

25. HAASE, G. R. "Diseases Presenting as Dementia," in C. E. Wells, ed., *Dementia*, pp. 163–207. Philadelphia: Davis, 1971.

26. HARMAN, D. "Free Radical Theory of Aging: Effect of Free Radical Reaction Inhibitors on the Mortality Rate of Male LAF Mice," *J. Gerontol.*, 23 (1968), 476–482.

27. HAYFLICK, L. "Human Cells and Ageing," *Sci. Am.*, 218 (1968), 32–37.

28. JACOBS, E. A., P. M. WINTER, and H. J. ALBIS. "Hyperoxygenation Effects on Cognitive Functioning in the Aged," *N. Engl. J. Med.*, 281 (1969), 753–757.

29. KAHN, R. L., A. I. GOLDFARB, M. POLLACK et al. "The Relationship of Mental and Physical Status in Institutionalized Aged Persons," *Am. J. Psychiatry*, 117 (1960), 120–124.

30. KRAMER, M., C. A. TAUBE, and R. W. REDICK. *Patterns of the Use of Psychiatric Facilities by the Aged—Past, Present and Future*, American Psychiatric Association Task Force on Aging. Washington, D.C.: APA, June 1971.

31. LEAF, A. "Every Day is a Gift When You Are over 100," *Natl. Geogr.* (Jan. 1973), 93–118.

32. MADDOX, G. L. "Self-Assessment of Health Status," *J. Chron. Dis.* 17 (1964), 449–460.

33. MARSHALL, J. *The Management of Cerebral Vascular Disease*. Boston: Little, Brown, 1965.

34. NEUGARTEN, B. L. et al. *Personality in Middle and Late Life*, pp. 189–190. New York: Atherton, 1964.

35. OBRIST, W. D. "Cerebral Physiology of the Aged: Influence of Circulatory Disorders,"

in C. M. Gaitz, ed., *Aging and the Brain*, pp. 117–133. New York: Plenum, 1972.

36. POST, F. *The Clinical Psychiatry of Late Life*. Oxford: Pergamon, 1965.

37. ————. *The Significance of Affective Symptoms in Old Age*, p. 10. Maudsley Monograph. London: Oxford University Press, 1962.

38. PRATT, R. T. C. "The Genetics of Alzheimer's Disease," in G.E.W. Walstenholme and M. O'Connor, eds., *Alzheimer's Disease and Related Conditions*. London: A Ciba Foundation Symposium, 1970.

39. PRYOR, W. A. "Free Radicals of Biological Systems," *Sci. Am.*, 223 (1970), 70–83.

40. SHTERNBERG, E. Y. and M. L. ROKHLINA. "Depression in Old Age," *Zh. Nevropatol. Psikhiatr.*, 70 (1970), 1356–1364.

41. SIMON, A. *Background Paper*, White House Conference on Aging. Washington, D.C.: U.S. Govt. Print. Off., 1971.

42. SMITH, K. U. and F. G. SMITH. *Cybernetic Principles of Learning and Education Design*, p. 29. New York: Holt, Rinehart, & Winston, 1965.

43. STREHLER, B. L. "Genetic and Cellular Aspects of Life Span Prediction," in E. Palmore and F. Jeffers, eds., *Prediction of Life Span*, pp. 31–49. Lexington, Mass.: Heath, 1971.

44. THOMPSON, L. W. *Effects of Hyberbaric Oxygenation on Psychological and Physiological Measures in Elderly Patients with Dementia*. Presented Gerontol. Soc., Miami, Nov. 1973.

45. THREATT, J., K. NANDY, and R. FRITZ. "Brain Reactive Antibodies in Serum of Old Mice Demonstrated by Immunofluorescence," *J. Gerontol.*, 26 (1971), 316–323.

46. TIME. "The Old in the Country of the Young," Aug. 3, 1970, pp. 49–54.

47. WANG, H. S. and E. W. BUSSE. "EEG of Healthy Old Persons—A Longitudinal Study. I. Dominant Background Activity and Occipital Rhythm," *J. Gerontol.*, 23 (1969), 419–426.

48. ————. "Dementia in Old Age," in C. E. Wells, ed., *Dementia*, pp. 152–161. Philadelphia: Davis, 1971.

49. WANG, H. S., W. D. OBRIST, and E. W. BUSSE. "Neurophysiological Correlates of the Intellectual Function of Elderly Persons Living in the Community," *Am. J. Psychiatry*, 126 (1970), 1205–1212.

50. WANG, H. S., W. D. OBRIST, C. EISDORFER et al. "Heart Disease and Brain Impairment in Community Aged Persons." Presented 23rd Ann. Meet. Gerontol. Soc., Toronto, October 1970.

51. WILKIE, F. L. and C. EISDORFER. "Intelligence and Blood Pressure in the Aged," *Science*, 172 (1971), 959–962.

52. WOLFORD, R. L. *The Immunological Theory of Aging*. Copenhagen: Muksgaard, 1969.

CHAPTER 4

THE NEUROPATHOLOGY ASSOCIATED WITH THE PSYCHOSES OF AGING

Armando Ferraro

⟮ Neuropathology of Cerebral Arteriosclerosis

To DESCRIBE the pathologic changes in cerebral arteriosclerosis accurately, it is necessary to separate the pathology of the large cerebral blood vessels from that of the small blood vessels, arterioles, and capillaries. In all the blood vessels involved, the ultimate result will be an obstruction to the blood supply of a given area, thus resulting in softenings of variable dimensions, or in the extravasation of blood leading to red softenings, or to the rupture of a blood vessel leading to massive hemorrhages.

Before describing the pathology of the vascular changes, it may be well to consider the fact that the clinical symptoms of cerebral arteriosclerosis are related to the extent of the branching of the blood vessels participating in brain-tissue damage caused by the softening or by the hemorrhage. Large softenings or hemorrhages are evidently more apt to result in neurological symptoms, whereas smaller softenings or blood extravasations are more apt to result in mental symptoms. Furthermore, from a neurological standpoint, the extent of the focal damage in the territory of the various blood vessels involved will determine the extent of the neurological symptoms.

It is not my task to discuss the clinical neurological and psychiatric aspects of cerebral arteriosclerosis, but it is not out of place here to mention briefly that the brain is supplied by the superficial and deep branches of the three main cerebral arteries, the anterior, the medial, and the posterior cerebral arteries, which represent the offshoot of the anatomical branching of the blood vessels participating in the formation of the circle of Willis. Very briefly, the superficial territory of vascular irrigation of the anterior cerebral artery covers in general the mesial surface of each cerebral hemisphere, that of the middle cerebral artery covers their external surface, and that of the posterior cerebral artery covers their basal surface. The neurological symptoms which follow softenings or hemorrhages in the territory of the superficial or deep branches of these arteries constitute the various clinical pictures of hemiplegia, monoplegia of the upper or lower extremities, hemianopsia, alexia, apraxia, aphasia and the like, according to the damaged cerebral territory.

I see no need to report the details of the macroscopic appearance of the brain damage in relation to the occlusion or rupture of each individual branch of the three main cerebral arteries, and will limit myself to illustrating the gross appearance of some of the focal softenings connected with the occlusion of some of the branches of the anterior, middle, and posterior cerebral arteries. Figure 4–1(a) illustrates the macroscopic appearance of a large area of softening in the region supplied by the calloso-marginal branch of the anterior cerebral artery; Fig. 4–1(b) the macroscopic appearance of a large area of softening in the region supplied by the anterior-parietal artery, a branch of the middle cerebral artery; and Fig. 4–1(c) the macroscopic appearance of a large area of softening in the region supplied by two other branches of the middle cerebral artery, the anterior temporal and the temporo-occipital arteries. Figure 4–2 illustrates the macroscopic appearance of a large bilateral area of softening in the region supplied by the parieto-occipital artery, a surface branch of the posterior cerebral artery.

Figure 4–3 illustrates, better than any description, the sclerotic appearance of some of the larger branches of both the anterior cerebral artery (Figure 4–1(a)) and the middle cerebral artery (Figure 4–1(b)) which discloses thickening of their walls, tortuosity, and nodosity. The pathologic process involving the large cerebral blood vessels is generally desig-

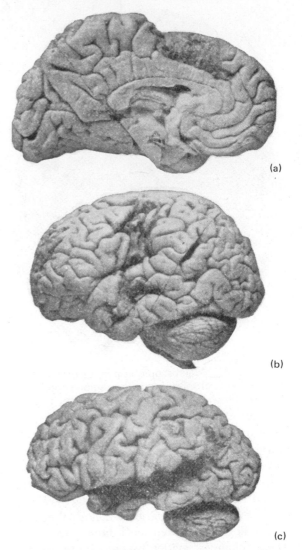

(a)

(b)

(c)

Figure 4–1. (a) Macroscopic appearance of a large area of softening in the region supplied by the calloso-marginal artery. (b) Macroscopic appearance of a large area of softening in the region supplied by the anterior parietal artery, branch of the middle cerebral artery. (c) Macroscopic appearance of a large area of softening in the region supplied by the anterior temporal and the temporo-occipital arteries, branches of the middle cerebral artery.

nated as "atherosclerosis" a process characterized by patches of yellowish material deposited along the internal surface of the artery, but often visible from the outside because of the translucency of the blood-vessel walls. These patches, which impart a beady nodular

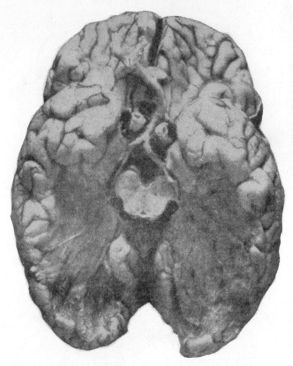

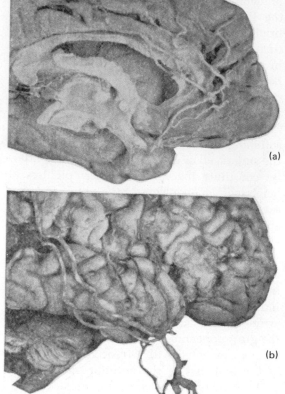

Figure 4–2. Macroscopic appearance of a large bilateral area of softening in the region supplied by the parieto-occipital artery, surface branch of the posterior cerebral artery.

Figure 4–3. (a) Macroscopic appearance of arteriosclerotic changes in branches of the anterior cerebral artery. (b) Macroscopic appearance of arteriosclerotic changes in branches of the middle cerebral artery. Note thickening, tortuosity, and somewhat nodular appearance of the diseased blood vessels.

appearance to the sclerotic vessels, result in various degrees of narrowing of their lumen, because of their projecting knobs under the intima layer of the vessel. Consequently the blood vessel walls become irregularly dilated and at the same time lose their normal elasticity. In addition to their local damaging effects, these changes evidently contribute to the wider disturbance of the cerebral hemodynamic equilibrium.

Microscopically the focal yellowish thickenings of the large blood vessels, also designated as "atheromas," consist of fatty substances, hyperplastic connective tissue, a thickened endothelial layer, and a thickened internal elastic membrane. The lipids in the intima consist predominantly of lipoproteins, cholesterol and its esters, 10 percent phospholipids and 30 percent natural fats.[55] Hyaline and calcium deposits may also be found in the midst of the atheromatous tissue undergoing necrosis. Figure 4–4(a) illustrates the fibrotic thickening of the walls of a sclerotic blood vessel and their fatty degeneration, and Fig.

4–4(b) the lumen of a vessel reduced by accumulated fat and elastic tissue, resulting from the splitting of its elastic membrane.

The atheromatous changes of the large blood vessels in humans are, with the exception of necrosis, quite similar to the changes produced experimentally in rabbits, hens, cockerels, and dogs fed high cholesterol diets, which result in a gradual shutting off of the blood circulation in the involved area.[9,79] However, this similarity of experimental pathology in humans and animals, resulting from high cholesterol diet, applies only to blood vessels outside the cerebral ones, inasmuch as, according to some investigators, the latter do not seem to participate in the pathologic process as do the blood vessels of other organs.

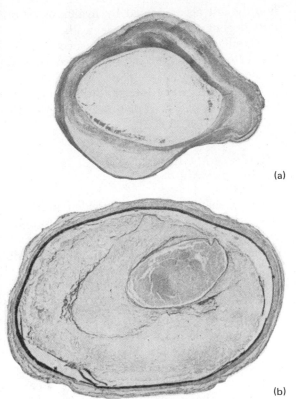

(a)

(b)

Figure 4–4.   Microscopic atherosclerotic changes in a large blood vessel. (a) Fatty degeneration and fibrotic thickening of the vessel walls. (b) Fatty degeneration, splitting of the elastic membrane, and marked reduction of the blood-vessel lumen.

Microscopic Changes in the Small Blood Vessels

In the small blood vessels the pathologic process has been designated not as atherosclerosis but as "diffuse hypertrophic arteriosclerosis" by Evans,[46] Ophuls,[113] and Moschkowitz,[105] or "arterio-capillary" fibrosis by Gull and Sutton,[69] or "arteriolosclerosis" by Neuburger,[110] Hall,[70] and others. In the diffuse hypertrophic type the early pathologic changes consist in the proliferation of the endothelial lining cells of the intima, followed later by an increase in the fibrous tissue and a delamination of the elastic membrane. In both small arteries and arterioles, the process is a diffuse one which may lead not only to a thickening of the media, but later to the

hyaline degeneration of the entire vessel wall. In this variety the increase in number of the cells of the intima, and their concentric lamellation, produce what has been referred to as "an onion-skin-like" appearance of the cross section of the vessel.

In the second variety of arteriosclerosis of the small blood vessels, the "arteriolosclerosis," Hall[70] described as the outstanding feature the hypertrophy of the muscular fibers of the media associated with increased collagen, resulting in the thickening of the vessel wall with the exception of the intima. A third variety is represented by "hyalinization" in which deposit of hyaline material in the subintimal layer is the primary feature. Hyalinosis may then extend gradually to the whole wall, leading at first to a decreased contractility of the small blood vessel and ultimately to the reduction of its lumen or even occlusion. According to Herburt,[71] hyaline degeneration, a frequent occurrence in cerebral arteriosclerosis, occurs when the arteriolar lesion develops slowly, and such a change may be seen associated at first with splitting, reduplication, and fragmentation of the internal elastic membrane.

Hyaline degeneration is, however, diffuse and prominent also in cerebral hypertension. Without entering into the discussion of the general relationship of hypertension to cerebral arteriosclerosis, the fact remains that it is in association with severe hypertension that the most severe and diffuse hyaline degeneration of the cerebral blood vessels has been reported and related to imbibition of the blood vessel walls by protein substances due to disturbed permeability of the vascular endothelium.

Anders and Eicke,[8] reviewing their cases of hypertension, stress that the occurrence of hyalinosis, which originates in the subendothelial layers, may invade the whole wall of the vessel, protrude in its lumen and end in a global fatty degeneration of the whole wall. They proposed for this condition the term "arteriopathia hypertonica." Rosenberg,[122] in his studies of the blood vessels in malignant hypertension, stresses however the point that a thickening of all three layers of the small blood vessels with splitting of the internal elastic membrane, and resulting reduction of the lumen of the blood vessel, is as frequent an occurrence. Because of the difficulty of drawing a distinct separation between hyaline degeneration, as an expression of cerebral arteriosclerosis, and severe hyaline degeneration related only to hypertension, one may consider general hyaline degeneration to be a variety of arteriosclerosis fitting into the general picture of cerebral arteriosclerosis. Figure 4–5 illustrates an advanced stage of hyaline degeneration in the midst of other vascular changes in a case clinically and pathologically diagnosed as cerebral arteriosclerosis.

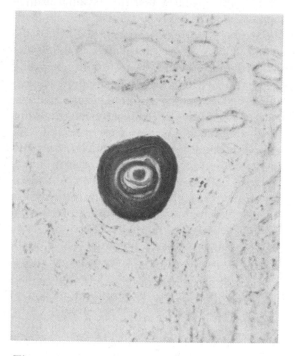

Figure 4–5. Marked hyaline degeneration of all the three layers of the walls of a blood vessel.

A fourth variety of arteriosclerosis of the small blood vessels is the one described by Scheinker,[131] as "obliterative cerebral arteriosclerosis" found particularly in older patients (sixty-eight to ninety-four years). He differentiated this condition from the "diffuse hyperplastic variety" because in obliterative cerebral arteriosclerosis, the pathologic changes are limited to the intima in terms of a proliferation of the subendothelial connective tis-

sue, though accompanied by hyalinosis or of fatty degeneration of the vessel walls.

"Capillary fibrosis," a special aspect of cerebral arteriosclerosis, has also been considered as being related to other specific endogenous or exogenous toxic or infectious diseases of the brain outside the field of cerebral arteriosclerosis.

Microscopic Changes in the Brain Parenchyma

Those changes could be divided into two categories: the changes following occlusion or rupture of large cerebral blood vessels, and the changes which follow the involvement of small blood vessels. However, this would repeat the basic description of the parenchymal change, which does not differ in the two categories, as far as softenings and hemorrhages are concerned, except in the severity and the extension of the lesions, the depth of the damage, and the degree of the reparative process. It goes without saying, that a large area of softening or hemorrhage is less apt to undergo repair capable of reestablishing the functionality of the damaged tissue and its continuity with the surrounding tissue.

Referring to a rather large area of softening of relatively recent occurrence, the basic microscopic changes consist in the presence, in that area, of a mixture of necrotic nervous tissue in the midst of which blood cells may still be found. If the lesion is an older one, blood cells may be absent, though residues of blood pigments may still be seen. If the softening is an older one, the progressive removal of the necrotic tissue may result in the formation of small or larger cavities in which remnants of the disintegrated tissue may still be present, most of it having been removed by phagocytosis. A certain amount of fluid may be present in such necrotic cavities. Figure 4–6 illustrates the microscopic appearance of such an area.

Without reference to the size of the ischemic softening, I may briefly state that an area of softening is characterized by a more or less complete process of disorganization or destruction of the nervous parenchyma. The destructive process involves all the neural ele-

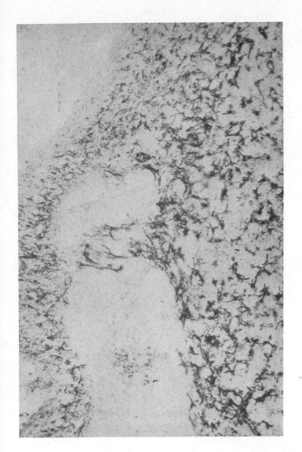

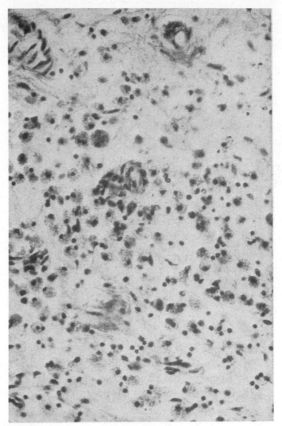

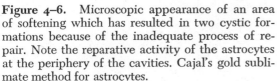

Figure 4–6. Microscopic appearance of an area of softening which has resulted in two cystic formations because of the inadequate process of repair. Note the reparative activity of the astrocytes at the periphery of the cavities. Cajal's gold sublimate method for astrocytes.

Figure 4–7. Microscopic appearance of an area of softening disclosing the presence of a large number of compound granular corpuscles. Nissl stain.

ments, nerve cells, nerve fibers, and glia cells, as well as the vascular and mesodermic elements of support. Nerve cells undergoing all gradations of degenerative changes may be seen, from the severe type of Nissl's "liquefaction," to the Spielmeyer "ischemic type" of degeneration. Reparative activities soon take place. They begin with the reaction of the microglia cells, which multiply, invade the degenerated tissue, and disclose all stages of transformation into compound granular corpuscles, intended to clear the disorganized areas from the remnants of degenerated tissue (Figure 4–7). Concomitantly the mesodermic elements of the nervous tissue, which constitute the blood vessel walls of the region, begin

to proliferate and gradually form a visible mesenchymal net.

In the first stage of the process of repair, the mesenchymal reaction is predominant. In a subsequent phase, the astrocytes participate very actively in that process through their hyperplasia and hypertrophy leading gradually also to the increased number of glia fibers, which, intermingling with the connective tissue elements, form the ultimate scar tissue. In the final phase of the process, the glia reaction is the dominant element, the scar tissue being ultimately formed by a preponderance of glial fibers.

On the other hand, if the vascular occlusion has been a minor one, or of a temporary nature as in the case of transitory vascular spasms, the structural damage is much less intense. As a matter of fact, morphologic evi-

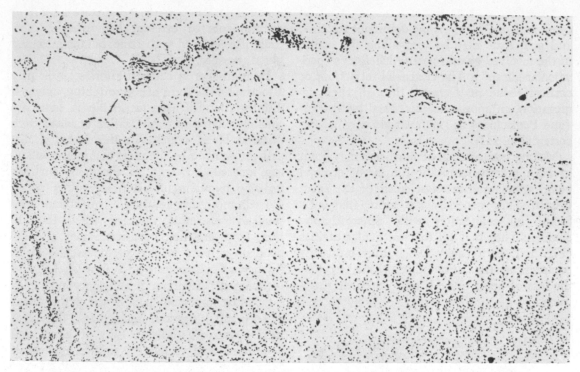

Figure 4–8. Microscopic appearance of spotty areas of cellular bleaching in the brain cortex resulting from rarefaction, and paling of most of the nerve cells which are undergoing an ischemic type of degeneration. Nissl stain.

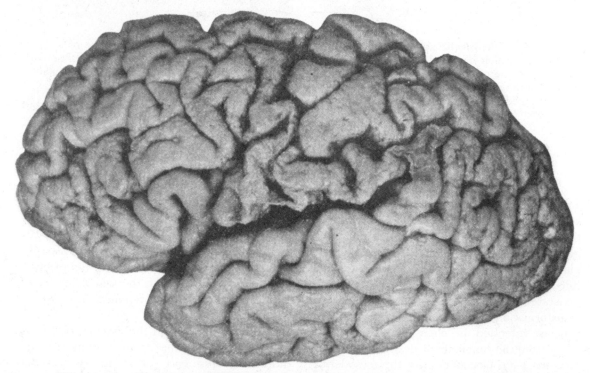

Figure 4–9. Macroscopic appearance of a diffuse "granular atrophy" of the cerebral cortex resulting from numerous cicatricial cortical retraction of the tissue.

dence of parenchymal destruction may be lacking completely, if the spasm was of a very short duration. Only if it lasts longer, will the blood deficiency result in irreversible structural changes, and in the case of the cortex, in small patches of the tissue, or in a more selective way in the involvement of individual nerve cells of a given cortical area. This "neuronal or selective neurosis," as Scholz[135] labeled it, is characterized mainly by the "ischemic type of degeneration" of individual nerve cells. Their collective presence may result in the formation of areas of different size and distribution in the midst of which bleaching of the nerve cells constitutes the only indication of the ischemic damage. Figure 4–8 illustrates the low-power microscopic appearance of spotty areas of bleaching in the brain cortex resulting from the paling of the nerve cells in the affected areas. At times the ischemia of a cortical area determines a necrosis of nerve cells along a certain well-defined cortical layer and is called "laminar necrosis." That transitory vasospasms may determine focal necrosis or laminar necrosis has been documented by Neuburger[109] in his cases of cardiac arrest of no more than a few minutes.

In cases of "patchy neuronal necrosis," the process of repair differs from the one taking place in larger or smaller areas of typical softenings. The reparative process in these cases is mainly one of glia repair, without participation of the mesodermic tissue. Glial proliferation of astrocytes and glial fibers represent the dominant elements in the resulting glia scars which can be observed along the course of individual vessels (Alzheimer's Perivascular Gliosis). Whatever the nature of the scar tissue affecting the cortex may be, the aggregation of several cicatricial areas may ultimately result in the macroscopic appearance of what Spatz[142] has described as "Granular Atrophy of the Cortex." Figure 4–9 illustrates the macroscopic appearance of a diffuse "Granular Atrophy of the Cortex" resulting from numerous minute cortical retractions due to scar tissue. The patchy type of ischemia, as well as the laminar type of cortical degeneration, are evidently of greater interest to the psychiatrist than to the neurologist, inasmuch as they generally are not accompanied by appreciable neurological signs but are more apt to result in mental symptoms.

Intracerebral hemorrhages may occur in both atherosclerosis of the larger blood vessels and arteriosclerosis of the small vessels. They generally are found more frequently in connection with atherosclerotic changes. They may fill the ventricular cavities (Figure 4–10) or a cavity which they create by compressing the surrounding tissue, so that the loss of brain tissue is only apparent.

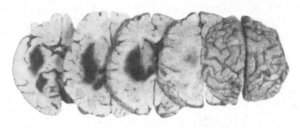

Figure 4–10. Macroscopic appearance of a massive hemorrhage in the left lateral ventricle.

In the past it was thought that massive hemorrhages in the brain were primarily the result of a ruptured blood vessel related to high blood pressure, or to a ruptured aneurysm. Later Rosenblath[123] refuting, as most other investigators did, the exclusive concept of Charcot, pointed to the coexistence of advanced renal diseases in cases of cerebral hemorrhages. He advanced the theory that under such circumstances an enzyme is elaborated, leading first to autolysis of the brain tissue around the blood vessels, which as a point of lowered resistance facilitates their rupture.

Westphal and Baer[158] felt that cerebral hemorrhages arising from diseased intracerebral arteries are the result of a progressive necrosis of the walls of the blood vessels themselves, a condition which they termed "angionecrosis." Globus and Strauss[63] and, later on, experimentally, Globus and Epstein[62] established the fact that ischemic changes surrounding diseased blood vessels are the important determinants of cerebral hemorrhages, especially if associated with a concomitant increased blood pressure.

Smaller hemorrhages in cerebral arteriosclerosis may also assume the form of what is termed "red softening" in which the disintegration of the nervous tissue is more intimately related to extravasation of blood from diseased vessels. In such instances, diapedesis seems to be the most important mechanism, related however to the same prehemorrhagic conditions of an altered perivascular tissue. Red softenings, which are generally related to a more general cardiovascular deficiency, occur indeed more frequently in connection with small arteriosclerotic vessels, as pointed out by Wilson et al.[160] and Neuburger.[110] Vascular insufficiency may play a far more important part in the pathogenesis of both softenings and hemorrhages than does local vascular pathology. Loss of blood and myocardial and circulatory failure may result in insufficient blood supply, resulting in a slowing down of the local circulation which creates a prestasis or stasis around the blood vessels, thus facilitating the development of white or red softenings. Red softenings are generally localized in the more richly vascularized gray matter where diapedetic hemorrhages take place not only from capillaries, but also from small veins, thus pointing out the importance also of the veinous circulation in the pathogenesis of hemorrhages.

Histopathogenesis of Cerebral Arteriosclerosis

Large Blood Vessels. Generally the accepted theories of atherosclerosis of the larger cerebral blood vessels are the same as those which apply to the other large blood vessels of the body. They stem mostly from the experimental work of Ignatowski,[74] Saltikow,[128] Wesselkin,[157] and Anitschkow,[10] who induced atherosclerosis in animals and related it to cholesterol deposits in the blood vessel walls. However, in 1856, Virchow[153] had already advanced the theory that atherosclerosis was related to fatty imbibition of the blood vessel walls, secondary to necrobiotic processes in the connective tissue cells and ground substance of the intima, a theory later on accepted by Aschoff,[11] Ignatowski,[74] Katz

and Stamler,[79] and most other investigators.

According to Wilens[159] both intimal thickening and lipids deposits are concomitant facts in atherosclerosis.

Klotz[82] believes that an increase, between the endothelial cells, of the ground substance which becomes hyaline-mucoid in character, precedes the deposits of lipids in the intima.

Leary[87] held that cholesterol-laden macrophages accumulate in the Kupffer's cells of the liver, and their analogues in the adrenals. These pass into the blood and lymph stream, through the lining filter, and become deposited in the intima of the arteries. From there they migrate through the endothelial cells into the subintima.

Duguid[44] held that cholesterol-laden macrophages accumulate in the intima of the arteries and remain in place, but soon become incorporated within the artery's walls by the endothelium growing over the cell mass, and give origin to intramural thrombi which may gradually increase in size.

Winternitz et al.[161] feel that the greater vascularity of the blood vessel's walls, resulting from local deposits of fats or intramural thrombi, is an important contributing factor to the production of atheromatous changes, a thesis upheld by Geiringer's[60] findings.

Hueper[73] contends that a film of fatty substances deposited on the surface of the intima, because of altered colloid composition, interferes with the proper oxidation metabolism of the intima, and results in changes which are secondary to nutritional deficiency.

Small Blood Vessels. The histopathogenesis of the arteriosclerosis of the small blood vessels may or may not have a direct relationship to the atherosclerotic changes reported in the large blood vessels.

Are the hyperplastic changes of the small vessels an integral part of atherosclerosis? It would be interesting, indeed, to investigate cases of cerebral arteriosclerotic changes of the small blood vessels, and relate them to the presence of severe or light atherosclerotic changes of the large arteries, or more so, to the absence of such changes. Unfortunately the various histopathogenetic theories of cerebral arteriosclerosis, mainly concerning studies of the small blood vessels, have been advanced without any attempt by their authors to correlate them with the pathology of the large blood vessels.

Thus, Eros,[45] studying the small cerebral blood vessels, with no reference to the large ones, emphasized that the primary and most important arteriosclerotic changes take place in the elastic tissue, especially in the internal elastic membrane. All other degenerative changes, such as fatty and mucoid degeneration, calcification, fibrous proliferation, and hyalinization, are only secondary to the changes in the elastic tissue. In general he distinguished two main types of the alterations of the elastic tissue: (1) the hyperplastic degenerative type; and (2) the hypoplastic degenerative type.

The hyperplastic degenerative type is characterized by the initial proliferation and splitting of the elastic membrane (Figure 4–11).

As the process advances, the elastic fibers gradually lose their individual outlines and tend to fuse with each other, giving the membrane a thicker appearance. While increased fibroblasts and collagenous fibers become more prominent, they are subsequently followed by fat and calcium deposits and by hyalinization and mucoid degeneration.

The hypoplastic degenerative type is characterized by either a very slight tendency to proliferation of the elastic membrane, or none at all. In the early stages the elastic membrane stains very poorly, loses its sharp outlines and soon fades out (Figure 4–12). No split in the membrane occurs, and there is only a slight tendency to fibrous proliferation of the intima proper. The secondary degenerative changes start early, with fat appearing in the loosened elastic membrane. Hyaline degeneration follows. Thrombosis is much rarer.

Bruetsch[29] makes a distinction between the

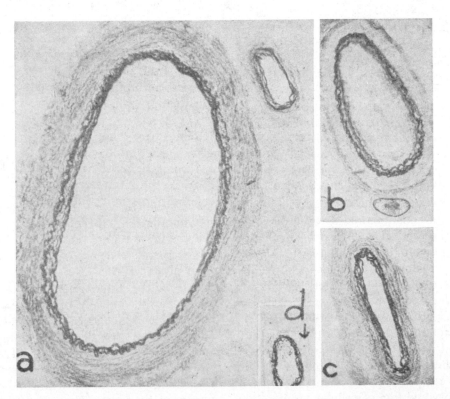

Figure 4–11. Hyperplastic type of cerebral arteriosclerosis; (a), (b), and (c) are pial arteries; (d) is an intracerebral artery. Note the proliferation of the elastica membrane, and the beginning degeneration of the hyperplastic tissue. Weigert stain for elastic tissue. (Courtesy Dr. G. Eros and the *J. Neurophatol. Exp. Neurol.*)

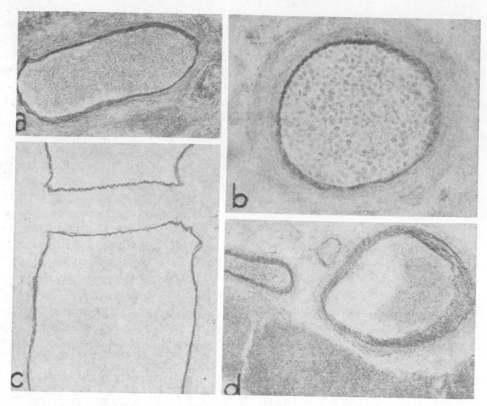

Figure 4–12.   Atrophic type of cerebral arteriosclerosis. Note the atrophic appearance, the thinning of the elastic membrane and the dilation of the blood vessel lumen, and the degeneration of the blood vessel walls. (Courtesy Dr. G. Eros and the *J. Neurophatol. Exp. Neurol.*)

histopathology of the large blood vessels of the circle of Willis and the histopathology of the small cerebral blood vessels. He does not however discuss the quantitative or qualitative relationship of the two pathologic changes. He stated that the lesions in the large cerebral arteries are predominantly fatty in type, owing to an accumulation of cholesterol and lipids in the arterial walls. In the small cerebral arteries, on the other hand, endothelial proliferation alone with lipids deposits predominates, while in the smallest blood vessels, hyaline degeneration often associated with endothelial and fibroblastic proliferation is a frequent feature (Figure 4–13(a)). In both large and small blood vessels, Bruetsch stressed the point that the fibroblastic proliferation is related to the presence of what he calls "embryonic foci of cellular proliferation" in all the involved blood vessels. These consist of a wall of loosely arranged cells, from one to fifteen deep, of a variety of cellular elements

(young fibroblasts, lymphocytes, or Maximow's undifferentiated mesenchymal cells) which may erupt at any time and lead to further fibroblastic growth (Figure 4–13(b)). Rapid proliferation of endothelial cells may entangle red cells and form an occluding mass, although not a true thrombus. According to Altschul,[5] the endothelial cells which line the inner wall of the arteries of all sizes—large, small, and even capillaries—are the progenitors of the foam cells found in the midst of the arteriosclerotic changes, cells which morphologically resemble closely mesenchimal or reticular cells if indeed they are not identical with them. The intima of the larger arteries shows an additional feature not clearly seen in the smallest vessels, namely thickening of the intima with consequent narrowing of the lumen. Formation of foam cells and of the mesenchimal and reticular cells must be considered together. The next stage of atheromatosis in the larger vessels is the

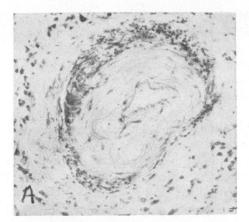

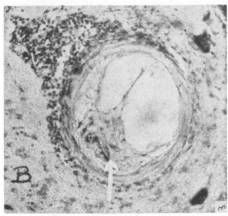

Figure 4–13. (a) Small cortical artery. The lumen is filled with hyaline tissue. Toluidine blue stain. (b) Small artery of the substantia nigra showing a focus of embryonic cellular proliferation, sending a tongue of cytoplasma containing minute hyperchromatic nuclei through the lumen. (Courtesy of Dr. W. L. Bruetsch.)

disintegration of the foam cells which help to form the atheroma proper.

Tuthill[148] contends that arteriosclerosis is not a disease of primary fat absorption. The first histopathological change is an increase in the height and extension of the areas of split elastica, and collagen increase at the specific sites of the branching of the large and of many small cerebral blood vessels. These primary areas are present from birth, and may remain unchanged through adult life. Deposits of fats and their absorption follow the primary process of the splitting of the elastica and of the increase of the collagen fibers. Hydrostatic changes at these levels of narrowing, related to the changes in blood volume, consti-

tute a contributing mechanical factor to the genesis of arteriosclerosis.

Relationship between the Arteriosclerotic Changes and the Clinical Symptoms

The important aspect of the clinico-pathologic relationship, particularly from the psychiatric standpoint, has been merely touched upon and by only a few authors, though if properly developed it might furnish us with valuable information. According to Eros,[45] focal neurological symptoms were more prevalent in cases of hyperplastic cerebral arteriosclerosis than in the hypoplastic type. Out of twenty-six cases of the hypertrophic type of arteriosclerosis, fifteen disclosed predominantly neurological focal symptoms, whereas predominantly mental symptoms were present in eighteen out of twenty-four cases of the hypoplastic type.

In the hypoplastic type the mental symptoms were usually much more severe than in the hyperplastic. Delusions and hallucinations were more often encountered in the hypoplastic type, while they were rather rare in the hyperplastic. In the hyperplastic type the more severe mental symptoms developed late in the course of the disease; at the beginning only irritability, nervousness and emotional instability were predominant. In the hypoplastic type, severe mental symptoms, often resembling schizophrenia, developed rather early.

In the earlier stages therefore, according to Eros, some indications as to the pathologic type of cerebral arteriosclerosis can be established on the basis of the presence of focal symptoms and the severity and character of the mental symptoms. In the later stages, when the damage of the parenchyma is already far advanced and deterioration sets in, the clinico-pathological distinction is difficult in the absence of focal neurological signs.

Physiopathology of Cerebral Arteriosclerosis

It has been assumed by most investigators that physiopathogenetic mechanisms determining atherosclerosis in the large cerebral blood vessels do not differ from the ones involved in atherosclerosis of the aorta, coronary arteries, and other important blood vessels.

A very comprehensive review of the whole subject can be found in Katz and Stamler's book *Experimental Atherosclerosis*.[79] These authors state that cholesterol is primarily and not secondarily involved in experimental atherogenesis. They feel that transintimal filtration from blood plasma is the mechanism whereby lipids (lipoprotein complex) enter the arterial wall. They also feel that the state of aggregation of cholesterol in plasma must be a key factor influencing the extent and rate of transudation of lipids into the arterial walls.

Although hypercholesterolemia is a factor in the production of the disease, an important element is the ratio between the cholesterol content of the blood and its phospholipids. The normal ratio in question is 0.8, i.e., 200 mg. of cholesterol per 100 to 250 cc. of phospholipids. The higher the ratio, the higher the incidence of atherosclerosis, especially of the coronary arteries. The lower the ratio, the more likely is the avoidance of atherosclerosis. Thus, the more the phospholipids are increased, as compared to the total cholesterol increase, the more protection exists against atherosclerosis. Without any altered lipid metabolism, little or no atherosclerosis develops, regardless of any other alterations of the arterial walls, including senescent changes.

That cholesterolemia alone is not responsible for atherosclerosis is indicated by the fact that hypercholesterolemia is not always found in atherosclerosis. This is why Katz and Stamler state that it is not only the level of cholesterol in the plasma that is important for atherogenesis, but also the quantity of exogenous cholesterol the body must transport, turn over and metabolize.

Further investigations on the relationship between cholesterol and atherosclerosis, carried on by Gofman and his associates,[64] established that in man, a high concentration of plasma cholesterol bearing lipoproteins (Sf 10–20) (Svedberg units of flotation) not directly correlated with the plasma total cholesterol concentration is associated with athero-

sclerosis. The Sf 10–20 constitute the less dense components, isolated by ultracentrifugation. These lipoproteins diminish on a restricted fat and cholesterol diet, even if no decrease of total cholesterol concentration follows.

The cholesterol is generally bound to the beta-lipoproteins. The more beta-lipoproteins, the more susceptibility to atherosclerosis. Kendall[81] and others feel, therefore, that atherosclerosis is the result of an elevated beta-lipoprotein level, perhaps combined with other localizing factors. Furthermore, individual situations as a result of which the plasma is unable to hold a greater concentration of sterols in solution, may lead to the precipitation of cholesterol in the blood stream.

Altered metabolism of lipids, so important in the production of atherosclerosis, cannot be separated from its interplay with other factors of exogenous or endogenous origin. Without entering into details, I will mention some which may lead to the precipitation or aggravation of either arteriosclerosis or atherosclerosis. They are: (1) hypervitaminosis D;[73,105] (2) pyridoxine deficiency;[121] (3) excessive vegetable proteins diet;[73] (4) adrenalinemia;[71] (5) excessive adrenal steroids;[2] (6) hypothyroidism;[73] (7) Diabetes mellitus;[91] and (8) hypertension.[39,51,73]

It has not yet been established whether the same physiopathologic mechanism or precipitating factors in the production of atherosclerosis in the large cerebral blood vessels apply also to the small and very small cerebral blood vessels. On the whole, with the exception of a few attempts on a small scale,[29] very little attention has been paid to the more general problem of the relationship of cerebral atherosclerosis to the lipid metabolism, and even less attention to the relationship of that metabolism to the arteriosclerosis of the small cerebral blood vessels. Investigations along such lines may furnish us with valuable data on the significance of the pathological lesions of the small blood vessels of the brain.

The various psychiatric hospitals all over the United States contain a wealth of clinical and autopsy material waiting to be studied by a well-organized team of research workers.

Beckenstein and Gold[16] reported that in 1942 at the Brooklyn State Hospital (New York) the number of deaths for arteriosclerosis and senile psychoses was 703, that is, 77.5 percent of the total number of deaths in the hospital for that same year. Out of these 703 deaths, 384 were cases of psychoses associated with cerebral arteriosclerosis.

Constitution and Heredity

Several investigators have pointed out that a certain constitutional physical makeup is more apt to be found among patients suffering from arteriosclerosis and hypertension. Moschkowitz[106] states that hypertensive patients are generally soft-muscled individuals, pudgy, short-necked, ungraceful, nonathletic, and overweight. Badia[12] found that the megalosplancnic type of Viola, or pycnic type of Kretschmer, discloses a tendency to chronic changes in the blood vessels of the heart, to hypertension, to precocious development of arteriosclerosis, and to cerebral hemorrhages. This view is shared by Larimore[86] and Fishberg.[51]

From the point of view of heredity, it has often been reported that siblings and parents of patients suffering from arteriosclerosis also disclose a history of cardiovascular disease. I will only refer to Allbutt's[3] case of a patient with hypertension, whose paternal ancestors for three generations had died of apoplexy—a total of four generations.

Studies by Boas et al.[20] of fifty families of arteriosclerotic patients whose cholesterol values in the blood exceeded 300 mg. per 100 cc., revealed the existence of abnormal cholesterol metabolism in 30 percent of all the families. Within these, all or most of the siblings showed an elevation of serum cholesterol. In addition, in nine of the fifty families, half of the examined members exhibited hypercholesterolemia.

Studies by Weitz,[156] Nador-Nikititis,[108] Curtius and Korkhaus,[38] and others on the occurrence of arteriosclerosis, hypertension, and cerebral hemorrhages in identical pair of twins reared in different environmental situations, support the contention that heredity plays an important part in this type of vascular pathology. Weitz[156] feels that the predisposition to hypertension behaves in the genetic sense as a Mendelian dominant character.

Differential Diagnosis from a Neuropathologic Standpoint

A few authors have been unwilling to accept a separation between psychoses associated with arteriosclerosis and senile dementia (Tanzi and Lugaro[146]), basing their view on the assumption that arteriosclerosis and senility are almost always associated. Meyer,[102] discussing arteriosclerosis and mental diseases, wrote that: "We have no means to speak of arteriosclerotic insanity, but only of insanity of senile or prematurely senile involution. . . . the real arteriosclerotic nature is only revealed by the course, and by the nervous and collateral symptoms, of focalized or general arteriosclerosis."

However, if one studies reports from clinical material, one does not encounter such a constant combination of senile dementia and arteriosclerosis. Simchowitz[138] in a study of twenty-three cases of senile dementia, found only eight in which well-developed arteriosclerosis was present. Bonfiglio[24] in a study of thirty-three cases of senile dementia, reported only eight in which well-developed arteriosclerosis was present.

From a pathologic standpoint, one must not consider as characterizing arteriosclerosis the mere presence, here and there, of small vessels disclosing changes assignable to this condition. If this were the case, one should diagnose as arteriosclerosis all sorts of mental disorders occurring in old age, and also the changes found in the brain of mentally normal individuals who die at an advanced age and whose vascular system shows occasional incipient sclerosis.

One must also keep in mind the fact that senile changes of the small blood vessels may lead ultimately to hyalinization and sclerosis of their walls. A certain amount of overlapping of vascular pathology is therefore to be expected. More characteristic of senile vascular changes are, according to Baker,[14] the splitting of the elastic membrane, a diminution of the muscular elements, and fibrosis of the media, with increased collagenous substance. Loss of elasticity, tortuosity, and dilatation of the blood vessels seem to occur more frequently in senility. Furthermore, one finds numerous senile plaques in senile psychoses, and also nerve cells disclosing the so-called Alzheimer's neurofibrillar disease—findings missing as a whole in cerebral arteriosclerosis. In arteriosclerotic brains, senile plaques were found in only one out of six cases by Simchowitz[138] and in two out of nine cases by Bonfiglio.[24]

Of additional assistance in the differential pathologic diagnosis between senile and arteriosclerotic psychoses, is the frequent finding in arteriosclerosis of vascular damage in the remainder of the cardiovascular system and in the kidneys (cardiac hypertrophy, myocardial infarcts, passive congestion of organs, and infarcts of the kidneys). Furthermore, the presence of cerebral red or white softenings of various intensity and extension, and involving well-known cerebral vascular territories, favors the diagnosis of arteriosclerosis.

(Neuropathology of Senile Psychoses

There is no direct correlation between cerebral pathological findings in senile psychoses, and the development of mental symptoms. Contrary to Simchowitz,[138] who believed that senile dementia was merely an exaggeration of the normal senium, Gellerstedt[61] has shown that anatomically it is not a simple quantitative difference which characterizes normal and pathological senium, an opinion shared by Grünthal,[66] Cerletti,[34] Critchley,[37] Bonfiglio,[26] Rothschild,[124] and others. Moreover, in cases of pathological senility, there is a lack of correlation between the severity of the cerebral structural change and the severity of the intellectual impairment. Conversely, marked alterations are occasionally found in the brains of old persons of normal mentality. Therefore,

tissue damage alone is not responsible for the onset of the psychosis.

The following macroscopic and microscopic changes are in general encountered in cases of senile psychoses:

Macroscopic Changes

Cranial Changes. The calvarium in old age is usually thicker than normal, the density being generally uniform. Atrophy of the skull bones, cranium, and face may be encountered much less frequently. Occasionally the process of atrophy is localized particularly in the parietal region, and hyperostosis of the inner table has been reported.

Brain. One of the general characteristics of the brain is a marked shrinkage resulting from both atrophy and loss of lymphatic fluid. Instead of an average weight between 1200 and 1400 g., weights of 1100 and 1000 g. are often reported. Weights as low as 912 g. and 815 g. have been reported by Grünthal[66] and by Critchley.[37]

Along with the shrinkage of the brain tissue, there follows a marked difference of 23 to 24 percent, between the volume of the brain and the volume capacity of the cranial cavity, instead of a normal difference of 12 percent. On the other hand, brains of normal old individuals may also undergo marked shrinkage and loss in weight (1002 g. in a case reported by Grünthal[66]), whereas brains of severe cases of senile dementia may differ only slightly from the normal average.

When shrinkage is present, as in most cases, the process is usually generalized, although at times it is more prominent in the frontal area, and the middle portion of the posterior area of the brain. The shrinkage of the nervous tissue itself is reflected in the widening of the brain sulci and thinning of the convolutions (Figure 4–14). As the result of a marked shrinkage of the brain parenchyma, an internal hydrocephalus may develop.

The dura matter is almost always thickened and, in many cases, adherent to the inner table of the skull. Longitudinal densification of that covering may be seen following the course of the external blood vessels. The pia is

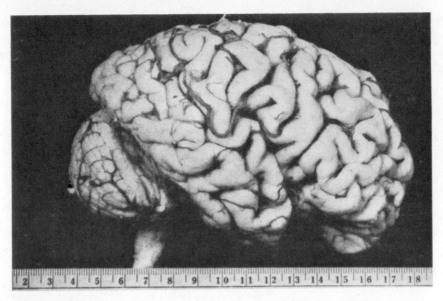

Figure 4–14. Macroscopic aspect of a senile brain in which shrinkage is moderate. The cerebral convolutions are thinned and the sulci are slightly widened.

generally three to four or more times thicker than normal.

Subdural hematomas are occasionally found in from 8 to 9 percent of the cases (Campbell[31]) and Leri[88] has reported occasional perforations of a thick and edematous pia.

Microscopic Findings

The brain cortex generally discloses a reduction in size because of an actual reduction in the volume of the nerve cells which appear smaller and closer to each other, and because of an actual loss in their number.

In general, phylogenetically older parts of the cortex, such as the motor areas, are less involved than are the parts developed later. The upper cellular layers of the cortex, particularly the third one, show the greatest damage in most cases, though not marked enough to disturb considerably the layering of the cortical lamination. In some cases that lamination is, however, greatly disturbed. In some areas the nerve cells still present may occasionally give the impression of being even more numerous because of the shrinkage of their interstitial tissue. In the same cortical convolutions, one may find areas of marked shrinkage, i.e.

volume reduction of most of the nerve cells and marked disturbed lamination, near-by areas in which the cells are better preserved, and the cytoarchitecture close to normal (Figures 4–15 to 4–18).

The pathological process which involves the individual nerve cells is generally known as "shrinkage" of the nerve cell. Shrunken nerve cells, which in the past were designated as "chronically diseased cells," are seen scattered in the various cortical areas. Most of the cells undergo a gradual process of necrobiosis, which leads to their gradual disappearance. Remnant shadows of such cells are dispersed here and there. Only occasionally, cells undergoing a simple acute swelling, or conversely the "acute severe type of degeneration" described by Nissl, are encountered. The shrinkage of the nerve cells which results in their deeply stained appearance is the most frequent finding.

Among the preserved nerve cells, many disclose an increase in pigmentation, particularly of the yellow type which may invade the whole of the cellular body, and at times spread into some of its processes. The extreme degree of such a change may lead to the "pigment atrophy" of the nerve cell, a patho-

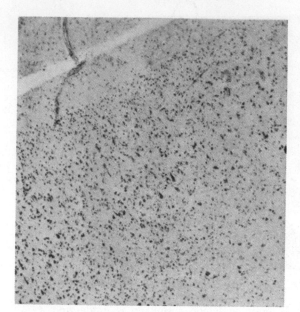

Figure 4–15. Reduction in the number of nerve cells and considerable shrinkage of their body, particularly in the inner cortical layers. Nissl stain.

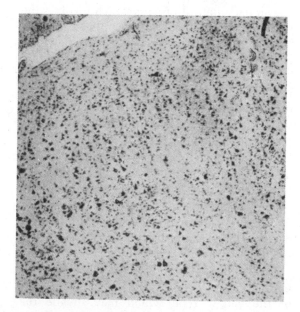

Figure 4–16. Patchy area, in which nerve cells are reduced in number, and reduction in the volume of the cell bodies is noticeable in the middle cortical layers. Nissl stain.

logic feature which seems to predilect the nerve cells of the inferior olivary bodies, and at times the nerve cells of the dentate nucleus. In contrast to the excessive pigmentation, a loss of the normal melanin pigment of the cells of the substantia nigra has been reported by Stief,[145] and by Grünthal.[66] In the basal ganglia, particularly in the striatum, a loss of

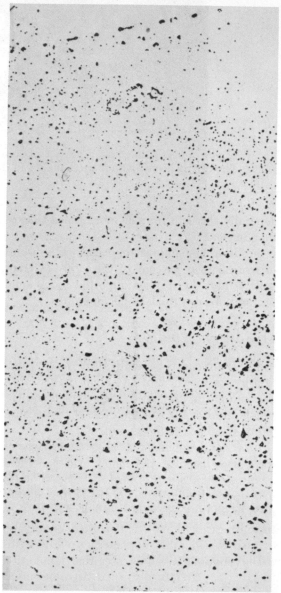

Figure 4–17. Marked reduction in the number of nerve cells in all of the cortical layers and marked shrinkage in the cell body of the remaining ones. Nissl stain.

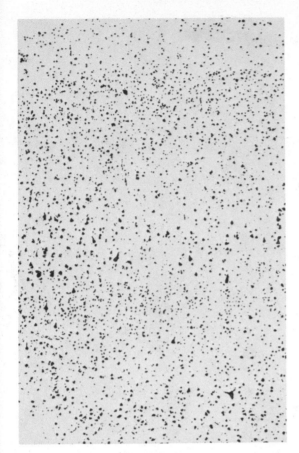

Figure 4–18. Uneven distribution of shrunken nerve cells and uneven reduction of their number, mostly in the middle and outer layers. Nissl stain.

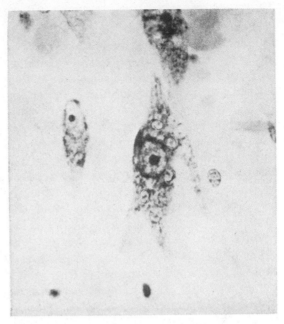

Figure 4–19. Nerve cells disclosing the granulo-vacuolar degeneration of Simchowitz; granules surrounded by vacuoles in the midst of the cellular cytoplasm. Nissl stain.

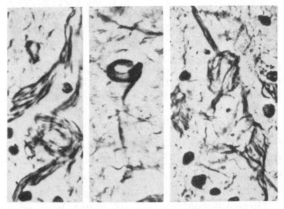

Figure 4–20. Various morphologic aspects of nerve cells disclosing the so-called Alzheimer neurofibrillar disease. Silver carbonate impregnation method of Del Rio Hortega.

the larger nerve cells has been reported, and in the cerebellum the Purkinje nerve cells appear diminished in size and in number.

A special type of nerve-cell pathology first described by Simchowitz,[138] the so-called "granulo-vacuolar degeneration" has been reported in cases of senile psychoses, particularly in the large pyramidal cells of the hippocampus, though present also in other cortical areas (Piazza[115]). The process consists in the appearance of granules scattered in the cytoplasm of the nerve cells, each granule being generally surrounded by a vacuole (Figure 4–19). According to Simchowitz[138] these granules do not contain fat tissue, a statement which is contested by Piazza.[115]

Another characteristic cellular change often found in senile dementia is the so-called "Alzheimer neurofibrillar disease of the nerve cells," a condition first described by Alzheimer in a variety of ageing diseases of the brain, but considered more closely related to that variety of presenile psychoses designated Alzheimer's disease. Within the nerve cells the neurofibrils coalesce and condense, thus as-

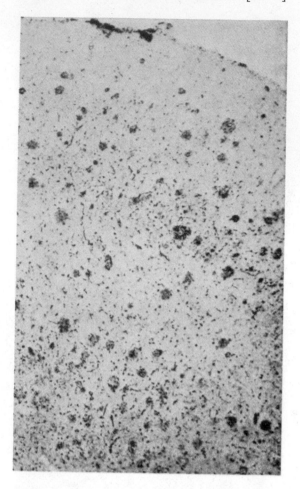

Figure 4–21. Numerous senile plaques distributed in various cortical layers. Silver carbonate impregnation method of Del Rio Hortega.

suming various peculiar aspects such as convolutions, spirals, loops, knots, and clumps within the cytoplasma (Figure 4–20), none of which are found in normal cells.

These unusual formations, which have also been described as surrounding certain nerve cells,[43] have been considered by the majority of investigators as resulting from degenerating neurofibrils within the nerve cells. However, this point of view is not shared by Achucarro and Gayarre,[1] Del Rio Hortega,[42] Lafora,[85] or Divry,[43] who have shown that the same changes occur in the pericellular, the neuroglial, and the syncytial reticulum of Held, and even in astrocytes, especially if undergoing

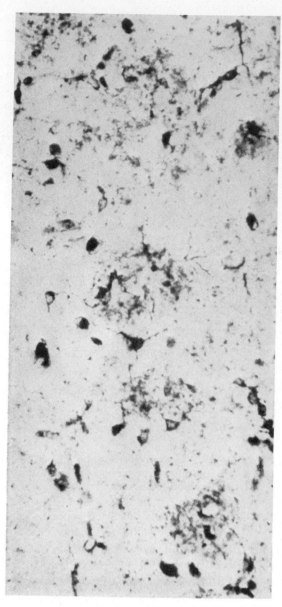

Figure 4–22. High-power magnification of senile plaques, illustrating their grandular and filamentous structure. Silver carbonate impregnation method of Del Rio Hortega.

ameboid degeneration, data which seem to point to a wider physicochemical disturbance of the amyloid and hyaline metabolism.

The association of Alzheimer's neurofibrillar disease with the other pathologic changes in the brain of senile psychotics occurs in 17 percent of the cases according to Simchowitz,[138]

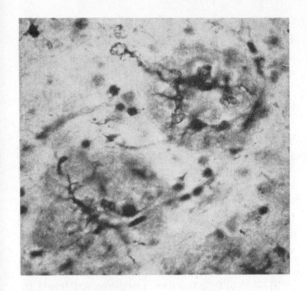

Figure 4–23. High-power magnification of two senile plaques in the midst of which reacting microglial cells are clearly visible. Silver carbonate impregnation method of Del Rio Hortega.

but in less than 6 percent according to Tiffany.[147] On the other hand, according to Cerletti,[33] Costantini,[35] Fuller,[57] Ley,[90] and Gellerstedt,[61] neurofibrillar change has been found in a few nerve cells of the brain of normal aged individuals.

Nerve cells showing the so-called Alzheimer's fibrillar disease are now, however, very numerous in senile dementia, and also in the presenile type of psychosis designated "Alzheimer's disease," where Perusini[114] first and Jervis[76] more recently, found that respectively one out of six and one out of two or three cells disclosed that change.

The most striking microscopic pathological feature in the brain in cases of senile psychosis is the presence of the so-called "senile plaques." These plaques were first described by Blocq and Marinesco,[19] in a case of epilepsy in 1892, as neuroglia nodules; in 1898, Redlich[118] called them miliary sclerosis, and Fisher,[52] in 1907, described them as "spherotrichia cerebri multiplex." It was Simchowitz who, in 1911, proposed the now generally accepted term of "senile plaques." They represent small areas of tissue degeneration, generally of a roundish aspect, in the midst of which granular or filamentlike detritus is recognizable in addition to other products of degeneration.

Senile plaques are scattered throughout the cortex from the frontal to the occipital pole, as shown in Figures 4–21 to 4–23. The frontal lobes and the Ammon's horn seem to be seats of predilection.[138] According to Tiffany,[147] senile plaques are found in the frontal, hippocampal, central, paracentral, occipital convolutions, and basal ganglia in that order of frequency. Rothschild[124] found them in abundance in the amygdaloid nucleus, in small numbers in the putamen and caudate nucleus, and less frequently in the thalamus and the substantia nigra.

According to Simchowitz,[138] the number of plaques is the best index of the severity of the senile process in the cortex. The more plaques, the more severe is the process. Such a contention, although generally accepted, is refuted by a few authors who feel that a pathological diagnosis of senile dementia may be acceptable even in the absence of senile plaques. Simchowitz[138] and Perusini[114] feel however, and I agree with them, that if a detailed examination of the brain of a senile psychotic is undertaken, one will never fail to find plaques, and their absence justifies a doubt as to the diagnosis of senile dementia.

An important corollary to that statement concerns the presence of plaques in normal senile brains. Such a question seems to have been disposed of, because normal senile brains do show senile plaques, occasionally in substantial numbers,[35,90] and sometimes as many as in senile dementia. Gellerstedt[61] detected senile plaques in 84 percent of normal aged brains, neurofibrillar alterations in 87 percent, and granulo-vacuolar degeneration in 40 percent. In each case, however, such findings were scarce, and at times detectable only after very careful examination.

The senile plaques have been considered as deriving from various individual structures of the nervous tissue. Some authors believe that they originate from neuroglia elements;[19,88,138,92] others consider them as derived from the nerve cells.[24,48] Still others assert that the disintegrated intercellular structure and the neuroglia reticulum constitute the elements from which senile plaques develop;[114,7,138] Marinesco feels that they originate from deposits of abnormal material.

In 1922, Ley[90] first expressed the opinion that in the formation of the senile plaques, microglia elements take part, a view later upheld by Verhaart,[151] and Urecchia and Elekes.[150] My own investigation on the histogenesis of the senile plaques has led me to conclude that senile plaques are formations that indeed may originate not only from degenerating microglia cells, but also from oligodendroglia cells and even directly from degenerating nerve cells (see Figure 4–24). A

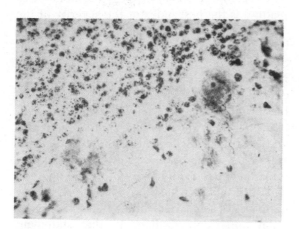

Figure 4–24. Two Purkinje cells of the cerebellum undergoing individual degenerative changes leading to the formation of senile plaques. Silver carbonate impregnation method of Del Rio Hortega.

detailed bibliography on the histogenesis of the senile plaques may be found in my paper on this subject.[48]

The histochemical process that governs the transformation of a cellular element into a senile plaque is as yet somewhat obscure. All that can be said is that it leads to the formation of a granular argyrophilic substance which according to Divry[43] represents a miliary hyalino-amyloidosis. The so-called nucleus of the plaques, that is, its central portion, shows the staining properties of an amyloid metachromatic substance which reacts in a brown-reddish color to Lugol's solution, which stains in red with Congo red, and which above all is birefringent at polarized light.

Divry[43] is also of the opinion that the so-called Alzheimer's neurofibrillar disease is the result of amyloid degeneration related to some colloidal disruption, that is, of a flocculation of the fibrinoplastic cellular substance, a process akin to syneresis. Morel and Wildi[104] felt that the amyloid degeneration in the plaques themselves, within the blood vessels or outside their walls, is the result of an altered protein metabolism (paraproteinemia) associated with impaired vascular permeability.

Free amyloid bodies are also frequently seen in senile dementia. They are scattered in various cortical areas, in the white substance, in the subependymal layer of the ventricular cavities, and more abundantly in the external lamina of the Ammon's horn. Various theories such as the neurogenic, gliogenic, lymphogenic, hematogenic, and postmortem, have been advanced for their histogenesis. After an investigation[49] which Damon and I carried out in this connection, we concluded that mostly microglial and oligodendroglial elements contribute to the origin of said bodies,

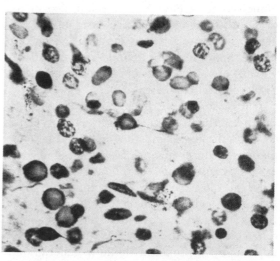

Figure 4–25. Numerous amyloid bodies diffusely distributed. Silver carbonate impregnation method of Del Rio Hortega.

through an amyloid degeneration of their cell bodies. Figure 4–25 illustrates amyloid bodies impregnated by the silver carbonate method in the course of their amyloid degeneration, and Figure 4–26 illustrates the genesis of amyloid bodies from clusters of oligodendroglia cells, which still retain some of their processes. An extensive literature on this subject is found in my publication on this subject.[49]

Neuroglial Tissue

With the atrophic process, which involves not only the cortex but also the white matter, there is a moderate neuroglia reaction of the progressive type—astrocytic reaction—which if present, is found in the outer layers of the cortex in the form of marginal gliosis. Hypertrophy of isolated astrocytes is observed here and there in the white and gray matter, but much less frequently an increase in their number (hyperplasia). Clasmatodendrosis of the glial fibers as well as reticulo-cystic degeneration of the astrocyte bodies is also found occasionally.

Deposits of free iron are common in the brain of aged people, localized particularly in the perivascular spaces of either the cortex or the white substance. A seat of predilection is generally the globus pallidus where free deposits of iron seem to be found, independently from their immediate relationship to the blood vessels. No specific relationship has been established from the quantitative standpoint between iron deposits in normal and pathological senility.

Myelin Sheaths and Nerve Fibers

In the brain cortex, the myelin sheaths do not seem to be substantially involved, except for a slight diminution of the myelinated fibers in the tangential layer, and a questionable diminution of fibers in the radiate and supraradiate layers. In the white matter, areas of patchy myelin rarefaction may be observed.

The axis cylinders, corresponding to the areas of myelin involvement, show occasional fragmentation, but nothing compared with that observed in the midst of the senile plaques and in their immediate vicinity.

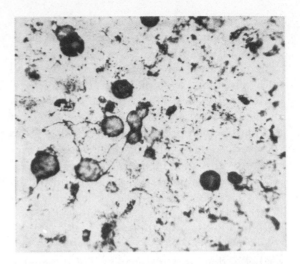

Figure 4–26. Oligodendroglial cells undergoing amyloid degeneration. Some of the cells still disclose a few of their disintegrating processes. Silver carbonate impregnation method of Del Rio Hortega.

Blood Vessels

Cerletti[33] first described in the senile atrophic tissue of the brain the presence of vascular loops and vascular knots, resulting from the elongation of the blood vessels which have lost their elasticity and which furthermore have to adjust themselves to the narrower space offered by the shrunken tissue. Aschoff[11] reports ectasia of the blood vessels, widening of their lumen, some increases of the internal elastic membrane and some twists in the course of the blood vessels which he attributed to fibrosis of the muscular elements.

Simchowitz[138] described what he termed "simple senile changes" of the small blood vessel: degenerative changes of the endothelial lining cells, fibrosis of the media, and slight reactive proliferation of the adventitial cells. According to Baker,[14] in old age the internal elastic membrane discloses fraying, and the muscular fibers of the media are replaced by connective tissue which later may become hyalinized. Hyalinization may, according to Binswanger and Schaxel,[17] spread to the adventitia. In the course of that process, the elastic fibers disappear first, followed by the muscular fibers of the media. Collagenous tissue is ultimately found surrounding the arterioles and the capillaries.

In eight cases of arteriosclerosis associated with pronounced senile changes, Eros[45] reported that in seven of them, the blood vessels showed hypoplastic degenerative changes of the elastic membrane. Recently Fisher[52] has reported, in cases of senile dementia, arteriosclerotic changes leading to more or less marked occlusion of the internal carotid arteries. He feels that a relationship may exist between these findings and the clinical picture exhibited by these patients.

In cerebral blood vessels, Scholz[134] has described a degenerative condition of the media, occurring in very old people, which he termed *Drusige Entartung*. This condition termed *degenerescence grumeuse* by Lafora,[85] consists on the infiltration of the media by a substance of homogeneous appearance, which according to the latter, shows the staining properties of the amyloid substance (Figures 4–27 and 4–28) and particularly of its birefringence.

In the choroid plexus the most common findings are the proliferation of the connective tissue, vacuolization and pigmentary degeneration of its epithelial cells, and the presence of calcareous hyaline and psammomatous bodies.

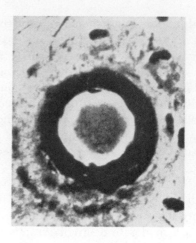

Figure 4–27. Amyloid degeneration within the walls of a blood vessel.

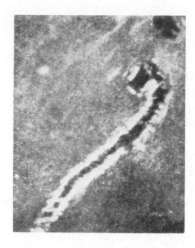

Figure 4–28. Birefringence of amyloid substance along the longitudinal course of a blood vessel.

SPINAL CORD

Its meninges are thickened and calcareous plaques may be seen attached to the pia arachnoid. Ossification is only rarely found. The spinal cord itself is generally shrunken and the myelin sheaths somewhat rarefied, particularly in the posterior and lateral columns. Astrocytic proliferation may be noticed around the blood vessels and in the areas of myelin involvement.

Accumulation of yellow pigment is often seen in the ganglion cells. Occasionally "Alzheimer's fibrillar disease" has been reported.[54]

The blood vessels may show a combination of simple senile degenerative and mild arteriosclerotic changes. Amyloid bodies generally surrounding the blood vessels seem to be prominent along the spinal cord septi and

mostly in the zone entrance of the posterior roots.

ELECTROENCEPHALOGRAPHIC STUDIES

Luce and Rothschild[94] reported a slowing of the predominant rhythm in their cases of senile psychoses, especially in those showing a more severe intellectual impairment. Diffuse dysrhythmia of brain waves in senile psychoses have been reported by Silverman, Busse, and Barnes.[137] These investigators found a correlation between diffuse dysrhythmias and decreased facility to communicate,

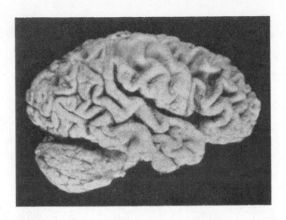

Figure 4–29. Macroscopic appearance of the right cerebral hemisphere in a case of Alzheimer's disease. Note the widely distributed shrinkage of the cerebral convolutions in most of the lobes and the markedly enlarged fissures and sulci.

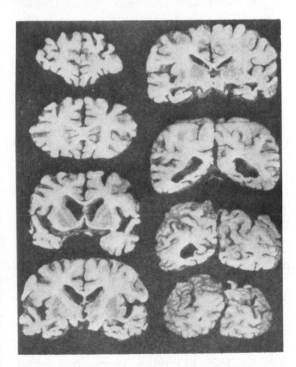

Figure 4–30. Macroscopic appearance of gross vertical sections of brain of Figure 4-29, illustrating the cerebral atrophy and the widening of the sulci from the frontal to the occipital pole and the dilatation of the lateral ventricles.

lower clarity of perception, increase in concrete concept formations, and greatly reduced psychomotor speed. When focal dysrhythmia was associated with diffuse abnormalities, or-

ganic deterioration was clearly noted. McAdam and McClatchey[96] felt that probably an impaired cerebral blood flow was the important factor in the abnormal electroencephalographic tracings. They too reported a high correlation between slow rhythm activity and intellectual deterioration.

⟨ Neuropathology of Presenile Psychoses

Alzheimer's Disease

It may be said in general that the same findings are reported in senile dementia and in Alzheimer's disease, a condition first described by Alzheimer[7] in 1907. Perusini[114] in 1910 and in 1911 contributed substantially to its clinical and pathological aspects, as a result of which the disease called Alzheimer's disease in Germany became known as Alzheimer-Perusini disease in Italy.

The atrophy of the brain tissue is more pronounced than in senile dementia, the reduction in volume of the convolution and the widening of the sulci being more marked (Figures 4–29 and 4–30). The process of atrophy, generally involving most of the lobes, is occasionally more pronounced in some of them—the frontal, temporal, parietal, or occipital. Circumscribed atrophy in one lobe only is rare, and cases of this type may constitute variants of Pick's disease rather than genuine cases of Alzheimer's disease.

Histologically the process of atrophy is represented by a diffuse disappearance of nerve cells and by a resulting disturbed cortical lamination. No particular cortical layers are involved, the cellular atrophy being more pronounced at times in the outer layers (Figure 4–31), at times in the middle layers, (Figure 4–32), and at other times indiscriminately in all cortical layers (Figure 4–33). On the whole, there seems to be no predilection for any special cytoarchitectural field; cortical areas of more recent ontogenetical development are as involved as are others of older organization. The involved areas are irregular,

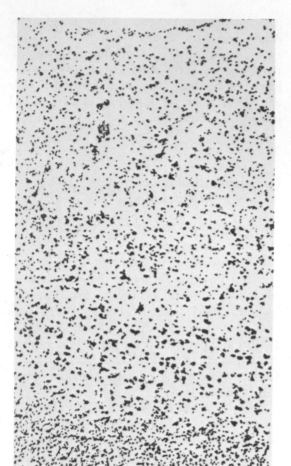

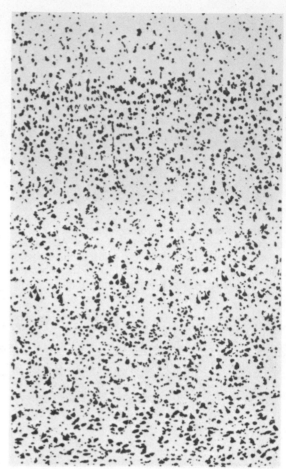

Figure 4–31. Shrinkage and disappearance of nerve cells involving mostly the outer cortical layers. Nissl stain.

Figure 4–32. Shrinkage and disappearance of nerve cells involving predominantly the middle cortical layers. Nissl stain.

and generally no clear-cut boundaries exist between normal and pathological areas. Occasionally, though, a sharp boundary is apparent between atrophic areas and the better preserved ones.

Corresponding to the areas of cortical cellular atrophy, there occurs an increase of glia cells. In the white matter, one finds also that increase which may represent an actual numerical increase in the number of the glia cells, or a relative one resulting from the shrinkage of the white substance. This glial increase may constitute one of the differential features from the senile psychoses, where gliosis, if present, rarely reaches an appreciable degree. Occasionally, fibrillar gliosis may be seen in some of the areas of the white substance, even

though in those areas the myelin sheaths appear to be preserved.

The most common individual type of the degenerative change of the involved nerve cells is that of shrinkage, or pyknosis; these nerve cells appear reduced in size, and deeply stained; their processes appear distorted and tortuous. Their intracellular pigment is generally increased, particularly in the lamina terminalis and the presubiculum of the Ammon's horn. However, one may also encounter a few nerve cells undergoing the severe acute type of degeneration of Nissl, consisting in their swollen appearance, poverty of the Nissl's substance, a marked vacuolization and peripheral disintegration. At times, a few nerve cells are encountered, undergoing the isch-

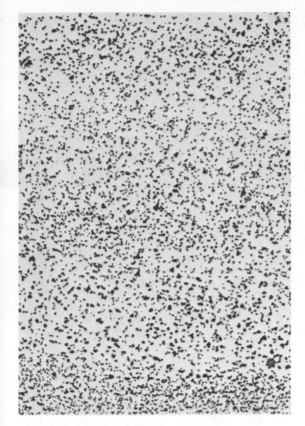

Figure 4–33. Shinkage and disappearance of nerve cells involving, indiscriminately, all cortical layers. Nissl stain.

emic type of cellular degeneration, particular in the vicinity of the blood vessels. Many distorted shadows, remnants of nerve cells, are detected, giving the impression that a slow progressive vascular mechanism contributes to the atrophic process. Only occasionally has the granulo-vacuolar degeneration of Simchowitz,[138] frequently encountered in the senile psychoses, been reported in Alzheimer's disease.

A most characteristic change of the nerve cells is the so-called Alzheimer's neurofibrillar disease. Contrasting with senile dementia, this type of cellular change has been reported by Lafora[84] as being always present in Alzheimer's disease. Figure 4–34 illustrates various aspects of Alzheimer's neurofibrillar disease in individual cortical nerve cells. Occasionally, round argyrophylic masses, resembling the inclusions described in Pick's disease,

have been reported in the cytoplasm of a few cortical nerve cells.

A diagnosis of Alzheimer's disease has been, however, considered compatible with the absence in the nerve cells of the characteristic neurofibrillar change, a statement contested by the majority of the investigators. Indeed, if one considers the difficulty of establishing a differential clinical diagnosis between senile dementia, Alzheimer's disease and Pick's disease, one is justified in insisting—for a correct diagnosis of Alzheimer's disease—on the presence in the brain of the whole typical pathology, including the Alzheimer's neurofibrillar changes.

The proportion of the nerve cells showing Alzheimer's neurofibrillar change to normal cells is as high as 1 to 2, or 1 to 3. It is precisely the large number of nerve cells disclosing that special intracellular change which characterizes Alzheimer's disease pathologically. There is, however, no parallelism between the number of nerve cells so diseased and the cortical atrophy, some severely atrophic areas lacking at times the presence of nerve cells disclosing the neurofibrillar changes. Such changes are infrequent in the basal ganglia (striatum and thalamus), but numerous in the Ammon's horn, particularly in the Sommer's sector.

The pathogenesis of the Alzheimer neurofibrillar disease is a debated question. Although the majority of the investigators still maintain that the Alzheimer's changes result from degenerated neurofibrils, others do not share this view,[1,41,85] having demonstrated that the same argyrophilic incrustation of the neurofibrils in the cells are seen in the pericellular reticulum of the nerve cells, in the neuroglia reticulum, in the sincytium of Held, in the protoplasma of the cells of the choroid plexus, in the ependymal glio-epithelial cells and even in the cytoplasm of astrocytes, especially of those undergoing the so-called ameboid degeneration. These incrustations may, therefore, originate not only from neurofibrils, but also from the thickening of the spongioplasm of many other cells in the nervous tissue.

Alzheimer's neurofibrillar disease, although generally essential for the pathologic diagnosis

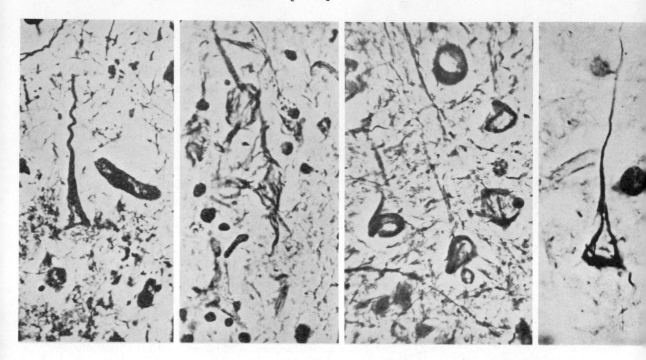

Figure 4–34. High power view of Alzheimer's neurofibrillary changes. Silver stain.

of Alzheimer's disease, is not pathognomonic of the latter. It may be found in senile dementia, particularly of the presbyophrenic variety. It has also been reported in other neuropsychiatric conditions, such as chronic epidemic encephalitis,[47,89] familiar spastic paralysis,[130] amyotrophic lateral sclerosis,[22] disseminated sclerosis,[95] involutional psychosis, Tay-Sachs disease,[100] and Pick's disease.[58,107] In all such conditions, the number of the nerve cells showing Alzheimer's changes is, however, very limited compared with the large number of cells involved in Alzheimer's disease. Furthermore, the neurofibrillar disease reported in these various human conditions as well as in some animals, may not be of the same nature as that reported in the Alzheimer disease proper.

SENILE PLAQUES

Senile plaques constitute an almost constant finding in Alzheimer's disease, rarely being absent in a typical case. According to Simchowitz,[138] in Alzheimer's disease the plaques are dominant in the occipital and parietal lobes, in contrast to their predominance in the frontal lobes in senile dementia. In general, however, they are distributed throughout the cerebral cortex, and more so in the subiculum of the Ammon's horn, although they have been reported in large number in the basal ganglia, the brain stem, and the cerebellum. The more diffuse are the senile plaques and the more severe and numerous the Alzheimer's neurofibrillar changes, the more severe, in general, are the clinical symptoms.

BLOOD VESSEL CHANGES

Most of the vascular changes reported in senile psychoses are generally found also in Alzheimer's disease. The senile atrophic angiopathy (the degenerative changes of the endothelial and aventitial cells of the blood vessel walls) and the so-called "dysphoric angiopathy" (Drusige Entartung of Scholz[134]) have been reported in Alzheimer's disease, although the latter seems commoner in very old patients. The character of the histo-chemical alterations in such angiopathy does not differ from those described by Divry[43] in senile psychosis, including the birefringence and the staining properties of the material deposited in the walls of the small blood vessels, capillaries and precapillaries and in their surrounding tissues, a material which possesses the properties of the amyloid substance. Even in the senile plaques themselves and in the argentophylic loops, spirals or baskets of the diseased Alzheimer cells, the same substance was detected by Divry,[43] thus pointing to a general metabolic disorder of which Alzheimer's disease of the brain may be a local expression.

PATHOGENESIS OF THE DISEASE

The close relationship of Alzheimer's disease to senile dementia, as first described by Alzheimer, was soon accepted by Perusini,[114] Bonfiglio,[26] Frey,[56] and Fisher.[53] Rheingold[120] and Reichhardt[119] consider the disease a variety of presbiophrenia.

Runge[127] considers Alzheimer's disease a special form of senility, occupying the same position among the senile psychoses that Lissauer's paralysis occupies in general paresis.

Hilpert,[72] Rothschild and Kasanin,[125] Malamud and Lowenberg,[99] and McMenemy and Pollack[97] consider Alzheimer's disease to be a syndrome which is due to various exogenous or endogenous factors. Senility may be only one of these factors.

Goodman[65] recently advanced the theory that Alzheimer's disease is related to devitalized microglia cells which are unable to fulfill their supposed trophic and nutritional functions. He related the devitalization to a disturbance in the cerebral metabolism of the iron which appears increased in practically all nerve cells.

Endocrine disturbances have also been thought to play a pathologic role in cases where myxedema was found associated with that condition.[7,80,133]

A common derivation for the senile and the presenile psychoses has been advocated by Braunmuhl,[27] on the basis of colloidal changes which are common in senile and presenile states. In his opinion, aging of the brain is the result of a change from a highly cellular colloid dispersion to a lesser one, resulting in condensation and coagulation. This process of "protoplasma hysteresis,"[126] which

may also occur in the presenile stages, does not differ from the one occurring in senility proper under the influence of various precipitating factors, which in Alzheimer's disease may act with greater intensity, thus leading to earlier and more extensive damage.

The vascular involvement, widely rejected in the past as a precipitating factor in presenile psychoses, seems at present to be less reluctantly accepted. Morel and Wildi[104] emphasize the importance of the altered vascular permeability. De Ajuriaguerra[40] speaks of circulatory changes leading to disturbed oxygen utilization, and Lafora[84] speaks of cerebral vascular pathoclisis. It is not, however, a matter of structural vascular damage, inasmuch as this may be absent, but of altered functionality, which may be transitory and recurrent (vasospasm). In Alzheimer's disease, vasospasm may constitute, indeed, a precipitating element which complicates the underlying senile process, and therefore precipitates and aggravates its expression. This contention is supported by the occurrence of nerve cell atrophy and gliosis, which at times are detected along the longitudinal course of a blood vessel. Furthermore the association of a mild arteriosclerosis with Alzheimer's disease has also been reported.

Von Bogaert[21] summarized the relationship of the vascular permeability to the presence of amyloid substance often reported in the brain in Alzheimer's disease. In his words: "In senile processes and therefore in Alzheimer's disease, an abnormal vascular permeability is found which allows the production of complex substances, which in some cases possess the attribute of the amyloid substance (amyloid angiopathy). If the deposit is limited to the walls of the blood vessel, it is referred to as 'congophilic angiopathy;' if it overflows into the adventitial space, welding it to the glio-adventitial structure and even penetrating into the nervous parenchyma, it is called 'dishoric angiopathy.' These discontinuous deposits tend to occur in areas differing from those where hyalinosis occur—both substances are often formed in the same brain, but in different parts. However, hyalinosis may be closer than is generally thought to the congophilic material." [p. 100] In his opinion, cerebral amyloid angiopathy is a sign of a more general humoral disturbance and of local tissue changes, which characterize "normal involution," but which become more pronounced in pathological senility and presenility.

RELATIONSHIP OF ALZHEIMER'S DISEASE TO THE SO-CALLED "JUVENILE TYPE"

The occurrence of Alzheimer's disease in early periods of life has created doubts as to the classification of the disease as a presenile psychosis. Similar doubts resulted also because of the occurrence of the disease in very old age. For the latter, a delayed pathological senility, triggered by delaying precipitating factors, may explain the occurrence of Alzheimer's disease in the course of advanced senium, and may preserve its relationship to it.

Concerning the so-called cases of "juvenile Alzheimer's disease," a critical review of some of these cases, undertaken by Jervis and Soltz,[78] brought out the following conclusions: Four of the ten cases reviewed[133,92, 84 and 85,155] disclosed insufficient pathological evidence and atypical clinical manifestations and therefore did not justify the original diagnosis of "juvenile Alzheimer's disease." In three other cases[15,99,93] although the pathology was characteristic, the clinical symptoms were atypical enough to exclude them from Alzheimer's disease. The four remaining cases[114,149,136,78] were typical from both the clinical and pathological standpoint. These cases occurred late in the fourth decade of life, instead of the fifth, in which presenile psychosis is more common. Jervis and Soltz concluded that this margin is evidently too narrow and insufficient to justify the differentiation of a nosological variety of a "juvenile type of Alzheimer's disease."

Also the "juvenile familial cases" disclosing a dominant genetic trait, described by von Bogaert et al.[23] and Worster-Drought et al.,[162] do not seem to belong to Alzheimer's disease. The paucity of the cerebral changes characteristic of that disease, the mental picture lacking the typical impairment of transcortical associative functions, and the presence of outstanding pyramidal, cerebellar, or extrapyramidal neurological symptoms, indicate a closer relationship of these cases to heredodegenerative diseases (spastic spinal paralysis, hereditary ataxia, hereditary chorea) than to Alzheimer's disease.

GENETIC FACTORS

Some cases have been described in support of a direct genetic hereditary link,[68,75,125] although serious doubts have been expressed as to their correct clinical diagnosis. Other cases of Alzheimer's disease show more of an indirect hereditary link, inasmuch as, in the same family, cases of senile dementia, schizophrenia, feeblemindedness, or alcoholism have been reported. Studying genetically and clinically sixty-nine cases of Alzheimer's disease, the Sjogrens et al.,[140] reported three secondary cases in three families among the parents of the patients, and three secondary cases among the siblings. The authors point out the possibility of a multifactorial inheritance in Alzheimer's disease, including genetic factors determining premature pathologic aging.

Pick's Disease

Pick's disease is an endogenous disease occurring in the presenile period of life, and is characterized clinically by a state of dementia, in addition to which, because of a primary circumscribed atrophy of the cerebral hemispheres, certain focal symptoms develop. This atrophy is the result of a slowly progressing degenerative process, lacking the character of inflammation or necrosis, and therefore disclosing no appreciable product of the disintegration of the involved tissue. Although Pick,[117] who first described this condition, considered it related to the senile psychoses, other investigators feel that the disease is an entity to be classified among the heredodegenerative processes.

The macroscopic appearance of the brain in Pick's disease reveals the presence of a circumscribed lobar atrophy, which is expressed in terms of shrinkage more or less pronounced, of the involved lobes, the marked shrinkage of the individual convolutions (knife-blade ap-

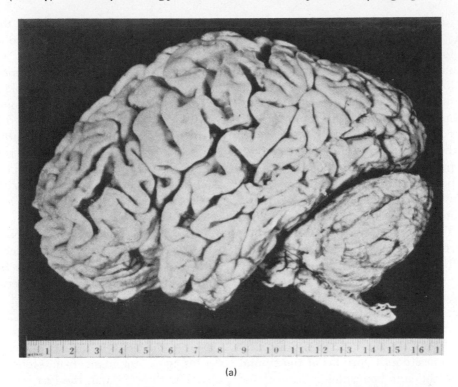

(a)

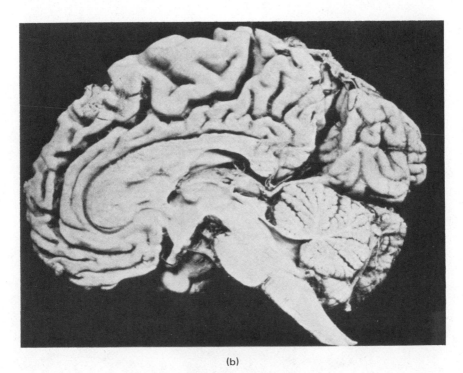

(b)

Figure 4–35. (a) Lateral view of a brain showing the atrophy, circumscribed mainly to the frontal and temporal lobes. (b) Medial aspect of the same brain. Note the well-preserved paracentral lobule.

pearance) and the broad widening of the cortical sulci.

The cerebral atrophy is generally circumscribed and localized in the orbitofrontal and temporal lobes. It is generally symmetrical but more pronounced over the left hemisphere. Frontotemporal-parietal localization is also encountered. Lobar atrophy limited exclusively to the occipital convolutions lacks postmortem pathological confirmation. In the frontal lobes, the frontal poles are more frequently involved. In the temporal lobes, the convolutions T2 and T3 are more frequently involved. The two posterior thirds of convolution T1 are generally preserved. In the parietal lobe, the gyrus supramarginalis is mostly affected.

According to Spatz[143] the most resistant cortical areas to the process of atrophy are the occipital convolutions, especially the calcarine area, the central convolutions, the paracentral lobule, the more dorsal portions of the frontal lobes, near the interhemispheric fissure, the temporal convolutions of Heschl, the caudal portion of the first temporal convolution and the Ammon's horn.

Spatz[141] also reports the presence of primary foci from where the atrophic process initiates, diffusing later to the surrounding tissue. One of these primary foci is to be found in the mediocaudal portion of the orbital lobes (gyrus rectus); a second focus he reported in the insula, a third in the fronto-opercular region, a fourth in the opercular portion of the precentral convolution, and a fifth in the frontal pole.

It is difficult to evaluate the report of Bonfiglio[25] who described a case of Pick's disease with atrophy limited solely to the basal ganglia, or the one of Verhaart,[152] where the predominance of the atrophy was in a cerebellar lobe.

Figure 4-35(a) illustrates the macroscopic aspect of the brain in a case of Pick's disease, disclosing a dominant fronto-temporal atrophy. The third frontal, the first temporal, and

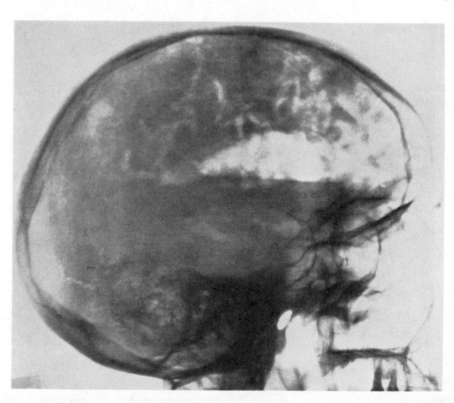

Figure 4–36. Pneumoencephalogram showing a large amount of air over the frontal lobes and the enlargement of the lateral ventricle.

the pre- and postcentral convolutions are well preserved. The Figure 4–35(b) illustrates the atrophy in the medial aspect of the same brain hemisphere. The frontal lobe is markedly atrophic, whereas the paracentral lobule is well preserved.

MICROSCOPIC CHANGES

The meninges appear thicker because of a more or less pronounced increase in the connective tissue. The main parenchymatous changes consist of a slow progressive process of atrophy of the neurons without appreciable disintegration or necrosis of the nervous tissue, but accompanied by hyperplasia of the glia fibers, and to a lesser degree of the astrocytes themselves.

Spatz,[141] Onari,[112] and Bagh[13] found the atrophy to be systemic, initiating at the distal end of the neuron, and progressing centripetally toward the nerve cell. The intensity and the diffusion of the involvement of the neurons determine the intensity of the shrinkage of the gray and white matter and of the subsequent dilatation of the cerebral ventricles.

Corresponding to the marked lobar atrophy, the encephalogram reveals a collection of air in the corresponding portion of the ventricular cavities. Figure 4–36 illustrates the pneumo-encephalographic findings related to the marked frontal atrophy in the case illustrated in Figure 4–35.

The degenerative process of the cortical nerve cells leads to their gradual rarefaction and complete disappearance. This process has no definite predilection, being at times more pronounced in certain cortical layers, and at others involving all of them. In certain cases the cellular atrophy from the outer layers of the cortex invades the middle layers (Figure 4–37); in others it is limited to the external layers; in still others it is more pronounced in the inner layers. In others it may unevenly involve most of the cortical layers (Figure 4–38). The boundaries between better-preserved areas and areas of major involvement are, at times, sharply demarcated while at others they fade gradually into well-preserved areas. At other times the disappearance of the nerve cells is patchy, and may

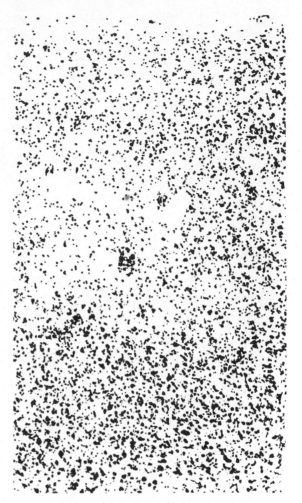

Figure 4–37. Extreme diminution of nerve cells and remnants of others, mostly in the outer cortical layers and extending into the middle layers.

be seen to follow the longitudinal course of a blood vessel (Figure 4–39).

The predominant type of the cellular involvement is the simple shrinkage of the cell body, with increased pigmentation so that it gradually becomes very pyknotic. Occasionally, however, vacuolation of its cytoplasm is observed, as well as the more specific type of granulo-vacuolar degeneration described by Simchowitz. In a few areas, the ischemic type of cellular degeneration described by Spielmeyer may also be encountered. Occasionally some of the degenerating nerve cells show increased content of fat products.

But the most characteristic aspects of nerve-

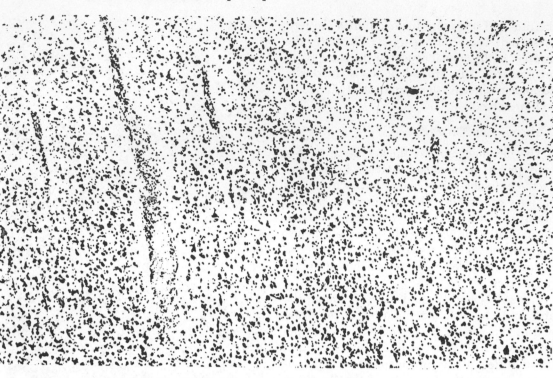

Figure 4–38.   Unevenly distributed nerve cells undergoing atrophy leading to cellular rarefaction in all the cortical layers.

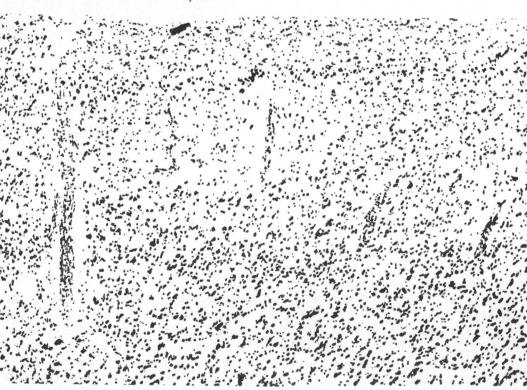

Figure 4–39.   Patchy areas of cellular atrophy and rarefaction of nerve cells along the longitudinal course of some blood vessels. Nissl stain.

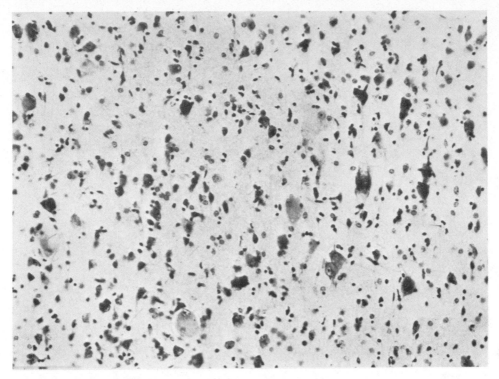

Figure 4–40. Nerve cells of the first temporal convolution undergoing the charactertistic swelling (Blähung). Nissl stain.

cell degeneration are two special ones which have been considered by some investigators as characteristic of Pick's disease. One type consists in the so-called "cellular swelling" (Blähung of Alzheimer) (Figure 4–40). Since the cytoplasm of these nerve cells has lost most of its Nissl's substance, these swollen cells appear poorly stained except for a thin peripheral chromatine band of the cytoplasm itself or of its nucleus. The nucleus, either swollen or distorted and pyknotic, is excentrically located. This type of cellular lesion seems to have a predilection for the less severely atrophic cortical areas, and recalls the type of cellular reaction described by Meyer[101] in various mental diseases as "central neuritis."

The other characteristic type of nerve cell change consists in the presence in the nerve cells of intracellular argyrophylic roundish inclusions, particularly numerous in the Ammon's horn. They are known as "cytoplasmic inclusions of Alzheimer" (Figure 4–41). These roundish bodies, which may displace the nucleus, possess metachromatic staining properties in addition to being argyrophylics. Though they do not stain with Congo Red, or show the optic birefringence of the amyloid substance, Divry[43] considers them to be the expression of colloidal condensation, an early stage of amyloid degeneration.

It is worthy of notice that nerve cells with cytoplasmic inclusions are found at times in large number in the areas where the atrophic changes are of a very moderate degree.

MYELIN SHEATHS

Involvement of axis cylinders and myelin sheaths varies from area to area, disclosing various aspects of early swelling, of fragmentation, and of granular disintegration accompanied by various degrees of demyelination. The demyelination may extend to the corpus callosum, while in the white substance it spares most of the so-called arcuate fibers. The sheaths of the optic nerves seem also better respected.

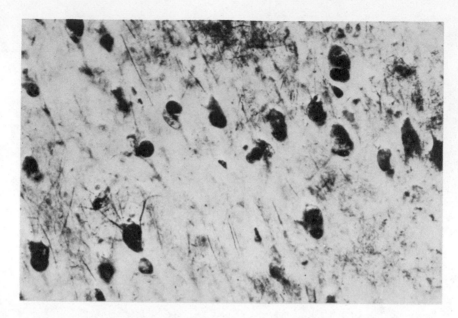

Figure 4–41. Characteristic argentophilic inclusions in the nerve cells of the Sommer sector of the Ammon's horn. Cajal silver stain.

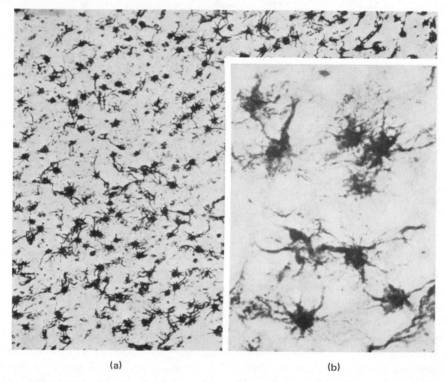

(a)   (b)

Figure 4–42. (a) Typical hypertrophy and hyperplasia of astrocytes. (b) Astrocytes undergoing degeneration (clasmatodendrosis). Cajal's gold-sublimate method.

GLIAL REACTION

The glial reaction in Pick's disease, as opposed to senile psychoses or Alzheimer's disease, is a major component of the histopathological process. At times there is a definite increase in the number of astrocytes and their related number of glia fibers, plainly visible with the Cajal method of gold sublimate impregnation. In the midst of such a glial astrocytic hyperplasia, hypertrophic cells are found disclosing at higher power, evident signs of clasmatodendrosis. Figure 4–42(a) illustrates an area of glia hypertrophy, and Figure 4–42(b) shows cells undergoing swelling and fragmentation of their processes (clasmatodenrosis). Oligodendroglia cells appear individually normal, but they give the impression of being abnormally numerous in the white matter. This is presumably related to the shrinkage of the white matter and does not necessarily represent an absolute numerical increase. As already mentioned in the definition of the disease, there are little or no fatty degeneration products in the atrophic areas, either free in the tissue or embedded in the microglia cells.

A common finding in relation to the reaction of the glia reaction in the areas disclosing a severe demyelinating process (Figure 4–43(a)) is the presence of an outstanding glial fibrosis (Figure 4–43(b)). Another impressive change is the very marked increase in the number of glial nuclei, detectable by the staining method, in the midst of some atrophic areas. Particularly interesting is the great increase of those nuclei which I have reported[50] in a typical case, along the course of various

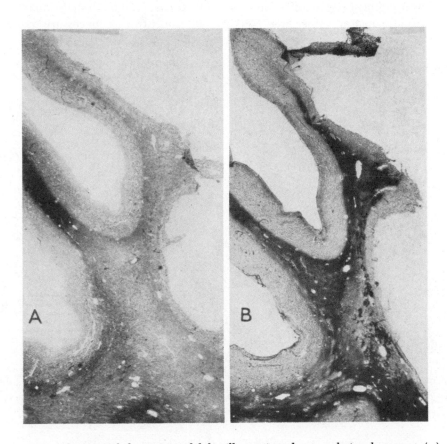

Figure 4–43. Section of the temporal lobe illustrating the correlation between (a) demyelination (Spielmeyer's method for myelin sheaths) and (b) fibro-glia proliferation on the same area (Holzer's stain for gliafibers).

small branches of small blood vessels which appear to be surrounded by a heavy collection of glial nuclei (Figure 4–44). Such a marked reaction surrounding the blood vessels seems to indicate the participation of a vascular factor in the pathogenesis of the disease.

BLOOD VESSELS

The blood vessels appear, at times, as if increased in number, though that appearance may be related to the shrinkage of the surrounding nervous parenchyma. Changes in individual blood vessels may run the gamut from a slight thickening of the adventitia, to minor proliferative changes of the lining endothelial cells, thus leading to an occasional slight endarteritis. Hyaline degeneration of small blood vessels has also been reported.

IRON PIGMENTS AND OTHER CHANGES

Increased iron pigment is generally found in the gray and white matter, either free in the tissue or embedded in the glia or nerve cells, more so at the boundaries between cortex and the white substance, and more so in the severely atrophic areas.

The participation of the basal ganglia and of the substantia nigra, in the pathologic process, thus leading to the development of extrapyramidal symptoms, has been emphasized by Ferraro and Jervis,[50] and confirmed recently by Spatz.[143] The latter stated that: "Our concept that extrapyramidal symptoms do not occur in Pick's disease must be revised." The atrophy reported in various nuclei of the thalamus has been interpreted by Simma,[139] as related to both a primary cellular atrophy of some of the thalamic nuclei, and to a secondary one resulting from the damage of the corresponding cortical areas where the thalamic fibers end.

Senile plaques and Alzheimer's neurofibrillar disease, although occasionally reported, do not constitute a necessary pathologic com-

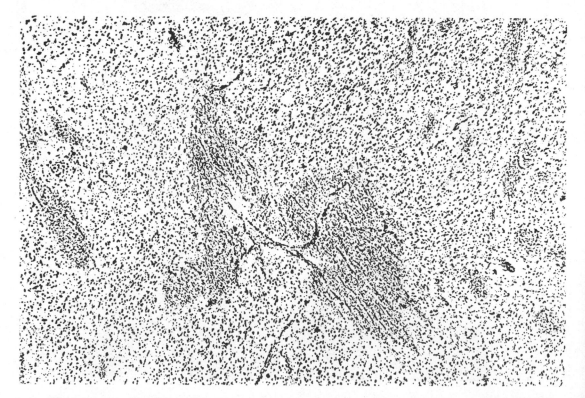

Figure 4–44. Small branches of a cerebral blood vessel, in the white matter, surrounded by a very marked increase of glia nuclei which outline the vascular course in an atrophic area.

ponent of the structural damage in Pick's disease.

An attempt by Neumann[111] to describe two different types of Pick's disease needs confirmation. The author feels that in one group there is a marked focal cortical devastation, with loss of nerve cells and axis cylinders. Demyelination and reactive gliosis parallel each other in severity. In the second group there is a widespread gliosis of the subcortex, out of proportion to the demyelination of these areas. Damage of cortical structures is less pronounced. Neumann suggests that these two types may have a different etiology.

Nosologic Position of Pick's Disease and Its Pathogenesis

That Pick's disease should be classified among the presenile psychoses, and thus related to senile psychoses, seems to be the opinion of a group of investigators. They believe that not only does the disease share some clinical features with Alzheimer's disease, but also that some of the characteristics of the circumscribed atrophy are similar pathologically to those of the more diffuse atrophy described in Alzheimer's disease. Furthermore, they feel that in cases of senile dementia there has been occasionally found a predominance of the senile atrophic process in one or more lobes. In addition, in Pick's disease, the same predominance of the cortical cellular atrophy in certain outer, middle, or inner layers, just as in senile psychoses and particularly in Alzheimer's disease, constitutes one more relationship between Pick's disease and the senile psychoses as maintained by Pick,[116,117] Fisher,[53] Altmann,[4] and Spielmeyer.[144]

Another group of investigators led by Spatz,[143] Onari,[112] and Bagh,[13] considers Pick's disease to be a member of the large group of progressive heredodegenerative systemic cerebral and spinal atrophies. They consider Pick's disease the result of a localized, premature cerebral senescence. The localized atrophy begins at the distal end of the neurons in the white substance, and progresses as a retrograde degeneration towards the nerve cells of origin, thus explaining the pathologic aspect of the swelling of the cortical nerve cells. This theory, which is an offshoot of Gower's concept of abiotrophy, implies that certain functional units are more apt to become diseased because of impaired congenital vitality.

This theory receives support from those who state that in Pick's disease only certain cytoarchitectural areas are involved,[58] that the third layer of the cortex is the predominantly diseased,[154] or that younger ontogenetical systems or associated areas, more recently myelinated, are the ones primarily involved.[141,143] Neuropathologic investigations do not always support this theory. Regions comparatively younger, such as Broca's area and the temporal gyri of Heschl, have been often reported spared, whereas regions phylogenetically older, such as the gyri hippocampi and the Ammon's horn, have been severely involved. Furthermore, involvement of regions corresponding to the associative areas of Flechsig, or to the third cortical layer, is not a constant finding. Finally the involvement of subcortical gray structures, a finding invoked in support of the theory that the disease is heredodegenerative in nature, might not be a primary involvement as maintained, but a secondary one, resulting at least in part from the atrophy of the corresponding cortical areas.

On the other hand, cases of Pick's disease in which genetic factors play a role, are undoubtedly on record.[26,28,51,152] Sjogren et al.,[140] in eighteen cases of Pick's disease confirmed by autopsy, have reported the occurrence in three families of three secondary cases among the parents, and in another family, one secondary case among the siblings. They feel that in Pick's disease the hypothesis of a major dominant gene, with modifying genes, appears somewhat acceptable. The report of Sanders et al.,[129] of a family in which seventeen members were apparently affected by the disease in the course of four generations, and the report of Malamud and Waggoner,[98] of another family with fifteen affected members in four generations, also support the Mendelian dominant character of the disease.

However, the fact that in Pick's disease, and to a lesser extent in Alzheimer's disease, the initial pathological involvement centers around the neurons (nerve cells and nerve fibers) with subsequent glial reaction, but no appreciable mesodermic involvement, seems to favor the concept of a close relationship between pathologic senility and presenility. If one considers that this same pathologic process of progressive atrophy affects all organs in the course of senility, one is tempted to see, in the general metabolic changes related to senility, the common pathogenic factor in the etiology of both senile and presenile psychoses. Genetic factors may, however, govern the premature development of the aging process as well as the structural makeup of the brain as a whole, or of certain portions of it.

This concept of a genetic premature senescence should not however diminish the importance of various exogenous factors—toxic, infectious, or endocrine—which have been considered by some investigators as the pathogenetic mechanisms in senility and presenility.[32] These exogenous environmental, and endogenous metabolic or endocrine or vascular factors are apt to accelerate the inherited process of aging. That a precipitating vascular factor may play an important part in determining some of the localized structural changes in Pick's disease has been hypothesized by several investigators, among whom are Schenk,[132] De Ajuriaguerra,[40] and Lafora.[85] The latter refers also to the possiblity of anoxia resulting from circulatory impairment, dependent on gradual occlusion of the internal carotid artery, as reported by Miller-Fisher.[103] However structural vascular structural changes are not essential in order to precipitate presenile changes. As Jervis and Ferraro[50] already reported in 1936, some of their findings, particularly in the white matter, were very suggestive of functional vasomotor imbalance, perhaps a vasospasm occurring repeatedly and followed in the long run by structural damage, i.e., nerve cell atrophy and their replacement by perivascular gliosis. Why repeated transitory angiospasms should affect only certain areas of the brain, remains to be investigated. Lafora[85] speaks of vascular pathoclisis as playing a role in senile and presenile dementias.

⟨ Bibliography

1. ACHUCARRO, N. and M. GAYARRE. "Contribucion al estudio de la Neuroglia en la corteza de la demencia senil y su participacion en la alteration celular de Alzheimer," *Trab. Lab. Invest. Biolog. Cajal*, 12 (1914), 67.

2. ADLESBERG, D., L. E. SCHAEFFER, and R. DRITSCH. "Adrenal Cortex and Lipid Metabolism; Effects of Cortisone and ACTH on Serum Lipids in Man," *Proc. Soc. Exp. Biol. Med.*, 74 (1950), 877.

3. ALLBUTT, C. Quoted by A. M. Fishberg, in *Hypertension and Nephritis*. Philadelphia: Lea & Febiger, 1939.

4. ALTMANN, E. "Ueber die Umschriebene Gehirnatrophie des Spaeteren Alters," *Zentralbl. Neurol. Psychiat.*, 83 (1923), 60.

5. ALTSCHUL, R. "Histologic Analysis of Arteriosclerosis," *Arch. Pathol.*, 38 (1944), 305.

6. ALTSCHUL, R., F. HOFFER, and J. D. STEPHEN. "Influence of Nicotinic Acid and Serum Cholesterol in Man," *Arch. Biochem.*, 54 (1955), 588.

7. ALZHEIMER, A. "Ueber Eigenartige Erkrankung der Hirnrinden," *Allg. Z. Psychiatr.*, 1907.

8. ANDERS, H. E., and N. J. EICKE. "Ueber Veranderungen an Gehirngefässen bei Hypertonie," *Z. Ges. Neurol. Psychiatr.*, 167 (1939), 562.

9. ANITSCHKOW, N. "Experimental Arteriosclerosis in Animals," n E. V. Cowdry, ed., *Arteriosclerosis*. Macmillan: New York 1933.

10. ANITSCHKOW, N. and S. SHALATOW. "Ueber Experimentelle Cholesterinsteatosis und ihre Bedeutung für die Entstehung Einiger Pathologisher Prozesse," *Zentralbl. Allg. Path.*, 34 (1913), 1.

11. ASCHOFF, L. "Ueber Arteriosklerose," *Z. Ges. Neurol. Psychiatr.*, 167 (1939), 214.

12. BADIA BRANDIA, M. "El Factor herencia en la etiologia de la hipertonia essencial," *Rev. Med. Barcelona*, 12 (1930), 3.

13. BAGH, K. VON. "Klinische und Pathologisch Anatomische Studien an 30 Faellen von Umschriebener Atrophie der Grosshirnrinde (Picksche Krankheit)," *Ann. Med. Int. Fennicae* (1946).

14. BAKER, A. B. "Structure of the Small Cerebral Arteries and Their Change with Age," *Am. J. Pathol.*, 13 (1937), 453.

15. BARRETT, A. M. "A Case of Alzheimer's Disease with Unusual Neurological Disturbances," *J. Nerv. Ment. Dis.*, 40 (1913), 361.

16. BECKENSTEIN, N. and L. GOLD. "Problems of Senile Arteriosclerotic Mental Patients; A Review of 200 Cases," *Psychiatr. Q.*, 19 (1945), 398.

17. BINSWANGER, O. and J. SCHAXEL. "Beitraege zur Normalen und Pathologischen Anatomie der Arterie des Gehirns," *Arch. Psychiatr.*, 58 (1917), 141.

18. BLEULER, E. *Textbook of Psychiatry.* New York: Macmillan, 1924.

19. BLOCQ, P. and G. MARINESCO. "Sur les lésions et la pathogénie de l'épilépsie dite essentielle," *Sem. Med.*, 12 (1892), 445.

20. BOAS, E., A. PARETS, and D. ADLERSBERG. "Hereditary Disturbance of Cholesterol Metabolism; A Factor in the Genesis of Atherosclerosis," *Am. Heart J.*, 352 (1948), 611.

21. BOGAERT, L. VON. "Cerebral Amyloid Angiopathy and Alzheimer's Disease," in G. E. W. Wolstenholme and M. O'Connor, eds., *Alzheimer's Disease and Related Conditions*, p. 95. A Ciba Foundation Symposium. London: Churchill, 1970.

22. BOGAERT, L. VON and I. BERTRAND. "Pathologic Changes of Senile Type in Charcot Disease," *Arch. Neurol. Psychiatry*, 16 (1926), 263.

23. BOGAERT, L. VON, M. MAERE, and T. DE SMEDT. "Sur les Formes familiales précoces de la maladie d'Alzheimer," *Monatsschr. Psychiatr. Neurol.*, 102 (1940), 249.

24. BONFIGLIO, F. L'Anatomia patologica delle psicosi dell'eta senile," *Riv. Sperim. Freniatria*, 45 (1921), 219.

25. BONFIGLIO, G. "Die Umschriebene Atrophy der Basalganglien," *Z. Ges. Neurol. Psychiatr.*, 106 (1937), 306.

26. ———. "L'Istopatologia delle psicosi dell'eta senile e presenile," *Proc. 1st Int. Congr. Neuropathol.*, Vol. II. Turin: Rosenberg & Sellier, 1952.

27. BRAUNMUHL, A. VON. "Zur Histopathologie der Umschriebenen Grosshirnrindenatrophie," *Arch. Pathol. Anat.* 270 (1928), 448.

28. BRAUNMUHL, A. VON and K. LEONHARD. "Ueber ein Schwesternpaar mit Pickscher Kranheit," *Z. Ges. Neurol Psychiatr.*, 150 (1934), 209.

29. BRUETSCH, W. L. "Arterioscelerotic Occlusion of Cerebral Arteries; Mechanism and Therapeutic Considerations," *Circulation*, 11 (1955), 900.

30. ———. "The Importance of Endothelial and Fibroblastic Cell Proliferation in Arteriosclerotic Occlusion of Cerebral Arteries," *J. Neuropathol. Exp. Neurol.*, 14 (1955), 348.

31. CAMPBELL, A. W. "The Morbid Changes in the Cerebro-Spinal Nervous System of the Aged Insane," *J. Ment. Sci.*, 40 (1894), 638.

32. CARDONA, F. "Sulla atrofia cerebrale circoscritta di Pick," *Riv. Patol. Nerv. Ment.*, 67 (1936), 70.

33. CERLETTI, U. "Nodi, treccie e grovigli vasali nel cervello senile," *Rend. Accad. Naz. Lincei*, (1909).

34. ———. "Una revisione del problema della degenerazione cosi detta senile," *Atti. Soc. Lombarda Sci. Med. Biol.*, 14 (1925), 2.

35. COSTANTINI, F. "Un senile normale 105 Anni," *Riv. Sperim. Freniatria*, 37 (1911), 510.

36. CRITCHLEY, M. "Discussion on Presenile Psychoses," *Proc. R. Soc. Med.*, 31 (1928), 1443.

37. ———. "The Neurology of Old Age," *Lancet* 1 (1931), 1221.

38. CURTIUS, F. and G. KORKHAUS. "Klinische Zwillingstudien," *Z. Ges. Anat.*, 15 (1930), 229.

39. DALEY, R. M., H. E. UNGERLEIDER, and R. E. GUBNER. "Prognosis in Hypertension," *JAMA*, 121 (1943), 383.

40. DE AJURIAGUERRA, J. "Discussion on the Pathology of Senility," *Proc. 1st Int. Congr. Neuropathol.*, Vol. 2. Turin: Rosenberg & Sellier, 1952.

41. DEL RIO HORTEGA, P. "Sobre la Formaciones fibrilares del Epitelio Ependimario," *Mem. R. Soc. Esp. Histo. Nat.*, 15, 1929.

42. ———. "Sobre la verdadera significacion de las cellulas neuroglixas llamada amiboides," *Bol. Soc. Biol.*, 1918. "Sobre las Formaciones fibrilares del epitelio ependimario," *Mem. R. Soc. Esp. Hist. Nat.*, 15, 1929.

43. DIVRY, P. "La pathochimie générale et cellulaire des processus séniles et préséniles," *Proc. 1st Int. Congr. Neuropathol.*, Vol. 2. Turin: Rosenberg and Sellier, 1952.

44. DUGUID, J. B. "Pathogenesis of Athero-sclerosis," *Lancet*, 257 (1949), 925.

45. EROS, G. "Observations on Cerebral Arterio-sclerosis," *J. Neuropathol. Exp. Neurol.*, 10 (1951), 237.

46. EVANS, G. "The Nature of Arteriosclerosis," *Br. Med. J.*, 1 (1923), 454.

47. FENYES, I. "Alzheimersche Fibrillenveraen-derungen im Hirnstamm einer in 28 Jaehri-gen Postencephalitischen," *Arch. Psychia-try*, 96 (1932), 700.

48. FERRARO, A. "The Origin and Formation of Senile Plaques," *Arch. Neurol. Psychiatry*, 25 (1931), 1042.

49. FERRARO, A. and L. A. DAMON. "The Histogenesis of the Amyloid Bodies in the Central Nervous System," *Arch. Neurol. Psychiatry*, 12 (1931), 229.

50. FERRARO, A. and G. JERVIS. "Pick's Disease," *Arch. Neurol. Psychiatry*, 36 (1936), 739.

51. FISHBERG, A. M. *Hypertension and Neph-ritis*, 4th ed. Philadelphia: Lea & Febiger, 1958.

52. FISHER, O. "Die Histopathologie der Pres-biophrenie," *Allg. Z. Psychiatr.*, 45 (1908), 500.

53. ———. "Ein Weiterer Beitrage zur Klinik und Pathologie der Presbiophrenie," *Z. Ges. Neurol. Psychiatr.*, 27 (1913), 397.

54. FLUEGEL, F. E. "Quelques recherches ana-tomiques sur la dégénérescence sénile de la moelle épinière," *Rev. Neurol.*, 34 (1927), 618.

55. FRENCH, J. E. "Atherosclerosis," in H. Florey, ed., *General Pathology*, 2nd ed. Philadelphia: Saunders, 1958.

56. FREY, E. "Beitrage zur Klinik und Patho-logische Anatomie der Alzheimerschen Krankheit," *Z. Ges. Neurol. Psychiatr.*, 27 (1913), 397.

57. FULLER, S. "Alzheimer's Disease; (Senium Praecox)," *J. Nerv. Ment. Dis.*, 39 (1912), 440.

58. GANS, A. "Betrachtungen ueber Art und Ausbreitung des Krankhaften Processes in Einem Fall von Pickscher Atrophie des Stirnhirns," *Z. Ges. Neurol. Psychiatr.*, 80 (1923), 10.

59. ———. "Fälle von Pickscher Atrophie des Stirnhirn," *Zentralbl. Neurol.*, 33 (1923), 516.

60. GEIRINGER, E. "Intimal Vascularization and Atherosclerosis," *J. Pathol. Bacteriol.*, 631 (1951), 201.

61. GELLERSTEDT, N. "Zur Kenntniss der Hirn-veränderungen bei der Normalen Alter-dissolution," Inaugural Dissertation, Up-sala University, 1933.

62. GLOBUS, J. H. and J. A. EPSTEIN. "Massive Cerebral Hemorrhage; Spontaneous and Experimentally Induced," *Proc. 1st Int. Congr. Neuropathol.*, Vol. 1. Turin: Rosen-berg & Sellier, 1952.

63. GLOBUS, J. H. and I. STRAUSS. "Massive Cerebral Hemorrhage," *Arch. Neurol. Psy-chiatry*, 18 (1925), 215.

64. GOFMAN, J. W., F. LINDGREN, H. ELLIOT et al. "The Role of Lipids and Lipoproteins in Arteriosclerosis," *Science*, 111 (1950), 166.

65. GOODMAN, L. "Alzheimer's Disease; A Clinico-Pathological Analysis of Twenty-three Cases," *J. Nerv. Ment. Dis.*, 118 (1953), 97.

66. GRÜNTHAL, E. "Klinish-Anatomisch Ver-gleichende Untersuchungen ueber den Greisenblödsinn," *Z. Ges. Neurol. Psy-chiatr.*, 3 (1927), 763.

67. ———. "Ueber Erblichkeit der Pickschen Krankheit," *Z. Ges. Neurol. Psychiatr.*, 136 (1931), 464.

68. GRÜNTHAL, E. and O. WEGNERT. "Nachweis von Erblichheit der Alzheimerschen Krankheit," *Monatsschr. Psychiatr. Neurol.*, 101 (1939), 8.

69. GULL, W. and H. SUTTON. "Arterio-Capil-lary Fibrosis," *Med. Chirurg. Trans.* 55 (1872), 273.

70. HALL, M. H. "The Blood and Lymphatic Vessels," in W. Anderson, ed., *Pathology*, 3rd ed. St. Louis: Mosby, 1957.

71. HERBURT, P. A. *Pathology*. Philadelphia: Lea & Febiger, 1955.

72. HILPERT, P. "Zur Klinik und Histopathologie der Alzheimershen Krankheiten," *Archiv. Psychiatr.*, 76 (1926), 379.

73. HUEPER, W. C. "Arteriosclerosis," *Arch. Pathol.*, 38 (1944), 162; 39 (1945), 51.

74. IGNATOWSKI, A. "Ueber die Wirkung des Tierischen Eiweisses auf die Aorta und die Parenchymatosen Organe der Kaninchen," *Arch. Pathol., Anat.*, 198 (1909), 245.

75. JAMES, G. W. B. Quoted by L. Bini in *Le Demenze Presenili*. Rome: Edizioni Italiane, 1948.

76. JERVIS, G. A. "Alzheimer's Disease," *Psy-chiatr. Q.*, 11 (1937), 5.

77. ———. "The Presenile Dementias," in O. J.

Kaplan, ed., *Mental Disorders in Later Life*, p. 262. Stanford: Stanford University Press, 1956.

78. JERVIS, J. and S. SOLTZ. "Alzheimer's Disease; The So-Called Juvenile Type," *Am. J. Psychiatry*, 99 (1936), 39.

79. KATZ, L. N. and J. STAMLER. *Experimental Atherosclerosis*, Springfield, Ill.: Charles C. Thomas, 1953.

80. KEHRER, F. "Die Psychoses des Um-und Rückbildungs Alters," *Z. Ges. Neurol. Psychiatr.*, 167 (1939), 35.

81. KENDALL, F. E. "Aging and Atherosclerosis," *Bull. N.Y. Acad. Med.*, 32 (1956), 517.

82. KLOTZ, O. "Compensatory Hyperplasia of the Intima," *J. Exp. Med.*, 12 (1910), 707.

83. KRAEPELIN, E. *Lehrbuch der Psychiatrie*. Leipzig: Barth, 1912.

84. LAFORA, G. R. "Zur Frage des Normalen und Pathologische Senium," *Z. Ges. Neurol. Psychiatr.*, 13 (1912), 460.

85. ———. "Valorisation critique des découvertes histopathologiques de la sénilité," *Proc. 1st Int. Congr. Neuropathol.*, Vol. 2. Turin: Rosenberg & Sellier, 1952.

86. LARIMORE, J. W. "A Study of Blood Pressure in Relation to Types of Bodily Habitus," *Arch. Intern. Med.*, 31 (1923), 567.

87. LEARY, T. "The Genesis of Atherosclerosis," *Arch. Pathol.*, 32 (1941), 507.

88. LERI, A. "Le cerveau sénile," Thèse, Université de Lille, 1906.

89. LEWY, F. "Primäre und Sekundäre Involutive Veränderungen des Gehirns," *Krankheitsforsch.*, 1 (1925), 164.

90. LEY, R. *Etude anatomique de la sénilité*. Brussels: Livre Jubilaire de la Société Belge de Neurologie, 1932.

91. LIEBOW, I. M. and H. K. HELLERSTEIN. "Cardiac Complications of Diabetes Mellitus," *Am. J. Med.*, 7 (1949), 660.

92. LOWENBERG, K. and D. ROTHSCHILD. "Alzheimer's Disease; Its Occurrence on the Basis of a Variety of Etiologic Factors," *Amer. J. Psychiatry*, 99 (1931), 289.

93. LOWENBERG, K. and R. W. WAGGONER. "Familial Organic Psychosis (Alzheimer's Type)," *Arch. Neurol. Psychiatry*, 31 (1934), 737.

94. LUCE, R. E. and D. ROTHSCHILD. "The Correlation of Encephalographic and Clinical Observations in Psychiatric Patients over 65," *J. Gerontol.*, 8 (1953), 167.

95. LUTHY, F. "Ueber Einige Bemerkenswerte Fälle von Multipler Sklerose," *Z. Ges. Neurol Psychiatr.*, 130 (1930), 219.

96. MCADAM, W. and W. T. MCCLATCHEY. "The Electroencephalogram in Aged Patients," *J. Ment. Sci.*, 98 (1952), 711.

97. MCMENEMEY, W. H. and E. POLLACK. "Presenile Diseases of the Central Nervous System," *Arch. Neurol. Psychiatr.*, 45 (1941), 683.

98. MALAMUD, N. and R. W. WAGGONER. "Genealogic and Clinico-Pathologic Study of Pick's Disease," *Arch. Neurol. Psychiatr.*, 50 (1943), 288.

99. MALAMUD, W. and K. LOWENBERG. "Alzheimer's Disease," *Arch. Neurol. Psychiatr.*, 21:805, 1929.

100. MARINESCO, G. "Contribution à l'etude anatomo-clinique et à la pathogenie de la forme tardive de l'Idiotie Amaurotique," *Bull. Acad. Med. Roumaine*, 9 (1925), 119.

101. MEYER, A. "On Parenchymatous Systemic Degeneration Mainly in the Central Nervous System," *Brain*, 92 (1901).

102. ———. "Arteriosclerosis and Mental Diseases," *Trans. Med. Soc. New York*, 1903.

103. MILLER-FISHER, C. "Discussion on Senility," *Proc. 1st Int. Congr. Neuropathol.*, Vol. 2. Turin: Rosenberg & Sellier, 1952.

104. MOREL, F. and E. WILDI. "General and Cellular Pathochemistry of Senile and Presenile Alterations of the Brain," *Proc. 1st Int. Congr. Neuropathol*, Vol 2. Turin: Rosenberg & Sellier, 1952.

105. MOSCHKOWITZ, E. *Vascular Scleroses*. New York: Oxford, 1942.

106. ———. "Hyperplastic Arteriosclerosis versus Atherosclerosis," *JAMA*, 143 (1950), 861.

107. MOYANO, A. "Dementia Presenile; Pick y Alzheimer," *Arch. Argent. Neurol.*, 7 (1932), 231.

108. NADOR-NIKITITIS, E. DE. "Sur l'etiologie de l'hypertension arterielle essentielle," *Arch. Mal. Coeur.*, 18 (1925), 582.

109. NEUBURGER, K. T. "Arteriosclerosis," in O. Bumke, ed., *Handbuch der Geisteskrankheiten*, p. 570. Berlin: Springer, 1930.

110. ———. "Summary and Critical Evaluation of Neuropathology of Vascular Diseases," *Proc. 1st Int. Congr. Neuropathol.* Vol. 1. Turin: Rosenberg & Sellier, 1952.

111. NEUMANN, M. A. "Pick's Disease," *J. Neuropathol. Exp. Neurol.* 8 (1949), 255.

112. ONARI, K. V. and H. SPATZ. "Anatomische Beitrage zur Lehre von der Picksche Krankheit," *Z. Ges. Neurol. Psychiatr.*, 101 (1926), 470.

113. OPHULS, W. "The Pathogenesis of Arteriosclerosis," in E. V. Crowdry, ed., *Arteriosclerosis*. New York: Macmillan, 1933.

114. PERUSINI, G. "Ueber Klinische und Histologische Eigenartige Psychische Erkrankungen des Spaetern Lebensalters," in F. Nissl and A. Alzheimer, eds., *Histologische und Histopathologische Arbeiten ueber die Grosshirnrinde mit Besonderer Beruechksichtigung der Pathologischen Anatomie der Geisteskrankheiten*, Vol. 3, p. 297. Jena: Fischer, 1910.

115. PIAZZA, U. "Contributo allo studio del nosografismo e del reperto istopatologico delle presbiofrenie," *Riv. Ital. Neurol. Psych.*, 5 (1912), 193.

116. PICK, A. "Senile Hirnatrophie als Grundlage von Herderscheinungen," *Wien. Klin. Wochenschr.*, 14 (1901), 403.

117. ———. "Ueber einen Symptomcomplex der Dementia Senilis durch Umschriebene Hirnatrophie," *Monatschr. Psychiatr. Neurol.*, 19 (1906), 97.

118. REDLICH, E. "Ueber Miliare Sklerose der Hirnrinde bei Seniler Atrophie," *Jahrb. Psychiatr. Neurol.*, 17 (1898), 208.

119, REICHARDT, M. Quoted by L. Bini in *La Demenze Presenili*. Rome: Edizioni Italiane, 1948.

120. RHEINGOLD, J. "Ueber Presbiophrenie Sprachstorungen," *Z. Ges. Neurol. Psychiatr.*, 76 (1922), 220.

121. RINEHART, J. F. and L. D. GREENBERG. "Arteriosclerotic Lesions in Pyridoxin Deficient Monkeys," *Am. J. Pathol.*, 25 (1949), 481.

122. ROSENBERG, E. F. "The Brain in Malignant Hypertension," *Arch. Intern. Med.*, 651 (1940), 544.

123. ROSENBLATH, E. "Ueber die Entstehung der Hirnblutung bei dem Schlaganfall," *Dtsch. Z. Nervenh.*, 61 (1918), 10.

124. ROTHSCHILD, D. "Senile Psychoses and Psychoses with Cerebral Arteriosclerosis," in O. Kaplan, ed., *Mental Disorders in Later Life*, p. 289. Stanford: Stanford University Press, 1956.

125. ROTHSCHILD, D. and J. KASANIN. "Clinico-Pathologic Study of Alzheimer's Disease," *Archiv. Neurol. Psychiatr.*, 36 (1936), 293.

126. RUCZIKA, V. "Beitraege zum Studium der Protoplasma-Histeretischen Vorgaenge," *Arch. Mikr. Anat.*, 101 (1924), 459.

127. RUNGE, W. "Die Geistesstorungen des Greisenalters," in O. Bumke, ed., *Handbook der Geisteskrankheiten*, Vol. 8. Berlin: Springer, 1930.

128. SALTIKOW, S. "Die Experimentelle erzeugten Arterienveranderungen," *Zentralbl Allg. Pathol. Anat.*, 19 (1908), 321.

129. SANDERS, J., V. W. SCHENK, and P. VAN VEEN. "A Family with Pick's Disease," *J. Nerv. Ment. Dis.*, 92 (1940), 684.

130. SCHAFFER, K. "Zur Normalen und Pathologischen Fibrillenbau der Kleinhirnrinde," *Z. Ges. Neurol. Psychiatr.*, 16 (1926), 263.

131. SCHEINKER, I. M. "Obliterative Cerebral Arteriosclerosis, A Characteristic Vascular Syndrome," *Am. J. Pathol.*, 22 (1908), 321.

132. SCHENK, V. W. D. "Maladie de Pick; Etude Anatomo-Clinique de 8 Cas," *Ann. Med. Psychol.*, 109 (1951), 574.

133. SCHNITZLER, J. G. "Zur Abgrenzung der Sogennanten Alzheimersche Krankheit," *Z. Ges. Neurol. Psychiatr.*, 7 (1911), 34.

134. SCHOLZ, W. "Die Drusige Entartung der Hirnarterien und Capillaren," *Z. Ges. Neurol. Psychiatr.*, 162 (1938), 694.

135. ———. "Les Nécroses parenchymateuses electives par hypoxémie et oligémie et leur expression topistique," *Proc. 1st Int. Congr. Neuropathol.* Turin: Rosenberg & Sellier, 1952.

136. SCHOTTKY, J. "Ueber Praesenile Verblödung," *Z. Ges. Neurol. Psychiatr.*, 140 (1932), 133.

137. SILVERMAN, A. M., E. W. BUSSE, and R. H. BARNES. "Studies in the Process of Aging; Electroencephalographic Findings in 400 Elderly Subjects," *Electroencephalogr. Clin. Neurophysiol.*, 7 (1955), 67.

138. SIMCHOWITZ, T. "Histologische Studien ueber die Senile Demenz," *Histol. Histopathol. Arb. Nissl.* 4 (1910), 268.

139. SIMMA, K. "Die Subcorticalen Veranderungen bei Pickscher Krankheit," *Monatschr. Psychiatr. Neurol.*, 123 (1952), 205.

140. SJOGREN, T. M., H. SJOGREN, and A. G. H. LINDGREN. "Morbus Alzheimer and Morbus Pick; A Genetic Clinical and Patho-Anatomical Study," *Acta. Psychiatr. Scand.* 82–1 (Suppl.), 1952.

141. SPATZ, H. "Ueber die Systematischen Atrophien," *Arch. Psychiatr.*, 108 (1937), 1.

142. ———. "Pathologisch Anatomie der Kreis-laufstörungen des Gehirn," *Z. Ges. Neurol. Psychiatr.*, 167 (1939), 301.

143. ———. "La Maladie de Pick et la sénescence cérebrale prematurée localisée," *Proc. 1st Int. Congr. Neuropathol.*, Vol. 2. Turin: Rosenberg & Sellier, 1952.

144. SPIELMEYER, W. "Ueber die Alterserkrankungen des Zentralnervensystem," *Dsch. Med. Wochenschr.*, (1911).

145. STIEF, A. "Beitrage zur Histologie der senilen Demenz," *Z. Ges. Neurol. Psychiatr.*, 91 (1924), 579.

146. TANZI, E. and E. LUGARO. "Trattato delle malattie mentali," *Soci. Editricie Milanese.* Milan, 1916.

147. TIFFANY, W. J. "The Occurrence of Miliary Plaques in Senile Brains," *Am. J. Insan.*, 70 (1913–14), 739.

148. TUTHILL, C. R. "Cerebral Arteries in Relation to Arteriosclerosis," *Arch. Pathol.*, 16 (1933), 453.

149. URECCHIA, C. T. and C. DANETZ. "Quelques Considérations sur la maladie d'Alzheimer," *Encéphale*, 19 (1924), 382.

150. URECCHIA, C. T. and N. ELEKES. "Contribution a l'etude des plaques séniles," *Bull. Acad. Nat. Med.*, 94 (1925), 795.

151. VERHAART, W. J. C. "On the Development of Senile Plaques in Alzheimer's Disease and Other Senile Cerebral Diseases," *Acta. Psychiatr. et Neurol.*, 4 (1929), 339.

152. ———. "Over die Ziekte van Pick," *Med. Tijasch Geneesk*, 74 (1930), 586.

153. VIRCHOW, R. *Die Cellularpathologie in ihrer Begrundung auf physiologischer und pathologischer Gewebelehre.* Frankfurt: Meidinger 1858.

154. VOGT, C. "Die Picksche Atrophie als Beispiel fur die Eunomische Form der Schichtenpatholise," *J. Psychol. Neurol.*, 36, (1928), 124.

155. WEIMANN, W. "Ueber eine Atypische Presenile Verblödung," *Z. Ges. Neurol. Psychiatr.*, 23 (1921), 355.

156. WEITZ, W. "Studien an Einetigen Zwillingen," *Z. Klin. Med.*, 101 (1925), 115.

157. WESSELKIN, N. W. "Ueber die Ablagerung von Fettartigen Stoffen in den Organen," *Arch. Pathol. Anat.*, 212 (1913), 225.

158. WESTPHAL, K. and R. BAER. "Ueber die Entstehung des Schlaganfalles Pathologischanatomische Untersuchungen zur Frage der Enstehung des Schlaganfalles," *Dsch. Arch. Klin. Med.*, 151 (1926), 1.

159. WILENS, S. L. "The Nature of Diffuse Intimal Thickening," *Am. J. Path.*, 272 (1950), 825.

160. WILSON, G., C. RUPP, and H. E. RIGGS. "Factors Influencing the Development of Cerebral Vascular Accidents," *JAMA*, 145 (1951), 1227.

161. WINTERNITZ, M. C., R. M. THOMAS, and P. M. LE COMPTE. *The Biology of Arteriosclerosis*, Springfield, Ill.: Charles C. Thomas, 1938.

162. WORSTER-DROUGHT, C., J. GREENFIELD, and W. MCMENEMEY. "A Form of Presenile Dementia with Spastic Paralysis," *Brain*, 63 (1940), 237.

CHAPTER 5

NEUROSYPHILITIC CONDITIONS: GENERAL PARALYSIS, GENERAL PARESIS, DEMENTIA PARALYTICA

Walter L. Bruetsch

Haslam,[39] an apothecary at Bethlem Hospital in London, is usually credited with having given the first description of general paralysis in 1798. In 1793, however, Chiarugi, the "Italian Pinel," had described some presumably genuine cases.

Haslam's thesis consisted of a report of twenty-nine consecutive cases of insanity which came to autopsy. Of the twenty-nine patients, four may conceivably have been cases of dementia paralytica. The credit for having described this disease is based chiefly on one report—that of a man, forty-two years of age. The mental illness had come on suddenly, while he was working in a garden. He believed himself to be the king of Denmark and at other times the king of France. He also professed to be the master of all dead and living languages and claimed that he had come to England with William the Conqueror. Later, he developed apoplectic phenomena. His speech was inarticulate. He became demented, bedridden, and emaciated, and his buttocks ulcerated. Eighteen months after the onset, he died. Postmortem examination revealed opaque and thickened meninges and enlarged ventricles. It is fair to say that Haslam unknowingly described in this report a typical case of general paralysis.

In the upsurge of syphilis during the Napoleonic wars, many former soldiers developed general paralysis, and French psychiatrists deserve credit for the elucidation of the disorder. Esquirol,[28] in 1814, directed attention to the slurred speech accompanying it. In 1822 Bayle,[5] a young physician at the insane asylum of Charenton in the suburbs of Paris, was the first to recognize general paralysis as a disease entity with characteristic symptoms and distinctive brain changes. The importance of this contribution lies in the fact that, for the first time, a group of patients whose disease could be recognized both clinically and anatomically as a distinct entity had been separated from the general run of mental cases.

In 1826 the French psychiatrist Calmeil[20] referred to the disease as *paralysie générale des aliénés* (the general paralysis of the insane). To this day, the term has been retained with slight variations in most countries.[59] Calmeil explained why he coined this term: The French clinicians were impressed by the fact that no other mental disease culminated so frequently in "general paralysis" of all the mental and physical faculties. In the advanced stage, the patients developed a generalized weakness of the entire muscular system. They became unable to move about and finally became bedfast. On the other hand, in the institutions there were many other cases of insanity with similar abnormal behavior and dementia, yet in spite of being there for twenty and more years, the patients did not develop this kind of general weakness.

(Etiology

There was much speculation as to the etiology of the disease. Calmeil only once referred to syphilis in the anamnesis of a known debauchee, saying only that he did not know whether this patient had a venereal disease and whether he had been treated with mercury. For many years, it did not enter the minds of psychiatrists that a "skin disease" could also be responsible for a mental disease. Most earlier authors believed that occupations in life which involved hardships, both mental and physical, favored the onset of the illness. As late as 1877, von Krafft-Ebing[48] gave the following etiologic possibilities: heredity, dissipation (Bacchus and Venus), smoking of ten to twenty Virginia cigars, excessive heat and cold, trauma to the head, exhaustive efforts to make a living, weak nerves, and fright. Among women the menopause was given as the most important factor because the onset of general paralysis was frequent between the ages of forty and fifty. Strikingly, von Krafft-Ebing in 1877 did not mention syphilis among the possible causes, although Esmarch and Jessen[27] had published their now famous paper on syphilis and insanity in 1857.

At about the same time, 1860, the Danish physician Steenberg also saw such a connection.[58] In his doctoral thesis entitled, "Syphilitic Brain Disease," Steenberg reviewed the hitherto assumed causes of dementia paralytica, such as heredity, psychic causes, overwork, and alcoholism. He showed that separately and collectively they were insufficient to explain dementia paralytica, but that, by assuming syphilis as the etiologic factor, a solution as to the cause of this disease was at hand. In 1874 Jespersen, among others, on the basis of a large amount of data, furnished the evidence that general paralysis resulted from syphilis.[58]

At the International Medical Congress in Copenhagen in 1884, where the question of syphilis in dementia paralytica was discussed, there occurred one of the last important disputes concerning the etiology of general paralysis.[58] The Danish physicians were outspoken in their assertion that dementia paralytica was a result of syphilis. Möbius (Leipzig) shared this view. Bajenoff (Moscow) discussed Maudsley's (London) absolute rejection of the theory of the syphilogenic origin of the condition. He himself was skeptical. Magnan (Paris) mentioned that at the mental hospital of St. Anne in Paris, where 300 general paralytics were admitted annually, only thirty to forty syphilitics were found among the cases of dementia paralytica. He again emphasized the role of alcohol. In France almost no one, with the exception of Fournier, believed at that time that there was a connection between general paralysis and syphilis. Shortly before the turn of the century, in 1898, no less an authority than Virchow,[72] in a discussion before the Berlin Medical Society, vehemently denied the syphilitic etiology of general paralysis, tabes dorsalis, tabetic optic atrophy, and aortic aneurysm.

At this stage, the trend of investigation shifted from the clinic to the laboratory. With the introduction of the newer methods of staining, histopathologic studies on the brain cortex of the mentally ill received a new impetus. In 1904 Nissl[60] and Alzheimer[3] gave a detailed description of the microscopic changes in the brain of general paralytic patients, which were uniform in all instances, including those without a history of syphilis. Furthermore, the Wassermann test, which had been devised about this time (1906), gave a positive reaction in blood and spinal fluid. Schaudinn, in 1905, had discovered the organism of syphilis, but, owing to technical difficulties, it was not until 1913 that Noguchi and Moore[61,62] were able to demonstrate spirochetes in the brain of general paralytics. The demonstration of *Treponema pallidum* in the cerebral cortex closed the chain of evidence concerning the syphilitic nature of the disease.

Frequency

Throughout the world, until the advent of penicillin, general paralysis was responsible for a high proportion of the admissions to mental institutions. Of the patients admitted to state hospitals for mental disease in the United States, between 5 and 15 percent were so afflicted. In the mental hospital Dalldorf, in Berlin, the admission rate of both men and women paralytics in the period from 1892 to 1902 varied between 22 and 32 percent of the total admissions.[45] In 1930 the number of general paralytics admitted to the Tokyo In-

sane Hospital constituted 30.7 percent.[53] In Batavia (former Dutch East Indies), one third of all Asiatic patients admitted to the psychiatric division of the General Hospital suffered from neurosyphilis.[71] At the Central State Hospital of Indianapolis, from 1927 to 1931, the admission rate due to general paralysis varied between 20.5 and 24.7 percent. By 1947 the figure had dropped to 12.2 percent, and in 1970 it had dwindled to less than 1 percent.

Most general paralytic patients now in mental institutions of the United States are carryovers from the previous decades of high-admission rates. They are patients who were treated with malaria or penicillin but in whom residual organic defects prevented a return to the community.

In a group of 241 patients with various types of neurosyphilis, there were twelve cases of general paralysis.[42]

Clinical Features

The clinical picture of general paralysis consists of a progressive deterioration, leading to a complete undermining of the whole mental and physical personality. It always terminates fatally if not properly treated.[47]

The symptomatology is varied, and general paralysis may produce any psychiatric syndrome, such as manic-like phases, severe depressions, schizophrenic symptoms, and, in the initial stage, a psychoneurosis.

The incubation period averages fifteen years, the lower limit being three years and the upper range approximately forty years.

◖ Mental Symptoms

The most outstanding feature of general paralysis is the progressive destruction of all mental functions. The central symptom of the disease is the dementia, around which are grouped a variety of accessory psychiatric and neurologic manifestations.

The onset of the mental disorder is often

difficult to ascertain. The history, as given by the patient, concerning the earliest symptoms is usually worthless. Of greater importance are the observations of close relatives, but even the patient's wife may fail to see the significance of the earliest changes, such as misplacing various articles and repeating the same story several times. One patient, an ardent card player, would sit up all night playing cards, and at other times would shuffle a deck of cards endlessly without playing.

Memory soon becomes affected. Recent events cannot be remembered, while remote happenings may still be recounted with accuracy. The patient forgets that he has just eaten his dinner, and he is confused about the time of day. Although the patient may do some minor erratic things, his personality may remain intact for a considerable length of time, and routine duties may be carried out remarkably well.

A disturbance of affect may set in relatively early. The patients become apathetic and dull, and remain unimpressed by tragedies that may strike their families. Sometimes, the incipient stage is characterized by anxiety and emotional instability. The appearance of euphoria is most characteristic. This feeling of well-being is difficult to differentiate from the peculiar stage of happiness in the manic phase of a manic-depressive psychosis. It may be a component of the loss of judgment.

With the advance of the illness, irritability, loss of memory, and slovenliness become more obvious. At this stage, gross mental abnormalities may suddenly appear. I knew a patient who drove at high speed through a red light, killing a pedestrian. When he was arrested, he did not comprehend the seriousness of the charge and told police in an excited manner that he was King Herod. Some patients commit sudden acts of violence. One patient at a public health center, where he was receiving weekly injections of tryparsamide, took the door of the waiting room off the hinges and tore the linoleum from the floor. A bartender entered his competitor's business place and, with an ax, hacked the furniture to pieces. Sometimes patients will do odd and silly things, such as going to the grocery store and walking away without paying the bill. One patient tried to buy a Buick automobile in a five-and-ten-cent store. A merchant created confusion in a bank, where he insisted on cashing a check for $25,000 without having funds on deposit. One patient forced his wife into the car and drove her to the local mental hospital, saying that she was insane. Another patient came home with a six-foot maple tree and tried to plant it on the windowsill.

Such acts are the result of gross loss of judgment, which is one of the basic symptoms of the disease and from which some of the delusions originate. Delusions, however, are not always present in the clinical picture. Some patients live merely in childlike contentment, manifesting boastful tendencies throughout the course of the disease. The content of the delusions is usually related to the educational background and to the news of the day. In the 1920s, when Henry Ford was in the limelight, many patients imagined themselves to be Henry Ford. At about the same time, the Prince of Wales, then a bachelor, visited the United States. An unmarried woman with general paralysis told me that she was engaged to marry the Prince. In 1933, when prohibition ended, one patient boasted of drinking several gallons of whisky a day. During World War II, a grandiose paralytic told medical students during a lecture that he was a dive-bomber pilot and that he had just returned from the battle of the Coral Sea, during which he had sunk several Japanese battleships and a dozen cruisers. His plane had had both wings shot off, but he returned safely to his base. Other patients during the war period claimed to own aircraft carriers and battleships. The records of the grandiose delusions often give a panorama of the historic and social background of a nation. In France the patients used to be Napoleon, in Germany they were the Kaiser, in Czarist Russia they were czars and grand dukes. But in Soviet Russia they are great engineers or inventors.[65] Grandiose delusions, as a rule, are transitory and disappear easily, even without treatment. On the other hand, in a few malaria-treated patients, exalted delusions persisted for years, although the serology had reverted to normal.

As the psychosis progresses, the mental deterioration becomes the outstanding symptom, and the original symptomatology recedes to the background. In the terminal stage the deterioration is profound. There is no other mental disease in which dementia is so complete. At this time there are often wild outbursts of destructiveness, and the strongest sedation is necessary to control the patient. The most absurd things may happen. One patient drove a pencil deep into the root of his tongue, "trying to dig out a bug which was under his molar teeth." Frequently, one observes prolonged grinding of the teeth which is almost pathognomonic of the disease. Finally, the patients become bedridden and develop a "general paralysis" of all the intellectual and physical functions. Bedsores over hips and buttocks may develop, which even the utmost care cannot prevent. In other instances, spasticity sets in, causing flexed extremities, and subsequent contractures of legs and arms. Following penicillin treatment, the physical condition of the patient is better maintained despite dementia, and distressing states such as these here described are now rarely seen.

❨ Psychiatric Syndromes

How frequently the various syndromes occur is difficult to estimate, because they cannot be sharply differentiated and often merge into one another. Bostroem's[9] figures, listed in Table 5–1, are possibly the most reliable.

TABLE 5–1

SYNDROME	PERCENT
Simple dementia	34.0
Euphoric dementia	29.0
Expansive type	10.0
Hypomanic form	0.5
Depressive form	7.0
Delirious and confusional state	11.0
Motor excitement	5.5
Schizophrenic syndrome	3.0

The Simple and Euphoric Dementias

The most common type of general paralysis is the gradually deteriorating form. A slowly advancing dementia occurs without delusions and excitement. Impairment of judgment, memory defects, and lack of insight are the principal symptoms. In half of the cases, the dementia is colored by a euphoric state.

The Expansive and Depressed Forms

The usual textbook picture of general paralysis represents the expansive type with delusions of grandeur. The exalted mood, the absurd delusions of wealth and power, and the happy, cheerful frame of mind make the diagnosis easy.

The depressed type may start with an attack of extreme worry lasting for months before other symptoms appear. The picture may resemble an agitated depression in middle life or an involutional melancholia. One of my patients believed that he was going to die and prayed in a loud voice for long periods of time. A fifty-year-old preacher threatened to chop off his head as a sacrifice for the sins which he had committed. Occasionally there are successful suicide attempts. The taking of poison was the first symptom of disease in one instance; in another, a patient jumped out of a third-floor hospital window.

The Schizophrenic Syndrome

About 3 percent of the cases of general paralysis present the schizophrenic form.[9] From South America a much higher rate has been reported.[7] Some patients in this group present paranoid delusions as the only outstanding clinical manifestation.[21] One patient told me that people were reading her thoughts; another accused relatives and physicians of trying to poison him to collect his insurance. A laborer brought a revolver to the factory and shot a fellow worker, imagining that the latter held a grudge against him. Paranoid delusions oecurring in general paralysis may be as fleeting and temporary as the grandiose delusions, and often disappear following therapy. Instances with the psychopathology characteristic of schizophrenia have been reported by the most experienced psychiatrists. Bumke[17] tells of a case with negativism from the pre-Wasserman days. For one year this patient was considered a catatonic schizophrenic, until he suddenly died of paralytic convulsions.

Hallucinations occur in about 6 percent of cases. Auditory and visual hallucinations are most common, but olfactory hallucinations have also been observed. At times, it is difficult to say whether one is dealing with true hallucinations or with confabulation. Hechst,[41] in a histologic study of the schizophrenic type of general paralysis, came to the conclusion that schizophrenic symptoms are not associated with any particular localization of the paralytic brain process.

The Senile Form

Until Nissl's[60] and Alzheimer's[3] histopathologic studies, senile general paralysis was in the main unrecognized, being diagnosed as senile or arteriosclerotic psychosis. In the aged, the disease is particularly difficult to diagnose without a spinal fluid examination. In most cases, argyrophil plaques in the brain are absent, but senile alterations are occasionally added to the paralytic process.[4] Contrary to prevailing opinion, excellent therapeutic successes have been obtained in old age.

The Taboparalytic Form

In the taboparalytic form there is a combination of general paralysis and tabes dorsalis (Figure 5–1). Some clinicians are willing to make a diagnosis of taboparalysis only if, in addition to the absent patellar reflexes, there is an ataxic gait or other tabetic symptoms, such as root pains, crises, etc. Absent knee jerks

without other symptoms of tabes are common, and these cases are not different from those of the usual general paralytic patient.

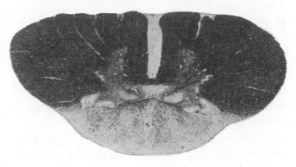

Figure 5–1. Spinal cord in taboparalysis. There is a degeneration of the posterior columns. Weil's myelin sheath stain.

Lissauer's General Paralysis

In 1901, Lissauer[49] called attention to an atypical type of general paralysis, characterized by epileptiform and apoplectiform attacks, followed by signs of a localizing nature, such as hemiplegia, aphasia, apraxia, or hemianopsia. Lissauer's general paralysis is rare.[57] At autopsy, there is extreme atrophy of an entire cerebral region, or of a group of convolutions, which far exceeds the generalized cortical atrophy of the brain in the average case.

Prepsychotic Personality

Most authors agree that, in general paralysis, the premorbid personality influences the clinical picture.[63] The cerebral process seems to serve as a release for personality trends, intensifying innate tendencies. If an individual with a cyclothymic constitution develops general paralysis, he will frequently show a manic or depressive reaction. If he has euphoric tendencies, he will become expansive and excited. Likewise, schizoid personalities are prone to show schizophrenic states. This relation, however, is not an absolute one. In some instances the clinical picture corresponds only slightly to the premorbid personality, and in others not at all.

⟦ Physical Signs

The important neurologic symptoms of general paralysis are the speech defect, pupillary abnormalities, handwriting disorders, changes in the tendon reflexes, convulsions, and apoplectic phenomena.[16]

In the incipient stage no physical signs may be present, and a most careful neurologic examination, including psychologic testing and electroencephalogram, may give no clue as to the organic nature of the illness. But an examination of the cerebrospinal fluid will, even at this early stage, reveal a typical "paretic" formula. In some instances, the nervous manifestations were attributed to stressful life experiences until, weeks later, more obvious symptoms became manifest or the spinal fluid was examined. On the other hand, the disease may begin with a sudden convulsion, a transient hemiplegia, or an aphasia preceding mental changes by several months.

The disorder of speech is so typical that a correct diagnosis can often be made as the patient talks. The disturbed articulation is manifested as hesitation and later as slurring. The speech defect used to be the main symptom on which the psychiatrists of the nineteenth century depended for diagnosis. If this particular speech involvement was present in an insane patient, he was considered incurable. It can often be recognized during conversation. Otherwise, test phrases such as "Methodist Episcopal Church," "army reorganization," "national hospital for the epileptics," and others have to be employed to reveal the disturbance. Later, the patient is unable to form sentences, and in the terminal stage, the speech is completely unintelligible. It should be added that cerebral arteriosclerosis with bulbar symptoms may cause a similar speech impediment.

The pupillary changes consist of irregularity of outline, inequality of size, and impairment (diminution or absence) of the light and convergence reflexes. Normal pupils are present in 5–10 percent of cases,[45] but toward the end of the illness almost all untreated paralytics have pupillary abnormalities. Following penicillin treatment, there is, at times, an improvement in the pupillary reactions. Of greatest importance is the Argyll Robertson pupil. The frequency of this sign depends on the stage of the disease. It is infrequent in incipient general paralysis; in the advanced stage, it is present in about 50 percent of cases. Pupils which are fixed to both light and accommodation are less frequent. The diagnostic value of absolute fixation of the pupils is not as great as that of the Argyll Robertson sign; the former may be observed in various other diseases, for example, cerebral arteriosclerosis, multiple sclerosis, or alcoholism.

Handwriting disturbance is manifested by misspelled words, omissions, misplacements, and repetitions of letters and syllables (Figure 5–2). Almost never does the patient recognize the mistakes. Occasionally, the outstanding feature of the handwriting disorder is the tremor. In the advanced stage, there is agraphia, the patient being unable to draw

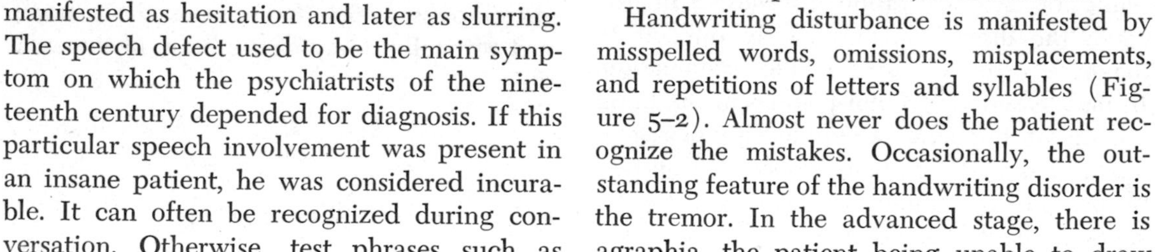

Figure 5–2.   Sample of handwriting in general paralysis. The patient was asked to write Central State Hospital, Indianapolis, Indiana, and the date, which was June 28, 1952.

more than a few wavering lines. The handwriting is normal in 10 percent of patients.

Junius and Arndt[45] reported on knee jerks in 992 untreated cases; patellar reflexes were normal in 16 percent, increased in 54 percent, and diminished or absent in 30 percent. The abdominal reflexes are occasionally absent; less frequently, the cremasteric reflexes are wanting.

A fine or coarse rapid tremor particularly of the extended fingers, tongue, and labial muscles is often present. The face becomes expressionless and devoid of normal mimic motions. There is flattening and smoothing out of the nasolabial folds.

The most important motor disturbances are convulsions and apoplectic phenomena. They appear in any stage of the disease and are present in 35–65 percent of cases. Psychomotor attacks or epileptic equivalents occur, manifested by sudden periods of excitement, extreme violence, and impulsive shouting. sodes. In successfully treated patients, the Some patients have died during these epiconvulsions, as a rule, cease entirely. Occasionally, however, the seizures persist indefinitely, despite disappearance of all other symptoms.[35] In a few otherwise completely recovered cases, convulsions made their appearance for the first time a few months or several years after malaria or penicillin therapy.

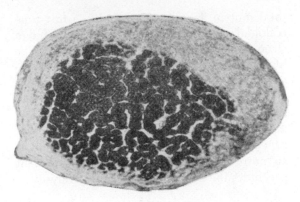

Figure 5–3. Partial syphilitic optic atrophy in general paralysis. The optic nerve reveals a large marginal area of demyelination. There was two-grade paleness of the optic disk and an irregular contraction of the visual field. (Courtesy of Charles C. Thomas, Publisher.)

composed of plasma cells and lymphocytes, extend from the periphery along the septa toward the interior of the optic nerves, first producing marginal degeneration. This manifests itself in a concentric and slowly advancing narrowing of the visual fields.

(Involvement of the Aorta

The most important and frequent extracerebral lesion of general paralysis is syphilitic aortitis,[14,73] having been observed at autopsy in 33–56 percent of cases.[50] Most instances are clinically asymptomatic, with the exception of the aortic aneurysm and aortic valve incompetency. In the author's own findings, a slight or moderate widening of the aortic arch, as revealed in X-rays, was present in 7 per cent. An insufficiency of the aortic valve was diagnosed by auscultation in 2 percent.

(Syphilitic Optic Atrophy

In about 2 percent of general paralysis there is complete or nearly complete blindness owing to optic atrophy.[15] If special attention is paid to the early stages of this complication, partial optic atrophy can be recognized in about one third of the cases (Figure 5–3).[64] The early signs consist of field defects, and somewhat later of pallor of the optic disks, reduction of visual acuity, and difficulties in distinguishing colors.[15]

Syphilitic optic atrophy is due to a chronic inflammatory process, followed by a slow degeneration of the nerve fibers.[15] Infiltrations,

(Laboratory Findings*

Cerebrospinal Fluid

The abnormalities of cerebrospinal fluid consist of an increase of cells, elevation of the

---

* Sparling's article[68] can be consulted for further details of laboratory findings in the diagnosis and treatment of syphilis.

total protein, increase in globulin, a first-zone colloidal gold curve (paretic curve), and a strongly positive Wassermann reaction. The blood Wassermann and Kahn tests are positive in 95 percent.

There are patients in whom only a complete spinal fluid examination permits a differential diagnosis between general paralysis and other psychiatric conditions. Negative spinal fluid in an untreated (but not in a treated) patient precludes the diagnosis of general paralysis.

Electroencephalogram

In untreated patients, abnormal or borderline tracings are observed in from 55–81 percent.[31,37] In general paralysis or in any other type of neurosyphilis, there is no characteristic electroencephalographic pattern. The more abnormal the electroencephalogram, the greater is the likelihood of a history of convulsions. The incidence of abnormal electroencephalograms, in cases of general paralysis with seizures, is 91 percent, as compared to 44 percent in those without convulsions.[37]

Following successful therapy, an improvement in the electroencephalographic tracings has been reported in most instances.[19] In the interpretation of an electroencephalogram the existence of organic alterations may be revealed, but an occasional absence of electroencephalographic abnormality does not exclude the presence of a cerebral lesion.

Pneumoencephalogram

Pneumoencephalography is not a delicate diagnostic method because of the limitations in the recognition of minor cortical atrophies.[25] It is of little auxiliary value in the diagnosis of early general paralysis. In advanced cases there is dilatation of the ventricular system and of the subarachnoid spaces.

(Pathology

Gross Changes

The macroscopic findings in general paralysis consist of cloudy and thickened meninges,

atrophy of the cerebral convolutions (Figure 5–4), enlargement of the ventricles, and granular ependymitis. In incipient cases there may be almost no gross changes in the brain. The turbidity of the meninges is the result of a

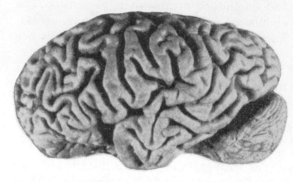

Figure 5–4. Brain in general paralysis. Marked atrophy of the cerebral convolutions. The sulci are gaping.

chronic syphilitic meningitis. Minor degrees of atrophy of the cerebral convolutions are difficult to discern. The decrease of weight due to the atrophic process may amount to 100 g., or more, although it is not rare to find brains with normal or even increased weight.

Microscopic Changes

The main histologic feature of general paralysis is a syphilitic meningoencephalitis. The meninges are infiltrated with plasma cells and

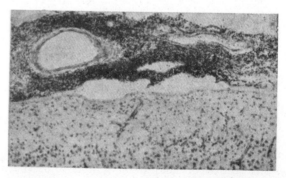

Figure 5–5. General paralysis. Syphilitic meningitis. The meninges are infiltrated with plasma cells and lymphocytes. Toluidine blue stain.

lymphocytes (Figure 5–5). In the cortex, and to a lesser degree in the white matter, there is

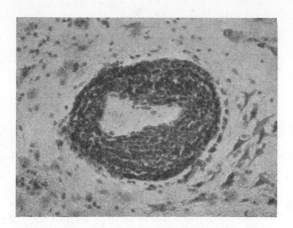

Figure 5–6. Perivascular infiltration of a cortical vessel in general paralysis. Toluidine blue stain.

perivascular infiltration (Figure 5–6). Some of the infiltrating cells in the vessel walls and the rod cells of Nissl, when stained by the Turnbull blue method, reveal blue pigment granules.[56] This pigment represents the so-called "iron of general paralysis." In the capillaries, multiplication of endothelial cells takes place, causing capillary obstruction. Moreover, there is new formation of capillary buds and of small blood vessels, most of which never become normally functional blood channels. These newly formed vessels pierce the parenchymatous tissue. They contribute to the subtle disorganization of the cortex and thus become an important factor in the causation of the ensuing dementia. Another alteration of the mesodermal tissue is the formation of rod cells, the *Stäbchenzellen* of Nissl. The rod cells are derivatives of Hortega's microglial cells, which assume the form of enlarged rod-shaped cellular elements. And finally, there is a diminution of the perivascular clasmatocytes (histiocytes), only seen on supravital study.[10]

The scarcity of the phagocytic elements in the general paralytic brain is linked to the question as to why only a small number (3–5 percent)[34] of all untreated syphilitics develop general paralysis. Clasmatocytes are generally identified with antibody formation and with local tissue immunity.

The ganglion cells show all degrees of changes, the majority of diseased nerve cells exhibiting the chronic type of cell degenera-tion. But normal-appearing neurons are found lying next to markedly degenerated forms. The myelin sheaths and the axis cylinders, as well as the neuroglia reveal minor alterations. Cajal[18] gave an excellent review of the glial changes in general paralysis.

The summation of the histopathologic changes in both the mesodermal and the ectodermal tissue leads to a disturbed cytoarchitecture of the cortex, in which the normal arrangement of the cell layers is lost (Figure 5–7).

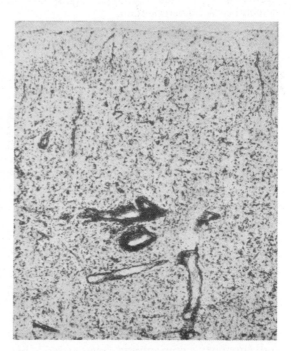

Figure 5–7. Disturbed cytoarchitecture of brain cortex in general paralysis. The normal arrangement of cell layers is lost, and the ganglion cells show all degrees of degeneration. Perivascular infiltration is pronounced. Toluidine blue stain.

Spirochetes in the Brain

In brains of untreated patients, spirochetes in great numbers may be present (Figure 5–8). In other brains a few or no organisms can be found, despite time-consuming search in many tissue blocks.[32,36,44] In his famous 1913 studies, Noguchi,[61,62] and all others after him, succeeded in finding *Treponema*

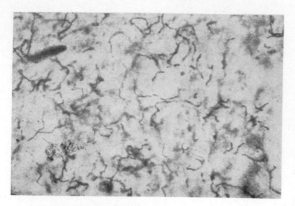

Figure 5–8. General paralysis. Spirochetes in cerebral cortex. Dieterle stain.

pallidum in approximately one fourth of the cases.[44] The high percentage of negative results is explained by a possible cyclic decrease, and by an increase in the number of organisms. During the phasic decrease, spirochetes rarely attain such numbers as to put themselves within easy reach of microscopic search. *Treponema pallidum* has a preference for the gray matter. In the white matter and in the meninges they are rare, if not completely absent.

(Treatment

After the syphilitic etiology of general paralysis had been established, antisyphilitic treatment with arsphenamine (salvarsan), bismuth, and mercury compounds was tried, but without success.

Malaria Therapy

For many years it had been recognized that mental patients improved occasionally after an intercurrent febrile disease, such as typhoid fever, malaria, erysipelas, and tuberculosis. In 1887, Wagner-Jauregg[74] proposed the idea of intentionally inducing a febrile disease for therapeutic purposes. He selected first the streptococcus of erysipelas, but this proved unsatisfactory. A simple fever-producing agent became available in 1890 with Koch's tuberculin. Wagner-Jauregg used tuberculin at first in all types of psychiatric patients. After observing improvement mainly among general paralytics, he concentrated on that mental disorder. Later, he used typhoid vaccines.

During World War I, a soldier who had contracted malaria on the Balkan Front was admitted by mistake to the psychiatric clinic of the University of Vienna. Wagner-Jauregg, then head of the clinic, seized this opportunity, and on June 14, 1917, inoculated three general paralytic patients with the blood from this soldier. This marked the beginning of malaria therapy. The first favorable reports of this mode of treatment were received with skepticism, but psychiatrists in Europe soon hailed the discovery. In 1927 Wagner-Jauregg was awarded the Nobel prize for this achievement.

Malaria therapy consisted of inoculating a general paralytic patient with 1–3 cc. of *Plasmodium vivax* (tertian) malaria blood, obtained from another patient who was undergoing this treatment. The patient was permitted to have eight to twelve malarial paroxysms with daily temperature elevations ranging from 103 to 105°F. Malaria fever was then terminated with quinine.

Penicillin Therapy

In 1943, when Mahoney[54] and co-workers suggested that penicillin had treponemicidal action, the National Research Council furnished the expensive new drug to a few psychiatrists (Dattner, Ebaugh, Solomon, and Bruetsch) for evaluation in the treatment of general paralysis. It soon became apparent that penicillin in the amount of 10 million units was equal to malaria therapy and would surpass it if given in still higher total dosage.[12] Although *Treponema pallidum* was extraordinarily sensitive to penicillin, it was possible to show that 10 million units were not sufficient because spirochetes persisted in some brains. A minimum of 15–20 million units was recommended for maximal results in general paralysis.[12]

Malaria therapy produced full recoveries in 35 percent of unselected patients. Penicillin, in the total dosage of 10 million units, raised the recovery figure to 50 percent.

Latin-American investigators[7] by using a combination of penicillins which maintain various levels of blood concentration, raised the recovery rate to 83 percent. The schedule consists of three injections of 2.4 million units of benzathine penicillin G (1.2 million units into each buttock) on the first, fifth, and ninth days, plus twenty injections of 500,000 units of procaine penicillin, administered every twelve hours.[70] The total dosage is 17,200,000 units, given within ten days.

The disappearance of mental symptoms may begin during therapy, or it may be delayed for several weeks or months. Within six to twelve months there will be an improvement in the nonspecific tests of the spinal fluid (cell count, globulin, total protein, and the colloidal gold reaction). But the Wassermann tests of blood and spinal fluid may not become negative for ten years or longer.[70] Persistence of positive serologic tests for syphilis, or progression of clinical symptoms, does not necessarily mean a continuation of infection. Treatment for the sole purpose of obtaining seronegativity is usually futile.

The favorable effect of penicillin is also reflected in the brain tissue. There is a reduction and final disappearance of the round cell infiltrations, of Nissl's rod cells, and of the iron pigment.[12,33]

The action of penicillin is on the syphilitic organisms themselves. Malaria therapy, on the other hand, stimulates the defensive powers of the host by activation of the reticuloendothelial cells (clasmatocytes, histiocytes).[10,11,13]

There is convincing evidence that penicillin alone is capable of curing general paralysis.[22] Where it fails, malaria therapy will also probably fail.[76]

To sum up, penicillin in the treatment of general paralysis is highly efficacious in large dosage. It is inexpensive and practically without risk, and the treatment is of short duration.

RETREATMENT

If the patient has received a minimum of 15 million units of penicillin, retreatment is usu-

ally not necessary. If there is no improvement after three months, another course of penicillin may be given, for the penicillin might have been absorbed poorly from the muscle depots.

PENICILLIN SENSITIVITY[*]

Penicillin allergy is now the most common of all drug allergies and the most frequent cause of anaphylactic shock in man.[43] In cases with a clear-cut penicillin allergy, penicillin should not be used. When the history of penicillin allergy is less clear-cut, consideration may be given to penicillin skin testing or hemagglutination tests.[24] Skin tests using nanogram amounts of penicilloyl polylysine and penicillin from the vial detect many, but not all, cases of penicillin allergy. Fatalities due to intradermal testing are extremely rare, but have been reported. Intradermal tests should be followed by intramuscular tests using minute amounts of penicillin. All penicillin allergy testing should be done in the hospital with resuscitation equipment at the bedside, experienced medical personnel, and a large-bore intravenous drip running.

Symptoms of anaphylaxis to penicillin include vertigo, nausea, flushing, pruritis, dyspnea, and abdominal pain. At the first sign, 0.5 cc. at 1/1000 epinephrine and 50 mg. Benadryl should be given IM, and an intravenous drip with large needle started. If severe dyspnea or hypotension occurs, intravenous vasopressors, air way, and assisted respiration will be necessary.

One complication of antibiotic treatment of syphilis is the Jarisch-Herxheimer reaction.[75] The reaction is presumed to be a response to antigens released from killed spirochetes. Fever appears within twelve hours of the onset of treatment and lasts up to 48 hours. Temperatures of 102°F are not rare and 104°F has been recorded. Aspirin and skin cooling measures may be used for treatment. In neurosyphilis, convulsions and increased agitation may appear. The patient must be sedated and restrained if necessary. Treatment should

---

[*] We are indebted to William T. Bachmann for editorial advice and help in revising this section on penicillin sensitivity.

be continued with no change in the original schedule.

If penicillin cannot be used, tetracycline is the drug of choice.[51,68] The drug should be given orally in divided doses of 2 g. per day for thirty to forty days for neurosyphilis. Follow-up spinal fluid analysis should be performed more frequently (at 1, 3, 6, and 24 months after treatment would be adequate for the usual case). Erythromycin is the drug of third choice. It should be given orally in the estolate form (Ilosone) in the same doses as tetracycline. Liver function must be monitored as hepatotoxicity has been reported with erythromycin estolate. Other forms of erythromycin are not absorbed from the gastrointestinal tract well enough to be used. Cephalothin is probably a good alternative to penicillin in the treatment of neurosyphilis. However, a significant number of people allergic to penicillin are also allergic to cephalothin, and treatment schedules for neurosyphilis have not been clinically evaluated.

(Psychotherapy

After successful treatment with penicillin, the patient becomes a well-adjusted personality without any psychotherapy whatsoever. If treatment with antibiotics should fail, psychotherapy will not benefit the patient either.

After the patient has gained insight, the problem should be frankly discussed with him and his relatives. Specific instructions as to medical checkups and the avoidance of hazardous occupations should be provided. Work around dangerous machines and the driving of trucks and buses should be prohibited, because a former general paralytic patient is never entirely safe from a seizure, although he may have been free of mental symptoms for years.[35]

The Fully Recovered Patient

The intelligence in this group shows no deviation from previous levels, and full working capacity is restored.[26] This is true not only of the simpler occupations, such as farming, but also of the professions. Kauders[46] reported a general paralytic patient who was treated in 1920 with therapeutic malaria and, twenty-seven years later, at the age of eighty, enjoyed full mental and physical health, being active as the manager of a circus.

The Partially Recovered Patient

In some cases the premorbid intellectual and emotional status cannot be restored. These patients require permanent institutional care. They constitute the bulk of the general paralytic patients who are at present in mental institutions. For example, hospitalization for approximately 5000 veterans of World War I, who developed insanity due to syphilis, has now been provided by the Veterans Administration.[69] In most of these patients, the delusions and the bizarre behavior have disappeared; they now represent all stages of mental deterioration. In some instances, cyclothymic manifestations have come into prominence, and others exhibit a schizophrenic picture with mannerisms and oddities which in no way can be differentiated from the classical type of schizophrenia. Since in some of these cases the spinal fluid abnormalities have reverted to normal and the pupillary reactions also have become normal, there are no longer clinical signs in the conventional sense of an organic psychosis.

Some authors attributed the new clinical picture to a concomitant affective or schizophrenic disorder.[66] The post-treatment psychiatric syndromes in general paralysis are complex exogenous reactions resulting from residual alterations of the brain cortex, which are so subtle that they do not reveal themselves with present methods of neurohistology.

Patients with residual brain damage at times have periods of acute agitation and require treatment with tranquilizing drugs.[40]

A paranoid-hallucinatory syndrome develops in a few patients during or after malaria or penicillin treatment.[21] Electroshock therapy is of benefit in this condition.

❲ Psychosis with Meningovascular Neurosyphilis

The term "meningovascular neurosyphilis" embraces syphilitic processes in the meninges and vessels of the brain. In contrast to general paralysis, which is always fatal if not treated, meningovascular syphilis frequently shows clinical and serologic improvement even without treatment.

The important anatomic feature is cerebral softening due to endarteritic occlusion of cerebral arteries. The common clinical manifestation is apoplexy resulting in a hemiplegia, which at times is associated with an aphasia. The hemiplegia often improves rapidly, without any therapy, and to a far greater degree than might be expected from the initial symptoms.

The focal lesions are sometimes associated with acute psychic disturbances, in which periods of confusion and delirious states are conspicuous. Clouding of consciousness develops in some patients, with complete disorientation of several months' duration. This may be followed by a rather sudden return to an almost normal mentality. In other instances, various degrees of emotional apathy or dementia may follow the stroke. Slight pupillary changes are frequently the only residual neurological signs.

The chronic mental disorders with meningovascular syphilis do not show any characteristic content and may resemble any psychotic state.[8]

Patients with gumma of the brain usually present mental symptoms, but a gummatous new growth is now a great rarity.[2,38]

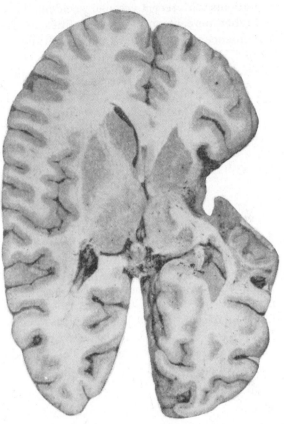

Figure 5–10. Meningovascular neurosyphilis. Large area of softening involving right internal capsule. Stroke at age of forty-one. The patient was hemiplegic and aphasic for the remainder of his life.

Laboratory Findings

Cerebrospinal Fluid Reactions

In the fluid, the cell count may vary between 5 and 500 cells per cubic mm. In half of the cases, the cell count is normal. The protein content ranges from normal values to 500 mg. per 100 cc. In a typical case, the colloidal gold reaction shows a mid-zone curve, but a first-

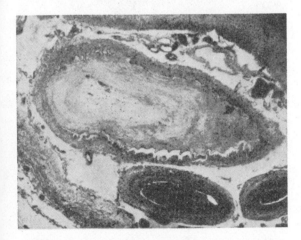

Figure 5–9. Syphilitic occlusion of artery in brain of patient with meningovascular neurosyphilis. Hematoxylin-eosin stain.

zone (paretic) curve is occasionally present. The Wassermann reaction in the spinal fluid is positive in two thirds of the cases, and in the blood in 80 percent. Occasionally, a positive Wassermann reaction of the blood or of the spinal fluid is the only abnormality.

ELECTROENCEPHALOGRAM

Patients with recent vascular accidents have a higher percentage of abnormalities in the electroencephalogram than those with old lesions.[37] In some patients with an old hemiplegia, the electroencephalogram is normal.

Therapy

In the treatment of meningovascular syphilis, a course of penicillin consisting of 10 million units is usually sufficient.

❰ The So-called "Tabetic Psychosis" Other Than Taboparalysis

In an occasional instance of tabes dorsalis, a psychotic state occurs, resulting from syphilitic endarteritis of the small cortical vessels. In 10 percent of tabes, general paralysis (taboparalysis) used to develop. This tragedy can now be prevented by penicillin therapy.

❰ Psychosis with Congenital Neurosyphilis

Juvenile General Paralysis

This form of general paralysis constituted 1.6–1.8 percent of all cases admitted to mental institutions.[55] In the great majority of cases, the illness begins around the age of fourteen or fifteen. In 10 percent the onset is before the sixth year of life, and in 3.6 percent mental symptoms begin after the twentieth year.

There are minor clinical variations from the adult form.[30] Mental retardation, which is present in about 40 percent, becomes appar-

ent soon after birth and is often associated with retarded physical development. Convulsions prior to the onset of juvenile general paralysis occur in one third of the cases, simulating idiopathic epilepsy. Optic atrophy is more frequent than in the adult form.

The psychiatric syndromes are less clearcut, with the exception of the dementing type. A schizophrenic picture with mutism, catatonic behavior, and negativism has been observed. One of my patients, a well-developed and intelligent seventeen-year-old Negro girl, without the physical stigmata of congenital syphilis and with normal pupillary reactions, was considered a catatonic schizophrenic, until a routine spinal fluid examination revealed findings characteristic of general paralysis. Following penicillin therapy there was complete recovery.

Stigmata of congenital syphilis are present in 75 percent and consist of Hutchinson's teeth (Figure 5–11), residue of previous interstitial

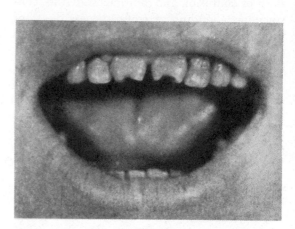

Figure 5–11. Juvenile (congenital) general paralysis. Hutchinson's teeth. Note notching of median incisors.

keratitis, and nerve deafness, listed according to their importance.

The anatomic changes in the brain are generally the same as in the adult type.

Juvenile Meningovascular Neurosyphilis

This type of congenital neurosyphilis is more frequent than juvenile general paralysis, but its diagnosis is infinitely more difficult because of the uncharacteristic clinical and serologic findings. Symptoms may be present at the time of birth or may make their appearance in infancy, puberty, or even later in life.[29]

Whenever congenital syphilis involves the central nervous system, it may cause arrest or deterioration of the intellectual development of the child.[6,23] Behavior disorders are occasionally observed in this type of cerebral involvement, which is usually stationary in nature. The abnormal behavior ranges from lying, stealing, and attacks of rage to impulsive acts. Irritability, restlessness, and depressive phases are often present. Two thirds of these problem children rate below average in intelligence, some being feeble-minded and others are borderline cases of mental deficiency. The remaining children possess normal intelligence.[52,67] Psychotic episodes may occur, associated with temporary confusion, periodic hallucinations, and pseudodementia.

Penicillin treatment shows particularly favorable results in progressive cases. In stationary cases with positive serologic reactions, therapy has a prophylactic effect in forestalling a new flare-up of the disease in later years.

(Bibliography

1. ALEXANDER, M. and J. TITECA. "L'Épilepsie post-malariathérapique," *J. Belge Neurol. Psychiatr.,* 36 (1936), 354.
2. ALPERS, B. J. "Gumma of the Brain," *Am. J. Syph.,* 23 (1939), 233.
3. ALZHEIMER, A. "Histologische Studien zur Differentialdiagnose der Progressiven Paralyse," in A. Alzheimer, and F. Nissl, eds., *Histologische und Histopathologische Arbeiten über die Grosshirnrinde, mit Besonderer Berücksichtigung der Pathologischen Anatomie der Geisteskrankheiten,* Vol. 1, p. 18. Jena: Fischer, 1905–1913.
4. ARIETI, S. "General Paresis in Senility; Critical Review of the Literature and Clinico-Pathologic Report of Six Cases," *Am. J. Psychiatry,* 101 (1945), 585.
5. BAYLE, A. L. J. *Recherches sur l'arachnitis chronique, la gastrite et la gastro-entérite chronique, et la goutte, considérées comme causes de l'aliénation mentale.* Paris: Didot le Jeune, 1822.
6. BENDA, C. E. "Syphilis in Serum Negative Feebleminded Children; A Histologic Study in Meningoencephalitis Syphilitica and in the Nissl-Alzheimer Endarteritis," *Am. J. Psychiatry,* 96 (1940), 1295.
7. BORGES FORTES, A. "Tratamento da Paralisia General pela Penicilina, *Arq. Bras. Neuriat. Psiquiatr.,* 51 (1956), 23. Penicilina e demência paralítica, O Hospital, Rio de Janeiro, November, 1956, pp. 645–673.
8. BOSTROEM, A. "Die Luespsychosen," in O. Bumke, ed., *Handbuch der Geisteskrankheiten,* Vol. 8, Spez. Teil 4, pp. 70–146. Berlin: Springer, 1930.
9. ———. "Die progressive Paralyse (Klinik)," in O. Bumke, ed., *Handbuch der Geisteskrankheiten,* Vol. 8, Spez. Teil 4, p. 248. Berlin: Springer, 1930.
10. BRUETSCH, W. L. "Activation of the Mesenchyme with Therapeutic Malaria," *J. Nerv. Ment. Dis.,* 76 (1932), 209.
11. ———. "The Histopathology of Therapeutic (Tertian) Malaria," *Am. J. Psychiatry,* 12 (1932), 19.
12. ———. "Penicillin or Malaria Therapy in the Treatment of General Paralysis? (A Clinico-Anatomic Study)," *Dis. Nerv. Syst.,* 10 (1949), 368.
13. ———. "Why Malaria Cures General Paralysis," *J. Indiana State Med. Assoc.,* 42 (1949), 211.
14. ———. "Penicillin Therapy of Cardiovascular Syphilis with Large Total Dosage; Its Rationale Based on Histologic Studies," *Am. J. Syph.,* 35 (1951), 252.
15. ———. *Syphilitic Optic Atrophy,* pp. 6, 57, 78. Springfield, Ill.: Charles C. Thomas, 1953.
16. ———. "Neurosyphilis: Symptomatology and Pathology," in A. B. Baker, ed., *Clinical Neurology,* Vol. 2, pp. 799–845. New York: Hoeber, 1955.
17. BUMKE, O. *Lehrbuch der Geisteskrankheiten,* p. 386. München: Bergmann, 1936.
18. CAJAL, S. R. "Neuroglia of the Cerebrum and Cerebellum in Progressive Paralysis with Technical Observations on the Silver Impregnation of Pathologic Nervous Tissue," *Z. Ges. Neurol. Psychiatr.,* 100 (1926), 738.
19. CALLAWAY, J. L., H. LÖWENBACH, R. O. NOOJIN et al. "Electroencephalographic

Findings in Central Nervous System Syphilis Before and After Treatment with Penicillin," *JAMA*, 129 (1945), 938.

20. CALMEIL, L. F. *De la Paralysie considérée chez les aliénés.* Paris: Baillière, 1826.

21. DATTNER, B. "Zur Frage der Paranoïd-Halluzinatorischen Paralysen," *Wien. Med. Wochnschr.*, 87 (1937), 278.

22. ———. "Treatment of Neurosyphilis with Penicillin Alone at Bellevue Hospital," *Am. J. Syph. Gonor. Ven. Dis.*, 32 (1948), 399.

23. DAYTON, N. A. "Degree of Mental Deficiency Resulting from Congenital Syphilis," *JAMA,* 87 (1926), 907.

24. DEWECK, A. L. in M. Samter et al., eds., *Immunological Diseases*, 2nd ed., p. 433. Boston: Little Brown, 1971.

25. EBAUGH, F. G., H. H. DIXON, H. E. KIENE et al. "Encephalographic Studies in General Paresis," *Am. J. Psychiatry*, 10 (1931), 737.

26. EPSTEIN, S. H. and H. C. SOLOMON. "The Effect of Treatment on the Mental Level of Patients with General Paresis," *Am. J. Psychiatry*, 95 (1939), 1181.

27. ESMARCH, F. and W. JESSEN. "Syphilis und Geistesstörung," *Allg. Ztschr. Psychiatr.*, 14 (1857), 20.

28. ESQUIROL, E. "Démence," in *Dictionaire des sciences médicales*, Vol. 8, p. 283. Paris: Panckoucke, 1814.

29. FERGUSON, F. R. and M. CRITCHLEY. "A Clinical Study of Congenital Neurosyphilis," *Br. J. Child. Dis.*, 26 (1929), 163.

30. ———. "A Clinical Study of Congenital Neurosyphilis. Part II. Congenital Tabes, Tabo-paresis and General Paralysis," *Br. J. Child. Dis.*, 27 (1930), 1.

31. FINLEY, K. H., A. S. ROSE, and H. C. SOLOMON. "Electroencephalographic Studies on Neurosyphilis," *Arch. Neurol. Psychiatry*, 47 (1942), 718.

32. FORSTER, E. and E. TOMASCZEWSKI. "Nachweis von Lebenden Spirochäten im Gehirm von Paralytikern," *Dtsch. Med. Wochnschr.*, 39 (1913), 1237.

33. GIANASCOL, A. J., G. D. WEICKHARDT, and M. A. NEUMANN. "Penicillin Treatment of General Paresis; A Clinicoanatomic Study," *Am. J. Syph.*, 38 (1954), 251.

34. GJESTLAND, T. "The Oslo Study of Untreated Syphilis; An Epidemiologic Investigation of the Natural Course of the Syphilitic Infection Based upon a Re-study of the Boeck-Bruusgaard Material," *Acta Derm. Venereol.*, Suppl. 34, 35 (1955), 1.

35. GOUGEROT, H. "Les Reliquats cicatriciels de la syphilis viscérale. Épilepsie résiduelle après guérison de la paralysie générale progressive," *Paris Méd.*, 1 (1929), 209.

36. GRANT, A. R. and H. T. KIRKLAND. "Spirochaetes in the Brain in General Paralysis," *J. Ment. Sci.*, 73 (1927), 595.

37. GREENBLATT, M. and S. LEVIN. "Factors Affecting the Electroencephalogram of Patients with Neurosyphilis," *Am. J. Psychiatry*, 102 (1945), 40.

38. GROSS, S. W., A. STEIN, and P. G. MYERSON. "Surgical Treatment of Gummas of the Brain," *Am. J. Surg.*, 58 (1942), 78.

39. HASLAM, J. *Observations on Insanity: with Practical Remarks on the Disease and an Account of the Morbid Appearances on Dissection.* London: Rivington, 1798.

40. HAYES, R. H. and I. WEBNER. "Chlorpromazine in the Treatment of Symptomatically Refractory Conditions in General Paretics," *Dis. Nerv. Syst.*, 17 (1956), 48.

41. HECHST, B. "Histopathologische Untersuchungen bei der Schizophrenen Form der Progressiven Paralyse," *Arch. Psychiatr.*, 102 (1934), 25.

42. HOOSHMAND, H., M. R. ESCOBAR, and S. W. KOPF. "Neurosyphilis: A Study of 241 Patients," *JAMA*, 219 (1972), 726–729.

43. IDSOE, O., T. GUTHE, R. P. WILLCOX et al. "Nature and Extent of Penicillin Side Reactions with Particular References to 151 Fatalities from Anaphylactic Shock," *Bull. WHO.*, 38 (1968), 159.

44. JAHNEL, F. "Die Spirochaeten bei der Paralyse," in O. Bumke, ed., *Handbuch der Geisteskrankheiten*, Vol. 11, pp. 498–538. Berlin: Springer, 1930.

45. JUNIUS, P. and M. ARNDT. "Beiträge zur Statistik, Aetiologie, Symptomatologie und pathologischen Anatomie der progressiven Paralyse," *Arch. Psychiatr.*, 44 (1908), 249.

46. KAUDERS, O. "Zur Klinik, Theorie und Geschichte der Malariabehandlung," *Wien. Z. Nervenheilkd.*, 1 (1947), 47.

47. KRAEPELIN, E. "General Paresis," Nerv. & Ment. Dis. Monogr., No. 14. New York: Nerv. & Ment. Dis. Publ. Co., 1913.

48. KRAFFT-EBING, VON, R. "Zur Kenntnis des Paralytischen Irreseins beim Weiblichen Geschlecht," *Arch. Psychiatr.*, 7 (1877), 182.

49. LISSAUER, H., and E. STORCH. "Uber einige Fälle Atypischer Progressiver Paralyse," *Monatsschr. Psychiatr. Neurol.*, 9 (1901), 401.

50. LÖWENBERG, K. "Syphilis of the Central Nervous System and of the Aorta," *Klin. Wochnschr.*, 3 (1924), 531.

51. LUCAS and PRICE. "Cooperative Evaluation and Treatment for Early Syphilis," *Br. J. Vener. Dis.*, 43 (1967), 244–248.

52. LURIE, L. A., J. V. GREENBAUM, and E. B. BRANDES. "Syphilis as a Factor in Behavior Disorders of Children," *Urol. Cutan. Rev.*, 45 (1941), 108.

53. McCARTNEY, J. L. "The Psychopathic Hospitals of Japan," *J. Nerv. Ment. Dis.*, 71 (1930), 640.

54. MAHONEY, J. F., R. C. ARNOLD, and A. HARRIS. "Penicillin Treatment of Early Syphilis; Preliminary Report," *Ven. Dis. Inform.*, 24 (1943), 355; *Am. J. Public Health*, 33 (1943), 1387.

55. MENNINGER, W. C. *Juvenile Paresis.* Baltimore: Williams & Wilkins, 1936.

56. MERRITT, H. H., M. MOORE, and H. C. SOLOMON. "The Iron Reaction in Paretic Neurosyphilis," *Am. J. Syph.*, 17 (1933), 387.

57. MERRITT, H. H. and M. SPRINGLOVA. "Lissauer's Dementia Paralytica; A Clinical and Pathologic Study," *Arch. Neurol. & Psychiatry*, 27 (1932), 987.

58. NEEL, A. V. and I. OSTENFELD. "Contribution to History of Dementia Paralytica with Special Reference to Contributions of Scandinavian, Particularly Danish Scientists," *Acta Psychiatr. Neurol.*, 21 (1946), 605.

59. NICOL, W. D. "General Paralysis of the Insane," *Br. J. Vener. Dis.*, 32 (1956), 9.

60. NISSL, F. "Zur Histopathologie der Paralytischen Rindenerkrankung," in A. Alzheimer, and F. Nissl, eds., *Histologische und Histopathologische Arbeiten über die Grosshirnrinde, mit Besonderer Berücksichtigung der Pathologischen Anatomie der Geisteskrankheiten*, Vol. 1, p. 315. Jena: Fischer, 1905–1913.

61. NOGUCHI, H. "Additional Studies on the Presence of Spirochaeta Pallida in General Paralysis and Tabes Dorsalis," *J. Cutan. Dis.*, 31 (1913), 543.

62. NOGUCHI, H. and J. W. MOORE. "A Demonstration of Treponema Pallidum in the Brain in Cases of General Paralysis," *J. Exp. Med.*, 17 (1913), 232.

63. ORLANDO, R. and M. ARNDT. *Paralisis General. Estado Actual y Problemas*, pp. 101, 179. Buenos Aires: Lopez & Etchegoyen, 1945.

64. ――――. "La atrofia óptica en la neurosífilis," *Neuropsiquiatría*, 1 (1950), 110.

65. PAGE, J. "Mental Disease in Russia," *Am. J. Psychiatry*, 94 (1938), 859.

66. ROTHSCHILD, D. "Dementia Paralytica Accompanied by Manic-Depressive and Schizophrenic Psychoses; the Significance of Their Co-existence," *Am. J. Psychiatry*, 96 (1940), 1043.

67. SCHULTE, H. "Klinischer Beitrag zur Kenntnis der Kongenitalluischen Störungen des Zentralnervensystems," *Z. Ges. Neurol. Psychiatr.*, 169 (1940), 250.

68. SPARLING, F. "Diagnosis and Treatment of Syphilis," *N. Engl. J. Med.*, 284 (1971), 642–657.

69. TAGGART, S. R., S. B. RUSSELL, and E. V. PRICE. "Report of Syphilis Follow-up Program Among Veterans After World War II," *J. Chron. Dis.*, 4 (1956), 579.

70. THOMAS, E. W. "Current Status of Therapy in Syphilis," *JAMA*, 162 (1956), 1536.

71. VAN WULFFTEN PALTHE, P. M. "Syphilis des Nervensystems bei Asiaten in Niederländisch-Indien (Java und Sumatra)," *Acta Psychiatr. Neurol.*, 12 (1937), 207.

72. VIRCHOW, R. "In Discussion of: Tabische Sehnerven Atrophie, Tabes, Progressive Paralyse und Aneurysma der Aorta," *Berl. Klin. Wochnschr.*, 35 (1898), 691.

73. VOLLAND, W. "Ueber das 'Paralyseeisen' und die Eisenablagerungen bei Mesaortitis Syphilitica unter Besonderer Berücksichtigung ihrer Herkunft und Spezifität (Histopathologische und Humoralpathologische Untersuchungen)," *Arch. Path. Anat.*, 309 (1942), 145.

74. WAGNER-JAUREGG, J. and W. L. BRUETSCH. "The History of the Malaria Treatment of General Paralysis," *Am. J. Psychiatry*, 102 (1946), 577.

75. WARRELL, D. A. "Physiologic Changes during the Jarisch-Herxheimer Reaction in Early Syphilis," *Am. J. Med.*, 284 (1971), 642–657.

76. WONG, Y. T. and H. PACKER. "Penicillin Versus Penicillin-Malaria in the Treatment of Dementia Paralytica," *Am. J. Syph., Gonor. Ven. Dis.*, 32 (1948), 212.

CHAPTER 6

POSTENCEPHALITIC STATES OR CONDITIONS

Henry Brill

❰ Postencephalitic States or Conditions

VARIOUS acute encephalitic syndromes have long been recognized[20] but postencephalitic states, as they are now understood, did not emerge as important until the 1916–1930 epidemic of encephalitis lethargica which showed that such a disease could do vast damage and that medicine was quite unprepared to cope with viral encephalitis. This experience had a profound impact on medical thinking and left great concern that this disease or even a more devastating one might break out again. This fear has now abated, but recent advances in general virology indicate that the concern was not without foundation. In an article entitled "Viruses may Surprise Us"[13] Sabin is quoted as saying that new syndromes may be caused by familiar viruses, by new ones, or by new antigenic variants as in the case of influenza. He feels that more study needs to be directed toward pre- and postnatal viral infections in

congenital defects. The potential scope of this problem is seen in his statement that "The viruses of the human heritage which maintain themselves in nature by passing from one human being to another, now number about 200—the vast majority identified during the last 10 years." He states, "In addition, studies mostly of recent years have revealed at least 200 distinct viruses in the arthropod-borne group."

It is clear that we live more intimately with the world of viruses than was previously realized and many of them are now known to attack the central nervous system. The resulting syndromes are described as meningitis, meningo-encephalitis, and encephalomyelitis, according to the pathology which tends to predominate, but there is a continuum among these pathological forms and mixed states are common.

Most of these infections, such as herpes simplex, Japanese B encephalitis, and St. Louis encephalitis, do not become chronic, and they leave residual central nervous system damage in only a minority of cases. Such damage can be severe and may be focal and/or diffuse, but it is not progressive. The acute infection may be marked by a well-defined febrile episode associated with the usual cerebral signs such as stiff neck, stupor, coma, convulsions, and myoclonia, but at least in some postencephalitic states there may be no such history.[10] One can only speculate what part such infections may play in the total psychiatric scene. So far we know only about cases where the damage is severe or the clinical syndrome is specific. It remains to be seen whether viral infections can also cause minor degrees of damage which lead to conduct disorders, hyperkinesis of children, and other syndromes now gathered under the controversial rubric of minimal brain dysfunction (MBD). For a time, the experience with Von Economo's encephalitis suggested that this was a distinct possibility, but most authorities now seem to reject this view.

To some extent, the question has been reopened by the discovery of chronic virus infections of the central nervous system, especially that of Kuru and slow measles in man, as well as scrapie and visna in animals (see p. 163). In addition it has been shown that viruses may multiply within morphologically intact neurons and produce disease through dysfunction of these neurons.[2] What may be the psychiatric significance of these data remains for future research to decide, but it is now certain that encephalitis lethargica is not the only chronic progressive viral infection of the brain.

Classification and Nomenclature

Terminology in this field makes use of anatomical, clinical, and etiological names but is actually controlled by usage. Thus the so called postencephalitic states following Von Economo's disease are, in fact, chronic encephalitic states, with pathological evidence of continued active inflammation alongside evidence of previous destruction. They were designated as postencephalitic because historically they were observed after acute infections and long before the chronic nature of the infection was fully understood; the term has now been established by usage. Usage has also decreed that the major postencephalitic and chronic encephalitic states, which were known before Von Economo's disease was discovered, should continue to be described separately under their old designations, and this includes such entities as rheumatic chorea, paresis, and rabies, as well as infantile cerebral palsy. On the other hand, the postencephalitic and chronic encephalitic disorders which were recognized after Von Economo's encephalitis tend to be classed with the postencephalitic states.

This is true even though postencephalitic residuals were recognized well before Von Economo's time. Oppenheim, as quoted by Mayer,[20] noted already in 1900 that such damage could be left after measles, scarlet fever, pneumonia, erysipelas, whooping cough, and mumps, and after the hemorrhagic encephalitis of influenza. These syndromes must, however, have been considered neurological rather than psychiatric because the prestigious Tuke's *Dictionary of Psychological Medicine* in 1892 does not even list a category of encephalitis.[25] It describes "inflammation of the brain" but only under the heading of "delirium." The *Dictionary* even mentions mental disorders following influenza but does not appear to relate them to brain damage.

Advance has been spectacular since the days of Oppenheim and even Von Economo, but many uncertainties still remain, and we still have no fully established system of classification of the syndromes now recognized as encephalitic or postencephalitic.

Some of the disorders are classified by their vectors as in the case of arthopod-borne viruses (arbo viruses); others are classified on the basis of pathology (hemorrhagic encephalitis); some by the distribution of pathology (leukoencephalitis), still others by geographical titles (Japanese B., Australian X, Russian summer encephalitis), and some by the host species (fox encephalitis, equine encephalitis). Finally, the classification by pathological syndrome is also of a multiple nature and may be based on the distribution of the reaction (leukoencephalitis), the location of the pathology as in encephalomyelitis, or the nature of response (inclusion body encephalitis).

As the etiological agents are identified, descriptive terms are becoming more specific, or are being displaced by terms derived from the etiological agent such as "encephalitis due to slow measles virus." Even an etiological classification must at this time, however, remain incomplete because the classification of the viruses themselves is still a matter of vigorous debate.[29]

Distinctions among the various forms of encephalitis and postencephalitic states, other than the Von Economo type, still remain of limited clinical importance, and a simple account of the major forms seems adequate for most purposes since they represent essentially chronic, static, nonspecific organic brain syndromes. Nevertheless, the clinician cannot ignore even the acute reactions, if only because he must usually diagnose the postencephalitic states retrospectively and on the basis of clinical history and hospital records of the initial infection.

(Encephalitis Lethargica (Von Economo's Disease)

History

In 1917 Von Economo described what seemed to be a new epidemic disease which he called encephalitis lethargica. During the next few years this disorder took on pandemic proportions and involved tens of thousands of victims leaving an estimated one third of them with permanent, progressive, bizarre neuropsychiatric residuals.[20,26] Decades of research have failed to resolve the mystery of the origin of this disorder or its mode of transmission. The etiological agent is presumed to be a virus, but it has not been isolated nor have specific immune bodies been identified, even though a considerable number of cases still survive with what appears to be a chronic active encephalitic process.

The original outbreak overlapped the 1919 pandemic of influenza and for a long time these two disorders were confused with each other, but they are now considered to be entirely separate.

During the epidemic and for some time thereafter scientific interest was intense, and it was hoped that this strange new disease would be a sort of a medical Rosetta Stone which would provide neurophysiological equivalents of somatic events and vice versa.[21] Many challenging questions were raised because of the close association of a well-defined neuropathology with classical functional disorders such as compulsive obsessive states, hysterical neuroses, and psychoses with severe conduct disorders, all of them intertwined with neurological and neurovegetative changes. Contemporary observers were firmly convinced that they were observing not simple release phenomena but specific reactions to the damage caused by encephalitis. For a time the issues which had been raised seemed to have good hopes of resolution, but research results were minimal, and scientific interest finally faded. It was not until the development of the major tranquilizers and the subsequent introduction of L-Dopa that such hopes were revived.

Epidemiology

The epidemiology of encephalitis lethargica has now receded into medical history. The disease may have been endemic in Eastern Europe, and Neal[21] quotes papers to that effect, but the first well-documented scientific report deals with the 1916–1917 epidemic which soon became pandemic and persisted for at least a dozen years as a disease of winter months. It involved persons of all ages, but mainly between ten and thirty. Direct transmission was not shown to be a factor, and the incubation period appeared to run from several days to two weeks. The total number of victims is unknown, although in Britain[15] the peak of the outbreak was reached with 5036 cases reported in 1924. In New York 1247 cases were admitted to mental hospitals between 1919 and 1939. Wilson[26] states that mental signs remained in over half the cases who had them during the acute phase and were seen in about a third of all survivors below the age of sixteen. Other authorities estimate that about a third of all the victims died, while another third suffered the progressive disorder and only a third recovered. Many of those subsequently disabled could give no history of an acute attack.

The subsequent course of the epidemic was no less mysterious than its origin. By 1930 it had apparently run its course, although sporadic cases were reported for the next decade or more and some authors were still reporting occasional cases in the 1960s.[8] The *Lancet* published such a paper and raised serious questions editorially as to the diagnosis, but still was moved to ask: "If the infection has not vanished, does it perhaps lurk under other guise . . . and is recrudescence still a possibility?"[15] This unanswered question still haunts the subject.

Pathology

The acute lesion is nonpurulent and nonhemorrhagic, which distinguishes it from the bacterial infections and influenza, respectively. It is located in the gray matter of the brain and the cord, which separates it from various types of leukoencephalitis (measles, mumps, vaccina). Inflammatory perivascular reaction is usually severe, and microscopic foci are widely disseminated, particularly in the cortex (Figure 6–1), basal ganglia (Figure 6–2), hypothalamus, and periaqueductal gray matter of the brain stem. The substantia nigra is especially damaged (Figure 6–3), and this damage remains a hallmark of the disease. In chronic cases the usual residuals of old inflammation are found, particularly in the basal ganglia and mesencephalon, but in addition, even after many years, new areas of active inflammation are to be seen in the same general distribution. The pathological findings are highly variable as to intensity and distribution, which is in striking contrast to the relative uniformity of the clinical typology.

Etiology and Pathogenesis

The etiology has always been assumed to be a filterable virus, even though no inclusion

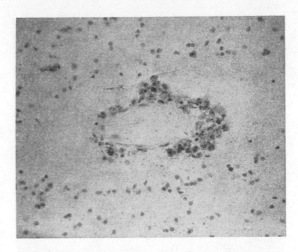

Figure 6–1. Cerebrum: White matter disclosing a blood vessel with enlarged perivascular space containing an inflammatory exudate (some macrophages are filled with yellowish or greenish pigmentation). Nissl stain; medium-power magnification.

bodies have been described, no virus isolated, and no specific immune bodies identified.

Originally, theories as to pathogenesis revolved about the location of the neuropathology and the nature of the underlying psychopathology of the individual. It is perhaps a measure of the state of medical thinking at that time that social issues received no attention. The neuropathology did indeed indicate that the central gray was important for psychic functioning, and the damage to the basal ganglia and substantia nigra was correlated with the Parkinsonian syndrome. Nevertheless, the available explanations were never adequate to account for the complex pattern of this disorder. Theories based on psychodynamics and personality studies were equally unsatisfying, and indeed most authors opposed the idea that this postencephalitic syndrome was simply a release phenomenon and an expression of underlying personality. As Rosner said, "The tragic feature is personality change, not personality exaggeration."[21] A new chapter in the understanding of the pathogenesis of this disorder was opened in the early 1950s, and some of the mystery was dispelled when it was found that full doses of the tranquilizing agents of the phenothiazine and Rauwolfia series can reproduce many of the

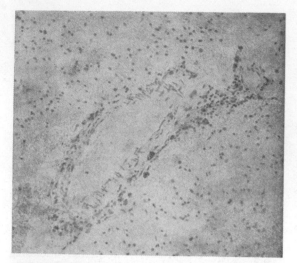

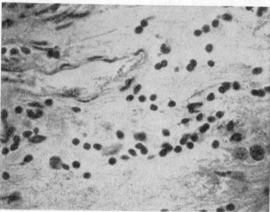

Figure 6–2. (top) An area in the globus pallidus revealing the presence of a perivascular inflammatory reaction. Nissl stain; low-power magnification. (bottom) Perivascular inflammatory exudate showing predominance of lymphocytes. Nissl stain; medium-power magnification.

features of the chronic encephalitic syndrome in a quantitatively controllable, reversible, and nonprogressive form. Such symptoms include Parkinsonian rigidity, masked facies, tremor, salivation, and on occasion even oculogyric crises, dystonia, torsion spasm, and akathesia. Use of these tranquilizers may also precipitate emotional complications, especially depression, restlessness, and tension, all of which are seen in the postencephalitic syndrome. One can even see some parallel between the rousable stupor of acute encephalitis and that produced by heavy phenothiazine dosage.

The significance of the curious parallelism

between the tranquilizer-induced reactions and those resulting from lethargic encephalitis has since been further clarified by observations of the action of another drug, L-Dopa. This drug was originally developed on the basis of a hypothesis that the Parkinsonian symptoms

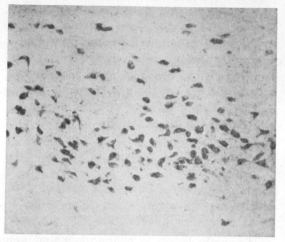

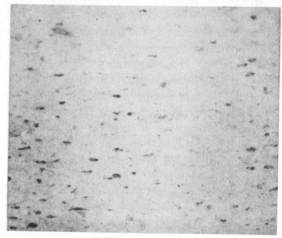

Figure 6–3. (top) Substantia nigra of an adult (control case). (bottom) Depigmentation and pronounced loss of neurons in the substantia nigra in a postencephalitic Parkinsonian syndrome. Nissl stain; medium-power magnification.

were related to the observed depletion of brain dopamine, especially in the basal ganglia and substantia nigra. Dopamine itself proved ineffective, but L-Dopa, which is converted to dopamine in the brain, proved to be of value. It is thought to act as a neurotransmitter of inhibitory impulses, and counterbalances the central acetylcholine which is excitatory. A lack of dopamine appears to release an overaction of acetylcholine, and this imbalance is thought to be a fundamental cause of Parkinson's syndrome. It is of great theoretical interest that the new drug can itself initiate a wide variety of dose-dependent reversible psychiatric and neurological symptoms, because this gives further evidence that dopamine is indeed important in psychic as well as neurological functioning. All this has again directed major scientific attention to a study of the Parkinsonian syndrome, but this time it is at the level of molecular biology.[19]

Psychiatric Symptoms

Perhaps the most difficult aspect of this singular disease to describe is the psychiatric symptomatology. To those who know the cases, chronic encephalitis has a high degree of specificity and a quality which can hardly be mistaken, but it is virtually impossible to identify and completely separate the components of the diagnosis. The physician's impression is constellative, global, and composed of a blend of psychiatric, neurological, and vegetative symptoms and signs, no one of which is specific in isolation from the others. The psychiatric symptoms are not typically organic in nature, since memory and intellect are not impaired, and when they occur in the absence of other findings, there is nothing to distinguish this disorder from personality disorder, neurosis, hypochondriasis, or functional psychosis. Many postencephalitics were indeed treated under other diagnoses during their pre-Parkinsonian phase and correctly classified only as neurological symptoms emerged, often an event of chagrin and surprise for the psychiatrist.

Wilson comments that "despite variations the generic picture is curiously precise, but none the less cumbersome to define."[26] This holds true of the psychiatric as well as the neurological aspects and, indeed, any separation between the two must be, to a large extent, artificial, since even the grossest postencephalitic Parkinsonian syndrome has functional components, while tics and character-istic compulsive and phobic symptoms are found so regularly associated with the disorder that it is hard to escape the conclusion that some organic factor underlies both. The view that symptoms are determined by both organic and dynamic factors as stated by Schilder[24] seems entirely tenable. We will now consider some of the commoner postencephalitic subsyndromes.

CONDUCT DISORDER

Especially in children, even before the onset of gross neurological symptoms, severe conduct disorder was a frequent sequel, beginning immediately after the acute infection or after a delay of months. Among the characteristics of the children, particularly the group aged three to ten years, were a marked destructiveness and impulsiveness, with a tendency to carry primitive impulses into headlong action. Children who had previously behaved normally, would lie, steal, destroy property, set fire, and commit sexual offenses, without thought of punishment. The motivation was even less comprehensible and less subject to immediate control than in the so-called psychopathies, but the capacity for real remorse was strikingly well retained. A characteristic instability of emotion, coupled with disinhibition of action, led to serious aggressions, usually against others, but occasionally against the patient himself, resulting in gruesome self-mutilations. Institutionalization of these cases was imperative and led to the development of some of the early units for inpatient care of emotionally disturbed children, notably the one at Kings Park State Hospital in New York, in 1924.

In adults, conduct disorder was also a serious problem, although not to the same degree as in children. Yet the results were a serious problem, and a famous virologist whose father was a victim of this disease once commented to me that it had changed him from a well-known academician into "an animal." Like the children, adults would express deep remorse and retained the capacity for self-criticism of their behavior, which seemed to have a compulsive quality. There was often a marked discrepancy between the good intellectual capacity and the primitive behavior. Such a patient was a "master of what he said" but, in his compulsive action, was a "slave of what he did." In the mental hospital these patients were known for their impulsive behavior and occasional aggressiveness, even though they usually made good emotional contact and could discuss things quite clearly. Lethargic encephalitis is described as being able to cause convulsive disorder in children; in very young patients mental deficiency is also a possible outcome.

Cases of conduct disorder due to Von Economo's disease are now no longer seen. They were usually at their worst before the onset of obvious neurological symptoms, and the behavior problems gradually disappeared as the neurological disability advanced. In addition, of course, childhood cases have long since ceased to appear.

Schizophrenic-like Reactions

Reactions similar to schizophrenia have been described, but true schizophrenia is quite unusual, and, on closer examination, these are seen to be pseudoschizophrenias. The emotional reaction is shallow and often dull and apathetic, but it is still postencephalitic and not schizophrenic. Delusions of reference and hallucinations may occur, but they are superficial and lacking in schizophrenic symbolism. Certain of the motor rigidities of encephalitis lethargica sometimes bear a superficial resemblance to catatonia, and various paranoid reactions, especially of transitory nature, also occur. Paranoid hallucinatory and delusional syndromes are sometimes due to atropine-type medications but are usually a part of the postencephalitic picture. They are distinguished from schizophrenia by the absence of the usual schizophrenic disorders of emotion and thought and the lack of autism. Actually, the postencephalitic patient tends to manifest strong dependency needs, and this leads to a clinging relationship which is quite the opposite of schizophrenic withdrawal, and his ability to discuss and control his problems is also different in quality from that seen in schizophrenia. This aspect of the chronic encephalitic reaction is well described by Schilder.[24]

Depression

A strong tendency to depression is reflected in the characteristic whining voice, clinging manner, and dependent and complaining attitude. Depression often centers about the physical symptoms, and is hard to distinguish from hypochondriasis. Self-accusations and delusions of guilt may take the form of a monotonous plaint whose pattern is perhaps so strongly colored by the facies, the voice, and the bradykinesis and bradyphrenia that it seems different from ordinary depressions. The pleading, demanding, and impatient clinging resembles what one sometimes encounters in epileptics. The content tends to be of an organic depressive nature. Euphoria is described but is relatively unusual.

In a review of 201 cases of postencephalitic Parkinsonism, Neal found pathological depression listed nine times, psychotic depression eight times, and hypomania eight times, but depression of the pattern described above is far more frequent.[21]

Hypochondriasis

Patients may complain of almost all forms of physical discomfort. These include pains, burning, tension, restless feelings, shooting sensations, and dead feelings, as well as hypochondriacal concern about heart, lungs, stomach, etc. Verbal productions are often marked by a compulsive quality and are full of expressions of frustration, impatience, and discomfort, but these are difficult to evaluate since the disease attacks neural elements throughout the central nervous system; often the patients leave the impression that they may be suffering from something akin to central pain.

The response to placebo is striking and could well shake the confidence of the strongest organicist; no patients are more suggestible or more readily pacified for a short time by a new therapy. Yet they are equally suggestible with respect to some of the gross neurological symptoms and can even be brought to suppress the Parkinsonian tremors for brief periods of time. In this connection they seem to be manifesting an organically determined disorder of volition.

EYE FINDINGS

Among the most common complaints are those centered about the eyes. The patients seem to be trying to verbalize some indescribable sense of discomfort, and indeed, their eyes often appear congested and uncomfortable. Some of this must be laid to loss of eye blink and the long periods of rigid stare with resultant fatigue and discomfort in the muscles and periocular tissues, but the oculogyric crisis as yet remains without full explanation of either functional or organic type. It is now reproduceable chemically with some of the phenothiazines and with L-Dopa. In postencephalitics it is strongly associated with other psychiatric symptoms such as forced thinking and stereotyped ideas or a compulsive preoccupation with the eyes of others. Attacks may be periodic and fairly regular but are usually irregular. They may be controlled for a time by an effort of will, but the patients do not consider the attacks as subject to volition since they complain, "My eyes turn up," and not "I have to turn my eyes up." The usual direction of gaze is upward, but variants include forced gaze in other directions and combinations with postural distortions. Attacks may last from minutes to hours and may be interrupted only by falling asleep.

Other ocular complaints include burning, blurred vision, photophobia, shooting pains, macropsia, micropsia, and visual distortion. Here too one can identify functional components, but disorder of the visual neurological apparatus is extensive, and these patients also suffer from various opthalmoplegias, often with diplopia, and show pupillary anomalies and accommodation difficulties. The staring, unblinking expression and masklike greasy facies may suggest the diagnosis at first glance.

Work Capacity

Loss of work capacity is sometimes given little emphasis in psychiatric descriptions, per-haps because it is not obvious in the examining room, and it often seems to be assumed that this impairment is, somehow, secondary to other factors. However, in a number of neuropsychiatric disorders and especially in the postencephalitic state, as well as in other conditions with brain damage, impairment of work capacity can be a leading symptom and a disability of its own, not strongly correlated with other signs or symptoms and highly resistant to therapy. As yet little studied, except in relation to vocational and other types of rehabilitation, this problem is prominent and persistent in postencephalitics, may antedate gross neuropsychiatric findings, and quite commonly continues after they are brought under control by medication; it may be related to the chronic sense of fatigue often described and to slowness of thinking or bradyphrenia.

Neurological and Vegetative Symptoms

Parkinsonism is by far the commonest finding. This is characterized by masking of the face, loss of blink, and in the extremities a characteristic rhythmical tremor, rigidity, and loss of associated reflexes. It is less frequent in children and has a marked tendency to progress. Onset is characteristically insidious, local and asymmetrical; it spreads gradually to other parts of the body, becoming more intense and more general, until the fully developed syndrome is present. The motor disability, even when severe, may be briefly reversible, sometimes in a spectacular manner. The author once saw a severely incapacitated former boxer, who had been annoyed for days by a fellow patient, suddenly recapture his motor capacity with great effect, and then lapse again into a full Parkinsonian state. On command, such patients can regularly suspend their tremor for a short time, and catch a ball or carry out some other brief coordinated task, but despite pride in their performance, they do not initiate it themselves. The moment they relax, the rigidity and rhythmical tremor take over again. Gait is characteristic and diagnostic. Associated movements of the arms and trunk are impaired or lost. The arms do not swing, and in the fully developed syndrome the body is carried "en bloc." In addition, there are almost always bizarre changes and motor distortions. The patient leans conspicuously, usually forward but sometimes backward or to the side; he sidles, or shuffles along with some typical oddity of movement; often it looks like a tic blended into the walk. Among the variants are propulsive gait, a tendency to lean forward and walk always faster in a half run which may not stop till the patient reaches a point of support, or retropulsion—a similar tendency to walk or run backward. The usual postencephalitic compulsive quality characterizes these symptoms too.

Rigidity is of cogwheel type and asymmetrical. Tics and mannerisms of many kinds are seen, among them torticollis, facial grimaces, and movements difficult to distinguish from torsion spasms. The tremor, which is a rhythmical rest tremor, ceases only during sleep; it is most often seen in the upper extremities but may involve other parts, especially the legs, jaw, and tongue, in various combinations. Among the rarer syndromes are cataplexies and myasthenoid disturbances as well as chorealike movements. All of these bear the stamp of the basic disease.

The speech of the well-developed case is highly characteristic, and the many varieties have a common denominator. The voice is monotonous, nasal and somewhat singsong, and often trails off into nothingness, as does the writing, because spasm increases as the activity progresses. Frequently observed is palilalia, a needless repetition of words or phrases. Sometimes dysarthria is prominent, and sometimes bradykinesis; often, refuge is taken in a few hastily spoken words, followed by staring silence.

Hypersalivation is the most prominent of the purely vegetative findings and, combined with the masking and stiffness of the face and lips, often leads to drooling. Among the wide variety of other neurovegetative disturbances are seborrhea of the face, irregularity of respiration often of bizarre form, marked adiposity (sometimes with polydipsia and polyuria), disturbances of appetite and of sleep, lability of temperature control, excess perspiration, and pupillary irregularities.

COURSE

The chronic syndrome may follow the initial infection immediately or after a latent period which may last for many years. Once neurological symptoms have been established, the usual course is irregularly progressive although static cases have been described. Pregnancy, trauma, infection, or other stress can produce exacerbations. A majority of the cases now seen in ordinary clinic and hospital practice give no history of acute encephalitis, although sometimes a story of illness with diplopia or hypersomnia can be elicited. In this respect the sequence is analogous to that of paresis.

Differential Diagnosis

Diagnosis rests on the neurological and neurovegetative findings and the history of progression. This disorder is distinguished from Parkinson's disease by the asymmetry and irregularity of the symptoms and the bizarre additional elements. The postencephalitic form is also to be distinguished from the many nonprogressive types of Parkinsonian syndrome. None of these has the vegetative findings or the typical encephalitic disturbances of gait, station, and behavior. Poisoning by carbon monoxide or manganese, cerebral trauma, and Wilson's disease may also produce basal ganglion symptoms, and these are similarly differentiated. Parkinsonism due to medication may combine with a neurological disability of other origin to produce puzzling syndromes, but the matter becomes clear when medication is withdrawn.

In the case of a child with pure behavior disorder, diagnosis poses a more difficult problem, and in the absence of at least minor specific progressive neurological findings, or of a known outbreak it would seem that the diagnosis of encephalitis lethargica should not be made.

⟨ Treatment

Treatment of the chronic encephalitic syndrome remains symptomatic. Medication, regimen, psychotherapy, and psychosurgery are all used, and effects in the psychic, somatic, and social spheres reinforce each other.

Medication

The pharmacological therapies are, in general, used according to schedules which call for titrating drugs against symptoms, the end point being a satisfactory effect, or symptoms of toxic overdose, whichever comes first, and often the two are not far apart. The topic is so complex as to forbid a complete review of all drugs in this paper, but drug-induced Parkinsonism has made this type of treatment commonplace, and there are many excellent descriptions; one example is Chap. 72 in the 1971 *AMA Drug Evaluations*.[1]

Three general classes of drugs are now available, the anticholinergic, the antihistamines, and the newer drugs levodopa and amantidine. The anticholinergic drugs tend to lose their effectiveness with continued administration, and for this reason a fairly complex pharmacy is necessary, but shifts from one to another medication should not be made abruptly.[7] The anticholinergic group produces atropinelike side effects and one must watch for such complications as prostatism, glaucoma, and serious loss of accommodation for near vision. Temperature control may also be impaired, and this is doubly important because it appears that this function is already weakened by the encephailitis, and deaths from heat stroke can occur. Fortunately, the newer anticholinergics have far less peripheral effect than the original drugs which they have now virtually replaced. The older drugs include atropine itself, scopolamine, hyoscyamine, stramonium, and bellabulgara. In addition, the amphetamines once had considerable vogue.

The anticholinergic drugs in current use are synthetic and include trihexyphenedyl HCl (Artane, Pipanol, Tremin HCl), biperiden (Akineton), cycrimine HCl (Pagitane) and procyclidine HCl (Kemadrin).[1]

The antihistamine-type drugs are of weaker action, have fewer side effects and are used chiefly to potentiate the effects of the anti-cholinergics or for patients who cannot tolerate the more potent drugs. They include diphenhydramine HCl (Benadryl), chlor-phenoxamine HCl (Phenoxene), and orphenadrine HCl (Disipal). Benztropine mesylate (Cogentin) is described as intermediate between the anticholinergics and the antihistaminics in therapeutic potency and side reactions.

Both L-Dopa and amantidine appear to be effective in postencephalitic Parkinsonism and seem to represent a distinct advance[3,22] in practice as well as theory. L-Dopa (levodopa) influences all the symptoms, akinesia, ridigity, and tremor being benefited in that order. Toxic effects are frequent and include mental symptoms and various types of involuntary movement.[3] It appears that in the present state of knowledge, L-Dopa is best reserved to treat the exacerbations of the postencephalitic state and to give relief in the intractable cases. Amantidine is also effective but far less dramatic. It has milder side effects, is additive to the anticholinergic drugs and does not appear to establish tolerance. Where, for any reason, the anticholinergic drugs are withdrawn, the process should be gradual to avoid serious aggravation of symptoms.[7]

Regimen

All authors acknowledge that the general management of the patient is important. Adequate nutrition, regular exercise within the limits of the patient's capacity, maintenance of interest and activity, moderate recreational interests and hobbies, physiotherapy, vocational training, and rehabilitation where indicated, are all important elements. On the other hand, overstress is harmful, and excess fatigue is to be avoided. Alcohol is usually poorly tolerated and is not advised. Above all, an optimistic constructive attitude on the part of the physician is crucial.

Psychotherapy

Complex psychotherapeutic techniques have been described by various authors, but I am inclined to agree with Rosner quoted by

Neal,[21] that "effective psychotherapy in chronic encephalitis still demands a rather primitive dependence on rapport between patient and doctor." While there are limitations, the psychotherapeutic modalities which are available should be tried. Used in conjunction with the drug therapy and regimen, they can produce marked amelioration of an otherwise intolerable existence.

Neurosurgery

Neurosurgery has been reserved for far advanced intractable cases of postencephalitic Parkinsonism. Destructive lesions of the globus pallidus,[18] the thalamus,[27] the subthalamic region, and even the internal capsule have all been reported as producing desirable results.[14] When successful, these procedures improve both rigidity and tremor on the opposite side of the body, with corresponding general improvement of symptoms. Bilateral operations are common. Among the earlier operations were cortical excisions to control tremor and rigidity, and nerve sections for torticollis.

([Other Postencephalitic States

The spectacular experience with encephalitis lethargica focused medical attention on encephalitis as a cause of neuropsychiatric disorders, and within a few years a number of new entities were identified. The first was St. Louis encephalitis described in 1933.[12] Others include Japanese B encephalitis, Australian X disease, and Murray Valley encephalitis.

The late 1960s have seen spectacular advances in virology due to such technical improvements as new methods of virus culture, the use of the electron microscope for identification, and the development of new immunological techniques, such as immunofluorescent staining methods. As a result the number of identified viruses has greatly increased and various types of viral encephalitis are being diagnosed and reported routinely. They re-main, however, more important from the point of view of public health than from that of psychiatry, because in most types the acute attack generally ends in complete recovery, although death rates are sometimes high. When residuals do occur they are nonspecific and nonprogressive, and their treatment belongs to that of the organic syndromes. Certain rare types of chronic progressive encephalitis have, however, been identified and because of this fact and because the various forms of encephalitis do represent a variety of central nervous system pathology, these viral infections do have some psychiatric interest. A brief discussion of several of the more important types of viral encephalitis is presented here. For a more exhaustive account of the virology, the reader is referred to the comprehensive report by Whitty et al.[28]

([Encephalitis Due to Arbo Viruses (Arthropod-Borne)

These include St. Louis, Japanese B, equine, and California encephalitis, and Colorado tick fever, some sixty types in all.[12] They vary widely as to morbidity and mortality; recovery with severe sequelae is not unusual.[9,23] The residual defect is nonspecific and therapy is that of the focal and diffuse syndromes which follow. Many of these disorders occur in epidemic form.[9]

([Hemorrhagic Encephalitis

Hemorrhagic encephalitis has been known for at least 200 years. It may complicate many types of infection but is most frequently associated with influenza. Recovery with serious damage is reported even in the older literature.[20,21] The lesion is nonprogressive, nonspecific, focal and/or diffuse, and the treatment of these postencephalitic states is that of the chronic brain syndrome which follows.[21]

Postinfectious Encephalitis (Leukoencephalitis)

Postinfectious encephalitis is a variety occasionally seen after many viral infections,[9] especially the exanthems, and the statement is often made that within recent years such reactions have become more frequent.

After infection with such viruses as varicella, variola, measles, mumps, vaccina, or after rabies vaccination, acute demyelinating encephalomyelitis may develop very rapidly. This is primarily in the white matter and tends to center about the venous system. The nature of the reaction remains obscure; it is not considered to be due to a direct attack of the virus on the nervous tissue but probably represents an immunologic allergic mechanism similar to that of experimental allergic encephalomyelitis. The location of the offending virus, the site of autoimmune body formation, and the nature of the reaction remain to be explored. Thrombosis of small vessels and areas of necrosis and hemorrhage are found. When recovery occurs, it is usually complete, but there may be severe residuals with hemiplegia, convulsions, mental defect, and behavior disorder. Such syndromes may be also due to vascular lesions of unknown mechanism which can complicate a wide variety of systemic infections in children.

Other Types

Among the types left to be discussed, the slow, latent, or chronic types[11] are especially interesting. The demonstration of "slow" measles virus as an etiological agent in encephalitis[2] of children is of great theoretical importance even though the condition is relatively rare. This virus attacks the parenchyma directly, invades the cells and replicates within them and is thus quite different in mechanism from the encephalitis which is generally caused by the exanthems. It is of insidious onset, and generally progresses with increasing cerebral symptoms such as mental deterioration and myoclonus to a fatal outcome within a year. Measles can also cause the usual leukoencephalitis like that following other exanthems.

Amantidine has been reported as checking[6] the spread of slow measles encephalitis, which is now thought to include several disorders previously known under such names as subacute sclerosing panencephalitis (SSPE) (Pette Dohring), subacute sclerosing leukoencephalitis (Van Bogaert), and Dawson's inclusion body encephalitis.[4] Another form of slow virus infection known as Kuru is found only in New Guinea among the Fore people where it appears to be of relatively recent origin. It takes the course of a fatal degenerative cerebellar disease, but it has been shown to be transmittable to chimpanzees.[5] Other forms of chronic virus encephalitis have been identified in humans and in animals (Cytomegalus virus, fetal rubella, visna and scrapie in sheep, mumps in hamsters, etc.[2] So far as is known today, such disorders are rare in humans, but the potential implications of these discoveries is obvious.

Another important recently discovered viral encephalitis is that due to herpes simplex. Now considered to be the commonest cause of nonepidemic encephalitis, it often leaves severe neuropsychiatric residuals. It does not belong to the "slow virus" group.

Finally, one may note that virus infections of the central nervous system may be not only latent or chronic, but they may also not be demonstrable by ordinary neuropathological techniques. Such viruses may produce disease by causing dysfunction in morphologically intact but infected neurons.[2]

What such findings may mean for neuropsychiatric practice remains to be seen.[9] At the very least, the door has been opened to diagnosis, prevention, and even treatment of some relatively rare obscure diseases which till now were thought to be degenerative.[6,14] The preponderance of evidence today seems to be against assigning a significant role to the virus infection with respect to major psychiatric problems such as the highly controversial MBD. But virus infections have surprised us before, and as Sabin has pointed out, they may do so again.[13] The scene for such a surprise may have been set by the laboratory demonstrations of chronic latent virus infection of the central nervous system. For this we find clinical support in the observation that clinical symptoms of viral encephalitis may break out when immunosuppressant drugs are used.[2]

It is to be expected that we shall hear much more on these issues in the near future. It does not seem likely that interest in the viral forms of encephalitis will again be lost as happened after the 1916–1930 epidemic.

❮ Bibliography

1. AMERICAN MEDICAL ASSOCIATION, Council on Drugs. *AMA Drug Evaluations*, 1st ed. Chicago: Am. Med. Assoc., 1971.

2. BRODY, J. A., W. HENLE, and H. KOPROWSKI. *Chronic Infections, Neuropathic Agents (China), and Other Slow Virus Infections.* New York: Springer Verlag, 1967.

3. CALNE, D. B., G. M. STERNE, D. R. LAURENCE et al. "L-Dopa in Post Encephalitic Parkinsonism," *Lancet*, 1 (1969), 744–747.

4. DE JONG, R., ed. *Yearbook of Neurology Psychiatry and Neurosurgery*, 1967–68, footnote p. 64. Chicago: Yearbook Medical Publishers, 1968.

5. GAYDUSEK, D. C., C. J. GIBBS, JR., and N. ALPERS. "Experimental Transmission of Kuru-Like Syndrome to Chimpanzees," *Nature*, 209 (1966), 794–796.

6. HASLAM, R. H. A., M. P. McQUILLAN, and D. B. CLARK. "Amantidine Therapy in Subacute Sclerosing Panencephalitis," *Neurology*, 19 (1969), 1080–1086.

7. HUGHES, R. C., J. G. POLGAR, and D. WEIGHTMAN. "Levodopa in Parkinsonism: The Effects of Withdrawal of Anticholinergic Drugs," *Br. Med. J.*, 2 (1971), 487–491.

8. HUNTER, R. and M. JONES. "Acute Lethargic-Type Encephalitis," *Lancet*, 2 (1966), 1023–1024.

9. JOHNSON, R. T. "Chronic Infections Neuropathic Agents: Possible Mechanisms of Pathogenesis," *Curr. Top. Microbiol. Immunol.*, 40 (1967), 3–8.

10. ———. "Neurologic Diseases Associated with Viral Infections," *Postgrad. Med.*, 48 (1971), 158–163.

11. JOHNSON, R. T. and K. P. JOHNSON. "Slow and Chronic Virus Infections of the Central Nervous System," in F. Plum, ed., *Recent Advances in Neurology*, pp. 33–78. Philadelphia: Davis, 1969.

12. JOURNAL OF THE AMERICAN MEDICAL ASSOCIATION, unsigned editorial. "St. Louis Encephalitis," 193 (1965), 150–151.

13. ———. "Current Viruses May Surprise Us," 197 (1968), 49–50.

14. KRAYENBUHL, H., K. AKERT, K. HARTMAN et al. "Study of Anatomico-Clinical Correlation in Patients Operated on for Parkinsonism," *Neurochirurgie*, 10 (1964), 397–412.

15. LANCET, unsigned editorial. "Encephalitis of a Lethargica Type in a Mental Hospital," 2 (1966), 1014–1015.

16. MALZBERG, B. "Age of First Admissions with Encephalitis Lethargica," *Psychiatr. Q.*, 3 (1929), 244.

17. MARSHALL, W. J. S. "Herpes Encephalitis Treated with Intravenous Idoxuridane and External Decompression," *Lancet*, 2 (1970), 579–580.

18. MARTIN, J. P. "Globus Pallidus in Post Encephalitic Parkinsonism," *J. Neurol. Sci.* 2 (1965), 344–365.

19. MARTIN, W. E. "Tyrosine Hydroxylase Deficiency, a Unifying Concept of Parkinsonism," *Lancet*, 1 (1971), 1050–1051.

20. MAYER, E. E., ed. *Oppenheim's Diseases of the Nervous System.* Philadelphia: Lippincott, 1900.

21. NEAL, J. B., ed. *Encephalitis: A Clinical Study.* New York: Grune & Stratton, 1942.

22. PARKES, J. D., K. J. ZILKA, P. MARSDEN et al. "Amantidine Dosage in Treatment of Parkinson's Disease," *Lancet*, 1 (1970), 1130–1133.

23. RICHTER, R. W. and S. SADATOMO. "Neurologic Sequelae of Japanese B Encephalitis," *Neurology*, 11 (1961), 553–559.

24. SCHILDER, P. (1953) *Brain and Personality*, reprint ed. New York: International Universities Press, 1969.

25. TUKE, D. H. *Dictionary of Psychological Medicine.* Philadelphia: Blakiston, 1892.

26. WILSON, S. A. K. *Neurology*, Vol. 1. Balti-

more: Williams & Wilkins, 1940.

27. WALTZ, J. M., M. RIKLAN, S. STELLAR et al. "Cryothalamectomy for Parkinson's Disease: Statistical Analysis," *Neurology*, 16 (1966), 994–1002.

28. WHITTY, C. W. M., J. T. HUGHES, and F. O. MacCALLUM, eds., *Virus Diseases and the* Central Nervous System. London: Oxford University Press, 1969.

29. WILDY, P., ed. Classification and Nomenclature of Viruses. Vol. 5. *Monograph of Virology*. First Report of the Int. Comm. on Nomenclature of Viruses. Basel: Karger, 1971.

CHAPTER 7

HEAD INJURY

Kenneth Tuerk, Irving Fish, and Joseph Ransohoff

THE INCREASING incidence of serious head injuries in the United States is a by-product of the rapid pace of urban life, as well as of the increasing use of high-speed transportation. Precise statistics are not available but the estimates are staggering. It is well known that accidents are by far the leading cause of death under the age of thirty,[38] over 100,000 annually in the United States. Approximately 50,000 deaths occur each year as a result of automobile accidents,[20,43] and of these, it is estimated that 60 percent of the victims (or 30,000) died directly as a result of head injury. Vehicular accidents account for about 3 million head injuries yearly, 750,000 concussions, 150,000 skull fractures and 150,000 significant brain injuries[20] (Figures 7–1 and 7–2).

Improved facilities, better understanding of the pathology of head trauma, and advancements in therapy have led to more successful treatment. Mortality has decreased, but as increasing numbers of patients are saved, the morbidity rate has increased. Not all patients are fortunate enough to recover without neurological sequelae.

Evaluation of a posttraumatic patient can be quite complex. Certain deficits, such as hemiparesis, and hemianopsia are obviously of an organic nature. Subtle mental changes may be either organic or functional, or represent a combination of both factors. At times, the symptoms may be only those of mild mental changes, such as irritability or forgetfulness, with or without such vague symptoms as headache and light-headedness. The skills of both the neurologist and psychiatrist may be taxed in evaluating and treating these patients with the ultimate goal of rehabilitation and return to a normal, productive position in society.

In evaluating the head injury patient, the examining physician should be aware of the possibility of preexisting disease of the central nervous system which may not come to light until an episode of trauma brings it to the patient's or the physician's attention. A slowly developing homonymous hemianopsia may go

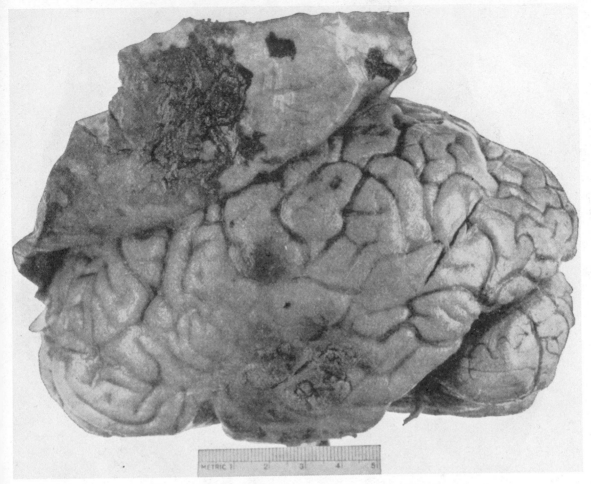

Figure 7–1. The brain of a thirty-year old male in a traffic accident. The dura is reflected from the left hemisphere to show a subdural hematoma. In the rolandic operculum there is contusion of the brain with subpial bloody discoloration of the cortex. Below in the temporal lobe there are contusion and laceration of the brain. The cut in the occipital lobe is an autopsy artifact. (Courtesy of Dr. Paul I. Yakolev, Warren Anatomical Museum, Harvard University.)

totally unnoticed by the patient, for example, until such time as he is involved in an auto accident when the other vehicle approaches from his "blind side." Similarly, the patient with developing cerebellar ataxia may not be conscious of his gait disturbance until a fall. Subsequently he may date all of his difficulties to that dramatic episode.

Similarly, in evaluating the patient for possible mental changes after head trauma, one must not only determine that trauma actually occurred, but also that it was significant, and that there was a cause-and-effect relationship between the trauma and the symptoms.

⟨ Significant Head Trauma

Significant head trauma is generally thought to be that which is followed either by alteration in the state of consciousness, focal neurological signs, or a skull fracture. Although the patient may appear absolutely normal in all respects, any of these conditions are grounds for hospitalization for at least a twenty-four-hour observation period.

In arriving at these criteria, one must remember that while injuries to the soft tissues of the head are not of neurological signifi-

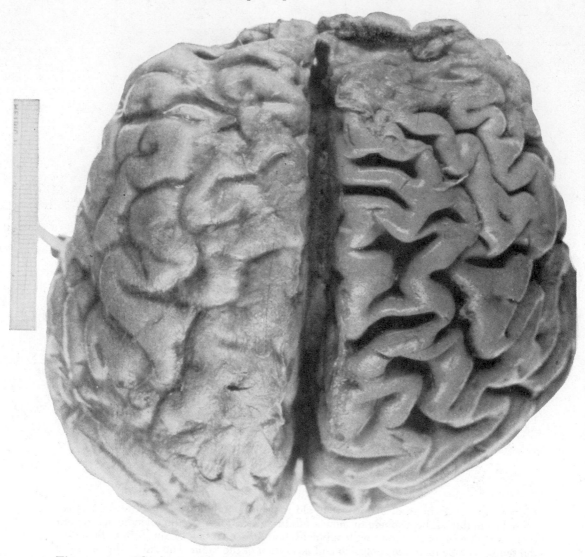

Figure 7–2.   The brain of a middle-aged man who suffered a head injury in an automobile accident several years prior to his death. He showed both intellectual and social deterioration and died in a state hospital. The frontal lobes show old traumatic destruction of convolutions, with atrophy and scarring of the brain. The pia-arachnoid is stripped off from the right hemisphere to show extensive corticomeningeal adhesions over the areas of the old cerebral trauma. (Courtesy of Dr. Paul I. Yakolev, Warren Anatomical Museum, Harvard University.)

cance per se, they do afford some indication of the forces applied to the head during the trauma, and can serve to alert us to the possibility of underlying brain damage. During the twenty-four-hour period of observation, evidence of acute intracranial changes generally appears. We must remember, however, that while these guidelines are helpful, it is certainly possible for delayed deterioration to occur after a period of observation, as in the incidence of chronic subdural hematoma, and can even occur without meeting any of the above criteria for admission to the hospital for observation. Figures 7–3 to 7–5 show various stages of brain damage after cerebral trauma.

Trauma, severe enough to cause alteration or loss of consciousness, is obviously significant. Indeed, the severity of the brain injury can be correlated with the length of time the patient remains unconscious.[31,32,38] Loss of con-

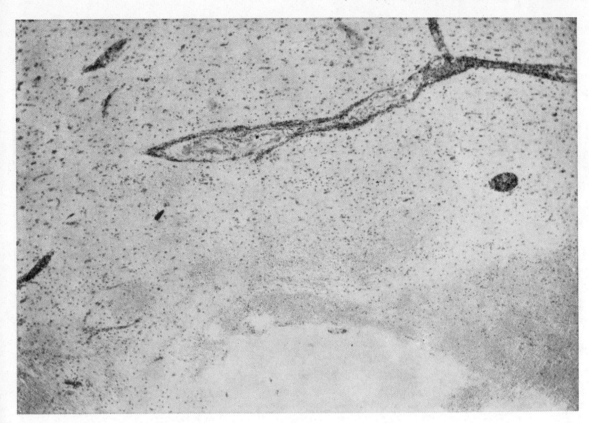

Figure 7–3. Cerebral Trauma. Contusion; two days old. Cortex. Hemorrhagic extravasate in the right lower corner of the field; hyperemia; perivascular infiltration ("cuffing") with inflammatory cells. Cresyl violet stain (X 80). (Courtesy of Dr. Paul I. Yakolev, Warren Anatomical Museum, Harvard University.)

sciousness for a few seconds to an hour may be empirically classified as mild, one to twenty-four hours as severe. This, however, is a rough guide and does not mean that a patient who was unconscious for only a few seconds (or not at all) cannot develop dangerous complications.

Patients with a history of unconsciousness often have a period of pre- and posttraumatic amnesia. Pretraumatic amnesia is defined as the time interval from the last moment remembered before injury to the time of injury. Posttraumatic amnesia is defined as the time interval from the moment of injury to the time when the patient remembers awakening. Again, a rough correlation can frequently be made between the severity of the intracranial injury, the length of unconsciousness and the extent of pre- and posttraumatic amnesia.[31,32,38]

Following head injury, the patient may be seen in either the acute or chronic stage. Although most patients will not be seen by a psychiatrist until the chronic stage, a brief discussion of the acutely injured patient is important to an understanding of the posttraumatic psychiatric sequelae.

⟮ Concussion

The definition and implications of the term "concussion" have undergone much change since the description of Wilfred Trotter in 1925. He felt that it was an "essentially transient state due to head injury which is of instantaneous onset, manifest widespread symptoms of purely paralytic kind, does not as such comprise any evidence of structural cere-

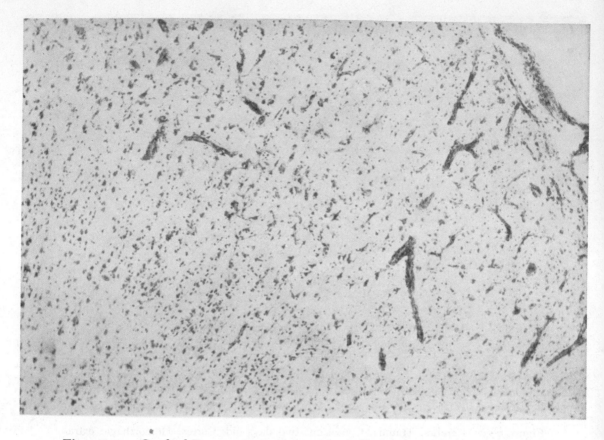

Figure 7–4. Cerebral Trauma. Contusion; six days old. Cortex. Intense proliferation of new capillaries; patchy areas of nerve-cell loss; beginning organization of the damaged tissue into future scar. Cresyl violet stain (X 80). (Courtesy of Dr. Paul I. Yakolev, Warren Anatomical Museum, Harvard University.)

bral injury and is always followed by amnesia for the actual moment of the accident."[42]

Some authors have included those patients who are dazed and confused, as well as those who have actually lost consciousness.[7] Clinically, a concussion with loss of consciousness is accompanied by flaccidity, abnormal brain stem reflexes, bradycardia, and apnea. If this state is prolonged, death may ensue, and autopsy may show few or no structural changes. These phenomena can be explained in only two ways: widespread simultaneous neural dysfunction or focal dysfunction in areas concerned with levels of consciousness, as well as respiratory and cardiac reflexes.

It has been shown by French and Magoun that destruction of the reticular formation can produce coma.[15] It has also been shown by Foltz and Schmidt that, following concussion

in monkeys, evoked potentials from peripheral stimulation are abolished in the reticular formation but not in other ascending pathways.[12] Finally, electrical action in the brain decreases markedly in many areas after concussion, but the most marked depression almost always occurs in the medial reticular formation. These physiological data, with marked dysfunction of the reticular formation, seem adequate to explain the clinical events during and after a concussion.

A search for a structural pathological explanation is still in progress. It is felt, at least by some schools of neuropathology,[39,40] that structural alterations do occur at the time of concussion and include changes in neurons as well as axons.[21,37] However, cause and effect have not been proved and these changes may be concomitant rather than causative. Indeed,

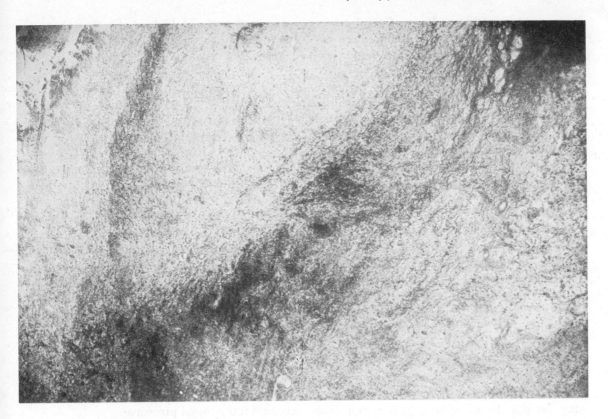

Figure 7–5. Cerebral Trauma. Contusion; several weeks old. Cortex. Organized scar; proliferation of mesodermal and neuroglial cicatricail tissue; the scar tissue is relatively avascular. Hematoxylin and eosin stain (X 40). (Courtesy of Dr. Paul I. Yakolev, Warren Anatomical Museum, Harvard University.)

it seems difficult to explain the phenomenon of concussion as anything other than brain-stem dysfunction and the absence of significant lesions is not surprising, as structural changes in this area are rarely compatible with survival. In any case, the term concussion comprises a convenient clinical category for the multitude of patients who have a head injury, a brief alteration in the state of consciousness and complete return to neurological normalcy after a relatively short period of time.

❨ Posttraumatic Syndrome

The arguments pro and con structural damage take on real significance in the consideration of the posttraumatic syndrome. This entity is defined as headaches, a feeling of unsteadi-

ness, at times true vertigo, and mental changes. These symptoms may occur alone or in combination, and they may or may not be associated with other more objective neurological signs. They may occur following minimal trauma as well as after a more severe injury. However, the degree of injury does not necessarily correlate with the severity of the posttraumatic syndrome. Headache is the most prominent symptom and is a complaint of most patients in the postconcussion state.[4,7,40] Giddiness and/or vertigo are about equally frequent, being present in approximately 50 percent of patients.[6,16] True vertigo usually indicates pathology and, when associated with postural nystagmus, is objective evidence of damage to the vestibular system.[3,17] Finally, the many mental symptoms which occur are the most difficult to characterize. Although a mild organic mental syndrome may, indeed, be present, normal results on formal testing are the rule.[39] The usual complaints are nervousness, irritability, impaired memory, and difficulty in concentration.

Although Russell found a slightly higher incidence of this syndrome in more severely injured patients,[31] there is truly no consistent relationship between the severity of postconcussion state and the extent of the injury. A mildly dazed patient may be disabled for years, while a comatose patient may recover without developing this syndrome. Taylor[41] argues convincingly for an organic etiology, expressing the opinion that this syndrome is present in the majority of patients following head injury and, if this is a functional disorder, then the majority of all postconcussion patients have disabling functional disorders. On the other hand, it is quite clear that there is a high incidence of this syndrome in industrial as opposed to recreational accidents, and a higher incidence of occupational incapacitation in cases involved in compensation or litigation actions.[23,31] These facts, however, may be due to secondary gain rather than being related to the organic or functional aspects of the syndrome.[41] In the follow-up study after the Korean War, 60 percent of the patients with long-term persistence of posttraumatic syndromes (four to six years) were competing as well as or better than before the injury.[6] Brenner et al.,[4] Symmons,[39,40] and Miller,[23] have all concluded that symptoms which persist for a long period of time are at least in part due to a significant functional overlay. Many investigators have felt that secondary gain plays an important role in the persistence of symptoms and that when financial matters are settled, the syndrome will subside.[4,23,40] Two long-term follow-up studies, however, do not bear this out[6,41] and in addition, the incidence of persistent and disabling symptoms is significantly higher in patients over the age of fifty.[31] This suggests that this syndrome cannot be totally accounted for on a functional basis. It would seem likely, in conclusion, that an organic substrate of a vasomotor nature affecting brain-stem functions plays an important part in the posttraumatic state. It also seems clear that there are non-organic functional factors affecting those individuals in whom the syndrome persists for months or years.

(Mental Changes Associated with Structural Injury

Patients with gross structural damage may have either contusions, lacerations, or hematomas. The hematomas may be either epidural, subdural, intracerebral or, commonly, combinations thereof. Brain swelling (cerebral edema) occurs in a high percentage of instances in association with these lesions and accounts for a significant degree of their morbidity and mortality. Neurological and neurosurgical evaluations are imperative and dictate the immediate medical or surgical treatment. The condition of the patient and his mental state will be determined by the extent of the injury to the brain, the intracerebral location of the injury and, finally, the degree of increased intracranial pressure.

Increased intracranial pressure will be relieved by either medical decompression with mannitol and/or steroids, or by surgical decompression. Early symptoms of increased intracranial pressure may include headache and increasing drowsiness, as well as progressive focal neurological deficits.

Once the pressure is controlled, the patient's clinical status will be a function of the extent and location of the intracerebral damage. Whether the insult be a contusion, laceration or hematoma, the degree of dysfunction should be maximal soon after the injury. At this point, the cerebral dysfunction is a result of: (1) dead and dying cells; (2) injured cells and connections which are not functioning, but will recover and function again; and (3) cells which are not functioning well because of pressure from either edematous brain or hematoma. Recovery begins soon after injury, as the edema subsides and the repair processes ensue. The final result, assuming optimal recovery, will depend on the amount of unavoidable damage which was sustained at the time of injury. Thus, whether the patient is first seen while comatose, lethargic, or normal, he should remain stable or improve. Any further significant deterioration in the clinical status heralds the onset of a new pathological process other than the original trauma. This may be a systemic problem such as hypoxia or sepsis, or a neurological one such as seizures, meningitis, or hydrocephalus. In any case, one should be alerted to possible deterioration in a patient who was stable or improving. The cause is often treatable and the deterioration reversible.

In addition to the extent of the injury, the mental status can also be determined by the location of the lesion. A very small lesion, strategically placed in the brain stem, produces a greater deficit than a much larger lesion in one of the "silent" areas of the brain. Other focal lesions may produce a neurological deficit, such as hemiparesis or hemianopsia, without any change in mental status.

Although contusions, lacerations, and hematomas may occur at any site, the anterior temporal lobes and the frontal lobes are most common, owing to the sharp bony prominence of the sphenoid ridge and the roof of the orbits.

(Focal Injury

There are two areas of focal injury of particular interest to the psychiatrist. The first is the area of the dominant hemisphere, where a lesion may produce disturbances in comprehension manifest by some degree of aphasia, either expressive or receptive. See Chapter 11, entitled "Aphasia," for a detailed description of these symptoms. When severe, there is no question about the diagnosis and its organic substrate. However, a minimal degree of receptive dysfunction following recuperation from a head injury may bring the patient to the attention of a psychiatrist. The presenting complaint may be "personality change" or "inability to function as before" the injury. Awareness of the condition and appropriate examination will demonstrate the true etiology and the simple "personality change" may become a focal deficit in expression or understanding or both.

The second area of focal lesions, which may require psychiatric consultation, are the frontal and anterior temporal lobes, particularly when the orbital and medial portions are injured. As noted before, the frontal and temporal lobes are preferred sites for injury in head trauma. The first, and perhaps still one of the best, descriptions of such a patient is that of Phineas T. Gage, who, in 1848, was injured with a crowbar in the left frontal lobe. He recovered and lived for many years, but underwent an extreme change in personality and behavior which was followed and reported by his physician.[36] Other reports have since appeared,[14] but most of the information on the effects of frontal lobe ablation has come from patients on whom it was surgically performed for therapeutic reasons. This technique was first employed by Moniz in 1936.[9,14,24,27] The patients with frontal lobe ablation are characterized by apathy and lack of foresight. Their affect is flat, anxiety is reduced, and there is a lack of concern for the consequences of their actions, both verbal and physical. This leads to inappropriate behavior, tactlessness, and a lack of concern for environment and personal appearance.

Extensive testing has been performed on patients before and after ablation.[9,14,27] Speech is particularly affected. There is a significant reduction in spontaneous speech. Verbal response to questions is delayed and reduced to phrases and short sentences. Intelligence tests are difficult to evaluate. They show definite reduction in verbal scores. Performance scores are about the same and may actually improve after frontal-lobe ablations. There is decreased facility for abstract thinking. However, part of the reduction in scores may be attributed to damages in personality.

(Organic Mental Syndrome (OMS)

The most common and disabling change in mental status after severe head injury is an organic mental syndrome. This is a condition resulting from any of a number of organic pathological processes, whether traumatic or not. The syndrome thus is a final common pathway of many organic diseases, one of which is trauma and its sequelae.

The hallmarks of the syndrome are dementia and loss of recent memory. In its mildest form, there are subtle changes in personality such as increased instability, decreased attention span, reduction in capacity for abstract thinking and, out of proportion to all other signs, a decrease in recent memory and recall. If the organic mental syndrome is more severe, an outright dementia may occur with disorientation, lack of personal care, incontinence, and severe lability of affect. The mood may be either manic or depressed but this is governed to some extent by the premorbid personality. Focal neurological deficits may or may not be present. However, attempts to correlate the OMS with a specific localization of brain injury have failed. It is best correlated with diffuse, bilateral cerebral dysfunction. The first and most common etiology of an OMS following head injury is diffuse, bilateral brain damage as a result of the trauma and secondary edema.

As his state of consciousness improves, the patient may pass through a stage of traumatic delirium characterized by excessive motor activity and confusion. He may scream, try to climb out of bed, and alternate between periods of spontaneous but inappropriate speech and sleep. Sedation and restraints may be necessary to prevent the patient from inflicting further injury upon himself.

Finally, continuing on the path of recovery, the patient manifests a severe organic mental syndrome which gradually becomes milder and finally disappears.

Depending on the severity of the injury, patients may pass through these stages in a few minutes, days, or months. Generally, the more severe the injury, the longer the period of unconsciousness and the more extended and gradual the recovery period. After very brief concussions, there may only be a few minutes of confusion before return to normal, and all these stages may not be evident.

Unfortunately, not all patients recover.

Those with a severe deficit may be considered for institutionalization. Those with a milder deficit may be discharged from the hospital only to arouse anxiety in the family by even moderate changes in their behavior and personality. This may create havoc within the family unit.

The first step in the evaluation of such patients is to confirm the diagnosis of organic mental syndrome, i.e., dementia and loss of recent memory. At times, psychometric evaluation may be helpful in establishing the diagnosis. In cases of a posttraumatic organic mental syndrome, the crucial questions to be asked are whether the process is the end result of the traumatic event, whether further recovery will occur and, finally, whether the arrest in recovery is the result of some intervening, superimposed disease or complication. These patients are often young and ambulatory with a long life expectancy. Therefore, particularly as the rate of recovery of mental function is decreasing or when the condition has stabilized, the physician must be absolutely sure that nothing further can be done to advance recovery before offering a final diagnosis and prognosis to the patients and their families.

⟨ Chronic Subdural Hematoma

A chronic subdural hematoma usually manifests itself by increased intracranial pressure and progressive focal neurological deficit. At times, and particularly in an injured brain, a progressive organic mental syndrome may be the earliest sign. If not corrected, this progression may continue until the patient becomes progressively obtunded and, finally, comatose. Headache, although usually present, may easily be overlooked. Focal neurological signs may not be present until late and papilledema may be present in 25 percent of cases. Skull X-ray may show the pineal gland to be shifted off the midline. Brain scan will be positive in 90 percent of cases. Lumbar puncture may show xanthochromia and increased protein in 50 percent of cases. Lumbar pressure is usually elevated, but a normal pressure does not exclude the diagnosis of hematoma. Echogram may show a shift of the midline structures, and cerebral angiography is diagnostic.

Early diagnosis and treatment is quite gratifying, with most patients returning to their previous neurological status. However, the diagnosis may be missed in a slowly deteriorating patient until coma and herniation ensue. Emergency surgery at this time, while often successful, does not always carry the same favorable prognosis.

(Communicating Hydrocephalus

Another complicating condition, which may produce an organic mental syndrome, is a secondary communicating hydrocephalus. It has been known for some time that head trauma with bloody CSF (cerebrospinal fluid) may produce a subacute hydrocephalus in the weeks following the injury. Moritz and Wartman, in 1938, discussed three cases with postmortem changes of arachnoiditis.[25] In 1956, Foltz and Ward reported the successful treatment of hydrocephalus after subarachnoid hemorrhage of diverse etiologies,[13] including trauma. In their cases, onset was between the second and tenth week after the hemorrhage. The important factor in all of these cases appears to be the arachnoidal reaction to the blood in the spinal fluid, producing an obstruction to the normal flow of fluid in the subarachnoid space. The obstruction is usually at the level of the tentorium but may, at times, be over the cerebral convexity. This obstruction results in communicating hydrocephalus with its attendant large ventricles and signs of diffuse cerebral dysfunction. Although this was once thought to be a rare occurrence, studies have shown that some degree of hydrocephalus, although not always clinically significant, is quite common after head injury with bloody CSF.

The clinical course of posttraumatic hydrocephalus may vary. In its mildest state the diagnosis may be an incidental finding when contrast studies are performed for other reasons. In other cases, there may be a mild organic mental syndrome or deterioration of a previously improving neurological state. After a few weeks, the mechanisms of production and resorption of spinal fluid equilibrate and the process may resolve spontaneously. Finally, in its most severe expression, the hydrocephalus is progressive and relentless, causing not only a plateau of mental recovery, but retrogression, leading at times to severe obtundation. Neurological and neurosurgical consultations are imperative as the situation may become reversible after a shunting procedure.

In 1965, Adams et al.[2] reported the syndrome of "normal-pressure hydrocephalus" (occult hydrocephalus, low-pressure hydrocephalus). These patients present with a progressive OMS, unsteady gait, urinary incontinence, and normal pressure on lumbar puncture. There is nothing particularly characteristic about the OMS but the gait disturbance is quite unusual. It is somewhat broad based and unsteady, although no cerebellar signs are present. There appears to be some difficulty with the initiation of walking movements and some patients have stated that "it feels as if my feet are glued to the floor." This has been characterized as "a magnetic gait." Onset of these symptoms may be months and even years after the injury. Skull X-ray and lumbar puncture are normal. Definitive diagnostic tools are RISA (radioactive iodinated scrum albumin) cisternogram and pneumoencephalogram. In the former, the I^{131} salt-free albumin is injected via lumbar puncture. Normally, the follow-up brain scans show activity in the basal cisterns in four hours. By twenty-four hours, there is diffuse activity over the cerebral convexities and sagittal sinus. In occult hydrocephalus, the activity enters the lateral ventricles within six hours and, even at the end of forty-eight hours, there is no activity over the convexities. The pneumoencephalogram shows enlarged ventricles with little or no air in the supratentorial subarachnoid space, indicating a block of the CSF pathways at the level of the tentorium. This condition must be differentiated from hydrocephalus ex-vacuo, i.e., cerebral atrophy. In this situation, the RISA scan is normal and, although the ventricles are large as a result of atrophy, air does pass over the convexities and demonstrates widened sulci and atrophic gyri. Although there are two contrary reports,[33,34] most observers feel that shunting is of no value in these patients, as the hydrocephalus is secondary to atrophy, in contrast to the results of shunting in patients with obstructive hydrocephalus secondary to trauma.

In addition to trauma, other etiologies accounting for occult hydrocephalus include subarachnoid hemorrhage, meningitis, and intracranial surgery.[1,26] The idiopathic cases are thought to be due to unrecognized or forgotten trauma or infection. The few pathologic studies performed have confirmed the presence of adhesions at the base of the brain.[18]

◖ Posttraumatic Epilepsy

Posttraumatic epilepsy is a disorder which, at first, may appear to be functional but is, on close examination, an organic sequela of head injury.[5,28,44] The incidence is quite low in closed head injuries, whether or not the patient has been unconscious. However, when the dura is penetrated, the incidence rises to about 50 percent.[5,44]

Posttraumatic seizures can be divided into two groups, depending on whether the onset is early or late. Of the patients who develop seizures, about 10–15 percent have their ictus within one month, often within the first forty-eight hours after injury. These seizures are secondary to an irritative process set off by cerebral contusion, laceration, or edema. The prognosis is good and after appropriate therapy, the seizures usually subside. Although the long-term prognosis is good, maintenance anticonvulsant therapy should be initiated and a baseline EEG (electroencephalogram) obtained. Therapy may be discontinued after two years if the EEG has reverted to normal.

About 85 percent of patients with posttraumatic epilepsy have a delayed onset. Of those who develop seizures, 50 percent do so within six months and 75 percent in two years. Because of the high incidence of posttrau-

matic seizures in penetrating wounds and the social stigmata accompanying these seizures, we feel that all such patients should be placed on prophylactic anticonvulsant therapy for at least two years. The medication may then be discontinued if the EEG is normal. The prognosis of all types of posttraumatic seizures is good.

The seizure itself, with its period of relative hypoxia and postictal confusion may interrupt the convalescence of the head-injured patient, particularly if repeated. Focal neurological deficits may become more pronounced postictally and, with lesions of the dominant hemisphere, aphasia may become exaggerated.

Approximately 80 percent of posttraumatic seizures have a focal component. At times, the seizure arising from a temporal lobe focus consists entirely of psychomotor phenomena. These patients, more than others, may be brought to psychiatric attention. The dreamy state, periods of amnesia, episodes of déjà-vu and sudden emotional outbursts may easily be mistaken for a functional disorder.

◖ Boxing Encephalopathy

Boxing encephalopathy (chronic progressive traumatic encephalopathy of boxing) has been associated with the injuries received in the ring.[19,20,35] The disease is characterized by a progressive OMS with both pyramidal and extrapyramidal signs. Symptoms do not usually occur until fifteen to twenty-five years after the onset of the boxing career. Only a few pathological examinations have been performed and these show atrophy with widespread areas of gliosis. The etiology is contested. It was long felt to be secondary to repeated trauma with each episode causing a bit more permanent damage. This hypothesis is contradicted by the fact that symptoms may not begin until long after retirement and are then progressive. Alcoholism has been invoked as a possible etiology but retrospective studies have shown that a significant number of these patients are not alcoholic.[19] The exact etiology remains to be clarified. It may simply be that the repeated episodes of trauma leave only a marginal reserve. As these patients become older, they develop an OMS at an early age.

(Head Trauma in Children

If the incidence of head trauma is high in adulthood, it is virtually 100 percent in childhood, multiple minor head injuries being a frequent occurrence in this age group. Approximately 200,000 children each year have head trauma severe enough for them to be hospitalized. About 5–10 percent of these exhibit neurologic findings at the time of admission.

The differences in the sequelae of head trauma in children as compared to adults, is related to two main factors: (1) The state of closure of the sutures of the skull at the time of injury, and (2) The state of development of the brain at the time of injury.

Sutures

At birth the sutures of the skull are not closed. This allows for the growth of the skull to accommodate the enlarging brain comfortably, without increasing the pressure within the cranium. The period of the most rapid postnatal brain growth is the first six months of life. At about six to nine months, the sutures begin to fuse. The anterior fontanelle is the last to close at about eighteen months of age. Fusion between the bones of the skull gradually becomes more firm over several years.

The nonfused or partially fused skull of the infant and young child is apparently better able to absorb the energy transmitted to it by external forces, molding or distorting with the blow, and protecting the underlying brain. The young brain with its higher water content is also better able to tolerate external forces than the older, more solid adult brain. Every summer we see in our large-city hospital emergency rooms innumerable instances of survival following falls from open windows four or five floors above the street. This is another evidence for the tolerance of the infant to head trauma.

Thus, the dynamics of increased intracranial pressure are different in early childhood than in adulthood, and the younger the child, the greater the difference. It was mentioned previously that brain dysfunction following head trauma is caused by (1) direct injury to the brain, e.g., laceration or contusion; (2) by edema; and (3) by increased intracranial pressure secondary to edema or blood which may be intracerebral or extracerebral (subdural or epidural hematoma). Increased intracranial pressure in adults causes downward herniation in the cerebrum through the tentorium, causing pressure on the brain stem which results in disturbances of consciousness, cranial-nerve dysfunction and abnormalities in cardiovascular and respiratory function. This threatens life and must be treated immediately by decompression as mentioned previously. Otherwise permanent brain-stem dysfunction can result, although the brain stem may not have been injured directly. In young children, with an open fontanelle and sutures that are not closed, supratentorial blood or edema causes enlargement of the skull and accommodation of the increased contents which result from the injury. Consequently, the brain has less of a tendency to "herniate down" into the brain stem. However, this can occasionally take place if the sudden increase in intracranial volume exceeds the expansion capacity of the skull. Obviously, the older the child, the more the dynamics approach those of adults, and therefore, the more danger of injury secondary to herniation.

Hydrocephalus may follow head trauma because of obstruction of the extraventricular spinal fluid pathways along the base of the brain. This results in an enlarged head and pressure on the white matter surrounding the ventricles. Treatment consists of shunting the fluid from the ventricles into another body cavity such as the atrium of the heart, the peritoneum, or the pleural space.

If subdural hematomas are very large, they may also cause enlargement of the head and pressure on the gray matter of the cerebrum. If the subdurals are small, they may resorb on their own without causing pressure sequelae. Sometimes repeated paracentesis of the subdural fluid is enough to prevent signs and symptoms. If the subdurals are very large, shunting of the fluid into another body cavity may be required.[2,4]

Brain Development

The second major factor which differentiates the prognosis and sequelae of head trauma in children from adulthood is the state of development of the brain at the time of injury. The newborn brain has fewer cells, less myelin, and a less well developed dendritic system than that of adults. The immature injured brain is able to compensate better. It is said to have more plasticity. Intact parts of the brain can "take over" an injured or destroyed area's function. For example, in an adult, an injury to the dominant hemisphere in the speech centers results in aphasia. In children under two this never happens, and even up to the age of five, "compensation" by the opposite side is frequently complete or almost complete. As the patient gets older, the ability to compensate decreases.

All of this means that a child with a brain injury secondary to head trauma has a far better chance for complete or satisfactory recovery than an adult with a comparable head injury. Also, the younger the child, the better the chances of satisfactory mental and motor recovery. Unfortunately, this does not mean that every child recovers satisfactorily from a head injury. Approximately 5–10 percent of childhood head injuries, which result in hospitalization, are severe. About 30 percent of children with severe head injury who survive, remain with neurological and/or mental dysfunction.[22]

The most accurate gauge as to whether a child will remain with a brain dysfunction is the same as that with adults, namely the longer the posttraumatic amnesia (PTA), the more likely the chance for a permanent deficit. However, at every phase of recovery, the degree is much better in childhood.

Richardson[30] studied ten children who were comatose from seven to forty-seven days after head injury. The PTA varied between twenty-five and sixty-five days. Only one patient was so incapacitated that he could not care for himself. Six others had motor or movement abnormalities. All had some intellectual and behavioral changes. Improvement in these patients continued for up to four years after the head injury.

An interesting study of patients who suffered less severe head trauma and were evaluated an average of ten years later, was performed by Dencker[10] in Sweden. These patients were twins, and the twin was used as control. She failed to find any significant differences in intellectual, personality, EEG, or performance between the "head injured" and the control groups.

Sequelae of Head Trauma in Childhood

The common neurologic and psychologic sequelae of head trauma may be listed in six categories.

MOTOR AND MOVEMENT DISORDERS

Focal damage in the pyramidal system gives rise to spastic hemiplegia or hemiparesis. If the lesion is bilateral, quadraparesis results. If the lesion involves the postcentral gyrus, sensory abnormalities result. Sensory impairment is usually incomplete. Destruction of the extrapyramidal system, such as the lenticular nuclei, may result in choreiform or athetoid movements, tremors, and rigidity.

POSTTRAUMATIC SYNDROME

The posttraumatic syndrome, seen so extensively in adults, occurs in only about 1–6 percent of children following head injury.[22] In children, headaches predominate, with giddiness and aesthenia being quite rare. The vast majority of patients with this syndrome have a self-limited course, usually lasting less than six months. The very few cases which persist beyond six months are usually early adolescents or preadolescents. The etiology and pathogenesis of this syndrome is discussed earlier in this chapter (p. 171).

POSTTRAUMATIC EPILEPSY

Posttraumatic epilepsy occurs in about 10 percent of children.[11] The lesions are usually located in the medial portion of the temporal lobe, the posterior frontal, or the anterior parietal lobes. Those children who suffer a seizure at the time of or very shortly after a head injury are *not* more likely to have post-traumatic epilepsy. Even an EEG which shows epileptiform activity soon after injury is an unreliable prognosticator, for over a period of several weeks the epileptiform activity gradually disappears. If permanent seizures occur, it is generally within the first two years after the acute head injury.

MINIMAL CEREBRAL DYSFUNCTION SYNDROME

Although many patients recover full motor and sensory functions, they may remain with signs and symptoms of minimal cerebral dysfunction. These include hyperactivity, easy distractibility, short attention span, visual motor-perception deficits, cognitive dysfunction, clumsiness, spatial disorientation, and learning disability. This syndrome is discussed fully in Chapter 8. Suffice it to say here that head injury is occasionally etiologic in this syndrome. Caution must be shown in ascribing head trauma as the etiology in too many patients with minimal cerebral dysfunction. Almost every child has had a significant bump on the head at one time or another. This does not mean that the etiology of the minimal cerebral dysfunction is necessarily related to the head trauma.

MENTAL RETARDATION

Mental retardation resulting from head injury is a result of diffuse brain injury. Generally, the more extensive the injury, the more severe the retardation. There are usually associated motor and/or movement disorders associated with the mental retardation secondary to head trauma. In these patients the head injury is usually severe and the PTA prolonged.

PERSONALITY CHANGES

Occasionally children have profound changes in personality that are beyond those which fit into the category of minimal cerebral dysfunction. In addition to hyperactivity and short attention span they become aggressive, destructive, lacking in judgment, and emotionally extremely labile. This can be severely incapacitating to the child and his family. These children usually respond poorly to psychotherapy and medication. It may or may not be associated with motor dysfunction.

Natural History of Children Suffering Head Trauma

As mentioned previously, most children who suffer head trauma do not show any adverse sequelae. When evaluating the patient who has deficits (neurologic, intellectual, or behavioral), we must keep in mind the fact that recovery can take place for a period of up to four years after the injury.[10,11,30] This means that we must not "give up" on a patient early or because he has severe deficits soon after head trauma. For example, passive exercises to prevent contractures should be continued. Educational and environmental manipulation should be instituted when necessary. There should be frequent reassessment because gradual improvement is the rule and what may have been appropriate educational placement at the time of initial evaluation may be inappropriate six or eight months later.

Finally, evaluation of therapy must be assessed in the light of the spontaneous improvement. Heroic claims have been made for several elaborate modes of therapy. They must be assessed with the natural history of spontaneous improvement of head injuries in children in mind.

❲ Bibliography

1. ADAMS, R. D. "Further Observations on Normal Pressure Hydrocephalus," *Proc. R. Soc. Med.*, 59 (1966), 1135–1140.
2. ADAMS, R. D., C. M. FISHER, S. HAKIM et al. "Symptomatic Occult Hydrocephalus with 'Normal' Cerebrospinal Fluid Pressure: a Treatable Syndrome," *N. Engl. J. Med.*, 273 (1965), 117–126.
3. BARBER, H. O. "Postural Nystagmus, Espe-

cially after Head Injury," *Laryngoscope*, 74 (1964), 891–944.

4. BRENNER, C., A. P. FRIEDMAN, H. H. MER-RITT et al. "Post-Traumatic Headache," *J. Neurosurg.*, 1 (1944), 379–391.

5. CAVERNESS, W. F. "Onset and Cessation of Fits Following Craniocerebral Trauma," *J. Neurosurg.*, 20 (1963), 570–583.

6. ———. "Post-Traumatic Sequelae," in W. F. Caverness and A. E. Walker, eds., *Head Injury Conference Proceedings*, pp. 209–219. Philadelphia: Lippincott, 1966.

7. COURVILLE, C. B. *Commotio Cerebir*. Los Angeles: San Lucas Press, 1953.

8. CRITCHLEY, M. "Medical Aspects of Boxing, Particularly from a Neurological Standpoint," *Br. Med. J.*, 1 (1957), 359.

9. CROWN, S. "Psychological Changes Following Prefrontal Lobotomy. A Review," *J. Ment. Sci.*, 97 (1951), 49–83.

10. DENCKER, S. J. "Closed Head Injury in Twins," *Arch. Gen. Psychiatry*, 2 (1960), 569.

11. DEVIVO, D. C. and P. R. DODGE. "Diagnosis and Management of Head Injury," *Pediatrics*, 48 (1971), 129.

12. FOLTZ, E. L. and R. P. SCHMIDT. "The Role of the Reticular Formation in the Coma of Head Injury," *J. Neurosurg.*, 13 (1956), 145–154.

13. FOLTZ, E. L. and A. J. WARD, JR. "Communicating Hydrocephalus from Subarachnoid Bleeding," *J. Neurosurg.*, 13 (1963), 546–566.

14. FREEMAN, W. and J. W. WATTS. *Psychosurgery*, 2nd ed. Springfield, Ill.: Charles C. Thomas, 1950.

15. FRENCH, J. D., and H. W. MAGOUN. "Effects of Chronic Lesions in the Cephalic Brain Stem of Monkeys," *Arch. Neurol. Psychiatry*, 68 (1952), 591–604.

16. FRIEDMAN, A. P., C. BRENNER, and D. DENNY-BROWN, "Post-Traumatic Vertigo and Dizziness," *J. Neurosurg.*, 2 (1945), 36–46.

17. GORDON, N. "Post-Traumatic Vertigo with Special Reference to Postural Nystagmus," *Lancet*, 1 (1954), 1126.

18. HEINZ, E. R., D. O. DAVIS, and H. R. KARP. "Abnormal Isotope Cisternography in Symptomatic Occult Hydrocephalus. A Correlative Isotope Neuroradiology Study in 130 Subjects," *Radiology*, 95 (1970), 105–120.

19. JOHNSON, J. "Organic Psychosyndrome Due

to Boxing," *Br. J. Psychiatry*, 115 (1969), 45–53.

20. KILBERG, J. K. "Head Injury in Automobile Accidents," in W. F. Caverness and A. E. Walker, eds., *Head Injury Conference Proceedings*, pp. 27–36. Philadelphia: Lippincott, 1966.

21. LINDENBERG, R. "Trauma of Meninges and Brain," in J. Minckles, ed., *Pathology of the Nervous System*, Vol. 2, pp. 1705–1765. New York: McGraw-Hill, 1971.

22. MEALEY, J., JR. *Pediatric Head Injuries*. Springfield, Ill.: Charles C. Thomas, 1968.

23. MILLER, H. "Accident Neurosis," *Br. Med. J.*, 1 (1961), 919, 992.

24. MONIZ, E. "Essai d'un Traitement Chirurgical de Cértaines Psychoses," *Bull. Acad. Med. Paris*, 115 (1936), 385–392.

25. MORITZ, A. R. and W. B. WARTMAN. "Post-Traumatic Internal Hydrocephalus," *Am. J. Med. Sci.*, 195 (1938), 65–70.

26. OJEMAN, R. G., C. M. FISHER, R. D. ADAMS et al. "Further Experiences with the Syndrome of 'Normal' Pressure Hydrocephalus," *J. Neurosurg.*, 31 (1969), 279–294.

27. PETRIE, A. *Personality and the Frontal Lobes*, Philadelphia: Blakiston, 1952.

28. PHILLIPS, G. "Traumatic Epilepsy after Closed Head Injury," *J. Neurol. Neurosurg. Psychiatry*, 17 (1954), 1–10.

29. RABE, E. F., R. E. FLYNN, and P. R. DODGE. "Subdural Collections of Fluid in Infants and Children," *Neurology*, 18 (1968), 559.

30. RICHARDSON, F. "Some Effects of Severe Head Injury. A Follow-up Study of Children and Adolescents after Protracted Coma," *Dev. Med. Child Neurol.*, 5 (1963), 471.

31. RUSSELL, W. R. "The After Effects of Head Injury," *Trans. Med. Chir. Soc. Edinburgh*, 113 (1933–1934), 129–144.

32. RUSSELL, W. R. and A. SMITH. "Post-traumatic Amnesia in Closed Head Injury," *Arch. Neurol.*, 5 (1961), 4–17.

33. SALMON, J. H. "Senile and Presenile Dementia. Ventriculoatrial Shunt for Symptomatic Treatment," *Geriatrics*, 24 (1969), 67–72.

34. SALMON, J. H. and J. L. ARMITAGE. "Symptomatic Treatment of Hydrocephalus Exvacuo. Ventriculoatrial Shunt for Degenerative Brain Disease," *Neurology*, 18 (1968), 1223–1226.

35. SPILLANE, J. D. *Five Boxers, Br. Med. J.*, 2 (1962), 1205–1210.

36. STEEGMAN, A. T. "Dr. Harlow's Famous Case. The Impossible Accident of P. T. Gage," *Surgery*, 52 (1962), 952–958.

37. STRITCH, S. J. "Shearing of the Nerve Fibers as a Cause of Brain Damage in Head Injury. A Pathological Study of 20 Cases," *Lancet*, 2 (1961), 443–448.

38. SYMONDS, C. P. "Concussion and Contusion of the Brain and their Sequelae," in S. Brock, ed., *Injuries of the Brain and Spinal Cord and Their Coverings*, 4th ed., pp. 69–117. Baltimore: Williams & Wilkins, 1960.

39. ————. "Concussion and Its Sequelae," *Lancet*, 1 (1962), 1–5.

40. SYMONDS, C. P. and W. R. RUSSELL. "Accidental Head Injuries: Prognosis in Service Patients," *Lancet*, 1 (1943), 7–14.

41. TAYLOR, A. R. "Post-Concussional Sequelae. *Br. Med. J.*, 3 (1967), 67–71.

42. TROTTER, W. "On Certain Minor Injuries of the Brain," *Lancet*, 1 (1924), 933–939.

43. Vital Statistics of the United States, Vol. 2, *Mortality*, Washington, D.C.: Nat. Center for Health Statistics, 1967.

44. WALKER, A. E. *Post-Traumatic Epilepsy*. Springfield Ill.: Charles C. Thomas, 1949.

CHAPTER 8

FUNCTIONAL
DISTURBANCES
IN BRAIN DAMAGE

Kurt Goldstein

OUR KNOWLEDGE OF FUNCTIONAL disturbances in brain damage is based on the patient's symptoms. Symptoms are modifications of behavior in various performance fields. If one considers the symptoms as directly dependent upon damage of the brain matter in various regions and as directly related to defects in different performance fields, one can draw some conclusions about the relationship between a disturbance of a particular performance and a specific brain damage. Although the results thus reached are useful for practical purposes, we learn little of how a lesion modifies the specific function, and of the origin of the symptoms.

First of all, the pathological-anatomical picture seldom indicates the degree of functional disturbance produced by the injury, since this depends primarily upon the extent and intensity of the injury—factors which cannot be correctly determined even by careful microscopic investigation. Furthermore, the difficulty is increased by the fact that the kind of damage—such as hemorrhage, tumor, inflammation, or intoxication—has a different effect on the functional disturbance.

The question of the relationship between the symptom and the disturbance of the brain matter's function is by no means as simple as has often been thought; indeed, one can say it has become increasingly problematical. The main difficulty consists in determining which of the observed phenomena are actually directly related to the defect of the brain— a question which is, as yet, far from clear. Increasingly, we have learned that, when we refer to disturbance of performance caused by a brain lesion, we must consider not only the disturbed performance but all the observable modifications of the patient's behavior. We know from Jackson's distinction between different groups of sequelae of brain damage (see p. 183), that this is a very difficult task. When one further realizes that, in a brain lesion, the symptoms can differ because of various conditions of the whole organism, and that they may become understandable only as phenomena depending also upon the organism's general condition, it is doubtful whether one can speak of symptoms as caused by brain lesion alone, or whether one can do so only in an abstract, theoretical consideration of the facts.

As clinicians, we cannot be satisfied with merely theoretical interpretations of the symptomatology—interpretations based not on clinical experience but derived from studies in normal physiology and psychology—as has frequently been tried in the past. We have to try to reach a better understanding of the functional disturbances in brain damage by taking into consideration all that we observe about the patient, his whole behavior at a given moment, especially its deviation from the norm. This is what I consider to be my task in this presentation.

The material available for this procedure is so vast that to discuss a considerable part of it here would be impossible. I shall therefore try to show, by use of typical examples of symptom complexes, which factors must be considered for an understanding of the structure of symptoms in brain damage, thus enabling the reader to apply our results to other symptom complexes.

❲ Previous Views Regarding Brain Damage

Until recently, the symptoms observed in damage of the brain cortex were considered to be expressions of a loss of so-called "images," the aftereffects of previous experiences deposited in different circumscribed regions of the brain cortex, according to the different performance fields. It was also postulated that the symptoms could not result exclusively from the effect of these circumscribed defects—that

additional factors must be involved; only thus could the variations, the alternation between normal and abnormal reactions of the patient in seemingly the same task, be understood. These other modifying factors were considered to be "general mental capacities" such as attention, memory, interest, and emotions. The additional factors were brought more or less into relationship to localized or general brain functions. The influence of the atomistic theory of brain function was so great that one overlooked the fact that, by introducing these general functions, nothing was gained. As a matter of fact, closer observation showed that these "general functions" varied in the same way as did the single performance. Attention, for instance, may seem to be sometimes grossly disturbed, and yet the same patient, under other conditions, may appear attentive or even abnormally so (see Goldstein,[13] p. 249). Thus we found ourselves in the same situation as before when we tried to understand the variations of the phenomena by assuming the influence of such general functions.

Today it is hardly understandable that the solution to the problem was not discovered earlier, namely: to consider the symptoms not only in relation to the dysfunction of limited parts of the brain but in relation to the individual in whom they appear; in other words, to consider them as performances of the sick individual. The concentration of study not on the single symptom but on the behavior of the total personality of the patient, during examination and in everyday life, made it more and more evident that the symptoms could only be correctly evaluated if one considered them in relation to the condition of the total psychophysical personality. This instigated an intensive study of each single symptom in relation to the behavior of the total patient at a given moment, which, in turn, became the point of departure for the concept of the so-called organismic approach to psychopathology in general (see in regard to this, Goldstein[19]). It is this organismic approach which is the basis for this presentation.

The new approach was not the result of a new theoretical concept but the outcome of better observation and investigation. Closer scrutiny led to the concept that the symptoms are consequences of the sick organism's struggle with the demands of the tasks confronting it; in other words, symptoms are forms of behavior by which the individal tries, in spite of his defect, to come to terms in the best way with the outer and inner world. The approach grew out of the necessities of neuropsychiatric practice, out of the task of retraining a great number of young men with brain injuries and different mental defects with which we were confronted during and after World War I, and out of the recognition that the psychopathological theories prevailing at that time, and the methods of training based on them, were insufficient to fulfill the task. There was an urgent need to find a more successful interpretation of the phenomena, particularly so because the subjects with whom we were dealing could not any more be considered as interesting objects for theoretical studies, as was often the case in psychopathology in earlier times. The disastrous condition of the young men confronted us with a strong challenge to help them in every way possible. The approach became particularly promising after the analysis of the symptomatology of a great number of patients with various brain injuries had revealed another point of view in the consideration of organismic life in general and of man's in particular, namely: that the basic motivation of the living being is to realize its own nature; that is, to realize all its capacities to the highest degree possible in a given situation. By applying this viewpoint, many seemingly contradictory symptoms became understandable, and much better results of retraining were achieved.

The structure of the organismic approach will become clearer when we consider individual symptoms in brain damage. We shall see, then, that phenomena which were once considered to be different, isolated defects appear now to be simply different expressions of the same brain damage under different conditions of the whole organism.

Before entering into the subject, I want to make a few general remarks about the period in which the organismic approach originated and the place of this new approach within the ideas of that time. It was related to the new "holistic" orientation in physiology and medicine in general, which finds its expression in such a saying as, "There is no sickness—there are only sick human beings." I refer in this connection to a congress held in 1932 under the topic *Einheitsbestrebungen in der Medizin*,[7] where men famous in anatomy, physiology, and different fields of medicine came together to discuss this question with great enthusiasm.

While the new approach brought deeper insight into the function of the organism and a better understanding of pathological phenomena, it confronted us with a number of new methodological problems. When one considers each symptom as dependent on the condition of the entire organism, great difficulty arises in determining the relationship of a symptom to the specific brain damage. This particular problem had been seriously considered fifty years before by the famous English neurologist and psychopathologist, John Hughlings Jackson, who reached a general point of view in psychopathology to which ours bears much similarity.

Jackson, as an outgrowth of his experiences with aphasic patients, emphasized that psychopathological phenomena can be understood only if one gives up the theory of images, and he stopped considering disturbances of images in brain defects as causes of symptoms. He believed that, in order to understand psychopathological phenomena, one has to begin by analyzing the modification —due to its damage—of the function of the brain, and by considering the different symptoms of aphasic patients as expressions of a disintegration of the brain matter; expressions of a lowering of the function of the brain to a level where automatic and emotional reactions still are possible, while the highest function, the propositional symbolic function, is more or less lost.

Jackson's ideas were so far ahead of his time that he found little approval. In the famous discussion between him and the French neurologist, Broca, at the British Association for the Advancement of Science in London in 1868 in which both men defended their contradictory theories about the function of the brain, Broca emerged as victor; afterward, Jackson had little influence on the work in psychopathology. Although some great men in the field at that time, A. Pick, C. von Monakow, Adolf Meyer, and others, stressed Jackson's great significance, referred to his ideas, and used them in their work, he was nearly forgotten for a long time. He had to be newly discovered. This rediscovery occurred during the period referred to previously when clinical practice demanded better procedures for helping brain-injured soldiers in England. It was the English neurologist, Henry Head, who based his treatments on Jackson's ideas and demonstrated their fruitfulness for understanding much of the aphasic symptomatology and for its treatment. A little earlier, other unbiased studies by Storch, Heilbronner, Pierre Marie, Lotmar, Boumann, Gruenbaum, Woerkom, and K. Goldstein, influenced more or less by Jackson, gave different new interpretations of psychopathological phenomena which can be considered as precursory to the organismic approach.

By stressing the organismic approach as the best one for an understanding of the symptoms in brain damage, I do not want to imply that this approach has found full acceptance. Although a considerable amount of psychopathological research is more or less influenced by it, certain men prominent in the field are strongly opposed to it, for example, in this country, Nielson and some others.

Adherents to the older "classic" theory, founded on associationism and the assumption of isolated, circumscribed disturbances, base their opposition primarily on the argument that the new approach is too general and does not therefore do justice to the problem of localization, and, even more important in respect to the problem with which we are dealing here, to the great variety of modifications of performance of the brain-damaged patient.

As to the opposition concerning the problem of localization, I would like to point to various papers of my own, particularly the presentation of the subject in the German *Handbuch der normalen und pathologischen Physiologie*.[16] There I have shown that this problem is by no means neglected by the new approach; moreover, *that the approach put it on a more realistic basis*, so that many mistakes originating from the old concept can be avoided.

Proof that the new approach emphasizes the great variety of symptoms and the problem of understanding them will become apparent when we now discuss the symptomatology of patients with severe damage of the brain cortex.

❪ Effect of Impairment of the Abstract Attitude Owing to Brain Damage

I shall not start with a description of patients with defects in special performance fields, such as speech, motility, vision, sensation, etc., but with patients who show disturbances in all these fields in such a way that some performances in each field are impaired and even lost, while others seem relatively well preserved. This clinical picture occurs particularly in severe lesions of the frontal lobes or in diffuse damage of the brain cortex by injury or intoxication, in general paresis, etc. It can be shown that the complex and outwardly very inconsistent symptomatology of the patient can be understood as an effect of the damage to a special mental capacity which we call the abstract attitude. Before going into this matter, it seems necessary to make some remarks concerning the concept of the human mind which underlies this interpretation.[24,25]

The normal individual displays two kinds of attitudes toward the world—the *concrete* one and the *abstract* one. In the concrete one we are given over passively and bound to the immediate experience of the very things or situations in their uniqueness. Our thinking and acting are determined by the immediate claims made by the particular aspect of the object or situation. For instance, we act concretely when we enter a dark room and turn on the light switch. If, however, we refrain from turning the switch, reflecting that we might awaken someone asleep in the room, then we are acting abstractly. We transcend the immediately given aspect of sense impressions, we detach ourselves from the latter, and consider the situation from a conceptual point of view, reacting accordingly. The abstract attitude corresponds approximately to what Henry Head has called—in relation to speech —symbolic behavior.

The healthy individual is able to shift voluntarily from one attitude to the other, according to the demands of the situation. Some tasks can be performed only by virtue of the one, some only by virtue of the other attitude. For the beginning of any activity, the abstract attitude is a presupposition. During activity, the concrete attitude is often dominant, but, should the course of action be interfered with or disrupted, abstraction is required to correct such disturbances and to continue the activity properly.

Patients with impairment of abstract attitude may not appear to deviate grossly from normals in everyday behavior, because many routine tasks do not require the abstract attitude once these tasks have been set going. During observation of the patient in a variety of situations, however, it becomes evident that he does not react like a normal individual; he appears more stereotyped and reserved. He seems to lack initative and spontaneity. Tasks which demand choice or shifting particularly reveal the defect.

From analysis of the behavior of a great number of such patients in various everyday and test situations, we[25] have compiled a list of modes of behavior in which the performances are disturbed owing to impairment of the abstract attitude.

The patient fails if he has:

1. to assume a definite mental set;
2. to give an account to himself for acts and for thoughts;
3. to shift reflectively from one aspect of a situation to another;
4. to keep in mind various aspects of a task or of any presentation simultaneously;
5. to grasp the essential of a given whole, that is, break it up into pieces, isolate them, and synthesize them;
6. to abstract common properties reflectively;
7. to perform concepts, symbols, to understand them;
8. voluntarily to evoke previous experiences, for example images;
9. to assume the attitude toward the "merely possible;" and
10. to detach the ego from the outer world or from inner experiences.

It has often been said that the defect of the patients consists of an inability to cope with new situations, but that they are able to proceed in an abstract way as far as old experiences are concerned. The fact, however, is that patients fail equally in familiar situations and in new ones, if the situations demand the abstract attitude. On the other hand, they can cope with new tasks successfully, but they can do so only as long as these do not require the abstract attitude. Indeed, patients are more likely to fail in new situations rather than in old ones because the former frequently demand new sets, in other words, the abstract attitude.

The analysis of many patients' failures in different tasks has shown that a great number of symptoms are explainable as the result of this one defect and that in the same way the variations of the patients' reactions in apparently the same task can be so explained. If the patient seems to be successful at one time and fails at another, this seeming inconsistency is resolved when we realize that the tasks which appear equal to us may (as a result of the disturbance of this function) not be at all the same for the patient. The following example may illustrate this. If we present to the patient an angle built of two little sticks, with the opening downward, and ask him to copy the presentation after it is removed, he produces the angle correctly. If we present the same angle with the opening upward, the patient, after the angle is removed, is not able to produce it. For us, the angles are not different; for him, they are not only different, they have nothing in common. He says that the one (with the opening downward) appears to him like a roof; the other structure does not mean anything to him. His correct response was determined by the fact that the first structure appeared to him as something which corresponds to concrete experience; he failed with the second structure because this was not the case, because he could not assume the abstract attitude which is necessary to fulfill this task.

This is one of numerous examples which definitely show not only that the patient can react only to (for him) concrete conditions, but also how careful we should be in our interpretation, since the task set before the patient may to him appear totally different from the way it appears to us.

A few further examples from different performance fields may illustrate the failures due to impairment of abstract attitude. Just as the patient cannot deal with figures when they do not represent concrete objects, he fails further when he is confronted with ideas, thoughts, and feelings when their handling presupposes abstract attitude. He is unable to shift from reciting one series (for instance, numbers) to another (days of the week), because active shifting is impossible for him. He can follow or even take part in a conversation about a familiar topic or a given situation, but if he has to shift to another topic—even one equally familiar—he is at a complete loss. He may be able to read a word and, at another time, spell it, but when asked first to read and immediately afterward to spell, he is unable to do so. The patient's speech in everyday life may not show much deviation from the norm. He may in certain situations have a great number of relevant words at his disposal; this is the case when the words belong concretely to the situation. He will fail concerning the same words, however, when the situation demands that he consider their meaning. His words fit only definite concrete situations. He cannot understand that the same word can have different meanings. In respect to learning, he has the greatest difficulty in rote learning and very quickly forgets what he has learned. The same difficulty exists in the behavior of the patient with regard to practical activities, such as handicraft and labor. (Concerning the symptomatology of such patients, see[11].)

I would like further to mention two important general points. The first is that loss of abstract capacity cannot be regained by retraining. Only improvement of the brain damage may more or less restore the impaired capacity. The second point is that there are different degrees of abstract behavior, depending on the extent of conceptional complexity which the performance in question involves. Thus the patient may be able to fulfill some performances which need abstract consideration. The highest degree of abstract behavior is required for the conscious and volitional act of forming generalized concepts or for thinking in terms of a principle and its subordinate acts and verbalizing these acts. Similar abstract behavior is the act of consciously and volitionally directing and controlling every phase of a performance and of accounting for it verbally.

A lower degree of abstraction is necessary in volitionally planning an act or series of acts without distinct awareness of or self-accounting for every phase of its further course. In some performance, as in intelligent behavior in everyday life, only the directional act is usually abstract, and the ensuing performance follows a concrete plan. Here the patient may be successful until difficulties arise. He may fail when the required shift demands the abstract, anticipatory deliberation. It is apparent that only careful analysis of each performance in respect to the degree of abstraction required for execution will allow us to decide whether or not the patient is disturbed. The decision is easiest if some tests which have been constructed for this purpose[25] are used.

We are inclined to believe with Jackson that the abstract capacity, the symbol function, being the expression of the most complex function of the brain, suffers first in damage to the brain cortex, while isolated lesions in the motor and sensory areas show only damage of the concrete performance "instrumentalities" (see p. 188). Not infrequently, the symptomatology consists of a mixture of damage to both parts, although the damage may not necessarily be equal in both. Thus we can get very complex clinical pictures.

The opponents to the organismic approach stressed that it took into consideration only symptoms belonging to the higher level, the abstract attitude. This criticism may appear to be justified, since some authors mentioned only these disturbances in aphasic patients, because they considered aphasia an expression of a damage of symbolic function or "intelligence." This holds true, for example, for Pierre Marie, Ludwig Binswanger, and Kronfeld and Sternberg. It is, from the organismic approach, not at all appropriate, however, to omit the symptoms belonging to defects in the lower-level function, the so-called motor and sensory instrumentalities, which are necessary for realization of the symbolic function in the performances of the organism. The very complex picture which aphasia represents, in which motor and sensory disturbances of letters, words, and other features of language not dependent on the defect of the symbolic function are often so completely mixed with those which are dependent on it, gives all the more reason to study carefully the structure of *all* abnormal phenomena. Otherwise, one cannot reach a correct conclusion as to the origin of the clinical symptoms. This is all the more necessary since defects in the instrumentalities *secondarily* influence the use of the symbolic function. Only by analysis of all symptoms can one clarify what is primarily due to the latter. Indeed, even Jackson showed insufficient interest in the effects of disturbances of the "instrumentalities," in the destruction of single words and letters, in the disturbances of grammar, of the finding of words, and of sentence formation which are related to dedifferentiation of the function of the motor and sensory apparatuses.[15]

The problem of the relationship between the disturbances in damage of the instrumentalities of language (the instrumentalities belonging to the concrete forms of behavior, see Goldstein,[11] p. 163) and those due to damage of the symbolic function interests us, particularly, because clarity concerning this relationship is essential for correct evaluation of the symptoms not only in aphasia but in all performance fields.

Jackson did not sufficiently evaluate the disturbances of the instrumentalities, because he considered the separation between the higher and lower functions of the brain cortex to be too absolute. There is no doubt that the processes in the higher and lower levels of the brain are, to some extent, associated; both belong to the "mental apparatus." The organismic approach assumes that any damage which concerns one part of an apparatus changes the function of the rest of the apparatus as well; the "parts" can be considered as only artificially separated "parts" of a whole. This is the case in the connection between the lower- and higher-level functions of the brain cortex. Under normal conditions all performances are determined by a working together of both functions as a unit. Under certain conditions, performances come into the fore which are related to the one level; under other conditions, those which are related to the other level. Such a preponderance of behavior related to one level exists if this level is important for the self-realization of the individual in a particular situation. Thus, for instance, if an individual is thinking with concentration, the concrete world is more or less forgotten; it is, so to speak, in the background (see[19] p. 109). The opposite holds true when an individual is totally involved in concrete behavior. The various abnormal performances correspond to the different ways in which the union of the two functions is impaired.

Jackson speaks of a disintegration from the voluntary to the automatic-emotional level. He goes so far in his separation of the two levels that he assumes, concerning language, that the lower-level activities are related to the "inferior" hemisphere, the right one, while the symbolic function is connected with the "superior" left hemisphere, an assumption which is not in accord with the newer concept of localization.[16] Indeed, Jackson has stressed, in general, the modification of the function of one apparatus owing to damage of another one connected with the first one. On this concept is based his distinction of positive and negative symptoms; the negative ones are an expression of the direct damage of an apparatus, the positive ones the effect of the modification of the function of an apparatus due to another one to which it is related. But he did not come, in my opinion, to a correct conclusion regarding the function of the lower-level apparatus separated from the function of the higher one in disintegration of brain function.

He assumed that defects in the higher level did not alter the behavior related to the lower level, in so far as the lower level continues to remain "integrated." We assume, too, that impairment of abstract attitude is an effect of a dedifferentiation of brain function, a reduction of the most complicated function to a simpler one; however, this does not imply that the undamaged lower-level apparatus remains unmodified in its way of functioning. Phenomena belonging to the lower level do *not* remain fully integrated, and the preserved automatic and emotional performances of the patient do *not* simply represent the effect of the lower-level function as it existed before. It is not enough to say that the function of the brain is *reduced* from a level corresponding to the voluntary activities to a lower one corresponding to emotional and automatic performances. The character of this reduction, of this modification of the brain function, has to be considered if one wants to understand behavior on the lower level in all its details. Neither the automatic nor the emotional reactions of patients with impairment of abstract attitude appear, on closer investigation, "normal."

◖ The Automatisms in Damage of the Higher Level of Brain Function

The automatic reactions in damage of the higher level of the brain function show definite deviations from the norm. They do not come so easily into action. Conditions in the outer world or within the individual, which usually instigate them, must now be present in a very "adequate" way; in even small deviations from the familiar conditions, the learned automatisms do not occur. So, for instance, it is not enough to ask the patient to utter the (very automatized) series of numbers; the first numbers often have to be presented orally; only then is the patient able to speak the rest of the series correctly. If the patient is interrupted at any point in the procedure, he will not be able to continue, as a normal person would. These and many other phenomena not only show that the automatisms also are

functionally modified in damage to the higher level, but also point to the fact that the automatisms are normally closely related to the higher level, more closely than one usually assumes.

The observable modifications of the automatic reactions are not fully explainable by the assumption of a lack of the influence of the higher-level function; only when one considers them as a change in the normal relationship between the figure and ground in the unit they represent can they be understood. Every process in a stimulated area is accompanied by a definite excitation in the part of the organism not directly stimulated. We call the excitation in the stimulated area the *figure* and the excitation in the rest of the organism the *ground*. All performances of the organism, as well as all experiences, are so organized. Figure and ground are intimately interconnected; to every figure belongs a definite ground. The phenomena corresponding to either one can be properly evaluated only by considering the other as well. What is meant by figure and ground is most obvious in visual experiences; however, all other experiences and performances, such as motor reactions, speaking, thinking, feeling, etc., are organized in a similar way. To this organization of the performances correspond equal organizations of the physiological processes in the nervous system.

All damage to the nervous system, especially brain damage, disturbs the figure-ground organization in general or in a part which belongs to a definite performance field. The sharp differentiation of figure from ground suffers, including a general leveling or intermingling of the phenomena belonging to figure and background. This can, at times, be carried to the point of inversion, so that what normally is figure becomes ground, and vice versa. We expect a definite figure as reaction to a definite stimulation, but the patient may respond according to the background. This change of the normal figure-ground organization is the basis of a great number of symptoms in damage of the nervous system and in neuroses and psychoses. It is clear that reactions in isolated parts will be deprived of the influences of the normal figure-ground organization which goes on within them, and that they will thus be changed, particularly in respect to their contents. Normal figure-ground organization is, like all performances, dependent upon processes belonging to the higher level as well as to those within the realm of the instrumentalities. It is determined by previous experience, by memory. Furthermore, one has to consider that figure-ground organization in one field is related to the figure-ground organization which the whole organism represents.

In all performances the whole unit is in action. According to the significance of one or the other part for the performance, this part is in the foreground, but the performance is correct only if it occurs in correct relationship to the background which the other part represents—which changes according to the demands of a definite task. If the lower-level function is somewhat separated from the higher-level function, this will come to the fore in modifications of the automatisms, according to the significance of the higher-level function in preserving the relationship of the two levels for definite tasks of the organism—in some tasks more, in others less. Thus the patient's difficulty in starting an automatic series shows that, for the setting in motion of an automatism, some higher-level function (I would say some abstract attitude) is necessary. What has taken place following disintegration of the brain function is a damage of the normal figure-ground relationships between the two levels, which may be observed in variations of the automatic activities under various conditions of the whole organism, by which the figure-ground relationship is determined. Normally, this figure-ground relationship exists which makes possible the fulfillment of the task to which the organism is exposed. After damage to the higher level function, the figure-ground organizations are disturbed—the most complicated ones more than the simpler ones. This shows that the automatisms are, in general, effective, but they are not normal, being modified by the disturbance of the more complicated figure-ground configurations in the

disintegration of the brain function involved.

This interpretation of the automatic performances in disintegration of the brain function corresponds to the general explanation of the automatisms and reflexes, to concrete behavior in general, which I have given on another occasion (see[18] Chap. 5). I tried to show that these phenomena are not the effect of isolated processes in the organism but represent figures in organizations of the whole organism which differ from those in normal performances only in the special form of the organization.

There is another factor which brings us further understanding of the modification of the behavior in damage of abstraction: the influence of isolation of the lower level in its function. The change of the function of one part of a unit owing to its separation from another part cannot be considered alone as the effect of a lack of influence of one on the other. The effect of isolation itself modifies the function of the separated part. Consideration of this factor has proved to be of the greatest significance for understanding many symptoms in pathology. It has shown that the modification follows definite laws which are equally discernible in each performance field which is in a state of isolation. The modification by isolation concerns particularly the dynamics of the processes. We shall consider them in more detail later, when we take up symptoms which are the effect of direct damage to the instrumentalities (see p. 195).

(Emotional Reactions in Disintegration of the Brain Function

For Jackson, the paradigm of the lower-level function was emotional, interjectional speech which is usually fully preserved in damage to the higher level, the symbolic function. Concerning this preservation of emotional, interjectional speech, we are confronted with a more difficult problem than in the automatisms—owing to the uncertainty of opinion about the nature of emotions. Jackson was inclined to consider emotional reactions as belonging to the same category of behavior as the automatisms, and thus to consider the preservation of both in disintegration of brain function as equal phenomena. It is doubtful whether it is justified to put the two groups of phenomena under the same heading. Normally, they show a number of differences, particularly a different relationship to the total personality and to the symbolic function. Automatic phenomena represent part processes of the voluntary activities and are dependent on them. They always occur under the direction of the latter or under the direction of outer-world influences. Emotional reactions are not voluntarily produced, but their connection with the abstract attitude differs essentially from the connection of the automatic activities with the latter. The emotional activities have something in common with the abstract activities in that both represent attempts of the personality to come to terms with the world, that both are emanations of a definite attitude toward the world. The emotional attitude differs from the abstract attitude, however, in that this coming together of personality and world is more immediate, more in relation to the existence of the individual, while the abstract attitude guarantees the organization of an ordered world separated from the individual. Because of this close connection to the existence of the individual, emotions play a particular role in all forms of self-realization and occur in concomitance with, and not in dependence on, the voluntary activities. One has often assumed that emotions are simply disturbing phenomena. This is most certainly wrong. I would like to refer in this respect to newer research published by Leeper[33] and K. Goldstein.[14] Success and failure in all performances are accompanied by definite emotions. Which kind of emotion arises depends on the implications of the situation with regard to the individual's way of realizing his nature in a particular case. The correct emotions—that is, those which help to achieve self-realization—are of great significance for executing correct performances.

The emotions are complex phenomena; they consist of inner experiences which are not conscious in the usual sense of the word, but of which we are well *aware* (see in regard to this Goldstein,[19] p. 34). They consist further of activities by which they are "actualized"— movements of the face and body, the so-called expressive movements of different kind; of linguistic utterances such as interjections, sounds, words, and sentences which are brought to the fore in characteristic intonations; and finally of physiological processes in the vegetative nervous system.

What has been called emotional language represents the linguistic part of the motor activities (instrumentalities) belonging to emotions. The activities in emotions—and so also the linguistic phenomena—are based on innate mechanisms acquired in experiences related to the world in general, and most particularly in relation to other human beings. These motor phenomena correspond to the other automatisms in so far as they are concrete activities and come to the fore in emotional situations, as the automatisms do in voluntary activities.

From this aspect it seems incorrect to speak of emotional language; it would at least be less prejudiced to speak of linguistic means, linguistic instrumentalities for realizing the emotional attitude which a situation provokes. They represent special linguistic phenomena, but they are not different in principle from those instrumentalities which are used in abstract attitude. Emotional language is a special, not a more primitive, form of language. The emotional attitude is not a more primitive attitude than the abstract one; it differs from it by another kind of relationship to the total personality, a closer one. It seems appropriate to assume that the greater significance of emotions for the existence of the personality in the world makes the substrata underlying them more resistant to damage of the brain function. It is for this reason that they are better preserved than those substrata underlying the symbolic attitude.

From our discussion it seems that we are not justified in considering that emotional reactions are equal to automatisms. We have mentioned that the automatisms show modifications in impairment of abstraction. Does that impairment not find expression also in differences between the emotional reactions of the patient as compared to those of normal individuals? I think it does. Clarification of this point seems to me important for a better understanding of the abnormally frequent occurrence of emotional reactions and their modifications in patients.

Considering the facts, we must stress the following: Emotional phenomena usually are more predominant in patients with impairment of abstraction than in normal people. Most probably the reason for this is that the world of the patient, owing to impairment of abstract attitude, is not organized normally and so makes many normal reactions impossible. The patient, when urged to react, tries to do what he is able to do, and he is most able to produce emotional reactions, and therefore also emotional language. The emotional activities, however, occur not only more frequently than normally but they are modified as well. They show the characteristics of *isolation* (see p. 194); the isolation is due to the lack of the normal relatedness to the reactions in the abstract world, by the impairment of the latter.

Thus we come to the following result: Preservation of the emotional language is an expression of the preservation of emotional reactions; in individuals with disintegration of the brain function, it is *not*—as is the case in preservation of the automatisms—a direct effect of an inferior brain function coming to the fore. Preservation of emotional reaction represents the maintenance of this attitude of man toward the world, which, in normal man, exists alongside the abstract attitude. Because the emotional attitude is more closely related to the personality and more important for its self-realization, it shows greater resistance toward damage of the brain function and thus may remain undisturbed when the abstract attitude is disturbed. The emotional instrumentalities are preserved in the same way as are the instrumentalities in general in impairment of abstract behavior. This shows in the possibility of using them in concrete behavior. The odd preservation of emotional language does not present a special problem. Whether a patient is able to produce language or not depends on the attitude under which such language is demanded in a given situation, that is, whether the abstract one or the emotional fits the situation. If the latter is the case, the patient will bring out words; in the former case, he will not. This could be demonstrated by a great number of examples which show that the patient is able to utter a word in an emotional attitude but is not able to do so voluntarily, that is, in the abstract attitude, even immediately afterward. One particularly instructive example concerning a patient of Jackson may illustrate this. The patient responded to the demand to say "no" by saying, "I cannot say 'no.'" He was not able, however, to repeat the word "no." The speaking of the word "no" in the sentence is not a voluntary act but belongs to the patient's concrete reactions. The repetition of the word "no" presupposes the voluntary attitude (see ref.[15] p. 71) which he could not assume, therefore he was unable to say the word on demand. From a superficial aspect this would seem to be a contradiction, since the patient was able to say the word "no" with great emphasis when asked to do something which he could not do, that is, when in an emotional attitude. This seeming contradiction is resolved when we realize that the words appear to be the same but actually are not the same, since they represent totally different reactions of the whole organism. The patient was able to utter the word only when the situation induced him to take an emotional attitude. It is obvious that wrong interpretations of the patient's capacities can easily occur if this difference in attitude is not taken into consideration.

I would like to mention, in the latter respect, another very instructive example: it concerns the difficulty in finding words, particularly names of even the most common objects. This is a very frequent symptom of aphasic patients. No matter how similar, on face value, failures of the patients may appear in respect to the finding of words, the defects can be due to a defect of an entirely different function. In one kind of patient, the inability to name is an expression of an impairment of abstraction; in another, it is a sequela of a defect in the instrumentalities of language, a memory defect. The patients of the first kind have not lost the words but are not able to utter them in naming, because naming, as analysis has revealed, presupposes the abstract attitude. The other kind of patients, with difficulty in finding the name, have no defect in abstract attitude, but their instrumentalities of language are damaged, and therefore they cannot find the words. Only when one considers the whole picture which the patients present does the difference of the origin of the symptom become apparent. As long as one pays attention only to the effective reaction, as has often been done—in this case the difficulty in naming objects—the underlying damage of the brain function may appear the same. This fallacy occurs particularly if one records the results of examination by the plus and minus method and considers the answers only in respect to success or failure. This conclusion from the effective answer, without analysis of the way in which the patient came to the answer, the "fallacy of effect," is the cause of many mistakes in the interpretation of psychopathological phenomena and in the building of theories. It shows up particularly in failures of retraining when the interpretation was wrong.

Similar observations, as we have mentioned, can be made not only concerning the language of the patients but in regard to other motor activities which belong to emotional situations. An example may illustrate this: The patient was asked to behave as he would in a situation in which he became angry with some one and was menacing him. He was not able to do so. When we demonstrated such behavior to him, he began to laugh, apparently perplexed, not quite sure what was meant. He was not able to perform the action on demand. But, observed in a situation in which he actually got angry, he behaved instantaneously like a normal individual as shown by the expression of his face, the action of his fists, etc. This example points to the important difference which often exists between the patient's behavior during special examination and during everyday life. Observation under

the latter condition, so often neglected, deserves the greatest attention.

([Symptoms Due to Direct Damage of the Instrumentalities

Up to now, our description of symptoms in damage of the brain cortex was concerned with effects due to disintegration of the brain function from the higher-level function to the lower one. We have discussed symptoms caused by impairment of the higher-level function, the abstract attitude, and have discussed the effect of the impairment of the abstract attitude on the lower-level function, the motor and sensory activities, the so-called instrumentalities, by which the higher-level function is actualized.

At this point we shall consider symptoms which are the effect of direct damage to the instrumentalities. We have to restrict ourselves here to a *survey* of the different ways in which damage of the function of the brain, concentrated in definite regions, is revealed in modifications of normal behavior. From this point of view, we have to classify the symptoms into two main groups.

Symptoms which Represent Direct Sequelae of Damage to the Substratum of a Definite Region

These sequelae rarely take the form of complete loss of a performance; more commonly, the performances affected undergo modifications. Such modifications can be considered as a result of a systematic disintegration of the concerned function. Structurally, this disintegration invariably exhibits the same features, regardless of the region involved, be it the spinal cord or the subcortical apparatus, and regardless of whether it concerns reflexes, motility, sensation, speech, thinking, or feeling. A particularly important consequence of this dedifferentiation is impairment of abstract attitude and abnormal concreteness of behavior, about which we have spoken before.

All direct damage causes a rise of the

threshold and a retardation of excitation. The receptivity of the patient is reduced in the involved sense organ. It takes him much longer to react. This manifests itself in the fact that patients may succeed perfectly in a task when they are given a sufficiently long time of exposure but fail in the same task when given only brief exposure, for example, when examined by the tachistoscope. (The tachistoscope is an instrument which allows exposure in different short lengths of time.) Pathology consists of a slowing down of the physiological process.

The patient may perceive when the stimulus is strong enough and presented long enough, but he may cease to see it after a certain time, in spite of continued stimulation. Later, the sensation may appear again; it seems that the threshold changes during stimulation. This is also true in stimulation of normal individuals, but it is far more apparent in brain damage.

When excitation takes place despite obstacles, it spreads abnormally and remains effective an excessively long time. This is due to disturbance of the process of "equalization" by which the effect of the stimulation is regulated (see Goldstein,[19] p. 113). Examples here are phenomena such as tonic innervation, repetition of the same movements, reiteration in reflexes (clonus), etc. A word grasped with great difficulty by an aphasic patient sticks, perseverates, and influences subsequent performances.

Another characteristic effect of the damage is the fact that performances are determined to a much greater extent than normally by stimulating influences, external or internal. We call this abnormal stimulus responsiveness.

Symptoms Due to a Separation of an Undamaged Area from a Damaged One

By such separation or, better, "isolation," the function of the undamaged area, and thus the performance, is modified in a definite way. The pathology can consist in an isolation of parts of the unit which the organism as a whole presents and an isolation of the subunits corresponding to definite performance

fields. Isolation can occur in gross anatomical separation or in functional separation; it can also occur in psychological conditions.

It seems useful to give here a brief summary of the functional changes caused by isolation (see Goldstein,[19] p. 133). The reaction appears modified in the following ways:

1. The effect of an adequate "stimulus" is abnormally strong.

2. The effect of an adequate stimulus is of abnormal duration.

3. The reaction is abnormally influenced by inadequate stimuli, external or internal. It is abnormally "stimulus bound."

4. The individual is forced to react. He appears to be easily fixated when his reaction to the present stimulus is completely successful. If his reaction, however, is not fully successful, he seems to be forced to react to another present stimulus. If, now, the correct reaction takes place, fixation will set in; if the correct reaction does not take place, the patient will again be forced to react to still another stimulus, etc. Thus he may appear very distracted. The patient seems to be driven to achieve an "adequate" reaction by which the entrance of "catastrophe" is eliminated (p. 197). Fixation and distractibility appear so as the two results of the same defect under different conditions.

5. As a result of loss of the normal influence of the rest of the organism on the activity in the isolated part, the reaction appears to be lacking special contents. It appears, or actually is, more "primitive" because it lacks properties belonging to the "nature" of the individual. The degree of primitivity and diminished appropriateness depends on the place and extent of the isolation, on how large a part of the whole organism is excluded from cooperating in the reaction (see[19] p. 148 ff.).

6. Isolation distorts the normal figure-ground organization which is of essential importance for the outcome of any normal reaction.

All the factors mentioned above are responsible for occurrences of abnormal performances, and all of them have to be considered in the evaluation of any one symptom in damage of the brain cortex.

(Symptoms Representing the Reaction of the Individual to the Defect

So far, we have discussed symptoms in brain damage only in their relation to defects of structure and function of the brain. Our results were still somewhat unsatisfactory, particularly in regard to *understanding the variability* of the symptoms. We must try, therefore, to go a step further, to regard the phenomena not only in their relation to the damage of structure and function but in their relation to the reaction of the individual and of the whole organism to the defect. Such a step corresponds to the procedure of the organismic approach and often leads to a better understanding of the patient's behavior.

Systematic investigation of the patient's general condition while he is able to fulfill a task and when he is unable to do so reveals another fallacy, which consists of only recording the effect of failure or success in the performance. One observes, particularly in patients with impairment of abstract attitude, that the patient, unable to fulfill a simple, seemingly unimportant task, may be completely changed in his total appearance. The same man who, shortly before, looked animated, calm, in good mood, well poised, collected, and cooperative, while successfully fulfilling a task, appears now to change color, to be agitated; he starts to fumble and becomes unfriendly, evasive, even aggressive. This overt behavior is very reminiscent of that of a person in a state of anxiety. The relationship of this general condition to the capacity of fulfilling a task becomes particularly evident from the fact that such a general condition can be experimentally produced, in some patients, by presenting them with a task which we know they will not be able to perform.

We call the state of the patient, when he is successful, an ordered condition; the state in a situation of failure, a disordered or catastrophic condition. In the latter condition the patient is incapable of performing tasks in which he is usually successful, which he is able to do very well when in the "ordered" condition. Such failure lasts for shorter or longer periods of time. One observes frequent catastrophic conditions, particularly in patients with impairment of abstract capacity. Since an individual with such impairment is unable to account to himself for what he is doing or experiencing we assume that he is not aware of his failure; as a matter of fact, he is unable to say, when questioned about it, whether or not he has been confronted with something frightening. Hence we come to the conclusion that the catastrophic condition is not a conscious reaction to the failure but, rather, belongs intrinsically to the objective situation of the organism in failure.

Even the smallest failure may have this effect on these patients, since they are unable to decide which failure might be dangerous for them and which might not. They are, so to speak, always endangered whenever their reaction is not adequate. Thus any objective failure can bring the organism into disorder, into catastrophe, into anxiety.

I cannot, in this presentation, discuss the consequences of our description of these phenomena for a theory of anxiety (see[18] Chap. 7). Here, we are interested only in the symptoms which these patients show, owing to the occurrence of anxiety, which are not directly related to the damage of the brain. If we do not pay attention to this, we may be deceived about the patient's brain defect and may consider symptoms as being related to it, when actually they are not. Consideration of the phenomenon of catastrophe explains the variability of symptoms under similar conditions.

One factor which is apt to modify the symptomatology considerably is the development of protective mechanisms by which the occurrence of catastrophes is eliminated or at least reduced. It is easy to understand that all patients, when they do not essentially improve, have the greatest desire to get rid of the anxiety, for otherwise they are prevented from using even their preserved capacities and thus from coming, at least partially, to a state of self-realization.

We realize that patients with even severe brain damage and impairment of abstraction show, after a certain time, a diminution of the disordered behavior, of catastrophic conditions and anxiety, and yet, examination reveals no change whatever in the damage to their mental capacities. In such cases this can occur only if the patient is no longer exposed to tasks he cannot cope with, or is able to take the failure without reacting with catastrophe. Concerning the first point, observation of his behavior in everyday life reveals that he lives apparently in a modified environment, an environment from which far fewer tasks arise which might lead to catastrophes. How does such modification of environment take place? Observation shows that the patient is withdrawn from the world around him so that a number of stimuli, including dangerous ones, do not arise. He avoids company. He is as much as possible doing something which he is able to do well. What he is doing may not have any particular significance for him, but concentration on activities which are possible for him makes him relatively impervious to dreaded stimulation. Particularly interesting is his excessive orderliness in all respects. Everything in the surrounding world has a definite place. Similarly, he is very meticulous in his behavior as to time, whereby the determination as to when he should do something is related to events and to activities of his which always occur at the same time, or to a definite position of the hands of a clock. This orderliness enables him to prevent too frequent catastrophes.

Another interesting protective mechanism is unawareness of the defect. We observe this particularly in patients with impairment of abstract attitude, but also in patients who are incapacitated in a special performance field without mental damage, for instance, in severe hemiplegia. This symptom, called Anton's symptom, described first by Anton in 1899,[2] occurs particularly when the incapacitation is total (see[39] p. 38), so severe that the patient is not able to use the disturbed capacity at all. The symptom may not take place if the defect is partial and if the patient is able to use the capacity at least to a certain degree, for example, if he can move his paralyzed leg somewhat. This protective mechanism has been described as denial, a procedure which would

demand a somewhat conscious activity. I do not think that such an interpretation is correct. Certainly, it can be rejected as far as it applies to patients with impairment of the abstract attitude, who are, owing to this defect, unable to do anything voluntarily. Whether the phenomenon becomes more understandable if one ascribes to it unconscious influences is doubtful. I think it is sufficient to consider it as an effect of a new organization of the behavior of the organism, which, though *not directly related to the defect*, occurs from the organism's tendency to realize the capacities which it has, in pathology those which are preserved. Within this new organization the effect of the disturbance does not become apparent. This would make it understandable that the patient is not only unaware of the defect, but that the defect is so arranged in his behavior, without his knowledge, that the disturbance does not show.

It is not the disagreeable experience of the failure itself which produces the new organization. This becomes evident when lack of awareness or other protective mechanisms disappear under the influence of the physician. As transference develops between patient and physician—when, for example, under the influence of the physician the patient learns to bear his disturbances and learns through his own experience that, by bearing them, his general contact with the world is improved—then he is more able to realize himself without the shelter of the protective mechanisms. With this added security, he is able to give up his safeguards. Indeed, the more the abstract capacity which makes such deliberation possible is preserved, the more is this the case.

We consider the organization of protective mechanisms as an expression of the attempt of the organism to come to terms with the demands made on it, in such a way that self-realization is guaranteed as much as possible. I would like to stress that these passively originating, protective mechanisms occur not only when the abstract attitude is impaired but also if it is by circumstances diminished, as, for example, in severe anxiety in normal individuals.

There is another way to eliminate danger to

self-realization which is produced more actively by conscious interference. One should distinguish these mechanisms, which occur particularly in neuroses, from the passively originating protective mechanisms by terming them differently—by calling them defense mechanisms.

In view of these facts, we should be very cautious in the interpretation of symptoms; the possibility that some phenomena observed in the patient might not be the effect of a damage but of a protective mechanism always has to be considered. This concerns also the absence of symptoms by "denial," which might be expected in a special damage of the brain.

Somatic symptoms, resulting from defects of the nervous system, can also bring the patient into general disorder. Here also, we observe after a certain time, a modification of behavior by which, even when the original damage is neither eliminated nor improved it is no longer effective. For instance, a patient may, after damage to one hemisphere of the cerebellum, suffer from disequilibrium, falling, deviations in walking, etc., and from different disturbances in general, subjectively and objectively, and so may be hindered subjectively or objectively in his self-realization. After a certain time the general disturbances improve, without improvement of the pathological condition (which special examination shows existent as before). Concomitantly with the general improvement, however, we see that a deviation of the body has occurred, which seems to bring about a new equilibrium, a better general condition, and thus a better possibility for self-realization. The patient, however, is not aware of his deviation.

That this general improvement is related to the deviation becomes apparent by the fact that improvement disappears immediately when one tries to eliminate the deviation; in other words, such action brings the patient into the previous condition, into catastrophe. We say that the deviation represents the individual's new, preferred condition (see[19] p. 340). The following few remarks may explain what is meant by this. If we consider an organism by the usual atomistic method as composed of parts, members, and organs which can be used in very different ways, and if we then look at the organism in its natural behavior, we find that many kinds of behavior which, on the basis of the first consideration can be conceived of as possible, are actually not realized. Instead, only a definite selective range of behavior can be observed. Normally, each performance is executed only in a definite or, as we say, preferred manner. Observation of the whole organism in a situation where one performance field—be it motility, perception, language, etc.—shows preferred behavior reveals that all other performance fields exhibit preferred behavior as well. In the above case we say that the organism is in an ordered condition; it performs all its activities in the best way; it can use all its capacities in coming to terms with the demands of the outer world; it has a definite constant visual acuity, an erect position of the body, is able to speak and to act according to its nature, that is, is able to realize itself in the best way.

The organism always tries to achieve such ordered behavior in spite of its defect. It can be reached only through modification of the behavior in the damaged performance field by finding a new preferred behavior which goes along with a somewhat modified but preferred behavior all over. This must be considered in our evaluation of deviations; we have to distinguish those which are the expression of the defect from those which are an expression of the new, preferred behavior; that is, from those which are means to guarantee the new order. This distinction demands careful study of the influence of the deviation on the behavior of the whole organism, that is, whether or not it is accompanied by order or disorder of the latter. A symptom belonging to a preferred condition is characterized by the fact that any voluntary change of the new preferred behavior brings the organism into general disorder and that it returns involuntarily to that very behavior. So, for instance, should the head be in a tilted position, any attempt to bring it to the normal erect state produces not only general disorder, but the head returns involuntarily to the new preferred condition, in this case a tilted position.

What we have described here concerning the effect of a cerebellar damage can be observed in damage of each performance field in the change of the direction of the performances toward a new preferred order. This new preferred condition can be achieved in two different ways.[22] One way consists of yielding, giving in to the defect; the other, of building a counteracting mechanism by which the effect due to an abnormal condition is compensated. These two ways of eliminating the danger to self-realization do not present equal effects. By the first, the normal functioning is, in principle, unchanged. It is the more "natural" procedure; it occurs more automatically, scarcely demands voluntary activity on the part of the individual, and therefore brings greater security. By the second way the normal form of functioning in the particular apparatus is changed. It is a more volitional type of behavior; it is not as secure, leads more readily to fluctuation, and admits greater possibilities for catastrophic reactions. Whether one or the other way of adapting to the irreparable defect occurs depends on which offers the best possibility for self-realization under the given conditions. If this is guaranteed by the first procedure, it will occur, since it is the more secure procedure; if, however, this is not possible, then the second way of adaptation occurs.

The significance of the preferred condition for the best performance must be considered most carefully in all therapy, even if that condition deviates from the "normal." Any attempt to bring the patient into the "normal" condition may make all treatment meaningless and inane. The similarity of this situation in organically disturbed patients and in neurotics is theoretically of the greatest interest. Unfortunately, we cannot even touch this point here.

We mentioned before that the symptomatology of a patient with brain damage can become more difficult to understand in direct relation to the defect because of a factor other than the protective mechanisms. This factor is the development of the relation between the physician and the patient. If this relationship is good, the patient will no longer become afraid so easily and the occurrence of catastrophes may be diminished; thus, many defects may come to the fore which the patient concealed simply by not reacting because he was afraid to let them appear. The development of a kind of transference between the patient and the physician is of the greatest significance for a correct examination, for finding the defects related to the damage, for evaluation of the symptoms, and, not least, for execution of correct therapy. This development of transference in organic patients has not had the attention it deserves. In this respect I would like to refer the reader to my article about organismic therapy.[26a]

❮ The Nature of "Distorted" Performances and Their Interpretation as Symbolic Phenomena

The discussion of the protective mechanisms, particularly their consideration as new preferred behavior, has some bearing on the understanding of phenomena which are usually called compensational or distortive. When we observe such phenomena, the question of whether we are actually dealing with pathology always arises. I have in mind particularly some reactions, unusual as to form and content, of aphasic, apraxic, agnostic patients. What does the material which the patient brings to the fore represent? Sometimes it certainly is the expression of disturbances in the field of the instrumentalities. Sometimes, however, one gets the impression that the material corresponds to activities and experiences which have played a particular role in the premorbid life of the personality, and which are now released, so to speak, through pathology. From this point of view such material has been considered as of particular significance for the study of the deeper level of the patient's personality. It seems to me important that we look at these phenomena a little more carefully than is usually done. They deserve attention not only in relation to their interpretative value as symptoms but from a more general point of view as well. They have suggested an interpretation as "symbolic" phenomena, which, in my opinion, is mostly wrong. The error originated because their relationship to the total condition and behavior of the patient was not fully considered.

Some utterances of aphasics, also of such whose symbolic function was generally disturbed, can easily give the impression of symbolic phenomena and often have been interpreted as such. I think they can be understood in various other ways as well which are not in contradiction to the existing basic defect, the defect of the symbolic function. Some are so-called "physiognomic phenomena"[42] and represent normal reactions which occur in a special concrete and not symbolic attitude of the individual. This is easily overlooked because these phenomena are not well known. In our culture particularly, they play a small part in everyday life and are not familiar except in the experience of artists. In normal life they are, so to speak, embedded in our realistic everyday attitude toward the world, and they come to the fore only in special situations. We do not have sufficient studies of the physiognomic behavior of our patients, but I feel justified in assuming, from my experience, that this behavior differs from normal physiognomic experiences which are related somewhat to the symbolic attitude. This relation is lacking in the physiognomic experiences of the patients. They appear particularly when the attitude of abstraction is diminished by pathology, and especially in patients with a premorbid inclination for the physiognomic attitude toward the world. Such utterances should not be considered as symbolic. For these patients, a shifting from the physiognomic attitude to the more usual attitude, which, for normal individuals is easy, becomes almost impossible. Their aspect is, so to say, fixated due to "isolation."

Other utterances are more difficult to evaluate and frequently give rise to symbolic interpretations. They are outstanding in the sense that they consist of poetic, symbolic, or even newly coined words; they may appear to be utterances of particularly intelligent, cultured, and erudite personalities. I have often observed such "quasi-symbolic" phenomena in aphasic patients. In a recent paper, W.

Riese[37] has stressed the occurrence of such phenomena. He has considered them as means "evidently to compensate the naming defect of the patients." The patients' neologisms "impress the listener by their descriptive and figurative power." The language of one of his patients, "a highly educated scientist and humanitarian" before his sickness, became "after a brief initial period of complete loss of speech, formal, solemn, poetical, dramatic, pathetic and 'Shakespearean,' frequently using quotations." He continues: "What the brain injury brought to the fore was that element in his nature which disease could not destroy, but rather released" and "I reached the conclusion that disease may occasionally reveal though in a distorted fashion what is great and noble in man's nature."[37] p. 11

It is true that such utterances and behavior may occur in patients with brain defects. I have noted that disease may emphasize the premorbid character of the patient, especially in the way the patient now bears the defect and in what way the untouched part of the personality helps him to overcome his failures. Whether in a patient with impairment of the abstract attitude an interpretation such as W. Riese suggests is justified, I would doubt. In such cases, I think, we are dealing with phenomena of "quasi-high" value, and I assume that the patient Riese describes belonged to that group. Closer consideration may show that the phenomena represent material which previously belonged to the behavior of a high-level personality, which appears now in the form of protective mechanisms and has lost their previous meaning for the particular individual. These utterances represent the undamaged remnants of the instrumentalities of speaking and thinking, which prevail now because the adequate activities due to the impairment of abstraction are impossible. The previous particular way of speaking, the previous rhythm and preference for poetic, dramatic, pathetic expression of the personality are preserved, but this material no longer is an expression of the attitude to which it originally belonged, the attitude which is lost through damage to the brain. Some abnormalities which these utterances show, and which Riese has carefully reported, reveal that we are no longer dealing with utterances prompted by the premorbid personality of the patient. They reveal "no planning, no effort, they occur passively, apparently without intent." In all this, they show the characteristics of isolated automatisms. The rapidity and fluence with which they are uttered (which Riese mentions, and which I have often observed on such occasions) may be even better described as being "thrust out." I think that the patient utters the words in this manner because he wants to get rid as quickly as possible of the distress in which he finds himself when he cannot react correctly but feels forced to do so. As one of my patients said: "If one is asked, one has to answer," and he brought out something which occurred passively in him by *association* of previous knowledge to the task he had to fulfill now. He said definitely that he did not know and could not say how it entered his mind, but that he was forced to utter it.

Such examples definitely point to the fact that these utterances are not related to the present personality. Certainly, their prominence is an indicator that we are confronted with experiences which the individual has had before, and therefore his utterances may reveal the premorbid character of the personality, but we cannot assume that they represent the old personality as released by pathology. In any case, we must be careful to see whether we are justified in so doing or whether these utterances do not belong to "quasi-high" behavior.

I have discussed these phenomena in some detail because I consider it important for the psychiatrist to be fully aware of this problem. We meet the same problem and the same wrong interpretation in the evaluation of utterances of schizophrenics, which have often been considered as symbolic, as expressions of deep insight into the essential things of human life, which disease has revealed. Here too, I do not want to deny that the particular premorbid personality of the schizophrenic patient may become apparent in some of his behavior. This is understandable, because we assume that the patient is not totally modified in the typical schizophrenic manner but is partially

normal, or, better, in some respects normal. (Federn has stressed this particularly. Compare[26a].) Thus he may show normal and even high-level personality behavior under some conditions, but I would deny that this particular high-level behavior is related to the schizophrenic condition. We shall understand the behavior of the patient only when we distinguish sharply between high-level behavior and "quasi" reactions which only appear to be of high-level nature. That the latter occur in schizophrenics is to be expected, particularly when we assume that the patient's behavior is frequently abnormally concrete.

We know, since Vigotski's[40] investigation, that thinking in concepts is disturbed in schizophrenic patients, at least in some groups of such patients. This was confirmed by the work of Hanfmann,[27] Kasanin,[31] Bolles and Goldstein,[5] and others. Storch[39] was already doubtful whether one is justified in considering schizophrenic behavior as symbolic. Beck[3] has stressed, on the basis of his Rorschach studies on schizophrenics, that it is an error to assume that the schizophrenic gives the world "a form and outline which the healthier do not see," that he has "a greater power or superior ability to transmute his experience into something richer." The author wonders "whether the general belief in the schizophrenic profuse fantasy life is not due to confusing distortion with fantasy." He adds: "Fantasy actually involves a *creating* of something totally new. . . . The schizophrenics' misconstructions take on fantastic form. But this is still not fantasy. It is inaccuracy. . . . Not having the power to apprehend the presented real world is what chiefly distinguishes the schizophrenic's percepts and his thinking."

I have come to the conclusion that in schizophrenia we are dealing not with an organic defect of abstraction but with a nonuse of abstraction which concerns only a definite part of the world, and that this is an effect of the anxiety which the schizophrenic experienced in early youth in relation to his personal environment. This nonuse of abstraction is a protective mechanism against the danger of catastrophe and anxiety.[26a]

The fact that the origin of the abnormal

concreteness in schizophrenics differs from the origin of such concreteness in organic patients becomes apparent in certain essential differences of the symptomatology. This can be seen, for instance, in the frequent appearances of physiognomic experiences. The schizophrenic's utterances sometimes yield "symbolic" interpretations but are often revealed, by analysis, to be only pseudo-symbolic phenomena. Such phenomena are here particularly suited to appear as symbolic, since the distortion of behavior brings out much of the instrumentalities belonging to the preschizophrenic condition of the patient where the symbolic attitude plays a more or less important role in the thinking of the patient. Further attention must be paid to the fact that schizophrenics often build complex mechanisms to cover their ideas, feelings, etc., which may easily appear to be of a high-level function, owing to their complexity, but which prove to be only complex associations built on a very concrete basis. This is often difficult to unveil, because the schizophrenic has not only passively originating protective mechanisms, like the organic patient, but also has defense mechanisms, which he produces intentionally, that may give the impression of higher-level function and sometimes may be also an expression of it. The picture of schizophrenic behavior is so complex that its origin may be understood only by a very detailed analysis. In this analysis the distinction between real symbolic and "quasi," pseudo-symbolic behavior has to be taken very seriously.

❨ The So-called General Mental Functions as Origin of Definite Symptoms

I stressed, in the beginning of my presentation, that in the interpretation of symptoms a distinction has often been made between defects in a special performance field and defects of so-called general functions, and that this distinction is not justified since the general functions appear changed in the same manner as do the specific performances. There is not enough space here to give detailed proof of

the correctness of my statement, but I would like to make a few remarks about the changes in these general functions, particularly those which are related to the personality change of the patient owing to impairment of abstract attitude. I have chosen these because analysis of this dependence may be especially useful for psychiatrists.

First, there is the problem of memory. Under certain circumstances the faculty for reproducing facts acquired previously may be about normal in patients with impairment of abstract attitude. Things learned in school, for example, may be recalled very well, but that is the case only in certain situations. The situation must be suited to the reawakening of old impressions. If the required answer demands an abstract attitude on the part of the patient, he may be unable to recollect. Therefore he fails in many intelligence tests which seem very simple to a normal person, and may be amazingly successful in others which appear complicated to us, namely in those which can be executed without the abstract attitude. He is able to learn new facts and to keep them in mind, but he can learn them only in a concrete situation and can reproduce them only in the same situation in which he has learned them. Because intentional recollection of experiences acquired in infancy requires an abstract attitude of the adult in relation to the situation at that time, and the events in infancy were not experienced abstractively, the patient is unable to recall experiences of infancy, but we can observe that aftereffects of such experiences appear passively, at times, in his behavior. He is incapable of recollecting when asked to recall things which have nothing to do with the given situation. He can recall only when he is able to regard the present situation in such a way that facts from the past belong to it. Repeated observation in many different situations demonstrates clearly that such memory failures are not caused by an impairment of memory content. The patient has the material in his memory, but he is not able to use it freely. He can use it only in connection with a definite concrete situation.[26a]

We arrive at the same results in testing attention. At one time the patient appears inattentive and distracted; at other times, he is attentive, even abnormally so. The patient's attention is usually weak in special examinations, particularly so at the beginning, when he has not as yet become aware of the approach to the whole situation, something he can get only through concrete activity. When he has done so, has entered the situation concretely, his attention is usually satisfactory, and he may even appear abnormally attentive, because under such circumstances he might often be totally untouched by other stimuli from the environment to which normal persons would unfailingly react. In other situations he will seem to be very distracted, as, for instance, in those which demand a change of approach. He seems distracted because he is incapable of making a choice. Consequently, it is not correct to speak of a change in attention in such patients in terms of plus or minus. The state of the patient's attention is but part of his total behavior and is to be understood only in connection with it.

Another important problem is judgment as to the patients' emotional experiences. Usually, the patients are considered emotionally dull, and often they appear so, but it would be incorrect simply to say that they are suffering from a diminution of emotions. The same patient can be dull under some conditions and very excited under others. This can be explained when we consider the patient's emotional behavior in relation to his entire behavior in a given situation. When he does not react emotionally in an adequate way, investigation may reveal that he has not grasped the situation in such a way that emotion could arise. The patient may have grasped only one part of the situation—the part which can be grasped concretely—and this part may not give any reason for an emotional reaction. His emotional reaction appears to us inappropriate because we grasp the whole situation to which the emotional character is attached, while he reacts only to a part of it. This connection between emotions and total behavior becomes understandable when we consider that emotions are not simply related to definite experiences but are, as I have stressed before (see p. 190), inherent aspects of all behavior, are part

and parcel of behavior. No behavior is without emotion, and what we call lack of emotion is a deviation from normal emotions corresponding to the deviation of behavior in general. From this point of view, the following modifications of reactions, which are of particular interest in respect to the problem of emotions in general, are interesting: We frequently see that a patient reacts either not at all or in an abnormally quick manner. The latter occurs particularly when the patient believes he has the correct answer to a problem. Although this quick behavior might seem to be simply an effect of a change in the time factor of his reactivity, it is actually the effect of an emotional factor. To some extent, the patients are always in danger of coming into catastrophic conditions, and the quick response is an effect of their tension, of which they want to rid themselves by all means. They are forced to release tension because they cannot handle it and cannot bear it. To bear tension presupposes deliberation, considering the future, etc., all of which is related to abstraction. The difference in behavior between these patients and normal people throws light on the nature of the trend to release tension. The patients must, so to speak, follow the "pleasure principle." They must, owing to their abnormal concreteness, react to the stimulus in a way which brings release. The trend to release tension thus appears as an expression of pathology, as an effect of a protective mechanism to prevent catastrophic conditions. The ability to speed up an activity or part of it, when this corresponds to the requirements of the task, belongs to normal behavior, but in the same way as the capacity to bear tension and even to enjoy it at times, when it is necessary to fulfill a particular task. In contrast to this, patients with impairment of abstraction are only able to experience the pleasure of release of tension. They never appear to enjoy anything, a fact which is often clearly revealed by the expression of their faces. This becomes understandable when we are aware of the fact that in any kind of joy immediate reality is transcended, that joy is a phenomenon which presupposes the abstract attitude and especially the category of possibility. Thus brain-injured patients who are impaired in this attitude cannot feel joy. Experience with brain-injured patients teaches us that we have to distinguish between pleasure through release of tension and the active feeling of enjoyment and freedom so characteristic of joy. Pleasure through release of tension is the passive feeling of being freed from distress, and therefore this feeling lasts, in normals, only until a new situation stimulates new activity. Joy, on the other hand, is something we try to extend, something which admits the possibility of infinite continuation.

The two emotions of joy and pleasure play essentially different roles in regard to self-realization. They belong to different performances or different parts of a performance. Pleasure may be a necessary state of respite, but it is a phenomenon of standstill. It is akin to death. It separates us from the world and the other individuals in it; it is equilibrium, quietness. In joy there is disequilibrium. But this disequilibrium is productive, leading toward fruitful activity and a particular kind of self-realization. This difference in the significance of the two emotional states for the normal person and the brain-injured patient is an expression of the essentially different behavior of the latter and of the different world in which he lives.

The drive toward release of tension is one of the causes for the strange behavior of brain-injured patients in friendship and love situations. The lack of the experience of future forces them to look for close relationships to other people and to maintain such relationships at all costs. At the same time, close relationships are terminated suddenly should their maintenance necessitate some bearing of tension, that is, should any difficulties arise in the relationship. The following example is illustrative: One of my patients, Mr. A., was for years a close friend of another patient, Mr. X. One day Mr. X. went to a movie with another man. Mr. X. had invited Mr. A. to go along with them, but the latter did not want to go, since he had seen the picture before. When Mr. X. returned, my patient was in a state of great excitement and refused to speak to Mr. X. He could not be quieted by any explanation. He was told that his friend had not meant to offend him and that his friendship had not changed, but these explanations made no impression at all. From that time on, Mr. A. was the enemy of his old friend, Mr. X. He was aware only of the fact that his friend had been companion to another man, and he felt himself slighted. The experience had produced great tension in him. He regarded his friend as the cause of that tension and reacted to him in a way which is readily understandable in terms of his inability to bear tension and to put himself in the place of someone else.

Another patient never seemed to be concerned about his family. He never spoke of his wife or children and was unresponsive when we questioned him about them. When we suggested to him that he should write to his family, he was utterly indifferent. He appeared to lack all feelings in this respect. At times, according to an established practice, he visited his family in another town and stayed there for several days. We learned that while he was at home he conducted himself as any man would in the bosom of his family. He was kind and affectionate to his wife and children, and interested in their affairs in so far as his abilities would permit. Upon his return to the hospital from such a visit, he would, when asked about his family, smile in an embarrassed way and give evasive answers; he seemed utterly estranged from his home situation. Unquestionably, the peculiar behavior of this man was not actually an effect of deterioration of his character on the emotional and moral side; his behavior was the result, rather, of the fact that, owing to his impairment of abstraction, he could not summon up the home situation when he was not actually there, and therefore he could not show adequate feeling and behavior. Lack of active imagination, which is so apparent in this example, makes such patients incapable of experiencing any expectation for the future. Active imagination depends on the abstract capacity.

This lack is apparent, for instance, in the behavior of a male patient toward a woman whom he later married. When he was with her, he seemed to behave in a friendly, affectionate way and to be very fond of the girl. But when he was separated from her, he did not care about her at all; he would not seek her out and certainly did not desire to have a love relationship with her. When he was questioned, his answers indicated that he did not even understand what sexual desire meant. He could not imagine any sexual situation and did not understand pictures which showed such situations. When he met the girl again, however, when she spoke to him, he was immediately able to enter into the previous relationship. He was as affectionate as before. When she induced him to go to bed with her, embraced him and put his penis into her vagina, he performed an apparently normal act of sexual intercourse, with satisfaction for both. She had the feeling that he loved her. She became pregnant, and they married. The above case also reveals the great significance of speech and voice for any relationship, particularly when other possibilities are destroyed by the defect of the brain function, as was the case here.

Some other so-called general factors which are often mentioned as obstacles to examining such patients consist of fatigue and perseveration. Here, also, observation shows that these phenomena are not always present in the same way, that they change according to the situation, as do all performances. Observation of our patients shows that fatigue is not a simple function of the duration of continuous performance but depends to a high degree upon whether or not the performance in question is within or somewhat above the capacity level of the patient. Thus a paradoxical situation may occur, where fatigue decreases as the activity continues. This happens, for instance, when a later task is "easy" to perform while the earlier tasks could be executed only with difficulty. Another point is the fact that fatigue does not express itself simply as a slowing down of performance but, especially at the beginning, as a fluctuation of performance (Goldstein,[20] p. 260). Subjectively, the individual feels not only incapacitation but also discomfort, uncertainty, and distress. The phenomena occurring in fatigue show great similarity to those observed in catastrophic condi-

tions and seem to be closely related to them. Patients with severe brain damage tire easily because many normal tasks represent difficult ones for them, thus producing distress. While fatigue in difficult tasks may thus be understandable, we may ask whether the same point of view is appropriate to explain the fact that fatigue occurs also in continuous work consisting of a task which is within the limits of the individual's capacity. I think that is the case. Continuation means consumption of energy which deteriorates the function of the substratum, so that a task which was previously easy to perform may be changed into a difficult one; therefore, mere continuation may produce catastrophe and fatigue. This becomes evident by the fact that fatigue does not set in as early when the task is varied. Boredom and interest influence the fatigue rate. This must be considered particularly in testing situations. If, after we recognize the onset of fatigue, we should change the task, the patient may then perform without fatigue and may do so better, both subjectively and objectively. This is particularly true if the succeeding task is within the capacities of the individual, and if the change does not demand a voluntary shifting on the part of the individual, which, as we have mentioned previously, is an especially difficult problem for many brain-injured patients. Automatized performances may be continued for a long time without the patient showing and experiencing fatigue. We frequently observe, however, severe breakdowns after excellent performances. This suggests that the symptoms of fatigue are not only signs of catastrophe but also indications of imminent catastrophe— warnings, which, thoroughly considered, may help to prevent the latter. Patients with a mental defect which appears in a lack of planning and foresight are particularly prone to fatigue, since they do not recognize the protective danger signals and thus become abnormally tired.

Perseveration is a frequent phenomenon in brain damage. I am inclined to assume that it is a secondary phenomenon due to incapacitation in some performances, and a means to avoid catastrophe occurring under such conditions. Perseveration occurs particularly when the patient is forced to fulfill tasks with which he is unable to cope. For instance, a patient who has difficulty with arithmetic may be able to answer promptly at long as he has to solve problems which are within his capacity. The moment he is given a problem which he is unable to fulfill, he may either be thrown into a catastrophic state and not react at all, or he may repeat the last correct result or a part of it, that is, he perseverates. If he is then given an example, however, which he is able to solve, he may again answer correctly, and all perseveration will disappear. The same patient may show perseveration under some conditions and distractibility under others, so that it becomes evident that we are not dealing with a primary defect of rigidity. As we have explained previously, the sick organism tries to react as well as possible to the task set before him. Confronted with assignments which he cannot fulfill, he tries to react to that part of the task in which he is able to succeed by means of his remaining capacity, and he sticks to that rigidly, because thus he can best avoid catastrophe. But under certain conditions he becomes aware that he has not fulfilled the task correctly. Then he gives up the first reaction, I think, because continuing it does not help in overcoming distress. He tries again and may become attached to another part of the situation to which he is able to react, but again may feel that he is not performing the task demanded. Thus he appears abnormally distractible. Neither rigidity, perseveration, nor distractibility is a defect per se; they are phenomena coming to the fore under special conditions which can be defined. They can be avoided—at least to a certain degree—by the same means by which abnormal fatigue can be avoided, because ultimately they originate from the same cause.

❲ Some Remarks Concerning the Method of Examination

I would like to conclude with some remarks concerning the method of examination which follows the rules prescribed by the organismic approach. From our discussion it is evident that only a method can be successful which takes the relationship of each performance of the patient, each success and each failure, to the whole behavior of the patient and the whole organism into consideration, and which particularly keeps in mind that a performance can be evaluated correctly only in respect to the trend of the organism for self-realization. The organismic approach by no means overlooks the significance of the study of details, correct reactions and failures, of the quantitative deviations from the average and the influence of previous capacities of the individual patient; it uses all available quantitative methods and applies statistics to the evaluation. But one should be aware that statistics can be really helpful only when we are confronted with quantitatively different material, and that, in the symptomatology of brain cortex damage, particularly those which are of interest for the psychiatrist, we are mostly dealing with qualitative deviations from the norm. Statistically valid results, therefore, are not too important for the increase of our knowledge of what pathology did to the patient and what we can learn from pathological findings for understanding normal behavior.

According to our evaluation of the significance of abstract attitude for all performances, the capacity of abstraction should be tested in the beginning of any examination. Whether the abstract attitude is impaired and how much it is impaired can be evaluated by observing the patient under the conditions of various modes of behavior which can be correctly executed only in this attitude. Some tests have been constructed which allow one to judge the patient's capacity in an easier and more correct way. The tests differ as to whether the material used is language or the execution of some performances—matching, sorting, making choices, etc. The results with the first group of tests are sometimes difficult to establish because of the ambiguity of language and because they are not always simple to apply when the patients are suffering from language defects. The advantage of the other group of tests is not only that they do not use language but also that they are so organized that judgment can be based directly on the results of the behavior of the subject in the test.

As an example of the first group of tests, the Proverb-and-Phrases tests by Hadlich, John Benjamin[4] may be mentioned; as an example of the other group, the Vigotski test should be mentioned, particularly in the presentation by Hanfmann and Kasanin;[27] further mention should be made of the various performance tests of Goldstein and Gelb,[24] Goldstein and Scheerer,[25] Weigl,[41] and others. (See also the papers by Von Domarus,[9] Beck,[3] Cameron,[7] and Angyal,[1] and the psychological monograph by Goldstein and Scheerer.[25])

The use of various tests in examining the same patient is recommended, since each test differs somewhat as to its applicability and definiteness in determining the impairment of abstraction and as to its ability to characterize the various forms of abnormal concreteness. The technique of the Goldstein-Gelb-Scheerer tests enables one, by the use of various materials and by the application of various specified subtests besides the main test, to determine whether or not a patient can assume the abstract attitude, to measure somewhat the degree of the impairment, and to find out the specific type of concreteness to which the patient is confined. This proved to be particularly helpful in distinguishing between the defect in organic patients and in schizophrenics.

(Bibliography

1. ANGYAL, A. "Disturbances of Thinking in Schizophrenia," in J. S. Kasanin, ed., *Language and Thought in Schizophrenia.* Berkeley: Univ. California Press, 1944.
2. ANTON, "Fehlende Selbstwahrnehmung des Defekts," *Arch. Psychiatr.,* 32 (1899).
3. BECK, S. J. "Errors in Perception and Fantasy in Schizophrenia," in J. S. Kasanin, ed., *Language and Thought in Schizophrenia.* Berkeley: Univ. California Press, 1944.
4. BENJAMIN, J. "A Method for Distinguishing and Evaluating Formal Thinking Disorders in Schizophrenia," in J. S. Kasanin, ed., *Language and Thought in Schizophrenia.* Berkeley: Univ. California Press, 1944.
5. BOLLES, M. and K. GOLDSTEIN. "A Study of Impairment of Abstract Behavior in Schizophrenic Patients," *Psychiatr. Q.,* 12 (1938), 42.
6. BOUMANN, L. and A. A. GRUENBAUM. "Experimentell Psychologische Untersuchungen zur Aphasie," *Z. Ges. Neurol. Psychiatr.,* (1925), 96.
7. BRUGSCH, T., ed. *Einheitsbestrebungen in der Medizin.* Leipzig: Steinkopf, 1933.
8. CAMERON, N. "Experimental Analysis of Schizophrenic Thinking," in J. S. Kasanin, ed., *Language and Thought in Schizophrenia.* Berkeley: Univ. California Press, 1944.
9. CRITCHLEY, M. *The Parietal Lobe.* London: Arnold, 1953.
10. DOMARUS, E., VON. "The Specific Laws in Logic in Schizophrenia," in J. S. Kasanin, ed., *Language and Thought in Schizophrenia.* Berkeley: Univ. California Press, 1944.
11. GOLDSTEIN, K. *Aftereffects of Brain Injuries in War.* New York: Grune & Stratton, 1942.
12. ———. "The Concept of Transference in the Treatment of Organic and Functional Nervous Disease," *Acta Psychother.,* 2 (3/4) (1954), 334.
13. ———. "The Effect of Brain Damage on the Personality," *Psychiatry,* 15(3) (1952), 245.
14. ———. "On Emotions," *J. Psychol.,* 31 (1951), 37.
15. ———. *Language and Language Disturbances.* New York: Grune & Stratton, 1948.
16. ———. "Die Lokalisation in der Grosshirnrinde," *Handbuch der Normalen und Pathologischen Physiologie,* Vol. 10, pp. 600–842. Berlin: Springer, 1927.
17. ———. "The Modification of Behavior Consequent to Cerebral Lesions," *Psychiatr. Q.,* 10 (1936), 586.
18. ———. "Naming and Pseudonaming." *Word.,* 2(1) (1946), 1.
19. ———. *The Organism.* New York: American Book, 1939.
20. ———. "Physiological Aspects of Convalescence and Rehabilitation Following Certain Nervous System Injuries," Symposium, K. Ancel, ed. Federation Proceedings, 1944.

21. ———. "The Significance of the Frontal Lobes for Mental Performance," *J. Neurol. Psychopathol.*, 17 (1936), 27.

22. ———. "Das Symptom, seine Entstehung und Bedeutung," *Arch. Psychiatr. Neurol.*, 6 (1925), 84.

23. ———. "The Two Ways of Adjustment of the Organism to Cerebral Defects." *J. Mt. Sinai Hosp.*, 9 (1942), 4.

24. GOLDSTEIN, K. and A. GELB. "Ueber Farbennamenamnesie," *Psychol. Forsch.*, 6 (1924), 127.

25. GOLDSTEIN, K. and M. SCHEERER. "Abstract and Concrete Behavior," *Psychol. Monograph*, 53 (1941), 239.

26. GOLDSTEIN, K. and J. STEINFELD. "The Condition of Sexual Behavior by Visual Agnosia," *Bull. Forest Lawn Series*, 1 (1942), 37.

26a. GOLDSTEIN, K. "The Organismic Approach," in S. Arieti, ed., *American Handbook of Psychiatry*, Vol. 2, 1st ed., pp. 770–797. New York: Basic Books, 1959.

27. HANFMANN, E. and J. KASANIN. "A Method for the Study of Schizophrenia," *Arch. Neurol. Psychiatr.*, 41 (1939), 568.

28. HEAD, H. *Aphasia and Kindred Disorders of Speech*. New York: Macmillan, 1926.

29. HEILBRONNER, K. "Die Aphasischen, Aphasischen und Agnostischen Störungen," *Handbuch der Neurologie*, Springer, Berlin, 1919.

30. JACKSON, J. H. "Croonian Lectures on the Evolution and Dissolution of the Nervous System," *Lancet* (1884), 535, 649, 739.

31. KASANIN, J. S., ed. *Language and Thought in Schizophrenia, Collected Papers*. Berkeley: Univ. California Press, 1944.

32. KRONFELD, A. and E. STERNBERG. "Der Gedankliche Aufbau der Klassischer Aphasiedehre, etc.," *Psychol. Medizin*, Vol. 2. Stuttgart: Enke.

33. LEEPER, R. W. "A Motivational Theory of Emotion, etc.," *Psychol. Rev.*, 55 (1948), 5.

34. LOTMAR, F. "Zur Kenntnis der erschwerten Wortfindung, etc.," *Schweiz. Arch. Neurol. Psychiatr.*, 5 (1919), 206.

35. MARIE, P. "Revision de la question de l'aphasie," *Semaine Medicale*, 1906.

36. NIELSON, T. M. *Agnosia, Apraxia, Aphasia*, New York: Hoeber, 1947.

37. RIESE, W. "Hughlings Jackson's Doctrine of Aphasia and Its Significance Today." *J. Nerv. Ment. Dis.*, 122(1) (1955), 1.

38. SCHACHTEL, E. G. "On Memory and Childhood Amnesia," *Psychiatry*, 10 (1947), 1.

39. STORCH. A. *The Primitive Archaic Forms of Inner Experiences and Thought in Schizophrenia*. Nerv. & Ment. Dis. Monog. No. 31. New York: Nerv. and Ment. Dis. Publ. Co., 1934.

40. VIGOTSKI, I. "Thought in Schizophrenia," *Arch. Neurol. Psychiatr.*, 31 (1934), 1063.

41. WEIGL, E. "On the Psychology of Socalled Processes of Abstraction," *J. Abnorm. Soc. Psychol.*, 36 (1941), 3.

42. WERNER, H., *Comparative Psychology of Mental Development*, p. 59. New York: Harper, 1940.

43. WOERKOM, W. VON. "Ueber Stoerung im Denken bei Aphasie-Patienten," *Monatsschr. Psychiatr. Neurol.*, (1925), 59.

CHAPTER 9

PSYCHIATRIC CONDITIONS ASSOCIATED WITH FOCAL LESIONS OF THE CENTRAL NERVOUS SYSTEM*

D. Frank Benson and Norman Geschwind

(Introduction

TRADITIONALLY, focal pathology which involves the central nervous system has been the concern of the neurologist and neurosurgeon. It has long been realized, however, that focal pathology can produce a great variety of behavioral changes, some of which may directly involve the psychiatrist and are the subject of this chapter.

Most abnormalities of behavior caused by focal brain disease involve malfunction of major motor and sensory systems and produce

little difficulty in diagnosis. Some behavioral manifestations, however, such as those involving the so-called higher functions, e.g., aphasia, memory loss, and attention, are sometimes not readily recognized and categorized. In addition, there is a group of behavioral disturbances produced by focal brain damage which are distinctly psychiatric in nature. The latter include such manifestations as aggressive behavior, compulsiveness, severe anxiety, euphoria, depression, paranoia, and others. This chapter will present some of the disturbances of the higher functions and psychiatric disorders produced by focal lesions. Admixture of symptoms is common and represents a considerable challenge to the diagnostician, par-

* The work reported here was supported in part by Grant NS-06209 of the National Institute of Neurological Diseases and Stroke.

ticularly when one realizes that many of the individual signs or symptoms seen with neurological disease also occur frequently in functional disorders.

Not all types of psychiatric symptomatology occur as the result of brain lesions, but the variety observed is extensive. Rejection of the possibility of organic causation because the clinical picture is, for example, typically schizophrenic, is unjustified. Furthermore, one should not automatically assume that psychiatric disorder is only indirectly related to an organic cause. Focal lesions often produce characteristic psychiatric disorders. For example, right hemisphere symptomatology is distinctly different from that of a temporal-lobe epilepsy, and Broca's and Wernicke's aphasics consistently show different emotional behavior.

It should be remembered that brain lesions causing psychiatric disorder may do so without producing any significant disturbance of cognitive function. The extensive literature on frontal lobotomy demonstrates that, despite dramatic changes in behavior, changes in cognitive function are not prominent. Failure of psychological test batteries to show signs of "organicity" does not exclude organic causation for psychiatric symptomatology.

The reader may well decide that the differential diagnosis between organic and functional disorder can be extremely difficult; we would agree. While organic causes of psychiatric complaints are less common than functional, their recognition is important both for theoretical reasons and because they open additional and specific therapeutic possibilities.

Certain general rules may be helpful. Hallucinations in childhood are far more suggestive of organic causation than when they occur in early adult life. A marked change in personality beyond the age of forty always suggests the possibility of organic disease. Meticulous history-taking may be needed to bring this out, however. If a change in personality occurs insidiously over several years, striking abnormalities may remain unnoticed by the family. Also, many people have a bias towards perceiving the personalities of their close associates as continuous. Thus the woman who has just been beaten by her husband may insist that there has been no change in his personality, yet admit, on direct questioning, that he had never struck her during the first ten years of their marriage.

One must be wary of sweeping statements such as: "Aggressiveness is characteristic of organic disease of the brain." The symptom of aggressiveness, in fact, differs sharply in organic disorders. Temporal-lobe epileptics often give elaborate justifications for aggressive behavior based on strongly held moral positions; the same sort of justification would be extremely unusual in a patient with a frontal lesion who had been aggressive. Of course, much aggressive behavior, particularly in the young, has no demonstrable pathology in the brain.

Finally, we must comment on the word "depression" which presents difficulties because of its ambiguous use. At present, it is used both as a diagnosis and as a description of behavior. Even when employed to describe behavior, the usage is ambiguous. The statement that a patient is "depressed" may mean that he is agitated, tearful, guilt-ridden, and suicidal. It may also mean that the patient is apathetic and suffers a psychomotor retardation. While psychomotor retardation may be the cardinal sign of a late-life depression,[54] it is also a characteristic of many organic behavioral disorders. The apathetic, depressed appearance of many cases of organic brain disorder merely reflects a shallowness of emotional expression. Agitated depression, on the other hand, is rare as an organic symptom and a psychogenic depressive illness almost never occurs in patients with severe organic brain disorder. The term "depressed" should therefore be avoided as a description of behavior and replaced by more precise descriptive terms.

⟨ Etiologic Factors

In general, the symptomatology produced by focal pathology of the central nervous system (CNS) depends on the anatomic locus of the lesion as well as the specific variety of pathology. The most frequent forms of focal pathology underlying behavioral symptoms are intracerebral space-occupying lesions, cerebrovascular disease, and trauma. Some manifestations of inflammatory disease, particularly abscess or granuloma, may produce focal symptomatology, but many varieties of central nervous system (CNS) disease (the degenerative, demyelinating, toxic-metabolic, developmental, and most inflammatory disorders) cause widespread CNS pathology (see chapter 3 for additional details). Even these disorders, however, often produce focal disturbances.

Most cerebrovascular and traumatic insults to the brain occur acutely, and the history suggests the probable source of behavioral changes. Many behavioral symptoms, however, do not occur immediately and differentiation from symptoms produced by a reaction to the diseased state may prove difficult. Premorbid personality structure is often retained but individual personality traits may become either exaggerated or damped. Changes in behavioral responses (mood, affect, interpersonal relations) which occur late after acute brain damage may not be manifestations of the original pathology. Additional organic disturbance or purely psychogenic reactions may underlie such changes. Both states are potentially correctable but all too frequently insufficient attention is given to these patients; the clinician tends to accept the original insult as the source of the late behavioral developments.

Space occupying lesions offer much greater diagnostic difficulty. The onset is usually insidious, often with vague behavioral changes, and the classic signs of CNS involvement frequently appear late. As emphasized by Mayer-Gross et al.,[122] the absence of organic clinical features does not exclude the possibility of organic disease; indeed, apparently functional disturbances are often the earliest manifestations of brain tumor. Many psychiatrists have had the sobering experience of misdiagnosing and offering psychotherapy to a patient subsequently proved to have a brain tumor. Abnormal behavior patterns which appear unrelated to present stress, personal or familial background, genetic processes or other positive indications of functional disorder should always arouse suspicion, particularly in the older patient.

Several inflammatory diseases may appear only, or primarily, as focal processes and produce behavioral symptomatology. For instance rabies, a virus infection, involving the hypothalamus and hippocampus, usually produces depression, anxiety, and apprehension initially, then advances to terrifying delusions and ideas of reference. Only later do physical signs, such as pharyngeal spasms, occur. Encephalitis caused by herpes simplex infection usually centers in one or both temporal lobes. Early symptoms may include disorientation, memory loss, and aimless wandering. Bizarre ideation and inappropriate actions may occur before delirium, fever, severe headache, and diminished state of consciousness announce the presence of encephalitis.[72,156] Most often the course of herpes encephalitis is fairly rapid and dramatic, but if slow and/or partial in development, it may offer a severe challenge for diagnosis. Intracerebral granulomas and abscesses often present the general signs of space-occupying lesions but, if the onset is insidious, strongly resemble deteriorating functional disturbances. Hypochondriasis, psychomotor retardation including apathy, cognitive deterioration, and loose thought associations may be the presenting signs.

(Subcortical Syndromes

One of the striking advances of the past two decades in the understanding of cerebral mechanisms concerns the effects, both facilitatory and inhibitory, of various subcortical structures. Most dramatic was the demonstration by Moruzzi and Magoun of the effect that lesions of the brainstem reticular substance had on sleep and consciousness.[127] In the cat, destructive lesions of the midbrain reticular substance produced a state of somnolence, both clinical and electrical (EEG). The animal would respond to sensory stimuli (noise and touch) and could move all limbs but remained asleep. In contrast, an animal with lesions involving the major motor and sensory pathways of the midbrain, but sparing the reticular substance, retained a normal ability to awaken. It is suggested that this central reticular core, through connections with many subcortical neural structures, acts to modulate and modify cerebral activity. The functions attributed to this system include the initiation and maintenance of wakefulness, the orienting reflex and the focus of attention, many sensory control processes including habituation and external inhibition, conditional learning, memory functions, and the management of internal inhibition including light and deep sleep.[116]

Another system, essentially antagonistic to the reticular system, has been demonstrated. This is usually called the nonspecific thalamocortical projection system,[37] but involves, anatomically, many subcortical centres including medullary and other brainstem centers, the caudate nucleus, hypothalamic and limbic structures, portions of the thalamus and selected areas of cortex. Identification of these two phylogenetically ancient and interlocking systems, both of which constantly modify cerebral activity, has allowed fuller understanding of complex mental symptomatology. In general, behavioral responses result from a composite of internal and external stimuli set against both of these internal regulating mechanisms. Many behavior modifiers, particularly drugs and the toxic states, are best understood as involving these subcortical systems. These behavior modifiers, while primarily affecting a single system, usually have a widespread (thus nonfocal or multifocal) distribution; there are, however, several focal disorders which produce major behavioral alterations by involvement of these subcortical systems and which will now be discussed.

Consciousness

Modifications of the state of consciousness may be produced by focal lesions involving specific subcortical areas. Thus the unconscious states, coma, stupor, and lethargy, produced by head injury, are often ascribed to focal involvement of the mesencephalic reticular substance.[56] At times gross pathology (i.e., hemorrhage, infarction, edema, or laceration) is present in the upper brainstem of patients who have suffered prolonged coma; other cases, however, show only minimal evidence of pathology, e.g., demyelination or lymphocytic clusters.[162] Often there is no pathological remnant, even in cases which suffered moderately prolonged unconsciousness. Other varieties of focal pathology may also affect this area and produce changes in the state of consciousness. Thus tumors, aneurysms, hemorrhages, and infectious processes (encephalitis) which involve the upper brainstem often produce a diminution of alertness.

Attention

Two clinically distinguishable varieties of attention abnormality can be ascribed to disorders in the subcortical alerting system. One is the type occurring in drug-intoxication states, head injury, increased intracranial pressure, etc., associated with the diminished state of alertness described above. These patients can be alerted but their attention rapidly wanes and they drift back into a somnolent state (accurately described as "drifting attention"). In these cases the "background" state of alertness is impaired while "phasic" alerting is relatively unaffected. This disturbance of attention usually indicates pathological involvement of the midbrain or thalamic portion of the reticular activating system.

In the second variety of attention disturbance the patient appears fully alert but has great difficulty maintaining attention on the immediate task (called "wandering attention"). While this patient is alert and attempts to be cooperative, his attention is distracted by almost any external stimulus. A coherent mental evaluation is extremely difficult because of this unpredictable irregularity of attention. Wandering attention may result from either focal or widespread CNS disease; if present, focal pathology is usually located higher in the neuraxis than that which produces the drifting attention state. Subfrontal tumors, CNS lues, and some tumors of the limbic system are characterized by this inability to inhibit external stimuli. Clinically similar defects of attention may be seen in the severely depressed patient (internal distracting stimuli) and the acute schizophrenic with grossly disturbed thought processing (distracted by either internal or external stimuli).

Thus when a patient with a behavioral problem manifests a disturbance of attention, the examiner should suspect pathology involving the two complex, subcortical neural systems which modify cerebral activity, the reticular activating system and the nonspecific thalamo-cortical projection system.

Akinetic Mutism

Akinetic mutism has been defined as a state of limited responsiveness to the environment in the absence of gross alteration of sensory-motor mechanisms.[151] Two varieties are recognized, a hyperpathic type (coma vigil) and an apathetic type (somnolent mutism). In the former variety there is a state of alert or vigilant coma in which the patient lies immobile but appears alert since there is free movement of the eyes in following visual stimuli. If stimulated sufficiently, this patient may become restless or even agitated and may even say a few words but soon settles back to a state of extreme inertia. In the second variety the patient is also immobile but with eyes closed. Only strong stimuli produce movement, including eye opening; vertical gaze palsy or even total ophthalmoplegia, including loss of pupillary light reflex, is usually present. After stimulation, this patient rapidly subsides into the lethargic state, so that this is an apathetic or somnolent variety of akinetic mutism.

The two varieties of akinetic mutism reflect separate neuroanatomical loci. In the apathetic type the lesion, as would be expected, involves the junction area of the mesencephalon and diencephalon and produces both a state of lethargy and occulomotor disturbances. The vigilant variety occurs with pathology higher in the neuraxis, usually involving the postero-medial and inferior aspects of the frontal (septal area) or the hypothalamus. Both varieties involve portions of the reticular activating and/or the diffuse thalamic projection systems. Many varieties of pathology may produce akinetic mutism, including tumor, granuloma, abscess, encephalitis, hemorrhage, trauma, vascular infarction, angioma, and occult hydrocephalus. Thus this specific behavioral disturbance is dependent on the location, not the nature of the pathology.

(Limbic System Syndromes

Since Papez's postulation[131] that portions of the rhinencephalon (limbic system) were important for emotion, there has been an increasing emphasis on the role played by these phylogenetically ancient structures in behavior.[57,112,149] For the present discussion the limbic system includes the hippocampus and hippocampal gyrus, the temporal pole, amygdala, fornix, hypothalamus, septal nuclei, certain thalamic nuclei (anterior, dorso-medial and intralaminar), cingulate gyrus, and parts of the orbital frontal cortex. The functions of these structures have been extensively reviewed[113,114] and need not be listed here. Many behavioral syndromes may result from disease involving the limbic system. It should be noted that most disorders which affect the limbic system also affect other structures. Since, anatomically the limbic system is spread through much of the brain it is often involved along with contiguous, nonlimbic structures. This combination of behavioral features produces a complex clinical picture. Focal involvement of limbic function does occur, however, and can produce striking behavioral pictures. When one considers the "four F's" of the limbic system, feeding, fighting, fleeing, and the undertaking of mating activity,[115] it is obvious that disorders of the limbic system will often come to the attention of the psychiatrist.

Emotional Disturbance

There has long been awareness that structural brain disorder could cause emotional disturbance and, since Papez, many investigators have considered damage to the limbic system as particularly important. Others have noted that pathology outside the actual limbic system may produce severe behavior disorder which they attribute to limbic release or disinhibition. Many of the emotional disturbances produced by damage to the limbic system are similar to those seen in "functional" disorders.

In 1937 Kluver and Bucy[100] demonstrated that bilateral anterior temporal-lobe resection produces a striking behavioral change in the monkey. Abnormalities included psychic blindness, abnormal tameness, hypersexuality, strong oral tendencies and hypermetamorphopsia, the tendency to shift attention frequently. Their work implied that bilateral limbic destruction (or release) could produce striking behavioral abnormality. Very few human cases which fit this description have been reported. The authors once cared for a university professor, severely injured in an auto accident. who was found at operation to have severe bilateral anterior temporal contusions. Necrotic tissue was removed from the anterior temporal regions on both sides. During recovery there was a phase, lasting over a month, in which he was fully conscious, and had no demonstrable paresis, primary sensory loss or visual field defect. He did not appear to understand language and spoke only a mumbled jargon. He apparently recognized no one (not even old friends) and could not, or would not, name objects placed in front of him or in his hand. He ate voraciously and showed a tendency to place everything in his mouth, even such things as the tea bags from his tray. He made sexual advances indiscriminately but otherwise had a flat affect. There was an almost constant shifting of attention and if restrained he would become agitated, only to calm down immediately if his attention was diverted. We believed he fulfilled the clinical criteria for the Kluver-Bucy syndrome at that time. He eventually made considerable recovery. Most reported cases of the human Kluver-Bucy syndrome[137,170] show some, but not all, of the features reported in the original animal experiments.

Flattening of affect (placidity) has also been reported,[138] in tumors and vascular disorders of the limbic system, particularly involving the anterior midline structures (septal area and hypothalamus). The affective change may vary from a mild indifference to a total akinetic mute state (see above). Malamud,[119] in his description of psychiatric symptoms produced by tumors involving the limbic system, described seven cases with anterior midline pathology, who showed affective changes (flattening, depression, manic outbursts, or instability) and who were originally diagnosed as either schizophrenic or neurotic. Severe depressive symptomatology including withdrawal, negativism, apathy, and even suicide attempts, has also been reported with limbic pathology.[123,160] Many of the objective findings of depression, are, however, also produced by bilateral brain pathology (see below, frontal lobes). As already noted, psychomotor retardation can be produced in many ways and deserves careful evaluation.

Agitated, aggressive, impulsive, and assaultive behavior have also been ascribed to pathological involvement of the limbic system.[121,134,169] Most of these reports suggest a relationship between violent behavior and temporal-lobe disorder, specifically seizures, and will be discussed under Temporal Lobe Syndromes.

Vegetative Disturbances

Pathology involving the limbic system can produce abnormalities in vegetative or endocrine function. When these symptoms are combined with the emotional disturbances described above, the resulting syndrome can readily be mistaken for psychosomatic or neurotic disturbance. Severe anorexia, clinically identical to anorexia nervosa, has been described frequently with hypothalamic disease including tumors.[187] The opposite, i.e., hyperphagia, associated with outbursts of rage, polydipsia, polyuria, and slowly progressive dementia has been reported[144] in a patient with a tiny tumor of the hypothalamus. Diabetes insipidus is a well known disorder resulting from pathology involving the anterior portion of the pituitary; it can be differentiated from "compulsive water drinking" only by carefully performed water loading tests.[42] Amenorrhea, impotence, sterility, and loss of libido[94,96] are reported with limbic pathology, particularly that affecting the midline structures. Conversely, hypersexual behavior has been reported following midline encephalitis[140] and abnormal sexual behavior has been reported in cases with seizures arising from temporal-lobe foci.[34,91]

Memory Disturbances

Another major neuropsychiatric aspect of limbic-system disease concerns memory. In the past two decades a fairly clear-cut clinical–anatomical correlation has been demonstrated for memory defects. Excellent reviews of this work are available[5,167,175,188] and only a synopsis will be presented here.

Many terms have been used to describe memory functions. Unfortunately, the usage of these terms in the literature has not been consistent. In general the functions called memory may be divided into three distinct categories: immediate recall (also called registration, short-term memory, immediate memory, minute memory, auditory attention); recent memory (consolidation, short-term memory, intermediate-term memory, ability to acquire new knowledge, learning, putting to memory); and remote memory (retrieval, long-term memory, store of information, ability to retrieve old knowledge). Note that "short-term memory" has been and still is used to refer to two different types of memory function, an unfortunate source of additional confusion. Clinical and pathological findings clearly demonstrate that one variety, i.e., recent memory or the ability to acquire new knowledge, depends upon intactness of limbic structures. The classic example of disordered recent memory is Korsakoff's psychosis incidental to thiamine deficiency (see Chapter 15). Similar mental pictures may occur after head trauma (posttraumatic amnesia), cerebrovascular disease, cerebral surgery, and, in a modified state, electroconvulsive shock therapy.

Korsakoff's psychosis is often called the amnestic-confabulatory syndrome to emphasize its two most conspicuous features. The amnesia has distinct clinical characteristics. There is excellent (sometimes supernormal) ability to attend to auditory stimuli, and tests such as digit span are usually normal. In contrast, newly learned material cannot be retained for even a few minutes. Thus the doctor's name is forgotten within minutes and there is disorientation as to time and place because the patient cannot "remember." The ability to retrieve old learned material is relatively preserved, but evaluation reveals a period of retrograde amnesia. Most often this period is at least several years before onset; often there are gross lacunae in memories for many additional years. The best retained memories are either those that are oldest and most overlearned (language, toilet training, feeding, dressing and grooming activities, and early life experiences) or those concerning emotionally significant occurrences (operations, death of a loved one, etc.).

Confabulation, often noted as the second major symptom of Korsakoff's psychosis, is not a constant feature and is not necessary for the diagnosis, but, when present, is remarkable. The patient answers all questions, often with bizarre responses. Thus, when asked where he is, he will offer an incorrect address or place name; if asked when he last saw the examiner he will give a response, again incorrect and often apparently bizarre; when asked the day and date he hesitates, then responds incorrectly; if asked what he did the previous day he often describes a job, a trip, a visit, or some other activity in considerable but incorrect detail. Careful study of confabulatory responses usually reveals that they represent material from the patient's past. Barbizet[4] has described the confabulatory state as one in which the patient cannot remember that he cannot remember; when asked a question he will offer the best answer available to him, something from his store of old, overlearned memories. Confabulations, then, represent old information offered in answer to a new question.

Recovery from Korsakoff's psychosis is variable, but at least some degree of improvement is usual. The first sign of recovery is realization that something is wrong with the memory. As this concept grows, the amount of confabulation decreases and within two to three months of onset, almost all patients with Korsakoff's psychosis cease confabulating. Some patients make considerable recovery, sufficient to allow them to return home and even to undertake a simple job.[175] Others, however, fail to recover, and must remain in custodial care. In general, the disability in acquiring new knowledge, as characterized by Korsakoff's psychosis, is accompanied by a striking personality change which usually includes passivity, indifference, apathy, and contentment. In the later stages of the illness, although apathy usually persists, some of the patients do express concern about their disorder and may even show episodes of anger.

Nutritional Korsakoff's psychosis is based on thiamine deficiency secondary to alcoholism or severe malnutrition. The onset is usually acute, with restlessness, confusion, and often an occulomotor abnormality signifying Wernicke's encephalopathy. With prompt treatment (thiamine by injection) the occulomotor disturbance can be corrected. The stage of acute alcohol withdrawal is passed in a few more days. Only then (usually five to ten days after onset) can the presence of Korsakoff's psychosis be ascertained with certainty.

There are many reports on the neuropathology of Korsakoff's psychosis[5,175,188] and all agree that bilateral pathology in the mammillary bodies (posterior hypothalamus) is almost always present. A recent study, based on fifty-three cases,[175] claims that degenerative changes in the dorsal medial nucleus of the thalamus were more important in the pathogenesis of memory disorder than those in the mammillary bodies.

Posttraumatic amnesia (PTA) is even more common than Korsakoff's psychosis but is usually accompanied by so many other signs and symptoms that the memory loss is often not clearly demonstrated. Pure posttraumatic amnesia and Korsakoff's psychosis present similar clinical pictures. Complete recovery, however, is much more likely after traumatic memory loss. During periods of PTA the patient exhibits a long retrograde amnesia amounting to at least several years; if the PTA clears this retrograde amnesia shrinks[7] and becomes very short, often involving only a few seconds preceding the head trauma. From this it would appear that the same structures that are necessary for learning new material are also necessary for retrieval of recently learned material. As head injury produces widespread effects, it is difficult to localise precisely the pathology responsible for PTA. Most investigators agree, however, that the temporal lobes, particularly the hippocampal regions, are the most likely sites of pathology underlying traumatic memory disturbance.

Clinical pictures similar to Korsakoff's psychosis have been reported following cerebrovascular disease.[36,176] In these cases bilateral posterior cerebral artery obstruction which produced infarction of the medial aspects of both the temporal and occipital lobes has been demonstrated. Unilateral infarction of the left hippocampal region may produce a memory loss similar to that of Korsakoff's psychosis except that it clears in a few months.[65]

Brain tumor with bilateral medial temporal involvement can cause an amnesic state.[159] Similarly, colloid cysts of the third ventricle and other tumors involving the walls of the hypothalamus can produce an amnestic state.[27] In these cases obstruction of CSF (cerebrospinal fluid) flow producing a hydrocephalus must be considered, but in some reported cases with memory loss this complication has been adequately ruled out.[191]

Typical Korsakoff-like states may occur after temporal-lobe surgery. Scoville[149,150] reports this finding after bilateral temporal-lobe resection, and a number of surgeons[125,154,178] have reported memory loss after unilateral temporal-lobe resection. In the latter, subsequent study usually demonstrated significant pathology in the unoperated temporal lobe. There are reports of amnestic state following bilateral surgical sectioning of the fornix[165] or bilateral fornix infarction[23] but most neurosurgeons quote other works[27,43] suggesting that there are no residua of bilateral fornix section.

Thus a severe memory disorder (inability to learn new material plus inability to retrieve recently learned material) appears after bilateral injury to central limbic-system structures (hippocampal region and mammillary bodies, possibly the dorsal-medial nucleus of the thalamus and the fornix). When this memory loss, with its strong element of disorientation, is combined with the emotional and vegetative disorders mentioned earlier, the resulting clinical picture presents many features commonly seen by the psychiatrist.

⟮ Syndromes of Unilateral Hemispheric Involvement

The cerebral hemispheres, comparatively massive in size, are the most striking anatomical feature of the human nervous system. These structures comprise a vast area of enfolded cortex with underlying white matter pathways and subcortical nuclear centers. The two hemispheres have often been considered mirror images of each other, but recent investigations[67,111,192] have demonstrated significant asymmetries. Certain behavioral tasks are dependent upon the function, solely or primarily, of only one of the two hemispheres. Language is the prime example of a strongly lateralized cerebral function (dominance), but some other behavioral tasks are, to a greater or lesser degree, also hemisphere-specific. While knowledge of these lateralized functions and of the significance of the interhemispheric connections remains incomplete, knowledge of the recognized hemisphere-specific syndromes is important to the student of behavior.

The dramatic loss of language following left hemisphere damage and the common preference for the right hand in skilled activities has emphasized the importance of the left hemisphere. This hemisphere is often called the dominant or major hemisphere and some investigators have considered that the right hemisphere acts only as a reserve, an area of cortex which performs only elementary activities but has the potential to take over many of the "higher" functions subserved by the left

hemisphere. The possibility that the right hemisphere is also dominant for specific functions has been promoted by the study of constructional disturbances following right hemisphere pathology.[108,135] Recent studies of behavior following temporal lobectomy[126] and callosal separation[18,63,66] have further demonstrated the functional importance of each of the hemispheres and the great importance of interhemispheric cooperation in carrying out complex behavioral tasks.

Left Hemisphere

The loss of language (aphasia) following focal damage to the left hemisphere and the absence of language problems following a similarly placed lesion in the right hemisphere are the most striking manifestations of lateralization of cortical function. Language function is frequently correlated with handedness and the two have been carefully studied.[8,146,163] Aphasia, the loss of language function, is the best studied of the lateralized hemisphere disabilities and will be reviewed below (and in Chapter 11). For most humans the left hemisphere appears essential for verbal tasks including speech, comprehension of speech, reading, and writing. The ability to name or describe a function is also specific for the left hemisphere. Studies of the syndromes of corpus callosum separation, first described by Liepmann[104] demonstrate this clearly.[59,66] Patients who have suffered separation of the corpus callosum neither name nor describe the function of objects placed in their left hand (when blindfolded) but can select the correct objects from a group (using the left hand). Recognition and memory of the palpated object is performed by the right hemisphere but translation into words is not. In contrast, objects placed in the right hand are immediately named and fully described. Somewhat analogous results are present after left-temporal lobectomy; there is a drop in verbal memory, both in comparison to premorbid scores and to the abilities of individuals who have undergone right temporal lobectomy.[125] Tests of callosally sectioned patients[60] have suggested the presence of some reading capability in the right hemisphere, but the reading level is rudimentary when compared to the function performed by the left hemisphere. Writing is also a strongly lateralized left-hemisphere function. Callosally disconnected patients can write legible sentences with the right hand but either cannot write (except for copying) or write aphasically with the left hand.[66]

Many skilled motor activities appear to be under left-hemisphere control. Actions performed to verbal command are directly dependent upon left-hemisphere function, but even imitation of movements is often difficult for patients who have suffered left-hemisphere damage. This asymmetry of motor function comprises most of the findings referred to as apraxia.[63,105]

Thus we see that focal damage in the left hemisphere may result in many symptoms related to language or motor control; this includes many of the varieties of aphasia, alexia, agraphia and apraxia. Left-hemisphere damage may be present without any of these symptoms, but their presence strongly suggests left-hemisphere involvement.

Right Hemisphere

Several comparatively rare behavioral abnormalities, e.g., dressing difficulty and prosopagnosia are traditionally linked to right hemisphere damage[20,21] and several other disturbances, such as constructional difficulty and unilateral neglect, are frequently reported after right-hemisphere damage. Some investigators suggest a single common factor, a disturbance of visual-spatial orientation and recent studies demonstrate that this function is more disturbed following right than left hemisphere damage;[3,14,35] visual-motor difficulties are however not confined to rightsided damage.

Constructional disturbance (often called constructional apraxia) denotes a difficulty in drawing, copying, or manipulating spatial patterns or designs. Both right[132] and left hemi-

sphere[109] focal damage are capable of producing constructional disturbance, but most authorities agree that the disturbance is greater in right hemisphere pathology.[83] Problems in construction are seen in a high proportion of cases with structural brain lesions,[129] and studies show that the disability demonstrated in constructional tasks correlates with both the specific demands of a given test and the locus of pathology.[6] In general the properties of constructional ability which deal with execution (e.g., drawing, manipulation) are more affected by left-hemisphere damage, while the properties dealing with visual-spatial orientation and recall are more affected by right-hemisphere damage.[180] Unfortunately almost all of the standard tests (Bender-Gestalt, Benton three-dimensional figures, etc.) combine both types of task and therefore act as screening tests. The presence of significant constructional disturbance strongly suggests an organic basis for a behavioral problem, and if constructional disturbance is the only significant neurological abnormality noted, a right-hemisphere locus should be suspected.

Prosopagnosia is a state in which there is difficulty in recognizing faces of individuals who are well known to the sufferer.[20] At the extreme, even the patient's own face cannot be recognized in a mirror and male-female distinction is dependent upon clothing or other nonphysiognomic features. Several investigators have suggested that facial recognition depends on subtle visual distinctions and consider that prosopagnosia represents a mild variety, almost a *forme fruste*, of visual agnosia. A number of recent studies[15,41,86] have demonstrated that patients with right-hemisphere pathology have greater difficulty in distinguishing facial features than those with left-hemisphere damage. None of their subjects, however, had true prosopagnosia. Prosopagnosia is rare but it is almost always reported in patients who have other evidence suggesting right-hemisphere pathology.[81] Recently Tzavaras et al.[173] reviewed all cases of true prosopagnosia with postmortem reports in the literature and found that each had bilateral pathology, suggesting that this disorder results, not from right-hemisphere damage alone, but from bilateral involvement of specific areas. This would explain the great rarity of prosopagnosia despite the common occurrence of right hemisphere pathology.

Dressing disturbance (apraxia) was first described in 1941[21] and has been described frequently since then. Two varieties have been distinguished.[9] One is dependent upon unilateral neglect in which the patient adequately grooms one side of the face and body while totally ignoring the other.[39] The second resembles a visual-spatial disturbance; when given an article of clothing the patient is unable to orient it correctly in space and, while attempting this, hopelessly tangles the article of clothing.[9] The first variety, like other examples of unilateral neglect, is more commonly, but not exclusively, associated with right-hemisphere damage; the visual-spatial type occurs in patients with severe right or bilateral posterior cerebral involvement.

Musical ability, at least that portion dealing with melody, rhythm, and inflection, appears to be a function of the right hemisphere. There are a number of cases of "amusia" recorded in the literature, some with right-hemisphere damage,[50,186] others with left.[88] A recent investigation[19] by Bogen and Gordon showed that after injection of sodium amytal into the left carotid artery, the patients could hum a melody but could not sing the words. After right sided injection the opposite happened, i.e., good ability to recite the words but without a recognizable melody.

Unilateral neglect is a fairly common expression of cerebral damage and frequently manifests itself through rather complex behavioral symptomatology. While neglect can occur after damage in either hemisphere, it is most frequent when the site of pathology is on the right. All behavioral symptoms to be mentioned here can occur following left brain damage, but are more common or severe with right-hemisphere involvement.

A great number of variations of unilateral neglect are recognized (see Critchley[32] for detailed classification), dependent on specific combinations of behavioral abnormality.

These variations can be considered points on a spectrum, not sharply distinct clinical entities, but to be understood they must be separated. For this purpose a simple classification will suffice:

1. Inattention to
2. Unconcern about } illness, blindness,
3. Unawareness of } paralysis, etc.
4. Denial of

The first and third categories indicate degrees of neglect, most often involving one side only, and are self-descriptive. Unawareness is a more severe degree of unilateral neglect and often indicates the presence of some degree of clouding of the sensorium. While the demonstration of inattention often demands some special examination technique (such as double simultaneous stimulation), simple observation of the patient with unawareness will show considerable decrease in use of the involved side or limb. When confronted, these patients admit that they have the difficulty demonstrated and also admit concern about the disabled state. They do not express concern, however, unless prompted, and attempt their routine activities as though they had no disability. The patient manifesting unconcern, on the other hand, shows evidence of inattention and/or unawareness coupled with an indifference for the disability. He also admits to the disability when confronted, but shows an inappropriate, flat, or facetious reaction. The final variety, in which there is overt denial of the illness, is the most severe. The patient will deny such obvious disabilities as unilateral paralysis or blindness, insisting that he can walk or run, or attempting to describe an unseen panorama in front of him. He often employs vague excuses for not performing the requested task (e.g., "I've been ill recently," "I don't have my spectacles here," "The light in this room seems very poor," etc.). The symptoms are bizarre and these patients always show some disturbance of mental status. This denial of illness must be differentiated from psychogenic denial, the strongly motivated attempt to downgrade the severity of an illness or situation (see below).

Each variety of unilateral neglect may involve impairment of any sensory or motor function. Denial and unawareness may also involve purely mental tasks (i.e., denial or unawareness of aphasia, memory loss, intellectual deterioration, etc.). Denny-Brown et al.[40] suggested an asymmetry of finely balanced hemispheric functions (*amorphosynthesis*) as the underlying factor in unilateral neglect. They postulated that a system attuned, through years of practice, to respond equally to balanced sensory stimuli reaching each hemisphere will respond most to the stronger signals arriving in the normal hemisphere and will neglect the weaker signals arriving in the damaged hemisphere. Amorphosynthesis appears to offer a basis (anatomically and functionally) for the common occurrence of inattention and unawareness after unilateral cortical damage. The greater prevalence of right- than left-hemisphere damage as the source of unilateral inattention, however, demands additional explanation. The possibility that there is a specific center for modulation (awareness) of this balance has been suggested. Damage to such a center, then, could weaken the ability to recognize unilateral inequalities. This intriguing hypothesis, however, remains totally unsubstantiated and additional factors must be considered.

Active denial of disease cannot be explained simply on the basis of amorphosynthesis. For instance, Anton's Syndrome, the denial of blindness, almost invariably occurs in the context of bilateral visual loss. Even the classic denial of hemiplegia (anosognosia of Babinski) appears to go beyond a mere inequality of stimuli reaching the cortex. This disorder occurs much more frequently in cases of left hemiplegia, and there is a tendency to treat anosognosia as a symptom of right-hemisphere (parietal) disorder. This doctrine has been questioned. Weinstein,[181,182] who has made extensive studies of the disorder, suggests that anosognosia is motivated, i.e., the patient shows evidence of awareness of the disability which he is denying. As evidence he cites the dying patient, denying illness, but revealing that he recognizes the situation by describing the hospital as "a slaughter-house" or as a final rest home. He also cites the frequent occur-

rence of reduplication of place, where the patient names the hospital correctly but locates it much closer to his own home town.[182] Weinstein records many patients who suffer anosognosia but do not have right hemisphere disease. While his own material did contain more left than right hemiplegias, we would agree that it is appropriate to consider other aspects of behavior when analyzing denial of illness.

The emotional behavior demonstrated in the milder disturbance, unconcern, is worthy of note. These patients exhibit shallow emotional reactions, often have a mildly euphoric affect, tend to flare up with outbursts of anger which recede rapidly. Often they are facetious and show inappropriate social behavior. In short, they resemble patients with frontal-lobe pathology (see below) and their unconcern about a unilateral neurological disability could be considered a combination of "frontal lobishness" and amorphosynthesis.

Another possible consideration would be that a disorder of memory had been added to the specific neurological loss. Patients may deny disease because they cannot remember that they have any difficulty. Indeed, this mechanism does occur in some cases of denial[7] and, when carefully sought, significant recent memory loss is present in many cases of denial associated with organic brain disease. There can be little doubt that disorder of memory is a frequent and important component of anosognosia, but there are cases in which it does not seem to be playing a role.

Another theory that has been advanced to explain the greater frequency of denial or unconcern with right rather than left hemisphere lesions is that right-hemisphere lesions produce a change in emotional responsiveness. Proponents of this view note the apathy, facetiousness, and mild euphoria of many left hemiplegics (right-hemisphere damage), contrasting this with the sadness and despair of many right-hemiplegic patients. If correct, this view would suggest right-hemisphere dominance for some aspects of emotion. The strongest evidence for this view is the very difference in the emotional responses of right and left hemiplegics. Evidence advanced from other types of data to support this concept is still controversial. Some investigators[79] assert that right unilateral ECT (electroconvulsive therapy) is more effective than left in the treatment of depression; this is not substantiated in other reports.[30] Some observers report that after left-carotid amytal injection patients show a right hemiplegia, aphasia, and weeping, while after right-carotid injection they are said to show left hemiplegia and euphoria, but others deny finding these results in their material. The patient composition of the various series may have been different, and this issue must remain open. Certainly, if a unilateral difference in emotional response does exist it would play a significant role in the response to neurologic disability.

A final possibility to be considered is the presence of a purely psychological source of the denial. Certainly psychogenic denial does exist (the repressions, sublimations, etc., of psychodynamics) and sometimes produces a denial of perfectly obvious illness. There are significant differentiating points, however, and the type of denial should always be ascertained. The organic variety of denial occurs only in the face of brain disease complicated by impairment of mental functioning; the functional variety, in contrast, occurs without evidence of coarse brain disease and in a clear mental state. The psychogenic type of denial is usually intellectualized, rationalized, and presented in a quasi-logical manner; in contrast, the denial of the brain-injured patient tends to be crude and concrete.

In summary, organic brain disorders exist in which the presence of disease is neglected or denied. These cases frequently show an inequality of basic sensori-motor function and, in the more severe syndrome of denial of disease, this inequality is complicated by a change in the mental picture, either a facetious, euphoric "frontal-lobe" type of behavior or a loss of recent memory.

⟦ Language Syndromes—Aphasia

Much more is known about abnormal language function than any of the other disorders of behavior produced by focal brain damage. Generally termed "aphasia," this subject has been intensively studied for over a century; unfortunately there are still many unsolved problems and a great deal of disagreement exists. When fully developed, aphasia usually presents little diagnostic difficulty and indicates focal brain disease. In more subtle forms, however, aphasia may prove difficult to recognize and is easily mistaken for a functional psychiatric disease. Also, several of the varieties of aphasia produce specific behavior patterns which merit psychiatric concern. A short review of aphasia will help in recognition of these problems.

Aphasia can be defined most simply as a loss or impairment of language caused by brain damage. This definition presupposes that normal language had once been present and excludes pure speech disturbance (i.e., bulbar palsy, Parkinsonian dysarthria, scanning speech, etc.). For the vast majority of people the function of language is performed almost exclusively by one hemisphere, the left, a factor of obvious significance in the study of focal brain disease. Specifically, over 99 percent of right-handed people have language dominance in the left hemisphere.[8] The picture is not so clear for the left-handed but increasing evidence suggests that some language function in each hemisphere is most common.[73,85] The presence of aphasia indicates left-hemisphere pathology in at least 95 percent of cases, regardless of handedness.

Further evaluation of the phenomenon of aphasia is dependent upon the classification of the varieties. Dozens of classifications of aphasia are currently in use, based on clinical, anatomical, neurological, psychological, linguistic, and even philosophical considerations. Careful evaluation demonstrates that the same or at least highly similar symptoms appear in many of the classifications, although under different names. The following list presents the classification developed at the Boston Veterans Administration Hospital,[9] which is a modification of several of the nineteenth-century continental classifications and is based on personal evaluation, by the authors, of over 1500 aphasics; it presents this classification of the aphasias as well as some significant related disorders.

Clinical Varieties of Aphasia

A.   Aphasia with repetition disturbance
    1.   Broca's aphasia
    2.   Wernicke's aphasia
    3.   Conduction aphasia
B.   Aphasia without repetition disturbance
    1.   Isolation of the speech area
    2.   Transcortical motor aphasia
    3.   Transcortical sensory aphasia
    4.   Anomic aphasia
C.   Disturbances primarily affecting reading and writing
    1.   Alexia with agraphia
D.   Total aphasia
    1.   Global aphasia
E.   Syndromes with disturbance of a single language modality
    1.   Aphemia
    2.   Pure word deafness
    3.   Alexia without agraphia

Two of the most popular simple classifications of aphasia deserve comment, if only to reject them. First, the popular expressive-receptive classification of Weisenburg and McBride[183] has serious shortcomings. Almost all aphasics have difficulty with language expression but there are important differences in the type of expressive disorder which this classification overlooks. The equally popular motor-sensory dichotomy, originally proposed in 1874 by Wernicke,[185] is unsuitable because, in great part, the original, specific meanings of these terms have been lost. Most often they are equated to the unsatisfactory expressive-receptive dichotomy. If these terms are to be used, the examiner must recognize that many forms of disordered expression are not "motor" disturbances.

Aphasia may be usefully subdivided into aphasia with normal repetition and aphasia with abnormal repetition. The latter category includes the classic varieties, Broca's and Wernicke's aphasias and a third distinct variety, conduction aphasia. Each variety will be described briefly and correlated with the usual anatomic locus of the causative lesion.

Broca's Aphasia

Originally described in 1861 by Broca[24] and subsequently described under many different names (motor aphasia, cortical dysarthria, verbal aphasia, efferent kinetic aphasia), this variety of language disturbance has a fairly consistent symptom picture. Conversational speech is nonfluent (dysarthric, sparse, dysprosodic, effortful, of short-phrase length, and consisting mainly of meaning-rich words); comprehension of spoken language is essentially normal; both repetition and naming ability are disturbed but are often better than spontaneous speech. Writing is almost always abnormal, whereas reading comprehension is often preserved. The causative lesion almost invariably involves the posterior-inferior portion of the third frontal convolution (Broca's area). Most patients with Broca's aphasia also have a right hemiplegia, and apraxia (the sympathetic dyspraxia of Liepmann) often affects the left limbs.

Wernicke's Aphasia

A second variety of aphasia, first described in 1874 by Wernicke[185] presents a strikingly different clinical picture. Conversational speech is distinctly fluent (well articulated, presented rapidly with normal melody and phrase length) but is often contaminated by word-finding pauses and paraphasias. The term "paraphasia" designates substitutions within language. This may involve phonemes (literal paraphasia) or words (verbal paraphasia) or may consist of completely incorrect utterances (neologisms). When multiple paraphasias are combined with a rapid output, the production becomes incomprehensible and is sometimes called "jargon aphasia." Since "jargon aphasia" may also be used to designate other types of disordered speech, one must be careful about its use. The verbal content of the output in Wernicke's aphasia is strongly biased toward relational, grammatical, and filler words and phrases; it is deficient in the meaningful nouns noted in Broca's aphasia. Other characteristics include severe disturbance of both comprehension and repetition of spoken language, inability to read or write, and usually a difficulty in word finding (naming). The causative lesion usually involves the posterior-superior portion of the first temporal gyrus. Often there are no overt neurologic signs (such as paralysis, sensory loss, or hemianopia) except for the language disturbance and, on the basis of his rapid, bizarre speech and poor comprehension, the patient may be misdiagnosed as confused or psychotic.

Conduction Aphasia

Originally characterized by Wernicke and eventually confirmed by a number of European neurologists, this variety still has not been accepted by many investigators. Much recent work[84,98] including our own[12] gives strong support to its existence and importance. Clinically these cases show fluent speech, often contaminated by paraphasia, with good comprehension but seriously disturbed repetition. Naming is disturbed, as is writing. Quite frequently reading comprehension is maintained, even though reading aloud is impossible. Paresis is minimal or absent, but cortical sensory loss on the right side of the body is often present. Classically, the causative lesion was described as lying deep in the white matter of the supramarginal gyrus, thus involving the arcuate fasciculus and acting to separate the temporo-parietal language area from the frontal language area. Individual cases of conduction aphasia, however, have been reported in which the significant pathology was a total destruction of the left first temporal gyrus; in other words, in some cases the picture of conduction aphasia rather than Wernicke's aphasia occurs with lesions in this site. Two different anatomical locations of pathology apparently can produce the same clinical syndrome.[12]

The second group of aphasias, those in which repetition is normal, are more difficult to diagnose, and patients with these disorders are frequently referred to the psychiatrist for behavioral investigation. While most often the result of focal brain disease, some of these syndromes can also derive from more widespread dysfunction, particularly degenerative or toxic-metabolic disorders, and, when seen in mild form, offer considerable diagnostic difficulty.

Isolation of the Speech Area

This striking clinical syndrome has only been reported a few times in pure form[68,74] but is not infrequent in less complete form. The patient with the isolation syndrome does not speak unless spoken to, and then repeats almost slavishly what has been said by the examiner (echolalia). There is no demonstrable comprehension of spoken or written language, no ability to write or name objects, but, in contrast, great ability to repeat even long and complex sentences, nonsense material, and foreign phrases. Usually these patients can complete stock phrases, e.g., grass is———; red, white and———. A severe degree of primary neurological disability is usually present and, in fact, almost the only useful function retained by these patients is the ability to repeat. The pathology has, in general, been caused by severe anoxia which has selectively involved the vascular border zone between the middle cerebral and anterior and posterior cerebral tributaries. This pathology spares the immediate perisylvian area but involves large areas of cortex in the frontal, temporal, and parietal lobes.

Transcortical Motor Aphasia

In this disorder the patient is nonfluent in conversational speech (except for a striking ability to echo), comprehends well, and repeats normally. Naming, reading, and writing are usually disturbed. Hemiplegia is present in most cases. The language output may resemble that of Broca's aphasia but is better described as a reluctance to speak. The comparative ease and clarity of repetition is all the more remarkable in contrast. The causative lesion involves the frontal association cortex anterior and/or superior to Broca's area, the frontal portion of the border zone.

Transcortical Sensory Aphasia

In pure from this disorder is rather uncommon, but it occurs fairly often in incomplete form and is often misdiagnosed. The patient speaks fluently but incoherently. He often repeats the examiner's questions (echolalia) but then produces totally unrelated answers. These answers, however, consist of real words, phrases, and sentences with proper intonation. Testing of comprehension shows remarkable disturbance, often a total inability to understand. Alexia and agraphia are present, in addition to a severe naming disturbance. Repetition is dramatically intact. These patients may have cortical sensory disturbance and/or homonymous hemianopsia but often have no paresis. The causative lesion involves the dominant parietal cortex, specifically the parietal border zone and/or the posterior temporal cortex.

Anomic Aphasia

Disturbances of word finding are certainly the most common finding in aphasia, and vary from mild to gross in degree. In the purest form, called anomic aphasia, conversational speech is fluent and somewhat paraphasic,

and comprehension of spoken language may be slightly disturbed but is usually adequate, and repetition is perfectly normal. Testing demonstrates some difficulty in word finding and writing, and often (but not always) some disturbance in reading. Usually there is no evidence of elementary neurological disorder. The clinical picture of anomic aphasia may be the result of focal vascular pathology in the posterior portion of the border zone area. A similar aphasic picture is often a prominent feature of biparietal degenerative disorders such as Alzheimer's Disease, and also appears in toxic or metabolic encephalopathy or raised intracranial pressure. Anomic aphasia also occurs in the recovery stage of many varieties of aphasia. Anomic aphasia, then, is seen frequently but, by itself, does not indicate a specific cerebral focus or particular etiology.

The clinical picture of any case of aphasia depends not only on the areas involved but also on the degree of involvement, the degree of language dominance, and differences in individual language development. Nevertheless, most cases of aphasia can readily be placed in this classification and the site of the underlying focal lesion can be localized with a high degree of accuracy.[11] Table 9–1 gives an outline of the primary differentiating findings of the major types of aphasia.

TABLE 9–1. **Clinical Aspects of Aphasia**

	SPON-TANEOUS SPEECH	COM-PRE-HENSION	REPE-TITION	NAMING	READING	WRITING
Broca's aphasia	NF	+	−	±	aloud − comp. +	−
Wernicke's aphasia	F	−	−	±	−	−
Conduction aphasia	F	+	−	±	aloud − comp. +	−
Global aphasia	NF	−	−	−	−	−
Isolation syndrome	NF	−	+	−	−	−
Transcortical motor	NF	+	+	−	aloud − comp. +	−
Transcortical sensory	F	−	+	−	−	−
Anomic aphasia	F	+	+	−	+	−

Legend: NF = non fluent; F = fluent; + = normal or mildly affected;   − = severely affected;
         ± = variable degree of involvement.

Several other varieties of aphasia deserve comment. Global aphasia refers to significant disturbance of comprehension with grossly nonfluent speech, usually caused by a large lesion in the sylvian region involving nearly all of the speech regions. Pure word deafness denotes a "pure" disturbance of auditory language comprehension; the patient understands written but not spoken language. Speaking and writing are essentially normal. Aphemia denotes a "pure" disturbance of spoken language, the patient retaining language comprehension and the ability to write. Alexia without agraphia denotes loss of the ability to read with no other language loss. These entities sometimes occur in "pure" form but, not infrequently, they are seen with only slight admixture of other disorders.

Psychiatric Features of Aphasia

Having considered briefly the clinical-anatomical outline of the aphasias recorded above, let us now turn to the behavioral features which may bring the patient to the attention of the psychiatrist. First we will note the problems that lead to diagnostic errors, then the specific reactions seen in aphasic individuals which demand psychiatric management.

ANOMIC APHASIA

Even a mild difficulty with word-finding (naming on visual or tactile confrontation, manufacturing word lists), suggests organic brain disease and warrants investigation of this possibility. In view of the large number of people using drugs, the possibility of toxic sources of anomia is important. It should be noted that a disproportionate degree of difficulty in writing (agraphia) is almost always present in patients with clinically significant toxic or metabolic disorders.

WORD SALAD

For many years psychiatrists[16] have described a severe disorganization of spoken and written language which occurs in degenerated schizophrenics, called "word salad" at its most extreme. It is generally recognized that im-proved treatment of the schizophrenic has made this disorder uncommon, but the diagnosis is still made occasionally. It has been our experience that every case of "word salad" which we have been asked to evaluate in ten years has had a demonstrable Wernicke's aphasia or, rarely, transcortical sensory aphasia with significant comprehension loss and marked neologistic paraphasia. A specific organic basis has always been demonstrable. Thus, before accepting the diagnosis of word salad on the basis of schizophrenia, patients should be carefully evaluated for evidence of aphasia. There should be little difficulty in making this distinction. Word salad is traditionally a disorder of the chronic, backward schizophrenic. Acute onset of fluent language output filled with paraphasic errors in a previously healthy individual in middle or late life almost invariably indicates the presence of aphasia. Even in the patient with well-established chronic schizophrenic disorder, the *acute* onset of "word salad" should suggest aphasia. The greatest problem occurs in the long-term patient who has been misusing language for many years. Even in this patient, language disorder should be considered and evaluated; there are instances of fluent aphasics misdiagnosed and treated for years as psychotic.

PARANOID REACTION

Among the many recognized sources of paranoid reaction, the psychiatrist should also be aware of the aphasias, particularly those with severe comprehension disturbance (Wernicke's aphasia, pure word deafness and transcortical sensory aphasia). These patients often ask the examiner to speak more clearly (they hear but cannot understand) and do not realize that they are speaking gibberish. They may believe that those around them are discussing them, possibly in a special code which they hear but cannot understand. They develop severe frustrations and suspicions because their questions or statements go unheeded. A very large number of patients suffering auditory comprehension disability in marked degree show some degree of paranoia (similar to the paranoia which occurs in some cases of long-standing deafness). Their suspicion may be so extreme that the patient becomes a danger to the hospital staff, his family, other patients, acquaintances, or himself. The majority of patients from our aphasia section needing seclusion care have suffered a paranoid reaction, complicating an aphasia with severe comprehension difficulty.

DEPRESSION, FRUSTRATION, AND THE CATASTROPHIC REACTION

In aphasia, as in all organic brain disease, the diagnosis of depressed affective state may be difficult. Many patients with organic brain disease, particularly those with anterior involvement, show a blunting of affect, psychomotor retardation, and diminished interest in their surroundings. Yet, when specifically questioned, they do not express depressive feelings. These objective signs of depression are commonly noted after frontal (see below) and certain subcortical (e.g., Parkinsonism) lesions but the appearance of apathy is not accompanied by a depressed affective state. Nonetheless, true depression can occur in aphasic patients, and is particularly common in Broca's aphasia. In contrast, the patient with a severe aphasia from a posterior lesion rarely exhibits depression; in fact, these patients often fail to recognize their problem and appear euphoric or unconcerned. We believe that the depressive reaction seen in Broca's aphasia is usually a normal response to his disability. The lack of concern of the patient with the posterior lesion, on the other hand, is abnormal and depends on the specific clinical qualities produced by a specifically located brain lesion.

Frustration is seen most frequently in the aphasic with an anterior lesion. While frustration can be unpleasant for the patient and a hindrance to therapy, it is actually a favourable prognostic sign; the patient shows that he cares, is more likely to make an effort, and is therefore a better candidate for therapy. Goldstein[74] described an extreme degree of frustration in aphasia under the term "catastrophic reaction." In this state the degree of frustration was overwhelming, leading to emotional breakdown with a combination of weeping, withdrawal, and anger. The catastrophic reaction is very rare and if the aphasic patient is handled with sympathy, frustration need not interfere with either evaluation or therapy.

In general, understanding, sympathy, and encouragement on the part of the examiner or therapist can overcome most of the complications of frustration in aphasia. This level of "supportive psychotherapy" is an integral part of the management of almost all victims of aphasia. Affective illness, on the other hand, is often difficult to manage and demands considerable attention. In our experience the depressed aphasic patient has not responded well to treatment with antidepressant drugs and we have been reluctant to use ECT on individuals who have recently suffered a major brain injury. Intensive supportive measures, preferably by someone experienced in communicating with aphasic patients, is usually helpful. We have found that a trained speech therapist, working under the guidance of a psychiatrist, is more useful than either alone or both working with the patient independently. Additional support can be gained by including these patients in a small group with others receiving aphasia therapy. Group therapy not only offers support and a relationship with others suffering a similar disability, but also offers practice in communication in a less stressful environment.

❨ Frontal-Lobe Syndromes

The frontal lobes are the largest divisions of the cortex, and with the Rolandic and sylvian fissures and the sagittal sulcus as boundaries, are also the best demarcated. The frontal lobes, however, are far from homogeneous. At least four distinct subdivisions, based on thalamic connections, can be specified, i.e., Rolandic, sylvian, limbic-temporal, and frontal proper,[38] and distinct neurological symptomatology has been suggested for each. In many cases, however, an admixture of symptoms referable to these four divisions is seen. In addition, frontal signs are often mixed with signs resulting from damage to other parts of the brain. Despite this common overlap of symptomatology, a clinical picture suggestive of frontal-lobe involvement has been recognized for many years.

Many of the changes produced by frontal-lobe pathology are neurological, (paralysis, aphasia, etc.). In addition, involvement of frontal association cortex can produce a transient total unresponsiveness to visual stimuli in the opposite field,[95] a transient sensory loss (inattention), and occulomotor disturbance;[184] some authors have even attributed a memory defect to frontal lesions.[38] Frontal pathology produces distinct changes in behavior and personality, often referred to as the "frontal-lobe syndrome." The literature contains many descriptions of frontal-lobe syndromes, with variations based on the type of pathological material evaluated or on the orientation of the investigator. To evaluate this we will briefly review reports of frontal head injury, of psychosurgery, and of brain tumors, with several other neurological disorders which primarily affect the frontal lobes.

Head Injury

Behavioral changes following frontal-lobe injury have been reported for over one hundred years. In 1868 Harlow[80] described his patient Phineas Gage, a previously neat, upright, and capable foreman, who sustained an injury in which a crowbar traversed the left frontal lobe. Following injury the patient was described as irresponsible, vacillating, and incapable of carrying out sequential activities. Many similar case studies have followed, one of the most notable being the patient of Brickner[22] who underwent bilateral frontal-lobe resection for treatment of a parasagittal meningioma. In addition to individual case studies, there are many group studies of patients with frontal-lobe war injuries.[48,177] Feuchtwanger[49] studied patients with frontal gunshot wounds and described changes in mood and attitude, including facetiousness, euphoria, irritability and apathy, defective attention, tactlessness and inability to plan ahead. Kleist[99] separated convexity lesions (motor and intel-

lectual abnormalities) and orbital lesions (emotional disturbances), a division confirmed by others. A third locale, called the basal area but actually indicating midline inferior frontal structures, has also been suggested as the source of specific symptomatology.[101] In general, these studies agreed that convexity lesions were characterized by a lack of drive, disinhibition, indifference, lack of productive thinking, euphoria, and incapacity to make a decision. Patients with orbital lesions were said to have normal intelligence on formal testing but severe personality changes; they were aggressive, disinhibited, demanding, interfering, and lacking in perseverance, with increased sexual libido and potency and proneness to criminal offences. With involvement of the basal area (hypothalamus and orbital frontal region) marked sluggishness and apathy were described, along with a disturbance of the fundamental drives such as appetite, thirst, and sleep.

While these studies suggest that differentiation of the psychiatric picture may be based on the site of focal injury, this division is somewhat artificial. Most head injuries are not well localized, and a broader definition of the frontal-lobe syndrome is needed. In a recent British review of head injury cases Lishman[106] included under the term "frontal lobe syndrome" all patients with one or more of the following psychic symptoms in severe degree: (1) euphoria; (2) lack of judgment, reliability, or foresight; (3) disinhibition; and (4) facile or childish behavior. To this list many investigators would want to add apathy, the loss of drive.

Psychosurgery

Psychosurgery, the attempt to control abnormal behavior through surgical attack on the brain, has produced a great deal of information on the functions of the frontal lobes. While there has been some disagreement in reported results, due in part to variation in the surgical procedure, there has been much agreement on the behavioral outcome of frontal lobectomy and leucotomy,[55] cingulotomy,[172] and orbital undercutting.[166] Greenblatt and Solomon[76] reviewed much of the pertinent literature and their own extensive experience up to 1956 and outlined four principal behavioral consequences of bilateral frontal lobotomy:

1. Reduced drive demonstrated by
   a. apathy, laziness, lack of initiative and spontaneity, and general contentment;
   b. decrease in suspicion, hostility, aggressiveness, violence, delusions, and fantasy.
2. Reduced self-concern demonstrated by
   a. decreased self-consciousness, less preoccupation with self, less sensitivity to criticism.
3. More immediate outward behavior demonstrated by
   a. less withdrawn, more notice of external activity;
   b. more outspoken, lack of tact, less concern for the future.
4. Superficial, shallow affective state
   a. quicker to become angry, but bear no grudge;
   b. general euphoria.

These behavioral changes are noticeably similar to the changes noted after severe frontal-lobe injury and can be said to characterize the "frontal-lobe syndrome."

Cerebral Tumor

A third source of study material, of more concern to the practicing psychiatrist, consists of tumors involving the frontal lobes. Onset is usually insidious and behavioral abnormalities often appear first, prompting early psychiatric evaluation. At first behavior may be poorly restrained and tactless, with decreased concern for family members and a mood of fatuous jocularity (*Witzelsucht*). The patient may become boastful or grandiose, but initiative is decreased; work quality deteriorates along with decreasing attentiveness and concern, and finally a state of apathy and indifference replaces the previous euphoria. Socially unacceptable disinhibition such as urinating in public, carelessness in dressing, or inappropriate sexual approach may occur. By this late stage there is often other evidence to suggest neurological disorder such as seizures, unilateral paresis, visual disturbance, headache, or aphasia. These findings may, however, first suggest psychiatric disorder. In a review of 250 cases operated on for frontal-lobe seizure foci, Rasmussen[143] noted six varieties of aura. Three were clearly neurological with combinations of unconsciousness, adversive turning, and generalized grand-mal seizures, but the other three consisted of behavioral symptoms. These included: (a) a vague epigastric sensation, i.e., a rising feeling beginning in the abdomen; (b) vague, poorly described sensations which involved the entire body, usually called "restlessness," "flush," "heaviness," etc.; and (c) sudden alterations in thought process, a forced thinking. The latter was described by the patients as "forced to think about something," "my thoughts suddenly became fixed," or "loss of thought control." The first sign of aphasia in frontal tumor is almost always a loss of word-finding ability (anomia), producing a rambling, circumlocutory speech pattern, difficult to recognize as aphasic. Thus, tumors of the frontal lobe often mimic psychiatric disorder and offer a formidable diagnostic problem for the psychiatrist.

Syphilis

Before the advent of penicillin, general paralysis of the insane (GPI) was one of the commonest forms of organic brain disease, affecting first, and usually most severely, the frontal lobes (see Chapter 5). Now a rare disorder, GPI still deserves consideration in the differential diagnosis of dementia, especially in the middle-aged. A considerable variation in the onset and course has been reported;[25] usually the onset is insidious with change of temperament and personality occurring before notable intellectual loss. Most often (in about two-thirds of cases) there is a gradual deterioration into a simple or euphoric dementia, characterized by impaired judgement, defective memory, and lack of insight. A much smaller group (about 10 percent) develop the classic expansiveness with a happy, exalted mood and delusions of superb health, fabulous sexual prowess, masterful artistic capabilities, or superhuman strength. Differentiation from true mania is necessary but usually easy; the GPI victim is childlike and naive and the presence of underlying dementia is often readily demonstrated. The opposite state, serious depression, occurs almost as frequently in the early stages of GPI, with hypochondriacal and nihilistic delusions and even suicide attempts. Again the presence of dementia and a shallow, blunted affective state help to differentiate GPI from true depression. Once suspected, the diagnosis of GPI is readily confirmed by neurological examination and laboratory studies. The outstanding success and comparative safety of penicillin therapy makes it virtually mandatory that any case with reasonable suspicion of GPI receive a full therapeutic course (12–16 million units in divided doses). Many such patients are restored to full mental health (up to 80 percent of cases treated early;)[171] others are left with a stable residual brain damage, usually a dementia with major frontal-lobe features.

Huntington's Chorea

A more generalized disorder of the CNS which often produces major frontal-lobe disturbance is Huntington's chorea (see Chapter 17). The earliest manifestations are usually psychiatric, with insidious but progressive personality deterioration, showing either of two pictures, i.e., irritability, morose discontent, and oversensitivity or apathy and social disinhibition. The further progression to chorea and dementia is uneven; some patients have severe movement disorder and little dementia, while others show the opposite. Severe personality deterioration, however, invariably occurs and may precede either state by many years. A distinctive feature of the dementia of Huntington's chorea is the relative preservation in most cases of new learning ability in the face of severe intellectual dysfunction and marked distractibility.[122]

Normal Pressure Hydrocephalus

Normal pressure hydrocephalus (NPH),[1], [168] a frequently reversible disorder of cerebrospinal fluid circulation, produces a dementia which features marked frontal-lobe symptomatology. Of the three cardinal symptoms of NPH, gait disturbance, incontinence, and dementia, the first two and at least part of the third appear to result from frontal-lobe dysfunction. In this disorder there is a tremendous overall increase in size of the ventricular system, but with the greatest enlargement demonstrable in the frontal horns.[10] Diagnosis, by intrathecal radioisotope study,[133] air encephalogram,[102] or both[10] can be followed by shunting, most often a ventriculoatrial bypass, which often produces a dramatic improvement in the entire picture.

Presenile Dementia

Of the presenile dementias (see Chapter 3), Pick's disease is characterized by early and marked changes in the frontal lobe in contrast to the early biparietal involvement of Alzheimer's disease. Pick's disease is well described as a "sloppy" dementia with crude, coarse social behavior, incontinence, and apathy. Alzheimer's disease can, in most cases, be termed a "neat" dementia featuring a remarkable preservation of social graces overlying a severe disturbance of cognitive functions. In late stages, with increased involvement of the frontal cortex, Alzheimer patients also develop a "sloppy" dementia. Occasionally, a patient with Alzheimer's disease shows early frontal signs and may be differentiated from patients with Pick's disease only by the greater intellectual disturbances.

Pseudobulbar States

A variable mixture of signs and symptoms is contained in the syndrome usually referred to as pseudobulbar palsy. The prefix "pseudo-" is used to indicate that bilateral upper motor neuron paresis is producing a false impression of lower brainstem (bulbar) pathology. Thus a flattened, expressionless face, lack of eye blinking, hoarseness, dysphagia, and drooling are common. In addition, there is often but not always evidence of bilateral upper motor neuron paresis of the limbs; incontinence, apathy, and disinterest are common but are not essential parts of the picture. The most characteristic finding is a disturbance in the control of behavior, correctly termed a "lability of emotional expression." These patients laugh or cry excessively, usually in response to an appropriate but trivial stimulus. In some cases an initial laughing expression can be seen to change slowly to unhappiness and then to agony. While the initial response may be appropriate to the stimulus, the degree of response is not; if asked, the patient will deny experiencing the degree of happiness or sadness that he is expressing and often feels distress because of his inability to control the response.

Recognition of the pseudobulbar state can help the psychiatrist avoid several misdiagnoses. The presence of an expressionless facies in a patient who manifests outbursts of severe weeping in response to appropriate but mild stimuli can easily lead to the diagnosis of a depressive reaction. The pseudobulbar state does not respond well to the present antidepressive drugs and ECT is quite likely to harm an already damaged brain further. The proper diagnosis can be made simply by noting the marked difference between the subjective and the objective expression of emotion, and the presence of bilateral motor involvement.

The drooling and expressionless patient who has outbursts of excessive laughing or crying is easily considered to be demented. It is true that many patients with pseudobulbar state do suffer intellectual deterioration but in some disorders, amyotrophic lateral sclerosis for instance, signs of the pseudobulbar state may coexist with an entirely intact intellect. Even cases of psuedobulbar palsy secondary to bilateral vascular disease may have considerable retention of intellect. The lability of emotional expression seen in the pseudobulbar state should be considered an example of disinhibition, not of intellectual impairment.

In summary, the behavioral symptomatology of frontal-lobe pathology is varied but can be characterized by: (1) some degree of poor judgment or foresight; (2) superficial or shallow affective state; (3) disinhibition; and (4) reduced drive and self-concern. When some combination of these findings is noted in a behavioral evaluation, organic pathology involving the frontal lobes should be suspected.

(Temporal-Lobe Syndromes

The temporal lobe, like the frontal lobe, has long been considered to have a symptomatology of its own but the anatomical demarcation of the temporal lobe is less exact. The sylvian fissure does separate the temporal lobe from the frontal and anterior parietal lobes, but the posterior boundary of the temporal lobe is indistinct. The supramarginal and angular gyri and the temporal-occipital junction are all transitional areas, both anatomically and functionally. Williams[190] suggested three discrete functional areas for the temporal lobe: (1) special sensory, i.e., primarily auditory but also containing cortical centers for taste, smell, and equilibrium; (2) association, i.e., not only auditory but also visual and possibly some somesthetic association areas which occupy much of the lateral surface of the temporal lobe; and (3) visceral, i.e., the medial and inferior aspects of the temporal lobe contain major structures of the phylogenetically ancient limbic lobe (hippocampus, amygdala, fornix, uncus, hippocampal gyrus). Pathology in the temporal lobe usually involves several of these areas simultaneously, producing a varied symptomatology. Many of the symptoms produced by temporal-lobe dysfunction have already been discussed (aphasia, memory loss, limbic disorders) but one aspect of great significance for the psychiatrist remains, the behavioral abnormalities associated with temporal-lobe seizures.

Temporal-Lobe Seizures

It is generally accepted that the temporal lobe contains the most epileptogenic tissue in the brain,[164] but only in recent years has the full implication of temporal-lobe seizures been realized.[58,69] Many varieties of motor seizures from short absences to full grand-mal convulsions are the result of temporal foci. Associated in some cases with seizures discharge, but often appearing to occur independently, are many varieties of aura, ictal manifestations and postictal activities which are behavioral acts. The following list outlines these symptoms.

Ictal Symptoms of Psychomotor Epilepsy

I. Sensory symptoms
    A. External: Olfactory, auditory, visual, somesthetic sensations
    B. Visceral: oropharyngeal, esophageal, abdominal sensations, etc. (i.e., nausea, palpitations, hunger, heat, cold, need to urinate, etc.)

II. Mental symptoms
    A. Consciousness: varies from fully normal to totally lost
    B. Perceptual:
        1. Illusions: micropsia, macropsia, metamorphasia, déjà vu, jamais vu, depersonalization, etc.
        2. Hallucinations: complex, dynamic, dreamlike
    C. Ideational: thought-blocking or interfering thoughts
    D. Temporal: time stands still (or rushes by)
    E. Affective: fear, depression, pleasant, unpleasant, anger

III. Motor signs
    A. Somatic:
        1. Simple: clonic contractions, unilateral or bilateral hypertonic: primarily axial, posturings
        2. Complex: orienting and investigatory actions; ambulation or flight; response to stimuli (scratching, putting hand to face, clearing throat, etc.);

confusional state gestures: palpation of body part, rearrangement of clothes, manipulation of objects, occupational activities
    B. Vegetative signs:
        1. Respiratory: apnea, polypnea
        2. Digestive: mastication, salivation, borborygmi
        3. Vasomotor: paleness, flushing
        4. Pupillary: usually mydriasis
    C. Speech disorders:
        1. Aphasia (indicative of left-temporal focus)
        2. Speech automatism (indicative of right temporal focus)

This classification was originally presented by Gastaut[58] from a study of several thousand temporal-lobe seizure patients. Several modifications have been made based on subsequent studies.[155,189] Unfortunately, this list can only offer an outline of the many behavioral disturbances that occur; it cannot provide the detailed clinical description that each variety deserves. For this the reader is referred to clinical studies.[120,153] Some aspects of temporal-lobe-seizure behavior have, however, received considerable attention in recent years and deserve to be discussed here.

The motor manifestations of temporal-lobe discharge may be extremely limited, often consisting of only a few seconds of absence, and are easily mistaken for the thought-blocking of a schizophrenic or a neurotic. Motor activity, such as movement of the jaw, mastication, licking of the lips, eye blinking, or the rhythmic jerking of a finger may be observed. A glassy-eyed, vacant stare and a total amnesia for the period of absence are common. Often, however, the patient resumes activity or conversation immediately after the short episode and continues as though nothing had happened. Thus, even an experienced observer may be unaware that he has witnessed an epileptic seizure.

Abnormalities of perception are frequent manifestations of temporal-lobe seizure. Micropsia or macropsia (changes in the size of objects seen) should always suggest temporal or temporal-occipital pathology. "Déjà vu" is a feeling that an episode occurring now has occurred in exactly the same fashion in the past (reexperience, familiarity). Efron[44] has suggested that this phenomenon is due to a delay in the callosal transfer of sensory impulses from the nondominant hemisphere to the dominant hemisphere. The delay could produce a repeated conscious experiencing of the single stimulus and thus a strong sense of familiarity. Déjà vu is experienced by almost everyone at some time but, if a frequent complaint, temporal-lobe pathology should be suspected. It is more common with right-hemisphere than left-hemisphere disease.[29]

The presence of an emotion, mood, or feeling tone as part of a psychomotor seizure has received attention. Williams[189] studied all descriptions of the emotional content reported as part of a convulsive episode by several thousand patients. Only one hundred of them described emotional experiences and only four states were noted (fear, depression, pleasantness, unpleasantness). Other observers[110] have confirmed this limited variety of ictal emotionality. Fear is reported most often (well over half in several series) and a report of paroxysmal unexplained feelings of fear should suggest the possibility of psychomotor seizures.

Serafetinides and Falconer[155] studied speech disturbances reported by one hundred patients treated surgically for temporal-lobe seizures, and found significant disturbance in sixty-seven. Dysphasic manifestations (inability to produce or comprehend speech) were associated with left-temporal lesions almost exclusively. Speech automatisms (recurrent utterances), on the other hand, occurred most often in cases with right-temporal-lobe pathology. The patients producing speech automatisms were always unaware (amnesic), while those with dysphasia were usually aware of their language difficulties.

Aggressive, violent behavior either ictal, postictal or interictal has recently received emphasis as part of the temporal-lobe seizure pattern.[45,164,169] Mark et al.[121] speak of a "dyscontrol syndrome" and outline four major symptoms: (1) unrestrained and senseless brutality (particularly wife- or child-beating); (2) manic behavior after limited alcoholic intake (pathological intoxication); (3) sexual assault; and (4) repeated serious traffic accidents. In addition to these symptoms they look for speech or reading defects, visual field defects, memory impairment, seizures, hallucinations "or other indications of schizophrenia," gross sleep disturbances, and episodic mood disturbances. Any combination warrants investigation by EEG and pneumoencephalogram; demonstration of a focal abnormality in the temporal lobe in either would be considered confirmation of psychomotor seizures as the source of behavioral dyscontrol. Mark et al. have recorded a number of carefully investigated cases[121,164] and their hypothesis has received additional support from other cases.[52] Other investigators, however, have disagreed; the role of temporal lobe seizures in violent behavior remains unsettled (see below).

A number of careful studies[70,89,157] have demonstrated that at least one type of serious interictal behavior disturbance may occur in patients with temporal-lobe-seizure disorder. This has been called a schizophrenia-like state and, indeed, is often indistinguishable from schizophrenia. In this condition there are frequent delusions—both primary and secondary—and hallucinations, mainly auditory, but occasionally mixed with visual, gustatory, or olfactory references. Paranoid states are common, as well as catatonic states and repetitive, stereotyped, ritualistic activities. Affective responses, however, are usually preserved; this preservation of affect and the ability to establish rapport are the major clinical points which differentiate the schizophrenia states from "true" schizophrenia.[157] Pond[141] found no deterioration to a hebephrenic state in the schizophrenia-like group, although partial mental and social incapacity was the long-term outlook. The quasi-schizophrenia state often appears at a time when the seizures decrease or are brought under control, usually many years after the onset of seizures.[157,161] In the majority (80 percent in Slater's series[157]) there is evidence of temporal-lobe pathology as the source of the seizure focus.

In addition to the schizophrenic-like state, many authors[17,51,128] suggest that other aspects of interictal behavior may be altered in patients with temporal-lobe seizures. Personality deterioration, dementing states, and paroxysmal mood changes are frequently reported. Many investigators state that psychomotor epilepsy produces behavior changes which are "clinically indistinguishable from purely psychiatric disorders" (Gibbs).[69,71] Some[121,164] feel that impulsiveness and aggressive behavior are common interictal phenomena and use this point to urge earlier and more radical treatment of temporal-lobe epilepsy.

The presence of psychiatric abnormalities in the interictal phase of psychomotor epilepsy, however, is not universally accepted. Guerrant et al.[78] reviewed the literature comparing the behavior of psychomotor and other seizure patients and found an absence of careful documentation. They then analyzed the psychiatric status of thirty-two psychomotor epileptics, twenty-six idiopathic grand-mal patients and twenty-six patients with chronic medical illness not involving the brain, utilizing both psychiatric and psychological evaluations. They found no differences in the incidence of psychiatric abnormality in any of the three groups, and concluded that psychomotor epilepsy did not produce a specific personality derangement. Their conclusion is seriously weakened, however, by the fact that over 90 percent of all three groups, including their "normal" control group, had psychiatric abnormality, and by their own finding that "psychotic" abnormalities were more common in the temporal-lobe group, while "neurotic" abnormalities were more frequent in the medical controls. Stevens[161] performed a similar study comparing psychomotor and grand-mal-seizure patients and found the incidence of psychiatric abnormality approximately equal in the two types, with a much lower incidence in focal nontemporal epileptics. She noted, however, that the prevalent psychiatric disabilities in the psychomotor group included "schizophrenia, mood disturbance, anxiety, and withdrawal" while the grand-mal group

showed apathy and mental slowing. Also, the psychomotor patients decompensated psychiatrically when they became seizure free whereas the grand-mal group decompensated in the face of more frequent seizures. Most recently Mignone et al.[124] analyzed the results of psychological tests given to seizure patients at the NIH and found no significant difference in Minnesota Multiphasic Personality Inventory (MMPI) profiles between psychomotor and nonpsychomotor epileptics. The profiles of both groups, however, were different from normal controls. There would appear to be an increased incidence of behavioral abnormality in patients with psychomotor seizures when compared to normal subjects; whether this behavioral abnormality differs either quantitatively or qualitatively from that of grand-mal epileptics remains unsettled.

The diagnosis of temporal-lobe disorder as the cause of bizarre or paroxysmal behavior depends on a healthy degree of suspicion on the part of the examiner. History of a major seizure occurring at any time of life in a patient with bizarre behavioral problems should arouse suspicion. Confirmation by laboratory studies is not always easy to obtain. Not only routine EEGs but one or more specialized studies such as sleep- or metrazol-activated tracings utilizing special leads (sphenoidal or nasopharyngeal) should be used. The presence of a temporal-spike focus, either unilateral or bilateral, would confirm a suspected temporal-lobe-seizure diagnosis. Air encephalography is often abnormal in patients with temporal-lobe-seizure disorder. This is a hospital procedure with distinct though transient morbidity, and is usually reserved for patients considered for surgery or where the presence of a tumor is suspected.

Treatment of temporal-lobe-seizure disorder is neither easy nor certain. Anticonvulsants, usually in large doses, are sometimes effective. Mysoline, Dilantin, and phenobarbital are most frequently recommended. Control of interictal symptoms may be aided by use of tranquilizers such as the phenothiazines, Valium or Librium. Successful control has occasionally been reported with other anticonvulsants; bromides, Phenurone, or Mesantoin have all been used but toxicity limits their use to exceptional cases under the closest supervision.

Surgery has proved beneficial in carefully selected cases of temporal-lobe seizures. If the focus for the seizure discharge is localized in one temporal lobe, removal of that lobe often produces improved seizure control, improved personality, and even improved intelligence.[46] Temporal-lobe amputation, however, is known to affect memory; verbal memory is disturbed if the left side is removed, and non-verbal memory by right-temporal amputation. The degree of memory loss, however, is mild and usually not significant to the patient. Bilateral temporal-lobe amputation, on the other hand, produces a severe memory disturbance resembling Korsakoff's psychosis.[150] Similar memory loss has occasionally been reported after unilateral amputation.[178] In this situation, pathology involving the other temporal lobe has been either demonstrated or conjectured. Temporal-lobe amputation does not appear to alter the schizophrenic-like behavior in most cases.[157] Most investigators agree that surgery has a limited place at present in the treatment of seizures but has been successful in selected cases, and with improving techniques—particularly specific stereotaxic procedures—may play an important role in the future.

(Parietal- and Occipital-Lobe Syndromes

The primary function of these posterior hemispheric areas is the reception and integration of extrinsic sensory stimuli. Somesthetic information first reaches the cortex in the post-Rolandic area, and visual stimuli are initially channelled to the calcarine cortex of the occipital lobe. Surrounding both of these areas of primary sensory cortex are large areas of sensory association cortex. In addition, a fairly large area of cortex at the temporo-parieto-occipital junction, the angular gyrus, appears to act as a secondary association area,[33] receiving and processing stimuli from visual, somesthetic, and auditory association areas. It is in this area that cross-modal associations (from one sensory sphere to another) are thought to occur.[26,62] Much of the clinical symptomatology of these two areas consists of demonstrable sensory deficit (e.g., decreased position sense, astereognosis, visual field defect) but some of the symptomatology can mimic psychiatric disturbance.

Intelligence

Damage to the parietal lobe, particularly the angular gyrus, which disrupts second-order associations, may affect certain aspects of intelligence. Involvement of the left angular gyrus usually produces a severe aphasia with constructional disturbance, right-left disturbance, acalculia, and other disturbances to be discussed; but despite these specific disturbances other aspects of intelligence may not be affected.[193] With bilateral parietal involvement, however, severe intellectual deterioration is noted. Alzheimer's disease usually starts with biparietal deterioration; depression of intelligence is an early clinical feature. Analysis of findings, however, demonstrates that specific abnormalities are notable (i.e., anomia, constructional disability, memory disturbance); it does not appear appropriate to consider the parietal lobes as centers for some overall faculty of "intelligence."

Body Image

Through the sensory channels entering the brain (vision, cutaneous sensibility, proprioceptive impulses, labyrinthine inputs, etc.) we are consciously aware of our own bodies, their component parts, and their constantly changing position in space. This complex function may be referred to as "body image" or "body scheme" and is subject to a number of disorders[32,53] (see Chapter 33). The most prominent disorders of body image are those producing neglect, unawareness, or even denial of a part of one's body, and have been discussed in the section on right-hemisphere disorders. While many reports link these disorders to parietal defects,[77,130] other studies suggest that lesions elsewhere may also be implicated.[174,182] Amorphosynthesis, the inequality of perceptual rivalry discussed earlier, usually indicates parietal or occipital locus of causative lesion.

The Gerstmann syndrome is often cited as an example of disturbance of body image. As originally defined,[61] this syndrome consisted of four components: finger agnosia, right-left disorientation, acalculia, and agraphia. To this complex Schilder[148] added a fifth component, constructional disturbance. There was general agreement that the Gerstmann syndrome indicated dominant (usually left) parietal pathology. Recent studies have questioned the syndrome as lacking in intersymptom correlation,[13,87,139] but there is still general agreement that the combination of all four of the originally listed components strongly suggests dominant parietal dysfunction.[9] The fifth component, constructional disturbance (see earlier discussion), while not soley produced by parietal dysfunction[6] is very severe, with biparietal pathology; this is often one of the earliest signs of a dementing process beginning with parietal degeneration.

Neuropsychological investigation of brain-injured individuals has demonstrated that parietal damage, far more than damage in other areas, produces a disturbance of topographical orientation.[136,152] Both route-finding and maze-learning were abnormal in many cases with parietal damage, but neither difficulty was related to defect in one hemisphere preferentially. The patient who tells of getting lost on the streets or is unable to find his way about the ward should be suspected of parietal disturbance. This deficit has been termed topographagnosia and may be investigated clinically by asking the patient to draw or locate significant features on a map of his state, country, home, or the hospital ward.

Visual Hallucinations

Most of the signs and symptoms produced by focal pathology in the occipital lobe are obviously neurological or ophthalmologic and are rarely considered functional. An exception, however, must be made for visual hallucinations. There are many varieties of visual hallucination, some associated with psychiatric disorders (e.g., schizophrenia) and some with obvious organic pathology (e.g., temporal or occipital tumor). Some occur in special stress situations without obvious alteration of nervous tissue (e.g., black-patch psychosis, the hallucinations of sensory deprivation) and some are the product of a transient functional alteration (e.g., a migraine aura). Visual hallucinations may occur in many nonfocal brain diseases such as delirium tremens, drug intoxications, febrile states, and encephalitis (see chapters 1 and 2). Often, however, the etiologic causation is not clear when hallucinosis is first investigated and a short review of some focal CNS lesion-producing hallucinations is indicated.

Tumors are well known as a source of visual hallucinations. In 1889 Jackson and Beevor[93] reported well-formed visual hallucinations in a case with a tumor involving the tip of the right temporal lobe. The next year Henschen[88] reported a case of visual hallucinosis in a patient with an irritative lesion of the occipital lobe. Most subsequent reports have confirmed the importance of the temporo-occipital axis in cases of visual hallucinations caused by tumor. There is also a relationship between the nature of the hallucinatory experience and the location of the tumor. With occipital involvement the visual imagery is often brightly colored, diffuse, and formless, usually involving only one half of the visual field. The images are described as floating stars, zig-zags, spots, or fire. When the tumor is more anterior, the hallucinatory images tend to be well formed and are sometimes accompanied by auditory hallucinations. Familiar individuals or objects, often in meaningful activity, have been reported in the visual hallucinations of temporal-lobe tumor cases.[174] Formed hallucinations may also occur in occipital lesions,[28] particularly if the right hemisphere is involved.

Not all visual hallucinations due to structural lesions involve cortical structures, however. There are reports of visual hallucinations occurring in patients subsequently proved to have pathology which involves the subcortical visual pathways.[103,158] In some the hallucinations consisted of poorly formed images, colored and in motion; in others the images were complex, with recognizable figures and faces. The latter occurred almost exclusively in patients who became recently blind and persisted after the onset of blindness.

Another type of visual hallucination, reported only rarely but likely to cause diagnostic confusion, is peduncular hallucinosis. Most patients with this disorder are elderly[103] and are usually described as being mildly confused; some complain of giddiness or vertigo, and blindness or severe diminution of vision is usually reported. The hallucinations tend to be persistent and well formed, frequently Lilliputian (little people, miniature animals, etc.), often brightly colored, and usually in rapid movement.[31] The affective response to these hallucinations is often one of pleasure; the patients are interested in and amused by the hallucinatory experience. Only rarely does the hallucination produce distress or alarm. In the cases first reported,[103] vascular pathology involving the mesencephalon was reported. More recently "peduncular hallucinosis" has been reported with mass lesions in the interpeduncular fossa (pituitary or hypothalamic tumors). The disturbance of vision may be due to pressure on the optic tracts, but may also be secondary to bilateral obstruction of the posterior cerebral arteries producing ischemia in the calcarine region,[147] or to other as yet unexplained mesencephalic mechanisms.

Focal causes of hallucinosis are exceptional; most individuals suffering hallucinations have a demonstrable toxic-metabolic or functional source. If the patient reports depression of visual acuity along with the hallucinosis, however, a focal disturbance should be sought.

❰ Brain Tumors

Of all focal neurological disorders producing psychiatric symptomatology, the most perturbing to psychiatrists is the brain tumor. As so cogently stated by Pool and Correll:[142] "There is a pathetic, poignant ineffectiveness about doing psychotherapy in the hope of exorcising an expanding brain tumor. We have become so enchanted with emotional factors in the production of symptoms that we sometimes forget organic components."

Brain tumor is not common in psychiatric practice and its rarity allows the physician to overlook this possibility when seeing a patient with clear-cut behavioral symptomatology. Hard statistics on the frequency of brain tumor in psychiatric practice are not available; several studies report the occurrence of brain tumor as ranging between 0.3 and 0.6 percent of new patients in general psychiatric practices.[90,145] Mental hospitals report that brain tumor is present in between 1.5 and 4.0 percent of their autopsies.

The classic signs and symptoms of brain tumor, i.e., headache, vomiting, and papilledema often occur too late to be helpful. Most earlier abnormalities such as seizures, hemiparesis, visual field defect, etc., indicate neurological disorder and patients with these findings are usually seen by neurologists or neurosurgeons. Many brain tumors do not produce elementary neurological findings initially, however, and may produce psychiatric symptomatology. In fact, most individuals with tumors seen by the psychiatrist have no elementary neurological signs or symptoms. The question of why the patient with a brain tumor is so often seen by the psychiatrist has been explored[145] and the following suggested:

1. Behavioral changes may be the only initial finding, but the organic nature of these symptoms may not be obvious.
2. A brain tumor may occur in a functionally psychotic individual.
3. The patient may develop functional symptoms secondary to a misdiagnosis and/or mismanagement of the unrecognized brain tumor.
4. The patient may develop functional symptoms secondary to subjective awareness of decreased function caused by brain tumor.

As the psychiatric symptomatology of the brain-tumor patient may be identical to that arising from psychogenic causes, psychiatrists must remain alert for other suspicious symptomatology. A persistent and increasing headache should always be considered suspicious. Most signs of increased intracranial pressure, however, occur late, often too late for optimal treatment. The most helpful symptomatology depends upon focal disturbances produced by the tumor, a subject already discussed in this chapter. While tumors producing motor, sensory, visual, or extraocular symptoms, seizures, etc., eventually become obvious, tumors occupying a so-called "silent area"—e.g., the anterior frontal, or posterior parietal regions of either hemisphere, or the right temporal lobe —do not. Psychiatric symptomatology may be the major abnormality.

While a high level of suspicion is the one indispensable tool for diagnosing brain tumors, one simple test may help. Reproduction (copying) of line drawings, including both two dimensional figures (square, daisy, clock, etc.) and three-dimensional figures (cube, house, etc.), are requested, and judgment is made concerning the quality of the reproduction. Poor reproductions may result from unilateral neglect, messiness of lines, alteration of angles, loss of the third dimension, disturbance of either internal or external configuration, etc.[129] Normal adults copy line drawings adequately as do persons with psychogenic disorders, but pathology in either hemisphere involving frontal, parietal, or occipital tissue usually causes difficulty in producing copies.[129] If there is uncertainty about the drawing ability, standardized psychological tests such as the Bender-Gestalt may be employed for confirmation. Almost any type of organic brain disorder including degenerative dementia, head injury, meningitis, etc., will produce abnormality. In contrast, most psychogenic disorders do not cause abnormalities and the tests are valuable as screening measures. While abnormal drawings do not specify location or type of pathology, poor ability to reproduce drawings should be looked upon with considerable suspicion. Note, however, that significant lesions of the temporal lobes may not cause any drawing problems.

Laboratory studies can be of help in diagnosing brain tumor, but they are only of value when the presence of brain tumor is suspected.

At present, both the electroencephalogram and the radioisotope brain scan offer nontraumatic evaluation for brain tumor and the new computerized axial tomograph (CAT) appears to perform this function even better. If these tests give equivocal or nondiagnostic results, additional testing may be necessary. Lumbar puncture is useful, elevated pressure or elevated protein being suggestive of brain tumor. Arteriography and pneumoencephalography are used frequently and are often mandatory in the full investigation for brain tumor. Each of the last three tests carries a small but real risk for the patient and should be performed under the supervision of a neurologist or neurosurgeon. Negative results are not necessarily useful. There are many reports of negative diagnostic tests in patients subsequently proved to have a tumor.[2]

As the brain is contained in a fixed structure, anything that takes up space acts as a tumor. The list of brain tumors, therefore, is extensive. The tumor most likely to produce psychiatric symptomatology is the meningioma because it grows slowly, often originates in silent areas and can become very large before producing recognizable neurological symptomatology. Similarly, slow growing members of the glioma family (oligodendroglioma and low-grade astrocytoma) often cause difficulty for the psychiatrist. Subfrontal tumors such as craniopharyngioma and supracellar cyst frequently present with psychiatric symptomatology. Rapidly growing gliomas, dependent upon their location, can also lead to behavioral changes. Hematoma, particularly chronic subdural hematoma of the elderly, and abscess often produce psychiatric symptomatology. Actually, almost anything which occupies space inside the skull can produce psychiatric findings and be mistaken for psychogenic disease. A strong level of suspicion remains the most valuable clinical tool available for this treacherous diagnostic problem.

Bibliography

1. ADAMS, R. D., C. M. FISHER, S. HAKIM et al. "Symptomatic Occult Hydrocephalus with 'Normal' Cerebrospinalfluid Pressure: a Treatable Syndrome," *N. Engl. J. Med.*, 273 (1965), 117–126.

2. ANGEL, R. W. and D. F. BENSON. "Normal Air Encephalogram in Patients with Tumor of the Brain," *Neurology*, 9 (1959), 426–429.

3. ARRIGONI, G. and E. DE RENZI. "Constructional Apraxia and Hemispheric Locus of Lesion," *Cortex*, 1 (1964), 170–197.

4. BARBIZET, J. "Defect of Memorizing of Hippocampal-Mammillary Origin," *J. Neurol. Neurosurg. Psychiatry*, 26 (1963), 127–135.

5. ———. *Human Memory and Its Pathology.* San Francisco: Freeman, 1970.

6. BENSON, D. F. and M. I. BARTON. "Disturbances in Constructional Apraxia," *Cortex*, 6 (1970), 19–46.

7. BENSON, D. F. and N. GESCHWIND. Shrinking Retrograde Amnesia. *J. Neurol. Neurosurg. Psychiatry*, 30 (1967), 457–461.

8. ———. "Cerebral Dominance and Its Disturbances," *Pediatr. Clin. North Am.*, 15 (1968), 759–769.

9. ———. "Aphasia and Related Cortical Disturbances," in A. B. Baker and L. H. Baker, eds., *Clinical Neurology*, pp. 1–26. New York: Harper & Row, 1971.

10. BENSON, D. F., M. LeMAY, D. H. PATTEN et al. "Diagnosis of Normal-Pressure Hydrocephalus," *N. Engl. J. Med.*, 283 (1970), 609–615.

11. BENSON, D. F. and D. H. PATTEN. "The Use of Radioactive Isotopes in the Localization of Aphasia-Producing Lesions," *Cortex*, 3 (1967), 258–271.

12. BENSON, D. F., W. SHEREMATA, R. BOUCHARD et al. "Conduction Aphasia," *Arch. Neurol.*, 28 (1973), 339–346.

13. BENTON, A. L. "The Fiction of the 'Gerstmann Syndrome'," *Neurol. Neurosurg. Psychiatry*, 24 (1961), 176–181.

14. ———. "Constructional Apraxia and Minor Hemisphere," *Confin. Neurol.*, 29 (1967), 1–16.

15. BENTON, A. L. and M. W. VAN ALLEN. "Impairment in Facial Recognition in Patients with Cerebral Disease," *Cortex*, 4 (1969), 344–358.

16. BLEULER, E. *Dementia Praecox.* Trans. by J. Zinkin. New York: International Universities Press, 1950.

17. BLOCH, S. "Etiological Aspects of the Schizophrenia-like Psychosis of Temporal Lobe Epilepsy," *Med. J. Aust.*, 1 (1969), 451–455.

18. BOGEN, J. E. "The Other Side of the Brain II: An Appositional Mind," *Bull. Los Angeles Neurol. Soc.*, 34 (1969), 135–162.

19. BOGEN, J. E. and H. W. GORDON. "Musical Tests for Functional Lateralization with Intracarotid Amobarbital," *Nature*, 230 (1971), 524–525.

20. BORNSTEIN, B. "Prosopagnosia," in L. Halpern, ed., *Problems of Dynamic Neurology*, pp. 283–318. Jerusalem: Jerusalem Post Press, 1963.

21. BRAIN, W. R. "Visual Disorientation with Special Reference to Lesions of the Right Cerebral Hemisphere," *Brain*, 64 (1941), 244–272.

22. BRICKNER, R. M. *The Intellectual Functions of the Frontal Lobes.* New York: Macmillan, 1936.

23. BRION, S., C. PRAGIER, R. GUERIN et al. "Korsakoff Syndrome Due to Bilateral Softening of Fornix," *Rev. Neurol. Paris*, 120 (1969), 225–262.

24. BROCA, P. "Remarques sur le siège de la faculté du langage articulé, suivis d'une observation d'aphémie," *Bull. Soc. Anat. Paris* (1861), 330–357.

25. BRUETSCH, W. L. "Neurosyphilitic Conditions," in S. Arieti, ed., *American Handbook of Psychiatry*, Vol. 2, 1st ed., pp. 1003–1021. New York: Basic Books, 1959.

26. BUTTERS, N. and B. A. BRODY. "The Role of the Left Parietal Lobe in the Mediation of Intra- and Cross-Modal Associations," *Cortex*, 4 (1968), 328–343.

27. CAIRNS, H. and W. H. MOSBERG, JR. "Colloid Cyst of the Third Ventricle," *Surg. Gynecol. Obstet.*, 92 (1951), 545–570.

28. COGAN, D. Personal communication.

29. COLE, M. and O. L. ZANGWILL. "Déjà Vu in Temporal Lobe Epilepsy," *J. Neurol. Neurosurg. Psychiatry*, 26 (1963), 37–38.

30. COSTELLO, C. G., G. P. BELTON, J. C. ABRA et al. "The Amnesic and Therapeutic Effects of Bilateral and Unilateral ECT," *Br. J. Psychiatry*, 116, (1970), 69–78.

31. CRITCHLEY, M. "Neurological Aspects of Visual and Auditory Hallucinations," *Br. J. Med.*, 2 (1939), 634–659.

32. ————. *The Parietal Lobes.* London: Arnold, 1953.

33. CROSBY, E. C., E. HUMPHREY, and E. W. LAUER. *Correlative Neuroanatomy of the Nervous System.* New York: Macmillan 1962.

34. CURRIER, R. D., S. C. LITTLE, J. F. SUESS et al. "Sexual Seizures," *Arch. Neurol.*, 25 (1971), 260–264.

35. DEE, H. L. "Visuoconstructive and Visuoperceptive Deficit in Patients with Unilateral Cerebral Lesions," *Neuropsychologia*, 8 (1970), 305–314.

36. DeJONG, R. N., H. H. ITABASHI, and J. R. OLSON. "Memory Loss Due to Hippocampal Lesions, Report of a Case," *Arch. Neurol.*, 20 (1969), 339–348.

37. DEMPSEY, E. M. and R. S. MORRISON. "The Electrical Activity of a Thalamo-Cortical Relay System," *Am. J. Psychol.*, 138 (1943), 283–296.

38. DENNY-BROWN, D. "The Frontal Lobes and Their Functions," in A. Feiling, ed., *Modern Trends in Neurology*, pp. 13–89. New York: Hoeber, 1951.

39. DENNY-BROWN, D. and B. Q. BANKER. "Amorphosynthesis from Left Parietal Lesion," *Arch. Neurol.*, 71 (1954), 302–313.

40. DENNY-BROWN, D., J. S. MEYER, and S. HORENSTEIN. "The Significance of Perceptual Rivalry Resulting from Parietal Lesion," *Brain*, 75 (1952), 29–471.

41. DeRENZI, E. and H. SPINNLER. "Facial Recognition in Brain Damaged Patients," *Neurology*, 16 (1966), 145–152.

42. DINGMAN, J.F. and G. W. THORN. "Diseases of the Neurohypophysis," in M. W. Wintrobe et al., eds., *Harrison's Principles of Internal Medicine*, 6th ed., pp. 435–443. New York: McGraw-Hill, 1970.

43. DOTT, N. M. "Hypothalamus—Surgical Aspects," in *The Hypothalamus.* London: Oliver and Boyd, 1938.

44. EFRON, R. "Temporal Perception, Aphasia and Déjà Vu," *Brain*, 86 (1963), 403–424.

45. ERVIN, F., A. W. EPSTEIN, and H. E. KING. "Behavior of Epileptic and Non-Epileptic Patients with 'Temporal Spikes'," *Arch. Neurol. Psychiatry*, 74 (1955), 488–497.

46. FALCONER, M. A. "Significance of Surgery for Temporal Lobe Epilepsy in Childhood and Adolescence," *J. Neurosurg.*, 33 (1970), 233–252.

47. FALCONER, M. A., E. A. SERAFETINIDES, and J. A. CORSELLIS. "Etiology and Pathogenesis of Temporal Lobe Epilepsy," *Arch. Neurol.*, 10 (1964), 233–248.

48. FAUST, C. "Die Psychischen Störungen nach Hirnträumen," in H. W. Gruhnle, ed., *Psychiatrie der Gegenwart*, Band 2, pp. 552–645. Berlin: Springer, 1960.

49. FEUCHTWANGER, E. *Die Funktionen des Stirnhirns.* Berlin: Springer, 1923.

50. ————. *Amusie.* Berlin: Springer, 1930.

51. FLOR-HENRY, P. "Schizophrenic-like Reactions and Affective Psychoses Associated with Temporal Lobe Epilepsy: Etiological Factors," *Am. J. Psychiatry*, 126 (1969), 400–403.

52. ————. "Psychosis and Temporal Lobe Epilepsy," *Epilepsia*, 10 (1969), 363–395.

53. FREDERICKS, J. A. M. "Disorders of the Body Schema," in P. G. Winken and G. W. Bruynm eds., *Handbook of Clinical Neurology*, Vol. 4, pp. 207–240. Amsterdam: North-Holland, 1969.

54. FREEDMAN, A. M. and H. I. KAPLAN. *Comprehensive Text Book of Psychiatry.* Baltimore: Williams & Wilkins, 1967.

55. FREEMAN, W. and J. W. WATTS. *Psychosurgery.* Springfield, Ill.: Charles C. Thomas, 1942.

56. FRENCH, J. D. "Brain Lesions Associated with Prolonged Unconsciousness," *Arch. Neurol. Psychiatry*, 68 (1952), 727–740.

57. FRIEDMAN, H. M. and N. ALLEN. "Chronic Effects of Complete Limbic Lobe Destruction in Man," *Neurology*, 19 (1969), 679–690.

58. GASTAUT, H. "So-called 'Psychomotor' and 'Temporal' Epilepsy," *Epilepsia* (3rd ser., 2 (1953), 59–99.

59. GAZZANIGA, M. S., J. E. BOGEN, and R. W. SPERRY. "Some Functional Effects of Sectioning the Cerebral Commissures in Man," *Proc. Natl. Acad. Sci. USA*, 48 (1962), 1765–1769.

60. GAZZANIGA, M. S. and R. W. SPERRY. "Language after Section of the Cerebral Commissures," *Brain*, 90 (1967), 131–148.

61. GERSTMANN, J. "Fingeragnosie und Isolierte Agraphie, ein Neues Syndrom," *Z. Ges. Neurol. Psychiatr*, 108 (1927), 152–177.

62. GESCHWIND, N. "The Development of the Brain and the Evolution of Language," in C. I. J. M. Stuart, ed., *Monograph Series*

on Languages and Linguistics, No. 17, report of the 15th Annual Round Table Meeting on Linguistic and Language Studies, April 1964, pp. 155–169. Washington: Georgetown University Press, 1964.

63. ———. "Disconnexion Syndromes in Animals and Man," *Brain*, 88 (1965), 237–294, 585–644.

64. ———. "The Apraxias," in E. W. Straus and R. M. Griffith, eds., *Proceedings of the Second Lexington VAH Conference on Will and Action*, pp. 91–102. Pittsburgh: Duquesne University Press, 1967.

65. GESCHWIND, N. and M. FUSILLO. "Color Naming Defects in Association with Alexia," *Arch. Neurol.*, 15 (1966), 137–146.

66. GESCHWIND, N. and M. KAPLAN. "A Human Cerebral Disconnection Syndrome," *Neurology*, 12 (1962), 675–685.

67. GESCHWIND, N. and W. LEVITSKY. "Human Brain: Left-Right Asymmetry in Temporal Speech Region," *Science*, 161 (1968), 186–187.

68. GESCHWIND, N., F. A. QUADFASEL, and J. SEGARRA. "Isolation of the Speech Area," *Neuropsychologia*, 6 (1968), 327–340.

69. GIBBS, E. L., F. A. GIBBS, and B. FUSTER. "Psychomotor Epilepsy," *Arch. Neurol. Psychiatry*, 60 (1948), 331–339.

70. GIBBS, F. A. "Ictal and Non-Ictal Psychiatric Disorders in Temporal Lobe Epilepsy," *J. Nerv. Ment. Dis.*, 113 (1951), 522–528.

71. GIBBS, F. A. and E. L. GIBBS. "Psychiatric Implications of Discharging Temporal Lobe Lesions," *Trans. Am. Neurol. Assoc.*, 73 (1948), 133–137.

72. GLASER, G. H. and H. J. PINCUS. "Limbic Encephalitis," *J. Nerv. Ment. Dis.*, 149 (1969), 59–67.

73. GLONING, I., K. GLONING, C. HAUB et al. "Comparison of Verbal Behavior in Right-Handed and Non Right-Handed Patients with Anatomically Verified Lesion of One Hemisphere," *Cortex*, 5 (1969), 43–52.

74. GOLDSTEIN, K. *Language and Language Disturbances*. New York: Grune & Stratton, 1948.

75. GOODGLASS, H. and F. QUADFASEL. "Language Laterality in Left Handed Aphasics," *Brain*, 77 (1954), 521–548.

76. GREENBLATT, M. and H. C. SOLOMON. "Studies of Lobotomy," in *The Brain and Human Behavior*, pp. 19–34. Proceedings of the Association for Research in Nervous and Mental Diseases (ARNMD), Dec. 7 and 8, 1956. New York: Hafner, 1966.

77. GRINKER, R. and A. SAHS. *Neurology*, 6th ed. Springfield, Ill.: Charles C. Thomas, 1966.

78. GUERRANT, J., W. N. ANDERSON, A. FISCHER et al. *Personality in Epilepsy*. Springfield, Ill.: Charles C. Thomas, 1962.

79. HALLIDAY, A. M., K. DAVISON, M. W. BROWNE et al. "A Comparison of the Effects on Depression and Memory of Bilateral ECT and Unilateral ECT to the Dominant and Non-Dominant Hemispheres," *Br. J. Psychiatry*, 114 (1968), 997–1012.

80. HARLOW, J. "Recovery from the Passage of an Iron Bar Through the Head," *Publ. Mass. Med. Soc.*, 2, 1868.

81. HÉCAEN, H. "Clinical Symptomatology in Right and Left Hemisphere Lesions," in V. B. Mountcastle, ed., *Interhemispheric Relations and Cerebral Dominance*, pp. 215–243. Baltimore: Johns Hopkins, 1962.

82. HÉCAEN, H. and J. DE AJURIAGUERRA. *Méconnaissances et Hallucinations Corporelles*. Paris: Mason, 1952.

83. HÉCAEN, H. and G. ASSAL. "A Comparison of Constructive Deficits Following Right and Left Hemispheric Lesions," *Neuropsychologia*, 8 (1970), 289–303.

84. HÉCAEN, H., M. B. DELL, and A. ROGER. "L'Aphasie de conduction," *L'Encéphale*, 2 (1955), 170–195.

85. HÉCAEN, H. and J. SAUGET. "Cerebral Dominance in Left-Handed Subjects," *Cortex*, 7 (1971), 19–48.

86. HÉCAEN, H. and A. TZAVARAS. "Etude Neuropsychologique des Troubles de la Reconnaissance des Visages Humains," *Bull. Psychol.*, 276 (1968–9), 754–762.

87. HEIMBURGER, R. F., W. DEMYER, and R. M. REITAN. "Implications of Gerstmann's Syndrome," *J. Neurol. Neurosurg. Psychiatry*, 27 (1967), 52–57.

88. HENSCHEN, S. E. *Klinische und anatomische Beitrage zur Pathologie des Gehirns*. Uppsala: Almquist and Wilsell, 1890.

89. HILL, D. "The Schizophrenia-like Psychoses of Epilepsy," (Discussion) *Proc. Roy. Soc.* 55 (1962), 315–316.

90. HOBBS, G. E. "Brain Tumors Simulating Psychiatric Disease," *Can. Med. J.*, 88 (1963), 186–188.

91. HOOSHMAND, H. and B. W. BRAWLEY. "Temporal Lobe Seizures and Exhibitionism," *Neurology*, 19 (1970), 1119–1124.

92. JACKSON, J. H. *Selected Writings*, Vol. 2, J. Taylor, ed. London: Hodder and Stoughton, 1932.

93. JACKSON, J. H. and C. BEEVOR. "Case of Tumor of the Right Temporal Sphenoidal Lobe Bearing on the Localization of the Sense of Smell and the Interpretation of a Particular Variety of Epilepsy," *Brain*, 12 (1889), 346–357.

94. JOHNSON, J. "Sexual Impotence and the Limbic System," *Br. J. Psychol.*, 111 (1965), 300–303.

95. KENNARD, M. "Alterations in Response to Visual Stimuli Following Lesions of the Frontal Lobe in Monkeys," *Arch. Neurol. Psychiatry*, 41 (1939), 1153–1165.

96. KIM, C., D. R. BONNETT, and T. S. ROBERTS. "Primary Amenorrhea Secondary to Non-Communicating Hydrocephalus," *Neurology*, 19 (1969), 533–535.

97. KIMURA, D. "Right Temporal Lobe Damage," *Arch. Neurol.*, 8 (1963), 264–271.

98. KINSBOURNE, M. "The Minor Cerebral Hemisphere as a Source of Aphasic Speech," *Arch. Neurol.*, 25 (1971), 302–306.

99. KLEIST, K. *Gehirnpathologie*. Leipzig: Barth, 1934.

100. KLUVER, H. and P. C. BUCY. "Psychic Blindness and Other Symptoms Following Bilateral Temporal Lobectomy in Rhesus Monkeys," *Am. J. Physiol.*, 119 (1937), 352–353.

101. KRETSCHMER, E. "Die Orbitalhirn- und Zwischenhirnsyndrome nach Schädelbasis Frakturen," *Allg. Z. Psychiatry*, 124 (1949), 358–360.

102. LEMAY, M. and P. F. J. NEW. "Radiological Diagnosis of Occult Normal-Pressure Hydrocephalus," *Radiology*, 96 (1970), 347–358.

103. LHERMITTE, J. *Les Hallucinations*. Paris: G. Doin & Cie., 1951.

104. LIEPMANN, H. *Das Krankheitsbild der Apraxie ('Motorischen Asymbolie')*. Berlin: Karger, 1900.

105. ———. "Das Krankheitsbild der Apraxie," *Monatsschr. Psychiatr. Neurol.*, 17 (1905), 289–311.

106. LISHMAN, W. A. "Brain Damage in Relation to Psychiatric Disability after Head Injury," *Br. J. Psychiatry*, 114 (1968), 373–410.

107. LURIA, A. R., K. H. PRIBRAM, and E. D. HOMSKAYA. "An Experimental Analysis of the Behavioral Disturbance Produced by a Left Frontal Arachnoidal Endothelioma," *Neuropsychologia*, 2 (1964), 257–280.

108. McFIE, J., M. F. PIERCY, and O. L. ZANGWILL. "Visual-Spatial Agnosia," *Brain*, 73 (1950), 167–190.

109. McFIE, J. and O. L. ZANGWILL. "Visual Constructive Disabilities Associated with Lesions of the Left Cerebral Hemisphere," *Brain*, 83 (1960), 243–260.

110. MACRAE, D. "Isolated Fear, A Temporal Lobe Aura," *Neurology*, 4 (1954), 497–505.

111. MACRAE, D., C. L. BRANCH, and B. MILNER. "The Occipital Horns and Cerebral Dominance," *Neurology*, 18 (1968), 95–98.

112. MACLEAN, P. D. "Psychomatic Disease and the Visceral Brain," *Psychosom. Med.*, 11 (1949), 338–353.

113. ———. "The Limbic System and its Hippocampal Formation, *J. Neurosurg.*, 11 (1954), 29–44.

114. ———. "The Limbic System (Visceral Brain) in Relation to Central Gray and Reticulum of the Brain Stem," *Psychosom. Med.*, 17 (1955), 355–366.

115. ———. "Contrasting Functions of Limbic and Neocortical Systems of the Brain and their Relevance to Psychophysiological Aspects of Medicine," *Am. J. Med.*, 25 (1958), 611–626.

116. MAGOUN, H. W. *The Waking Brain*. Springfield, Ill.: Charles C. Thomas, 1963.

117. MALAMUD, N. "Psychiatric Symptoms and the Limbic Lobe," *Bull. Los Angeles Neurol. Soc.*, 22 (1957), 131–139.

118. ———. *Atlas of Neuropathology*. Berkeley: University of California Press, 1957.

119. ———. "Psychiatric Disorder with Intracranial Tumor of Limbic System," *Arch. Neurol.*, 17 (1967), 113–123.

120. MARGERISON, J. H. and J. A. N. CORSELLIS. "Epilepsy and the Temporal Lobes: A Clinical, Electro-encephalographic and Neuropathological Study of the Brain in Epilepsy, with Particular Reference to the Temporal Lobes," *Brain*, 89 (1966), 499–530.

121. MARK, V. H., W. H. SWEET, F. R. ERVIN

et al. "Brain Disease and Violent Behavior," presented at the Society for the Advancement of Behavioral Therapy (in conjunction with the Am. Psychiatric Assoc.), Sept. 3, 1967, Washington, D.C.

122. MAYER-GROSS, W., E. SLATER, and M. ROTH. *Clinical Psychiatry*, 3rd ed., London: Baillière, 1969.

123. MICHAEL, R. P. and J. L. GIBBONS. "Some Inter-Relationships between the Endocrine System and Neuropsychiatry," *Int. Rev. Neurobiol.*, 5 (1963), 243.

124. MIGNONE, R. J., E. F. DONNELLY, and P. SADOWSKY. "Psychomotor and Non-Psychomotor Epileptics," *Epilepsia*, 11 (1970), 345–359.

125. MILNER, B., and W. PENFIELD. "The Effect of Hippocampal Lesions on Recent Memory," *Trans. Am. Neurol. Assoc.*, 80 (1955), 42–48.

126. MILNER, B. "Visual Recognition and Recall After Right Temporal Lobe Excision in Man," *Neuropsychologia*, 6 (1968), 191–200.

127. MORUZZI, G. and H. W. MAGOUN. "Brain Stem Reticular Formation and Activation of the EEG," *Electroencephalogr. Clin. Neurophysiol.*, 1 (1949), 455–473.

128. MULDER, D. W. and D. DALY. "Psychiatric Symptoms Associated with Lesions of Temporal Lobe," *JAMA*, 150 (1952), 173–176.

129. NAHOR, A. and D. F. BENSON. "A Screening Test for Organic Brain Disease in Emergency Psychiatric Evaluation," *Behav. Psychiatry*, 2 (1970), 23–26.

130. NIELSON, J. M. *Agnosia, Apraxia and Aphasia: Their Value in Cerebral Localization.* New York: Hafner, 1936.

131. PAPEZ, J. W. "A Proposed Mechanism of Emotion," *Arch. Neurol. Psychiatry*, 38 (1937), 725–743.

132. PATERSON, A. and O. L. ZANGWILL. "Disorders of Visual Space Perception Associated with Lesions of the Right Cerebral Hemisphere," *Brain*, 67 (1944), 331–358.

133. PATTEN, D. H. and D. F. BENSON. "Diagnosis of Normal-Pressure Hydrocephalus by RISA Cisternography," *J. Nucl. Med.*, 9 (1968), 457–461.

134. PETERS, U. H. "Pseudo-psychopathic Emotion Syndrome of Temporal Lobe Epileptic," *Nervenarzt*, 40 (1969), 75–82.

135. PIERCY, M. and V. O. G. SMYTH. "Right Hemisphere Dominance for Certain Non-Verbal Intellectual Skills," *Brain*, 85 (1962), 775–790.

136. ———. "The Effects of Cerebral Lesions on Intellectual Function: A Review of Current Research Trends," *Br. J. Psychiatry*, 110 (1964), 310–352.

137. PILLERI, G. "The Kluver-Bucy Syndrome in Man," *Psychiatry Neurol.*, 152 (1967), 65–103.

138. POECK, K. "Pathophysiology of Emotional Disorders Associated with Brain Damage," in P. J. Vinken and G. W. Bruyn, eds., *Handbook of Clinical Neurology.* Vol. 3, pp. 343–367. Amsterdam: North-Holland, 1969.

139. POECK, K. and B. ORGASS. "Gerstmann's Syndrome and Aphasia," *Cortex*, 2 (1966), 421–437.

140. POECK, K. and G. PILLERI. "Release of Hypersexual Behavior Due to Lesion in the Limbic System," *Acta. Neurol. Scand.*, 41 (1965), 233–244.

141. POND, D. A. "The Schizophrenia-like Psychoses of Epilepsy," *Proc. R. Soc. Med.*, 55 (1962), 316.

142. POOL, J. L. and J. W. CORRELL. "Psychiatric Symptoms Masking Brain Tumor," *J. Med. Soc. N.J.*, 33 (1958), 4–9.

143. RASMUSSEN, T. "Surgical Therapy of Frontal Lobe Epilepsy," *Epilepsia*, 4 (1963), 181–198.

144. REEVES, A. G. and F. PLUM. "Hyperphagia, Rage and Dementia Accompanying a Ventromedial Hypothalamic Neoplasm," *Arch. Neurol.*, 20 (1969), 616–624.

145. REMINGTON, F. B. and S. L. RUBERT. "Why Patients with Brain Tumors Come to a Psychiatric Hospital: A Thirty Year Survey," *Am. J. Psychiatry*, 119 (1962), 256–257.

146. ROBERTS, L. "The Relationship of Cerebral Dominance to Hand, Auditory and Ophthalmic Preference," in P. J. Vinken and G. W. Bruyn, eds., *Handbook of Clinical Neurology*, Vol. 4, pp. 312–326. Amsterdam: North-Holland, 1969.

147. ROZANSKI, J. "Peduncular Hallucinosis Following Vertebral Angiography," *Neurology*, 2 (1952), 341–349.

148. SCHILDER, P. "Fingeragnosie, Fingerapraxie, Fingeraphasie," *Nervenarzt*, 4 (1931), 625–629.

149. SCOVILLE, W. B. "The Limbic Lobe in Man," *J. Neurosurg.*, 11 (1954), 64–66.

150. SCOVILLE, W. B. and B. MILNER. "Loss of

Recent Memory after Bilateral Hippo-campal Lesions," *J. Neurol. Neurosurg. Psychiatry*, 20 (1957), 11–21.

151. SEGARRA, J. M. "Cerebral Vascular Disease and Behavior. I. The Syndrome of the Mesencephalic Artery," *Arch. Neurol.*, 23 (1970), 408–418.

152. SEMMES, J., S. WEINSTEIN, L. GHENT et al. "Correlates of Impaired Orientation in Personal and Extrapersonal Space," *Brain*, 86 (1963), 747–772.

153. SERAFETINIDES, E. A. and M. A. FALCONER. "The Effects of Temporal Lobectomy in Epileptic Patients with Psychosis," *J. Ment. Sci.*, 108 (1962), 584–593.

154. ———. "Some Observations of Memory Impairment After Temporal Lobectomy for Epilepsy," *J. Neurol. Neurosurg. Psychiatry*, 25 (1962), 251–255.

155. ———. "Speech Disturbances in Temporal Lobe Seizures. A Study of 100 Epileptic Patients Submitted to Anterior Temporal Lobectomy," *Brain*, 86 (1963), 333–346.

156. SHEARER, M. L. and S. M. FINCH. "Periodic Organic Psychosis Associated with Recurrent Herpes Simplex," *N. Engl. J. Med.*, 271 (1964), 494–497.

157. SLATER, E., A. W. BEARD, and E. GLITHERO. "The Schizophrenia-like Psychoses of Epilepsy," *Br. J. Psychiatry*, 109 (1963), 95–150.

158. SMITH, R. A., D. B. GELLES, and J. J. VANDERHAGEN. "Subcortical Visual Hallucinations," *Cortex*, 7 (1971), 162–168.

159. SMITH, R. A. and W. A. SMITH. "Loss of Recent Memory as a Sign of Focal Temporal Lobe Disorder," *J. Neurosurg.*, 24 (1966), 91–95.

160. SPILLANE, J. D. "Nervous and Mental Disorders in Cushing's Syndrome," *Brain*, 74 (1951), 72–94.

161. STEVENS, J. R. "Psychiatric Implications of Psychomotor Epilepsy," *Arch. Gen. Psychiatry*, 14 (1966), 461–471.

162. STRITCH, S. J. "The Pathology of Brain Damage Due to Blunt Head Injuries," in A. E. Walker and W. F. Caveness, eds., *The Late Effect of Head Injury*, pp. 501–526. Springfield, Ill.: Charles C. Thomas, 1969.

163. SUBIRANA, A. "The Relationship Between Handedness and Language Function," *Int. J. Neurol.*, 4 (1964), 215–234.

164. SWEET, W. H., F. ERVIN, and V. MARK.

"The Relationship of Violent Behavior to Focal Cerebral Disease," in S. Garattini, and E. B. Sigg, eds., *Aggressive Behavior*, pp. 336–352. Proceedings of the Symposium on the Biology of Aggressive Behavior, Milan, May 1968. Amsterdam: Excerpta Medica, 1969.

165. SWEET, W. H., G. A. TALLAND, and F. R. ERVIN. "Loss of Recent Memory Following Section of the Fornix," *Trans. Am. Neurol. Assoc.*, 84 (1959), 76–82.

166. SYKES, M. K. and R. F. TREDGOLD. "Restricted Orbital Undercutting," *Br. J. Psychiatry*, 110 (1964), 609–640.

167. TALLAND, G. A. *Deranged Memory: A Psychonomic Study of the Amnesic Syndrome.* New York: Academic, 1965.

168. TAVERAS, J. M. "Low-Pressure Hydrocephalus in Neuro-Ophthalmology," in J. L. Smith, ed., *Symposium of the University of Miami and the Bascom Palmer Eye Institute*, Vol. 4, pp. 239–309. St. Louis: Mosby, 1968.

169. TAYLOR, D. C. "Aggression and Epilepsy," *J. Psychosom. Res.*, 13 (1969), 229–236.

170. TERZIAN, H. and G. DALLE-ORE. "Syndrome of Klüver-Bucy Reproduced in Man by Bilateral Removal of the Temporal Lobes," *Neurology*, 5 (1955), 373–381.

171. THOMAS, E. W. "Current Status of Therapy in Syphilis," *JAMA*, 162 (1956), 1536–1539.

172. TOW, P. MacD. and C. W. M. WHITTY. "Personality Changes After Operations on the Cingulate Gyrus in Man," *J. Neurol. Neurosurg. Psychiatry*, 16 (1953), 186–193.

173. TZAVARAS, A., H. HÉCAEN, and H. LeBRAS. Le Problème de la Spécificité du Déficit de la reconnaissance du visage humain lors des lesions hémisphériques unilatérales," *Neuropsychologia*, 8 (1970), 403–416.

174. ULLMAN, M. *Behavioral Changes in Patients Following Strokes.* Springfield: Charles C. Thomas, 1962.

175. VICTOR, M., R. D. ADAMS, and G. H. COLLINS. *The Wernicke-Korsakoff Syndrome.* Philadelphia: Davis, 1971.

176. VICTOR, M., J. ANGEVINE, E. MANCALL et al. "Memory Loss with Lesions of Hippocampal Formation," *Arch. Neurol.*, 5 (1961), 244–263.

177. WALCH, R. "Über die Aufgaben der Hirnverletztenheime nach dem Bundesver-

sorgungsgesetz," in E. Renwald, ed., *Das Hirntrauma*, pp. 461–468. Stuttgart: Thieme, 1956.

178. WALKER, A. E. "Recent Memory Impairment in Unilateral Temporal Lesions," *Arch. Neurol.*, 78 (1957), 543–552.

179. WALSHE, F. G. and W. F. HOYT. *Clinical Neuro-Ophthalmology*, 3rd ed. Baltimore: Williams & Wilkins, 1969.

180. WARRINGTON, E. K. "Constructional Apraxia," in P. J. Vinken and G. W. Bruyn, eds., *Handbook of Clinical Neurology*, Vol. 4, pp. 67–83. Amsterdam: North-Holland, 1969.

181. WEINSTEIN, E. A. and M. COLE. "Concepts of Anosognosia," in L. Halpern, ed., *Problems of Dynamic Neurology*, pp. 254–273. Jerusalem: Jerusalem, 1963.

182. WEINSTEIN, E. A. and R. L. KAHN. *Denial of Illness: Symbolic and Physiologic Aspects*. Springfield, Ill.: Charles C. Thomas, 1955.

183. WEISENBURG, T. S. and K. E. McBRIDE. *Aphasia*. New York: Hafner, 1964.

184. WELCH, K. and P. STUTEVILLE. "Experimental Production of Unilateral Neglect in Monkeys," *Brain*, 81 (1958), 341–347.

185. WERNICKE, C. *Der aphasiche Symptomencomplex*. Breslau: Franck & Weigert, 1874.

186. WERTHEIM, N. and M. I. BOTEZ. "Receptive Amusia: A Clinical Analysis," *Brain*, 84 (1961), 19–30.

187. WHITE, L. E. and R. F. HAIN. "Anorexia in Association with a Destructive Lesion in the Hypothalamus," *Arch. Pathol.*, 68 (1959), 275–281.

188. WHITTY, C. W. M. and O. L. ZANGWILL. *Amnesia*. New York: Appleton-Century-Crofts, 1966.

189. WILLIAMS, D. "The Structure of Emotions Reflected in Epileptic Experiences," *Brain*, 79 (1956), 29–67.

190. ————. "The Temporal Lobe and Epilepsy," in D. Williams, ed., *Modern Trends in Neurology*, 2nd ser. pp. 338–352. London: Butterworth, 1957.

191. WILLIAMS, M. and J. PENNYBACKER. "Memory Disturbances in Third Ventricle Tumors," *J. Neurol. Neurosurg. Psychiatry*, 17 (1954), 115–123.

192. YAKOVLEV, P. I. and P. RAKIC. "Patterns of Decussation of Bulbar Pyramids and Distribution of Pyramidal Tracts on Two Sides of the Spinal Cord," *Trans. Am. Neurol. Assoc.*, 91 (1966), 366–367.

193. ZANGWILL, O. L. "Intellectual Status in Aphasia," in P. J. Vinken and G. W. Bruyn, eds., *Handbook of Clinical Neurology*, Vol. 4, pp. 105–111. Amsterdam: North-Holland, 1969.

CHAPTER 10

THE NEURAL ORGANIZATION OF LANGUAGE: APHASIA AND NEUROPSYCHIATRY*

Jason W. Brown

. . . the thought which only seemed naked was but pleading for the clothes it wore to become visible, while the words lurking afar were not empty shells as they seemed, but were only waiting for the thought they already concealed to set them aflame and in motion.

—Vladimir Nabokov

⟨ The History of Aphasia

From Gall to Wernicke

Although there are references to speech loss from cerebral lesions dating as far back as the *Hippocratic Corpus* of 400 B.C., the modern era is usually taken to begin with the phrenology of Franz Joseph Gall in the early 19th century. His work[39] had far-reaching implications,[109] but for the still unborn field of aphasia research it signalled a shift in attention away from the holistic approach which was current at the time to the possibility of a cerebral localization of speech. Gall reasoned specifically from a single instance in which large eyes and a prodigious verbal memory happened to occur in the same individual, a childhood acquaintance, that speech was a function of the frontal lobes. The French neurologist Bouillaud was so impressed by this assertion

* Supported in part through a grant from the Foundations' Fund for Research in Psychiatry.

that he offered an award of 500 Frs. to anyone who could disprove it. Bouillaud[15] also wrote an historically important paper in which he distinguished between the sign function of speech and its articulatory apparatus (i.e., between internal and external speech), and on the basis of a few cases argued that the "legislative organ of speech" resided in the anterior (frontal) lobes of the brain.

Paul Broca, a student under Bouillaud at Bicêtre Hospital, could not fail to be influenced by the exciting debate stimulated by these ideas. An opportunity to settle the issue finally occurred when a fifty-one-year old patient with excellent comprehension but almost complete loss of speech was admitted to the ward. The postmortem examination, from which date one can ascribe the beginnings of the science of aphasia, demonstrated, as predicted by Bouillaud, a large Sylvian lesion in the left hemisphere, the center of which was in the third, and partly the second, frontal convolution. Broca[17] conceived the speech loss, aphemia, to be a kind of ataxia of those movements which served for the articulation of words. In subsequent papers[18,19] he defined the "motor speech area" as consisting of the posterior part of the third or inferior frontal convolution (F_3), and by 1865 sufficient data had been collected to suggest a possible relationship, in right handers, to the left hemisphere.[20*] It is of interest that the term "aphemia," chosen by Broca for this disorder, was criticized by Trousseau[10] on the grounds that it connoted infamy (i.e., unspeakableness), rather than lack of speech. Gradually it has become customary to use the term "aphasia" for loss of speech *and* writing, and "aphemia" for loss of speech alone.

Certainly it can be said that at that time the various approaches to the problem of aphasia had not yet hardened into the distinct schools of thought that so characterized later work in the field. While Broca is often represented as the earliest "localizer," an impartial reading of his papers gives a very different impression. For example, his treatment of "aphemia" as a return to a childhood stage in speech development foreshadows modern accounts of agrammatism and phonemic disintegration. Moreover, Broca stressed that aphemia was a type of motor speech disorder, and distinguished it, as had Bouillaud before him, from the true language disturbance of verbal amnesia.

Hughlings Jackson[59] was generally sympathetic to Broca's work, though he disapproved of the distinction between articulation and word memory, these being just different aspects of the capacity to produce words. Following J. G. F. Baillarger, Jackson stressed the common dissociation between voluntary and involuntary performances in motor aphasia, and suggested a special relation of the latter to minor hemisphere. In later writings Jackson emphasized that the aphasic, though speechless, was not wordless, and that aphasia consisted not of a loss of speech but a loss of the ability to "propositionize," defining a proposition as a relation of words such as to make one new meaning. Perhaps Jackson's chief contribution to aphasia theory, and particularly to what was later to become psychoanalytic theory, was his evolutionary account of levels of function. According to this view, successively higher levels of functional organization were laid down in the course of encephalization, each new level suppressing and having a degree less automatization than that which came before. This conception had a clear impact on Freud's early thinking and without doubt figured prominently in the topographic theory and the account of repression.

The ontogenetic interpretation of Broca, and the phylogenetic account of Jackson, were destined to survive but a short time in neuropsychology. In 1874 Carl Wernicke, after six months on an aphasia service, published his monograph *Der aphasische Symptomenkomplex*.[108] Following T. Meynert's demonstration of the central terminations of the auditory nerve, Wernicke argued that destruction of the sound images of words, laid down adjacent to the acoustic projection zone in the posterior part of the superior temporal convolution (T_1), should result in an inability to understand or repeat speech. Since patients with impaired speech comprehension ap-

* For additional early historical information see references 10, 22, 52, 53, and 90.

peared to recognize objects, and could express some needs by mimicry, the concepts corresponding to these sounds images were thought to be intact. Thus, three forms of aphasia could be distinguished: (1) motor or Broca's aphasia; (2) sensory aphasia (with destruction of the auditory sound images); and (3) verbal amnesia, due to involvement of the posterior concept field (Begriffsfeld). Moreover, Wernicke also commented that a lesion *between* the "sensory" and "motor" zones should produce a condition in which comprehension was preserved, speech was intelligible though paraphasic, and repetition was selectively impaired. This latter disorder, described on a theoretical basis only, was termed conduction aphasia, (Leitungsaphasie) (see p. 262). The simple diagrams which Wernicke employed to illustrate these aphasic disorders (Figure 10–1) lead to the brain maps of L. Lichtheim and others, achieving in the latter part of the 19th century an almost baroque complexity, as in the ornate but wholly imaginary diagram of Charcot[30] (Figure 10–2).

The association theory of Wernicke, in providing a reductionistic alternative to the genetic accounts of Broca and Jackson, had an enormous appeal at the time and continued to dominate thinking until the critique of Pierre Marie in 1906. However, the Wernicke-Lichtheim model was challenged in one short but important monograph.

The Contribution of Freud to Aphasia

In 1891, when Freud's modest study of aphasia first appeared,[37] the school of Wernicke was the most influential in Europe. It is only against this background that one can sense the daring—indeed, revolutionary—flavor of Freud's work.* The book is chiefly concerned with a refutation of the localizationist (centers and pathways) model in favor of a concept of a unitary cortical speech zone:

* Years later Freud was to write to Binswanger[11] that Wernicke was ". . . an interesting example of the poverty of scientific thought. He was a brain anatomist and could not help dissecting the soul as he had the brain."

Our concept of the organization of the central apparatus of speech is that of a continuous cortical region occupying the space between the terminations of the optic and acoustic nerves and of the areas of the cranial and certain peripheral motor nerves in the left hemisphere. . . . We have refused to localize the psychic elements of the speech process in specified areas within this region . . . (and) the speech centres are, in our view, parts of the cortex which may claim a pathological but no special physiological significance. [p. 67][37]

In relation to this speech zone, language was built up through a process of *psychological* association (Figure 10–3). Accordingly:

From the psychological point of view the "word" is the functional unit of speech; it is a complex concept constituted of auditory, visual and kinaesthetic elements. [p. 73][37]

It follows that:

. . . all aphasias originate in interruption of associations, i.e., of conduction. Aphasia through destruction or lesion of a centre is to us no more and no less than aphasia through lesion of those association fibres which meet in that nodal point called a centre. [pp. 67–68][37]

On this basis Freud attempted a reclassification of the aphasias, an attempt far from successful, for even he had to confess that:

I am well aware that the considerations set out in this book must leave a feeling of dissatisfaction in the reader's mind. I have endeavored to demolish a convenient and attractive theory of the aphasias, and having succeeded in this, I have been able to put into its place something less obvious and less complete. [p. 104][37]

The reader does sense, however, that the work on aphasia served to liberate Freud's thinking from the anatomically bound dogmas of the time, and encouraged him to proceed into psychological speculation without the gnawing feeling that anatomy—at least the anatomy of the day—must always have the last word. There is, moreover, much in this monograph which presaged his later formulations. Specifically, one notes the application of the Jacksonian concept of dissolution to the pathology of learned associations; there is the

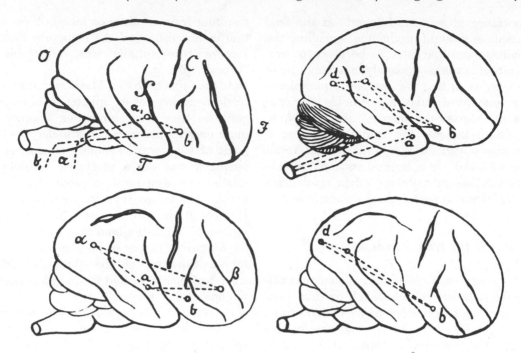

Figure 10–1. Diagrams from Wernicke[108] representing hypothetical sensori-motor centres and conducting pathways.

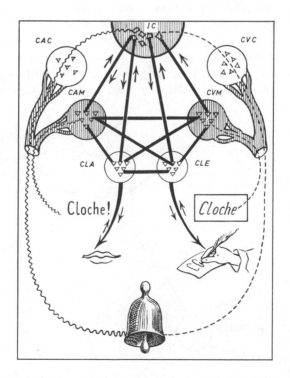

Figure 10–2. Charcot's illustration of mechanisms involved between hearing the sound of a bell, and producing the word "bell" in speech and writing. (Reprinted with the permission of Butterworth & Company.)

importance given to the "word" as the final segment in thought production, signalling the prominent position later to be given to verbalization in the psychoanalytic method; there is a suggestion that the analysis of paraphasic errors may have played a part in his later concept of "slips-of-the-tongue;" and chiefly, to my mind, there is the central idea that if neuropsychological symptoms could result from a breakdown in learned associations, psychological symptomatology might result from the formation of pathological associations.

A Search for New Formulations

Whereas Freud's lucid and meticulous criticism of the classical school fell on deaf ears, Pierre Marie's aggressive paper of 1906 came like a bombshell.[76] The very subtitle of this paper "La troisième circonvolution frontale gauche ne joue aucun rôle spécial dans la fonction du langage," was an indication of Marie's extreme dissatisfaction with the excessively localizationist approach to aphasic disorders. Marie held that the expressive defect in motor "aphasia" was actually an anarthria due to involvement of the zone of the lenticular nucleus (Figure 10–4). Wernicke's, or true, aphasia was a kind of intellectual defect

resulting from a posterior lesion. A combination of anarthria and the comprehension defect of true aphasia was responsible for "Broca's aphasia."

At the same time that Marie was attempting to rid neurology of its aphasia brain maps, as naive as they were numerous, another and more constructive trend was under way. The point of view was beginning to emerge that language was not a piecemeal assembly of smaller units but rather a productive activity within a cognitive matrix. The influence of Humboldt was still present in the developing science of linguistics, and this, combined with the hierarchic theory of Jackson and the mental structuralism of the Würzburg school, came together in Arnold Pick's new concept of the aphasias.

For Pick[87,88] the aphasias were disruptions at sequential stages in the realization of speech out of thought. He described four stages in the transition of thought to speech: an early stage (1) in which thought is formulated with increasing clarity out of memory in such a way that its partial contents are combined to a type of schematic or structural whole; the second stage (2), that of structural thought, is prior to linguistic formulation; there is a preparation toward a predicative arrangement, and elements of tone, tempo, and

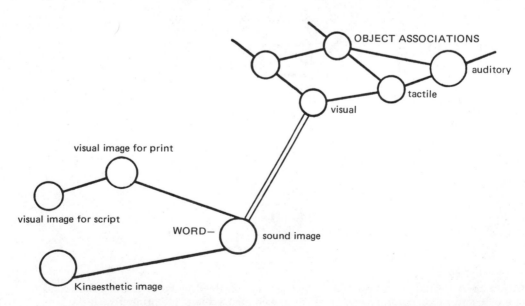

Figure 10–3.   Schema of the formation of a word concept, from Freud.[37]

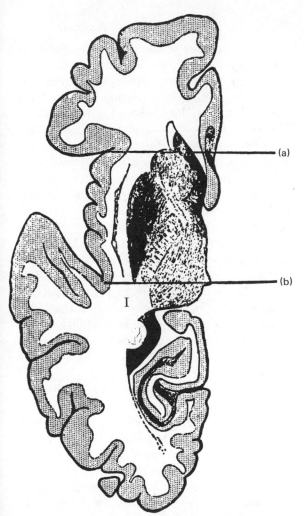

Figure 10–4. A lesion of the quadrilateral space of Marie,[76] lying between the anterior (a) and posterior (b) extent of the lenticular nucleus, produces an anarthria, while a lesion at I, involving the lenticular zone and also interrupting temporo-parietal fibers, accounts for true aphasia.

grammar come into play; the next stage (3), that of the sentence pattern, develops under the influence of an emotional factor, and leads (4) to the automatic choice of words. There is a correspondence between Pick's account of intuitive (1) and structural (2) thought, and the *Bewusstseinslage* and *Bewusstheit* of the Würzburg school, as well as with the (later) "sphere" and "concept" of Paul Schilder. Moreover, the possibility that language issued out of a prefigurative ideational stage embedded in a spatial attitude leads to the con-

cept of spatial defects in the semantic aphasia of Head[52] (see p. 257), as well as the more recent notion that the memory trace may be integrated in the space-coordinate system.[70] Pick's work has been discussed in recent publications by Spreen[98] and Brown.[23]

In England, Head,[52] who was familiar with Pick's writings, attempted to incorporate them with personal observations of aphasic patients. His classification of verbal, syntactic, nominal, and semantic aphasia represents an advance only in the postulation of the final of these forms, semantic aphasia. Even here, however, the effort to bring this disputed "deep-level" aphasia into relation with disorders of spatial-constructional thought tended to weaken the force of Head's argument.

The two other major figures of the time, Karl Kleist[66–68] and Kurt Goldstein,[44–47] were unable to resolve their dynamic psychological point of view with a localizationist mentality. Kleist,[66,68] for example, attempted to translate Pick's classification into an extreme form of (myeloarchitectonic) cortical localization. While there is much of value in Kleist's work, a cursory glance at his pathological specimens is enough to dissuade even the most sympathetic reader from too ready an acceptance of his anatomical theories. On the other hand, Goldstein[47] did not even attempt to superimpose his view of the psychology of language on a pathological anatomy, but wisely elected to treat the psychological and pathological aspects separately. With regard to the former, his contribution has to be measured by the exhaustive scholarship which was brought to bear on every phase of his work, the Gestalt orientation, and emphasis on organismic factors. The cognitive basis of language was always in the foreground of his work. Perhaps the one concept for which he is best known is the distinction of "abstract" and "concrete" behavior. However, most workers now recognize that disorders which were attributed to alteration of the abstract attitude, e.g., anomia, occur without such alteration, while concrete thinking occurs in the absence of true anomia. For this reason, a classification of aphasia based on the concept of "abstraction" and "concreteness" does not have wide appeal. According to Goldstein,[45,47] anomia (anomic or amnesic aphasia) was a disorder of thought (i.e., of abstraction), while Broca's aphasia was chiefly a defect of the final stages of word production. Central (conduction) aphasia was a disturbance *between* the two, at the transition of thought to speech, viz., a defect of "inner speech." To some extent this classification recalls the microgenetic account of Pick, though Goldstein's pathological descriptions, and his interpretations of the pathological anatomy, did not deviate greatly from the original views of his teacher, Wernicke.[41]

In addition to this line of study, which was fundamentally a continuation of certain trends in the early German school of aphasia, there were also during this time several other noteworthy contributions. Weisenberg and McBride[107] introduced American readers to the historical debate surrounding various issues in the field, and provided a healthy—even if somewhat vacuous—alternative to the rigid classifications then available. Johannes Nielsen[80] was for many years one of the principle authorities on aphasia in the United States. His work, like that of Kleist, was characterized by erudition and a dynamic point of view not readily apparent on superficial reading. Penfield and Roberts[84] gave valuable descriptions on the effects of stimulation of speech cortex in waking subjects, and argued, chiefly from negative extirpations, that thalamo-cortical connections played a central role in the anatomical organization of language. Some of these traditions have been carried on in England, by Brain[16] and Critchley[34] among others. In Germany, the Gestalt approach has been furthered by the work of Bay[8,9] and Conrad,[33] and in France the best known authors are Alajouanine,[2] Lhermitte and coworkers,[72] and Hecaen.[54]

❨ Status of the Field

There are two major orientations in modern aphasia research, both of which have grown out of the classical tradition: the argument from the psychological point of view, and the argument from the point of view of anatomy.

Psychological Accounts of Aphasia

A great number of distinct theories fall into this category. Of these, one of the more progressive is the current attempt to bring linguistic description into relation with aphasic symptomatology. Psycholinguists have shown increasing interest in aphasic language and the term neurolinguistics is often taken as a designation of this new synthetic approach.

One of the earliest attempts in this direction was Jakobson's[61] study of aphasic breakdown and correspondences with language acquisition in the child. More recently,[60] utilizing Luria's classification and the distinction implicit in this system of posterior spatial (simultaneous) and anterior temporal (successive) processes, two major categories of aphasic disturbance have been distinguished, a *similarity* disorder, characterized by an inability to select and identify, and a *contiguity* disorder, characterized by an inability to combine and integrate.

There have also been attempts to demonstrate correspondences between aphasic language and expectations of distinctive feature theory.[62] Especially important in this regard are studies by Blumstein[13] and Lecours and Lhermitte.[71] The transformational grammar of Chomsky[31,32] has been tested against aphasic language in studies by Weigl and Bierwisch.[104] In this respect, the reader is referred to studies by Goodglass,[48,49] and Zurif[111] on agrammatism; Green,[51] Kreindler,[69] and Kertesz[64] on jargonaphasia; and Marshall and Newcombe,[77] and Rinnert and Whitaker[91] on semantic paraphasia. A review of work in psycholinguistics and aphasia was published in 1973.[50]

The term "neurolinguistics" appears to have been introduced by Henri Hecaen, who has also developed a linguistic typology of the aphasias.[54] Accordingly, three major aphasic groups, expressive, amnesic, and sensory, are distinguished. Within the expressive group, there are three forms: (1) an impairment of phonemic realization (motor aphasia); (2) an impairment of syntactic realization (agrammatism); and (3) an impairment of programming at the level of the phrase (conduction aphasia). Amnesic aphasia is a selectional disorder, often linked to other aphasic forms. Within the group of sensory aphasia, three elements can be isolated: word deafness, impaired verbal comprehension, and a disorganization of attention. These elements often occur together in varying degree, and determine the pattern of expressive language.

The classification of Luria[75] is a departure from standard works chiefly in the functional approach toward each aphasic syndrome, and not in the description of the symptom complex per se. The following six forms are distinguished: (1) *sensory* aphasia, in which the expressive pattern is attributed to impaired phonemic discrimination; (2) *acoustic-amnestic* aphasia, which differs from the above chiefly in the improved repetition; (3) *afferent* and (4) *efferent* motor aphasia, which incorporate distinct aspects of Broca's aphasia; (5) *semantic* aphasia, which seems to include amnestic aphasia, and is similar to Head's account; and (6) *dynamic* aphasia, with reduced spontaneity of speech, similar to a mild transcortical motor aphasia. However, objections can be raised against this classification on several counts. For example, the impairment of phonemic discrimination, central to the sensory forms, is tested chiefly through productive systems; phonemic discrimination is an extremely resistant ability in a wide range of aphasic patients with disturbed speech comprehension; evidence for the kinaesthetic basis and postcentral localization of afferent aphasia is wanting; dynamic aphasia seems to merge with the reduced speech picture of dements and various types of partial mutism. Moreover, as suggested by the syndrome designations, there is assumed to be a specific functional impairment in each disorder, i.e., in verbal memory, acoustic sensation, the evidence for which is at best controversial. Finally, the pathological account of primary and secondary cortical "analysers" in relation to these disorders does not take us very far beyond classical speculations regarding a similar role for primary (projection) and secondary (association) cortex. Nonetheless, Luria's work is extremely valuable for the ingenious testing methods and careful clinical observation, the thorough study of individual cases and the application of an experimental approach to traditional "bedside" technique. From the point of view of theory, the major contribution is the concept of aphasia as a disturbance in cognitive function. Thus, speaking of language organization, Luria has written that the system of semantic codes "possesses a complex hierarchical structure. It begins with the system of words, behind each of which there stands not only a unitary image, but a complex system of generalizations of those things which the word signifies." Similarly, perception is studied not as a simple receptive function but as an active process, comparable to speech and motility. Perception involves ". . . the recognition of the dominant signs of an object, the creation of a series of visual hypotheses or alternatives, the choice of the most probable of these hypotheses, and the final determination of the required image . . ." The reader will note that this sequence is identical to other descriptions of stages in the course of problem-solving behavior, i.e., thinking.

Eberhard Bay[8,9] has also viewed aphasia as a disturbance in concept formation. However, Bay's model is incomplete and to a degree expedient, and exception can be taken to many interpretations, e.g., the account of agrammatism as an economy of effort or the explanation of paraphasia as secondary to lack of speech awareness and logorrhea.

Klaus Conrad[33] conceives aphasia as an arrest or interruption in the microgenesis of cognition. An aphasia is a pregestalt (Vorgestalt) stage in the process of language formation. Conrad has distinguished four levels of pathophysiological change which, from the highest to the lowest are, respectively, *Strukturwandel, Gestaltwandel, Funktionswandel,* and *Formwandel.* Pathology induces a change in functional level, not a loss of function. The reduced level then determines the symptomatology. However appealing this approach, the discussion of aphasia is not altogether successful, for a general theory of regression does not account for the diversity of aphasic symptoms. Conrad has also helped to clarify the problem of "severity" in hierarchical systems. In Conrad's view, the lower (i.e., word close) the lesion, the more severe, but more restricted, the local effect, while higher (i.e., thought close) defects produce a slight impairment in more widespread functions, and involve more of the patient's native personality.

Anatomical Theories of Aphasia

Psychological studies of aphasia have not yet succeeded in the formulation of a unitary theory of these disorders, nor are such theories commonly attempted. However, caution has not been the most distinguishing·characteristic of the anatomical school. Although there continue to be minor disputes over the specific role in language of one or another anatomical structure, the basic approach, on which there is, regrettably, essential agreement, has remained unchanged for a century after Wernicke's monograph. The position has been summarized by Geschwind.[42]

According to this view (Figure 10–5)

speech is perceived by way of (left) Wernicke's area, and from there conveyed to "Parietal association" cortex for comprehension. Language is presumed to be formed in some way in the posterior part of the brain and passed forward to Broca's area for articulation. Repetition is accomplished through a cortical reflex circuit, comprising Wernicke's area, Broca's area, and the *fasciculus arcuatus* between, though this pathway is not usually specified as that underlying the postero-anterior flow (development) of spontaneous speech. The aphasias represent disruptions of these processes (actually, the processes are inferred from their pathology to be localized to these areas). Thus, a lesion of left posterior superior temporal gyrus is said to produce Wernicke's (sensory, receptive, jargon) aphasia, lesion of the posterior inferior frontal gyrus, Broca's (motor, expressive, anarthric) aphasia, and lesion of the *fasciculus arcuatus*, conduction (central, repetition) aphasia.

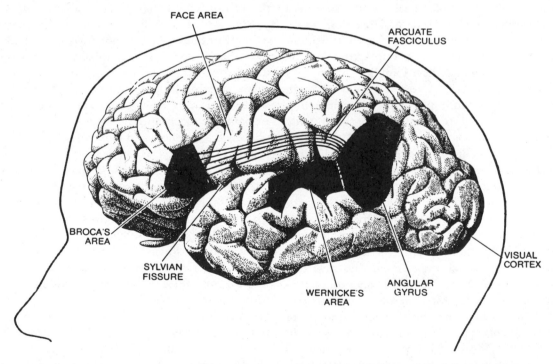

Figure 10–5. A contemporary diagram of speech cortex,[42] illustrating structures which are presumed to be involved in the production of aphasia, i.e., Broca's area in motor aphasia, Wernicke's area in jargonaphasia, angular gyrus in anomia, and arcuate fasciculus in "conduction" aphasia. (From "Language and the Brain," by N. Geschwind. Copyright © 1972 by Scientific American, Inc. All rights reserved.)

Anomia (amnestic, nominal aphasia) is due to lesion of parietal cortex (angular gyrus), but does not have the strong localizing features of the other syndromes. The transcortical aphasias occur with selective preservation of the primary speech zone. Disorders of reading, writing, and praxis are aligned with this anatomical account through interpretations based on the effects of lesion of the *corpus callosum*. For example, the syndrome of "pure alexia" or word blindness is explained through the destruction of the left occipital cortex and the splenium of *corpus callosum*, which produces a state in which the patient presumably can see written words in the intact left visual field but is unable to read because of interruption of callosal fibers conveying the perception of these words to "speech cortex" for language analysis (Figure 10–6).

This classical account of aphasia has been reinforced through findings in patients undergoing complete surgical section of the *corpus callosum* as a form of treatment for epileptic seizures. Two recent reviews by Dimond[35] and Gazzaniga[40] are available. Following this operation, patients demonstrate a relative inability to name objects tactually with the left hand, or read material presented tachistoscopically to the left visual field, nor can they carry out to command skilled actions with the (distal) left extremities. However, patients are able to identify the tactual or visual object or word by selecting it (the appropriate object) from an assortment, if this is done nonverbally and with the left hand. This has led to the conclusion that right-hemispheric contents are isolated from dominant left-hemispheric, and that, to some extent, one can speak of a separate consciousness in each hemisphere. Evidence for a left-hemispheric priority in verbal tasks, and a right-hemispheric priority on visual-spatial performance, has given rise to speculations regarding different forms of thought in each hemisphere. Such considerations range from the improbable[14,95] (Figure 10–7) to the absurd. The wide interest in studies of this type, and the readiness with which many students accept the simple interpretations offered, suggests that we are at the beginning of a wave of neophrenology that

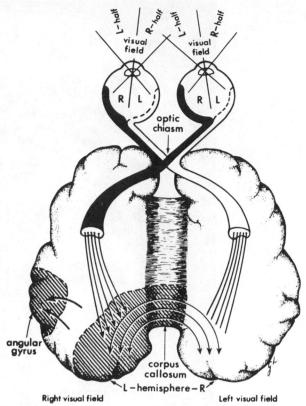

Figure 10–6. According to the classical account of *pure* alexia, a lesion of left occipital cortex and splenium of corpus callosum results in an interruption in the flow of visual information to left speech cortex, while lesion of angular gyrus leads to alexia *with agraphia*. This condition, however, can be explained on a perceptual basis through a reduced functional level in right occipital lobe.[22]

could lead to a long unproductive period in neuropsychology.

Comment. There is no question but that the introduction of linguistic concepts and methods has had a profound effect on research in aphasia. In particular, interest in transformational grammar, and experimental studies stimulated by this model, have helped to bring about a considerably more dynamic approach to the problems of aphasia than has characterized the field in the past. There is also increasing dissatisfaction with previous theories of aphasia. This includes those on the one hand in which some common element is isolated from the symptomatology and then employed to explain all the other symptoms, e.g., as has occurred in regard to "abstract attitude," Gestalt formation, etc., as well as, at the other

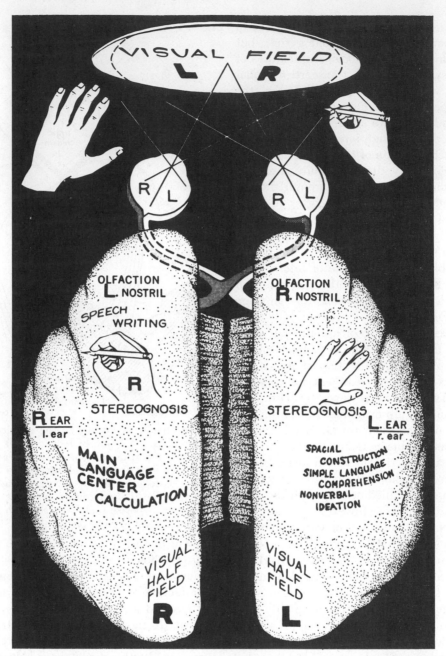

Figure 10–7. A more extreme representation of left and right hemispheric functional asymmetry.[96] (From "Perception in the Absence of the Neocortical Commissures," in D. A. Hamburg, K. Pribram, and A. Stunkard, eds. *Perception and Its Disorders*. New York: Williams & Wilkins. Reprinted with the permission of the publisher and the Association for Research in Nervous and Mental Disease.)

extreme, accounts in which a specific (disordered) function is proposed for each element of the symptom complex, e.g., as in stimulus response or association theories of aphasia.

Psychological models of aphasia must, it would seem, conform to the constraints imposed by pathological correlations of aphasic syndromes. The pathology of aphasia is neither obvious nor random but is a subtle clue to the anatomy and organization of normal language. Both language production and the anatomical structure by which it is supported develop in an orderly way. In pathology, the change in language and the change in structure are inseparable and equally lawful. Structure is not a rigid skeleton on which function is superimposed, but is an organic form created by the continuous flow of process. Seen in this light, the *combined* study of aphasic language and of its correlated brain pathology appears to be the most trustworthy guide to an understanding of the structure of real language.

❨ Typology of Aphasia

Introduction

Language develops through a formative or microgenetic process as a component of cognition. There are several more or less arbitrary stages in this process, though normally we are aware of only the final product. In various states, for example during sleep or hypnagogy, one may see these earlier, otherwise concealed (i.e., traversed), levels appearing as pathological speech forms. Generally this is a transient phenomenon. However, with structural brain lesion the "earlier" stage, the aphasic syndrome, may become the final speech product and this product may persist indefinitely as a relatively stable form. Each type of aphasia, therefore, can be conceived as a preliminary level in normal language which pathology has brought to the fore. Moreover, at each of these levels, the "pathological" language form,

the aphasia, also points to a corresponding level in cognitive development. Thus we may study an aphasia both from the point of view of language, as a manifestation of a prefigurative stage in the normal process, and from the point of view of cognition, as exhibiting features characteristic of whatever cognitive stage happens to be realized in the momentary language level.

When we look at aphasia from this standpoint, questions arise concerning some of the most basic aspects of brain study. For example, the view that an aphasic syndrome is the result of a combination of two or more discrete defects must be treated with great caution. Wernicke's aphasia is not word deafness *plus* verbal paraphasia *plus* anosognosia *plus* euphoria, but rather is a defect in cognition at some level where processes underlying these disorders (rather, achievements) are coextensive. The aphasic syndrome represents a molar level to which the patient has been reduced and is not a compilation of disorganized functions.

This, in turn, has implications for our understanding of *severity*. Within the posterior or fluent aphasias, for example, it would be misleading to speak of a severe jargon or a mild paraphasia. This ignores the change in the *qualitative* aspects of the jargon, or the paraphasia. When semantic jargon deteriorates it may become neologistic; when verbal paraphasia deteriorates it may approach semantic jargon. The central point is that an alteration of one element in the disorder, say in comprehension or in repetition, will always be accompanied by a change in other elements as well. If there is sufficient change the result is a new syndrome and not just a more severe manifestation of the original condition. We may say that severity in a microgenetic system always entails a difference of kind as well as degree.

In the classification that follows, the aphasias are arranged in such a way as to reflect the sequence of stages in normal language production (Figure 10–8). This sequence unfolds on an axis between a semantic or selectional process and a stage of phonemic encod-

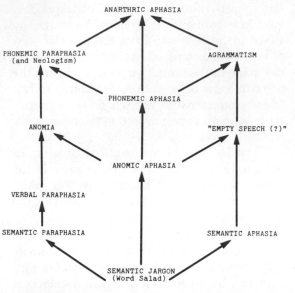

REFERENTIAL —— BOTH —— EXPOSITIONAL

Figure 10–8. The aphasias can be aligned in a transitional series corresponding to the sequence of stages in normal language production. These relationships are especially evident in the course of recovery or deterioration. In pathological states the arrows are to be considered bidirectional. A distinction is made as to whether there is preferential involvement in referential or expositional speech (partial aphasic forms) or both (major syndromes). Neologistic jargon is not depicted but represents involvement of both the semantic and phonemic levels.

ing. The precursors of the words, the forms or clusters of the utterance-to-be, emerge through a semantic operation by means of which the developing utterance is shaped in the direction of the final performance. At this stage, there is a "noun priority" in the entry of lexical items into the forming sentence pattern. A transition then occurs from the ordered abstract-sentence frame to the phonemic representatives of the constituent words in preparation for articulation. At this stage, the small (function) words are introduced. In the course of this process both a referential (i.e., nominative) and an expositional (i.e., discursive) orientation can be discerned, a discovery which has helped to clarify some of the complex interrelationships between these forms.

Apart from its linguistic character, each of the aphasias incorporates aspects of a corresponding level in cognition. A change in awareness or in affect, the presence or absence of delusional or hallucinatory phenomena, these are not additions to the clinical picture but have an inner bond with the aphasic form. These alterations in cognition will be briefly noted in the description of each syndrome and more fully discussed in the final section. Reference will be made to the pathological "locus" of each type of aphasia, reserving a more thoroughgoing discussion for the following section.

Description of the Aphasias

SEMANTIC DISORDERS

Semantic Jargon. This is basically a disorder of word meaning that involves both naming and conversational speech in the presence of moderate loss of oral comprehension. The disorder is associated with a lesion of the posterior-middle and superior-temporal gyrus (posterior T_2 and T_1), often bilaterally. In older patients the lesion is more commonly unilateral and on the left side. Semantic jargon is one form of Wernicke's (receptive, sensory) aphasia. Such patients produce good words and sentences, but with defective meaning. An example from Alajouanine et al.[3] is a patient who described a *fork* as ". . . a need for a schedule" or another who defined a *spoon* as ". . . how many schemes on your throat." Another patient, asked about his poor vision, said "My wires don't hire right." A case of Kreindler et al.[69] replied to a question about his health with: "I felt worse because I can no longer keep in mind from the mind of the minds to keep me from mind and up to the ear which can be to find among ourselves." A patient of Heilbronner responded to a similar question with "Yes, I think that I am now so safe than now much with others to some extent directly." Occasionally, neologisms are present which may lead to strikingly bizarre utterances. Thus an aphasic physician, asked if he was a doctor, said "Me? Yes sir. I'm a male demaploze on my own. I still know my tubaboys what for I have that's gone hell and some of them go."

Speech production is fluent, there is no word search, in spite of incorrect choices, and vocabulary use is fairly good, at times even pretentious. There is semantic or verbal paraphasia on tests of naming and repetition. This refers to a substitution of one word for another, e.g., "table" for "chair." However, in semantic jargon the link between the substitution and the target word is often not so clear as in the "in-class" substitution of this example. Rather, a patient might call a chair an "engine," or an "Argentina." The term *semantic paraphasia* can be used for this latter type of substitution, and *verbal paraphasia* for categorical substitution.

Comprehension is moderately impaired, though ordinarily some understanding is possible, while reading aloud and writing show alterations parallel with speech. About 20 percent of such patients are hemiparetic, the rest often ambulatory and with few or no "hard" neurological findings. In such patients, a distinction from psychotic language or thought disorder is frequently difficult. This is particularly so in view of the fact that there is commonly a euphoric, even manic, mood elevation or aggressivity, and auditory hallucinations may occur during the course. A paranoid state is not uncommon, and may make speech therapy difficult or impossible. Patients tend to be logorrheic, and show partial or complete absence of awareness of their defective speech. However, they usually reject jargon spoken by the examiner, and resist efforts at correction of their own speech. The awareness of speech content, as with all other elements of the syndrome, may change from moment to moment. Awareness appears to be inversely related to the semantic "distance" of the utterance from its presumed goal.

This stage of unintelligible semantic jargon may resolve in one of two directions, to involvement of expositional speech with intact naming, or involvement of referential speech (naming) with preserved conversation. The former is termed "semantic aphasia," the latter (pure) "semantic paraphasia." Both of these disorders occur with bilateral temporal-lobe pathology.

Semantic Aphasia. This disorder was first described by Head[52] as an interruption at a prelinguistic phase in the thought-speech transition. Patients demonstrated a want of recognition of the full significance of words and phrases apart from their verbal meaning. There was a failure to comprehend the final aim or goal of an action and an inability to clearly formulate a general conception of what was heard, read or seen in a picture, although many of the details were enumerated. Memory and intelligence were relatively intact, counting was possible, but calculations were impaired and there was a failure to understand jokes, games, and puzzles. In Head's descriptions the recorded statements and short letters of his cases do not always convey to the reader the full flavor of the defect as emphasized in the commentary. Nor did his spatial tests clearly illustrate the specific nature of the disorder. However, most of his cases demonstrated some grammatical disturbance. Thus one patient wrote: "Just a few lines to let you know that I am getting on all right and I shall will be home again. I must tell you that Uncle George and Aunt Ann cane (came) and see me yesterday and more so Bob Higgins so I am very Lucky for getting friends." On another occasion, this patient remarked, "I was worked for . . ." Another patient wrote: ". . . one could spend one's time in a more profitably . . ." and another said: "If I pay too much attention I get wrong with what I've got to do." Another patient said: "My son is just home from Ireland. He is a flying man. Takes the ship about to carry the police to give information, to carry the letters of the police."

More recent studies[22] show that in semantic aphasia there is a disturbance of contextual meaning, through which utterances of *skewed meaning* are produced. The disorder is especially prominent in proverb, story, or picture interpretation. Consider this example of a patient's written description of his speech (patient's capitals and punctuation).

Speech that could be found as a Type of speed I believe. I possible mood of my own maybe because of misunderstanding. Possibly because of my own thought In a certain way. a friend of mine told myself. I had a "cast Iron Fact" especially during a conversation. [p. 45]22

The disorder is apparent in speech and writing. Speech is fluent and somewhat logorrheic, and may have a confabulatory flavor (see below). Comprehension may be quite good, while naming, reading aloud, and repetition are intact. Spatial-constructional difficulty may or may not be present, and the neurological examination can be normal except for the aphasia. Patients tend to be euphoric with partial insight into their disability. Paranoia and hallucination are not prominent features, but too few cases have been described to be more precise on this point.

Semantic Paraphasia. In this disorder which has been (incorrectly) termed "nonaphasic misnaming,"105 conversational speech is fairly well preserved but errors occur on tests of object naming. These take the form of "associative" responses, e.g., a pipe is called a *smoker*, glasses a *telescope*. The pretentious and facetious quality of the paraphasia appears when a doctor is called a *butcher* or a syringe a *hydrometer to measure fluids*. The paraphasia affects about 10–15 percent of names produced, depending upon test item. Although the object-naming difficulty may follow a word-frequency distribution, this not true for the paraphasic response.

The disorder usually occurs in the context of diffuse disease, drowsiness, or confusion. Speech is fluent, at times logorrheic, but not clearly aphasic. Comprehension is good and repetition is preserved. Patients show euphoria, reduced speech awareness, and/or denial. There is a similarity with certain Korsakoff patients who may also show semantic paraphasia restricted to naming tasks, as in the Korsakoff patient who referred to the examiner as "Herman Joseph Prince Macaroni."103

Mechanism of the Semantic Disorders. Three disorders of semantic origin have been described: (1) semantic aphasia, when context (expositional speech) is primarily affected; (2) semantic paraphasia, with distur-

bance in referential speech; and (3) semantic jargon, when both reference and context are involved. The fact that the first and second forms occur independently indicates that neither is a partial expression of the other, though semantic jargon may be taken as a combination of the two. The mechanism which accounts for the disorder is similar in both the expositional and referential forms. In semantic aphasia the speaker is unable to use the verb or predicate of the forming utterance as a free unit to which the subject and object only partially relate. A combination of any two of these elements (e.g., subject and verb, or verb and object) tends to determine the third. The direction of this pressure is not invariably subject → verb → object, but is often the reverse. All lexical items may be affected, and it may be difficult to determine which element of the phrase is defective (if content words, paraphasia; if function words, paragrammatism). In the above example, "speech that could be found . . ." acceptable bondings occur between individual words (speech that, that could, could be found) but not between the initial and latter segments of the phrase. The disorder has a close relation to schizophrenic speech. Consider an example from the study of paralogic by von Domarus, quoted by Arieti:4

$$\begin{array}{c}
\text{Certain Indians (A) / are / swift (x)} \\
\text{Stags \quad (B) / are / swift (x)} \\
\therefore \text{Certain Indians (A) are stags (B)} \\
\text{Here, A} \cong \text{x becomes A} = \text{x} \\
\text{B} \cong \text{x becomes B} = \text{x} \\
\text{A} \cong \text{x} \cong \text{B becomes A} = \text{x} = \text{B}
\end{array}$$

This is quite similar to what occurs in semantic aphasia. In the following example from a Cloze test22 an aphasic patient was required to insert words deleted from a test phrase. The patient's solution is in brackets. Test phrase is "The baby—something that he had—done before." [p. 49]22

A.	x.	B.
The baby	[was]	something
that he had	[been]	done before

Here A $\cong$ x and x $\cong$ B becomes A $=$ B

The inserted word agrees with those in its immediate surround (e.g., baby *was, was* something; had *been, been* done) and a partial fit is accepted as satisfactory. Responses to proverb tests show identical errors, the patient generally interpreting one component of the proverb partially and then attempting to consolidate it obliquely to the other components.

In semantic aphasia the noun phrase tends to become stabilized at the expense of its predicative relationships. Context is adapted to subject. One might say that the noun phrase conditions the predicate rather than being contained within, or defined by, it. This has a determining effect upon utterances in which topics are developed within understood contexts. In semantic paraphasia (see below), misnamings show the influence of implicit contexts derived from the examiner's knowledge of the object to be named. However, predicative or contextual function is otherwise adequate and acts to normalize noun production in conversational speech.

In semantic paraphasia there is an identification of two otherwise disparate subjects (e.g., "doctor" and "butcher") on the basis of one or two shared attributes (e.g., white coat, cutting, etc.). Consider the following example:

misnamings of schizophrenic patients, as in "le song" for bird, "le kiss" for mouth.[46] Similarities between schizophrenic and aphasic speech have also been discussed by Schilder,[95] Critchley,[34] and Alajouanine.[2] Arieti[4] has given a full and lucid discussion of the problem of schizophrenic language, and has demonstrated the central position of paralogical thinking.

Kleist[66] commented that paralogia was a confabulation within the verbal sphere. This concept is probably identical with the "confabulation d'origine verbale" of catatonic patients. If paralogia is a kind of "verbal" confabulation, it may be asked to what extent this relates to the confabulation of Korsakoff's syndrome and related confusional states. Language of this type has been described in Korsakoff's syndrome, as in the response of a patient to the proverb *Safety First*, "It's rather a lateral term which means it could apply to a host of things. A road for one thing." Victor[102] has commented that aphasic errors are common during the confusional prelude of the amnestic syndrome.

It is likely that an inner bond exists between the semantic aphasic complex and confabulation. Confabulation is no more the "filling in of a gap in memory" than is paraphasia a

Task	Presented object A	Shared predicate C	Paraphasic response B
Naming	bedpan	stool, sitting, etc.	"piano stool"

Mechanism

$$A \cong B$$
$$B \cong C$$
$$\therefore A = C$$

Related Disorders. Similar language disturbances have been noted in schizophrenic patients. For example, the utterance "A boy threw a stone at me to make an understanding between myself and the purpose of wrongdoing."[28] is similar in structure to that of semantic aphasia, while Arieti's example[4] of word salad, "The house burnt the cow horrendously always," is very close to semantic jargon. The disorder of semantic paraphasia is recalled in the "associative"

compensation for a memory loss. In confabulation there is substitution *of* a semantic field, in semantic paraphasia, there is substitution *within* the semantic field. The two speech forms reflect the microgenetic *level* of disruption and are not unrelated psychological deficits. In this respect it is of interest that patients with semantic jargon have often been described as having features of the Korsakoff syndrome.[106] Moreover, the possibility that an inner relationship exists between amnestic confabulation and schizophrenic paramnesia has not received sufficient attention.

NOMINAL DISORDERS

The developing linguistic form, having more or less successfully traversed the semantic or selectional stage, proceeds toward the "abstract representation" of the (correct) lexical item. Disorders at this level are, therefore, characterized by improved control of word-meaning but inability to evoke the intended word. As with the preceding stage, anomia is not a single entity but is rather a series of (pathological) speech forms which point to one or another segment or phase of the process of language production. A disturbance at this stage may occur to some extent independently in referential speech (as in anomia proper, i.e., word-finding difficulty) and in expositional speech (so-called *empty speech* of anomia, circumlocution). Verbal paraphasia occurs as well, and is to be distinguished from semantic paraphasia, with which it has generally been equated, on the basis of the "in-class" substitutions ("shaver" for razor, "green" for red). Verbal paraphasia is to be conceived as an intermediate stage between semantic paraphasia and anomia proper.

Background. The concept of verbal amnesia as a defect in the mental evocation of words was an early development in aphasia study. As a distinction was drawn between internal and external speech, verbal amnesia, as a disturbance of the internal phase of language, came to be set against motor aphasia, which was a disturbance of the external phase. This early view gave way to a division of anomia into specific visual, auditory, tactile, and motoric forms, and for a time the concept of a pure anomia regardless of sensory modality was abandoned (see Pitres,[89] for a review of the historical period). The modern conception of anomia dates from the papers of Kurt Goldstein.[45,47]

According to Goldstein, the difficulty in naming objects derived from an inability to assume an "abstract attitude" with regard to the item being tested. Words which could not be produced as names, or which could be produced but not brought into relation with the object designated, appeared spontaneously in conversation. This indicated that word memory was preserved. Thus it must be the conditions under which the word *is evoked* that are altered, viz., a loss of the ability to apply words as symbols for objects, i.e., as word concepts. This difficulty became even more apparent if the patient was asked to sort objects according to various attributes such as color, size, or shape. The inability to give the name of a single object reflected a disturbance of the word concept of that object, and this disturbance was exaggerated by the requirement that diverse objects be categorized according to shared attributes.

Goldstein's description of amnesic aphasia (anomia) achieved wider acceptance than his psychological account. It was pointed out that abstraction was frequently impaired in the absence of anomia, and that anomia occurred with categorical behavior that was not strikingly abnormal, or if so, no different from that seen in other aphasic syndromes. Also to be included in this period are works by Heilbronner[55] and Lotmar,[74] particularly as concerns verbal paraphasia. Lotmar especially discussed the spheric nature of word substitution, and attempted to show how apparently random substitutions occurred through intermediate links.

Recent studies have shown that word frequency is an important factor in the anomic defect. It has been shown in normal subjects, in dysphasics,[57,92] and in patients with organic dementia, that word-finding difficulty relates to the vocabulary frequency of the target item, i.e., the object or action to be named. In a study deriving from this work, A. Wingfield, cited by Oldfield,[81] demonstrated that perceptual identification does not show the same frequency dependency as does object naming. This led Oldfield[81] to propose a two-stage model of naming, an initial stage of perceptual identification and a second stage of word finding, only the latter of which is dependent on word frequency. There is some evidence[22] that the specific anomias (e.g., "visual" or "tactile" anomia), and true or aphasic anomia relate to involvement at each of these respective stages.

Verbal Paraphasia. This disorder refers to a stage where the lexical item, the word, has realized (been selected to the point of) a categorical approximation, e.g., "shaver" for razor, "green" for red. There is some ability to self-correct, i.e., some awareness of speech error, but this may differ from one moment to the next, depending on the nature of the substitution. Although the difficulty in naming may have a relationship to the vocabulary frequency of the target word, i.e., patients having more difficulty with rare than common words, the paraphasic errors do not appear to show this effect. Thus, patients may say "spectacles" for glasses, or "fuchsia" for red. While this form of language is often admixed with other anomic features (see below), the absence of verbal paraphasia in anomia proper should not be interpreted as a reluctance to speak or a more careful search for words. Verbal paraphasia is not a reflection of personality type; rather it reflects a cognitive level around which the "personality" is organized. Features of this cognitive level include some degree of euphoria, a more active, though not logorrheic, speech flow than in anomia, and partial awareness of the disorder.

Anomic Aphasia (anomia, amnesic or nominal aphasia). Patients of this type have difficulty in word finding which affects nouns preferentially. Typically, such patients can point to the correct object when it is named, can repeat the object name, and can select the correct name from a group, although they are unable to name the object directly. This is true for "visual naming," as well as naming through other perceptual modes, e.g., touching the object, hearing the sound of the object, etc. Patients are also unable to name from a description or definition of the object, e.g., "what do you use to sweep the floor?" The word-finding difficulty may be akin to the common phenomenon of word lapse or the forgetting of a name or place in the speech flow. Not uncommon is the incipient "tip-of-the-tongue" nature of the needed word.[7] Patients may be able to give the initial letter of the target word or the

number of syllables, and can use the test object appropriately. These features suggest that word meaning is relatively well preserved and that some "skeleton" or abstract frame of the intended word is available. The disorder may be limited to referential speech, or may appear in conversation with circumlocution and emptiness of speech. The true anomic who does not produce verbal paraphasias has a more acute awareness of his difficulty and may show frustration and catastrophic reactions.

The difficulty in word finding tends to occur in the following direction: nouns → verbs → grammatical (function) words. Abstract nouns may be more difficult than concrete nouns. When the disorder involves both referential and expositional speech, a "nonfluent" state can result. Such patients have greatly reduced speech with only a starter phrase or a stereotypy available, such as "Well I . . ." or "It's a . . ." Speech tends to be limited to small grammatical words and simple verbs. This condition can be distinguished from anterior nonfluency (i.e., Broca's aphasia) by the reciprocal order of word loss. In the anomic, the small verbs and function words are the last, not the first, to disappear.

Word-finding difficulty occurs in various organic and nonorganic states. Anomia and circumlocution have been described in schizophrenia.[12] Chapman[29] has emphasized that schizophrenic patients "have a true difficulty in word finding, although it tends to be episodic in occurrence and very similar to the paroxysmal dysphasia which occurs in temporal lobe epilepsy." Anomic errors are also common in fatigue and distraction, and in sleep and transitional utterance.

Anomia tends to be associated with either unilateral or diffuse lesions. In anomia and in verbal paraphasia, lesions may occur outside the classical speech areas. The more severe "nonfluent" anomia occurs with unilateral (left) temporo-parietal lesion. Lesions of the posterior middle-temporal gyrus (T2) and its continuation to angular gyrus appear to be highly correlated with this form. The more fluent the anomia, the more likely is diffuse pathology or lesion outside the speech area.

Anomia occurs in dementia, increased intra-cranial pressure, postanaesthetic or confusional states, as well as with subcortical or thalamic lesion, where it is most likely due to a referred effect on cortex.

Comment on the Semantic and Anomic Disorders. The various disorders which have thus far been discussed can be aligned in a series which retraces the microgenetic development of normal language. The sequence of semantic jargon, through associative and then categorical substitution to true anomia, corresponds to stages in the normal productive process. Within the semantic "segment," the progression is through systems or fields of word meaning of wide "psychological distance." These lead to more narrow "associative" responses which represent an intermediate stage between semantic jargon and correct word selection. Anomia points to a stage where the correct word has been all but selected but cannot yet be fully realized in speech. The anomic stage corresponds to the emergence of the correct lexical item preparatory to phonemic encoding.

In addition to this linguistic change, there is an evolution of other aspects of cognition. Thus, in semantic jargon there is euphoria, at times mania, often with a paranoid trend. There is logorrhea and a lack of awareness of speech error. This picture gives way in semantic aphasia and semantic paraphasia, to a mitigation of logorrhea and euphoria, with patchy but still incomplete awareness of difficulty. This continues into verbal paraphasia where incorrect words (e.g., "table" for chair) can often be rejected. There is a transition from active, but not logorrheic, speech to hesitancy, and finally to an inability to speak at all. The transition from one state to another occurs *pari passu* with increasing awareness of speech errors, improved self-correction, and step-by-step transformation from one affective and behavioral form to another.

PHONEMIC DISORDERS

These disorders point to a stage in the production of language where the intended word, having been properly selected, does not achieve correct phonemic realization. Accord-ing to whether the defect is expressed primarily in referential or expositional speech, we can distinguish, respectively, phonemic paraphasia and phonemic aphasia. Ordinarily these are included together in the syndrome of central or conduction aphasia.

Background. The phonemic disorders were originally defined on an anatomic basis by Wernicke[108] without regard to the qualitative aspects of the speech of such patients. The disturbed function of repetition was gradually singled out as central to the syndrome and attributed to damage to a pathway between the posterior and anterior speech areas (see Brown[22] for further discussion). Kurt Goldstein[47] argued against an interruption of a conducting pathway in favor of a more dynamic interpretation. Goldstein believed the condition represented an impairment at the thought–speech transition, and termed it "central" aphasia, placing emphasis on the paraphasia as reflecting a disturbance of inner speech. Goldstein's comments regarding a possible relationship between anomic aphasia and central (phonemic) aphasia are worth quoting in full:

A combination of amnesic aphasia with symptoms of central aphasia is frequent. There arises the question of whether we are dealing with an accidental combination due to similar locality of the underlying lesion, or whether there is an inner relationship between both defects. As little as we are able to say now, the latter possibility is worth pondering in respect to the closeness of the phenomenon of inner speech to the nonspeech mental process. [pp. 277–278][47]

Phonemic Paraphasia. In this disorder, the disturbance chiefly affects nouns and is apparent on tests of object naming. Spontaneous speech is often quite good with few or rare paraphasias. Patients make errors of the type: "cable" for table, or "predident" for president. Repetition may be involved in a similar manner. Comprehension may be quite good. Such patients are usually classified as mild "conduction" aphasics or resolving "motor" aphasics.

Phonemic Aphasia (central, conduction aphasia). When conversational speech shows a picture of fluent phonemic paraphasia with phonemic errors on naming and repetition tasks and good comprehension, the diagnosis of phonemic aphasia is in order. There is a close resemblance to phonemic paraphasia, the distinction resting on the improved speech and defective naming and repetition of the former, and the more impaired spontaneous speech of the latter, where naming may be relatively well preserved and repetition is involved at the phrase, rather than single-word, level. This disorder may be present at the start and may appear in the course of a deteriorating anomia and as a stage in the recovery of a neologistic jargon (see below). An example of such speech is that of a patient who, when asked where she lived, said: "I have been spa staying with a friend of mine but I do hate to imp impose on her. I want to pay my own way. Do they have some sort of chart where you can take this tee tee . . ." When phonemic aphasia develops out of a neologistic jargon (q.v.), speech is more active with some neologism and comprehension is less well preserved. Such a patient described his speech difficulty as: "Well it's very hard to because I don't know what it would my pi why what's wrong with it, but I can't food, it's food and rood to read the way I used to do all right off . . ."

The disturbance is equally present in naming and repetition and in a manner generally comparable to conversational speech. This is particularly evident when phonemic aphasia appears in the deterioration of an anomia. Thus, if an anomic patient is asked to name an ashtray, the word is not produced but can be repeated. In the regression of the anomia, the patient will first fail to cue with the initial sound of the word, i.e., when the examiner says "ash . . . ," but will still repeat the word "ashtray." At a later stage failure will occur in spite of a strong phonemic cue, e.g., "ashtr . . . ," in which all but the final syllable of the word is given, but the word "ashtray" can still be repeated. Ultimately a stage is reached where the patient can neither cue nor repeat. At this point the patient is a phonemic (conduction) aphasic. In this example we can see that the *disorder of repetition is only a failure to name given the whole word as a cue.* The transition from the *anomic*, who repeats the

word but fails to name with a cue up to the penultimate syllable, and the *phonemic aphasic* who fails given a cue including the final syllable (i.e., on repetition) establishes a functional continuity between these two disorders. There is a different speech form in these patients since the phonemic aphasic has achieved a linguistic level beyond that of the anomic. There is also a heightened awareness of speech content. Circumlocution has given way to deficient production, frustration to self-correction.

With regard to anatomical correlation, the evidence suggests that dominant posterior-superior temporal gyrus and its "parietal continuation" as supramarginal gyrus are chiefly involved. Cases with a lesion of angular gyrus have been reported, as well as instances in younger patients with a lesion limited to the left Wernicke's area.

Phonemic aphasia is uncommon in non-organic states, but phonemic errors may occur in speech during fatigue or distraction. An example of such errors in normal sleep utterance is the following: "David, I day (?say) David . . . that's you that day dated day dravid Dave dravid about 25 or 30 noked naked day dreams." The "clang association" is more prominent than is generally seen in phonemic aphasia, although clang errors are prominent in neologist jargon (see below).

THE PROBLEM OF NEOLOGISM

Aphasic jargon with neologism is a disturbance altogether different from semantic jargon, although both disorders are often treated as different manifestations of Wernicke's aphasia. As in the semantic, nominal, and phonemic disorders, there may be two expressions of the defect, in referential speech, as neologistic paraphasia, and in both referential and expositional speech, as neologistic jargon.

Neologistic Paraphasia. In this disorder, speech is generally comprehensible with occasional neologism, often in the context of fluent phonemic paraphasias. The neologism appears especially when a highly specific response is demanded, e.g., on proverb interpretation, and under the conditions of naming. An example is the following, from a patient who was questioned about his work: ". . . it was my job as a convince, a confoser, not confoler but almost the same as a man who was commersed." Another patient described her accident in this way, "So when I passed drive I told him let me drive. I had go so he let me go, so I went, wen in and went in on the semidore." The neologism primarily affects content words with relative sparing of the small grammatical words. The disorder is probably closely allied to phonemic aphasia and paraphasia, the neologism at times appearing as a phonemic error severe enough to render the word unintelligible.

Neologistic Jargon. This disorder refers to speech so pervaded by neologism that it is no longer intelligible. The neologisms may range from wordlike products to a series of clang contaminations. Thus, one patient responded to the idiom "swell-headed" with the interpretation, "She is selfice on purpiten," while at another time, asked about her speech problem, she said: "Because no one gotta scotta gowan thwa thirst gell gerst derund gystrol that's all." A progression may be seen from fluent, logorrheic neologistic speech with few clang associations, to reiteration of certain neologisms and perseverations on the basis of sound similarity to clang association so intense that it seems to determine the jargon output, e.g., "Then he graf, so I'll graf, I'm giving ink, no, gefergen, in pane, I can't grasp, I haven't grob the grabben, I'm going to the glimmeril let me go."

In such patients, comprehension is severely impaired. Naming and repetition are characterized by neologistic responses, e.g., "galeefs" for comb, "errendear" for yellow. There is a lack of awareness of speech errors, and patients will gesture actively, seemingly convinced that they are communicating something to the examiner. There is heightened affectivity, often with euphoria and exaggerated expression. It is of interest that patients will appear to accept their own jargon if it is recorded and played back to them, but will reject the same (transcribed) jargon if it is spoken to them by an examiner.

The pathological location of the lesion is in the dominant posterior superior temporal region. There is evidence[65] that the lesion incorporates both Wernicke's area proper and supramarginal gyrus.

In schizophrenia, neologisms are more often of the "portmanteau" type, either as fusions of separate words, e.g., "mondteufel," "cage-weather juice," "snowhousehold," or assimilations of otherwise recognizable components of separate words, e.g., "enduration" for *endure* plus *concentration*. These forms can perhaps be explained along the lines suggested for semantic paraphasia. Occasionally, unintelligible utterances may occur, e.g., "I have seen you but your words alworthen" (Question: What does alworthen mean?) "Ashers guiding the circumfrax." (see Bleuler[12] for other examples). In schizophasic jargon, one may encounter utterances of the type: "Ulrass Asia peru arull pelhuss Pisa anuell pelli." Similar types of jargon may be seen in transitional states,[38] e.g., "amarande es tifiercia," and sleep speech, e.g., "she shad hero sher sher sheril shaw takes part . . ." A form of aphasic jargon referred to as undifferentiated or phonemic jargon[3] may resemble such utterances, e.g., "Eh oh malaty, eh favility, abelabla tay kare abelabla tay to po sta here, aberdar yeste day (?yesterday)."

Interpretation of Neologistic Jargon. Although the place of neologistic jargon in the aphasias is uncertain, there is evidence that, at least in the most florid cases, it may represent a combination of semantic jargon and phonemic aphasia. In such cases, semantic paraphasias would be produced which would not achieve correct phonemic realization, the result being a phonemic distortion superimposed on a semantic paraphasia. This is consistent with the fact that neologistic jargon tends to improve to either semantic jargon or phonemic aphasia. Thus, if the semantic disorder clears, the patient is left with a phonemic defect, while clearing of the phonemic disorder would reveal the underlying semantic disturbance. In other (milder) cases, however, the neologism probably consists of a normal underlying word frame which is distorted to the point of unintelligibility by phonemic paraphasia. In addition, there are certainly many instances, as illustrated above, where the neologism is a result of clang associations and/or word fusions.

ANARTHRIC APHASIA

Included in this group are disorders at the final stage in speech production, disturbances affecting expositional speech primarily—as in agrammatism—and disturbances affecting both referential and expositional speech, anarthric or Broca's aphasia. While these disorders are considered *as if* they were impairments at a stage in advance of that involved in phonemic aphasia, viz., at the terminal grammatization and articulation, it may well be that they represent alterations in a motoric or action system organized, not in sequence, but in parallel with posterior linguistic structures.

Background. The historic period (discussed on pp. 243–244) during which the symptomatology and pathological correlative features of Broca's aphasia were worked out, gave way to a series of analytic studies which began with investigations of agrammatism.[58,87] Isserlin[58] and Pick[87] noted a gradation in Broca's aphasia from mild hesitation and stammering in speech, through agrammatism to a stage of near muteness. The agrammatic stage, characterized by a predominance of nouns and verbs (especially infinitives), lack of prefixes and suffixes, and pronoun confusion closely resembled an early stage of childhood speech.

More recently, Alajouanine[1] has made important contributions to our understanding of stereotypies and speech awareness in the Broca's aphasic. Following the approach and classification of Hughlings Jackson, Alajouanine has emphasized the automatic nature of the stereotypy and the lack of awareness which accompanies it, and he has distinguished four stages through which the stereotypy resolves. There is an initial stage of modification in which, through intonational adjustments, the stereotypy comes to express a wide variety of emotional states; then a stage of checking the stereotypy which signals the patient's first awareness of the utterance, followed by a transitional period in which other expressions, automatic or not, come to accompany the original, but now impersistent stereotypy; finally, there is abolition of the stereo-

typy with gradual return of speech into an agrammatic phase.

Sabouraud et al.[93] have characterized the fundamental defect in Broca's aphasia as an inability at different levels to pass from one complete utterance to another. This results from a loss of contrasting features in the expression; i.e. those oppositions which provide for lexical definition are conserved while contextual contrast is lost. Luria[75] has distinguished two forms of frontal aphasia, a kinetic or efferent motor aphasia, and a kinesthetic or afferent motor aphasia. He argues that these two independent conditions constitute what is usually called Broca's aphasia.

Agrammatism (telegrammatism). This disorder is characterized by relatively good use of nouns or substantives and a loss of the small function or grammatical words. This is especially prominent in conversational speech, but is generally present in repetition, reading aloud and writing as well. The disturbance may be present from the start, as in the so-called one-word or holophrastic sentence, e.g., the patient saying "water" or "glass, water" instead of "May I have a glass of water?" This may improve to more typical agrammatic speech:[48]

> My uh mother died uh, me uh, fifteen uh, oh I guess six months my mother pass away . . . my brother in uh Baltimore an stay all night an 'en I lef' for Florida, Mammi Beach, an uh, an uh, anen uh, Mammi Beach an stay all night and back again. Hitch hike.

With continued improvement this leads to a stage of relatively good speech with loss of inflections, restriction of verbs to the infinitive or present tense and an absence of unstressed grammatical words. Agrammatism has been considered a kind of speech economy, an articulatory defect primarily affecting grammatical words, and a true grammatical deficit. In our view the problem may be considered a deficiency in phonemic realization affecting grammatical words primarily. Since there is a graded entry of nouns, verbs and function words into the forming sentence, i.e., leading from an initial noun priority to the final grammatization, there is preservation of these content words which have already achieved a stage of phonemic encoding. For this reason it is the still developing function words, and particularly the late-added inflections, which are preferentially involved. This helps to explain why the order of word loss in agrammatism (grammatical words → verbs → nouns) is reciprocal to that of anomia (nouns → verbs → grammatical words). In the latter, the nouns are the first to appear and are therefore the first to be lost, whereas in agrammatism the nouns have completed their development and are therefore the most resistant.

Agrammatism is the commonest form of aphasia in dextrals with right hemispheric lesions[27] and is probably more common in aphasic lefthanders regardless of side of lesion. In such patients, language organization is similar in some respects to that of children in whom, next to muteness, agrammatism is the most common aphasic form. It is also of interest that agrammatism has been described in catatonic schizophrenia,[67] though it is by no means common in this disorder. The pathological localization of agrammatism is presumably the same as for anarthric aphasia.

Anarthric Aphasia (Broca's, motor, expressive aphasia). In this form the usual picture is one of nearly total speech loss, often with no verbalization apart from a stereotypy or automatism. Comprehension may be well preserved but other speech performances are about equally impaired. At times, naming and repetition may be slightly better than conversational speech. Such patients may improve to phonemic paraphasia or to agrammatism, depending on whether the content words or the terminal grammatization is chiefly affected. Less commonly there is recovery to dysarthria with abolition of the stereotypy and the gradual return of labored but nonaphasic speech.

In addition, the majority of patients are hemiplegic, and most have facial and left-sided apraxia. Writing is impaired to the same extent as speech. In cases where writing is markedly superior to speech, a diagnosis of "pure" motor aphasia may be considered, although the existence of this form is now held in some doubt. The term "nonfluency" is often used in relation to such patients. This concept includes a number of disturbances, however, such as dysprosody, dysarthria, agrammatism, and short "phrase length," so that unless the precise characteristics of the nonfluent condition are specified, the concept itself is of little value. Patients with anarthric aphasia tend also to be somewhat apathetic and passive in their behavior. Some writers have commented on the loss of volition or will (*Willenlosigkeit*), an attitude which is, in fact, more common than the frustration or despair often identified with this disorder. At times, one may see apathy give way to euphoric elation or labile crying during the stereotypic utterance. Awareness of the difficulty may change from moment to moment in relation to the dominant speech form, i.e., volitional or automatic speech.

Although there has been much controversy over the exact borders of Broca's area, there is general agreement on the central importance of the posterior part of the inferior or third frontal convolution (F_3). Goldstein[47] cited evidence for a more extended speech zone, involving the precentral operculum and mechanisms in this latter area for movement of the mouth, tongue and larynx.

Comment. In the preceding discussion, the major aphasic disorders have been reviewed from the point of view of a model of normal language production. Accordingly, the aphasias represent disruptions of (actually, a coming-to-the-fore of) earlier or prefigurative stages in the formative process. It now remains to bring the transcortical aphasias and the so-called isolation syndrome into relation with this model.

"TRANSCORTICAL" APHASIA

Background. This group of disorders comprises three major forms, transcortical motor aphasia (TMA), transcortical sensory aphasia (TSA), and combined transcortical aphasia (CTA) or "isolation" syndrome. Common to all forms is the occurrence of good (echolalic) repetition. In respect of the above forms, this occurs in the context of impaired speech, impaired comprehension, or impairment of both speech and comprehension. Historically the concept of a speech area separated from other portions of the cortex was first suggested by Huebner[56] in 1889, on the basis of a single case with loss of speech and comprehension, but relatively good writing, both spontaneous and to dictation, reading aloud and repetition. The brain showed two principal lesions (Figure 10–9), softening around the posterior part of T1, presumably interrupting connections between Wernicke's area and the parietal-concept field, and a small area of softening in F3 considered (in my view, incorrectly) to be of no importance.

Subsequently, cases of echolalia with temporal-lobe atrophy were described by Pick[86] and Liepmann.[73] The chief clinical feature of these and all subsequent cases is echolalia. This is characterized not simply by the ability to repeat but by compulsive and automatic repetition.

The echo response is a brief, precise and often explosive utterance which differs from the approximations of childhood imitation. Echolalia is not a parrotlike reflex function. There is often "personalization" of the content,

e.g., the patient asked "How are you?" echoes "How am I?" Moreover, it invariably has a social character, the response occurring only when the patient is addressed. There is also a completion effect,[99] patients finishing incomplete rhymes or phrases, e.g., "ham and . . . (eggs)." Patients may also correct in the echo an incorrect grammatical form in the presentation.[5]

In dementia, echolalia occurs with widespread but predominantly temporal-lobe atrophy. In aphasic states, there may be partial lesion of either anterior (TMA) or posterior (TSA) speech areas, or both (CTA) (see Figure 10–10). Echolalia may result from a predominantly posterior lesion assumed to interrupt parietal associations when there is diffuse atrophy or a smaller anterior lesion; or there may be a large infarct in the center of the dominant Sylvian speech zone.[99] Geschwind et al.[43] have described a demented echolalic with diffuse pathology sparing the Sylvian speech area. These authors argued that the *intact* portion of cortex and intervening arcuate

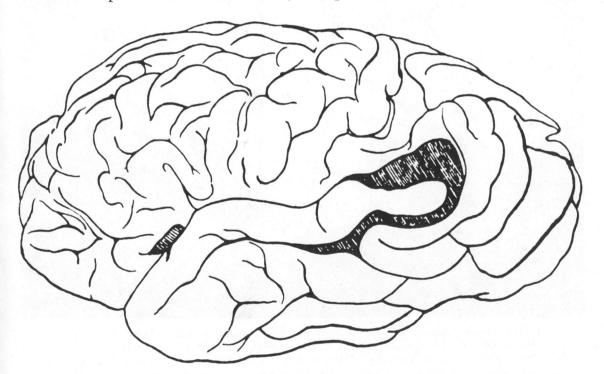

Figure 10–9. Heubner's[56] drawing of the major lesions in a case of echolalia with markedly reduced speech and comprehension (combined transcortical aphasia, "isolation syndrome").

fasciculus mediated the echolalic repetition, speech initiation and comprehension having been lost as a result of destruction of the remainder of the cortex. Echolalia is a symptom in a variety of late-stage dementias. It occurs in schizophrenia and mental deficiency. In the latter, it may represent the furthermost stage of language acquisition.

Interpretation of Echolalia. In aphasic states it is not uncommon to have echolalia at the level of single words or very short phrases. This may occur in phonemic and in jargon aphasia, and is a partial expression of the more pronounced echo response seen in the so-called transcortical aphasia. In the *motor* form of transcortical aphasia, echolalia stands out

against a background of reduced spontaneous speech. The pathology of this disorder is incompletely understood, but often there is a partial involvement of Broca's area. In transcortical *sensory* aphasia, there is a more automatic echo response appearing in the context of reduced comprehension. In this disorder the pathology appears to be the subtotal involvement of Wernicke's area. The isolation syndrome may correctly be conceived as a *combined* (motor and sensory) transcortical aphasia.

The anatomical limits of Broca's and Wernicke's areas are defined on an arbitrary basis so that it is unclear how a pathological lesion can be said to "surround" or lie on the periph-

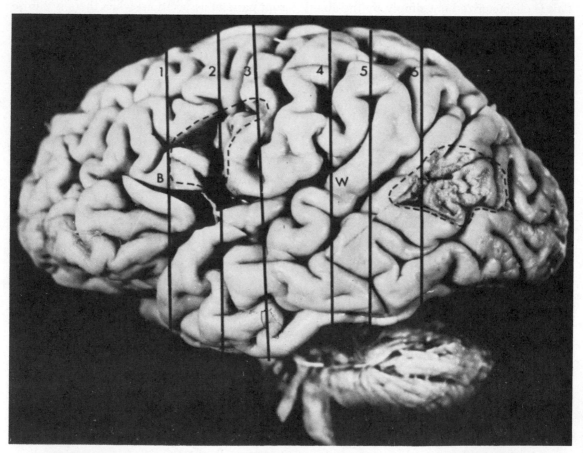

Figure 10–10. A personal case of combined transcortical aphasia (CTA). There is a large cystic infarct in the left posterior inferior frontal region, destroying much of Broca's area and extending subcortically to involve the region of traversal of the arcuate fasciculus. There is another area of superficial softening in posterior middle temporal gyrus. The pathology of CTA is a partial lesion of the anterior and posterior speech zone, bringing about a reduced functional level in performances supported or mediated by these areas.

ery of these areas. It is more likely that there is a *partial* lesion of either the anterior or the posterior speech zone, or both, and that this pathology brings about a deterioration or regression of function within those damaged areas. There is evidence for such partial lesions in all cases described, not only in the two focal cases but in a variety of diffuse atrophies as well.

The need for a more dynamic account of this disorder is emphasized by cases such as that of Stengel (and one of my own cases) where CTA occurs with destruction of the entire (left) Sylvian area. To say that the echo response derives from the opposite hemisphere is not to solve the problem but only to transfer it to the other side, for it is impossible to say whether the echo response reflects the degree to which the left hemisphere has been reduced or the highest level of which the right hemisphere is capable. Both arguments, in fact, amount to the same thing, since echolalia, like every other aphasic syndrome, is determined by the *combined performance of both residual left and intact right hemispheric capacity.* This concept of a linguistic regression induced by partial (or complete) damage to both of the (left) cortical speech zones, and of the resultant symptom, echolalia, as an *achievement* of the combined action of both hemispheres, helps to bring this disorder into relation with other conditions, e.g., dementia or mental retardation, where echolalia occurs, respectively, as a final stage in deterioration or as an endpoint in development.

⟦ The Neural Organization of Language

In historical writings on aphasia, it was generally maintained that the localization of a specific function could be inferred from an impairment of that function with focal pathology, that a lesion of a specific area gave rise to a symptom through disruption of the normal mechanism localized in, or mediated by, the area in question. Gradually, however, it has become clear that the anatomical structure which mediates language and cognition is as dynamic as the psychological systems which it supports. The "centers" of traditional aphasiology may rather be considered as *levels* by means of which language is carried one stage further. Similarly, the conducting pathways of the classical theory are not to be conceived as channels for the association of ideas, to link up perceptions to movements, or written words to spoken sounds, but are more likely concerned with temporal interrelationships between various levels in the cognitive structure.[25] The nature of the anatomical organization underlying language production can best be understood through a consideration of the process of cerebral dominance or lateralization.

Dominance

Although estimates differ, it is generally assumed that about 85 percent of the population is right-handed, and of these nearly all have left-hemispheric dominance for language. Among left-handers, there is a slightly greater tendency for left-hemispheric language dominance than right. In a large group of unselected patients there is about an 80 percent chance of developing some degree of aphasia with a left-hemispheric lesion regardless of handedness, and conversely, if one looks at an unselected population of right and left handed aphasics, about 95 percent have a left-hemispheric lesion. Furthermore, studies by Brown and Wilson,[27] suggest that hemispheric dominance for speech may be independent to an extent from hemispheric dominance for praxis, and that degree of speech lateralization may be inversely related to the priority of the opposite (usually right) hemisphere in spatial performance. Among the procedures currently being used to study hemispheric dominance are selective intracarotid amytal injection, dichotic listening and unilateral ECT (electroconvulsive therapy).

Lateralization and the Formation of the Speech Area

Hemispheric dominance or lateralization for language is not a state which is achieved at a certain time, say by age five, ten, or twenty, but is rather a process which, in a normal brain, may continue throughout life.[26] Moreover, there is fundamentally no difference between lateralization and "localization." Rather they are different aspects or phases of a unitary process. The initial phase, *interhemispheric specification* (lateralization), leads to a diffuse language organization in the left hemisphere. This is followed by a second phase of *intrahemispheric specification* ("localization") in which progressive differentiation occurs within the wider speech zone of that (the dominant) hemisphere.[25]

If we examine the effects of a lesion of left Wernicke's area (posterior T1), we discover that the form of aphasia produced by this lesion differs according to the age of the patient. Such a lesion in a five-year-old child produces a "motor" type of aphasia, with mutism or agrammatism. In a ten-year-old child, one sees an anomic aphasia, while at that same age and on into middle life, a phonemic (conduction

or central) aphasia may result. Finally, in late life, this lesion produces a jargonaphasia. Thus, four different types of aphasia can occur with the same lesion, depending on the age of the patient. At the very least this is persuasive evidence against a naive function localization.

Our knowledge that the process of *inter-* and *intra*hemispheric language specification takes place during the life span helps to account for this phenomenon. In the young child, an initial diffuse left-hemispheric language organization accounts for the fact that a lesion of frontal, parietal, or temporal lobe (including Wernicke's area) produces a "motor" form of aphasia. Subsequently, within this wider area a new region will emerge (Figure 10–11(a)), a lesion of which (incorporating Wernicke's area) produces an anomic aphasia. Gradually into middle life, a still smaller region is differentiated within the previous zone, a lesion of which (again, including Wernicke's area) produces phonemic paraphasia and

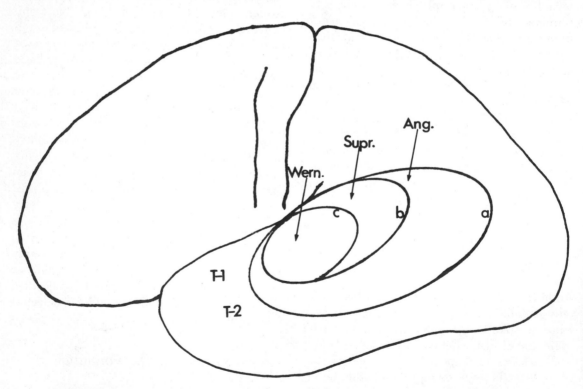

Figure 10–11. An illustration of zones of core differentiation in the posterior language area.[25] The angular (Ang.) and supramarginal (Supr.) gyri, and Wernicke's area (Wern.) represent ontogenetic levels in an evolving structural form, and are not the discrete anatomical loci of traditional cortical morphology.

phonemic aphasia (Figure 10–11(b)). Finally in late life there is gradual differentiation of a still smaller zone (Wernicke's area proper), lesion of which produces jargonaphasia (Figure 10–11(c)). Consistent with this is the fact that jargonaphasia is unusual in young adults where it generally requires bilateral lesions, possibly of limbic structures. The central point is that a two-phase developmental sequence, lateralization followed by intrahemispheric specification, creates a dynamic emergent structure which then supports the process of language production. At each stage in this process, involvement of the residual area of each preceding stratum produces the form of aphasia identified with that stratum when it represented the dominant level in ontogenesis.

Moreover, these strata are not to be conceived solely as neocortical differentiations, but as representatives of more widely distributed levels in cerebral phylogenesis. Further, the levels correspond to the three major sequential stages of language production which have been revealed in the study of the posterior aphasias:

progression from a limbic, through a generalized-neocortical to a specialized (asymmetric) neocortical level provides a dynamic, emergent structure mediating corresponding stages in the microgenesis of language and cognition.

There is a close relationship between this ontogenetic process which builds up the speech area, and the process of encephalization. In fact, the asymmetric structure of the speech area is a continuation of a similar trend in phylogeny. In this respect, the old theory of encephalization as a series of levels of progressively higher functional organization has been reexamined by Sanides,[94] who has demonstrated that brain expansion occurs through a process of "core differentiation." According to Sanides, in the phylogeny of neocortex ". . . ever new waves of growth and differentiation evolved, and each time a new cortex developed as a core, displacing the previous core to a ringlike structure." There is a striking correspondence between this account and the description of differentiation within the posterior, and by implication, the anterior speech areas in the course of maturation. Sanides[94] has also demonstrated that the "association" or

Phonemic	(specialized neocortical)	asymmetric, localized
Nominal	(neocortical)	unilateral but poorly localized
Semantic	(limbic)	bilateral

The semantic disorders are associated either with bilateral temporal lesions or unilateral (left) temporal lesion in the presence of mild generalized involvement. There is evidence in such disorders of bilateral limbic system lesion[106] or involvement of the cortical representatives of limbic structures. The nominal disorders (anomia and verbal paraphasia) occur with either diffuse or focal involvement of neocortex; however, focal lesions cannot be accurately localized, and anomia can also result from subcortical lesion, probably through a referred effect on generalized neocortex. The phonemic disorders are strictly associated with asymmetric focal lesions. Neologistic jargon is also asymmetric and focal, as it concerns, either directly or in combination, a disruption at the phonemic level. This morphogenetic

"integration" cortex in man is not, as traditionally believed, the "highest" region of the brain, but *precedes* the "primary" or "projection" cortex in evolution. This is consistent with the idea that lesions of "integration" cortex produce, as in anomia, a disorder microgenetically prior to disorders produced by lesion of "primary" cortex and immediate surround, e.g. phonemic aphasia and neologistic jargon. It is likely, therefore, that asymmetric neocortical organization, i.e., hemispheric specification for language, represents an ontogenetic solution to a phylogenetic problem, that of size limitations imposed upon an expanding brain in the course of evolution.

There have also been important recent findings with regard to cortico-cortical connections.[63,82,85] There is evidence (in subhuman primates) that the frontal "integration" cortex receives projections from the various "sensory" cortices and that it is in relation to limbic system by way of cingulate gyrus and lateral temporal lobe, and to thalamus via nu. dorsomedialis. Similarly, the temporo-parietal "integration" cortex receives short fiber connections from the various "sensory" cortices, and is also in relation to the limbic system via lateral temporal cortex and cingulate gyrus, and to the thalamus by way of lateralis posterior and pulvinar. Moreover, there are connections between parietal lobe and ·frontal granular cortex. These facts suggest that in primates, anterior and posterior "integration" cortices, i.e., regions homologous to the corresponding speech zones in man, are organized in a similar if not parallel fashion. Both areas are in relation to the parasensory cortices, both connect to medial and lateral limbic structures and have comparable thalamic representations.

These findings are of significance with regard to the problem of the relationship between the posterior and anterior speech areas. While it is generally believed that language is formed posteriorly and somehow conveyed, by way of the thalamus, insula or association pathways, to Broca's area for motor speech, there is, in fact, little evidence for this view.[25a] Rather, it may well be that a simultaneous realization occurs out of a common deep structure into the final linguistic and motoric components of the language act.

Comment. The neural organization of language is characterized by an evolving structural form which is built up during the course of life by a continuous two-stage process, that of *inter-* and *intra*hemispheric specification. The process through which the language structure develops, moreover, is only a prolongation into ontogeny of an identical trend in phylogenesis. This genetic approach to the problem of language organization can recapture the dynamic element which is ignored by older static concepts of "centers" and conducting pathways.

The term *microgenesis* has been proposed for the continuous formative activity which underlies cognition. It is implicit that the process of microgenesis recapitulates the sequence of phylo- and ontogenetic forms. The described series of evolutionary and developmental levels supports this process of cognitive formation. Language, that is, the series of levels through which language develops, may be thought of as a final ontogenetic "sensorimotor" differentiation within the neocortical ground supporting cognition up to a prelinguistic phase.

❨ General Aspects of Aphasia

Denial

Denial or lack of awareness of disease is a common manifestation in both organic and functional disorders. The first description was by von Monakow[78] in 1885 in respect to two cases of cortical blindness, while the term anosognosia, often applied to this phenomenon, was coined ·by Babinski[6] for lack of awareness of hemiparesis. Lack of awareness is also characteristic of several aphasic forms, e.g., jargon, stereotypy, and echo responses. In general, three types of denial are recognized: (1) partial or complete unawareness of a deficit; (2) explicit denial of the deficit, or, in the case of hemiplegic denial, of the very existence of the hemiparetic limbs; and (3) denial associated with distortions, hallucinations, or other illusory phenomena referrable to the impaired body zone (e.g., phantom or reduplicated limbs, visual hallucination). The view that denial is a reaction of the personality as a whole to the disorder is contradicted by the selective nature of the symptom. Thus, patients with left hemiplegia may deny weakness in the arm but admit to weakness in the leg. This occurs when there is a return of threshold sensory or motor function in the lower extremity while the arm ,remains fully paralyzed. Similarly, there may be catastrophic depression over subtotal cortical blindness with persistent denial of a hemiplegia. One patient with a left hemiplegia and previous amputation of the first two fingers of the left hand was able to correctly explain why he could not move his amputated fingers, but when asked to move the other (para-lyzed) fingers of the same hand, he refused to admit the paralysis. In a case of cortical blind-ness,[100] there was denial for the totally blind right visual field and awareness of visual loss on the left side where only minimal vision re-mained (motion and light perception). Thus, denial may spare a less recent disorder, may involve one of two (usually the more severely involved) hemiparetic limbs, and may spare deficient performances referrable to the same body zone, depending on the reason for the deficiency.

In patients with denial there is commonly some degree of disorientation, recent memory loss, and a confabulatory trend. There appears to be a relationship between the severity of the perceptual deficit and the confabulation. Cases of denial with fair visual or somaes-thetic perception have a marked Korsakoff syndrome, whereas the more severe the per-ceptual impairment, the less prominent the Korsakoff and confusional state. This inner bond between the severity of the perceptual disturbance and the occurrence of confabula-tion is an important clue toward an under-standing of the mechanism of denial.[22]

Those forms of language accompanied by deficient insight, the stereotypy, the echo re-sponse, and certain types of jargon are not isolated problems but are part of a continuous series across the spectrum of linguistic change. A transition has been demonstrated between the stereotypic and the volitional utterance (see p. 265). Patients who recover from a Broca's aphasia do not recall the stereotypic content, but may painfully recollect their ini-tial attempts to produce their own name. In echolalia, there is commonly an inverse rela-tion between the fidelity of the repetition and the degree to which it is understood. Such pa-tients may show echolalia for nonsense words or a foreign language, and paraphasic repeti-tion for their mother tongue. In some patients, a transition occurs between the echo and nor-mal repetition. This takes place over four stages: (1) initial brief latency, explosive echo responses accompanied by euphoria or labile emotionality, and lack of awareness for the echoed content; (2) echolike responses with

surprise or uncertainty (partial awareness) of the performance; (3) repetitions with par-aphasia, especially phonemic paraphasia, with moderate awareness, and efforts at self-correc-tion; and (4) complete failure of an anomic type, with acute self-awareness, frustration, and at times catastrophic reactions. These forms of repetition may coexist and alternate in a single patient, just as the Broca's aphasic may have concurrent stereotypy and volitional speech. In each instance, awareness can only be described in terms of a momentary state, as a part of a general attitude bound up with an utterance in the process of formation.

Affective Changes in Aphasia

It has long been recognized that aphasic pa-tients tend to show different affective features according to the nature of their language dis-order. Schilder wondered whether the apathy and/or depression of Broca's aphasia and the euphoria of Wernicke's aphasia were intrinsic to the speech disturbance rather than a sec-ondary reaction. A study of linguistic change in aphasia suggests that the affective picture is indeed an inner component, not something "added on" to the language disturbance. Moreover, the affective state is not specific to the "syndrome" but to the cognitive level, or speech content manifesting that level, which is in the foreground at the precise moment dur-ing which the affect is displayed. This helps to account for the fluctuation in affective state that occurs in aphasic patients, since this is correlated with a similar fluctuation in the lin-guistic-cognitive level.

In general, the semantic disorders are char-acterized by varying degrees of euphoria and excitement. In anomia, there is an improved awareness of the speech disorder, frustration, and some degree of self-correction and censor-ship. In phonemic aphasia, there is a more acute insight into the speech content, with improved self-correction. Marked alterations in affect are usually not apparent. In Broca's aphasia, there is apathy, dullness, and some depression. Frustration and catastrophic reac-tion are not as common in this group as in anomia. Patients with neologistic jargon may be euphoric and excited. At times there is a definite paranoid trend, though systematized delusions are unusual. Paranoia may also occur in semantic jargon but is less common. In the rare disorder of word deafness, a condition characterized by impaired speech perception despite good hearing and nonaphasic speech, the presentation is almost invariably characterized by an acute psychosis with marked paranoid ideation and auditory hallucination. Many of these patients are initially hospitalized on a psychiatric service until diagnosis becomes clear. The etiology of paranoia in aphasia is uncertain, though there are at least three possible explanations: (1) it might reflect a lesion of temporal lobe independent of the aphasia; (2) it might relate to impaired speech perception and in that respect would be comparable to the "paranoia of the deaf"; or (3) it might have an inner relationship with the language form of the aphasia.

Hallucination

Hallucination does occur in aphasia, chiefly, if not exclusively, with the temporal-lobe disorders, word deafness and (less commonly) jargon. In the former, auditory hallucination tends to appear at the onset, while in jargon it may intervene after several days. These hallucinations may consist of noises, single words, or sentences, e.g. the patient of Ziegler[110] who heard such phrases as "Carl, we're going this way" and "It will be all right." As in other perceptual spheres, e.g., vision or somaesthesis, there is a relation between the density of the perceptual deficit and the likelihood of hallucination. In organic disease, hallucination often points to a lesion of the cortical projection zone of the hallucinated modality.

In schizophrenic patients, there is impaired comprehension during a bout of auditory hallucination. This has been attributed to inattention or distraction. Yet a similar phenomenon occurs in organic cases, where the hallucination seems to "fill the void" created by the loss of the perceptual channel. In general, there is a striking similarity between functional and organic hallucination.[79] The fact that in the former there may be a higher incidence of auditory than visual content, or that organic hallucination is less systematized, may reflect, respectively, only fortuitous anatomical factors (e.g., the rarity of a focal lesion restricted to auditory cortex) and duration, i.e. that systematization requires a more prolonged hallucinatory state than is generally seen in organic conditions. In fact, in some instances where hallucination may persist for several years, e.g., in "peduncular hallucinosis," patients may develop a hallucinatory psychosis with marked organization and systematization of the hallucinatory ideation. One difference between organic and functional cases in this respect may be the fact that the former do not show the same degree of fear or panic at the onset of the hallucinatory state; in fact, some organic patients appear to be entertained by their hallucinations. Certainly, this seems to be true for some cases of organic *visual* hallucination, but probably does not hold for auditory hallucination.

❲ Toward a Unitary Model of Organic and Functional Disorders

Every symptom in an aphasic disorder points to a level in cognition. The change in affect or in awareness, the occurrence of delusional or hallucinatory states, the appearance of concrete or paralogical thinking, these are not, so to say, outside the aphasia but are a reflection of that cognitive level of which the aphasic speech form is one element.

A study of the aphasias suggests that the pattern of symptom formation is identical in organic and functional disorders. An aphasia represents a disruption in, i.e., a coming-to-the-fore of, higher levels in the linguistic component of cognition. Agnosia and apraxia are parallel disorders in the spheres of perception and action. The asymmetric organization of these "higher" levels accounts for their special relationship to organic, i.e., unilateral, pathology. In functional states, the picture also corresponds to a "coming-to-the-fore," but of lower levels in cognition. Symptoms may appear preferentially in the affective, motoric, perceptual, or linguistic components of cognition. Similar symptoms can be produced by organic lesions, if bilateral and precisely localized.

An approach to the aphasias, as well as to all psychopathological disorders, from the point of view of cognition can reveal this inner bond between organic and functional change.

◖ Bibliography

1. ALAJOUANINE, T. "Verbal Realization in Aphasia," *Brain,* 79 (1956), 1–28.
2. ———. *L'Aphasie et le Langage Pathologique.* Paris: Baillière, 1968.
3. ALAJOUANINE, T., O. SABOURAUD, and B. DE RIBAUCOURT. "Le Jargon des aphasiques," *J. Psychol.,* 45 (1952), 158–180, 293–329.
4. ARIETI, S. *Interpretation of Schizophrenia,* 1st ed., New York: Brunner, 1955; 2nd ed., New York: Basic Books, 1974.
5. AVAKIAN-WHITAKER, H. "On Echolalia." Paper presented at the Academy of Aphasia. Rochester, 1972.
6. BABINSKI, J. "Contribution à l'étude des troubles mentaux dans l'hémiplégie organique cérébrale (Anosognosie)," *Rev. Neurol. (Paris),* 27 (1914), 845–848.
7. BARTON, M., M. MARUSZEWSKI, and D. URREA. "Variation of Stimulus Context and Its Effects on Word-Finding Ability in Aphasics," *Cortex,* 5 (1969), 351–365.
8. BAY, E. "Aphasia and Non-verbal Disorders of Language," *Brain,* 85 (1962), 411–426.
9. ———. "Present Concepts of Aphasia," *Geriatrics,* 19 (1964), 319–331.
10. BENTON, A. and R. JOYNT. "Early Descriptions of Aphasia," *Arch. Neurol.,* 3 (1960), 205–222.
11. BINSWANGER, L. *Sigmund Freud: Reminiscences of a Friendship.* New York: Grune & Stratton, 1957.
12. BLEULER, E. *Dementia Praecox.* New York: International Universities Press, 1950.
13. BLUMSTEIN, S. "Phonological Aspects of Aphasic Speech," in C. Gribble, ed., *Studies Presented to Professor R. Jakobson by His Students,* pp. 39–43. Cambridge: Slavica, 1970.
14. BOGEN, J. "The Other Side of the Brain," *Bull. Los Angeles Neurol. Soc.,* 34 (1970), 73–105, 135–162.
15. BOUILLAUD, J. "Réchèrches cliniques propres à demontier que la perte de la parole, etc., *Arch. Gen. Méd.,* 8 (1825), 25–45.
16. BRAIN, R. *Speech Disorders.* London: Butterworths, 1961.
17. BROCA, P. "Remarques sur le siège de la faculté du langage articulé," *Bull Soc. Anat.,* 36 (1861), 330–357.
18. ———. "Nouvelle observation d'aphémie produite par une lésion de la moitié postérieure des deuxième et troisième circonvolutions frontales," *Bull. Soc. Anat.,* 36 (1861), 398–407.
19. ———. "Localisation des fonctions cérébrales siège du langage articulé," *Bull Soc. Anthropol.,* 4 (1863), 200–204.
20. ———. "Sur le Siège de la faculté du langage articulé," *Bull. Soc. Anthropol.,* 6 (1865), 377–393.
21. BROWN, J. "Hemispheric Specialization and the Corpus Callosum," in C. Gunderson, ed., *Present Concepts in Internal Medicine.* San Francisco: Publ. Letterman Hospital, 1969.
22. ———. *Aphasia, Apraxia and Agnosia: Clinical and Theoretical Aspects.* Springfield, Ill.: Charles C. Thomas, 1972.
23. ———. "Introduction," in: A. Pick, *Aphasia.* (English translation), Springfield, Ill.: Charles C. Thomas, 1973.
24. ———. "Language, Cognition and the Thalamus," *Confin. Neurol.,* 36 (1974), 33–60.
25. ———. "The Neural Organization of Language," *Brain Lang.,* 1 (1975), in press.
25a. ———. "The Problem of Repetition," *Cortex* (1975–76) in press.
26. BROWN, J. and J. JAFFE. "Hypothesis on Cerebral Dominance," *Neuropsychologia,* (1975), 107–110.
27. BROWN, J. and F. WILSON. "Crossed Aphasia in a Dextral," *Neurology,* 23 (1973), 23–30.
28. CAMERON, N. "Experimental Analysis of Schizophrenic Thinking," in J. Kasanin, ed., *Language and Thought in Schizophrenia,* pp. 50–64. New York: Norton, 1964.
29. CHAPMAN, J. "The Early Symptoms of Schizophrenia, "*Br. J. Psychiatry,* 112 (1966), 225–251.
30. CHARCOT, J.-M. "Des Variétés de l'aphasie,"

Prog. Méd., 11 (1883), 487–488, 521–523.

31. CHOMSKY, N. *Syntactic Structures.* The Hague: Mouton, 1957.

32. ———. *Aspects of the Theory of Syntax.* Cambridge: M.I.T. Press, 1965.

33. CONRAD, K. "Strukturanalysen hirnpathologische Fälle, I: Über Struktur und Gestaltwandel." *Dtsch. Z. Nervenheilk.*, 158 (1947), 344–371.

34. CRITCHLEY, M. *Aphasiology and other Aspects of Language.* London: Arnold, 1970.

35. DIMOND, S. *The Double Brain.* Edinburgh: Churchill Livingstone, 1972.

36. DOMARUS, VON E. "The Specific Laws of Logic in Schizophrenia," in J. Kasanin, ed., *Language and Thought in Schizophrenia,* pp. 104–114. New York: Norton, 1964.

37. FREUD, S. *On Aphasia.* Translated by E. Stengel. New York: International Universities Press, 1953.

38. FROESCHELS, E. "A Peculiar Intermediary State between Waking and Sleep," *J. Clin. Psychopathol.*, 7 (1946), 825–833.

39. GALL, F. and C. SPURZHEIM. *Anatomie et Physiologie du Système Nerveux en Général et du Cerveau en Particulier.* Paris: Schoell, 1810–1819.

40. GAZZANIGA, M. *The Bisected Brain.* New York: Appleton-Century-Crofts, 1970.

41. GESCHWIND, N. "The Paradoxical Position of Kurt Goldstein in the History of Aphasia," *Cortex*, 1 (1964), 214–224.

42. ———. "Language and the Brain," *Sci. Am.*, 226 (1972), 76–83.

43. GESCHWIND, N., F. QUADFASEL and J. SEGARRA. "Isolation of the Speech Area," *Neuropsychologia*, 6 (1968), 327–340.

44. GOLDSTEIN, K. *Die Transkortikalen Aphasien.* Jena: Fischer, 1915.

45. ———. "Das Wesen der amnestischen Aphasie," *Schweiz. Arch. Neurol. Psychiatr.*, 15 (1924), 163–175.

46. ———. "The Significance of Psychological Research in Schizophrenia," *J. Nerv. Ment. Dis.*, 97 (1943), 261–279.

47. ———. *Language and Language Disturbances.* New York: Grune & Stratton, 1948.

48. GOODGLASS, H. "Redefining the Concept of Agrammatism in Aphasia," Proc. 12th Int. Speech Voice Ther. Conf., Padua, 1962, pp. 108–116.

49. ———. "Studies on the Grammar of Aphasics," in S. Rosenberg and J. Kaplan, eds., *Developments in Applied Psycholinguistic Research.* New York: Macmillan, 1968.

50. GOODGLASS, H. and S. BLUMSTEIN. *Psycholinguistics and Aphasia.* Baltimore: The Johns Hopkins University Press, 1973.

51. GREEN, E. "Phonological and Grammatical Aspects of Jargon in an Aphasic Patient," *Lang. Speech*, 12 (1969), 103–118.

52. HEAD, H. *Aphasia and Kindred Disorders of Speech.* New York: Macmillan, 1926.

53. HECAEN, H. and J. DUBOIS. *La Naissance de la Neuropsychologie du Langage.* Paris: Flammarion, 1969.

54. HECAEN, H., J. DUBOIS, and P. MARCIE. "Critères Neurolinguistiques d'une Classification des Aphasies," *Acta Neurol. Psychiatr. Belg.*, 67 (1967), 959–987.

55. HEILBRONNER, K. Zur Symptomatologie der Aphasie. *Archiv. Psychiatr. Nervenheilk.*, 43 (1908), 234–298.

56. HEUBNER, O. "Über Aphasie," *Schmidt's Jahrb.*, 224 (1889). 220–222.

57. HOWES, D. "Application of the Word-Frequency Concept to Aphasia," in A. V. S. De Reuck and M. O'Connor, eds., *Disorders of Language.* London: Churchill, 1964.

58. ISSERLIN, M. "Aphasie," in O. Bumke and O. Foerster, eds., *Handbuch der Neurologie*, Vol. 6, pp. 627–806. Berlin: Springer, 1936.

59. JACKSON, H. *Selected Writings of John Hughlings Jackson*, Vol. 2, J. Taylor, ed., London: Hodder & Stoughton, 1932.

60. JAKOBSON, R. "Towards a Linguistic Typology of Aphasic Impairments," in A. V. S. De Reuck and M. O'Connor, eds., *Disorders of Language.* London: Churchill, 1964.

61. ———. *Child Language, Aphasia and Phonological Universals.* The Hague: Mouton, 1968.

62. JAKOBSON, R. and M. HALLE. *Fundamentals of Language.* The Hague: Mouton, 1956.

63. JONES, E. and T. POWELL. "An Anatomical Study of Converging Sensory Pathways Within the Cerebral Cortex of the Monkey," *Brain*, 93 (1970), 793–820.

64. KERTESZ, A. "A Linguistic Analysis of Fluent Aphasia," *Brain Lang.*, 1 (1974), 43–62.

65. KERTESZ, A. and F. BENSON. "Neologistic Jargon," *Cortex*, 6 (1970) 362–386.

66. KLEIST, K. *Gehirnpathologie.* Leipzig: Barth, 1934.

67. ———. "The Classification of Schizophrenia," *J. Ment. Sci.*, 103 (1957), 443–463.

68. ———. *Sensory Aphasia and Amusia*. Oxford: Pergamon, 1962.

69. KREINDLER, A., C. CALAVREZO, and L. MIHĂILESCU. "Linguistic Analysis of One Case of Jargon Aphasia," *Rev. Roumaine Neurol.*, 8 (1971), 209–228.

70. LASHLEY, K. "The Problem of Serial Order in Behavior," in L. Jefress, ed., *Cerebral Mechanisms in Behavior* (Hixon Symposium), pp. 112–136. New York: Wiley, 1951.

71. LECOURS, A. and F. LHERMITTE. "Phonemic Paraphasias: Linguistic Structures and Tentative Hypotheses," *Cortex,* 5 (1969), 193–228.

72. LHERMITTE, F. "Sémiologie de l'aphasie," *Rev. Praticien*, 15 (1965), 2255–2292.

73. LIEPMANN, H. "Ein Fall von Echolalie," *Neurol Zentralbl.*, (1900), 389–399.

74. LOTMAR, F. "Zur Kenntnis der erschwerten Wortfindung und ihrer Bedeutung für das Denken des Aphasischen," *Schweiz. Arch. Neurol. Psychiatr.*, 5 (1919), 206–239.

75. LURIA, A. *Higher Cortical Functions in Man*. New York: Basic Books, 1966.

76. MARIE, P. "Révision de la question de l'aphasie," *Sem. Méd.*, 21 (1906), 241–247, 493–500, 565–571.

77. MARSHALL, J. and F. NEWCOMBE. "Syntactic and Semantic Errors in Paralexia," *Neuropsychologia*, 6 (1966), 169–176.

78. MONAKOW, C. VON. "Experimentelle und Pathologische-anatomische Untersuchungen über die Beziehungen der sogennanten Sehsphare zu den infrakortikalen Opticuscentren und zum N. Opticus," *Arch. Psychiatr.*, 16 (1885), 151–199.

79. MORSIER, G. DE. "Les Hallucinations," *Rev. Otoneurophtalmol.*, 16 (1938), 241–352.

80. NIELSEN, J. *Agnosia, Apraxia, Aphasia*. New York: Hafner, 1965.

81. OLDFIELD, R. "Things, Words and the Brain," *Q. J. Exp. Psychol.*, 18 (1966), 340–353.

82. PANDYA, D. and H. KUYPERS. "Cortico-Cortical Connections in the Rhesus Monkey," *Brain Res.*, 13 (1969), 13–36.

83. PANDYA, D. and F. SANIDES. "Architectonic Parcellation of the Temporal Operculum in Rhesus Monkey and Its Projection Pattern," *Z. Anat. Entwickl. Gesch.*, 139 (1973), 127–161.

84. PENFIELD, W. and L. ROBERTS. *Speech and Brain Mechanisms*. Princeton: University Press, 1959.

85. PETRAS, J. "Connections of the Parietal Lobe," *J. Psychiatr. Res.*, 8 (1971), 189–201.

86. PICK, A. *Beiträge zur Pathologie und pathologischen Anatomie des Centralnervensystems*. Berlin: Karger, 1898.

87. ———. *Die agrammatischen Sprachstörungen*. Berlin: Springer, 1913.

88. ———. *Aphasia*. Translated by J. Brown. Springfield, Ill.: Charles C. Thomas, 1973.

89. PITRES, A. "L'Aphasie amnésique et ses variétés cliniques," *L'Echo Méd.*, 24 (1898), 276–281, 289–294, 301–306, 313–317, 325–332, 337–342, 351–352, 373–378, 385–390, 397–405, 409–425, 433–437.

90. RIESE, W. "The Early History of Aphasia," *Bull. Hist. Med.*, 21 (1947), 322–334.

91. RINNERT, C. and H. WHITAKER. "Semantic Confusions by Aphasic Patients," *Cortex*, 9 (1973), 56–81.

92. ROCHFORD, G. and M. WILLIAMS. "Studies in the Development and Breakdown of the Use of Names," *J. Neurol. Neurosurg. Psychiatr.*, 25 (1962), 228–233.

93. SABOURAUD, O., J. GAGNEPAIN, and A. SABOURAUD. "Vers une Approche linguistique des problèmes de l'aphasie (II). L'Aphasie de Broca," *Rev. Neuropsychiatr. l'Ouest.*, 2 (1963), 3–38.

94. SANIDES, F. "Functional Architecture of Motor and Sensory Cortices in the Light of a New Concept of Neocortex Evolution," in C. Noback and W. Montagna, eds., *The Primate Brain*, p. 183. New York: Appleton-Century-Crofts, 1970.

95. SCHILDER, P. and N. SUGÁR. "Zur Lehre von den schizophrenen Sprachstörungen," *Z. Neurol Psychiatr.*, 104 (1926), 689–714.

96. SPERRY, R. "Perception in the Absence of the Neocortical Commissures," in D. A. Hamburg, K. Pribram, and A. Stunkard, eds., *Perception and Its Disorders*, Vol. 28, pp. 123–138. Association for Research in Nervous and Mental Disease. New York: Williams & Wilkins, 1970.

97. SPREEN, O. "Psycholinguistic Aspects of Aphasia," *J. Speech Hear. Res.*, 11 (1968), 467–480.

98. ———. "Psycholinguistics and Aphasia: The Contribution of Arnold Pick," in H. Goodglass and S. Blumstein, eds., *Psycholinguistics and Aphasia*, pp. 141–170. Baltimore: The Johns Hopkins University Press, 1973.

99. STENGEL, E. "A Clinical and Psychological

Study of Echo-Reactions," *J. Ment. Sci.*, 93 (1947), 598–612.

100. STENGEL, E. and G. STEELE. "Unawareness of Physical Disability (Anosognosia)," *J. Ment. Sci.*, 92 (1946), 379–388.

101. TROUSSEAU, A. "De l'Aphasie, maladie décrite récemment sous le nom impropre d'aphémie," *Gaz. Hôpitaux*, 37 (1864).

102. VICTOR, M. Personal communication to author, 1973.

103. VICTOR, M., ADAMS, R., and G. COLLINS. *The Wernicke-Korsakoff Syndrome*. Philadelphia: Davis, 1971.

104. WEIGL, E. and M. BIERWISCH. "Neuropsychology and Linguistics: Topics of Common Research," *Found. Lang.*, 6 (1970), 1–18.

105. WEINSTEIN, E. and N. KELLER. "Linguistic Patterns of Misnaming in Brain Injury,"

Neuropsychologia, 1 (1964), 79–90.

106. WEINSTEIN, E., O. LYERLY, M. COLE et al., "Meaning in Jargon Aphasia," *Cortex*, 2 (1966), 165–187.

107. WEISENBURG, T. and K. E. McBRIDE. (1935) *Aphasia: A Clinical and Psychological Study*; reprint ed. New York: Hafner, 1964.

108. WERNICKE, C. *Der aphasische Symptomenkomplex*. Breslau: Cohn and Weigart, 1874.

109. YOUNG, R. *Mind, Brain and Adaptation in the Nineteenth Century*, Oxford: Clarendon, 1970.

110. ZIEGLER, D. "Word Deafness and Wernicke's Aphasia," *Arch. Neurol. Psychiatry*, 67 (1952), 323–331.

111. ZURIF, E. Paper presented at International Neuropsychology Society, Boston, 1974.

CHAPTER 11

APHASIA:

BEHAVIORAL ASPECTS*

J. P. Mohr and Murray Sidman

⟨ Introduction

THE SUBJECT MATTER of aphasia encompasses a spectrum ranging from the practical assessment of an acutely brain injured patient to the abstract theory of language. Since definitions of aphasia vary with the approach to the subject matter, descriptions adequate for one purpose are often inappropriate for another. This chapter is oriented toward the behavioral features of aphasia deficits.

Any understanding of aphasia requires consideration of the roles played by individual variables in the performance profile observed in a given patient at a given time. In roughly descending order of importance, these variables include the methods used to delineate the deficit, the site of the brain injury, the

* The preparation of this manuscript was supported in part by Grants number: HL 14888 from the National Heart and Lung Institute and Public Health Service Grants HD 05124 and HD 04147 from the National Institute of Child Health and Human Development.

patient's age and handedness, the rapidity of onset, duration, causative agent, the size of the brain injury, and coexisting motor and sensory deficits. Singly, and in combination, they can account for many seemingly contradictory or only loosely comparable features of different cases of aphasia.

A theoretical structure is helpful, but not a prerequisite in approaching the subject of aphasia. The spectrum of traditional and current theories of aphasia can be accommodated within the following elementary summary. At the lowest level of complexity,[26,30,50] the basic instrumentalities subserving discrimination, replication, and production of verbal stimuli, the phonologic aspects of language,[52] are considered to require the proper functioning of the cortical surface and subcortical white matter structures grouped around the Sylvian fissure of the left cerebrum. Auditory inputs from the brain stem pass via white matter pathways to the primary auditory cortex (Heschl's transverse gyri) located in the superior temporal lobe at the posterior region of the Sylvian fissure. Vocal outputs are controlled by the primary motor cortex (Rolandic fissure), subserving movements of the oropharynx, larynx, and resipiratory apparatus. Control of the individual movements, transitions of movements, and melodic sequences[29] involved in speaking aloud is exerted via the adjacent premotor cortex in the inferior frontal region (Broca's area).[6] Fiber pathways in the arcuate fasciculus, deep to the insula, may link the auditory and vocal motor regions to permit repeating aloud from dictation.[14] At a level of greater complexity, organization and comprehension of conversational speech, especially its semantic and syntactic aspects,[52] are traditionally thought to reflect activity of the inferior parietal and posterior temporal regions adjacent to the auditory cortex, the combination usually referred to as Wernicke's area.[50] Combined lexic and graphic activity is also thought to involve inferior parietal activity,[10] especially those portions adjoining the more posteriorly situated occipital lobe, whose main function involves processing of visual inputs. The most complex, abstract, and theoretical levels of language activity are considered to involve preverbal thought, i.e., the formulation of the basic message to be conveyed;[7,37] posterior and deep temporal-lobe functions may underlie these processes, the documentation for which remains theoretical and introspective at best.

Two main variations of the foregoing underlie most writings in the field of aphasia, even though they are not always explicitly stated. In the first variation,[26,27,50] brain mechanisms underlying language behavior are seen to reflect the interaction of relatively autonomous cerebral regions, i.e., auditory, visual, and motor. Constellations of individual findings (syndromes), which constitute clinical aphasia, reflect focal brain injuries (lesions) of varying origin, involving the cortical surface "centers" or the white matter pathways, separately or in various combinations. In the second variation,[30] only one cerebral region, situated in the posterior portion of the Sylvian fissure, is crucial for language behavior. The cerebral regions serving sensory input and motor output are seen functionally as essentially centripetal or centrifugal, respectively, to this central zone. Syndrome analysis is directed toward discovering evidence of deficits thought to reflect damage to the central language mechanism, irrespective of the input or output channels involved in the behavior being tested. Such deficits are considered aphasic, while involvements reflecting only damage to the centrifugal or the centripetal functions are not.

The basic theoretical formulations outlined above have served as the foundation for most of the many different viewpoints toward aphasia. It is all the more unfortunate, in view of the enormous amount of study given the subject, that basic ambiguities still prevent a clear understanding of the subject.

◖ Testing for Aphasia

The major aphasic syndromes were originally described from clinical observations. Although ingenious tests were often used in assessing the classic cases, the data now available are in most cases summary notes which reflect the investigator's interpretation of the behavior more than they do the actual behavior itself. The subsequent development of methods for analyzing behavior has resulted in a continual updating of the components of individual aphasic syndromes, with some divergence from previous interpretations.

Much of the controversy in the field of aphasia stems from clinical differences among patients with apparently similar lesions. Much of this variability reflects the selection of the aphasic population to be tested, the actual tests administered, and the methods of test administration.

Case Selection

A variety of approaches has been used in the selection of cases. Historically, the report of a single case or a few cases showing virtually identical findings, has set the precedent still favored by many investigators. Reports of one, or of a limited number of cases, generally include anatomic findings proved by autopsy, and involve intensive study for varying periods of time, and/or show singular or unique findings bearing on aphasia theory, all encompassed in a readably brief account. Taken together, fewer than one hundred such cases have contributed the majority of the data upon which the major current ideas on aphasia depend. Yet even these intensively studied single cases have undergone only a limited number of tests. It has been argued[18] that such cases are so rare and unusual that they are not representative of the field of aphasia in general. This contention has been countered[51] by the point that the combined factors of anatomy and pathologic processes in naturally occurring illness usually result in brain injuries whose location and extent encompass so many important regions simultaneously that most cases are too complex to permit a detailed analysis. The rare case of sharply specifiable deficits is of value as the exception that helps clarify the rules.

Another approach to case selection has been to study a large group sharing in common some major variables, such as site of lesion, etiology, age, etc. War injuries are a prototype of this approach.[40] These studies provide corroboration for the individual case reports. They suffer from the statistical summary approach in which details of individual cases can get lost in group averages.

In yet another approach, the purpose has been to screen an unselected population using a single test[4] or series of tests.[49] Separation of the case material in the groups is then based on the responses made by individuals. Such collections of cases seem to show the most general, and least specific, findings. Critics contend that the nonspecificity of the findings reflects the inclusion of cases differing widely in type, whose individual differences disappear when the data are averaged together. Supporters point to the need to establish an approach to deficit profile without dependence on these traditional criteria, so as to permit some validation of the traditional means of classifying cases.

Test Methods

The authors believe that the methodology used to approach a case of aphasia is basic to all other considerations, since it provides the data from which the theories should be derived. Accordingly, test methodology will be discussed before taking up the analysis of aphasia.

In his monograph on aphasia in 1874, Wernicke[50] noted a tendency for patients to seize upon any kind of cues available to them when they experienced difficulties with the tests designed to assess their language behavior. Although he recorded this observation—that patients may use any of a number of possible means to approach a task—in his early monograph on aphasia, deliberate specification of individual parameters in aphasia testing has received intensive attention only in recent years. As late as 1966[47] proposals could still be found calling for standardization of the stimulus, response, and other variables involved in aphasia testing.

At the present time, since major research centers tend to maintain and use their own methods, data from different centers are often not strictly comparable. Ambiguities and differences in the observation of aphasic behavior are a paramount source of disagreement, and a review of the major methods used to evaluate aphasia patients seems justified.

BEHAVIORAL

Although all aphasia tests are behavioral, few investigators explicitly and systematically use the principles and techniques that stem from objective behavioral science. We have, therefore, used the term "behavioral" to characterize our own approach.[44]

With some oversimplification, we can specify three major classes of behavioral variables which may interact with physiological processes to govern a person's interaction with his environment. First, all behavior, including that exhibited in aphasia tests, is governed by its consequences. Rather than depend solely on a patient's presumed motivation to do well in our tests, we provide explicit positive reinforcement, i.e., to encourage correct responses. Behavioral deficits, aphasic or other, may result from the breakdown of the controlling relation between behavior and its consequences, and the terms, "motivational" or "reinforcement deficit," are often applied. Little is known about such clinical deficits in humans; it need only be said here that a patient is likely to exhibit no consistent behavior if presumed reinforcers in the test situation are ineffective, and any conclusions about aphasia will be untenable in such patients.

A second class of variables is subsumed in the term, "stimulus control." Appropriate behavior occurs in response to stimuli which set the occasion for reinforcement, as determined by a person's behavioral history. When we observe that a particular stimulus occasions a response, and that its absence fails to do so, we have a controlling relation between stimulus and response. An example of the complexity involved in stimulus control is the relation between traffic lights and a driver's behavior. We have achieved considerable initial support for the notion that many aphasic deficits represent breakdowns of stimulus control; for example the controlling relation between printed words and oral naming (speech deficit), between pictures and written naming (writing deficit), or the nonverbal selection of appropriate pictures in response to printed words (reading comprehension).

The third class of variables may be termed "instructional." These include the constant stimuli of the test environment, the test procedures themselves, and the specific instructions given to the patient about what he is expected to do. Clearly, a patient who is not sensitive to instructional factors will exhibit test behavior that is unrelated to the purposes of the tests. Like motivational deficits, instructional deficits invalidate any conclusions specific to aphasia. Since aphasia, by its very nature, represents a communication disorder, instructional deficit is often difficult to circumvent in aphasia evaluation. The problem can be overcome by appropriate use of effective reinforcers, which function nonverbally to inform the patient when he is performing as requested.

Controls for reinforcement and instructional deficits are built into the procedures of the tests, which are, themselves, oriented toward the analysis of stimulus-control deficits characteristic of aphasia. The sequence of tests, furthermore, has been designed to reveal intact forms of stimulus control, thereby reducing the number of factors that must be considered to play a role in the patient's deficit. The tests themselves simply required the patient to name orally, write, or match (select from a number of alternatives) visual, auditory, or palpated test stimuli, such as single letters, three-letter picturable nouns and their pictures, color names and their colors, digit names and their digits, and manipulable objects. These tests demonstrate the control exerted by each stimulus (visual, auditory, or palpated) over each type of response (oral, naming, writing, and matching). The test battery yields a stimulus-control matrix in which stimulus (input) channels, response (output) channels, and controlling stimulus-response or stimulus-stimulus relations can be evaluated.

Such systematic behavioral evaluation has revealed six large groups of patients, five of which have not yet been extensively studied. The first group includes patients whose deficit is so mild as to escape detection by simple tests. These cases are frequently considered normal on initial brief bedside examinations. It remains to be seen whether more complex materials, at the sentence, paragraph, and syntactical level, will reveal deficit constellations similar to those shown in other patients tested with the simpler materials.

The second two groups are at the other end of the scale, and completely new test procedures will be required to study them effectively. The most severe deficits are those in which reinforcement is inadequate to maintain behavior, thereby precluding the delineation of a deficit profile. The few such patients we have tested have been those with medially placed frontal lesions exhibiting symptoms of hydrocephalus, clinical states of delirium, and dementia. This is a potentially fruitful area for the application of Pavlovian conditioning techniques. Also untestable by the present methods are patients with deficient instructional control, for their test behavior is completely unrelated to our test materials and procedures. These patients include a number of cases exhibiting the bedside syndrome of central, or Wernicke's, aphasia. Instructional deficits can be differentiated from reinforcement deficits only if reinforcement can be shown to be effective in some other kind of test, such as a less demanding visual or auditory discrimination, in which the need for instructional control is minimal.

The fourth and fifth groups are those who show deficient input (stimulus)[33] or output (response) channels.[36,37] These two groups include the vast majority of cases labelled in a brief bedside examination as showing "agnosia," "pure" word blindness, deafness, mutism, etc. Input deficit reveals itself when a particular type of stimulus fails consistently to control *any* type of response. Output deficit reveals itself when a particular type of response consistently fails to occur in the presence of *any* stimulus. The functions of the input and output channels are assessed by identity tests. These involve a response which is physically identical to the test stimulus. For example, repeating dictated words aloud, copying printed words, and choosing from among a visually presented set of words one which is typed and spelled exactly like the test stimulus, are all examples of responses which are physically identical to the test stimulus. These identity tests require no previous experience with the stimuli and serve principally to test the adequacy of stimulus discrimination and response production in the input and output channels used for testing.

Once these identity tests have shown the adequacy of the input and output channels, those channels and stimuli found adequate can then be used to explore the specificity of stimulus control in "nonidentity" tasks. In these tests, the response required is not physically identical to the test stimulus. Examples include spoken responses to visual stimuli, written response to dictated stimuli, selection of choices (matching) in which, for example, the test stimuli are pictures, and the comparison stimuli are words.

The sixth group of patients, with intact input and output channels, display differential relational deficits between otherwise normally functioning stimulus and response systems. This group, which includes the vast majority of patients whose conventional clinical bedside evaluation reveals clear evidence of aphasic disorder, has revealed a number of deficit profiles. Some include classical syndromes, some appear to be previously undescribed, and some are mainly of methodological and interpretive interest.*

Other investigators have independently devised methods similar in principle to our behavioral model. The principle of using common manipulable object stimuli presented separately in visual, auditory, and palpated form for separate spoken and written naming responses began with Head's six objects.[17] It was popularized in the United States,[8] was increased to twenty objects,[48] is found in modified form as a basis for a currently popular aphasia test battery,[38] and, in reduced form, is present as a subtest in many other aphasia test batteries. Extensive use has been made of the matching-to-sample paradigm as a means of "facilitating" correct responses on verbal tests requiring spoken or written responses where errors appeared.[21,22,48]

Similar procedures have seen extensive use in production examinations of inter- and intramodality performances in cases of surgical sections of the corpus callosum.[13,14]

TRADITIONAL TEST BATTERIES

Another major approach to delineation of aphasic deficits involves the presentation of a wide variety of individual tests, each designed to assess a given aspect of behavior, without deliberate continuity of stimulus material, input and response channels, or reinforcement across the spectrum of tests. Each test in the subgroups is constructed to stand individually and have its own validity. The performance profile that results for a given patient is compared with that obtained in normals and in other aphasic patients.

The corpus of tests included in these traditional batteries appears to have arisen from the large variety of individual tests created by

* See references 23, 24, 33, 34, 43, and 44.

previous aphasiologists,[4] to which modifications have steadily been added. Credit is given to Weisenburg and McBride[49] for the first systematic use of standard clinical psychological tests, including IQ tests, in the evaluation of aphasia. Several major groups of investigators have developed and validated systematically constructed batteries of individual and separate tests to an impressive level of complexity and reliability.[12,39,41]

Many of these test batteries contain an almost panoramic array of individual tests, covering virtually every theoretical aspect of speech function. Under circumstances of increasing complexity in succeeding trials, the subject may be asked to: name visually displayed manipulable objects, pictures, colors, forms, pictures reduced in size, numbers, letters, printed words, printed sentences; recognize sounds such as clapping made by the examiner; point to body parts on command; name a manipulable object placed unseen in either hand; indicate which one of several visually displayed printed words corresponds most closely to dictated sentences; point to the one of several visually presented words which matches the answer to a visually presented question after dictated paragraphs have been read to the subject; silently read printed questions and point to the visually presented words which answer the question; silently read paragraphs and answer printed questions by pointing to the correct printed alternative; count from one to twenty; name the alphabet from A to Z, the days of the week, the months of the year; write numbers, letters, words, and sentences to dictation; answer visually presented or dictated sentences in the form of questions by speaking aloud or writing the answers spontaneously; perform various computations on paper; press buttons which ring a bell or buzzer to indicate which among several alternatives is the principle that underlies a variety of pictures; place unseen objects into unseen holes conforming to the same shape; indicate which tapped rhythm matches the one originally presented; select the printed speech sounds dominant in the spoken form of visually presented words; tap with the index finger of each hand as rapidly as possible; reset a moving clock after it has completed ten cycles; speak aloud the word which is opposite in meaning to that spoken by the examiner or presented visually by the examiner; match spoken words to the correct one of several visually presented words which differ from one another in minor spelling or in similarities of sound or meaning; read a complicated paragraph silently and draw a line through a given letter each time it occurs in the paragraph; copy on paper complex visually presented forms; sort colors according to a previously dictated underlying principle; draw a man; find a figure hidden in a larger visually displayed figure; assemble blocks and other components to match visually displayed models; trace through a visually presented maze; recall a dictated short sentence after the passage of a short period of time; interpret proverbs dictated by the examiner; sing familiar songs; explain the difference between a father's brother and a brother's father, name items missing in a picture which are ordinarily expected to be present; describe the absurdity in a picture deliberately drawn to show an incongruous situation; take up a number of complex bodily positions demonstrated by the examiner seated facing the patient; name pictures presented as line drawings overlapping one another, up to four or five or a greater number of individual line drawings; indicate the direction the arrow should move in a drawing demonstrating a series of levers connected together with an arrow at one end and a handle at the other end; repeat from dictation a long series of complicated and closely related sound sequences; spell words forward and backwards; supply captions for complicated pictures. . . . The individual tests detailed above in simple descriptive form by no means encompass the vast spectrum available.

The brief enumeration of tests available in traditional test batteries points up a commonly noted problem with the utilization of many of these tests: the patient must show by behavior that instructions on the tasks have been sufficient before the examiner is free to conclude or undertake analysis as to reasons for failure. As a consequence, these tests are of value chiefly in demonstrating that the patient is capable of accomplishing them correctly. Reasons for failure can only rarely be analyzed on an individual test basis. Instead, the analyses of the syndromes delineated by these test batteries depend principally upon a comparison of the overall test scores among patients of differing focal brain injury and/or common etiology for their validity and for their value in assessing a deficit in aphasia. As a tool for analyzing the individual deficits or the range of deficits, there is so little deliberate continuity of test stimulus material, or input, or response channels utilized for such testing, as to make the individual tests virtually noncomparable with one another.

However critical our remarks may be concerning the analytic shortcomings of the tests, their value in predicting site and type of brain injury has been empirically validated. The question of which tests are critical, and why, and their relations to language or other behavioral processes have yet to be clarified.

THEORY-CORROBORATING TESTS

A number of individual tests used and popularized by famous investigators[16,17,29,30] were designed to demonstrate a particular point concerning the nature of aphasia, or to corroborate particular theories. Like many of the individual tests in the traditional test batteries, these theory-corroborating tests frequently are of greatest clinical value in demonstrating that the patient is capable of the tested performance, thereby indicating that the individual parameter which the test allegedly assesses is intact. The extent to which the data provided by the aphasic patient corroborate the test originator's views on aphasia is now mainly only a subject of historical interest.

These tests include the well-known three-paper test of Marie:[4] The patient is presented with a piece of paper on which the examiner, in his own handwriting, has written an instruction to the effect that, "When you have finished reading this page, tear the page into three parts. Give one to me. Throw a second

on the floor. Put the third in your pocket." The capacity of the intact patient to translate the examiner's handwriting style and follow this three-step command goes a long way towards settling any issue regarding the presence of aphasia. Goldstein[16] proposed another variety of tests to assess impairment in "abstract attitude." In these tests, the patients were asked to select from among a variety of stimuli the one which did not match the remainder of the group in terms of some functional principle, or to name the overall categorical word which would best describe the functional class of which the demonstrated materials were members, for example, tools. As a later development, Luria[29] has devised a variety of tests of increasing complexity which utilize essentially Pavlovian methods, but which have not yet been popularized in the West.

([Analysis of Aphasia

Despite its clinical frequency and the relatively large number of investigations into its properties, aphasia has proved a difficult subject for study. Definitions of terms remain unagreed upon even at the present time. The use of familiar but poorly defined eponyms, such as Broca's aphasia, to characterize clinical syndromes makes it frequently impossible to determine whether an aspect of aphasic behavior that emerges from detailed analysis is actually a component of the syndrome. Everyday clinical cases regularly provide more exceptions than do illustrations of the rules predicted by the all-encompassing theories of aphasia.

Despite its limitations, the behavioral approach to aphasia provides quantitative assessment of a variety of responses to a range of stimulus materials; it determines the state of individual input and output channels as a prerequisite for the identification of deficient input-output relations; it follows the evolution of syndromes over time; and its data are available for interpretation by any theories. It provided the nucleus of the material detailed below for the analysis of aphasia.

General Properties of Aphasia

Cases of aphasia share many general features of behavior with normal subjects, especially when the latter are tired or tested under difficult conditions. Reinforcement that is inadequate to maintain behavior in the face of frequent errors commonly leads to breakdown of the control exerted by the test procedures. This state of affairs is revealed in a number of ways. The patient may simply stop responding. He may perseverate previously correct responses, even though these responses are complex, i.e., writing whole words. At times, long delays occur before he responds. He complains of being tired or uncomfortable; lame excuses of poor vision, inadequate education, unfamiliarity with the tests, etc., are common. Occasionally, outbursts of anger occur, with the patient scattering the test stimuli around, rising and leaving the test site, turning away, or even assaulting the examiner. Control over the patient's behavior can usually be reestablished by changing to a task he can easily accomplish, increasing the reinforcement, slowing the rate of testing, and similar devices. The patient's ability to return to the task, and perform reliably over a long test session, suggests that "fatigue," traditionally considered a major variable in aphasia, is a reflection of the test procedures. Signs of fatigue are mostly evident when the patient is having difficulty with the test.

The errors occurring when the test situation maintains adequate control over the patient's behavior take three main forms,[24] which are also common with normal subjects. Repetition of a previous response or portion thereof (perseveration) is common. In many instances, a correct response given previously is repeated on a subsequent trial when the patient is having trouble with the test. At times, the source of this repetitious response (perseveration) is less clear. Many nonperseverative errors, such as literal or verbal errors, also show evidence of control exerted by the test situation. Literal errors approximate the desired response along some physical parameter, and take the form of similar sounds ("tog" for "dog") or shapes ("d" for "b"), etc. The response may bear so little physical resemblance to the one desired as to be characterized as neologism or jargon. Verbal errors share some functional class with the desired response; "cow" for "dog," "green" for "orange," and occasionally, "grass" for "green." At levels more complex than words, errors may appear in word sequence or sentence structure (semantic errors); grammatical construction may become simplified (agrammatism); the patient may accept as correct familiar sequences of words into which the examiner has deliberately substituted unexpected words or even neologisms;[52] other forms of errors may occur which become more and more difficult to separate from performances which characterize normal people deficient in education.

As patients and normal cases are retested over extended periods of time, general improvements in performance occur.* In oral and written naming, verbal paraphasic errors continue but are increasingly represented by names within the test set and decreasingly by names not in the test set. Even the patients' spontaneous responses gradually become restricted to words that are involved in the test itself. Presentation of the first letter or two letters of short words frequently used in the tests are sufficient for the experienced patient to respond correctly; introduction of novel stimulus materials prompts a dramatic reduction in the rate of performance and an increase in errors. Repeated testing with stimuli previously found difficult is associated with considerable evidence of patient dissatisfaction as soon as the first trial occurs, demonstrating his learned familiarity with the components of the test. In addition to gradual learning, some of the improvements are sudden, even after long periods of poor performance on a given test, and appear to represent newly discovered abilities, whose origins remain obscure.[35] In most instances, however, the performance improves in a slow but steady fashion.

A dichotomy in performance between identity and nonidentity tests[44] also characterizes

* See references 17, 23, 24, 33, 35, and 44.

aphasic and normal cases. Scores on tests for which identity responses are available equal or exceed those tests for which these responses are not available (nonidentity). Identity tests (see the section on test methods, p. 281) must be subdivided into first- and second-order identities for this rule to hold. In first-order identity tests, the patient need only indicate the physical identity of the same stimulus presented twice in the same modality. For example, a patient points to the blue color identical to the blue test stimulus, palpates a skeleton key exactly as he palpated the same key just before, nods when he hears the same word heard earlier as the test stimulus, etc. In second-order identity tests, the patient is required to cross a modality or to produce a response which takes a physical form identical to the test stimulus. Examples include repeating from dictation, copying on paper from sight or touch, and matching palpated manipulable objects to visual manipulable objects. Such tests, although they do not involve actual physical identities, can nevertheless be done correctly by normal subjects even if they have had no previous experience with the stimuli. No exception occurs to the rule that first-order identity performances equal or exceed nonidentity performances on equivalent tests, but an occasional deficit in performance of second-order identity tests may occur in aphasic patients when the equivalent nonidentity test is intact. For example, when presented with a series of dictated letters spelling a word, the patient may succeed in pronouncing the word at a time when he experiences difficulty repeating the sequence of individual letters. In general, however, both first- and second-order identity tests are accomplished successfully at times when the nonidentity forms of the test are not.

When identity tests are done poorly, input or output deficits must be suspected. When identity tests are done well, poor performances on nonidentity tests reveal relational disorders, i.e., responses are deficient only in relation to certain stimuli, or stimulus control is deficient only when certain responses are called for. Relational disorders, i.e., impaired performance on tests in which the correctly spoken, written, or matching-to-sample response requires previous experience with the test stimulus, prove to be critical components of syndromes that have classically emphasized input or output deficits, and may be taken to define the most interesting aspects, at least, of aphasia.

Syndromes with Greatest Emphasis on Output Channel Deficits

VOCAL OUTPUT CHANNEL AND GENERAL RELATIONAL DISORDER

Behavioral studies of cases which initially appear to typify the clinical bedside syndrome of total aphasia, and later are consistent with Broca's aphasia,[6] have corroborated traditional features, but, in addition, have revealed a number of findings hitherto undescribed in these syndromes.[35] These new findings prompt a reconsideration of the anatomical mechanisms and explanations.

The deficit profile has four main components.[35] A double deficit is found in oral naming; first, the patient is mute and produces no vocal responses on either identity or nonidentity tests. Later, the mutism clears away, as indicated by satisfactory oral naming in identity tests of repeating from dictation. From that point on, the second disorder, a relational deficit, is revealed: impaired performance in nonidentity oral naming tests. In contrast with oral naming, the performance on identity tests of written naming and matching-to-sample are intact from the beginning. Later, when oral-naming identity performance becomes adequate, so that anarthria can no longer account for poor scores on nonidentity oral naming tests, nonidentity written and oral naming can be compared in response to the same stimuli. At this point, the third deficit component appears, i.e., superiority of nonidentity written naming over nonidentity oral naming. The fourth component is demonstrated in all response forms and stimulus materials in nonidentity tests, namely, performance on tests involving the sounds of words exceeds performance on tests involving the sounds of single letters. This component is demonstrated by better scores in matching and writing of dictated words than of single letters, and better scores in the oral naming of visually presented words than of single letters. By contrast, most wholly visual tests are performed satisfactorily for both materials: The patient can match dissimilarly shaped upper- with lower-case letters having a name in common (i.e., E—e), and even can match scrambled words with pictures. Interestingly, one test ostensibly involving wholly visual functions, matching visual letters with homonymous visual words that do not contain the letter (c—sea, q—cue, i—eye), is done poorly. The time required for the delineation of each of the main features of the syndrome varies from a few weeks to several years in individual cases.

The initial mutism is severe. Only a few noises are made in forced exhalation. With time, vocalization emerges to testable levels. It shows elements of dyspraxia, revealed by improper setting of the oropharynx, and impaired coordination of respiration with vocalization, resulting in lack of smooth speech melody i.e., dysprosody. Despite traditional emphasis on the attributes of the vocal response,[1,15,27] performance on the identity tasks in repeating from dictation follows the expected patterns of exceeding that of the nonidentity tasks of producing the same names in response to appropriate visual, palpated, or even nonverbal sound stimuli.

The duration of the mutism is variable. In a few right-handed cases, the deficit ameliorates in a dramatically brief period—days to one or a few weeks.[32] Such rapid amelioration in a right-handed patient with left inferior frontal infarction has been considered a sign of superficial involvement of a cortical surface.[16] The intact intrahemispherical pathways (arcuate fasciculus) through which the central language zone (Wernicke's) is considered to relate to the ipsilateral inferior frontal region (Broca's area), and thence transcallosally to the nondominant inferior frontal region, have traditionally[16] been presumed sufficient to permit the nondominant inferior frontal region to mediate the vocal responses and permit the "recovery." Recently,[32] righthanded cases have been followed through this period of dramatically rapid amelioration of vocal speech deficit. Detailed autopsy evidence showed major damage to the dominant inferior frontal region, including the pathways considered necessary to mediate "recovery." Traditional formulations do not explain these cases, and alternative pathways, as yet undelineated, must be considered. The findings suggest the need for revision of current notions of cerebral "dominance" for speech, and indicate that the degree to which the inferior frontal regions share the mediation of vocal speech is only poorly understood.

The superiority of written over oral naming, when identity responses for both are intact, calls into question some notions of how writing behavior is mediated. Most classic[26] and many modern[25] accounts indicate that the deficit in written naming is a reflection of that in oral naming, and is at least as severe, usually more so. Accounts of aphasic deficits consider that writing reflects two components. In the first component, the morphology of the individual letters and digits is believed to depend on a direct pathway from visual to motor regions which guide hand movements.[26] Until recently, no theory has challenged the classic notion that the second component, the verbal content of the writing, depends upon pathways which pass through Broca's area, and presumably utilize it as a way station: "one speaks as one writes."[25] The only quantitative study[35] of this important subject, revealing a superiority of nonidentity written naming over nonidentity oral naming when both were adequate on identity tests, challenges this classical interpretation. The independence of written and oral naming suggests a new view,[35] which does not assume an obligatory relation between written and oral naming based on a unitary brain mechanism. Instead, the coexistence of superficially similar deficits in written and oral naming may merely reflect anatomical proximity of the two regions subserving these separate motor responses, favoring their common involvement by a single pathological lesion. Such anatomic proximity implies no functional interdependence between the two areas.

The more severe deficit with letter rather

than with word sounds, common to written and oral naming, appears also in matching-to-sample behavior. The emphasis in traditional formulations,[9,26,27,50] which envisioned the two naming deficits as reflecting correlated output disorders, can be properly shifted to include all forms of behavior. As a result, the deficit can be considered central to the input and output channels, per se. It must be pointed out, however, in anticipation of the following section on central aphasia, that the deficit profile in which nonidentity tasks show better scores with words than letters is opposite to that commonly found in cases conforming to traditional criteria for central aphasia.[44] Instead, this disproportionate deficit in nonidentity tasks involving the sounds of letters appears unique to this syndrome.[35]

Explanation of the data requires still further revision of accounts of both Broca's and total aphasia. Classical writings have explained the syndrome of total aphasia as a combination of Broca's and Wernicke's (central) aphasia.[27] The syndrome outlined above, although it conforms to classical clinical bedside criteria for total aphasia, is not explainable as a simple combination of Broca's and central aphasia. In addition, the complexity of the satisfactory responses in many nonidentity tasks suggests that the term, "total aphasia," is misleading. The deficit appears highly specific to certain verbal tasks, with disproportionately better performances on others of seemingly similar or greater difficulty.

Definitions of Broca's aphasia have given greatest attention to the disorder in oral speech,[2] with emphasis on the dyspraxic, dysprosodic, dysgrammatic components; on the issue of coexisting dyspraxias for nonvocal movements involving the same oropharyngeal musculature; on the coexistence of facial, lingual, and palatal paresis; on the issue of cerebral dominance; and on the exact location and depth of the lesion. Scanty information exists on the writing deficit, which is usually explained on the basis of the presumed dependence of verbal content on vocal speech, implicit or explicit. Broca's two cases[6] appear to have had principally disorders of vocalization. Unsettling reference,[5,27,49] however, has al-

ways been made to mild or moderate impairments in "comprehension," which occur in tests of silent reading and in performance of multistep dictated or printed commands. Ingenious tests with normals,[29] in which the tongue has been restrained, have shown impairments in reading, implicating vocal speech deficit as a partial explanation for the otherwise unaccountable deficits in comprehension in Broca's aphasia. Such explanations, however, do not account for the deficiencies in response to auditory dictated commands. Another approach has been anatomical,[30] suggesting that clinically unsuspected posterior extension of the lesion has occurred along the postcentral and parietal operculum, accounting for the minor central aphasia impairments. As emphasized above, however, the behavioral deficit in response to dictated stimuli in this syndrome is not typical of central aphasia. Finally, little or no qualitative differences separate the vocal and graphic behavior in total and Broca's aphasia.

The ambiguities surrounding the definition of Broca's aphasia have not been clarified over the years. Considering the great similarity between later cases of the traditional bedside syndrome of total aphasia, the uncertain status of "comprehension" in cases of Broca's aphasia, the anatomic problems surrounding the extent of the lesion in autopsied cases, and the wide variation in the course of the deficit, one might ask whether actual deficit features or mere historical precedent substantiate the syndrome of Broca's aphasia. The present authors suspect that the understandable desire to honor Broca's efforts at anatomicopathologic correlation serve as the chief basis for continued recognition of a separate syndrome referred to as Broca's aphasia. Further analysis of the syndrome of which the classical Broca's and total aphasia appear to be elements may be expected to modify views concerning the function of the anterior Sylvian operculum and the cerebral organization of language.

Disproportionate Literal Paraphasia

In this syndrome,[29] errors appear in both identity and nonidentity oral naming tasks, but not in equivalent tasks involving matching-to-sample. Although this syndrome is classified as both an identity and nonidentity output disorder of oral naming, the patient shows none of the mutism characteristically observed in the syndrome described above. Instead, vocalizations occur readily, but are equally erroneous on identity and nonidentity tasks. For example, repeating aloud, reading from text, and oral naming of visual, auditory, or palpated stimuli show similar scores with similar errors. In contrast to the deficit in oral naming, tasks not involving a spoken response, such as matching-to-sample, are done extremely well, and written naming is often quite satisfactory. The patient's exasperation and efforts at self-correction of his oral naming errors attest to his ready awareness of the deficit. The patient's errors include a disproportionate number of literal paraphasias, involving close anatomic approximations of the oropharyngeal positions required to produce the correct responses in each of the articulatory classes from lip to pharynx position. Errors increase with the rate of speech and with the proximity of the oropharyngeal settings required to produce the sequences of syllables.

In Wernicke's original scheme,[50] the term "conduction aphasia" was proposed for the syndrome, which could be considered to reflect interruption of the pathways from the "sensory" (Wernicke's) speech region to the "motor" (Broca's) regions. As originally constructed, the syndrome contained three elements. First, comprehension would be intact, since Wernicke's region was preserved. Second, the motor elements of speech (articulation, prosody) would be intact, reflecting the spared motor-speech regions. Third, content of speech would be paraphasic, as tested by spontaneous speech, reading aloud, and repeating from dictation. This third feature, the only real deficit to be found, was the expected result of the pathologic interruption of pathways linking Wernicke's region to the motor (Broca's) speech region. It is important to stress that the deficit was to take the form of paraphasic oral speech. Only the motor elements—articulation and speech melody—were considered to be normal, indicating that the deficit in speech does not merely reflect involvement of the inferior frontal (Broca's) region.

Cases frequently appear clinically which exhibit paraphasic, normally articulated, and normally melodic speech, with superficially intact comprehension, and are considered to satisfy the criteria for conduction aphasia. In most such cases, however, deficits in comprehension can readily be brought out by testing silent reading or matching-to-sample, which do not involve oral speech. These cases are more frequently better reclassified as examples of mild central (Wernicke's) aphasia.

The search for cases defined by the more stringent criterion of no demonstrable deficit in comprehension, has yielded few cases of conduction aphasia.[16,20,28,36] Awareness of this interesting syndrome has increased only in the 1960s,[14] but most reports are in the early literature.[16,20,28,36] Presumably, their rarity reflects the greater likelihood that pathologic injuries to the fiber pathways connecting the Wernicke and Broca regions would not be as discrete as required. Instead, the injury is more likely to involve larger areas, and result in more traditional syndromes of central, motor, or total aphasia.

Even fewer cases satisfying the clinical criteria have provided autopsy data. Meager though these data are[20,28,36] they pose a problem in interpretation by classic theory, which predicts that the main lesion should lie in the pathways linking the auditory with the motor-speech regions. Attempts[14] to identify these pathways have focused on the arcuate fasciculus, a white matter bundle which appears to pass between the posterior superior temporal plane (Wernicke's region) and the inferior frontal region (Broca's region), and satisfies the gross anatomic requirements. Autopsy cases[20,28,36] of "conduction" aphasia, however, have shown cortical surface infarction, apparently of embolic origin, without necessary involvement of the more deeply situated arcuate fasciculus. To date, no cases have been reported that show pure involvement of the arcuate fasciculus. The clinical setting for such a lesion occurs occasionally in putamenal hemorrhage, in which the hemorrhagic mass is limited to the posterior lateral putamen and the immediate surrounding area, which includes the arcuate fasciculus. In the one such case that has come to light,[31] the clinical syndrome was more of a central than a conduction aphasia.

Luria[10] has described a syndrome of *afferent motor aphasia*. In contrast with the usual form of motor aphasia, which he has referred to as "efferent," literal paraphasic errors in oral speech are attributable to anatomic settings of the oral apparatus that are imprecise but closely approximating those required. The lesion is presumed to lie in the postcentral region, interfering with sensory kinesthetic feedback from the oral cavity. The clinical findings agree with those delineated by behavioral methodology, adhering closely to classically defined conduction aphasia, but pointing clearly to mechanisms different in principle from those proposed classically.

The extent to which literal and verbal paraphasias occur independently of one another, as well as the basic deficit(s) reflected by literal paraphasia, remain important unclarified issues. Literal paraphasias that prove principally to reflect oropharyngeal anatomic approximations point to sensory and/or motor Rolandic deficits.[29] Traditionally,[19] by contrast, literal paraphasias are considered to take the form of homonyms of the desired response, and to reflect auditory input deficits. Verbal paraphasias, by contrast, are traditionally thought of as synonyms. However, few studies specify the relative frequency of each type. Furthermore, literal and verbal paraphasias are considered to occur together with such regularity as to suggest some mechanism in common, yet even fewer studies document the frequency with which they occur in the same case, especially a case with autopsy material. As a result, the theories on either form of paraphasia are largely speculative.

GENERAL RELATIONAL DISORDERS

A surprising proportion of cases tested by behavioral methods show deficits only on nonidentity tasks. No deficits are found for a given test stimulus on identity tests of repeating the stimulus from dictation, copying at sight, or matching the stimulus to its exact duplicate in the same modality. These intact performances permit the assertion that sensory discrimination and response production are adequate for these stimulus materials, and preclude an explanation of the impairments that is based on deficient input and output channels.

Although deficit profiles observed on nonidentity tests across the various stimulus materials take several forms, one in particular typifies that predicted by traditional formulations of central, or true, aphasia.[43,44] This profile shows a similar deficit in response to each of the classes of test stimuli. For example, in response to the same stimuli, whether they are single letters, words, pictures, color names, colors, digit names, digits, or manipulable objects, scores on nonidentity tasks of matching-to-sample exceed those for oral naming, which exceed those for written naming. Improvement occurs gradually with time and more or less equally with all types of test stimuli. At any point in time, errors may occur in response to any individual stimulus, but no individual stimulus reliably sets the stage for an error each time it is presented.

The traditional formulation[46,50] of the true or central deficit in aphasia involves disruption of a supramodal function whose normal role is to relate physically dissimilar stimuli which are verbally equivalent. This function was held to be accomplished by the "concept center."[26,50,51] Wernicke,[50] among others, considered this function actually to be performed by the portion of the brain outside those pathways subserving the instrumentalities of language.

Wernicke[50,51] argued that the initial acquisition of language is probably an auditory experience. Learning to speak aloud would involve auditory modulation of vocal efforts. Reading aloud would involve acquisition of an auditory-visual link between sounds and graphic stimuli, establishing pathways which would then permit instructions to the vocal apparatus for reading aloud utilizing the auditory region as an intermediate. A similar link would modulate graphic motor behavior. Lesions of the auditory region and connections would be expected to disrupt these relations.

The added assumption was that these separate behaviors permanently depend upon the auditory region. This dependence would account for the overall deficit in the utilization of the instrumentalities of language in lesions affecting the auditory region and related pathways.

Wernicke was careful to separate the essentially servile performances utilizing the instrumentality of language from the more abstract and poorly understood aspects of brain function involving "concepts." Diagrammatically,[50],[51] his scheme showed pathways from the ear to the superior temporal lobe serving auditory speech discrimination; pathways from the superior temporal lobe to the inferior frontal region serving to convey the instructions for vocalization to the motor region; pathways from the inferior frontal region to the brain stem serving to innervate the bulbar apparatus to produce speech sounds; pathways from the superior temporal lobe to the occipital region linking auditory with visual functions to subserve reading. None of these pathways necessarily serves "understanding" or "central language function." Instead, pathways from the superior temporal lobe to the remainder of the brain were considered to permit the auditory experiences, and those visual and palpated sensory experiences translated into auditory equivalences, to arouse associations in the remainder of the brain which provide "meaning" to the stimuli. Similarly, pathways outside the main speech zone were considered to converge upon the motor speech regions (Broca's area) to permit "meaning" to be given to vocal utterances. Without challenging the notions in principle, Dejerine[9] added the angular gyrus as a word center, whose supramodal function was to relate auditory and visual lexical stimuli as verbal equivalents, and to guide the motor regions for graphic responses. Recent arguments[14] have modernized the proposal of the angular gyrus as exerting a supramodal function relating physically dissimilar but verbally equivalent stimuli. Others[11],[29] have proposed essentially similar translatory functions for the inferior parietal regions, of which the angular gyrus is a component. These views argue that integration, or morphosynthesis,[11] is the basic

function to be expected of the inferior parietal region, since its anatomic position lies between the main primary sensory receiving areas in the cerebral cortex.

Emphasis on this region as central to language function helps encompass many aspects of behavior in such cases. The patients exhibit a remarkable unawareness of the extent, the time, even the existence, of their deficit. Both literal and verbal errors (especially verbal) occur in all forms of language usage, in tasks involving comprehension, and in language formulation, with scarcely a pause for correction. Oral speech tends to contain far more words than expected or required for efficient communication. The term "logorrhea,"[7] also referred to as augmentation and press of speech,[16] denotes the tremendous barrage of vocalizations that frequently characterizes these cases of central aphasia. In addition, efforts to instruct the patient to modify his response for different tests frequently are unsuccessful;[16] they are often met with perseveration of previous responses or principles of response, even though the tests have changed. Particularly frustrating to the examiner is the frequent tendency of patients to respond to commands only by acknowledging that a command was given; efforts to vary the command by adding, "please," "I would like you to . . . ," etc., are frequently met by a reply like "O.K., I will," but with no actual performance. Even more suggestive of a unitary deficit is the all pervasive nature of the deficit in language usage, which appears in tests involving spoken, written, and matching-to-sample responses.

Despite the many indices favoring these all-encompassing views of language function, a series of findings, both anatomic and behavioral, remain unaccounted for. Anatomically, an occasional case whose deficit profile suggests the traditional syndrome of total aphasia is shown at autopsy to have a lesion wholly confined to the dominant temporal lobe.[16] The temporal-lobe mutism in these cases contrasts sharply with the logorrhea usually characterizing such lesions. While temporal-lobe mutism suggests that the posterior Sylvian regions exert the major controlling function over the output of the inferior frontal region, such findings pose the difficult problem of explaining opposite observations by the same anatomic lesion. Suggestions that the more commonly observed logorrhea represents a release effect in which the inferior frontal region "runs on unchecked," seem less tenable in view of the existence of temporal-lobe mutism. Another suggestion is that logorrhea may represent a functional sign of decreased awareness by the patient of the extent of his deficit.

Another major anatomic question remains on how limited a lesion may produce the syndrome.[45] Autopsies commonly show infarction which varies considerably from case to case, spreading over variable distances from the superior temporal plane to the parietal, occipital, and temporal regions. There are only a few well-studied cases of focal lesions confined to the superior temporal plane. As a consequence of the wide differences in the neuropathologic basis for the clinical syndrome, there is considerable variation in what different authors accept as the anatomical boundaries of Wernicke's area. For some, the area is considered to be confined strictly to the superior temporal plane just posterior to Heschl's transverse auditory gyri, and ending before or at the inferior parietal lobules posteriorly and the second temporal convolution inferiorly. Other authors consider that the region is simply the large posterior Sylvian territory, encompassing all the previously mentioned areas and extending as far back as the anterior occipital region. This lack of universal agreement as to the extent of Wernicke's area has led to considerable ambiguity in the components of the individual syndrome.

Behavioral findings provide yet another series of problems for unitary views of language function, as well as the opportunity to test a number of predictions implicit in traditional theses. As alluded to above under Vocal Output Channel, demonstration of opposite relational deficits in test scores with words and single letters between cases clinically classified as total aphasia or as central aphasia, respectively, leads to the realization that the relational deficit in total aphasia is not identical to that in central aphasia, and forces the abandonment of the assumption that a common

deficit profile encompasses all relational performances in cases of aphasia. However, the coexistence of the severe output channel deficit in oral naming in total aphasia dilutes the significance of the findings somewhat, since other large differences separate the two types of cases.

The demonstration of differential deficits among patients who show only relational deficits further dispels notions of a unitary hierarchical deficit profile in aphasia. For example, some cases perform better in nonidentity tasks involving matching than in oral naming, and better in oral than in written naming,[43] while others show a superiority of nonidentity oral naming over both matching-to-sample and written naming for a given class of stimulus materials.[44] With different classes of stimulus materials, exceptions have been documented in which scores in nonidentity tasks with one material exceed those in another with one patient, while the opposite hierarchy of scores with these materials is seen in another patient.[44]

Evidence of still greater complexity in relational deficit profiles is provided by examples of different deficits with different materials in the *same* patient. One patient,[44] for example, experienced more difficulty in naming (reading) visual picture names than in naming the pictures; with colors and color names, however, the opposite was true—he had more trouble naming colors than visual color names.

Evolution of the deficit profiles across time also reveals a number of surprising changes. A smooth evolution sometimes occurs,[35] all scores rising uniformly and gradually to approximate satisfactory levels. In a number of cases, however, improvements occur gradually in one or more test stimulus materials, input, or response channels, leaving others essentially unchanged or improving at a much slower rate.[44] As a consequence of these unequal changes, the later profile is quite different from that predicted by the initial assessments. Autopsied cases[33] present anatomic findings for which a decision has to be made regarding the behavioral correlation. Failure of investigators to follow these evolutions has probably contributed significantly to interpretive problems in retrospective reviews of clinical anatomical studies.

One byproduct of the systematic behavioral approach is the opportunity to assess predictions of deficit profiles based on traditional syndrome formulation. The behavior presumed to be involved in spelling, in particular, proved of interest.[34,43] The steps involved in pronouncing words in response to dictated spelled words, or conversely, in spelling aloud in response to dictated words, have been held to require, first, the "mental" transfer of auditory to visual images, and then the "reading" aloud of these mental images as words or sequences of single letters.[14] These views are the basis for explaining the impaired performance on spelling tasks by patients with the syndrome of dyslexia and dysgraphia. Destruction of the angular gyrus, held responsible for the mental transformations, would be expected to result in spelling deficits. By transforming the presumed mental operations into observable behavior, it was possible to test these predictions, and to find them unsupported by data. Patients who could pronounce dictated spelled words, and spell dictated pronounced words were, nevertheless, deficient in writing the dictated spelled words, that is to say, in explicitly demonstrating transformation of the auditory stimuli to their visual graphic equivalents. Nor could they read visually presented words aloud, the second presumed component of the mental task. Thus, explicit behavioral analysis revealed patients who could perform both spelling tasks, yet were unable to perform the tasks whose "mental" accomplishment was supposed to make spelling possible. Verifiable behavioral alternatives to such mentalistic mechanisms appear warranted if we are to avoid the postulation of plausible-sounding anatomic correlations to explain nonexistent behavioral processes, or vice versa.

The problems posed above for unitary notions of aphasia remain unsolved; the behavioral data are not as yet sufficient in scope to supplant traditional formulations in their entirety. Perhaps the major value of the behavioral observations at present is to call attention to the usefulness of the methodology. By delineating individual components of the deficit profile, some understanding of the hierarchies of relevant variables can be achieved. Behavioral studies also suggest that one should approach aphasia by emphasizing techniques which are most likely to reveal behavior that is still available to the patient, rather than design tests to promote errors. It may even become feasible to measure the deficits in aphasia by the lengths the examiner must go to provide a setting for the patient to accomplish the desired behavior. By placing the burden on the examiner to find the patient's capacities, deficits reflecting artifacts of the test situation would be reduced, and emphasis would shift to the delineation of variables which permit the patient to acquire new behavior, and perhaps mitigate his aphasia.

(Approach to a Clinical Case of Aphasia

The concern of the clinician approaching a case of aphasia is to clarify the syndrome presented sufficiently to make judgments on the likely anatomic regions affected and on the etiology of the brain injury.

The clinical situations where assessment of aphasia is needed generally fall into four large groups. (1) The patient appears intact and the question arises whether there is any deficit in interpersonal communication at all. Examples include patients who have suffered traumatic head injury, are recovering from suspected encephalitis, or are in the early stages of suspected brain tumor or degenerative brain disease; (2) The patient is grossly aphasic. The approach in such a case involves the attempt to establish what positive behavior, of any kind, is available to the patient, so as to assess what regions of the brain can be inferred to have survived. Examples include patients suffering massive traumatic head injury, devastating strokes, serious encephalitis, and the like; (3) Aphasia may form an important part of the clinical picture and analysis of the positive and negative features of the aphasic deficit may provide diagnostic considerations not available by other means; and (4) There is a heterogenous group of aphasic syndromes which frequently pass unnoticed in the general physical and sometimes even in the neurologic examination. The alert consultant can find a fair percentage of such cases by constant readiness to pursue the required tests.

When the patient appears intact, he has to be presented with the most difficult of aphasic tests. The purpose is not to analyze errors, but to anticipate satisfactory performance. If the patient performs well, such tests should put questions of aphasia to rest. If he does poorly, little or no information regarding the nature of the aphasia has been provided. In such an instance, the examiner has learned merely that tests which do permit analysis of errors will be necessary. An example of a complex test is Marie's three-paper test.[4] Others include a complex picture of incongruous situations used in standard IQ tests, dictated or printed familiar metaphors (a rolling stone gathers no moss, etc.) and word problems from many of the standard IQ tests; the patient is required to describe or write his explanation or solution. In special situations, when the patient's deficits preclude lengthy written or spoken responses, difficult tests involving several steps can be created to permit a minimal motor response to reflect a great deal of complex unobservable behavior. For example, when a patient is asked to hold up the number of fingers that correspond to the position in the alphabet occupied by that letter in the alphabet sequence that comes immediately after the first letter in the name Boston. If he immediately puts up three fingers to correspond to the letter "C," a great deal of behavior has been assessed and the question of aphasia is largely settled. Clearly, these complex tests are of value only in saving examination time in the intact case.

Cases presenting a gross severe aphasia pose almost the opposite problem. In this situation, one attempts to determine what behavior, if any, is available to the patient. The patient should be roused to a state of full alertness, if necessary, before concluding that the patient is untestable. Then, initial attempts should be made to use the simplest and most direct commands, with simultaneous demonstrations of the desired movements. Should some response be forthcoming, it must be determined whether the patient is mimicking the movements or is responding to the content of the command. For spoken responses the examiner can dictate short sounds (ah) and encourage repetition. For graphic responses, simple shapes (circle), etc.; for motor responses, simple movements (wave) may serve to establish some behavior. Any identity tests performed satisfactorily serve to indicate that the input and response channels function per se.

Cases not coming under any form of identity test control can still be profitably examined by using aversive stimuli. Inferences regarding right hemisphere function can be gained in the patient for whom simple avoidance behavior can be conditioned by preceding a noxious stimulus delivered to the left side with a visual, auditory, or somesthetic stimulus. Some assessment of memory can also be made by repeating these tests at regular intervals without retraining.

If the simple identity tests can be performed, then simple nonidentity forms of the same tasks can be done. Advantage should be taken of any incidental movement by the patient, since such occurrence is proof of their availability as behavior per se. Examples include coughing, smiling, turning over in bed, etc. The words involved in commands for these movements should be used for the tests of repeating from dictation and copying from sight. Then these words can be used as dictated commands to try to elicit written responses, and as visual commands for praxic motor or spoken response. Should this much behavior be accessible, the patient can then be further analyzed as outlined in the next section.

Whatever data are obtained provide a baseline for observation of later changes. Declines in the behavioral state may prompt a change in the therapy, or improvement may demonstrate the effectiveness of treatment.

Should the tests described above demonstrate some nonidentity behavior, further analysis of the case is justified. The case may be one for whom analysis of the aphasic syndrome will help clarify the diagnosis. Such efforts can be expected to take time. It will be necessary to use a variety of stimulus materials, to attempt to establish some form of behavioral control with reinforcement techniques (using spoken words, such as good, money, food, etc.), and the identity, then nonidentity, behavior with the various input, and response modalities.

A gratifying by-product of such an analysis is a surprising number of instances in which some differential performance profile emerges that permits a diagnosis of one of the less severe aphasia syndromes. Most frequently observed is a case whose deficit was initially interpreted as motor aphasia or even total aphasia, and for whom analysis permits classification as pure word mutism. Similarly, the rarer cases of pure word deafness usually are considered initially to reflect central, or Wernicke's, aphasia. In the more severe syndromes, the main purpose of such analysis is to establish a baseline for further changes. For example, a hypertensive hemorrhage frequently evolves from a syndrome of minimal central aphasia to fully developed total aphasia, as may temporal-lobe abscess and deep-seated primary or metastatic brain tumor. By contrast, embolic involvement of the cerebrum rather frequently begins as total aphasia only to change to motor aphasia or central aphasia, and finally to a syndrome of amnestic aphasia. Evolution toward or away from more serious deficits is frequently of great value in establishing the etiologic diagnosis in an individual case.

The last group of patients are those for whom the diagnosis of a specific syndrome may be overlooked in more routine clinical medical or neurologic examination. These syndromes require the use of special techniques for their delineation, but depend chiefly upon the awareness of the examiner that these syndromes can exist in a patient whose conversational behavior appears essentially normal. The syndromes include those of the pure alexias with or without agraphia, amnestic aphasia, and the syndromes of nondominant hemisphere ideomotor apraxia (not discussed in this chapter). More exotic behavioral syndromes include "simultanagnosia"[53] and Balint's syndrome.[3] The failure of spontaneous speech with preserved repeating from dictation which can transiently characterize involvement of the anterior cerebral artery territory in the dominant hemisphere,[42] and the syndromes of grossly inappropriate factual content of conversation which may occur in states of increased intracranial pressure and/or unilateral or bilateral frontal disease,[29] are all uncommon, and are beyond the scope of this chapter.

❰ Bibliography

1. ADAMS, R. D. and J. P. MOHR. "Affections of Speech," in M. M. Wintrobe et al., eds., *Harrison's Principles of Internal Medicine*, 7th ed., pp. 137–148. New York: McGraw-Hill, 1974.

2. ALAJOUANINE, T., A. OMBREDAME, and M. DURAND. *Le Syndrome de Désintégration Phonétique dans l'Aphasie*. Paris: Masson, 1939.

3. BALINT, R. "Seelenlähmung des 'Schauens,' Optische Ataxie, Räumliche Störung der Aufmerksamkeit," *Monatsschr. Psychiatr. Neurol.*, 25 (1909), 51.

4. BOLLER, F. and L. A. VIGNOLO. "Latent Sensory Aphasia in Hemisphere-Damaged Patients: An Experimental Study with The Token Test," *Brain*, 89 (1966), 815.

5. BRAIN, R. *Speech Disorders*. London: Butterworths, 1965.

6. BROCA, P. "Remarques sur le siège de la faculté du langage articulé; suivies d'une observation d'aphémie," *Bull. Soc. Anat.*, 6 (1861), 330.

7. BROWN, J. W. *Aphasia, Apraxia, and Agnosia*. Springfield, Ill.: Charles C. Thomas, 1972.

8. CHESTER, E. D. "Aphasia," *Bull. Neurol. Inst.*, 6 (1937), 134–144.

9. DEJERINE, J. and C. MIRALLIE. *L'Aphasie Sensoriélle*. Paris: Steinheil, 1896.

10. DEJERINE, J. and N. VIALET. "La Localisation anatomique de la cécité verbale," *C. R. Soc. Biol. (Paris)*, 4 (1891), 61.

11. DENNY-BROWN, D. and R. A. CHAMBERS.

"The Parietal Lobe and Behavior," *Res. Publ. Ass. Res. Nerv. Ment. Dis.*, 36 (1958), 36.

12. EISENSON, J. *Examining for Aphasia.* New York: The Psychological Corporation, 1954.

13. GAZZANIGA, M. S., J. E. BOGEN, and R. W. SPERRY. "Observations on Visual Perception after Disconnection of the Cerebral Hemispheres in Man," *Brain*, 88 (1965), 221.

14. GESCHWIND, N. "Disconnection Syndromes in Animals and Man," *Brain*, 88 (1965), 237, 585.

15. ———. "Focal Disturbances of Higher Nervous Activity," in P. B. Beeson and W. McDermott, eds., *Cecil-Loeb Textbook of Medicine*, 13th ed., pp. 99–102. Philadelphia: Saunders, 1971.

16. GOLDSTEIN, K. *Language and Language Disturbances.* New York: Grune & Stratton, 1948.

17. HEAD, H. *Aphasia and Kindred Disorders of Speech.* New York; Macmillan, 1926.

18. HOWES, D. "Application of the Word-frequency Concept to Aphasia," in A. V. S. de Reuck and M. O'Connor, eds., *Disorders of Language*, pp. 47–75. Boston: Little, Brown, 1964.

19. JAKOBSON, R. "Towards a Linguistic Topology of Aphasic Impairments," in A. V. S. de Reuck and M. O'Connor, eds., *Disorders of Language*, pp. 2–42. Boston: Little, Brown, 1964.

20. KLEIST, K. *Gehirnpathologie.* Leipzig: Barth, 1934.

21. KREINDLER, A. and A FRADIS. *Performances in Aphasia.* Paris: Gauthier-Villars, 1968.

22. KREINDLER, A. and V. IONASESCU. "A Case of 'Pure' Word Blindness," *J. Neurol. Neurosurg. Psychiatry*, 24 (1961), 257.

23. LEICESTER, J., M. SIDMAN, L. T. STODDARD et al. "Some Determinants of Visual Neglect," *J. Neurol. Neurosurg. Psychiatry*, 32 (1969), 580.

24. ———. "The Nature of Aphasic Responses," *Neuropsychol.*, 9 (1971), 141.

25. LHERMITTE, F. and J. C. GAUTIER. "Aphasia," in R. J. Vinken and G. W. Bruyn, eds., *Handbook of Clinical Neurology*, Vol. 4, pp. 84–104. Amsterdam: North-Holland, 1969.

26. LICHTHEIM, L. "On Aphasia," *Brain*, 7 (1887), 433.

27. LIEPMANN, H. "Diseases of the Brain," in

C. W. Burr, ed., *Curschmann's Textbook on Nervous Diseases*, Vol. 1, pp. 467–80, 518–51. Philadelphia: Blakiston, 1915.

28. LIEPMANN, H. and M. PAPPENHEIM. "Über einen Fall von Sogenannter Leitungsaphasie mit Anatomischem Befund," *Z. Neurol. Psychiatr.*, 27 (1914), 1.

29. LURIA, A. *Higher Cortical Functions in Man.* New York: Basic Books, 1966.

30. MARIE, P. "Révision de le quéstion de l'aphasie," *Sem Méd.*, 26 (1906), 241, 493, 565.

31. MASSACHUSETTS GENERAL HOSPITAL. *Case Records*, Autopsy No. 31772. Boston: 1968.

32. MOHR, J. P. "Rapid Amelioration of Motor Aphasia," *Arch. Neurol.*, 28 (1973), 77.

33. MOHR, J. P., J. LEICESTER, L. T. STODDARD et al. "Right Hemianopia with Memory and Color Deficits in Circumscribed Left Posterior Cerebral Artery Territory Infarction," *Neurology*, 21 (1971), 1104.

34. MOHR, J. P. and T. R. PRICE. "An Unusual Case of Dyslexia with Dysgraphia," *Neurology*, 21 (1971), 430.

35. MOHR, J. P., M. SIDMAN, L. T. STODDARD et al. "Evolution of the Deficit in Total Aphasia," *Neurology*, 23 (1973), 1302.

36. PERSHING, H. "A Case of Wernicke's Conduction Aphasia with Autopsy," *J. Nerv. Ment. Dis.*, 27 (1900), 369.

37. PICK, A. *Die Agrammatischen Störungen.* Berlin: Springer, 1913.

38. PORCH, B. *Porch Index of Communicative Abilities.* Palo Alto: Consulting Psychologist Press, 1970.

39. REITAN, R. "The Significance of Dysphasia for Intelligence and Adaptive Abilities," *J. Psychol.*, 50 (1960), 355.

40. RUSSELL, W. R. and M. L. E. ESPIR. *Traumatic Aphasia.* London: Oxford, 1961.

41. SCHUELL, H., J. J. JENKINS, and E. JIMENEZ-PABON. *Aphasia in Adults.* New York: Hoeber, 1964.

42. SCHWAB, O. "Über Vorübergehende Aphasische Störungen nach Rindenexcision aus dem Linken Stirnhirn bei Epileptikern," *Dtsch. Z. Nervenkeilk.*, 94 (1926), 177.

43. SIDMAN, M. "The Behavioral Analysis of Aphasia," *J. Psychiatr. Res.*, 8 (1971), 413.

44. SIDMAN, M., L. T. STODDARD, J. P. MOHR et al. "Behavioral Studies of Aphasia: Methods of Investigations and Analysis," *Neuropsychol.*, 9 (1971), 119.

45. STARR, M. A. "The Pathology of Sensory Aphasia with an Analysis of Fifty Cases in

Which Broca's Centre was not Diseased,"
Brain, 12 (1889), 82.

46. TEUBER, H. L. "Lacunae and Research Approaches to Them," in C. H. Millikan and F. L. Darley, eds., *Brain Mechanisms Underlying Speech and Language*, pp. 204–216. New York: Grune & Stratton, 1967.

47. WEIGL, E. "On the Construction of Standard Psychological Tests in Cases of Brain Damage," *J. Neurol. Sci.*, 3 (1966), 123.

48. WEIGL, E. and A. FRADIS. "Semiologische Untersuchungen der Alexie," *Zh. Nevropatol. Psikhiatr.*, 59 (1959), 1425.

49. WEISENBURG, T. and K. E. McBRIDE. *Apha-*

sia. New York: Hafner, 1964.

50. WERNICKE, C. *Der Aphasische Symptomencomplex*. Breslau: Cohn & Weigert, 1874.

51. ———. "The Symptomcomplex of Aphasia," in A. Church ed., *Modern Clinical Medicine*, pp. 265–324. New York: Appleton, 1908.

52. WHITAKER, H. A. "Neurolinguistics," in W. O. Dingwall, ed., *A Survey of Linguistic Science*, pp. 136–252. College Park: University of Maryland Press, 1971.

53. WOLPERT, I. "Die Simultanagnosie—Störung der Gesamtauffassung," *Z. Neurol. Psychiatr.*, 93 (1924), 397.

CHAPTER 12

PSYCHIATRIC DISTURBANCES ASSOCIATED WITH ENDOCRINE DISORDERS*

Edward J. Sachar

⟨ Introduction

THE EVALUATION of psychopathology in patients with endocrine disorders poses problems for the psychiatrist, especially in determining what specific relation the endocrine disease has to the psychiatric abnormalities. In such disorders, there are many nonspecific factors which can affect mental functioning. Obviously, the mental status of the patient needs to be interpreted in the light of his premorbid functioning. Beyond

that, it should be noted that endocrine disease is often a severe stress involving loss of functions, feelings of illness, and changes in appearance, as well as sometimes posing a threat to life itself; the vulnerable personality may well decompensate under these conditions.

Furthermore, endocrine diseases have widespread biochemical and physiological consequences, and it is often difficult to determine whether the mental changes noted are due to direct hormonal influences on the brain, or to associated disturbances in electrolyte metabolism, blood sugar, renal function, and so forth. Unfortunately, much of the literature is obscure on these important points. Furthermore,

* Supported in part by NIMH Career Scientists Grant K2–MH–22613 and NIMH Project Grant MH–13402.

Peter Gruen assisted in the bibliographical review.

systematic psychiatric assessments have not been reported as frequently as one would like. For example, a description of a patient as being "agitated, confused, and delusional," leaves it unclear as to whether one is dealing with an organic mental syndrome or another type of psychotic reaction. In addition, because of the great difficulty of assembling nonbiased series and adequate control groups, precise data about the incidence of mental dysfunction specifically due to endocrine diseases are hard to gather. Elucidation of some of these issues is provided by observation of patients receiving hormone therapy, although here too consideration must be given to the mental effects of the medical illness being treated. It is with these limitations in mind, then, that this summary of the current status of knowledge about psychiatric disturbances in endocrine disorders is presented.

For a full medical discussion of the endocrine disorders, as well as a summary of related mental disturbances, the reader is referred to Williams' *Textbook of Endocrinology*.[92] For a recent comprehensive survey of the psychiatric aspects of endocrine disease, with an extensive bibliography, see Smith et al.[76]

(Adrenal Disorders

Cushing's Syndrome

Cushing's syndrome is produced by excessive secretion of corticosteroids from the adrenal cortex. In about 70 percent of cases, the adrenocortical hyperplasia is secondary to hypersecretion of ACTH (adrenocorticotropic hormone) from the anterior pituitary, either because of a tumor or a hypothalamic neuroendocrine disturbance. In these latter cases, then, both ACTH and cortisol are secreted excessively. In the remainder of cases, there is a secreting tumor of the adrenal cortex, with secondary suppression of ACTH. Because of the effects of cortisol on intermediary metabolism and electrolyte regulation, the illness is usually associated with hyperglycemia, truncal and facial obesity, osteoporosis, muscle wasting and weakness, and hypertension.[25] Hypersecretion of adrenal androgens may lead to hirsutism and intensification of libido in women (the latter probably related, in part, to local effects on the clitoris).

The occurrence of significant mental disturbance in Cushing's syndrome has been noted since Cushing's original paper[17]—indeed, one of his cases was found in a mental hospital. For reasons noted before, the precise incidence of significant psychopathology in Cushing's syndrome is hard to determine, but it is quite high, perhaps up to half the cases, and the range of psychological disturbances which occur is unusually wide. Rough estimates from the literature (reviewed by Smith et al.)[76] suggest that about 15 percent of untreated cases become frankly psychotic, with another 35 percent experiencing a significant mental disturbance of other types.[78,79,84] The literature, does not, however, distinguish between the aberrations seen in primary pituitary from those seen in primary adrenocortical Cushing's syndrome.

Depression (beyond the fatigue typical of the disease) is the most commonly occurring symptom ranging from a moderately depressed mood and overreactions to distressing life events, to severe depressive illness with delusions. Suicidal attempts occur in about 10 percent of cases.[78,83] Elation is also occasionally observed, at times closely mimicking naturally appearing manic psychoses, with grandiosity, mental and physical overactivity, sleeplessness and inappropriate behavior. Irritability, anxiety, insomnia, difficulty with concentration, and spells of agitation often occur. Paranoid states, sometimes with hallucinations, are not uncommon. Patients may also experience periods of amnesia, episodes of confusion, and outbursts of temper. The mental changes may be quite fluctuant, with, for example, periods of elation, depression, irritability, and lucidity rapidly succeeding each other. Organic mental syndromes are sometimes seen, but they are more likely to be associated with the medical complications of

Cushing's syndrome, e.g., severe hypertension with encephalopathy or congestive heart failure, uncontrolled diabetes, and electrolyte disturbances.

Prolonged corticosteroid therapy can induce somatic changes like those seen in Cushing's syndrome. Early psychiatric reports describe psychological responses to ACTH and cortisone, which were very similar to the wide range of mental disturbance seen in endogenous Cushing's syndrome, although not as common.* At present, potent steroid analogues, like prednisone, have generally replaced ACTH and cortisone in medical practice, but the types of psychiatric complications appear to be the same,[55,74] although some clinicians have the impression that depression was more common with ACTH therapy. Depression is much less commonly associated with steroid treatment than with endogenous Cushing's syndrome and elation seems much more common. True organic mental syndromes (in the absence of medical complications) probably are not common, and the confusional states appear to be primarily experiences of depersonalization and unreality, with perceptual distortions.[26]

Even with small doses of prednisone, mild changes of mood are frequent, especially elation. Occasionally, patients accustomed to the mild elation associated with steroid treatment become depressed after steroid withdrawal. From our review of recent medical literature, major psychiatric disturbances appear to be more likely in dose ranges above 20 mg. of prednisone a day. But beyond that, a clear relation of psychiatric risk to dose has not been established. The same dose may be well tolerated on one occasion and not on another.[61] Sometimes it is hard to separate the psychological effects of the illness being treated from the drug effects themselves, especially in steroid treatment of disseminated lupus erythematosus with CNS (central nervous system) involvement.[27]

As noted before, some of the psychological disturbances in Cushing's syndrome can be attributed to associated metabolic, cardiovascular, and electrolyte complications; some of the depression, for example, may be associated with hypokalemia. However, there appears little doubt that much of the psychopathology is due to the effects of ACTH and corticosteroids on the brain, although the mechanisms remain unclear. Corticosteroids have important effects on intracellular sodium content, and on the excitability of neural tissue, with alteration of the EEG (electroencephalogram) and lowering of seizure thresholds.[24,94,95] Both ACTH and corticosteroids exert influences on the enzymes involved in the metabolism of catecholamines and serotonin,[4,53,88] biogenic amines which have been implicated in naturally occurring affective disorders.[20] Interesting effects of hyperadrenalcorticism on sensory threshholds in taste, hearing and smell have been noted in patients with Cushing's disease.[31] Cortisol also increases the reuptake of norepinephrine by rat-brain tissue.[41] Maas has recently reviewed the literature on the effects of corticosteroids and ACTH on catecholamines and electrolytes, and suggests a mechanism by which these effects may mediate depressive states when the hormones are hypersecreted.[42] In hypophysectomized animals, corticosteroids prolong the extinction of learned avoidance behavior, while the opposite is true of ACTH.[6,22]

This experimental demonstration that ACTH alone has significant psychological effects which differ from those of corticosteroids may have important implications for understanding the differences in the psychological concomitants of Cushing's syndrome, Addison's disease, ACTH therapy, and corticosteroid therapy. It is possible, for example, that excess ACTH itself exerts primarily a depressing effect on mood, while excess corticosteroids may tend to produce mostly elation. This would account for the higher frequency of depression in pituitary Cushing's disease compared to steroid therapy, and the preponderance of depressive symptomatology in primary adrenal Addison's disease (see below) in which ACTH is hypersecreted. It is unfortunate that the older literature did not

* See references 12, 26, 38, 61, 66, 74, and 76.

systematically and clearly differentiate the psychiatric complications of ACTH therapy from that of corticosteroid therapy; if ACTH is "depressogenic," one would expect more depressions with ACTH therapy. Similarly, the literature generally does not distinguish between the psychological concomitants of primary hypothalamo-pituitary from primary adrenal Cushing's syndrome; one might expect a higher incidence of depression in the former, if ACTH is "depressogenic." It also should be considered that in all three forms of Cushing's syndrome—hypothalamic, pituitary, and adrenal—a variety of corticosteroids are hypersecreted, while in exogenous steroid therapy, a single synthetic steroid is administered. It may be that certain corticosteroids differ in their euphoric or depressive effects, and such differences may account for the differences in psychological responses to exogenous and endogenous steroids. These could be useful areas for future clinical investigation.

The treatment of choice for the psychiatric disturbances associated with Cushing's disease or corticosteroid therapy is to correct the disease or to reduce or temporarily discontinue the hormone medication. When the surgery must be delayed, or the medication continued for pressing medical reasons, however, the problem of controlling the psychiatric state by other means arises. We know of no definitive studies of the effectiveness of phenothiazines or antidepressants in such situations. Our own experience suggests that psychotropic drugs are often palliative, but rarely induce complete remission of the mental symptoms, as long as the hyperadrenalcorticism continues.

It should also be noted that certain naturally occurring psychotic states, particularly acute schizophrenia with emotional turmoil and severe depressive illnesses, are associated with excessive secretion of cortisol,[70–72] probably due to hyperactivity of the hypothalamic neuroendocrine cells controlling the secretion of ACTH. Such patients never show the physical stigmata of Cushing's syndrome, but it remains a possibility that the increased ACTH and cortisol secretion may have a secondary effect on CNS function, perhaps aggravating the existing psychopathology.[42]

Addison's Disease (Hyposecretion of Cortisol)

While acute failure of the adrenal cortex is a medical emergency, chronic adrenocortical insufficiency may lead to symptoms which are more subtle. The main clinical features include weakness and fatigue increasing as the day progresses; pigmentation of the skin; hypotension with associated dizzy spells and fainting; hypoglycemia with associated periods of headache; sweating; hunger; and gastrointestinal disturbances, including anorexia, weight loss, and diarrhoea.[25] In primary adrenocortical failure, there is a secondary hypersecretion of ACTH in the absence of feedback inhibition by cortisol.[54]

The mental symptoms are now seen as an "integral part of the disease syndrome."[94] Apathy and negativism are present in most cases, with depression and irritability occurring in substantial numbers (although one German report describes euphoria as a common complication).[84] Delusions occur in a small but significant percentage. Disorientation, confusion, delirium, and convulsions are features of severely advanced Addison's disease. As in Cushing's syndrome, the symptoms may fluctuate in intensity and gradually alter in type.[13,14,23,77]

There are several possible mechanisms for the psychiatric disturbances. Profound debilitation and weakness certainly play a role in the depression of many patients. The hypoglycemia (which, in the absence of cortisol, does not have to be great) may also contribute to the confusion and irritability, as may the decreased cerebral blood flow associated with marked hypotension. Correction of the electrolyte disturbances only partially alleviates some of the psychic disturbances.[94] Because of the similarity of many psychic symptoms to those of hypercalcemia, it is worth noting that Addison's disease is on rare occasions associated with elevated serum calcium levels.[58,75] Prerenal azotemia may also play a role.

Not all of the psychiatric abnormalities can be directly related to the severity of these metabolic complications, however, and there are significant effects of both cortisol deficiency and of ACTH excess on the brain. These include the previously mentioned effects on excitability of brain tissue, on intracellular electrolytes, and on the metabolism of biogenic amines. The paradox that depression is a common feature both of Cushing's and Addison's disease could possibly be related to the fact that in both conditions ACTH can be hypersecreted. With appropriate corticosteroid therapy (which also suppresses the excessive ACTH secretion) the physical and mental disturbances are nearly always reversed.

Adrenogenital Syndrome

In the adult, androgen-secreting tumors of the adrenal cortex produce pronounced virilizing effects in the female, with intensification of libido and associated psychological responses to the change in physical appearance.

It is in the virilized female infant, however, that the most enduring effects on the psyche may be noted. An adrenogenital syndrome at birth may be the result of inborn enzymatic defects in the synthesis of cortisol, or may be secondary to the use of androgenic progestins in the treatment of the pregnant mother to forestall impending abortion. Since there are frequently marked effects on secondary sex characteristics, especially in the female, the infant may be assigned to the wrong sex. The evidence, well reviewed by Money,[46] raises the possibility that gender identity is greatly influenced, perhaps fixed, by the nature of the sex assignment and associated social and psychological upbringing in early childhood, and that after gender identity is formed, it is unwise to reassign the child to his "correct" chromosomal sex.

Of further interest is the evidence that even transient fetal androgenization may have effects on the developing brain of the female, leading to enduring psychological traits in childhood and adolescence. Such effects were first noted in fetally androgenized female monkeys, who after birth were significantly more aggressive in play and in other social situations than their nonandrogenized female cohorts.[28] There is some preliminary evidence that there are analogous effects of fetal androgenization in human females, who have been reported to be more tomboyish in interests and behavior in childhood.[45,49] More controversial are preliminary data, suggesting that fetal exposure to androgens may be associated with a significant increase in intelligence;[19,47] artifacts in the sampling of the population may account for these latter results.

(Klinefelter's Syndrome

This genetic disorder (XXY) of males is associated with hypogonadism and decreased testosterone secretion. At puberty, testosterone secretion does not increase, with resultant eunuchoid appearance and impotence.

For many years, an apparent increase in psychopathology in these patients has been reported, well reviewed by Swanson and Stipes.[53] The available evidence (not conclusive) suggests that the average IQ of these patients is less than would normally be expected, and that the incidence of a variety of psychotic states is increased. The most common psychiatric disturbances, however, are severe character disorders of several types, especially schizoid withdrawal and antisocial psychopathy. It is not clear to what extent the psychopathology is due to the patient's psychological response to his sexual disorder; however, the physical disability does not become clinically manifest until puberty, and most psychological theories of psychosis and severe character disorders predicate traumata in *early* childhood. If indeed in such patients the IQ is lower and the incidence of psychosis and severe character disturbance is higher, one must consider the possibility of associated genetically determined mental aberrations, or of effects of testosterone deficiency on the developing brain.

Testosterone replacement therapy in the adult appears to be of little value in the treatment of either the impotence or the mental disturbance, although it may possibly be of value in the child or adolescent.

⟨ Thyroid Disorders

Hyperthyroidism

Excessive secretion of thyroid hormone may be due to tumors of the thyroid gland, or to excessive stimulation of the thyroid by extrathyroid agents. Graves's disease is an example of the latter and, in its clinically fully manifest form, is characterized by thyrotoxicosis, goitre, and exophthalmus. The disease is much more common in women. Recent evidence relates Graves's disease to the presence of an immunological blood factor of extrapituitary origin, of which long-acting thyroid stimulator (LATS),[35] may be an example.

The chief symptoms of thyrotoxicosis include an increase in metabolic rate, with excessive heat production, and associated heat intolerance and sweating; an increase in cardiac rate and output; weight loss despite increased appetite and caloric intake; muscular weakness and easy fatiguability.[35]

Mental symptoms are practically always present, with nervousness, emotional lability, and hyperkinesia characteristic of most patients.[35,44,65,89] To quote Ingbar and Woeber, "The nervousness of the thyrotoxic patients is not that of the patient who is chronically anxious, but rather is characterized by restlessness, shortness of attention span, and a need to be moving around and doing, despite a feeling of fatigue."[35] Other clinicians have noted that the warm dry hands of the nervous hyperthyroid patient distinguish her from the anxiety neurotic, whose hands tend to be cold and clammy. Crying spells, irritability, and excessive startle reactions are also typical. (In older patients, the muscular weakness may be so great as to preclude hyperkinesia, leading to a predominantly apathetic picture.)[30] Paranoid trends and suspiciousness occasionally are present. Nevertheless, more severe psychiatric illness in chronic hyperthyroidism is rare, except in the psychosis prone person.[15,44]

The so-called thyroid "crisis" or "storm" is rarely seen since the advent of modern antithyroid therapy. This fulminating attack of hyperthyroidism is usually characterized by extreme hyperpyrexia, anxiety, and tachycardia; delirium, coma, and even death may ensue. It may be precipitated by an episode of anxiety, especially presurgically.

The mental symptoms of hyperthyroidism are evidently related to the direct effect of thyroid hormones on the brain, and the symptoms can be partially reproduced in normal subjects by the administration of thyroid hormone,[90] but the mechanism is not clear. Thyroid hormone increases the sensitivity of neuroreceptors to catecholamines, decreases monoamine oxidase activity, and decreases the turnover rate of norepeinephrine;[3,86] these actions may play a role in the mental states associated with thyrotoxicosis.

Recent investigations have raised questions about once prevalent theories that Graves's disease is likely to be precipitated by emotional stress, especially object-loss,[37] or that it is more likely to occur in patients with specific personality types characterized by premature assumption of responsibility and a martyrlike suppression of dependency wishes.[2] Retrospective evaluations, always difficult, have not reliably replicated these psychological formulations.[32,65] A prospective study has shown increased activity of subclinical, but radiologically demonstrable, thyroid "hot spots" in association with nonspecific life stress;[86] the relation of these subclinical "hot spots" to the etiology of Graves's disease is unknown, however, and whether they even have a role in the pathogenesis of toxic nodular goitre is not established. The role of psychological factors in the etiology of hyperthyroidism remains, then, an open question.

Hypothyroidism

Hypothyroidism in the adult is commonly caused by surgery or radioactive-iodine therapy. The spontaneous form is usually secondary to atrophy of thyroid tissue, probably due to an autoimmune thyroiditis. The spontaneous disease usually has an insidious onset, and the changes may not be noticed by the patient until the disease is far advanced. With the deficiency of thyroid hormone the metabolic rate is markedly reduced, and nearly all hypothyroid patients experience cold intolerance, decreased sweating, and generalized weakness and lethargy. In addition, speech is slowed, eyes and face become puffy, and the skin coarse and dry.[35]

Mental symptoms are very common. Thinking is slowed in the great majority, and memory is impaired in about two-thirds of the cases.[35] Depressed mood is typical[89] although clinical depressive illness probably is not. Psychological testing confirms the impression that the majority of myxedematous patients suffer from at least a mild organic mental syndrome.[9,89] The psychoses which have been reported ("myxedema madness") occur in a small percentage of patients and appear to be mostly more dramatic and severe organic mental syndromes, with the typical symptoms of confusion, memory loss, and agitation, and occasionally paranoid ideas, delusions and hallucinations.

Unfortunately, while appropriate thyroid-hormone-replacement therapy reverses most of the clinical stigmata of myxedema, the organic mental deficit does not always fully remit, especially in cases of long standing hypothyroidism. In cretinism the prognosis is especially poor, with the degree of permanent intelligence loss roughly correlated with the duration of the untreated illness.[45]

❰ Parathyroid Disorders

Hyperparathyroidism

Parathyroid hormone promotes the absorption of calcium from the gastrointestinal tract, the resorption of calcium from bone, and the excretion of phosphate from the kidney, all of which actions increase the concentration of circulating calcium ion. Chronic hypersecretion of the hormone, due to tumor or neoplasia of the parathyroid gland, produces clinical symptoms related to the disturbances in bone metabolism and the effect of hypercalcemia on various organ systems: skeletal pains, anorexia, nausea, constipation, muscular weakness, polyuria, renal calculi with renal colic, and cardiac irregularities.[64]

Mental symptoms are present in at least half the cases, the most common being lassitude and depressive mood, with loss of interest and anhedonia.[64] A minority of patients develop organic mental syndromes, with memory impairment, confusion, paranoid ideas, and hallucinations.[1,59] In an outstanding study of fifty-four cases, Petersen[59] showed that the severity of mental symptomatology increases with the blood calcium level, with organic brain syndromes occurring primarily at concentrations of about 14–16 mg. percent and above. Parathyroid hormone itself appears to have no mental effects, since lowering blood calcium by dialysis (which does not affect parathyroid hormone itself) immediately reverses the mental disturbances, and patients with hypercalcemia due to other causes show similar mental aberrations.

Calcium ion plays a significant role in altering permeability and excitability of the nerve membrane, and also promotes the discharge and depletion of norepinephrine and its biosynthetic enzyme, dopamine beta hydroxylase, from nerve granules.[3] It is not unlikely that these actions play some role in the mental aberrations noted in hypercalcemia.

Hypoparathyroidism

Hypoparathyroidism is most commonly secondary to damage or surgical removal of the thyroid gland. About 200 cases of idiopathic hypoparathyroidism had been reported in the literature by 1962. In both conditions symptoms develop which are closely related to the lowered blood calcium concentration characteristic of the illness. Seventy per cent of cases present manifestations of tetany, such as numbness, tingling, and cramps in the extremities, leading to carpopedal spasm. In milder forms of the illness, the patient complains of fatigue, weakness, and tingling sensations.[63]

Mental symptoms are common. In an extensive review, collecting data from 258 papers, Denko and Kaelbling[21] attempted to classify the psychiatric disturbances occurring in patients with both idiopathic and surgical hypo-parathyroidism. Because the disease is rare, and cases have generally been reported by nonpsychiatrists, a clear picture of the psychiatric symptomatology is difficult to form. In idiopathic hypoparathyroidism, about one-third of the cases appeared to suffer intellectual deterioration, in many instances reaching levels of mental retardation. At least a third also showed symptoms of organic mental syndromes of various types, with some patients experiencing both intellectual deficit and organic mental syndromes. There also appear to be additional psychiatric disturbances which are hard to classify, described as "nervousness," "emotionality," etc. In idiopathic hypoparathyroidism, treatment of the endocrine disorder often leaves the individual with intellectual deficit. In surgical hypoparathyroidism organic mental syndromes also occur but intellectual deficit is seen less frequently. A variety of other psychotic states are noted, but their vague descriptions leave it unclear as to whether these are also organic mental syndromes or psychoses of other types. Treatment of the endocrine disorder in surgical hypoparathyroid cases (by Vitamin D) generally leads to complete remission of symptoms.

◖ Pancreatic Disorders

Diabetes

Diabetes in its usual form is believed to involve a genetic predisposition and an evolution which goes through several stages before the manifest clinical illness appears. Initially, the central disturbance may be a defect in the metabolic action of insulin; during this latent period insulin may actually be hypersecreted. In the later stages, when the disease is manifest, insulin secretion is deficient, and the clinical symptoms are secondary to this disturbance. As sugar fails to be metabolized, blood sugar rises and is excreted in the urine, with secondary polyuria and polydipsia. Proteins and fats are metabolized in excess, with associated weight loss, ketosis, ketonuria, and po-

tassium loss. Susceptibility to infection is increased, especially in the skin and genital tract. The patient feels chronically weak and fatigued and may complain of mental dullness and depression.[90]

The mental symptoms become especially prominent in severe untreated diabetic acidosis, which is associated with somnolence, difficulty in thinking, confusion, obtundation, and eventually, coma and death.[90]

The mechanism of the mental dysfunction in diabetic acidosis is partially understood. The deficiency of insulin per se is not responsible, since the brain does not require insulin to metabolize glucose, and although the patient is severely dehydrated, cerebral blood flow is not decreased. However, as shown in the classic study by Kety et al.,[36] cerebral oxygen consumption is substantially reduced, the decrement correlated closely with degree of stupor and also with the extent of ketosis. In all likelihood, certain of the blood-borne ketones act like ether anesthetics on the CNS.

Physiological stress such as infection, fever, and obesity may precipitate the onset of clinical diabetes, as well as exacerbate the established disease. There is some evidence that emotional stresses may play a similar role.[5,34,80] For example, in a study of adult diabetics on a metabolic ward, emotional stresses were shown to be associated with temporary increases in metabolic indices of diabetes.[34] The pathophysiological mediating mechanisms have not yet been demonstrated. One possible pathway is the hypersecretion of cortisol and adrenalin associated with severe emotional distress, since increases in both cortisol and adrenalin secretion antagonize the action of insulin. In support of the role of adrenalin, one study indicates that beta adrenergic blocking agents can be helpful in stabilizing the medical management of brittle juvenile diabetics,[5] who show increased FFA (free fatty acids) and ketonuria during stress interviews. It also may be relevant that nondiabetic patients who develop depressive illnesses are noted to have a relative insulin resistance, which reverts after recovery.[10,52,69]

Although it is beyond the scope of this discussion, it should be noted that severe diabetes poses a major burden on the psychological adaptative mechanisms of many patients, particularly juvenile and adolescent diabetics who must rigorously control diet and insulin dosage at a time when there is a great need not to feel different from their peers. Other patients may improperly manage their regimens in the context of periods of depression, struggles with significant objects, needs for secondary gain, and so forth. The fear of developing major medical complications from chronic diabetes also may shadow the outlook of many patients. The need for psychological sensitivity and understanding on the part of family members and primary physicians is accordingly great.

Hyperinsulinism

Hyperinsulinism spontaneously occurs with insulin-secreting islet-cell tumors of the pancreas, and more rarely, with insulin-secreting extrapancreatic tumors. In patients with adrenocortical insufficiency, the normal secretion of insulin is functionally excessive, giving rise to the symptoms of hypoglycemia. There is also a group of patients who appear to secrete excessive insulin postprandially with a drop to unusually low concentrations of blood sugar two to four hours after meals. Most commonly, however, hyperinsulinism occurs in diabetic patients who take more than their metabolically required dose of insulin.[91]

All of these states lead to hypoglycemia, and since brain metabolism is completely dependent on glucose, the primary symptoms of hypoglycemia are due to CNS glucose starvation, similar in its effects to cerebral anoxia. Indeed, the degree of depression of CNS oxygen utilization in hypoglycemia has been shown to be closely correlated with the CNS symptomatology.[33] As would be expected, preexisting brain damage or cerebrovascular insufficiency significantly increases the sensitivity to the effects of hypoglycemia. The initial effects are due to cortical depression and a concomitant release of epinephrine from the adrenal medulla. The cortical symptoms include headaches, faintness, confusion, restlessness, somnolence, hunger, irritability, and vis-

ual disturbances. Adrenergic symptoms include anxiety, tremor, perspiration, tingling of the fingers and around the mouth, tachycardia, and pallor.[33,91]

In patients with insulinomas or massive insulin overdose, progressive CNS depression may occur: the patient loses consciousness, and often manifests sucking, grasping, and grimacing movements, along with twitching and clonic spasms. Further CNS depression leads to the neurological signs associated with the involvement of deeper brain structures, such as Babinski signs, inconjugate ocular deviation, tonic and extensor spasms, and so forth.[33,91] Death may ensue.

Administration of glucose promptly reverses the acute symptomatology. However, those patients who suffer repeated or extended periods of severe hypoglycemia frequently suffer some degree of irreversible brain damage. The pathological and mental changes are similar to those seen after chronic CNS anoxia.

(Menstrual Disorders

Premenstrual Tension

Several systematic studies have confirmed what clinicians and women have long believed, that the menstrual cycle is frequently associated with definite changes in mental state, significant enough in some women to be termed a premenstrual syndrome.[18] Psychological assessments of large samples of women reveal that, for the groups as a whole, negative affects begin to increase about a week before menstruation, reaching a peak on the day of menstruation, and then falling after the menstrual phase, reaching a minimum during the middle portion of the cycle.[51,56] One study also indicates that positive pleasant feelings follow an inverse pattern, reaching a peak in midcycle.[56] The premenstrual feelings noted by the women included irritability, hostility, depressed mood, emotional overreactions to trivial incidents, crying spells, anxiety and tension, and mood swings. In addition, many women note difficulties with concentration, forgetfulness, and judgment. Behavioral changes, such as lowered school or work performance and withdrawal from social activities, also occur.[21,50] Other features of the premenstrual period are fatigue, bodily aches, particularly headaches and backaches, as well as water retention with uncomfortable feelings of distention. Moos[50] has noted that the psychological symptoms can be grouped in several categories (negative affects, concentration disturbances, behavioral changes, and pain) of varying prominence in different women, sometimes occurring together and sometimes not.

What is of further significance to the psychiatrist is the evidence that psychopathological disturbances of many types can be intensified during the premenstrual and early menstrual phases. One study, for example, suggests that preexisting neurotic traits become more prominent in the premenstrual period.[16] Others have noted that the incidence of suicide[43] and hospitalization for acute psychiatric illness[18] is disproportionately great during this phase.

The pathophysiological mechanisms underlying the various premenstrual syndromes are becoming clearer. While water retention accounts for the bloating, swelling, and painful distention troublesome to many women, it is not closely correlated with the onset and disappearance of many of the psychological symptoms, and diuretic medication is not particularly effective in relieving the purely psychological symptoms.[64]

On the other hand, there is a growing body of circumstantial evidence that progesterone, which is increasingly secreted in the premenstrual phase, may play a primary role in the psychological symptomatology. Regimens of combination-type oral contraceptives, which contain fixed doses of progestogens and estrogens, are associated with a greater incidence of those mental symptoms typically seen in the premenstrual syndromes, but also, as might be expected, the fixed dose of progestogens throughout the cycle appears to eliminate the psychological fluctuations seen during the normal cycle. On the other hand, the oral contraceptive regimens which administer only estro-

gens until the final five days of the cycle, at which point progestogen is added (sequential type), are associated with fewer emotional complications, although a premenstrual increase in symptomatology is once again apparent.[56]

A possible mechanism for the apparent mental effects of progesterone is an influence on monoamine oxidase activity (MAO). Grant and Pryse-Davies[29] reported that increased uterine MAO activity normally occurs in the premenstrual (progesterone) phase. Contraceptive agents which contain strongly progestational compounds markedly increase uterine MAO activity much earlier in the cycle, while agents that are primarily estrogenic in action tend to inhibit uterine MAO activity. The incidence of depressive symptomatology in their study roughly correlated with the effects of contraceptives on MAO activity.[29] If brain MAO is similarly affected, it is possible that increased catabolism of biogenic amines may be involved in the psychological symptoms, since such a neurochemical disturbance has been proposed to occur in clinical depression.[20]

These theories remain unsupported, however, and there are some defects. The synthetic progestogens in oral contraceptives differ in several ways from endogenous progesterone, and in some respects, resemble androgens in their biological activity. Furthermore, a clear hormonal difference between women with premenstrual tension and those without has yet to be demonstrated. Finally, for some women with premenstrual tension, progesterone administration appears to be helpful.

Functional Amenorrhea

It has long been recognized that under conditions of emotional stress women frequently fail to menstruate for one or two months. As an extreme example, a high incidence of amenhorrea was reported in women on imprisonment in concentration camps during World War II, even before starvation became a factor.[62] Similar observations have been made in less grim settings, however, for example among adolescent girls adjusting to boarding school, summer camp, etc.[39,62]

The mechanism appears to be a failure of ovulation,[39] associated with an absence of the usual midcycle burst of LH (luteinizing hormone) secretion by the pituitary.[7,67,85] Presumably, emotional stress in some way inhibits the hypothalamic neuroendocrine cells producing LH releasing factor.

In anorexia nervosa, amenhorrea also typically occurs, not necessarily associated with malnutrition.[68]

There is also a group of women who fail to ovulate for long periods of time in the absence of any demonstrable endocrine or gynecological abnormality, other than the absence of the surge of secretion of LH (luteinizing hormone) and related hormones at midcycle.[7,67,85] In the past the diagnosis of "functional" amenorrhea was made by exclusion of obvious anatomical or endocrine pathology. Recently it has been possible to re-establish ovulation by the use of such agents as clomiphene.[7,67,85] There are very few systematic psychological studies reported on such women, however, to support the idea, once widespread, that the disturbance is primarily psychogenic. The existing psychiatric case reports suggest in certain women the prominence of conflicts over masculine and feminine strivings, and also around separation-dependency issues with their mothers.[40,82] It should be noted, however, that these are common conflicts in women, while chronic functional amenorrhea is relatively rare.

(Failure-to-Grow Syndrome

Among children who fail to grow normally, a subgroup has been identified in which psychosocial issues appear to play a significant role. Frequently there is evidence of parental neglect, with associated behavioral disturbances of many types in the children, including the syndrome of anaclitic depression.[57] Endocrine studies on the children have demonstrated a failure to release growth hormone in response to the usual stimuli, such as insulin-induced hypoglycemia.[60] The disturbance appears likely to be in the hypothalamus, involving the neural influences which normally control secretion of growth hormone releasing factor or inhibiting factor from the median eminence neuroendocrine cells. What is especially striking is that after a period of emotionally supportive hospital care, behavior, growth, and growth hormone secretion all frequently return to normal.[55,60] Since growth hormone secretion appears to be closely related to the metabolism of brain catecholamines,[8] and since these neurotransmitters also mediate mood,[20] it is possible that emotional deprivation alters growth hormone secretion via these neurochemical mechanisms. In this respect, it is interesting to note that depressive illness in adults is frequently associated with an inhibition of growth hormone release.[11,69,73]

(Concluding Remarks

A review of the psychiatric disturbances associated with the major endocrine disorders (excessive or deficient secretion of the adrenal cortex, thyroid, parathyroids, and pancreatic islet cells) reveals a wide variety of psychopathology. Certain mental symptoms appear to be especially common, however, such as fatigue, depression, diffuse anxiety, and organic mental syndromes. While the fully developed endocrine disease is usually quickly recognizable by the psychiatrist, the early stages can frequently pass unnoticed, leading to incorrect diagnoses and treatment. Since endocrine disease is probably as frequent a cause of psychiatric disturbance as brain tumor, it would seem appropriate for the psychiatrist to be as alert to the possibility of the former as the latter, particularly in the presence of the symptoms noted above. A definitive diagnosis requires a full endocrine workup, of course, but screening information could easily be obtained by a group of morning blood tests readily analyzed by any good commercial laboratory: a fasting blood sugar, protein-bound iodine, calcium, cortisol, sodium, and potassium. Such a battery of tests probably should be considered as often as an electroencephalogram in the evaluation of the patient presenting with psychiatric disturbance.

Finally, as has been indicated, the mechanisms by which hormonal disturbances lead to mental aberration are in many instances still unclear. Further research in this area not only offers the potential for clarifying the pathophysiological effects of endocrine disease on the central nervous system, but may also illuminate significant neurochemical and neurophysiological aspects of primary psychiatric disorders as well.

❰ Bibliography

1. AGRAS, S. and D. C. OLIVEAU. "Primary Hyperparathyroidism and Psychosis," *Can. M. Assoc. J.*, 91 (1964), 1366–1367.
2. ALEXANDER, F., ed. *Psychosomatic Specificity*, Vol. 1. Chicago: University of Chicago Press, 1968.
3. AXELROD, J. *Neural and Endocrine Control of Catecholamine Biosynthesis*. Proc. 4th. Int. Congr. Endocrinology. Amsterdam: Excerpta Medica, 1973. In Press.
4. AZMITIA, E. C. and B. McEWEN. "Corticosterone Regulation of Tryptophan Hydroxylase in Midbrain of Rat," *Science*, 166 (1969), 1274–1276.
5. BAKER, L., A. BARCAI, R. KAYE et al. "Beta Adrenergic Blockade and Juvenile Diabetes: Acute Studies and Long Term Therapeutic Trial," *J. Pediatr.*, 75 (1969), 19–29.
6. BOHUS, B. "Central Nervous System Structures and the Effect of ACTH and Corticosteroids on Avoidance Behavior," in D. De Wied and J. A. W. M. Weijnen, eds., *Progress in Brain Research*, Vol. 32, pp. 171–184. Amsterdam: Elsevier, 1970.
7. BOON, R. C., D. S. SCHALCH, L. A. LEE et al. "Plasma Gonadotropin Secretory Patterns in Patients with Functional Menstrual Disorders and Stein-Leventhal Syndrome: Response to Clomiphene Treatment," *Am. J. Obstet. Gynecol.*, 112 (1972), 736–748.
8. BROWN, G. and S. REICHLIN. "Psychological and Neural Regulations of Growth Hormone Secretion," *Psychosom. Med.*, 34 (1972), 45–61.
9. BROWNING, T. B., R. W. ATKINS, and

H. WEINER. "Cerebral Metabolic Disturbances in Hypothyroidism," *Arch. Intern. Med.*, 93 (1954), 938–950.
10. CARROLL, B. J. "Hypothalamic Pituitary Function in Depressive Illness: Insensitivity to Hypoglycemia," *Br. Med. J.*, 3 (1969), 27–28.
11. ———. "Studies with Hypothalamic Pituitary-Adrenal Stimulation Tests in Depression," in B. Davies, B. J. Carroll, and R. M. Mowbray, eds., *Depressive Illness: Some Research Studies*, pp. 149–201. Springfield, Ill.: Charles C. Thomas, 1972.
12. CLARK, L. D., W. BAUER, and S. COBB. "Preliminary Observations on Mental Disturbances Occurring in Patients under Therapy with Cortisone and ACTH," *N. Engl. J. Med.*, 246 (1952), 205–216.
13. CLEGHORN, R. A. "Adrenal Cortical Insufficiency. Psychological and Neurological Observations," *Can. Med. Assoc. J.*, 65 (1951), 449–454.
14. ———. "Psychological Changes in Addison's Disease," *J. Clin. Endocrinol.*, 13 (1953), 1291–1293.
15. CLOWER, C. G., A. J. YOUNG, D. KEPES. "Psychotic States Resulting from Disorders of Thyroid Function," *Johns Hopkins Med. J.*, 124 (1969), 305–310.
16. COPPEN, A. and N. KESSEL. "Menstruation and Personality," *Br. J. Psychiatry*, 109 (1963), 711–721.
17. CUSHING, H. "Basophil Adenomas of the Pituitary Body and their Clinical Manifestations," *Bull. Johns Hopkins Hosp.*, 50 (1932), 137–195.
18. DALTON, K. *The Premenstrual Syndrome*. Springfield, Ill.: Charles C. Thomas, 1964.
19. ———. "Antenatal Progesterone and Intelligence," *Br. J. Psychiatry*, 114 (1968), 1377–1382.
20. DAVIS, J. "Theories of Biological Etiology of Affective Disorders," *Int. Rev. Neurobiol.*, 12 (1970), 145–175.
21. DENKO, J. D. and R. KAELBLING. "The Psychiatric Aspects of Hypoparathyroidism," *Acta Psychiatr. Scand.*, 38 (1962), 7–70.
22. DE WIED, D., A. WITTER, and S. LANDE. "Anterior Pituitary Peptides and Avoidance Acquisition of Hypophysectomized Rats," in D. De Wied and J. A. W. M. Weijnen, eds., *Progress in Brain Research*, Vol. 32, pp. 213–220. Amsterdam: Elsevier, 1969.
23. ENGEL, G. L. and S. G. MARGOLIN. "Neuro-

psychiatric Disturbances in Internal Disease," *Arch. Intern. Med.*, 70 (1942), 236–259.

24. FELDMAN, S. and N. DAFNY. "Effects of Adrenocortical Hormones on Electrical Activity of the Brain," in D. De Wied and J. A. W. M. Weijnen, eds., *Progress in Brain Research*, Vol. 32, pp. 90–101. Amsterdam: Elsevier, 1969.

25. FORSHAM, P. H. "The Adrenal Cortex," in R. H. Williams, ed., *Textbook of Endocrinology*, pp. 287–379. Phildelphia: Saunders, 1968.

26. FOX, H. M. and S. GIFFORD. "Psychological Responses to ACTH and Cortisone," *Psychosom. Med.*, 15 (1953), 631–641.

27. GANZ, V. H., B. J. GURLAND, W. DEMING et al. "Study of the Psychiatric Symptoms of Systemic Lupus Erythematosus," *Psychosom. Med.*, 34 (1972), 207–220.

28. GOY, R. W. and J. A. RESKO. "Gonadal Hormones and Behavior of Normal and Pseudohermaphroditic Nonhuman Female Primates," in E. B. Astwood, ed., *Recent Progress in Hormone Research*, Vol. 28, pp. 707–733. New York: Academic, 1972.

29. GRANT, C. and J. PRYSE-DAVIES. "Effects of Oral Contraceptives on Depressive Mood Changes and on Endometrial Monoamine Oxidase and Phosphates," *Br. Med. J.*, 28 (1968), 777–780.

30. HARE, L. and J. RITCHEY. "Apathetical Response to Hyperthyroidism: Report of Two Cases," *Ann. Intern. Med.*, 24 (1946), 634–637.

31. HENKIN, R. "Effects of Corticosteroids and ACTH on Sensory Systems," in D. De Wied and J. A. W. M. Weijnen, eds., *Progress in Brain Research*, Vol. 32, pp. 270–294. Amsterdam: Elsevier, 1969.

32. HERMANN, H. T. and C. QUARTON. "Psychological Changes and Psychogenesis in Thyroid Hormone Disorders," *J. Clin. Endocrinol.*, 25 (1965), 327–338.

33. HIMWICH, H. E. *Brain Metabolism and Cerebral Disorders.* New York: Waverly, 1951.

34. HINKLE, L. E. and S. WOLF. "Importance of Life Stress in the Course and Management of Diabetes Mellitus," *JAMA*, 148 (1952), 513.

35. INGBAR, S. H. and K. A. WOEBER. "The Thyroid Gland," in R. H. Williams, ed., *Textbook of Endocrinology*, pp. 105–286.

Philadelphia: Saunders, 1968.

36. KETY, S. S., B. D. POLIS, C. S. NADLER et al. "The Blood Flow and Oxygen Consumption of the Human Brain in Diabetic Acidosis and Coma," *J. Clin. Invest.*, 27 (1948), 500–510.

37. LIDZ, T. "Emotional Factors in the Etiology of Hyperthyroidism," *Psychosom. Med.*, 11 (1949), 2.

38. LIDZ, T., J. D. CARTER, B. I. LEWIS et al. "Effects of ACTH and Cortisone on Mood and Mentation," *Psychosom. Med.*, 14 (1952), 363–377.

39. LOESER, A. A. "Effect of Emotional Shock on Hormone Release and Endometrial Development," *Lancet*, 1 (1943), 518.

40. ——. "Behavioral and Psychoanalytic Aspects of Anovulatory Amenhorrea," *Fertil. Steril.*, 13 (1962), 20.

41. MAAS, J. W. and M. L. MEDNIEKS. "Hydrocortisone Effected Increase in the Uptake of Norepinephrine by Brain Slices," *Science*, 171 (1971), 178.

42. ——. "Adrenocortical Steroid Hormones, Electrolytes, and the Disposition of the Catecholamines with Particular Reference to Depressive States," *J. Psychiatr. Res.*, 9 (1972), 227–241.

43. MANDELL, A. and M. MANDELL. "Suicide and the Menstrual Cycle," *JAMA*, 200 (1967), 792.

44. MICHAEL, R. P. and J. L. GIBBONS. "Interrelationships Between the Endocrine System and Neuropsychiatry," in C. C. Pfeiffer and J. R. Smythies, eds., *International Review of Neurobiology*, Vol. 5. New York: Academic, 1963.

45. MONEY, J. "Psychological Studies in Hypothyroidism," *Arch. Neurol. Psychiatry*, 76 (1956), 296–309.

46. ——. *Sex Errors of the Body: Dilemmas, Education, Counselling.* Baltimore: Johns Hopkins, 1966.

47. ——. "Pituitary-Adrenal and Related Syndromes of Childhood: Effects on I.Q. and Learning," in D. De Wied and J. A. W. M. Weijnen, eds., *Progress in Brain Research*, Vol. 32, pp. 295–304. Amsterdam: Elsevier, 1970.

48. ——. "Gender Dimorphic Behavior and Fetal Sex Hormones," in E. B. Astwood, ed., *Recent Progress in Hormone Research*, Vol. 28, pp. 735–763. New York: Academic, 1972.

49. MONEY, J. and A. EHRHARDT. "Prenatal Hormonal Exposure: Possible Effects on Behavior in Man," in R. Michael, ed., *Endocrinology and Human Behavior*, pp. 32–48. London: Oxford University Press, 1968.

50. MOOS, R. "Typology of Menstrual Cycle Syndrome," *Am. J. Obstetr. Gynecol.*, 103 (1969), 390–402.

51. MOOS, R., B. KOPELL, F. MELGES et al. "Fluctuations in Symptoms and Moods During the Menstrual Cycle," *J. Psychosom. Res.*, 13 (1969), 37–44.

52. MUELLER, P. S., G. R. HENINGER, and R. K. MacDONALD. "Insulin Tolerance Test in Depression," *Arch. Gen. Psychiatry*, 21 (1969), 587–594.

53. MUELLER, R. A., H. THOENEN, and J. AXELROD. "Effect of Pituitary and ACTH on the Maintenance of Basal Tyrosine Hydroxylase Activity in Rat Adrenal Gland," *Endocrinology*, 86 (1970), 751–755.

54. NELSON, D. H., J. W. MEAKIN, and G. W. THORN. "ACTH-Producing Pituitary Tumors Following Adrenalectomy for Cushing's Syndrome," *Ann. Intern. Med.*, 52 (1960), 560–69.

55. NELSON, J. B., A. DRIVSHOLM, F. FISCHER et al. "Long Term Treatment with Corticosteroids in Rheumatoid Arthritis," *Acta Med. Scand.*, 173 (1963), 177–183.

56. PAIGE, K. E. "Effects of Oral Contraceptives on Affective Fluctuations Associated with the Menstrual Cycle," *Psychosom. Med.*, 33 (1972), 515–537.

57. PATTON, R. G. and L. I. GARDNER. "Short Stature Associated with Maternal Deprivation Syndrome: Disordered Family Environment as Cause for So-Called Idiopathic Hypopituitarism," in L. Gardner, ed., *Endocrine and Genetic Diseases of Childhood*. Philadelphia: Saunders, 1969.

58. PEDERSON, K. O. "Hypercalcemia in Addison's Disease," *Acta Med. Scand.*, 181 (1967), 691.

59. PETERSEN, P. "Psychiatric Disorders in Primary Hyperparathyroidism," *J. Clin. Endocrinol.*, 28 (1968), 1491–1495.

60. POWELL, G. F., J. A. BRASEL, S. RAITI et al. "Emotional Deprivation and Growth Retardation Simulating Idiopathic Hypopituitarism," *N. Engl. J. Med.*, 276 (1967), 1279–1283.

61. QUARTON, G. C., L. D. CLARK, S. COBB et al. "Mental Disturbances Associated with ACTH and Cortisone: A Review of Explanatory Hypotheses," *Medicine*, 34 (1955), 13–50.

62. RAKOFF, A. E. "Endocrine Mechanisms in Psychogenic Amenorrhea," in R. Michael, ed., *Endocrinology and Human Behavior*, pp. 139–160. London: Oxford University Press, 1968.

63. RASMUSSEN, H. "The Parathyroids," in R. Williams, ed., *Textbook of Endocrinology*, pp. 847–965. Philadelphia: Saunders, 1968.

64. REES, L. "The Premenstrual Tension Syndrome and Its Treatment," *Br. Med. J.*, 1 (1953), 1014–1016.

65. ROBBINS, L. R. and D. B. VINSON. "Objective Psychological Assessment of the Thyrotoxic Patient and the Response to Treatment," *J. Clin. Endocrinol.*, 25 (1965), 327–338.

66. ROME, H. P. and F. J. BRACELAND. "The Psychological Response to ACTH, Cortisone, Hydrocortisone, and Related Steroid Substances," *Am. J. Psychiatry*, 108 (1952), 641–651.

67. ROSS, G. T., C. M. CARGILLE, M. B. LIPSETT et al. "Pituitary and Gonadal Hormones in Women During Spontaneous and Induced Ovulatory Cycles," in E. B. Astwood, ed., *Recent Progress in Hormone Research*, Vol. 26, pp. 1–47. New York: Academic, 1970.

68. RUSSELL, G. and J. BEARDWOOD. "The Feeding Disorders, with Particular Reference to Anorexia Nervosa and Its Associated Gonadotrophin Changes," in R. Michael, ed., *Endocrinology and Human Behavior*, pp. 310–329. London: Oxford University Press, 1968.

69. SACHAR, E. J., J. FINKELSTEIN, and L. HELLMAN. "Growth Hormone Responses in Depressive Illness. I. Response to Insulin Tolerance Test," *Arch. Gen. Psychiatry*, 25 (1971), 263–269.

70. SACHAR, E. J., L. HELLMAN, D. K. FUKUSHIMA et al. "Cortisol Production in Depressive Illness," *Arch. Gen. Psychiatry*, 23 (1970), 289–298.

71. SACHAR, E. J., L. HELLMAN, H. P. ROFFWARG et al. "Disrupted 24-Hour Patterns of Cortisol Secretion in Psychotic Depression," *Arch. Gen. Psychiatry*, 28 (1973), 19–24.

72. SACHAR, E. J., S. S. KANTER, D. BUIE et al. "Psychoendocrinology of Ego Disintegration," *Am. J. Psychiatry*, 126 (1970), 1067–1078.

73. SACHAR, E. J., G. MUSHRUSH, M. PERLOW et al. "Growth Hormone Responses to L-Dopa in Depressed Patients," *Science*, 178 (1972), 1304–1305.

74. SAYERS, G. and R. H. TRAVIS. "Adrenocorticotropic Hormone, Adrenocortical Steroids and Their Synthetic Analogs," in L. Goodman and A. Gilman, eds., *Pharmacological Basis of Therapeutics*, pp. 1604–1642. New York: Macmillan, 1970.

75. SIEGLER, D. I. M. "Idiopathic Addison's Disease Presenting with Hypercalcemia," *Br. Med. J.*, 2 (1970), 522.

76. SMITH, C. K., J. BARISH, J. CORREA et al. "Psychiatric Disturbance in Endocrinologic Disease," *Psychosom. Med.*, 34 (1972), 69–86.

77. SORKIN, S. A. "Addison's Disease," *Medicine*, 28 (1949), 371–425.

78. SPILLANE, J. D. "Nervous and Mental Disorders in Cushing's Syndrome," *Brain*, 74 (1951), 72–94.

79. STARR, A. M. "Personality Changes in Cushing's Syndrome," *J Clin. Endocrinol.*, 12 (1952), 502–505.

80. STEIN, S. P. and E. CHARLES. "Emotional Factors in Juvenile Diabetes Mellitus: A Study of Early Life Experience of Adolescent Diabetics," *Am. J. Psychiatry*, 128 (1971), 700–704.

81. STOLL, W. A. *Die Psychiatrie des Morbus Addison.* Stuttgart: Thieme, 1953.

82. STURGIS, S. H., ed. *The Gynecologic Patient: A Psychoendocrine Study.* New York: Grune & Stratton, 1962.

83. SWANSON, D. and A. STIPES. "Psychiatric Aspects of Klinefelter's Syndrome," *Am. J. Psychiatry*, 126 (1969), 814–822.

84. TRETHOWAN, W. H. and S. COBB. "Neuropsychiatric Aspects of Cushing's Syndrome," *Arch. Neurol. Psychiatry*, 67 (1952), 283–309.

85. VAN DE WIELE, R. L., J. BOGUMIL, I. DYEN-FURTH et al. "Mechanisms Regulating the Menstrual Cycle in Women," in E. B. Astwood, ed., *Recent Progress in Hormone Research*, Vol. 26, pp. 48–62. New York: Academic, 1970.

86. VOTH, H., P. HOLZMAN, J. KATZ et al. "Thyroid 'Hot Spots': Their Relationship to Life Stress," *Psychosom. Med.*, 32 (1970), 561–580.

87. WALDSTEIN, S. S. "Thyroid Catecholamine Interrelationships," *Ann. Rev. Med.*, 17 (1966), 123–132.

88. WEINSHILBAUM, R., and J. AXELROD. "Dopamine Beta Hydroxylase Activity in the Rat after Hypophysectomy," *Endocrinology*, 87 (1970), 894.

89. WHYBROW, P. C., A. J. PRANGE, and C. R. TREADWAY. "Mental Changes Accompanying Thyroid Gland Dysfunction," *Arch. Gen. Psychiatry*, 20 (1969), 48–63.

90. WILLIAMS, R. H. "The Pancreas," in R. H. Williams, ed., *Textbook of Endocrinology*, pp. 613–802. Philadelphia: Saunders, 1968.

91. ———. "Hypoglycemia and Hypoglycemoses," in R. H. Williams, ed., *Textbook of Endocrinology*, pp. 803–846. Philadelphia: Saunders, 1968.

92. WILLIAMS, R. H., ed. *Textbook of Endocrinology.* Philadelphia: Saunders, 1968.

93. WILSON, W. P., J. E. JOHNSON, and R. B. SMITH. "Affective Change in Thyrotoxicosis and Experimental Hypermetabolism," in J. Wortis, ed.. *Recent Advances in Biological Psychiatry*, Vol. 4. New York: Plenum, 1961.

94. WOODBURY, D. M. "Relation Between the Adrenal Cortex and the Central Nervous System," *Pharmacol., Rev.*, 10 (1958), 275–357.

95. WOODBURY, D. M. and A. VERNADAKAS. "Effects of Steroids on the Central Nervous System," *Methods Hormone Res.*, 5 (1966), 1–57.

CHAPTER 13

EPILEPSY: NEUROPSYCHOLOGICAL ASPECTS

Gilbert H. Glaser[*]

❦ Introduction

EPILEPSY, as a state of disordered cerebral function, is derived from the Greek "epilepsia," meaning "a taking hold of or a seizing." Because of the existence of many kinds of seizures which appear in human disease under numerous and varied abnormal circumstances, designation as "The epilepsies" would be more appropriate.

The first definitive descriptions of both major and minor epileptic seizures are found in the Hippocratic writings[69] of the fifth century B.C., *The Sacred Disease*. These actually localized the disturbances in the brain and revealed such aspects as the premonitory experi-

* The assistance of Helen Sanders Brittain in the preparation of portions of this chapter is gratefully acknowledged.

ences or auras, the differentiation between so-called idiopathic and symptomatic epilepsy and the important influences of age, temperament, and menstrual cycles. These earliest considerations of human beings with epilepsy recognized the profound emotional experiences which in many different ways are associated with seizure phenomena. For example, in *The Sacred Disease* Hippocrates says:

Patients who suffer from this disease have a premonitory indication of an attack. In such circumstances they avoid company, going home if they are near enough, or to the loneliest spot that they can find if they are not, so that as few people as possible will see them fall . . . Small children, from inexperience as being unaccustomed to the disease, at first fall down wherever they happen to be. Later, after a number of attacks, they run to their mothers or to someone who they know well when they feel one coming on. This is through fear and fright at what they feel, for they have *not yet learnt to feel ashamed.* [Sect. 15, p. 189][69]

... as follows: ... uffered ... which ... uld not ... from a ... either". ... is point ... personal- ... They be- ... man, un- ... urse, nor ... less, sub- ... appetite ... en colour, ... nderstand- ... anifest by ... convulsive ... vely early. ... bed such a ... t the attack ... ecessary for ... a wall or ... face, and it ... idn't have to

ceased. ... lean, he was seized by a confusion in the head, and darkness in the eyes, and feeling it beforehand, he said an "Ave Maria" and before it had finished, the paroxysm had passed. He spat once and it was all over, but it came frequently during the day. There are some people who after the paroxysm have absolutely no memory of their falling down or of their affliction, whilst there are others who remember and *feel ashamed.*" Throughout the Middle Ages there was fixation on the relationship between epileptic phenomena and various magical, mystical, and religious philosophies.[162] These led to the inappropriate reactions to the epileptic as being "possessed" and worsened the already existing fears, anxieties, and feelings of shame and inadequacy in the afflicted individual. Many of the present-day stigmas and the psychological and social problems of the epileptic patient have their origins in this unfortunate history.

Beginning with the Renaissance, increasing insight and medical understanding of epilepsy gradually developed,[162] but it was not until the mid-nineteenth century with its anatomical and physiological approaches to the problem that the modern era began. Hughlings Jackson[78] developed the first comprehensive understanding of seizure origin from an abnormal focus of excessive discharge of brain gray matter, with especially pertinent descriptions of the "dreamy state" and uncinate-temporal lobe seizure, differentiating these from major convulsive activity. Gowers,[63] detailed the extensive variety of clinical epileptic symptoms even further, and emphasized states which he regarded as in a "borderland" between actual epileptic seizure and certain psychological phenomena. Actually, it was gradually recognized, during the 19th century, particularly by workers in France, e.g., Falret,[32] that psychological disturbances may occur in the epileptic subject as part of the seizure complex itself, i.e., ictal, or as an interictal disturbance involving various behavioral and cognitive functions. Disruptions of mental functions of severe degree such as psychoses were found, when brief and paroxysmal, to be ictal, but being more often of long duration, as part of an interictal state. The recognition of psychological precipitating factors both in a direct emotional or affective way, as in relation to various sensory stimuli, began in part with Richer of the Charcot school,[135] leading to a differentiation between "hystero-epilepsy" and what could be called "actual" epilepsy. Problems still remain, however, in delineating the role of the epilepsy in relation to mental disorder, and in separating out factors due to specific brain lesion.

The twentieth century has seen extensive research in this field: in-depth studies of the life history of the patients; finer neuropathological, neurophysiological, and biochemical correlations; the use of electroencephalography in diagnosis and in studying, in a concomitant way, relationship between seizure discharges and psychological functions; neuropsychological tests of increasing sophistication in delineating specific brain dysfunctions; antiepileptic drugs with increasing knowledge of

---

DR. JAMES E. WASSENMILLER

ADDRESS 720 WINTER STREET SE

PHONE 364-5757 DATE

seen the same day unless a true emergency exists. ALSO, PLEASE KEEP YOUR APPOINTMENT ONCE YOU HAVE MADE IT; otherwise, you will lose the right to be seen their effects on seizures and mental functions correlated with blood levels; and, finally, the combined approaches of both medical-pharmacological and psychological-social management in the treatment of many epileptic patients, leading to rehabilitation and placement in an effective role in society.

(Incidence

It has been difficult to determine an accurate epidemiology of epilepsy, particularly because of the increasing diagnostic awareness of the paroxysmal, but nonconvulsive, types of seizure disorders, especially those involving behavioral changes. The incidence may well be over 1 percent in the general population. Epileptic seizures appear in all age groups from the newborn to the elderly, but with different causes. There is a differential sex ratio of 140 males per 100 females. There are variations with different phenomena, for example the sex ratio with regard to the occurrence of chronic epileptic psychoses is about equal.

Only when seizures recur is the designation epilepsy appropriate. Not all epilepsy can be described in terms of convulsions, but the terms "fit," "attack," or "spell" are considered vague and inappropriate. Any disorder affecting brain function may result in seizures and the process must be considered in terms of various factors which may or may not be present in any individual instance, such as an anatomic substrate or actual physical lesion of brain tissue, the development of physiological disturbance, and biochemical and metabolic correlates. Genetic background and constitutional predisposition may be significant, and psychological determinants or "triggering" factors may be contributory.

(Mechanisms and Etiology

Basic Mechanisms[81]

Any neuron or aggregate of neurons may be made to discharge abnormally, by electrical stimulation, by alterations in basic metabolic environment, or by excitatory drugs. Thus, even a normal brain, may be made to develop either generalized or focal seizures. The various pathological disorders that produce recurrent seizures or epilepsy operate upon factors in terms of basic predisposition, specific abnormal process and precipitating or triggering circumstances. Certain regions of brain are considered seizure-sensitive, with low threshold and high susceptibility. These are especially related to motor and autonomic functions, such as motor cortex and the complex of the "limbic" system. The temporal lobe and its deeper limbic nuclear aggregates, the amygdala and hippocampus, are particularly involved in the development of seizures.[98] Their vascularity is vulnerable to compression, and the neuronal structures in these regions are very sensitive to metabolic disturbance such as hypoxia. It is difficult to separate cause and effect in this regard, since structural lesions in these regions may be the result of seizure activity with secondary vascular insufficiency and hypoxia; however, such lesions, following severe convulsions or *status epilepticus* in infancy, may themselves become epileptogenic and lead to further "limbic" seizure activity.

Factors of age and development are important from the perinatal period onwards. There often is a little-understood delay between the event of a lesion (i.e., as due to trauma or encephalitis), and the appearance of seizure. Certain seizure types are more common in infants, e.g., massive spasms; petit-mal seizures appear in childhood after the age of four or five rather than later in life. The occurrence of seizures with high fever is almost exclusively a phenomenon of early childhood.

Seizure activity may develop from an abnormal focus or a number of foci or may be generalized from the onset, seemingly without focal origin. However, generalization of paroxysmal discharge throughout the brain may occur from a focus so rapidly that the focal origin may be obscured. Many patients with an epileptogenic cerebral lesion, especially in a temporal lobe, are in this category. Certainly, however, major convulsions caused by such metabolic distortions as hypoglycemia, hypocalcemia, water intoxication, or the withdrawal of sedative drugs are examples of those generalized from the onset. In these instances the initiation of the seizure may be in the subcortical mesodiencephalic nonspecific reticular systems, with diffuse propagation bilaterally into cerebral cortex, especially motor and autonomic pathways. The rapid loss of consciousness which occurs first and the marked amnesia for the seizure afterwards can be related to this type of patterned spread.

However, it is reasonable to consider, as did Jackson, that most other seizures develop from a focus or aggregate of abnormally excitable neurons. The neuronal disturbances involved are those of intrinsic membrane instabilities related to both intra- and extracellular chemical derangements.[59,81] These produce excessive paroxysmal potential discharges, spreading then through essentially normal neural pathways away from the focus. Thus, the clinical manifestations of a particular seizure state depend upon both the focus of origin and the region of brain involved in the propagated discharge.

However, epilepsy as a clinical phenomenon is a discontinuous process. Seizures of any type have varying periodicity in any particular patient and may relate to the sleep cycle, the menstrual cycle, or to unpredictable body rhythms. Certain seizures may occur one or more times a day in some subjects, but at much longer intervals in others. Yet, the clinical "interseizure" state may be characterized by more or less continually abnormal electrical activity as seen in the EEG. There are, therefore, two clinical states of the epileptic, i.e., the actual overt seizure or ictal disturbance, and the interictal state. Under certain circumstances the interictal state may be manifest by subtle difficulties in cerebral function, such as in memory processing and learning, or in behavioral distortions. Whether these, too, might be related to actual subclinical ongoing seizure or ictal discharge remains a problem for continued investigation (see below).

Much attention now is paid to "reflex" or sensory precipitating factors in the production of seizures.[50,149] These often are quite specific for individual patients such as light flickering, i.e., photic sensitive and TV epilepsy, visual patterns, reading, and sound (musicogenic).

Both physiological and biochemical processes must be considered not only in our understanding of how epileptogenic neurons develop, but of how such seizure activity ceases. A property of "neuronal exhaustion" may be physiological, yet in some way due to depletion of metabolic substrates, along with ionic shifts. Such a secondary clinical concomitant of generalized convulsive activity as apnea contributes to cerebral hypoxia, if not controlled. Actually cerebral blood flow does increase initially to meet cerebral oxygen demands during such seizures, decreasing only later if the seizure is severe and prolonged as in *status epilepticus*.

Etiology in Epilepsy

IDIOPATHIC EPILEPSY

Epilepsies, or recurrent seizures, appear in man in a great variety of situations, and consideration of etiology must involve factors which may be genetic and constitutional, or acquired and symptomatic. In individual patients certain precipitating or contributing factors, while not specifically causative, may be highly important. A major problem in the understanding of epilepsy by the patient, his family, and even the physician, is the failure to find a specific cause, such as a structural or biochemical lesion, in a large number of patients (up to 75 percent). Even if such lesions are not found by the finest diagnostic techniques, it is indeed possible that a minute epileptogenic lesion could be present in a highly sensitive area of brain. One merely might consider the relatively high incidence of unrecognized encephalopathies in childhood associated with exanthema or head trauma to realize the possibility of production of such a lesion. Therefore, we can divide epileptics into two categories etiologically, the idiopathic and the secondary or acquired. Idiopathic epilepsy is diagnosed when no specific cause can be found. In acquired epilepsy such a cause is determined. Petit-mal epilepsy in childhood is regarded as the classic example of an idiopathic disorder, yet some cases are known to be associated with actual brain lesions.

The important question of genetics and heredity must be considered, particularly since it often plays a significant role in reactive psychological problems of the patient and his family.[2,9,117] A genetically transmitted predisposition for seizure tendency is present in certain families, especially involving patients with onset of seizure in early life, as petit mal. There also are families with a high incidence of febrile seizures in infants. Even some familial focal patterning may occur. It has been determined that the relatives of some epileptic patients have a 3–5 percent incidence of epilepsy and an even higher incidence of electroencephalographic abnormality. This is seen particularly in studies of monozygotic twins in whom such abnormalities may reach a correlation of over 40 percent. There may be a constitutional susceptibility for seizure associated with a head injury or brain tumor. Yet, since epilepsy is a symptom often associated with other neurologic abnormalities such as motor disturbance and mental subnormality due to various underlying cerebral diseases, an inheritance pattern for such specific cerebral disease must be considered as well. In addition, there are a known number of indirect factors, nongenetic, such as cerebral birth trauma secondary to narrow maternal pelvis, which can be related to seizure incidence in siblings.

Acquired or Symptomatic Epilepsy

Any disease or structural abnormality of the brain may be associated with seizures, as well as other neurological dysfunctions including those producing perceptual and intellectual disorders. These are listed below.

Congenital malformations of the brain cause varying incidence of epilepsy, depending upon degree, location, and general genetic factors. These include microgyria, porencephaly, hemangiomas, and Down's syndrome. Multiple anomalies may be associated with maternal rubella. Prematurity, breech delivery, and neonatal asphyxia all may be important factors in epileptogenesis.

Acute, subacute, and chronic infections are productive of epilepsy both during the active process and later due to residual lesions. The incidence of cerebral neurosyphilis has decreased. However, viral encephalitis, acute and subacute, is increasingly prominent. Certain of these, such as acute herpetic encephalitis, tend to localize in a temporal lobe.

Head injury is a major cause of acquired epilepsy, acutely and as a chronic residual effect. Posttraumatic epilepsy may develop within three years in up to 10 percent of cases after a closed head injury, and between 30 and 40 percent after open injuries. The seizure incidence depends upon the severity of the wound, dural penetration, and location.

Brain tumors (gliomas, meningiomas, metastatic) are associated with seizures, especially focal, in 30–40 percent of cases, the seizure being the first sign in 15–20 percent. The incidence is highest in supratentorial convexity tumors. Progression of symptoms from focal seizure to hemiparesis and organic mental dysfunction should be highly suggestive of tumor.

Cerebral vascular disease is a cause of epilepsy more frequently than usually realized, especially in older age groups. Seizures may occur in up to 25 percent of such patients due to localized vascular insufficiency and acute ischemic hypoxia, as well as secondary to the lesions of embolism, hemorrhage, and thrombosis. Prolonged syncope as in carotid sinus sensitivity and Adams-Stokes syndrome may develop into seizure. Diffuse cerebral arteriosclerosis, often associated with hypertensive disease, can produce a syndrome of dementia and focal or generalized seizures.

Cerebral degenerative and demyelinating diseases have a significant incidence of seizures. This reaches 5 percent in multiple sclerosis. The incidence is relatively high in the presenile dementias (Alzheimer, Pick) with both myoclonic and generalized seizures.

Toxic and metabolic cerebral disorders are associated with both seizures and encephalopathy (dementia, stupor, precoma, coma). Various drug intoxications as with alcohol, barbiturates, and other sedatives or tranquillizers produce seizure induction usually in a withdrawal phase, within forty-eight to seventy-two hours, often with delirium. Carbon monoxide intoxication, hypoxia, water intoxication, lead poisoning, hypoglycemia, hypocalcemia, and porphyria may cause seizures in individual instances.

In many cases a combination of factors may be playing a role, such as genetic predisposition, a toxic metabolic disturbance, a focal brain lesion, vascular insufficiency and a nonspecific trigger such as an emotional crisis or a flickering light. Each patient, therefore, must be evaluated diagnostically from many different aspects in order to establish etiology on the different levels leading to appropriate total therapy.

(Clinical Epileptic Manifestations with Emphasis on Neuropsychological Phenomena

Generalized Seizures

MAJOR OR GRAND MAL EPILEPSY

Within the major generalized seizure, a complex series of events occurs which the patient usually does not remember. A description must be obtained from witnesses, especially experienced, if possible, since details are extremely important, particularly in relation to establishing focal origin or in differentiation from a major hysterical state.

Such seizures usually start with a prodromal phase lasting minutes or even hours, with a change in emotional reactivity or affective responses, such as the appearance of increasing tension or anxiety, depression or elation. This initial phase may be difficult to recognize, and more often the onset of the seizure is regarded as the aura. This usually is a brief sensory experience directly related to the locus of origin of the seizure. Frequently experienced auras are a sense of fear and dread, a peculiar upper visceral epigastric sensation welling up into the throat, an unpleasant odor, various formed and unformed visual and auditory hallucinations and peculiar sensations in an arm or leg. At times, localized movements of an extremity or portions of the face precede the generalized seizure. The aura, as the initial phase, may allow distinction between seizure generalized from the start or generalized with focal onset. The convulsion itself often begins with sudden vocalization (the "epileptic cry"), loss of consciousness, tonic extensor rigidity of trunk and extremities, then clonic movements, impaired breathing with brief apnea, cyanosis, and stertor. Incontinence of bladder and bowels, biting of the tongue and inside of cheeks ensue in the clonic phase. Examination may reveal marked pupillary inequality and extensor plantar responses. After some minutes the excessive motor activity ceases, breathing becomes more normal and consciousness gradually returns. However, a postictal state is frequently present with confusion, general fatigue, headache, and at times residual neurologic signs, such as hemiparesis, sensory disturbances, and dysphasia. Postictal paralysis (Todd's paralysis) may last from several minutes to hours after the seizure. In general, there is complete amnesia for the major events of the seizure, with the exception of possible recollection of the prodromal phase and the aura.[155] Knowledge and familiarity of this entire sequence of events will help the physician to distinguish between actual epileptic seizure and "functional" seizurelike states.

The EEG pattern associated with generalized seizure, during the seizure itself, is difficult to distinguish from movement artifact, but otherwise may be seen to consist usually of bilateral discharges from all areas with patterns of high amplitude spikes and slow waves. These discharges may be present intermittently in the interseizure state. However, between seizures many patients (up to 25 percent) may have an EEG characterized by nonspecific generalized slow wave changes or even essentially normal patterns. Localized slow waves or discharges are suggestive of a focal cerebral lesion.

Generalized seizures appear in all etiologic circumstances and in all age groups. The frequency may vary greatly, with about 20 percent of patients only having nocturnal convulsions. In females, a cyclic occurrence may appear with the menses. The designation "fragmentary seizure" may be utilized for the occurrence of brief phases of the generalized complex, i.e., only auras (frequent epigastric "butterflies") or brief, abortive movements and disturbance of consciousness. These may occur in some patients during therapy with anticonvulsant drugs and relatively incomplete control.

PETIT MAL EPILEPSY

The seizure of "absence," a minor form of "generalized" epilepsy, is characterized primarily by a brief lapse of consciousness usually lasting 5–10 sec. but occasionally up to 30 sec. The petit-mal seizure ordinarily appears in childhood, with onset between the ages of three and ten years. Usually no specific cause is found, and this form of epilepsy is regarded as classically idiopathic. It tends to diminish in incidence after puberty and persistence into adult life is unusual, being quite infrequent after the age of thirty. In rare instances a specific brain lesion, such as a frontal calcified tumor or diffuse lipidosis, has been reported with petit mal.

Clinically, the patient is seen to have a sudden cessation of activity and to stare, without any gross movements. However, blinking of the eyelids is common and occasionally slight deviation of the eyes and head, along with brief minor movements of the lips and hands may occur. When more complex behavior alterations with motor acts are present, the pattern should be regarded as a brief automatism or minor motor seizure. The term "akinetic attack" refers to a generalized seizure with simple falling and loss of consciousness. It may be accompanied by an absence seizure and minor movements, but usually there is but a marked diminution of general postural tone. Afterwards, the patient recovers normal posture and mental clarity, though there may be a slight period of confusion.

The electroencephalographic correlate of petit-mal or absence seizure is a rhythmic 3-Hz. spike-and-wave discharge appearing from all regions synchronously both during and between seizures in about 85 percent of patients. Usually a discharge of more than two seconds is associated with a clinical seizure. Akinetic and myoclonic seizures may be associated with atypical spike-wave discharges, often slower than 3 Hz.

Photic sensitivity is present in a number of patients and may be familial. Flickering light at 12–14 Hz. most commonly triggers these seizures. In some patients, mere exposure to bright sunlight may precipitate seizures; in others the flickering of a television screen is effective. The phenomenon of self-induction of seizure[3,4,36] appears in this context, the patients inducing absence seizure by looking at a light and passing a hand in front of the eyes. Self-induced television epilepsy has been described.[3] Apparently, in these instances, a peculiar pleasurable sensation accompanies the experience of the seizure. The incidence of absence attacks varies from very few, often in the morning, to a great many, up to 100 or more per day ("pyknolepsy"). As the frequency increases, the child may develop difficulties in continuing certain tasks and in developing complex learning functions, since there may be a defect in memory patterning induced by the absence. The designation "petit-mal status" or "absence status" refers to many such attacks occurring close together in time, lasting from minutes to several hours and producing clouding of consciousness with marked confusion and disorientation. Close observation may reveal minor twitching of the eyelids and upper limbs along with a dull facial expression. The state is associated with prolonged EEG discharge of the 3-Hz. spike-wave type as well as more irregular complex slower and faster components with polyspikes. Instances of even more prolonged mental dullness with profound psychic disturbances, a change in personality, motor agitation, dreamy states, delusion and "dementing" syndrome have been found associated with this type of EEG abnormality.[49]

Myoclonic seizures as related seizure phenomenon in this group may be localized or generalized and when severe are often associated with impairment of consciousness. They involve sudden integrated contractions of a single muscle or many muscle groups producing relatively simple arrhythmic jerking movements of one or many joints or a body segment. They can exist as an independent entity, as a phenomenon preceding a generalized seizure, usually with a build-up in severity, or in association with petit mal absence. They often are sensitive to sensory influences and may be precipitated by light or sound stimuli, change in posture or movement of a limb, by drowsiness or an emotional upset. In some instances cerebellar dysfunction with ataxia may be present in an associated syndrome. The myoclonus epilepsy of "Unverricht" refers to generalized myoclonus and mental deterioration due to a diffuse degenerative metabolic disorder. Myoclonic seizures associated with other signs of diffuse cerebral dysfunction (confusion, stupor, dementia) occur in uremic encephalopathy, subacute encephalitis, Creutzfeldt-Jakob chronic viral encephalitis, and cerebral lipidoses.

A severe myoclonic seizure disorder appearing in the first eighteen months of life and usually associated with general cerebral deterioration and marked mental retardation is called infantile massive spasms or jackknife seizure. The infant develops marked flexion spasms of head, neck, and trunk, and extension of legs and arms. This probably is the most common major seizure pattern in infancy. Some known causes of this disorder are phenylketonuria, tuberous sclerosis, Down's syndrome, bilateral subdural hematoma, and marked porencephaly. However, the cause is often not determined.

The EEG correlates of myoclonic seizures usually are synchronous 2–3 Hz. spike-wave complexes in bursts, with clear EEG patterns interspersed. The massive spasm seizures are more associated with hypsarrhythmia, or relatively asynchronous, asymmetric slow spike-wave and slow-wave discharges.

Perceptual Functions during Seizures and EEG Discharges

A relatively controllable way of evaluating perceptual abilities during epileptic activity has been to study the ability of patients to perceive and react during overt electroencephalographic discharges. Because the petit-mal absence type of epileptic seizure has a high degree of correlation (over 85 percent) with the typical 3 Hz. paroxysmal spike-and-wave activity in the electroencephalogram,

such studies were first carried out in subjects with this disorder. Initially, Schwab[143] was able to demonstrate that patients with petit-mal seizures displayed a disturbance in response to auditory stimuli; the responses were delayed during attacks lasting about five seconds, and in those lasting more than eight seconds no response occurred. This was regarded as due to the distorted awareness or "unconsciousness" caused by the petit-mal seizure. Since that time, there have been a number of other investigations of this phenomenon of delayed or disturbed reactivity correlated with electroencephalographic discharges in subjects with petit mal and other forms of epilepsy. This subject is of great importance in our understanding of psychological disturbances in epilepsy and will be discussed in some detail.

A high degree of variability has been reported, but the experimental designs themselves have been very different, particularly in the types of tests performed by the subject. Not all investigations utilized tests of actual perceptual functions, although many cognitive elements were involved. Kooi and Hovey[89] studied the performance of standard psychological tests (i.e., Wechsler-Bellevue, particularly picture completion and digit symbol) during continuous EEG recording of patients with mainly grand-mal or psychomotor epilepsy, but with intermittent bilateral spike-wave discharges in the EEG. The test performances always were impaired, often with nonanswer responses during the EEG discharges. Similar results were reported by Davidoff and Johnson.[22] Visual motor continuous-performance tests showed greater deficiencies during suppressed or flattened periods in the EEG, in an unusual study by Prechtl et al.[124] Courtois et al.[19] reported an unequal affection during petit-mal attacks of somatosensory modalities, i.e., light touch most readily, then passive movement, and pain perception least. Goode et al.[61] and Mirsky and Van Buren[110] have demonstrated that patients with petit-mal epilepsy performed more poorly on a test of sustained attention, i.e., the continuous-performance test, than did patients with focal motor epilepsy. This test utilized a repeated specified visual signal, and it was found that the ability to execute the simple repetitive discriminative response was lost if the stimulus fell within a burst of spike-and-wave activity in the electroencephalogram. Actually, the interpretation of the mechanism of this disturbance still is not definite because it may be due (as Mirsky and Tecce[109] have emphasized) to reduced sensory input or reduced perception, to weakened motor effective capacity, to temporary impairment of the central integrative or decision-making process, to temporary forgetting of the task instructions, or to a combination of these factors. Mirsky and Van Buren suggested that both input and output might be affected by whatever produces the spike-and-wave discharge, although reduced input or reduced perception seemed to be more obviously disturbed than a weakened or reduced output. Thus, in the sensory task the subject was presented with a visual auditory stimulus with the instruction to hold it in mind until questioned by the examiner. When stimuli were presented during the spike-and-wave burst and the patient questioned a few seconds later, recall was severely impaired; the degree of impairment was generally less than that seen with the ordinary continuous-performance test. However, the interpretation of this as a "purely" sensory perceptive impairment remains equivocal. The patient may have registered the stimulus, but it may have been expunged from his memory by the physiological phenomenon manifested by the spike-and-wave burst. Alternatively, it may not be possible under these conditions to maintain a stimulus trace without some initial subvocal verbalization or rehearsal; there may be a subtle but important motor component even in this pure sensory perceptive task. It should be mentioned that these workers found that electroencephalographic bursts which were symmetrical, regular, and bilaterally synchronous tended to produce more deficit in these tasks than other less extensive EEG discharges. The interjected problem of memory disturbance has been emphasized by the work of Hutt et al.,[74,76] who showed that children with light-sensitive epilepsy demonstrated impaired recall of digits during bioelectric paroxysms in the EEG evoked by stroboscopic light stimulation.

Further analysis of this phenomenon has been carried out by Tizard and Margerison.[163] They showed that patients with petitmal epilepsy worked more slowly during the performance of various tests and made more errors during electroencephalographic spikewave discharges. Even very brief bursts of one to one-and-one-half second's duration, without overt behavioral accompaniments, were shown to be associated with significantly slowed response times. The psychological tests utilized by these workers were simple, repetitive, and continuous, and involved responses to various perceptual stimuli, such as auditory, visual, and tactile. The auditory stimuli were of both numbers and tones, the visual stimuli were of different combinations of numbers of lights and colors, and the tactile stimuli were those of a tickling stimulus applied to the hand. In six patients studied, all but one had an amnesia for the events occurring during clinical attacks or correlated electroencephalographic discharges. Even this patient, however, had some disturbance of recall. All of the patients exhibited defects in performance in all tests during the discharges. The phenomenon was not regarded as one merely of a loss of "consciousness" during spike-wave discharges of sufficiently long duration. When the discharge lasted longer than six to eight seconds, the disturbance of performance was much greater; however, the important finding in this study[163] is the demonstration of disturbed performance during the very brief discharges of around one to two seconds in duration, even though no clinical seizure or other behavioral abnormality was observed. The implication from all of these studies is that both perception and memory are disturbed during even brief seizure activity, and that both of these processes probably interact in developing the actual experience of the subject.

In many instances similar impairments of cognitive functions may be present between bursts of paroxysmal EEG discharge, implying a more persistent disturbance of integrating cerebral circuits. Another clinically highly significant observation, often of practical significance in patient management, is the frequently found suppression or limitation of paroxysmal seizure activity (especially petit mal) during states of attention, stimulation, concentration, and motor activity, particularly during periods of interest and high motivation.* However, periods of inactivity, boredom, and irritability may trigger even more seizures. The use of EEG telemetry on patients, especially school children in various task settings[66] is increasing our information and understanding of such psychological factors in the triggering of epileptic discharges in the EEG and actual seizures.

Sensory-Evoked Potentials during Epileptic Discharges

Disturbances of sensory perception already described as occurring in epileptic patients and often correlated with electroencephalographic discharges vary from simple to complex, and clearly involve different portions of the sensory perceiving and analyzing cerebral structures. The epileptic discharges may involve only certain systems or portions of systems and produce the changes that vary in their complexity of expression. Not all neuronal populations seem to participate fully in the different kinds of seizure activity, even those characterized by the generalized high-amplitude synchronous discharging seen during prolonged absence attacks.

Attempts have been made to study these phenomena by investigating cerebral sensory-evoked potentials in epileptic subjects in the interseizure state and during epileptic discharges. Cernacek and Ciganek[17] found a decreased amplitude of the earlier components of visual-evoked responses, i.e., presumably that portion related to primary receiving activity, and an increase in certain of the later secondary waves (especially their wave V), in patients in the interseizure state. This effect was more pronounced at lower frequencies of stimulation than at higher. Photogenic epileptic subjects did not differ from those with psychomotor and grand-mal epilepsy. Potentials

* See references 29, 40, 41, 83, 90, 94, and 134.

from occipital cortex were not specifically enhanced. However, Gastaut et al.[47] studied hemianopic subjects with visual epileptic seizures in the blind field and found, from the involved occipital regions, higher amplitude late components of visual-evoked responses. Similarly, Bacia and Reid[6] described an increase in amplitude of somatosensory-evoked potentials on the side of the epileptogenic focus in patients with focal epilepsy. They did not elicit altered responses in patients with "centrencephalic" epilepsy, with a prolonged high amplitude after discharge phenomenon. Gastaut and Regis[48] found the greatest changes in photosensitive generalized epileptics, with markedly increased secondary components (especially wave V) being evoked, correlated with the degree of photic sensitivity and seizure frequency. In general, similar findings were reported by Morocutti and Sommer-Smith,[112] Hishikawa et al.,[70] and Green.[64] The enhancement of the secondary component of the evoked response is thought to be due to the related phenomena of neuronal facilitation and recruitment at subcortical and cortical levels, greater postinhibitory rebound, and hypersynchronization of neuronal activity in cortical areas associated with epileptogenic activity.

Visual-evoked responses have been studied during physiological sleep in "centrencephalic" epileptics.[10] During the slow wave (first and second phases), the responses are similar to those in the waking state with greater amplitude of later components. In the paradoxical or REM sleep the responses show less reactivity and late waves of longer duration and later peaking in amplitude.

Rodin et al.[139] investigated visual-evoked potentials during epileptic discharges characterized as "petit-mal status," classical petit mal seizure, and tonic seizure with unresponsiveness. Evoked responses were "suggestively present" in three subjects during grand-mal seizure discharges. The evoked potentials were present in relatively unchanged fashion during petit-mal seizure induced by bemigride activation. At times "some change in latencies" during seizure activity was reported, but a quantitative analysis of these data was not given. During grand-mal-seizure activity in man the elements of evoked visual response were distinguishable during tonic and clonic phases, but not clearly in the immediate post-ictal phase; this latter deficit was related to hypoxia. These investigators also showed that photic responses could be evoked unchanged from cat cerebral cortex during seizure discharges produced by bemigride administration. The evoked responses could be elicited immediately postictally in these experiments. The animals were receiving artificial respiration and, therefore, the factor of hypoxia probably did not play the apparent significant role that it did with humans. The authors emphasized the importance of the elicitation of evoked responses during the clonic portions of seizure activity, and suggested that a process of generalized inhibition probably was not playing a significant role during such an epileptic phase.

Mirsky and Tecce[109] have conducted more elaborate investigations of visual-evoked potentials during electroencephalographic spike-and-wave activity in man. They demonstrated that the enhancement of the voltage of the evoked potential was least evident from the parietal-occipital region and more prominent from the anterior region, an effect which seemed to mirror the distribution of voltages of the spike-wave discharge itself, which is maximal in the frontal and less pronounced in the posterior region. Also, the form of the average evoked potential appeared to be influenced by the particular part of the spike-wave complex within which the stimulus was administered. However, the nature of these changes is not clear. These investigators also studied visual-evoked potentials during spike-wave discharges produced by the administration of chlorambucil to monkeys. This substance produced epileptiform activity thought to be similar to that associated with petit-mal absence in man. In these experiments, visual-evoked potentials were recorded during the spike-wave discharges; however there was an apparent reduction in amplitude of the potentials from areas associated with visual perception in the monkey including optic nerve and chiasm, lateral geniculate, and occipital cor-

tex. The reduction in evoked potential amplitude was absent from regions usually not associated with visual functions, such as the midline thalamus, frontal cortex, and pons. In fact, there was probably an enhancement of the potential from these regions. These results suggested to Mirsky and Tecce[109] that "if the size of the evoked potential reflects the amount of sensory information being transmitted, then there is actually less visual input (as seen in visually related structures) during spike and wave activity." The interpretation of the enhancement, if it be such, in nonvisual areas is problematical: "It may reflect differential inhibitory and/or disinhibitory effects during spike and wave seizure activity or some effect which serves to compensate for reduced information flow in the primary receptor." The other question suggested by this work is related to the influence on the evoked visual potential of the specific period in the development in the spike-and-wave burst into which the stimulus falls. These authors indicate that there are behavioral data to suggest that the period just prior to the appearance of the epileptiform burst is deleterious to performance in any continuous-performance test and that absence-seizure phenomenon may antedate the appearance of the paroxysmal burst in the electroencephalogram.

Focal or Partial Seizures

Focal or partial seizures are characterized by manifestations indicating involvement of a specific region of brain, and therefore usually represent an acquired epilepsy. Rapid secondary generalization of seizure may develop from a focus, but more usually the attack remains limited. Although any region of cortex or subcortex may develop excitatory seizure activity, certain regions are more frequently involved. Total loss of consciousness is uncommon, but usually there is some altered conscious awareness with varying degrees of amnesia for the events of the seizure.[155] This is particularly true when portions of the limbic system (i.e., hippocampus and amygdala) and associated diencephalic structures are involved in seizure production.[98]

The EEG concomitants of focal seizures including the psychomotor-temporal-limbic variety are characterized by discharges of spikes, complexes, and slow waves localized from the particular region involved in at least 75 percent of instances. Frequently, however, the discharges may be bilateral and asynchronous, representing transmission and diffusion of the focal abnormalities. This is especially true in the EEGs of children with focal seizures. Also, at times, deeply situated lesions produce only minimal or no significant scalp-recorded electroencephalographic abnormality. In adults, recording during sleep may evoke focal discharges, especially from patients with temporal-lobe limbic seizures.

Focal motor seizures are produced by lesions in any of the motor regions of the brain, especially the motor (pre-Rolandic) cortex. The classic Jacksonian motor seizure begins as a repetitive movement of a distal portion of an extremity, such as fingers or toes, and then spreads by a march of clonic contraction up the extremity toward the trunk. Consciousness seldom is altered unless spread occurs contralaterally. Focal motor seizures may affect speech production with even an arrest of speech.

Focal sensory seizures may be Jacksonian with lesions in the sensory (post-Rolandic) cortex producing a march of abnormal sensations, such as numbness and tingling, spreading up an extremity. Seizures derived from other sensory and receptive analysing areas contain more complex visual, auditory, olfactory, gustatory, and vertiginous components in varying degrees of organization (see below).

Autonomic seizures are produced from cerebral foci associated with autonomic functional representation, such as deep temporal-limbic or diencephalic-hypothalamic. Many of the symptoms are associated with other focal or generalized seizures, but, especially in children, they may exist more or less by themselves as paroxysms of abdominal pain, sweating, piloerection, incontinence, salivation, and fever.

Psychomotor-temporal-lobe (limbic) seizures represent the most prominent and common form of focal or partial epilepsy. The temporal lobe and its deeper nuclear masses, the amygdala and hippocampus and their associated limbic structures, as indicated previously, are particularly vulnerable to many pathological processes from the perinatal period onwards throughout life.[117,118] Such seizures may represent at least 25 percent of all seizures in childhood and well over 50 percent in adult life, often coexisting with grand-mal seizures. In over 60 percent of cases a definite structural lesion may be found, secondary to trauma, encephalitis, ischemia, hypoxia, or tumor (vascular malformation, hamartoma, glioma). The latter may be so small as to escape detection by neurodiagnostic radiological methods and may only be found within a temporal lobe resected for intractable incapacitating seizures. Even when focal frontal lesions or diffuse cerebral disease are present, for example, it is likely that clinical manifestations are evoked by propagation of the discharge through temporal-limbic structures.[99]

The most simple, but relatively rare, type of temporal-lobe seizure is manifest by a paroxysmal dysphasic speech disturbance when the dominant lobe is involved. This is usually an inability to form speech components, but may be experienced as a blocking of the ideation necessary to produce speech.[118] It has been associated with visual hallucinations.[36]

The clinical manifestations of psychomotor-temporal-limbic seizures are characterized by an initial aura most frequently consisting of anxiety and visceral symptoms, especially a peculiar epigastric sensation welling up into the throat.* This is followed by an alteration—not a loss—of consciousness, associated with many varied, complex mental states and automatic somatic and autonomic motor behavior. These phenomena are associated with at least a partial amnesia, particularly for automatisms. Recollection of sensory experiences of an aura, or of certain perceptual distortions early during the seizure, may be obtained.[155]

During the seizure itself, there is often arrest or suspension of ongoing activity at first, then simple movements such as lip-smacking, chewing, swallowing, sucking, and aimless

---

* See references 8, 30, 31, 45, 51, 63, 93, 118, and 171.

motions of the arms and legs. These are followed by repetitive stereotyped automatisms of varying complexity and involving partially purposeful or inappropriate and bizarre behavior. The latter can be associated with the environment and occasionally influenced by psychological factors related to unresolved conflicts. For example, one of our patients recited the "Apostles Creed" during his seizure. The activities in this phase of the seizure may merge into normal behavior.

The occurrence of olfactory hallucinations—usually unpleasant—associated with lesions of the mesial portions of the temporal lobe, the uncus, was called "uncinate" seizure by Jackson,[78] who also described the "dreamy" state of the patient during the seizure, occasionally prolonged postictally. He also reports the complex case of a physician with a temporal-lobe lesion who was, however, capable of organized, appropriate activity, i.e., examination of a patient, diagnosis, and prescription, with no recollection of these activities.[79]

In children with this type of seizure there is emphasis on visceral manifestations[53,55] with expressions of hunger, nausea, retching, vomiting, and abdominal pain. Spitting automatism[67] is an unusual expression of temporal-limbic seizure. Epileptic laughter or gelastic epilepsy[44] may be part of this complex.

Destructive, aggressive behavior occasionally occurs, but is not usually purposeful.* The possibility of paroxysmal, ictal violence leading to homicide is a problematic matter still under intensive investigation. The implication of actual temporal-lobe seizure in a specific directed violent attack remains difficult to prove.

Affective disturbances, particularly expressions of fear, anger, and depression may be present ictally.[31,142,170,171] Occasionally, prolonged fuguelike states with running or wandering about may last many minutes. A fugue of longer duration with the patient moving some distance and with amnesia for the experience is more likely a postictal automatism.

During many seizures of this type, patients are involved in experiential hallucinations,[118,]

* See references 31, 34, 43, 147, 157, and 164.

[119] both visceral and auditory, as well as interpretive illusions involving their own bodies or the immediate environment (i.e., micropsia, macropsia). These symptoms are frequently associated with ideational blocking and forced thinking. Common symptoms are the peculiar experiences of false familiarity with places and people (déjà vu), thoughts (déjà pensée), and voices (déjà entendu).

Ictal Perceptual Disturbances in Limbic Epilepsy

Ever since the fundamental descriptions of Jackson[78] and Gowers[63] the occurrence of perceptual disturbances during epileptic seizures has been studied particularly in patients with psychomotor-psychosensory seizure complex originating from the temporal lobes or limbic system as listed in Table 13–1. There

TABLE 13–1. **Perceptual Disorders in Limbic Epilepsy**

SOMATIC	VISCERAL
Olfactory	Gastric, epigastric
Visual	nausea
illusions	hunger
déjà vu	thirst
hallucinations	
Auditory	Abdominal
illusions	Pharyngeal
déjà entendu	Precordial
hallucinations	Respiratory
Vestibular	Genital, urinary
vertigo	Vasomotor
movement	
loss of equilibrium	
Gustatory	
Somesthetic sensations of	
face (nose, mouth)	
half of body	
extremities	

have been many clinical investigations of these ictal perceptual phenomena, with striking instances of both correlation and noncorrelation with either focal or generalized electroencephalographic discharges.[56] However, it is well known that scalp electroencephalographic recordings may give only incomplete or occasionally no reflection at all of abnormal discharge activity present in deep cerebral nuclear structures.[1,60]

To circumvent this problem, Penfield and his group[118,119] in many thorough and sustained investigations, have utilized electrical stimulation of temporal-lobe structures in conscious patients to reproduce the psychological disturbances experienced ictally. Similar methods and results have been described by others. Penfield[119] has classified the disordered perceptual phenomena as follows:

1. Psychical hallucinations or experiential seizures: the recall of past experiences in detail, with all the imagery that fell within the patient's attention at the time.

2. Psychical illusions: misrepresentations or altered interpretations of present experience, better called illusions of comparative interpretation or interpretive illusions. These are quite common, appearing in at least one third of the patients studied, either spontaneously as part of the seizure or as a result of temporal-lobe stimulation. During the illusory experience there is no depersonalization or loss of identity; although a voice may sound remote or a room may appear distorted and unfamiliar, the patient is usually able to distinguish reality from unreality.

The perceptual illusions have been classified further as follows: (1) auditory illusions, with sounds seeming louder or clearer, fainter or more distant, nearer or farther; (2) visual illusions, with objects appearing clearer or blurred, nearer or farther, larger or smaller, fatter or thinner, and so forth; and (3) illusions of recognition, the present experience seeming familiar, strange, altered and unreal. This includes the experience of the déjà-vu phenomenon. Less common illusions of perception are those of an increased awareness of surroundings, illusions of alteration and speed of movement and vestibular-visual disturbances in which objects appear tilted, along with vertiginous sensations.

Penfield and his group[119] found that auditory illusions could be produced by cortical temporal-lobe stimulations bilaterally, but visual illusions mainly from stimulations of the minor hemisphere. The latter finding may be correlated with a number of psychological studies which were able to show evidence of impaired eye–hand coordination, with difficulties in such tests as trail making and picture completion, particularly in cases with epileptic dysfunction of the nondominant temporal lobe.

Peculiar illusions of familiarity or of strangeness of the environment also are frequent in these patients, and are predominantly associated with epileptic discharge or electrical stimulation from the minor hemisphere. Distortions of the body image involve experiences of feeling disconnected, fragmented, malformed, or incomplete. A sensation of fear also is frequently associated with perceptions of peculiar bodily sensations involving thoracic and abdominal structures. Often feelings of lonesomeness, sorrow, absurdity, and disgust have been recounted, but it is remarkable that pleasant sensations are extremely rare.

In general, it is felt by these workers that the temporal-lobe functions involved are largely devoted to comparative interpretations of perceptions of the present environment and the analysis of the components of the different sensory perceptions, comparing them with previous experiences; these functions of analysis and comparison then transmit the experience into consciousness of the present and immediate significance. These functions become altered during states of seizure, producing the perceptual disturbances as experienced by the patient. Penfield has used the term "interpretive cortex" as applied to these regions of temporal lobe.

The disturbed perceptions in experiential hallucinations derived from temporal-lobe epileptic activity occur also in at least 10 percent of patients. These are similar to "flashback" phenomena which are past experiences and happenings incorporated into the patient's seizure pattern. They are more usually produced by stimulation of the involved cortex and only relatively infrequently are recalled otherwise by the subject. The phenomenon varies from fragmentary to extensive elaboration of various sights, sounds, and other perceptual experiences along with accompanying emotions, and the patient usually recognizes these as coming from his past. Again, these states appear almost twice as frequently in association with lesions of the nondominant temporal lobe as compared with the dominant; auditory experiences are about half as common as visual. Most such responses have been produced by stimulations of the lateral and superior surfaces of the first temporal convolution, and some can be produced by stimulations of the medial border of the hippocampal gyrus. The hallucinations involving somatic sensory perceptions are often associated with epigastric and other general visceral sensations and it is not unusual for some patients to have an abortive attack consisting of visceral experience alone. In many cases there is an association with sensory or psychic precipitation as a form of reflex epilepsy.[50,149] For example, attacks beginning with hand tingling may in some instances be precipitated by touching the hand, and certain attacks with visual hallucinations by utilizing light stimuli. There may be a lower threshold and a facilitation for these phenomenon in epileptogenic cortex involving these functions.

The effects of seizure activity on perceptual functions and memory processes reach profound complexities in relation to the temporal-lobe-limbic epilepsies. It does seem likely that abnormal bioelectrical excitatory states developing in and propagating through limbic-system structures can interfere with perceptual functions of patients during overt clinical seizure, but also in apparently interseizure states (see below) with no overt seizure actually observable or experienced (i.e., subictal excitation).[156]

Cortical sensory-evoked potentials during experimental limbic seizures have been studied. Flynn et al,[38,39] reporting a series of experiments on the performance and acquisition of a conditioned avoidance response during hippocampal after-discharge in cats, noted, in passing, that the potentials evoked by the clicks which preceded the shock continued to arrive at the cortex during the seizure. Experiments carried out by Prichard and Glaser[126] utilized auditory click and visual flash stimuli evoking cortical potentials in cats, unanesthe-

tized and with chronically implanted electrodes, during sleep, wakefulness, and bilateral limbic seizures. The seizures were induced by stimulation unilaterally across amygdala and hippocampus, which produced propagated bilateral seizure activity. The evoked cortical potentials to both auditory and visual stimuli during such seizures were of normal configuration and amplitude and were undistinguishable from those recorded during the waking state. There were no significant changes in the evoked responses even during marked behavioral limbic seizures characterized by behavioral changes in the animal which included alterations in posture, facial twitching, pupillary dilatation, drooling, and some vocalization. There were no differences either behaviorally or with regard to the evoked potentials whether stimulation was begun with the animals awake or asleep. These results indicated that during widespread limbic seizures the auditory and visual systems were in a functional state, at least with regard to the pathways generating the evoked potential to these sensory stimuli, similar to that present during wakefulness. The findings are consistent with clinical observations that some patients with psychomotor epilepsy can perform certain complex integrated acts involving perception during their seizures (even though the perceptions may be distorted), and with the studies of Flynn et al.[38,39] that cats could perform a conditioned leg withdrawal after a training period in which the conditioned stimulus was paired with an unconditioned stimulus only during hippocampal after-discharge. Further investigation, with patients in a clinical setting, is necessary in this area.

Thus, it does seem clear that under certain conditions sensory information presented to the brain only during limbic seizures can influence both immediate and subsequent behavior, and that such seizures need not disturb the occurrence in the cortex of the usual configuration of potentials evoked by auditory and visual stimuli. On the other hand, the fact that psychomotor epileptics are almost always at least partially amnesic for their seizures implies a defect of storage, if not of actual reception of sensory information, and the performance of certain previously conditioned responses actually may be disrupted during limbic seizures. All these clinical and experimental observations do present the consideration of a boundary between what a brain can do and what it cannot do during seizure discharge occurring in the involved cerebral structures, such as those regarded to be within "limbic," "centrencephalic," or other epileptogenic aggregates. The actual anatomical and physiological substrates finally responsible for the perceptual distortions are less clear. The more precise definition of these boundaries in both electrophysiological and behavioral terms, along with the correlation with the nature and extent of seizure activity, are among the avenues to a clearer understanding of epileptic processes in man.

The Interseizure State

The intellectual performance and behavior of a patient with epilepsy between obvious clinical attacks, whatever the type, characterize the interseizure or interictal state.* Generalizations are difficult, but since the etiology is specific in up to 25 percent of cases, certain points may be made. The interseizure disorder in a patient with a progressive degenerative cerebral disease, encephalitis, or an expanding brain tumor who develops changes in behavior, personality and intellectual-cognitive functioning is probably not due to any seizure activity but to the underlying brain disease. This applies as well to the child with extensive cerebral damage or malformation.

However, the larger group consists of patients with seizures and an otherwise presumably normal functioning brain at onset. A major question, then, concerns the potential influence of the recurrent seizure state (clinical and subclinical) upon total brain functioning. In the past, much attention was paid to the possibility of a specific personality distortion in epileptic patients, stated to be manifested by excessive irritability, arrogance, paranoid ideation, religiosity, and often social

* See references 12, 25, 27, 32, 37, 42, 52, 58, 65, 68, 71, 84, 95, 96, 117, 121–123, and 154.

withdrawal. This led to the persistence of inappropriate restrictive actions by society[9] and to general stigmatization.[169] However, the severe emotional problems and disturbances in the patients have been found to develop most often as a reaction to such restrictions— to the presence of an uncontrollable, overwhelming seizure disorder, and also, at times even more common, intrafamilial denigration.[125] Severely neurotic, maladjusted behavior then developed into the so-called "epileptic personality," which is just a collection of secondary reactive psychological phenomena. In Taylor's sample of 100 patients[161] with temporal-lobe epilepsy, only thirteen were considered psychiatrically normal; thirty were diagnosed "neurotic;" forty-eight "psychopathic" (e.g., aggressive, immature and inadequate, paranoid, antisocial, cyclothymic, schizoid, or sexual deviationist); sixteen "psychotic" (with eight of "schizophreniform psychosis," five with paranoid-hallucinatory psychosis, and one each with abrupt onset catatonic psychosis, "organic" psychosis, or simple schizophrenia). Two children were called "psychotic." Other patients were described as showing psychomotor retardation in depressive psychosis. In twelve cases two diagnoses were made. Five patients had an "epileptic personality," in one instance prior to onset of florid psychosis. Thus, practically all types of mental disorders may accompany epilepsy. The specific relationships between the two conditions require detailed psychiatric analysis by careful psychological testing, especially of cognitive neuropsychological components. These evaluations have practical therapeutic significance, since increasing psychological difficulties often lead to increased seizure activity more difficult to control. Yet, upon reviewing large populations of epileptic patients, one finds that most do have, or are capable of, normal behavior and intellectual functions, and can develop controlled personality characteristics which can lead to appropriate, effective adjustments in society. History and the literature is replete with descriptions of such individuals contributing to our civilization in all walks of life.[93]

A significant number of patients with frequent recurrent generalized seizures, especially *status epilepticus* and excessive numbers of absences, and particularly those with psychomotor-temporal-limbic seizures, may develop disturbances of cognitive intellectual functions, including memory and learning, and, at times interictal severe behavioral disorders and psychotic states.* The actual definitive role of the seizure disorder itself and its potential specificity in relation to these developments is difficult to analyze. The effects on mental function of prolonged administration of anticonvulsant drugs, and their resulting folate deficiency remain to be clarified.† In many patients, secondary social and psychological factors assume primary importance with the production of withdrawal, depression, neurotic symptoms and apparent impairment of intellectual performance of varying severity. Severe hyperkinetic states may develop in epileptic children.[115]

As described above, frequent absence attacks may interfere with tasks requiring repetition and which may be involved in learning and memory processing. This is unusual in most children with petit-mal seizures; in general, they have no significant intellectual difficulties or personality disturbance.

Certain patients with frequent grand-mal and/or psychomotor-temporal-lobe seizures may develop a slowly progressive intellectual disturbance. How often this occurs is not yet determined, nor is the general distribution of these difficulties known. In some instances the chronic effects of drugs such as phenobarbital and diphenylhydantoin may be important. In clinical experience these changes in overall brain functioning may be quite subtle in the early years of the epileptic disorder in a particular patient, and would be most recognizable in individuals of high intellectual attainment. There is increasing evidence that progressive damage in, or disturbed function of, certain susceptible brain areas, particularly in the deep temporal regions, occurs in association with poor seizure control (and perhaps increasing dosages of medication) over a period of several years (i.e., "epileptogenic encephalopathy"). The mechanism of this process is not clear; a concept of "consumptive hypoxia" of overactive cells leading to neuronal cell loss has been invoked.[117] In these patients, appropriate neuropsychological tests reveal progressive impairment of concentration and attention, memory defects, word finding distortions and subtle losses in ability to associate and to track patterns (i.e., perceptual disorders). However, it must be emphasized that the majority of patients with epileptic seizures under adequate control escape these difficulties and retain normal intellectual function.

(Neuropsychological Testing in Epilepsy

The effects of epileptic activity, both in the ictal and interictal states, on intellectual performance, learning and memory, have not yet been clearly elucidated.‡ Perhaps more important to the patient is the fact that anticonvulsant drugs still are administered over a long period of time without clear knowledge of effects on such functions. Most studies thus far have used a standard intelligence test such as the WAIS (Wechsler Adult Intelligence Scale), to provide for some measure of mental status, together with the Minnesota Multiphasic Inventory (MMPI),[82,103] or, in earlier years, the Rorschach test,[23] as an estimate of personality traits. These tests of relatively random populations of patients have demonstrated that there is a tendency for the distribution of simple scores, especially in clinic groups, to be skewed towards the lower end of the scale. Some authors have shown a discrepancy between verbal and performance IQ figures, and have attributed the finding to "organicity." A few longitudinal studies indicate that this finding may be true only for the patient at that particular time of testing.[137] There is a lack of good controlled testing, with age, sex, seizure history and frequency, anticonvulsant drug

---

* See references 12, 14, 18, 20, 24, 27, 32, 37, 52, 54, 62, 68, 77, 87, 117, 122, 128, 137, 161, and 172.
† See references 15, 16, 57, 96, 133, and 137.

‡ See references 18, 21, 24, 33, 65, 71, 87, 93, 100, 103, 128, 144, 145, 153, and 172.

levels and types, etc., taken into account.

More specific neuropsychological testing, using the more subtle techniques devised for the assessment of localized brain damage, can aid understanding of the epileptic patient at two levels.[120,165] The first is a knowledge of the general intellectual level, specific impairment associated with focal dysfunction, learning and memory difficulties—often consequences of poor attention and concentration—which may give invaluable help in vocational guidance and specialized teaching. The epileptic is often an "underachiever," since much school time may be missed and social factors make job finding difficult. It also can be important to find out how anticonvulsant drug therapy is influencing mentation, especially since many such drugs have a sedative effect. Thus, Cereghino and Penry[16] note that brain damage may make the patient susceptible to "mild depression and impairment of performance secondary to drug administration (that) may go unnoticed." One hopes that neuropsychological tests not only are able to "notice" such impairments, but also help balance the effects of maximum seizure control against possible dulling of intellect due to drug effects, by reassessments at different doses of the drugs. The now available sophisticated measures of anticonvulsant blood levels may not be relevant unless an overall measure, at the same level of sophistication, of the efficacy of the drug can be made. There has been but one such controlled (but acute) study relating impairment in perceptual-motor behavior distortion to blood phenobarbital level;[75] a detailed study of chronic effects needs to be performed with this and other drugs such as diphenylhydantoin.

The other level at which neuropsychological testing can function has been developed within the last thirty years. The neuropsychologist is concerned with the relationship between psychological function and cerebral structure. The effects on behaviour of localised lesions in the cerebrum have been studied extensively, in the hope that this will lead to a better understanding of the functions of these areas.[120,165] The interpretation of these studies is always subject to the limitations imposed by looking at a malfunctioning system in order to understand the normal. However, any theory of brain function must be able to account for changes observed during pathological behaviour. Thus, the closer study of psychological function in the epileptic—especially with focal seizures—may lead to a better idea of how the brain functions.

A clearer idea of the effects of repeated focal and generalised seizures on the specific areas involved, as well as on the ability of other areas of the brain to compensate, may be found. How far does such interruption of normal function give rise to permanent malfunction? How much compensation takes place in such a situation? To what extent does a faulty input (perceptual disorders in all modalities, often interrupted by ictal behaviour) give rise to faulty output and inappropriate responses, seen as personality disturbances? Does the clue to abnormal behaviour lie in the study, in particular, of temporal-lobe or limbic epilepsy? Do changes in EEG activity, such as spike-wave discharges, correlate with changes in mental activity? Does good seizure control prevent intellectual deterioration, as has been suggested in some studies (see above), or is some other variable more important?

The solution to these and many other problems may be found in part by the application of neuropsychological measurement in which specific tests for focal dysfunctions, using knowledge acquired through the study of localised cerebral lesions, may lead to a better understanding of brain function, and the means to achieve better treatment of the epileptic. A brief comment concerning these tests follows. As has been noted previously, in most studies in which the psychological aspects of epilepsy have been commented upon, the Wechsler Adult Intelligent Scale (WAIS) and Wechsler Memory Scale have been used.[129, 168] Neither of these two tests really gives a good indication of more subtle disturbances in brain function. The WAIS is a battery of tests in which two IQ scores are obtained, one verbal and one performance.[168] A simple statement of these two scores, or one of the "full scale IQ" which is a combination of the two, may obscure specific deficits. Thus, individually lower scores on one of the subtests may show only in the overall figure, without making it clear where the lower figure arose. Memory and concentration difficulties may lower some scores, particularly on arithmetic and digit span, not necessarily a purely verbal loss. Likewise, some of the tests on the performance scale (which ostensibly measures nonverbal, nondominant-hemisphere abilities) are not purely nonverbal or not purely performance verbal, thus rendering the distinction between the two IQ scores less significant. There is no valid reason why a lower score on the performance scale should mean "organicity" as has been stated by some authors. The WAIS has two "hold" tests, vocabulary and picture completion, from which an estimate of deterioration can be computed. But the bluntness of the total scores as instruments for measuring specific deficits may be the reason for the discrepant findings obtained with the use of the WAIS to distinguish groups of epileptics from each other and from control groups. It is not a test battery which enables one to show objectively, that which has been noted clinically.

Attempts to measure brain damage by the application of such tests have not been very useful, since there is an underlying assumption that Lashley's law of mass action stands, and is mensurable.[114] It is, however, possible to measure some aspect of intelligence commensurate with Spearman's g factor. The discrepancy between scores on a standardised vocabulary test (such as the WAIS or the Mill Hill), and the score on Raven's matrices, may give a good basic idea of dementia.[130] Vocabulary tests reflect acquired information, and are held to be good indicators, together with education and job history, of the level which an individual can attain. Raven's matrices* are held to measure a subject's ability to "develop a systematic method of reason-

* Raven's matrices consists of a graded series of patterns in which one part is missing and the correct missing part is chosen by the subject from a collection of six (or later in the test eight) alternatives. At its simplest, the task requires only matching a pattern, but at its most complex, the grasp of a subtle relationship between the parts of the system is required.

ing," not subject to previous training, cultural background, etc. Such a test can provide a useful baseline from which specific difficulties can be assessed, and some idea of the degree of dementia can also be found.[131]

❲ Memory and Temporal-Lobe Epilepsy

It has been shown repeatedly that the temporal lobe and related structures are involved in memory.† Not only has it been shown that bitemporal lobectomy produces a dense amnesia, both retrograde and anterograde (as in the well-known case[107,146] of H.M.) but much attention has been given to laterality effects. Thus, anterior lobectomy in the dominant hemisphere for speech, causes a lasting impairment in memory for verbal material.[101] [102,104] This is independent of whether the presentation be auditory or visual, and also of the recall technique used.[105,106] Removal of the nondominant hemisphere, or damage to it, gives an impairment in memory for visual material, such as places, faces, nonsense designs, and music, i.e., material that is not easily coded verbally.[86,166,167] A double dissociation effect between visual perception and visual memory has also been demonstrated in the nondominant hemisphere.[167] Apart from simple free recall experiments using verbal and nonverbal material, more complex paradigms using learning also show laterality effects. Left-temporal lobectomized patients show a deficit on Hebbs Digit Sequence task, right-temporal lobectomized patients do not.[106]

Experimental psychologists have also studied the various components of memory, three of which are now generally distinguished: (1) immediate or iconic memory having very limited capacity and a rapid decay of the stored material of about one second; (2) short-term memory (STM) or primary memory, having a trace of slightly longer but still limited duration (20–30 sec.) and with a slightly larger capacity; and (3) long-term memory (LTM) or secondary memory, in which a stable trace

† See references 13, 26, 28, 105, 146, and 169.

or engram exists and may remain permanently.[7,169] Evidence exists that the anatomical localisation of these memory systems may be different. Thus the amnesic syndrome, characterised by severe LTM loss in the presence of intact immediate and STM and intellect, is thought to be a concomitant of bilateral lesions of the diencephalon, thalamus, and hippocampus structures closely related to the temporal lobe.[13] A situation in which STM, particularly for auditorally presented material, is grossly impaired in the presence of intact LTM has been described.[150] The critical lesion is thought to be in the dominant parietal lobe, in the region of the supramarginal and angular gyri.

It thus is clear that the temporal lobes are important to the proper functioning of memory in man, as shown by a fairly extensive literature concerning subjects with brain lesions. It is, therefore, surprising that the problem of memory impairment in patients with epilepsy, especially temporal-lobe epilepsy, has not yet been analysed in the same depth, even given the evidence that lack of any structural damage to the temporal area is not always evident. Milner[105] has pointed out that care must be taken to distinguish between impairment of memory and impairment of attention or vigilance. Thus "absence" in petit mal may be interpreted later as producing memory loss, and generalised intellectual impairment may appear to the patient as memory loss. Given that such situations exist, there remains a need to study the memory problems that may be associated with epilepsy. Examples of dense amnesia seen after bitemporal lobectomy for epilepsy (H.M.),[107] or in one case after right-temporal lobectomy[26] have been studied. The episodes of déjà vu in temporal-lobe epilepsy have been interpreted as abnormal activity in the temporal lobe, giving rise to a false sense of memory, analogous, perhaps, to Penfield's stimulation studies.[118,119]

There have been studies of memory impairment in epilepsy, and many workers have sought to find both the differentially affected temporal-lobe epileptic, and the predicted laterality effects. Thus, Horowitz and Cohen[72] in a follow-up study of patients after surgery for temporal-lobe epilepsy, did not find any consistent memory impairment (using the Wechsler memory scale and Benton visual retention test, amongst other general tests of intellectual performance such as the WAIS). They do not accept the view that psychologists are able to demonstrate laterality effects, and argue that temporal lobectomy merely leads to impairment of "organization."

Serafetinides and Falconer[148] studied thirty-four patients with right anterior temporal-lobe ablations and showed that only two had some brief postoperative memory impairment; six had persistent memory deficits, but the authors state that "the type of memory deficit did not correlate with the more formal psychometric test results." They suggest that these six subjects must have had bilateral temporal-lobe dysfunction. Meyer[101,102] studied similar patients and found that nondominant lobectomies produced no change, and that dominant lobectomies produced auditory verbal learning difficulties. Many studies have made comparisons between various types of seizure patients. Guerrant et al.[65] found no overall significant differences in any of their groups of grand mal, petit mal and psychomotor (temporal-lobe) epileptics, with respect to memory functioning, using the memory span for objects and the Wechsler memory scale.

Mirsky, Primac et al.[108] found no significant group differences on memory tests between subjects with temporal-lobe epilepsy (TLE) of a focal and nonfocal nature. Scott, Moffett et al.[145] tested subjects with and without epilepsy, matched for age and IQ and found no differences in their performance on nonverbal tests in three modalities. Quadfasel and Pruyser[128] predicted a greater impairment in verbal skills and some memory difficulty in patients with TLE, and Fedio and Mirsky[33] and Dennerll[24] demonstrated some laterality effects in TLE patients.

Thus there is some confusion as to the precise nature of the memory impairments in the epileptic patients. Memory tests have not differentiated adequately between STM (short term memory) and LTM (long term memory) components; indeed, there is little indication that very remote memory has been tested at all. Although some studies have considered laterality effects, more subtle tests have not been used. Thus, the use of tests of nonverbal memory cannot be described as such, unless it is clear that no verbal labels can be applied to the stimulus to be remembered, at least during the time of presentation to the subject. Horowitz[71,72] is of the opinion that no gross differences between right and left foci in the temporal-lobe epileptic have yet been demonstrated. It has yet to be proved definitively that the lack of differentiation in these studies is a result of test inefficiency, or whether temporal-lobe disturbances in epilepsy really do produce a different type of dysfunction from other types of lesions, where perhaps the disturbance may be more continuous. Lack of direct information about the true origins—i.e., perhaps subcortical—of discharges in many patients with temporal-lobe epilepsy adds to the difficulties.

It has been noted that there is often a discrepancy between the observed clinical findings, the patient's subjective impression of memory impairment, and psychological test findings. Since memory is so vital an element in adequate functioning, good evaluation is important. More discriminating tests, such as have been employed in other memory studies, may improve the evaluation of this function in epilepsy. There is also a need for more careful control of other influences, such as anticonvulsant levels, seizure frequency, and the overall psychological state of the patient (i.e., level of anxiety, depression, etc.).

Interictal psychotic states can develop, especially in certain patients with psychomotor-temporal lobe epilepsy, and may be correlated with long-standing disturbances in intellectual function, particularly in perceptual-cognitive areas. The overall incidence of psychosis is relatively small and difficult to determine, yet significant; if psychotic states in epileptic patients are considered as the starting point of any study of this problem, then it is likely that their coincidence is not just a matter of chance.*

A fluctuating episodic behavioral and per-

* See references 14, 27, 37, 54, 121, and 152.

sonality disorder other than actual seizure can exist in a patient. At times an alternation between seizure and overt psychosis can be observed, especially in patients under medication. However, it is often difficult to distinguish an ictal or postictal psychotic episode from an interictal state. Ever since the mid-nineteenth century,[32] so-called acute epileptic psychotic reactions have been recognized as part of what is now regarded as the psychomotor-temporal-lobe seizure complex, and more prolonged psychotic disturbances with schizophreniclike manifestations have been differentiated from actual seizure in some patients. Epileptic "furor," fugue, twilight and depersonalization[85] phenomena have been described in both settings.

The electroencephalogram has aided somewhat in these considerations. Confusional states have been found to be more common in patients with bilateral spike-wave discharges and prolonged petit-mal seizures.[91,97,132] More complex psychotic disturbances of schizophreniclike qualities in patients with psychomotor seizures have been found with unmodified EEG rhythms, desynchronization of the EEG, "forced normalization" with disappearance of abnormal discharges[91] or a reinforced temporal abnormality.

The interictal psychotic states may appear early in the history of the patient, even at the onset of seizures, but more often some years later varying from six to 14 years.[37,54,152] The psychotic episodes may last from one to many days. Reactions are paranoid, depressive, confusional, and hallucinatory along with bizarre behavior. Episodes of self-mutilation have been reported. There usually is little or no occurrence of otherwise goal-directed destructive, violent behavior in these patients and no indications of major withdrawal or atavistic mechanisms. Affect is often warm and appropriate with much reality testing, a major difference from schizophrenic psychosis occurring in other spontaneous circumstances. Affective flattening is unusual. Catatonic disorders appear, but are usually transitory. Religious preoccupations are frequent, as well as related obsessional activities. Impulsive, compulsive eating and drinking may occur. Somnambulism has been reported. In some patients, acute disorganization of verbal productions is present along with bizarre distortions and many somatic delusions. Pregnancy fantasies have existed in some females. Diminished libido and sexual functions are found in some patients with temporal-lobe epilepsy[11,46,158] Hypersexuality is unusual. Sexual deviation, such as fetishism, has been reported in association with temporal-lobe epilepsy,[73] relieved, in one instance, by temporal lobectomy.[111]

Over half the patients have fluctuating memory disturbances with mild to moderate impairment, difficulty in attention and concentration and disorientation to time.[58] Extreme confusion occasionally appears, often lasting several hours and not associated with the usual manifestations of seizure with motor-sensory or visceral components. Partial to complete amnesia, often for the psychosis, suggests subclinical "seizure" activity; in some of the cases with confusion, bilateral EEG discharges suggesting subcortical origin may be correlated.

Psychological testing of such patients requires not only scoring, but also observation of performance and response.[54,58] There is evidence of loss of trains of association along with word finding and tracking difficulties, vacillation of alertness, and fluctuation in the accuracy of perceptions. Looseness of associations without bizarre content or mode of thought is common, along with indications of concreteness. However, there is usually no clear sign of autism or withdrawal; many patients make continued attempts to be in contact with reality. There are usually no signs of archaic thinking or autistic fantasy elaboration as would be found in more typical schizophrenic subjects.

Mild to moderate memory disturbances are frequent in these patients, with both retention and recall difficulties in both short- and long-term memory. Mere scoring of IQ levels is not very meaningful. Many patients express concern over problems in the clarity of their thinking and make concerted efforts to control, restrict, and contain emotions and actions in order to become clear, accurate, and realis-

tic. Misperceptions and arbitrary thought processes usually involve relatively benign, neutral content, although themes of religiosity are frequent. A degree of word-finding difficulty is often apparent, and distinct dysphasia is occasionally present (in over 10 percent of Slater's cases[152]). Flor-Henry[37] and others have emphasized the correlation of dominant temporal-lobe focal involvement and schizophreniclike psychosis in these patients. Some patients experience weakness of spatial orientation and fluctuating motor incoordination. Difficulty in arithmetic is sometimes present.

The paranoid elements involve projection of thoughts and feelings, but well-organized delusions of persecution, for example, are relatively uncommon. Indications of contamination and feelings of depersonalization and unreality are frequent. Disturbances of body image involve feelings of being disconnected, fragmented, malformed, awkward, or incomplete.

Most epileptic patients with interictal psychosis are found to have psychomotor temporal-lobe seizure disorders.[37,54,152] The classification of the seizure disorder must be on the basis of the clinical signs, not of the EEG, since the latter might show fluctuating bilaterality of discharge. The onset of the psychotic reaction does not appear to be clearly related to specific psychological triggers in many instances, but often does follow increasing build-up of tension and anxiety. Gradual intellectual disorganization, often subtle at first, may initiate the process. Some patients remain in an impulsive, aggressive, unstable, obsessional state without actual psychotic break. It should be stated that the actuality of a "true" or non-directly related schizophrenia could develop in patients with epilepsy,[153,154] but the above described schizophrenialike phenomena are qualitatively different.[54,68,121]

Taylor[159] has recently emphasized that, from the clinical point of view, the epileptic schizophrenialike psychoses emerge as a group of disorders following largely on psychomotor-temporal-lobe epilepsies involving mainly the left temporal lobe[161] either alone, or as part of a more generalized seizure disorder, emerging mainly in the second and third decades, where mesial temporal sclerosis is an improbable pathological substrate, to which females are more prone, but in whom half the risk to psychosis is past by the twenty-fifth year. Of interest is the increasing evidence that a number of cases of childhood psychosis or "autism" follow episodes of infantile epilepsy, especially of the myoclonic spasm type.[88]

The therapeutic implications of these considerations are yet to be fully realized. It might be expected that a psychotic reaction associated with a seizure disorder would regress as seizures respond to treatment. Although this does happen, the interictal behavioral disturbance occasionally persists and may increase as seizures are controlled. Anticonvulsant drugs are to be used, and the administration of certain psychotropic drugs such as "alerting" phenothiazines (i.e., fluphenazine) might be helpful.[25] In selected cases with intractable seizures and well-defined focus, temporal lobectomy has produced some improvement in "schizophrenic" symptoms, but this is unpredictable and does not correlate well with the response of the seizures.[31,71,161]

⟮ Clinical Evaluation of the Patient

The patient with epilepsy should receive a thorough diagnostic evaluation in order to determine the relative significance of the possible etiologic factors as well as precipitating circumstances. This requires thorough history taking, physical, medical, and neurologic examinations, and selected laboratory investigations with particular reference to blood chemistry studies, cerebrospinal fluid analyses, and electroencephalography; special radiologic studies may be required. The collected data may lead to the diagnosis of either a specific medical illness associated with seizures or a focal cerebral lesion.

History

In order to establish whether recurrent seizures are being experienced, a careful history should contain detailed descriptive material, usually from sources other than the patient. Eye-witness accounts are helpful. As much recollection as possible should be obtained from the patient, particularly of experiences of the aura or the onset of the seizure. The patterning or course of events during and after seizure episodes should be documented with special attention to phenomena which might be of localizing significance. Other information of great importance with regard to treatment concerns the circumstances under which the seizure occurs, e.g., time of day or night, frequency of attacks, and the influence of medication, menstrual cycle, pregnancy, food intake, sound or light stimulation, intake of alcohol, and psychological stress. Additional indications of neurologic disturbance should be described, e.g., headache, hemiparesis, hemisensory symptoms, dysphasia, and visual difficulties, especially loss of acuity and hemianopsia, and vertigo.

A family history may reveal data of importance, particularly with regard to susceptibility to seizure. In a significant number of families a history of febrile seizure in early childhood may be obtained, as well as seizures of both generalized and focal types extending into later life. In addition, since a number of genetically determined cerebral disorders may be associated with seizure as well as other neurologic abnormalities, the family history may include phenomena other than seizures as indications of brain disorder related to structural or metabolic abnormalities.

The general medical history is significant, since seizure may be associated with cardiovascular disease, various blood dyscrasias, and metabolic and endocrine disorders; for example, the history of neoplasm anywhere in the body is important, since a focal seizure may be the first manifestation of a cerebral metastasis.

The past medical and developmental history of the patient is of great significance in attempting to determine etiology; information concerning pregnancy, delivery, the neonatal period, and the developmental neurological milestones should be obtained. The position of the child on the developmental scale should be determined, particularly with regard to motor and intellectual skills. Past history should also include information regarding head injuries, reactions to immunizations, childhood diseases such as measles, mumps, and chickenpox, and any severe illness with delirium or coma that might be considered related to an encephalitis. A history of exposure to toxic substances is important, as well as the possibility of drug intake, particularly in adults suspected of taking barbiturate or tranquilizing drugs.

A detailed survey of the patient's social development and behavior in and out of the family setting is relevant, including an evaluation of intellectual performance at school and vocational performance. Attention should be paid to alteration in any of these phases of existence in relation to seizure occurrence, as well as between seizures, and also to possible effects of medication on seizure incidence or behavior.

Physical and Neurological Examination

Clinical examination of patients with seizures may not reveal significant physical or neurologic abnormality in 75 percent or more of cases. However, thorough physical examination is necessary to establish whether a general medical disorder is present; even examination of the skin may produce the requisite information for diagnosis of tuberous sclerosis, neurofibromatosis, or cerebral hemangioma. Examination of the lungs may provide the background for consideration of metastatic tumor or abscess; evaluation of the peripheral circulation and blood pressure may give indication of the possibility of the various types of cerebral vascular lesions, or aid in differential diagnosis of syncope and seizure.

The neurological examination serves two functions: (1) to give indication of general cerebral disorder, and (2) to demonstrate whether focal signs are present, indicative of a localized cerebral lesion. Neurological examination at the time of or shortly after a seizure may be important, since hemiparesis and related signs may be revealed. Psychological testing may be useful in the assessment of

general intellectual status, possible deterioration from a previously higher level of functioning, and the possibility of focal cerebral damage. As discussed previously, the WAIS and Wechsler Memory Scale give a very broad idea of the patient's functioning, but more careful evaluation of learning, memory, and perception is needed to distinguish subtler disturbances, as discussed above. The Rorschach and other projective tests have been used to demonstrate both "organicity" and the epileptic personality, but doubt has been cast on the validity of such techniques for this purpose. Attention should be paid to the patient's performance during these tests as well as to the actual scores.

Laboratory Investigations

Each patient with recurrent seizures, regardless of age, should be subjected to selected laboratory investigations at least once during the course of his history, particularly if changes in seizure patterns or neurologic signs develop. There are no routines, but at different age levels certain tests are more apt to produce results leading to specific etiologic diagnosis. In addition, certain studies are necessary for the evaluation of the general health of the patient and in following the effects of medication which may be toxic to various body systems. Aside from electroencephalographic abnormalities, there are no abnormal laboratory findings characteristically associated with the seizure process. Urinalysis is important to determine the state of kidney functioning, which, if abnormal, may preclude the use of certain drugs or may suggest a specific diagnosis. Similarly, a complete blood count is necessary, particularly if a blood dyscrasia is suspected. Severe seizure states, such as *status epilepticus*, may be associated with proteinuria, leukocytosis, and fever as secondary manifestations. In certain instances, special blood chemistry studies are important, e.g., blood sugar and glucose-tolerance test in the diagnosis of hypoglycemia and in the evaluation of a difficult-to-control diabetic. Determinations of serum calcium are necessary in the evaluation of infants and young children with seizure states, since hypocalcemia may cause generalized seizures, distinct from tetany. Evaluation of serum electrolytes and acid–base balance is extremely important in the study of both children and adults with metabolic encephalopathies and seizures in various disorders of the kidney, liver, heart, and lungs. As yet, no specific patterns of electrolyte distortion are associated with seizures, but at times variations in these can be so correlated. Determination of serum enzymes is mainly important in establishing the presence of general medical disorders, and serologic tests are helpful in the diagnosis of past infectious states.

The cerebrospinal fluid is apt to be normal except in a minority with certain neurological disease. Following severe seizures there may be a slight increase in cerebrospinal fluid protein and white cell counts, but this is usually transitory. In structural neurological disorders with concomitant seizures, the protein or pressure or both may be persistently elevated and the diagnosis is then dependent on other tests, such as contrast radiologic studies. Chronic infection of the nervous system can be associated with increase in white cell count in the cerebrospinal fluid, and occasionally the presence of cerebral neoplasm may be shown by neoplastic cells in the fluid, diagnosed by cell block and appropriate histologic examination.

Radiologic Studies

All patients should have an X ray of the skull and chest. The plain X-ray film may show abnormal calcifications and shift of the pineal or other signs of increased intracranial pressure. The X ray of the chest is of two-fold importance: (1) in the evalution of any anomalous cardiopulmonary status in an adult or a child; and (2) to reveal possible primary tumor in an adult.

The so-called contrast radiological studies of the intracranial contents are extremely useful diagnostic procedures, but since they have a certain morbidity they must be selected with great care and be performed when they can be expected to be most informative. Certainly, such procedures must be considered when there is suspicion of a focal intracranial lesion.

If there is increased intracranial pressure, particularly if there may be a lesion involving the posterior fossa, ventriculography may be the procedure of choice; however, this procedure generally gives incomplete information with regard to the subarachnoid spaces. Ordinarily, if the pressure is normal, a fractional pneumoencephalogram gives more information with regard to a lesion occupying space in the brain substance or distorting the ventricular or subarachnoid system. In addition, the presence of focal brain atrophy may be shown by differential enlargements of specific spaces such as the temporal horns of the ventricles.

Cerebral arteriography is useful in patients with and without evidence of increased pressure, and may give important information, particularly if there are focal or lateralizing signs. Abnormal vascular patterns are found in particular types of tumors, intracranial hematomas, and vascular malformations; the location of vascular occlusions may be found by arteriography as well. There are instances when such studies are negative but reveal a lesion when repeated later; occasionally such tests may be worthwhile in initial base-line investigations of a case.

The use of brain scanning with radioactive isotopes requires more evaluation, but there is increasing regard for these procedures as a means of determining the presence of certain types of tumors, either single or multiple, and of vascular lesions. In some instances a negative brain scan may eliminate the necessity, for the moment, of a contrast radiological procedure. Also, a significantly lateralized pickup in scanning may indicate the preferred side for an arteriogram, an indication which otherwise might not be clear from the neurological evaluation and the EEG.

Electroencephalography

The various electroencephalographic correlates of the different types of seizures have been described above. The EEG, however, must be regarded only as an indicator of a certain kind of cerebral activity determined by the recording method using electrodes upon the scalp. This is important to realize, since the EEG from a patient with known seizures of any type might be normal, as it is the case in a single-sample recording in 25 percent of such patients. Depth electrode recording techniques have shown that, in some of these instances, there may be abnormal discharges in the deeper structures such as the amygdala and hippocampus, while the electrical activity of the cortex shows no change. The EEG, therefore, has limited diagnostic applications, and it must be considered only as a reflection of certain cerebral functions to be correlated with other information obtained from physical and neurological examinations. The electroencephalographic findings are of varying usefulness in the diagnosis of epilepsy, depending on their nature and the circumstances under which they are obtained.

The EEG may be utilized as an aid in the confirmation of the presence of a seizure state, particularly if paroxysmal discharges are recorded during and correlated with a seizure; for example, in the petit-mal absence, up to 85 percent of children have the typical 3 Hz. spike-and-wave discharges both between and during seizures. In addition, these may be precipitated by overventilation and light stimulation. The EEG may merely contain generalized nonspecific slow-wave discharges, which may be considered only as an indicator of cerebral dysfunction, but not necessarily of a definite seizure disorder. Focal slow-wave abnormality is suggestive of a localized structural lesion and indicates the need for further investigations. In certain forms of focal epilepsy the EEG may show focal discharges of spikes, sharp waves, and complex components indicative of the epileptogenic nature of the focus. However, in some of these instances such abnormality might be transmitted from deeper, even centrally disposed, lesions.

In most laboratories of electroencephalography the procedure includes recordings in the waking state and during hyperventilation. Frequently, however, attempts are made to provoke generalized and focal paroxysmal discharges by means of sleep, sensory stimulation with light or sound, or certain metabolic and pharmacologic adjuvants. The EEG during sleep is useful to demonstrate focal discharges in patients with psychomotor-temporal-lobe epilepsy. Such discharges are increased during sleep in 50–75 percent of adults. The results in children are less definitive; in 25–35 percent of young patients the temporal activity becomes more prominent during sleep. However, in some patients sleep tends to produce increased bilaterality of abnormal temporal discharges. The use of sphenoidal electrodes is occasionally helpful in lateralizing temporal-lobe discharge, particularly when patients are being evaluated for surgery. At times barbiturate-induced fast-wave activity is found to be less marked in the involved temporal lobe. Photic stimulation detects patients with light-sensitive epilepsy and occasionally evokes lateralized discharges in patients with a sensitive focus.

There have been many attempts to alter the electrical activity of the brain in susceptible patients by inducing metabolic changes, such as hydration, following an injection of vasopressin or the induction of hypoglycemia with small doses of insulin. Various stimulant drugs have been used, e.g., pentylenetetrazol and bemegride. All of these methods, particularly the use of drugs, may precipitate paroxysmal discharges as well as clinical seizures; the latter are usually generalized, but occasionally activation of a focus occurs. Attempts to measure seizure discharge threshold have been largely unsuccessful because of great variability; in addition, many otherwise normal subjects respond to these procedures with seizure activity. For these reasons this approach is not recommended for general use in the diagnosis of an epileptic state. Occasionally, however, it may be desirable to view in detail the clinical phenomena of the seizure and to determine focal components either in the EEG or clinically. At times this can be accomplished by the administration of a controlled dose of a seizure-producing drug.

The degree of electroencephalographic abnormality, especially in its paroxysmal characteristics, may be regarded as an objective indicator of the severity of a particular seizure state in a patient; this may fluctuate with the clinical behavior of the seizure disorder. However, the use of the EEG to follow patients with epilepsy is limited since in many instances some degree of electroencephalographic abnormality persists even when seizures are controlled. This occurs most often in patients with psychomotor-temporal-lobe epilepsy and least often in children with petit-mal and myoclonic seizures.

Differential Diagnosis

The implications of a diagnosis of an epileptic disorder are so significant both medically and psychologically that the diagnosis must be positive and specific, excluding other disturbances characterized by similar transitory abnormalities of neurological function that are not seizures. Consciousness may be disturbed episodically by limitations of cerebral blood flow, either generally or locally, e.g., in instances of cerebral vascular insufficiency and syncope of various types, particularly the vasodepressor form. Disturbances of cerebral circulation occur frequently in older age-groups; there is usually evidence of hypertension and cerebral arteriosclerosis. Periodic blackouts and general confusional states may result from basilar artery insufficiency; however, there are usually other signs of brainstem and cerebellar dysfunction. Patients with deficient carotid circulation may have transitory hemiparesis and hemisensory disturbances along with dysphasia. Electroencephalographic findings of paroxysmal discharge may suggest the presence of a seizure state; however, rhythmic discharges may be related to lesions of vascular origin in the upper brainstem. The differential diagnosis in these patients involves careful evaluation of the history and general medical state of the patient; arteriographic confirmation of a vascular lesion may be necessary.

Syncopal episodes may resemble akinetic or minor motor seizure; actually, prolonged syncope can develop into convulsions due to the persistence of cerebral ischemia and hypoxia. The patient with syncope usually has some indication of disturbed vasomotor reactivity with excessive sweating, pallor, and tachycardia. Specific precipitating factors often are present, such as fear or other psychological upset; the confusion, headache, and drowsiness which occur after a generalized seizure do not usually appear. During a simple syncopal episode the EEG consists of diffuse asynchronous slow waves without paroxysmal or focal discharges.

Various disturbances of consciousness, from confusion to coma, may be produced by metabolic. disturbances not necessarily leading to seizures. These conditions are important in the differential diagnosis, since in specific instances of metabolic encephalopathy seizures may be only a minor clinical concomitant, and the overall distortion of general cerebral function may be of major concern. These clinical abnormalities appear in hypoglycemia, hyponatremia, kidney failure with uremia, hepatic insufficiency, and pulmonary insufficiency (with hypoxia and hypercarbia). The EEG in these states contains generalized, often intermittent, intermediate (4–7 Hz.) and very slow waves 1½–3 Hz.). Rhythmic components (such as the triphasic complexes in hepatic encephalopathy) may be present, but paroxysmal discharges are unusual unless actual seizures are occurring. Hypocalcemia, as in hypoparathyroidism, may produce tetanic spasms throughout the somatic musculature; occasionally these may be unilateral and suggestive of localized seizure, but consciousness is not lost and actual clonic contractions do not occur. However, as mentioned previously, hypocalcemia may precipitate actual convulsive seizures. Fluctuating distortions in behavior are also characteristic of many endocrine disorders, e.g., hypoadrenalism and hyperadrenalism, hypopituitarism and hyperpituitarism, and myxedema. In none of these states are seizure disorders particularly prominent.

Certain psychogenic disorders may resemble epileptic states and be difficult to distinguish from them. Hysterical "seizures" may occur independently, but are occasionally seen in patients with known seizures, i.e., so-called hystero-epilepsy. The clinical problem in these patients is often difficult to solve because of the interrelationships between the seizure state and the reactive development of the psychological disturbance. The hysterical seizure is not associated with neurological signs of reflex abnormality; the EEG contains no paroxysmal discharges. The hysterical seizure pattern is bizarre and not a sterotyped tonic-clonic movement sequence, and self-injury does not occur during, or as a result of, the hysterical seizure. The postictal states of confusion, headache, and drowsiness are absent. The diagnosis of hysterical seizure requires careful psychiatric evaluation because of the deep-seated and severe neurotic process involved. Similarly, certain hysterical or psychotic fugue disturbances and dissociative reactions may need to be distinguished from psychomotor-temporal-lobe seizures.

Treatment

The treatment of a patient with an epileptic disorder must take into account not only the patient and his disorder, but also his family and life situation. Much depends on the diagnostic evaluation and the etiology or precipitating factor. This can be clearly defined where a metabolic disturbance is obvious, e.g., in a hypoglycemic or hypocalcemic patient cured of seizures by administering glucose or calcium. Operable cerebral tumors represent another such situation. However, in many cases of acquired epilepsy the cause of the seizure cannot be treated directly, and symptomatic therapy with anticonvulsant drugs together with the total management of the patient are necessary. This may be true even in certain cases in which the precipitating factor is known, e.g., an anticonvulsant drug may be temporarily necessary in hypocalcemia, since a delayed response to calcium may be present. Seizures may continue even after surgery for a brain tumor due to postoperative scarring or incomplete excision. Immediate specific therapy is not always indicated in patients with acquired epilepsy. Only a limited number of patients with posttraumatic epilepsy are amenable to surgery for a localized meningo-cerebral scar. For these reasons, only a relatively small number of patients with seizures do not require anticonvulsant drugs and a general psychosocial rehabilitative program.

MEDICAL THERAPY WITH ANTICONVULSANT DRUGS

Drugs commonly used in the treatment of epilepsy are listed in Table 13–2 together with recommended dosage, indications, and toxic effects.

TABLE 13–2.   **Medical Therapy in Epilepsy: Anticonvulsant Drugs**

Bromides	
Daily dosage	Adults: 1.0–3.0 g. (not recommended for children)
Symptoms	All types of seizures, especially grand mal and psychomotor; may be combined with hydantoins
Toxic effects	Drowsiness, dulling, rash, psychosis; *rarely used now.*
Celontin (methsuximide)	
Dose	0.3 g. capsule
Daily dosage	Children: 0.6 g.; adults: up to 1.5 g.
Symptoms	Petit mal, psychomotor seizures, myoclonic seizures, massive spasms
Toxic effects	Ataxia, drowsiness, rarely blood dyscrasias, anorexia
Dexedrine (dextroamphetamine)	
Dose	5 mg. tablet; 10 and 15 mg. spansules
Daily dosage	Children: 5–15 mg.; adults: 15–50 mg.
Symptoms	Hyperkinetic behavioral disturbances in children, narcolepsy, to counteract sedative effects
Toxic effects	Anorexia, irritability, sleeplessness

TABLE 13–2.   **Medical Therapy in Epilepsy: Anticonvulsant Drugs** (*cont'd*)

Diamox (acetazolamide)

Dose	250 mg. tablet
Daily dosage	Children: 0.75–1.0 g.; adults: 1.0–1.5 g. Use intermittently, as an adjuvant in all types of seizures, especially those in females related to menstrual cycles; tolerance may develop
Toxic effects	Anorexia, acidosis, drowsiness, numbness of extremities, rare blood dyscrasia

Dilantin (diphenylhydantoin)

Dose	0.03 g. and 0.1 g. capsules; 0.05 g. tablet; 0.25 g./ml. suspension; 0.1 g. in oil capsule; 0.25 g. ampul for parenteral use
Daily dosage	Children: 0.1–0.3 g.; adults: 0.3–0.6 g. Effective blood level 10–20 μg/ml.
Symptoms	Grand mal, psychomotor, and focal seizures; most useful in combination with phenobarbital or primidone
Toxic effects	Rash, fever, gum hypertrophy, gastric distress, diplopia, ataxia, hirsutism (in young females); drowsiness uncommon; lymphadenopathy, rare megaloblastic anemia, secondary folate deficiency, "encephalopathy," hepatitis rare, aplastic anemia, agranulocytosis rare

Gemonil (metharbital)

Dose	0.1 g.
Daily dosage	Children: 0.1–0.3 g.; adults: 0.3–0.6 g.
Symptoms	Mainly in children with petit mal, myoclonic seizures, massive spasms, occasionally in grand mal
Toxic effects	Drowsiness, rash

Mebaral (mephobarbital)

Dose	0.03 g., 0.1 g. tablets. Demethylated to phenobarbital.
Daily dosage	Children: 0.06–0.3 g.; adults: 0.3–0.6 g.
Symptoms	Grand mal, petit mal, psychomotor, focal seizures; most useful in combination with hydantoins
Toxic effects	Drowsiness, irritability, rash

Mesantoin (methylphenylethylhydantoin)

Dose	0.1 g.
Daily dosage	Children: 0.1–0.4 g.; adults: 0.4–0.8 g.
Symptoms	Grand mal, psychomotor, focal seizures
Toxic effects	Rash, fever, drowsiness, ataxia, gum hypertrophy, (less than dilantin), neutropenia, agranulocytosis, aplastic and megaloblastic anemia.

Milontin (methylphenylsuccinimide)

Dose	0.5 g. capsules; 250 mg./4 ml. suspension.
Daily dosage	Children: 0.25–1.5 g.; adults: 2.0–4.0 g.

Symptoms	Petit mal, myoclonic, akinetic seizures, occasionally psychomotor seizures
Toxic effects	Nausea, dizziness, rash, hematuria (may be nephrotoxic)

Mysoline (primidone)

Dose	0.25 g. tablets; 250 mg./5 ml. suspension
Daily dosage	Children: 0.25–1.0 g.; adults: 0.75–2 g. The daily dosage should be built up very slowly. Blood levels: therapeutic range 5–15 μg/ml.
Symptoms	Grand mal, psychomotor, focal seizures, occasionally petit mal; useful in combination with Dilantin
Toxic effects	Drowsiness, ataxia, dizziness, rash, nausea, leukopenia rare

Paradione (paramethadione)

Dose	0.15–0.3 g. capsules; 0.3 g/ml. solution.
Daily dosage	Children: 0.3–1.8 g.; adults: 1.2–2.4 g.
Symptoms	Petit mal, myoclonic and akinetic seizures, massive spasms, occasionally psychomotor seizures (in children); often useful in combination with Dilantin and phenobarbital; somewhat less effective and less toxic than Tridione
Toxic effects	Rash, gastric distress, visual symptoms (glare, photophobia), neutropenia, agranulocytosis

Peganone (ethylphenylhydantoin)

Dose	0.25–0.5 g. tablets
Daily dosage	Children: 0.5–1.5 g.; adults: 2.0–3 g.
Symptoms	Grand mal, psychomotor, focal seizures
Toxic effects	Similar to Dilantin but less severe; may be substituted for Dilantin, but is generally less effective

Phenobarbital

Dose	0.015, 0.030, 0.060, and 0.1 g. tablets; 4 mg./ml. elixir. Therapeutic blood level 10–30 μg/ml.
Daily dosage	Children: 0.45–0.1 g.; adults: 0.1–0.3 g.
Symptoms	All seizure states; grand mal, petit mal, psychomotor, and other focal; most useful in limited dosage in combination with other drugs such as Dilantin
Toxic effects	Drowsiness, dulling, rash, fever; irritability and hyperactivity in some children

Phenurone (phenacemide)

Dose	0.5 g. tablet; 0.3 g. enteric coated tablet.
Daily dosage	Children: 0.5–2.0 g.; adults: 1.5–3.0 g.
Symptoms	May be effective in all types of seizures, especially focal temporal-lobe or other psychomotor seizures; should be used only in very resistant cases
Toxic effects	A *highly* toxic drug, producing liver damage, agranulocytosis, psychotic reactions, and rashes

TABLE 13–2.   **Medical Therapy in Epilepsy: Anticonvulsant Drugs**   (*cont'd*)

Tridione (trimethadione)	
Dose	0.15 g. tablet; 0.3 g. capsule; 0.15 g./4 ml. solution
Daily dosage	Children: 0.3–1.8 g.; adults: 1.2–2.4 g.
Symptoms	Petit mal, myoclonic and akinetic seizures, massive spasms, occasionally psychomotor seizures (in children); often useful in combination with Dilantin and phenobarbital
Toxic effects	Rash, gastric distress, visual symptoms (glare, photophobia), neutropenia, agranulocytosis
Zarontin (ethosuximide)	
Dose	0.25 g. capsule
Daily dosage	Children: 0.75–1.0 g.; adults: 1.5 g.
Symptoms	Petit mal seizures (the drug of choice, now); use with Dilantin in mixed seizure states
Toxic effects	Blood dyscrasias (pancytopenia, leukopenia), dermatitis, anorexia, nausea, drowsiness, dizziness, euphoria; disturbance of mental functions reported in some patients

The following drugs may be used in the emergency treatment of status epilepticus:

Drug	*Dose*
Sodium phenobarbital:	0.25–0.50 g., IV
Sodium amytal:	0.25–0.50 g., IV
Paraldehyde:	3.0 –5.0 g., IV diluted in saline, or 10–20 ml. IM
Dilantin sodium: (parenteral prep.)	0.25 g., IV or IM (to 0.5 g./24 hours)
Valium (diazepam)	10 mg., IV

More general anesthetics, such as ether, avertin, and xylocaine, have a limited usefulness in treatment of status epilepticus. Careful nursing and attention to fluid and electrolyte balance, airway, cardiac, and renal functions, and temperature control are essential. Adrenocorticotrophic hormone (ACTH) and adrenocortical steroids are used as anticonvulsants in treating massive spasm epilepsy in infancy associated with the "hypsarhythmic" electroencephalogram. A "ketogenic" diet may be helpful in certain children and young adults, with intractable seizures.

The basic mechanisms of anticonvulsant drugs are not clearly understood. Most such drugs are neuronal depressants with certain variations in action. The hydantoin drugs have been found to reduce the synaptic activity of posttetanic potentiation; the oxazolidine (trimethadione) drugs decrease transmission during repetitive stimulation. Increased stabilization of excitable neuronal membranes probably takes place by action upon electrochemical characteristics involved in ion permeability and membrane polarization. These stabilizing effects presumably decrease the activity of the abnormal hyperexcitable neuronal aggregates in an epileptogenic focus and, more importantly, generally prevent the spread of discharge through normal neuronal circuits.

While there are many anticonvulsant drugs, none is capable of total seizure control in all patients. However, careful selection and utilization in each individual case often leads to optimal results. Each physician should learn to use a number of these drugs and to recognize disturbing side effects as early as possible. Periodic blood counts, urinalyses, and liver-function tests are necessary during administration of many of these drugs.

The majority of the anticonvulsant drugs are administered to achieve a desired effect and the dosage must be increased to the point of tolerance without untoward toxic reactions.

Blood levels should be followed (see Table 13–2). It is best to start with a drug of choice; however, a single drug does not usually achieve the desired degree of control and a second may be necessary; two drugs may be indicated initially in patients with two different types of seizure, e.g., grand mal and petit mal. The process may require weeks of adjustment and during this time the patient's and family's cooperation in reporting effects on seizure frequency or side reactions is most important. Frequent changing of drugs is to be avoided.

Unfortunately, there is no specific anticonvulsant drug for each type of seizure. However, there is one major therapeutic axiom; the petit-mal absence does require a special anticonvulsant drug, either a succinimide (Zarontin) or an oxazolidine (trimethadione). Ethosuximide (Zarontin) is generally the drug of choice for this seizure state. This group of drugs is not effective in the treatment of major generalized seizures; conversely, the hydantoins are not generally effective in petit mal. Some authors state that the drugs effective in petit mal may worsen a generalized seizure state and vice versa; adequate evidence for this generalization has not been reported to date.

Generalized seizures, grand mal, and minor motor seizures are best treated with diphenylhydantoin sodium and phenobarbital. Initially, either drug may be administered to patients with infrequent attacks, but generally the combination of diphenylhydantoin and phenobarbital will achieve control of seizure in up to 85 percent of patients. Dosages should vary as indicated in Table 13–2. The average dose of diphenylhydantoin is 0.3–0.4 g. per day, usually administered as 0.2 g. in the morning after breakfast and 0.2 g. after dinner. The use of diphenylhydantoin has been enhanced by the determination of blood levels of the drug. The effective therapeutic range is between 10 and 20 μg/100 ml. Toxic effects usually appear at levels above this. The dosage of phenobarbital is initially 60 mg. at bedtime, with 30-mg. increments during the day if necessary; dosage is limited by its sedative effect.

Patients with psychomotor-temporal-lobe epilepsy are often more difficult to control. In these instances many trials may be necessary; the best results are to be expected with diphenylhydantoin and either phenobarbital or primidone. Although in some clinics the latter two drugs are used together, their sedative effects combine to make such administration difficult. Actually a significant amount of primidone is metabolized into phenobarbital. When employing primidone it is very important to start with doses ranging from 50 to 125 mg. per day, increasing slowly at weekly intervals to a maximum of 0.75 or 1.0 g. per day. If untoward side effects occur with diphenylhydantoin, substitution with the less reactive ethylphenylhydantoin is sometimes successful, although this drug has a weaker anticonvulsant effect. Mephenytoin and phenacemide are useful in difficult cases, but must be utilized with extreme care because of their high toxicity.

Occasionally, a paradoxical reaction to diphenylhydantoin occurs, at a time when a high or toxic blood level is reached, or, in some instances, even at a level regarded as nontoxic but relatively high for the particular patient.[57] This clinical state is characterized by a lapse of seizure control with actual increase in seizures, worsening of the EEG with increased paroxysmal discharges and background slow waves, and a dulling of perceptual-cognitive functions (with poor school or work performance, for example). Occasionally, focal neurological signs, such as hemiparesis, appear. There may be no usual "toxic" signs of diphenylhydantoin excess such as nystagmus or ataxia. Photic stimulation or other "alerting" stimuli may actually reduce the EEG phenomena. The term "diphenylhydantoin encephalopathy" has been applied to this state, but the mechanism of its production remains unclear. It is clinically significant, and can be treated by reduction of dosage.

Disturbances of intellectual function, along with psychotic states, reported in children treated with ethosuximide[141] have been difficult to evaluate in relation to the seizure process and interictal state.[15]

Certain stimulating drugs such as the amphetamines may be useful adjuncts in the therapy of certain patients, particularly to counteract sedative effects of phenobarbital or primidone without interfering with anticonvulsant action.

It is of interest that certain drugs interfere with the metabolism of diphenylhydantoin and increase its blood levels; these include dicoumarol, phenylbutazone, disulfiram, p-aminosalicylate, and isoniazid.

Acetazolamide is (Diamox) an important adjuvant in some patients with any type of seizure state, since it seems to have a general effect upon hyperexcitable cerebral neurons because of its inhibition of carbonic anhydrase or production of an acidosis. Since tolerance develops, the drug should be administered intermittently; it is occasionally useful, for example, in helping to control seizures occurring prior to or during the menstrual cycle. Under these circumstances acetazoleamide is administered for a week before and during the menstrual period. Some patients require its administration continually; tolerance does not develop in all patients.

The results of drug therapy are difficult to predict. With careful attention to individual details and general patient management, the patient with occasional generalized and psychomotor seizure can achieve effective control of seizure frequency. In children with petit-mal absences, the results are generally quite satisfactory. There are in each group of patients, however, a refractory number with increasing psychological and social problems as the years go by. This is the group which requires frequent changes in drugs and in which side effects become most troublesome.

Problems relating to drug withdrawal appear when patients achieve complete seizure control for a number of years; after two years the question of drug withdrawal is usually raised.[137] However, in most adults with grand mal and psychomotor epilepsy, continued therapy is necessary. In relatively few patients can drug withdrawal be accomplished even after freedom from seizures for three to five years; seizures usually recur. As has been pointed out, the EEG may remain abnormal in clinically seizure free patients, indicating seizure potentiality; and even in cases in which the EGG reverts to normal, drug withdrawal may be unsuccessful.

However, a calculated risk of drug withdrawal should be considered in some patients, since successful withdrawal could represent an important psychological achievement. Drug withdrawal should be attempted extremely carefully with small decrements over many weeks. Drug withdrawal can be expected to be more successful in children with controlled petit-mal epilepsy, particularly since there is a natural tendency for petit mal to diminish with age and maturity. However, in some of these patients generalized convulsions appear even after the absences have ceased.

DIETARY TREATMENT

In general, there are no dietary restrictions for the patient with epilepsy, nor is there a specific diet capable of aiding most patients. However, a diet high in fat content producing significant ketosis, i.e., the "ketogenic diet," is occasionally helpful in young children, particularly those with intractable absences and minor motor seizures. Anticonvulsant drugs usually have to be continued and the diet is difficult to maintain because of its lack of appeal.

PSYCHOLOGICAL THERAPY AND SOCIOLOGICAL MANAGEMENT

Even though drugs may achieve a significant degree of seizure control in individual patients, there are many problems related to the life and adjustment of the patient that need additional management. These are generally less marked when the seizures are under control, and require greater attention when seizures create continued problems. There are certain patients, particularly some children and adults with psychomotor-temporal-lobe seizures, who develop increased personality and behavioral disorders after seizure control; the reasons for this are not clear. In many patients, the coexistence of seizure and personality problems requires a combination of medical anticonvulsant therapy and psychologically oriented management.

Although many anticonvulsant drugs have sedative properties, these usually are not used directly. The so-called tranquilizing drugs have limited usefulness in the management of seizure patients. Chlordiazepoxide and diazepam may reduce disturbed behavior, particularly in children. The phenothiazine drugs have variable effects; the alerting phenothiazine, fluphenazine, is of some use in controlling abnormal behavior in certain patients with psychomotor seizures. However, other drugs in the chlorpromazine group are known to provoke paroxysmal discharges in the EEG and seizures.

In most patients there is a direct interplay of emotional disturbances with clinical seizure activity; patients in a state of psychological turmoil have increased seizure susceptibility and often require greater amounts of anticonvulsant drugs. The achievement of psychological adjustment often reduces seizure frequency and intensity, and lessens drug requirement. This fact must be considered in relation to the individual patient, the age, family, and social circumstances. Family understanding is of primary importance, since the child with seizures must live, insofar as possible, as a normal individual within home and school settings. A great problem, still to be overcome, is the stigma attached to epilepsy and the lack of understanding which exists not only among people in general but in relation to various restrictive legal and social practices. Most children with seizures can attend schools and vocational programs successfully; most adults with seizures can develop productive careers and engage in activities, such as marriage, childbearing, obtaining an education, driving an automobile, traveling, and working successfully in business and industry; while so engaged they can and should be protected by insurance and workmen's compensation programs. Only few patients require a protected environment in schools or "colonies" specifically developed for the epileptic. Even these should not be institutions in which many hundreds of epileptic patients are kept under essentially custodial care. Special treatment units or "colonies" in Great Britain, Holland, Denmark, and France are relatively small and homelike; they are designed to provide care for usually small numbers of patients at a time, involved in intensive programs of medical therapy, psychological management, education, and vocational training. From these units increasing numbers of adequately controlled patients are sent out into the general community where they can live well-adjusted and productive lives.

There are only a few occupations contraindicated for patients with a tendency toward seizures; these include activities of potential danger to either the patient or others, e.g., work requiring climbing to great heights, using heavy power equipment, or perhaps dangerous chemical substances; there may be exceptions in individual cases.

There is no medical reason to restrict driving an automobile if the patient has been seizure-free for at least two years. Furthermore, the work records of many patients with a history of seizures show that they are seldom involved in industrial accidents because they realize how important it is to their welfare to be most careful.

In a family situation, therefore, the person with epilepsy must be accepted on as normal a basis as possible; restrictive situations must be minimal, if needed at all, and a regular program of education and vocational planning should be developed. School officials frequently need appropriate orientation; most children and young adults with seizures are accepted without question by their associates.

In individual instances, both informal and formal psychotherapeutic measures can be undertaken in order to reduce emotional disturbances. The role of the family physician is all-important; often he alone can judge the problems in a family, school, or social setting and can, by his guidance and understanding, help the patient and his family overcome the feelings of despair, anxiety, fear, and self-consciousness that interfere with everyone's normal adjustment. It is only when anxieties and depressive tendencies develop into more severe reactions, associated with perhaps paranoid states, increased withdrawal, and excessive obsessional tendencies, that more intensive psychiatric treatment may become necessary. Occasionally, it is found that brief periods of appropriately oriented hospitalization with psychotherapy can help readjust or control such patients. This may also be required to evaluate the intensity of the psychological disturbance and the apparent intellectual difficulties that may be interfering with the patient's performance. Adjustment of drug schedules may be carried out at the same time. With increased experience even the child with epilepsy and behavioral disorder can be cared for best if he can attend a normal school with an understanding environment and, in addition, be associated with a clinical outpatient service in which the functions of the physician and social service department work together with the child and the family. It is becoming less necessary to arrange for either home tutoring or placement of such children into special schools or other facilities for the maladjusted.

"CONDITIONED INHIBITION" OR "DESENSITIZATION" THERAPY

There has been much interest, in recent years, in attempting to reduce or control seizures, particularly those triggered by sensory or reflex stimuli, by "desensitization" techniques. Whether these represent "true conditioning" in the Pavlovian sense remains problematic. However the results have sometimes been interesting and therapeutically successful. Olfactory stimuli have been known to arrest uncinate seizures since the time of Jackson,[78] and were studied in detail by Efron.[29,30] Forster and his group have been involved in a number of "conditioning" therapeutic trials in patients with various kinds of sensory or reflex-induced epilepsies (reading, photic, audiogenic, especially musicogenic).[40,41] These phenomena have led to experimental studies as well.[94,113] In specifically selected patients, therefore, such techniques, utilizing the known stimulus in a "desensitization" or "conditioning" paradigm, may lead to effective therapy.

SURGICAL THERAPY

There is no question that a patient with a lesion such as a brain tumor should be considered for operation, regardless of the state of the seizures. Surgical intervention with removal of a focus of abnormal discharge is considered an appropriate treatment for certain patients who have intractable focal epilepsy, after adequate trial of intensive medical care. The evaluation of such a patient, therefore, must consist of careful medical and neurological studies which should include a psychological consideration, since rehabilitation may be affected by the procedure. A focally discharging area should be determined by serial electroencephalographic studies as being fixed, and the region of brain considered for excision must be such that the patient will not be left with a severe speech, memory, or other neurological deficit.

Patients so evaluated often do not have obvious brain tumors, but the epileptogenic region involved as the discharging focus may contain a small tumor, a vascular lesion, or a scar secondary to trauma or previous encephalitis. This approach has been particularly used in patients with focal motor seizures, especially psychomotor-temporal-lobe or limbic seizures. It must be realized that even though many patients are considered for surgical therapy, few are chosen; the number of surgically treated epileptic patients is still only in the hundreds. Yet, the occasional patient carefully selected for such surgical therapy may achieve significant control of seizures. In some series good results have been reported in up to 50 percent; unfortunately, this means that an equal number are not better controlled postoperatively. In some cases, however, less anticonvulsant medication may be required. Occasionally, generalized seizures appear instead of previous psychomotor-temporal-lobe seizures. In most of these patients it would seem that the regions of brain involved are too widespread for limited excisions to be practicable. A small number of patients have experienced relief from severe personality disturbances, particularly aggressive psychotic behavior, but the surgical intervention usually has not been primarily directed toward this end. Bilateral operations on the temporal lobe have only limited effectiveness and may produce severe memory disturbances. The use of stereotaxic neurosurgical techniques to destroy epileptogenic regions deeply seated in brain, i.e., amygdala and hippocampus, has been recommended, particularly for certain patients with psychomotor-temporal-lobe epilepsy where there is such evidence from depth electroencephalographic studies. In a small number of carefully selected children with severe infantile hemiplegia, intractable convulsions, and behavior disturbance, cerebral hemispherectomy has been performed with improvement in seizure state and behavior despite the persistence of neurologic disability.

CONCLUDING REMARKS

Much more must be learned about the natural history of the epileptic in order to evaluate thoroughly the different therapies.[137] The question of treating the young child who has had a single febrile convulsion is typical of the problems involved. There is accumulating evidence that recurring seizures (especially with *status epilepticus*) do produce cerebral damage which may eventually cause clinical neurological dysfunction and further severe seizures. On the other hand, many infants and young children have one or a few seizures and then no more.

Proper medical therapy adequately controls most seizure states in over 60 percent of patients and partially controls an additional 25–30 percent. The drugs involved are decreasingly toxic, although anticonvulsant medication remains essentially nonspecific and broadly directed against mechanisms of neuronal hyperexcitability that are little understood. The remaining intractable patients may be considered for surgical therapy; such procedures are applicable, however as stated, to only a very small selected group. Surgical therapy is effective in only about 50 percent of those chosen. It is hoped that combined physiological and biochemical studies of disturbed cerebral and general bodily functions in epilepsy will lead eventually to more rational and effective therapy.

(Bibliography

1. ABRAHAM, K. and C. AJMONE MARSAN. "Patterns of Cortical Discharges and Their Relation to Routine Scalp Electroencephalography," *Electroencephalogr. Clin. Neurophysiol.*, 10 (1958), 447–461.

2. ALSTROM, C. H. "A Study of Epilepsy in its Clinical, Social and Genetic Aspects," *Acta Psychiatr. Neurol. Scand. Suppl.*, 63 (1950), pp. 1–284.

3. ANDERMANN, F. "Self-Induced Television Epilepsy," *Epilepsia*, 12 (1971), 269–275.

4. ANDERMANN, K., F. BERMAN, P. M. COOKE et al. "Self-Induced Epilepsy," *Arch. Neurol.*, 6 (1962), 49–65.

5. ARETAEUS. *The Extant Works of Aretaeus, The Cappadocian. Libri Septema.* Translated by Francis Adams. London: Sydenham Society, 1856.

6. BACIA, T. and K. REID. "Visual and Somatosensory Evoked Potentials in Man, Particularly in Patients with Focal Epilepsy," *Electroencephalogr. Clin. Neurophysiol.*, 18 (1965), 718.

7. BADDELEY, A. and K. PATTERSON. "Relation Between Long-term and Short-term Memory," *Br. Med. Bull.*, 27 (1971), 237–242.

8. BALDWIN, M. and P. BAILEY, eds. *Temporal Lobe Epilepsy.* Springfield, Ill.: Charles C. Thomas, 1958.

9. BARROW, R. L. and H. D. FABING. *Epilepsy and the Law,* 2nd ed. New York: Harper & Row, 1966.

10. BERGAMINI, L. and B. BERGAMESCO. *Cortical Evoked Potentials in Man,* pp. 49–52. Springfield, Ill.: Charles C. Thomas, 1967.

11. BLUMER, D. and A. E. WALKER. "Sexual Behavior in Temporal Lobe Epilepsy," *Arch. Neurol.*, 16 (1967), 37–43.

12. BINGLEY, T., "Mental Symptoms in Temporal Lobe Epilepsy and Temporal Lobe Gliomas," *Acta Psychiatr. Neurol. Scand. Suppl.*, 120 (1958), 151.

13. BRIERLEY, J. B. "Neuropathology of Amnesic States," in C. W. M. Whitty and O. L. Zangwill, eds., *Amnesia*, pp. 150–180. London: Butterworths, 1966.

14. BRUENS, J. H. "Psychoses in Epilepsy,"

Psychiatr. Neurol. Neurochir., 74 (1971), 175–192.

15. BUCHANAN, R. A. "Ethosuximide Toxicity," in D. M. Woodbury, J. K. Penry, and R. P. Schmidt, eds., *Antiepileptic Drugs*, pp. 449–454. New York: Raven, 1972.

16. CEREGHINO, J. J. and J. K. PENRY. "Testing of Anticonvulsants in Man," in D. M. Woodbury, J. K. Penry, and R. P. Schmidt, eds., *Antiepileptic Drugs*, pp. 63–73. New York: Raven, 1972.

17. CÈRNACĚK, J. and L. CIGÀNEK. "The Cortical Electroencephalographic Response to Light Stimulation in Epilepsy," *Epilepsia*, 3 (1962), 303–314.

18. COLLINS, A. L. and W. G. LENNOX. "The Intelligence of 300 Private Epileptic Patients," *Res. Publ. Assoc. Res. Nerv. Ment. Dis.*, 26 (1947), 586–603.

19. COURTOIS, G. A., D. H. INGVAR, and H. H. JASPER. "Nervous and Mental Defects During Petit Mal Attacks," *Electroencephalogr. Clin. Neurophysiol. Suppl.*, 3 (1953), 87.

20. CURRIE, S., K. W. G. HEATHFIELD, R. A. HENSON et al. "Clinical Course and Prognosis of Temporal Lobe Epilepsy—A Survey of 666 Patients," *Brain*, 94 (1971), 173–190.

21. DALLABARBA, G. "Mental Capactities of Epileptics at Intelligence Test 1," *Arch. Psycol. Neurol. Psychiatr.*, 18 (1957), 459–488.

22. DAVIDOFF, R. A. and L. C. JOHNSON. "Paroxysmal EEG Activity and Cognitive-Motor Performance," *Electroencephalogr. Clin. Neurophysiol.*, 16 (1964), 343–354.

23. DELAY, J., P. PICHOT, T. LAMPERIERE et al. *The Rorschach and the Epileptic Personality.* New York: Logos, 1958.

24. DENNERLL, R. D. "Cognitive Deficits and Lateral Brain Dysfunction in Temporal Lobe Epilepsy," *Epilepsia*, 5 (1964), 177–191.

25. DETRE, T. and R. G. FELDMAN. "Behavior Disorder Associated with Seizure States," in G. H. Glaser, ed., *EEG and Behavior*, pp. 366–376. New York: Basic Books, 1963.

26. DIMSDALE, H., V. LOGUE, and M. PIERCY. "A Case of Persisting Impairment of Recent Memory Following Right Temporal Lobectomy," *Neuropsychologia*, 1 (1964), 287–298.

27. DONGIER, S. "Statistical Study of Clinical and Electroencephalographic Manifesta-

tions of 536 Psychotic Episodes Occurring in 516 Epileptics Between Clinical Seizures," *Epilepsia*, 1 (1960), 117–142.

28. DRACHMAN, D. A. and J. ARBIT. "Memory and Hippocampal Complex," *Arch. Neurol.*, 15 (1966), 52–61.

29. EFRON, R. "The Effect of Olfactory Stimuli in Arresting Uncinate Fits," *Brain*, 79 (1956), 267–281.

30. ———. "The Conditioned Inhibition of Uncinate Fits," *Brain*, 80 (1957), 257–262.

31. FALCONER, M. A. "Some Functions of the Temporal Lobes with Special Regard to Affective Behavior in Epileptic Patients," *J. Psychosom. Res.*, 9 (1967), 25.

32. FALRET, J. "De l'Etat Mental des Epileptiques," *Arch. Gén. Méd.* 16 (1860), 666–679; 17 (1861), 461–491; 18 (1861), 26–37.

33. FEDIO, P. and A. F. MIRSKY. "Selective Intellectual Deficits in Children with Temporal Lobe or Centrencephalic Epilepsy," *Neuropsychologia*, 7 (1969), 287–300.

34. FENTON, G. W. and E. L. UDWIN. "Homicide, Temporal Lobe Epilepsy and Depression: A Case Report," *Br. J. Psychiatry*, 111 (1965), 304–306.

35. FERGUSON, S. M. and M. RAYPORT. "The Adjustment to Living Without Epilepsy," *J. Nerv. Ment. Dis.*, 140 (1965), 26–37.

36. FISCHER-WILLIAMS, M., R. G. BICKFORD, and J. P. WHISNANT. "Occipito-parieto-temporal Seizure Discharge with Visual Hallucinations and Aphasia," *Epilepsia*, 5 (1964), 279–292.

37. FLOR-HENRY, P. "Ictal and Interictal Psychiatric Manifestations in Epilepsy: Specific or Non-specific. A Critical Review of Some of the Evidence," *Epilepsia*, 13 (1972), 772–783.

38. FLYNN, J. P., P. D. MACLEAN, and C. KIM. "Effects of Hippocampal After-discharges on Conditioned Responses," in E. D. Sheer, ed., *Electrical Stimulation of the Brain*, pp. 380–386. Austin: University of Texas Press, 1961.

39. FLYNN, J. P., M. WASMAN, and D. EGGER. "Behavior During Propagated Hippocampal After-discharges," in G. H. Glaser, ed., *EEG and Behavior*, pp. 134–148. New York: Basic Books, 1963.

40. FORSTER, F. M. "Clinical Therapeutic Conditioning in Reading Epilepsy," *Neurology*, 19 (1969), 717–723.

41. FORSTER, F. M. and G. B. CAMPOS. "Conditioning Factors in Stroboscopic-induced Seizures," *Epilepsia*, 5 (1964), 156–165.

42. FREUD, S. (1923) "A Seventeenth-Century Demonological Neurosis," in J. Strachey, ed., *Standard Edition*, Vol. 19, pp. 72–105. London: Hogarth, 1955.

43. ———. (1928) "Dostoevsky and Parricide," in J. Strachey, ed., *Standard Edition*, Vol. 21, pp. 177–194. London: Hogarth, 1955.

44. GASCON, G. G. and C. T. LOMBROSO. "Epileptic (Gelastic) Laughter," *Epilepsia*, 12 (1971), 63–76.

45. GASTAUT, H. "So-called 'Psychomotor' and 'Temporal' Epilepsy," *Epilepsia*, 2 (1953), 59–96.

46. GASTAUT, H. and H. COLOMB. "Etude du comportement sexual chez les epileptiques psychomoteurs," *Ann. Méd. Psychol.*, 112 (1954), 657–696.

47. GASTAUT, H., G. FRANCK, W. KROLIKOWSKA et al. "Phénomènes de Déafferentation sensoriélle spécifique decélés par l'enregistrement transcranien des potentials évoqués visuels chez des sujets présentant des crises épileptiques visuelles dons leur champ hemianapsique uni-ou bilateral," *Rev. Neurol. (Paris)*, 109 (1963), 249.

48. GASTAUT, H. and H. REGIS. "Visually Evoked Potentials Recorded Transcranially in Man," in L. D. Proctor and W. R. Adey, eds., *Symposium on the Analysis of Central Nervous System and Cardiovascular Data Using Computer Methods*, pp. 8–34. Washington: NASA, SP72, 1964.

49. GASTAUT, H., J. ROGER, R. SOULAYROL et al. "Childhood Epileptic Encephalopathy with Diffuse Slow Spike-waves (Otherwise known as "Petit Mal Variant") or Lennox Syndrome," *Epilepsia*, 7 (1966), 139–179.

50. GASTAUT, H. and C. A. TASSINARI. "Triggering Mechanisms in Epilepsy: The Electroclinical Point of View," *Epilepsia*, 7 (1966), 85–138.

51. GASTAUT, H. and M. VIGOROUX. "Electroclinical Correlations in 500 Cases of Psychomotor Seizures," in M. Baldwin and P. Bailey, eds., *Temporal Lobe Epilepsy*, pp. 118–128. Springfield, Ill.: Charles C. Thomas, 1958.

52. GIBBS, F. "Ictal and Non-ictal Psychiatric Disorders in Temporal Lobe Epilepsy," *J. Nerv. Ment. Dis.*, 113 (1951), 522–528.

53. GLASER, G. H. "Visceral Manifestations of Epilepsy," *Yale J. Biol. Med.*, 30 (1957), 176–186.

54. ———. "The Problem of Psychosis in Psychomotor Temporal Lobe Epileptics," *Epilepsia*, 5 (1964), 271–278.

55. ———. "Limbic Epilepsy in Childhood," *J. Nerv. Ment. Dis.*, 144 (1967), 391–397.

56. ———. "Epilepsy and Disorders of Perception," *Assoc. Res. Nerv. Ment. Dis.*, 48 (1970), 318–333.

57. ———. "Diphenylhydantoin Toxicity," in D. M. Woodbury, J. K. Penry, and R. P. Schmidt, eds., *Antiepileptic Drugs*, pp. 219–226. New York: Raven, 1972.

58. GLASER, G. H., R. J. NEWMAN, and R. Schafer. "Interictal Psychosis in Psychomotor-Temporal Lobe Epilepsy. An EEG-psychological Study," in: G. H. Glaser, ed., *EEG and Behavior*, pp. 345–365. New York: Basic Books, 1963.

59. GLASER, G. H. and E. C. ZUCKERMANN. "Potassium Accumulation in Extracellular Spaces of Brain as a Possible Cause of Epileptogenic Activity," in G. Alemà, G. Bollea, V. Floris et al., eds., *Brain and Mind Problems*, pp. 309–329. Rome: Il Pensiero Scientifico, 1968.

60. GOLDENSOHN, E. S. "EEG and Ictal and Post-ictal Behavior," in G. H. Glaser, ed., *EEG and Behavior*, pp. 293–314. New York: Basic Books, 1963.

61. GOODE, D. J., J. K. PENRY, and F. E. DREIFUSS. "Effects of Paroxysmal Spike-wave on Continuous Visual-Motor Performance," *Epilepsia*, 11 (1970), 241–254.

62. GOODGLASS, H., M. MORGAN, A. T. FOLSOM et al. "Epileptic Seizures, Psychological Factors and Occupational Adjustments," *Epilepsia*, 4 (1963), 322–341.

63. GOWERS, W. R. (1881) *Epilepsy and other Chronic Convulsive Disorders*. London: Churchill, 1881; reprinted New York: Dover, 1964.

64. GREEN, J. B. "Reflex Epilepsy. Electroencephalographic and Evoked Potential Studies of Sensory Precipitated Seizures," *Epilepsia*, 12 (1971), 225–234.

65. GUERRANT, J., W. W. ANDERSON, A. FISCHER et al. *Personality in Epilepsy*. Springfield, Ill.: Charles C. Thomas, 1962.

66. GUEY, J., M. BUREAU, C. DRAVET et al. "A Study of the Rhythm of Petit Mal Absences in Children in Relation to Prevailing Situations," *Epilepsia*, 10 (1969), 441–451.

67. HECKER, A., F. ANDERMANN, and E. A.

RODIN. "Spitting Automatism in Temporal Lobe Seizures," *Epilepsia*, 13 (1972), 767–772.

68. HILL, D. "Psychiatric Disorders of Epilepsy," *Med. Press*, 229 (1953), 473–475.

69. HIPPOCRATES. Translated by J. Chadwick and W. N. Mann. *Medical Works of Hippocrates*, Sect. 15, p. 189. Oxford: Blackwell, 1950.

70. HISHIKAWA, Y., J. YAMAMOTO, E. FURIJA et al. "Photosensitive Epilepsy: Relationships Between the Visual Evoked Responses and Epileptiform Discharges Induced by Intermittent Photic Stimulation," *Electroencephalogr. Clin. Neurophysiol.*, 23 (1967), 320–334.

71. HOROWITZ, M. J. *Psychosocial Function in Epilepsy. Rehabilitation after Surgical Treatment for Temporal Lobe Epilepsy.* pp. 180. Springfield, Ill.: Charles C. Thomas, 1970.

72. HOROWITZ, M. J. and F. M. COHEN. "Temporal Lobe Epilepsy. Effect of Lobectomy on Psychosocial Functioning," *Epilepsia*, 9 (1968), 23–41.

73. HUNTER, R., V. LOGUE, and W. H. McMENEMY. "Temporal Lobe Epilepsy Supervening on Longstanding Transvestism and Fetishism," *Epilepsia*, 4 (1963), 60.

74. HUTT, S. J. "Experimental Analysis of Brain Activity and Behavior in Children with 'Minor' Seizures," *Epilepsia*, 13 (1972), 520–534.

75. HUTT, S. J., P. M. JACKSON, A. BELSHAM et al. "Perceptual-motor Behavior in Relation to Blood Phenobarbitone Level. A Preliminary Report," *Develop. Med. Child Neurol.*, 10 (1968), 626–632.

76. HUTT, S. J., D. LEE, and C. OUNSTED. "Digit Memory and Evoked Discharges in Four Light-Sensitive Epileptic Children," *Develop. Med. Child Neurol.*, 5 (1963), 559–571.

77. IVES, L. A. "Learning Difficulties in Children with Epilepsy," *Br. J. Disord. Commun.*, 5 (1970), 77–84.

78. JACKSON, J. H. *On Epilepsy and Epileptiform Convulsions.* Vol. 1, Selected Writings, J. Taylor, ed., London: Hodder and Stoughton, 1931.

79. JACKSON, J. H. and W. S. COLMAN. "Case of Epilepsy with Tasting Movements and 'Dreamy State' A Very Small Patch of Softening in the Left Uncinate Gyrus," *Brain*, 21 (1898), 580–590.

80. JASPER, H. H. "Some Physiological Mechanisms Involved in Epileptic Automations," *Epilepsia*, 5 (1964), 1–20.

81. JASPER, H. H., A. WARDS, and A. POPE. eds. *Basic Mechanisms of the Epilepsies.* Boston: Little, Brown, 1970.

82. JORDAN, E. J. "MMPI Profile of Epileptics: A Further Evaluation," *J. Consult. Psychol.*, 27 (1963), 267–269.

83. JUNG, R. "Blocking of Petit-mal Attacks by Sensory Arousal and Inhibition of Attacks by an Active Change in Attention During the Epileptic Aura," *Epilepsia*, 3 (1962), 435–437.

84. KARAGULLIA, S. and E. E. ROBERTSON. "Psychical Phenomena in Temporal Lobe Epilepsy and the Psychoses," *Br. Med. J.*, 1 (1955), 748–752.

85. KENNA, J. C. and G. SEDMAN. "Depersonalization in Temporal Lobe Epilepsy and the Organic Psychoses," *Br. J. Psychiatry*, 111 (1965), 293–299.

86. KIMURA, D. "Right Temporal Lobe Damage," *Arch. Neurol.*, 8 (1963), 264–271.

87. ———. "Cognitive Deficit Related to Seizure Pattern in Centrencephalic Epilepsy," *J. Neurol. Neurosurg. Psychiatry*, 27 (1964), 291–295.

88. KOLVIN, I., C. OUNSTED, and M. ROTH. "Cerebral Dysfunction and Childhood Psychoses," *Br. J. Psychiatry*, 118 (1971), 407–414.

89. KOOI, K. A. and H. B. HOVEY. "Alterations in Mental Function and Paroxysmal Cerebral Activity," *Arch. Neurol. Psychiatry*, 78 (1957), 264–271.

90. KREINDLER, A. "Active Arrest Mechanisms of Epileptic Seizures," *Epilepsia*, 3 (1962), 329–337.

91. LANDOLT, H. "Serial Electroencephalographic Investigations During Psychotic Episodes in Epileptic Patients and During Schizophrenic Attacks," in A. M. Lorentz De Haas, ed., *Lectures on Epilepsy*, Suppl. 4, pp. 91–133. Amsterdam: Elsevier, 1958.

92. LENNOX, W. G. "Bernard of Gordon on Epilepsy," *Ann. Med. Hist.*, 3 (1941), 372–383.

93. LENNOX, W. G. and M. A. LENNOX. *Epilepsy and Related Disorders.* Boston: Little Brown, 1960.

94. LOCKARD, J. S., W. L. WILSON, and V. UHLIC. "Spontaneous Seizure Frequency and

Avoidance Conditioning in Monkeys," *Epilepsia*, 13 (1972), 437–444.

95. LORENTZ DE HAAS, A. M. and O. MAGNUS. "Clinical and Electroencephalographic Findings in Epileptic Patients with Episodic Mental Disorders," in A. M. Lorentz De Haas, ed., *Lectures on Epilepsy*, pp. 134–167. Amsterdam: Elsevier, 1958.

96. LOVELAND, W., B. SMITH, and F. FORSTER. "Mental and Emotional Changes in Epileptics on Continuous Anticonvulsant Medication," *Neurology*, 7 (1957), 856–865.

97. LUGARESI, E., P. PAZZAGLIA, and C. A. TASSINARI. "Differentiation of 'Absence Status' and 'Temporal Lobe Status,'" *Epilepsia*, 12 (1971), 77–87.

98. MacLEAN, P. D. "The Limbic System and Its Hippocampal Formation. Studies in Animals and Their Possible Application to Man," *J. Neurosurg.*, 11 (1954), 29–44.

99. MARGERISON, J. H. and J. A. CORSELLIS. "Epilepsy and the Temporal Lobes," *Brain*, 89 (1966), 499–530.

100. MATTHEWS, C. G. and H. KLØVE. "Differential Psychological Performance in Major Motor, Psychomotor, and Mixed Seizure Classifications of Known and Unknown Etiology," *Epilepsia*, 8 (1967), 116–128.

101. MEYER, V. "Cognitive Changes Following Temporal Lobectomy for Relief of Temporal Lobe Epilepsy," *Arch. Neurol. Psychiatry*, 81 (1959), 299–309.

102. MEYER, V. and A. YATES. "Intellectual Changes Following Temporal Lobectomy for Psychomotor Epilepy," *J. Neurol. Neurosurg. Psychiatry*, 18 (1955), 44–52.

103. MIGNONE, R. J., E. F. DONNELLY, and D. SADOWSKY. "Psychological and Neurological Comparisons of Psychomotor and Non-psychomotor Epileptic Patients," *Epilepsia*, 11 (1970), 345–359.

104. MILNER, B. "Psychological Defect Produced by Temporal Lobe Excision," *Res. Publ. Assoc. Res. Nerv. Ment. Dis.*, 36 (1956), 244–257.

105. ———. "Alteration of Perception and Memory in Man: Reflections on Methods," in L. Weiskrantz, ed., *Analysis of Behavioral Change*, pp. 268–375. New York: Harper & Row, 1968.

106. ———. "Interhemispheric Differences and Psychological Processes," *Br. Med. Bull.* 27 (1971), 272–277.

107. MILNER, B., S. CORKIN, and H. L. TEUBER. "Further Analysis of Hippocampal Amnesic Syndrome: 13 year Follow-up of H. M.," *Neuropsychologia*, 6 (1968), 215–234.

108. MIRSKY, A. F., D. W. PRIMAC, C. A. MARSAN et al. "A Comparison of the Psychological Test Performance of Patients with Focal and Non-focal Epilepsy," *Exper. Neurol.*, 2 (1960), 75–89.

109. MIRSKY, A. F. and J. L. TECCE. "The Analysis of Visual Evoked Potentials During Spike and Wave EEG Activity," *Epilepsia*, 9 (1968), 211–220.

110. MIRKSY, A. F. and J. M. VAN BUREN. "On the Nature of the 'Absence' in Centrencephalic Epilepsy: A Study of Some Behavioral, Electroencephalographic and Autonomic Factors," *Electroencephalogr. Clin. Neurophysiol.*, 18 (1965), 334–348.

111. MITCHELL, W., M. A. FALCONER, and D. HILL. "Epilepsy with Fetishism Relieved by Temporal Lobectomy," *Lancet*, 2 (1954), 626–630.

112. MOROCUTTI, C. and J. A. SOMMER-SMITH. "Etude des Potentials evoqués visuels dans l'epilepsie," *Rev. Neurol.*, 115 (1966), 93–98.

113. NAQUET, R. "Conditonnement de décharge hypersynchrones epileptiques," in J. F. Delafresnaye, ed., *Brain Mechanisms and Learning*, pp. 625–640. Oxford: Blackwell, 1961.

114. NEWCOMBE, F. "Memory for Designs Test," *Br. J. Soc. Clin. Psychol.*, 4 (1965), 230.

115. OUNSTED, C. "The Hyperkinetic Syndrome in Epileptic Children," *Lancet*, 2 (1955), 303–311.

116. OUNSTED, C., D. LEE, and S. J. HUTT. "Electroencephalographic and Clinical Changes in an Epileptic Child During Repeated Photic Stimulation," *Electroencephalogr. Clin. Neurophysiol.*, 21 (1966), 388–391.

117. OUNSTED, C, J. LINDSAY, and R. NORMAN. *Biological Factors in Temporal Lobe Epilepsy*, p. 135. London: Heinemann, 1966.

118. PENFIELD, W. and H. JASPER. *Epilepsy and the Functional Anatomy of the Human Brain*, p. 896. Boston: Little, Brown, 1954.

119. PENFIELD, W. and P. PEROT. "The Brain's Record of Auditory and Visual Experience," *Brain*, 86 (1963), 595–696.

120. PIERCY, M. "The Effects of Cerebral Lesions

on Intellectual Function: A Review of Current Research Trends," *Br. J. Psychiatry*, 110 (1964), 310–352

121. POND, D. A. "Psychiatric Aspects of Epilepsy," *J. Indian Med. Profess.*, 3 (1957), 1441–1451.

122. ———. "Psychiatric Aspects of Epileptic and Brain-damaged Children," *Br. Med. J.*, 2 (1961), 1377–1382, 1454–1459.

123. ———. "Psychological Disorders of Epileptic Patients," *Psychiatry Neurol. Neurochir.*, 74 (1971), 159.

124. PRECHTL, H. F. R., P. E. BOCKE, and T. SCHUT. "The Electroencephalogram and Performance in Epileptic Patients," *Neurology*, 11 (1961), 296–304.

125. PRICE, J. C. and T. J. PUTNAM. "The Effect of Intrafamily Discord on the Prognosis of Epilepsy," *Am. J. Psychiatry*, 100 (1944), 593–598.

126. PRICHARD, J. W. and G. H. GLASER. "Cortical Sensory Evoked Potentials During Limbic Seizures," *Electroencephalogr. Clin. Neurophysiol.*, 21 (1966), 180–184.

127. PUTNAM, T. J. and H. H. MERRITT. "Dullness as an Epileptic Equivalent," *Arch. Neurol. Psychiatry*, 45 (1941), 797–813.

128. QUADFASEL, A. F. and P. W. PRUYSER. "Cognitive Deficit in Patients with Psychomotor Epilepsy," *Epilepsia* (Ser. 1), 4 (1955), 80–90.

129. RAPOPORT, D., M. GILL, and R. SCHAFER. *Diagnostic Psychological Testing.* London: University of London Press, 1970.

130. RAVEN, J. C. *Guide to Using the Mill Hill Vocabulary Scale with Progressive Matrices.* London: Lewis, 1948.

131. ———. *Guide to Using Progressive Matrices.* London: Lewis, 1949.

132. RENNICK, P. M., C. PEREZ-BORJA, and E. A. RODIN. "Transient Mental Deficits Associated with Recurrent Prolonged Epileptic Clouded State," *Epilepsia*, 10 (1969), 397–405.

133. REYNOLDS, E. H. "Mental Effects of Anticonvulsant Drugs and Folate Metabolism," *Brain*, 91 (1968), 197–214.

134. RICCI, G., G. BERTI, and E. CHERUBINI. "Changes in Intrictal Focal Activity and Spike-wave Paroxysms During Motor and Mental Activity," *Epilepsia*, 13 (1972), 785–794.

135. RICHER, P. *Etudes Cliniques sur L'Hystéro-épilepsie ou Grande Hystérie.* Paris: Adrien Delahaye et Emile Lecrosnier, 1881.

136. ROBERTSON, E. G. "Photogenic Epilepsy: Self-Precipitated Attacks," *Brain*, 77 (1954), 232–261.

137. RODIN, E. A. *The Prognosis of Patients with Epilepsy.* Springfield, Ill.: Charles C. Thomas, 1968.

138. RODIN, E. A., R. N. DEJONG, R. W. WAGGONER et al. "Relationship between Certain Forms of Psychomotor Epilepsy and 'Schizophrenia,'" *Arch. Neurol. Psychiatry*, 77 (1957), 449–463.

139. RODIN, E. A., S. GONZALEZ, D. CALDWELL et al. "Photic Evoked Responses During Induced Epileptic Seizures," *Epilepsia*, 7 (1966), 202–214.

140. RODIN, E. A., D. W. MULDER, D. L. FAUCET et al "Psychologic Factors in Convulsive Disorders of Focal Origin," *Arch. Neurol. Psychiatry*, 74 (1955), 365–374.

141. ROGER, J., H. GRANGEON, J. GREY et al. "Psychiatric and Psychological Effects of Ethosuximide Treatment in Epileptics," *Encephale*, 57 (1968), 407–438.

142. ROTH, M. and M. HARPER. "Temporal Lobe Epilepsy and the Phobic-Anxiety Syndrome, Part 2," *Compr. Psychiatry*, 3 (1962), 215–226.

143. SCHWAB, R. S. "Method of Measuring Consciousness in Attacks of Petit Mal Epilepsy," *Arch. Neurol. Psychiatry*, 41 (1939), 215–227.

144. SCHWARTZ, M. L. and R. D. DENNERLL. "Neuropsychological Assessment of Children with, without and with Questionable Epileptogenic Dysfunction," *Percept. Mot. Skills.*, 30 (1970), 111–121.

145. SCOTT, D. F., A. MOFFETT, A. MATHEWS et al. "Effect of Epileptic Discharges on Learning and Memory in Patients," *Epilepsia*, 8 (1967), 188–194.

146. SCOVILLE, W. B. "Amnesia after Bilateral Mesial Temporal-lobe Excision: Introduction to Case H.M." *Neuropsychologia*, 6 (1968), 211–213.

147. SERAFETINIDES, E. A. "Aggressiveness in Temporal Lobe Epileptics and Its Relation to Cerebral Dysfunction and Environmental Factors," *Epilepsia*, 6 (1965), 33–42.

148. SERAFETINIDES, E. A. and M. A. FALCONER. "Some Observations on Memory Impairment after Temporal Lobectomy for Epilepsy," *J. Neurol. Neurosurg. Psychiatry*, 25 (1962), 251–255.

149. SERVIT, Z., J. MACHEK, A. STERCOVA et al.

"Reflex Influences in the Pathogenesis of Epilepsy in the Light of Clinical Statistics," *Epilepsia*, 3 (1962), 315–322.

150. SHALLICE, T. and E. K. WARRINGTON. "Independent Functioning of Verbal Memory Stores: A Neuropsychological Study," *Q. J. Exp. Psychol.*, 22 (1970), 261–273.

151. SHIMAZONO, Y., T. HIRAI, T. OKUMA et al. "Disturbance of Consciousness in Petit Mal Epilepsy," *Epilepsia*, 2 (1953), 49–55.

152. SLATER, E., A. W. BEARD, and E. GLITHERO. "The Schizophrenia-like Psychoses of Epilepsy," *Br. J. Psychiatry*, 189 (1963), 95–150.

153. SMALL, J. G., V. MILSTEIN, and J. R. STEVENS. "Are Psychomotor Epileptics Different?" *Arch. Neurol.*, 7 (1962), 187–194.

154. STEVENS, J. R. "Psychiatric Implications of Psychomotor Epilepsy," *Arch. Gen. Psychiatry*, 14 (1966), 461–471.

155. STEVENS, J. R., G. H. GLASER, and P. D. MacLEAN. "The Influence of Sodium Amytal on the Recollection of Seizure States," *Trans. Am. Neurol. Assoc.*, 79 (1954), 40–45.

156. SYMONDS, C. "Excitation and Inhibition in Epilepsy," *Brain*, 82 (1959), 133–146.

157. TAYLOR, D. C. "Aggression and Epilepsy," *J. Psychom. Res.*, 13 (1969), 229–235.

158. ———. "Sexual Behavior and Temporal Lobe Epilepsy," *Arch. Neurol.*, 21, (1969), 510–516.

159. ———. "Ontogenesis of Chronic Epileptic Psychoses: A Reanalysis," *Psychol. Med.*, 1 (1971), 247–253.

160. ———. "Psychiatry and Sociology in the Understanding of Epilepsy," in E. M. Mandelbrote and M. G. Gelder, eds., *Psychiatric Aspects of Medical Practice*, pp.

161–187. London: Staples Press, 1972.

161. ———. "Mental State and Temporal Lobe Epilepsy. A Correlative Account of 100 patients Treated Surgically," *Epilepsia*, 13 (1972), 727–765.

162. TEMKIN, O. *The Falling Sickness*, p. 380. Baltimore: The Johns Hopkins Press, 1945.

163. TIZARD, B. and J. H. MARGERISON. "Psychological Functions during Wave-Spike Discharge," *Br. J. Soc. Clin. Psychol.*, 3 (1963), 6–15.

164. WALKER, A. E. "Murder or Epilepsy?" *J. Nerv. Ment. Dis.*, 133 (1961), 430–437.

165. WARRINGTON, E. K. "Neurological Deficits," in P. Mittler, ed., *The Psychological Assessment of Mental and Physical Handicaps*, pp. 261–287. London: Methuen, 1971.

166. WARRINGTON, E. K. and M. JAMES. "Disorders of Visual Perception in Patients with Localised Cerebral Lesions," *Neuropsychologia*, 5 (1967), 253–266.

167. WARRINGTON, E. K. and P. RABIN. "A Preliminary Investigation of the Relation between Visual Perception and Memory," *Cortex*, 6 (1970), 87–96.

168. WECHSLER, D. *The Measurement of Adult Intelligence*, 3rd ed., Baltimore: Williams & Wilkins, 1944.

169. WHITTY, C. W. M. and O. L. ZANGWILL, eds. *Amnesia*. London: Butterworths, 1966.

170. WILLIAMS, D. "The Structure of Emotions Reflected in Epileptic Experience," *Brain*, 79 (1956), 29–67.

171. ———. "Man's Temporal Lobe," *Brain*, 91 (1968), 639–654.

172. YEAGER, C. L. and J. S. GUERRANT. "Subclinical Epileptic Seizures: Impairment of Motor Performance and Derivative Difficulties," *Calf. Med.*, 86 (1957), 242–247.

CHAPTER 14

PSYCHOSES ASSOCIATED WITH DRUG USE

Malcolm B. Bowers, Jr. and Daniel X. Freedman

⟨ Introduction

THIS CHAPTER deals with the genesis of psychotic behavior in which intake of a pharmacologic compound plays a significant role. As used here, *psychosis* refers to an experience of self and external world, which, for a significantly prolonged period, is at marked variance with generally accepted notions of reality and which is not under individual control. Psychotic behavior may become manifest at a variety of stages in the course of drug use: during acute or chronic drug ingestion, during drug withdrawal, or at varying intervals following drug use. In the latter instance the contribution of the drug to the genesis of the psychotic behavior is often hard to assess.

The phenomena of drug-induced altered states of consciousness which involve marked but usually temporary distortion in self-image, feeling states, and perception of external reality, remind psychopathologists that one component of many major psychiatric syndromes are just such alterations in consciousness. In the naturally occurring psychotic reaction such states of mind may be long lasting, recurrent, evoked in response to individually perceived experience, and with time variously assimilated or rejected by the individual. The fact that the same or similar statements can currently be made about many drug-related states encountered clinically indicates just how instructive the drug model has become.

Psychotic behavior is more likely to occur in a higher dose range and following prolonged use of a given compound with psychotogenic potential. When such behavior occurs at a lower dose, is not associated with delirium, and extends beyond the known period of drug action, one suspects the presence of other factors which may have predisposed the individual to such a response. Such factors may include a broad range of conscious and unconscious situational or maturational stresses—psychosocial stresses, which might threaten the coping capacities of the individual. Such stresses may have been involved in the original motivation to use the drug in question.

A classification of syndromes produced by drugs with psychotogenic potential with regard to the presence or absence of delirium, the contribution of psychosocial stress, and relative similarity to naturally occurring states is somewhat arbitrary. However, the classification proposed by Brawley and Duffield[22] in their review of hallucinogenic drugs, has some utility for the purposes of this survey.

Many active drugs, administered long enough and in sufficient quantity, produce psychotic behavior as part of a more extensive spectrum of general metabolic, neurologic, or toxic effects. The psychic syndrome thus produced is usually associated with some evidence of intellectual impairment, such as restricted consciousness, memory loss, or disorientation. Thus many of the symptoms of acute toxic psychosis are those of acute brain syndrome. We recognize in reality that a continuum exists between compounds which produce psychotic phenomena in a clouded as opposed to a clear sensorium. With some exceptions, compounds which produce primarily acute brain syndrome or neurotoxic effects usually do not produce psychotic syndromes akin to the naturally occurring psychoses nor do their effects usually persist after the drug has been withdrawn, unless damage to the central nervous system has occurred. Brawley and Duffield refer to these compounds as "poisons," though actually they represent a heterogeneous group.[61]

A group of drugs with anticholinergic properties tends to produce delirium without extensive toxic effects on other systems. This clinical syndrome is characterized by restricted consciousness; disorientation to time, place, and person; impairment in recent memory; visual hallucinations; and some degree of retrograde amnesia. Yet a third group of drugs—the psychotomimetic hallucinogens—can produce acute psychotic states without markedly clouding consciousness or producing other signs of intellectual impairment. These states resemble more closely some manifestations of the naturally occurring psychoses but are usually approximately limited in time by the duration of drug action. However, in some instances, use of these compounds is coincidental with or effective in precipitating extended psychotic states in some vulnerable individuals. Neither the nature of such vulnerability nor the role of drug effects interacting with such factors has been defined.

❮ Psychotogenic Drugs with Generalized Metabolic or Toxic Effects

Almost any potent pharmaceutical agent can potentially be placed in this category. Drugs which mimic or alter hormonal systems seem particularly likely to produce psychotic reactions in some individuals. High doses of adrenal steroids and ACTH are noted for their potential psychotomimetic effects.[28,82,85] Although the literature is not in complete accord, many psychotic reactions produced by these agents have not been associated with delirium and have resembled so-called schizoaffective reactions. There is no mandatory mood change contingent upon hormonal excesses or deficiencies but euphoria as a component of mood change with steroid medication is not uncommon; perceptual changes with reference to the body and the environment can accompany any of these mood changes. We are aware of a few instances of self-medication with drugs such as prednisone in order to enhance affect. Psychosocial factors contributory to psychotomimetic reactions may be important when the steroid treatment is administered for life-threatening illness (for instance, systemic *lupus erythematosus*) or produces gross weight gain and change in facial appearance. In the case of systemic *lupus erythematosus* vascular changes in the central nervous system may be contributory to behavioral change. In the treatment of thyroid dysfunction a variety of behavioral reactions may ensue contingent upon thyroid status, treatment agent, or change in psychological organization.[13,20,59] Psychotic reactions have been reported in association with the administration or withdrawal of oral contraceptive preparations.[31,65]

Although little used today, bromide preparations used to be a major cause of psychotic reactions. Usually such psychoses were associated with significant disorientation, but Levin[74,75] has described a "bromide schizophrenia" which he feels differs from bromide delirium in that clouding of consciousness was not a symptom in the former condition, and differential diagnosis on admission for such disorders presented a challenge to the astute clinician. The variety of psychological states which bromides can produce are not familiar to many clinicians today, but Levin's studies document an array of syndromes more prominent when bromides were more readily available in proprietary sedative preparations. Replacement of retained bromide with saline was a useful therapy.[51] Bromides are still present in a few over-the-counter preparations, but they have largely been replaced by belladonna alkaloids.[101]

Acute inhalation of a variety of volatile organic solvents can result in unusual states of consciousness. These agents vary in their toxicity.[72] Gasoline, toluene, ethyl acetate, and trichlorethylene are among the compounds which can produce "inhalation psychoses."[15] Some individuals may develop habituation to such practices and polyneuropathy has been reported.[54] Most of these compounds are anesthetics and acute inhalation in poorly ventilated surroundings can result in unconsciousness and death from suffocation (glue sniffing) or a primary cardiac toxicity from fluorinated hydrocarbons in aerosols (freon).[10,45,46] The acute brain syndrome produced by inhalation of organic solvents is usually attended by clouding of consciousness and terminated soon after the offending compound has been removed.

Unique psychopharmacological properties have been described for the anesthetic phencyclidine (Sernyl) now primarily used in veterinary medicine. Extensively studied by Domino, Luby, and their colleagues,[33,34,78] this compound in subanesthetic doses produces a unique picture of dissociation of consciousness akin to sensory isolation in which the individual may experience a variety of distortions in body image.[79] Although clouding of consciousness may be present, cognitive and body image changes produced by phencyclidine have reminded some investigators of the primary clinical symptoms of schizophrenia. This compound has recently been found extensively on the illicit drug market (known as PCP) and often is an unexpected adulterant of material sold as LSD or mescaline.

Use of the antimalarial drug atabrine was associated with psychotic reactions during World War II. Most of these cases were apparently characterized by disorientation but several were quite prolonged.[80] Some correlation with accumulated drug or metabolite was apparent and paranoid features were prominent, presenting problems for differential diagnosis.

Psychosis may occur as part of a syndrome of withdrawal from drugs which produce tissue dependence such as the major narcotics and sedative antianxiety drugs, including ethyl alcohol, barbiturates, meprobamate, and the benzodiazepines. Withdrawal from sedative compounds generally produces neurological symptoms such as tremor and convulsions but, as classic studies have shown, hallucinations and delirium can be a prominent aspect of the syndrome of sedative withdrawal.[102] As is generally known, the onset of all or part of this syndrome may be delayed following withdrawal of sedative compounds. In part, this phenomenon is related to a long half-life of certain drugs such as meprobamate or chlordiazepoxide. The classic state of sedative withdrawal (delirium tremens) which occurs following ethyl alcohol is not considered a specific indication for antipsychotic phenothiazine drugs. In fact under certain conditions such drugs may be contraindicated[100] as they are in belladonna delirium (central anticholinergic syndrome).

❪ Deliriants-Atropinelike Drugs

Many drugs used in medical practice have atropinelike properties. In general these compounds are quite potent and may produce psychotic effects at doses of a few milligrams. The psychosis thus produced is the typical "belladonna delirium" or central anticholinergic syndrome characterized by disorientation, dry skin, mydriasis, tachycardia, visual hallucinations, amnesia, and slowing of the electroencephalogram.[43] This clinical picture usually subsides within twenty-four hours after the offending drug or drug combination has been discontinued. Older individuals with chronic brain syndrome or other factors predisposing to delirium are usually susceptible to psychotic reactions produced by these compounds. This syndrome can be specifically reversed by the administration of physostigmine,[30,35] but conservative management is usually sufficient once the atropinelike drug has been withdrawn. Phenothiazines (which possess anticholinergic properties) have been reported to exacerbate atropinelike psychosis so that differential diagnosis of this state from psychosis related to amphetamine or LSD-like drugs is essential, for in the latter cases phenothiazines and sedative antianxiety compounds, respectively, are usually helpful. The atropinelike psychosis frequently emerges in clinical psychiatric practice when a patient is receiving a combination of drugs which have anticholinergic properties such as phenothiazines, tricyclic antidepressants, and anti-Parkinsonian compounds.[9,108] It is generally believed that these psychotic reactions are related to the interruption of function in the central cholinergic neuronal systems. However, it is unclear why higher psychic function is affected early in the dose-response spectrum of the centrally acting anticholinergics, whereas anticholinesterase compounds tend to produce more widespread and life-endangering neurotoxic effects and a different pattern of altered psychic function with some similarities to depressive states.[19]

❪ Psychotomimetic Drugs

Amphetaminelike Drugs

Compounds with actions similar to amphetamine (methamphetamine, cocaine, methylphenidate, phenmetrazine, and diethylproprion) may produce psychotic reactions without marked clouding of consciousness.[4,7,95] Three years after the first use of amphetamine in the treatment of narcolepsy, psychotic reactions were reported.[110] These authors also speculated on the possible vulnerability of persons with psychopathic traits to such drug use and reactions. In more recent years, the use of amphetaminelike drugs for appetite suppression and psychomotor stimulation has led to periodic occurrence of such reactions.

At higher doses and with continuing use amphetaminelike drugs reliably produce psychotic symptoms which often cannot be distinguished from those of naturally-occurring paranoid psychoses.[29] It has been recently shown under certain experimental conditions that these compounds regularly produce a syndrome of psychotic suspiciousness and ideas of reference.[5,57] These clinical studies, in which amphetamine has been repeatedly administered to volunteer subjects so a relatively large cumulative intake is achieved over a few days, suggest that virtually all subjects will eventually become psychotic on such a regimen. Since the subjects have been amphetamine users, the factor of prior state (including personality) must be considered as a component in the response. Many investigators consider this high-dose amphetamine reaction the closest experimental analogue of the naturally-occurring psychoses. Bell, however, has recounted administration of higher doses of intravenous methamphetamine in amphetamine addicts.[11,12] He frequently observed very prompt onset of symptoms. These, however, are initially changes in perception, illusions, tension, and difficulty in locating the source and meaning of such changes. Paranoid interpretations followed later, as did the more typical ideas of reference and delusions. He observes this pattern in one group of cases encountered clinically whose symptoms eventually subsided while another group with auditory hallucinations had persisting symptoms.[11] These changes are not unlike the sequence of events observed with the psychotomimetic indoles (LSD, psilocybin, DMT [N,N[1]-dimethyltryptamine]) and phenylethylamines (mescaline).[48] Indeed sharp observation and reconstruction of the early onset of amphetamine psychoses indicate sensitivity to lights and reflections; perceptual changes precede and are later "explained," resulting in the more characteristic clinical signs (paranoid delusions) by which the amphetamine reaction is generally compared to acute schizophrenia.[18,83]

The fact that clinically effective antipsychotic compounds can antagonize the effects of amphetamine, and the differential effects of stereoisomers of this drug upon catecholamine systems[8,64] strengthens the argument that the effects of amphetamine may be a clue to neuronal mechanisms involved in some manifestations of the naturally-occurring psychoses. This subject has recently been reviewed by Snyder.[91,92] Many similarities exist between experimental amphetamine intoxication in animals and the clinical behaviors which are encountered, notably stereotypy. Ellinwood and his coworkers have analyzed amphetamine intoxication in several species from behavioral, histochemical, neurophysiological, and neuropathological points of view.[38–42,44]

Even at low doses amphetaminelike compounds may occasionally produce psychotic states and such psychoses may be prolonged, resembling naturally-occurring paranoid psychosis.[29] Under these circumstances one may speak of a drug-precipitated or drug-induced psychosis, the assumption being that amphetamine ingestion facilitated some process already moving the individual in the direction of a psychotic state. The following case illustrates the way in which amphetaminelike drugs may act synergistically to exacerbate a nascent psychotic state.

A twenty year-old woman, socially undeveloped and insecure, began her first job in a clothing store following graduation from high school. She became self-conscious when male employees made sexually provocative remarks. Soon she began to believe that other employees were saying and doing things designed to tell her that she should "grow up and masturbate." In this context she took one 5-milligram amphetamine tablet furnished by her brother. Her thought processes accelerated greatly, and her self-experience rapidly became severely disorganized. In a few days she was admitted to a hospital with a diagnosis of acute schizophrenia. Four months of hospitalization and phenothiazine drugs were required to bring her psychotic state under control.

It has become common practice for psychiatrists to assert that individuals who suffer prolonged psychotic reactions following low doses of amphetamine, cannabis, or LSD-like drugs were "already schizophrenic" or "latent schizophrenics." This judgment is always made retrospectively and involves some assumptions about schizophrenia which are unproven, including the idea that the preschizophrenic state can be characterized and recognized. The implication in these instances that the drugs play a relatively unimportant role in the emergence and perpetuation of psychotic symptoms may be unwarranted.

Several interesting clinical interactions of amphetamine with schizophrenia add to the puzzles as to underlying mediating systems that might be common to drugs and naturally occurring syndromes. There are some instances of amphetamine psychoses which persist and can be explained very much as persisting hallucinosis as explained in alcoholism, i.e., the evocation of or unmasking of some prior psychotic disorder or symptom.[11] When amphetamine was given to catatonic schizophrenics, they showed a "paradoxical" reaction of drowsiness and unresponsiveness (also seen in delirium tremens), whereas amytal "awoke" the catatonic patients and seemed to relax them sufficiently to relate with some degree of normalcy for a brief period.[37] When methylphenidate was given to persons recovering from acute schizophrenic episodes, the schizophrenic behavior was observed to recur, but when sufficient time for remission had taken place, the methylphenidate no longer evoked schizophrenic symptomatology.[68] The utility of these various cross comparisons probably lies in the spur they give to empirical research both at the clinical pharmacological and observational levels and in animal brain-behavior research: it is as if one is constantly narrowing down a focus upon the differentiating mechanisms.

Amphetaminelike drugs have recently been extensively used by the illicit drug community.[90] High doses are frequently administered orally or intravenously. In such a setting, brief psychotic reactions are common and often accompanied by dangerously aggressive behavior. Such amphetamine abuse can also be associated with consequences which are life-threatening to the user, including subarachnoid hemorrhage and the usual serious medical complications of intravenous drug abuse.[77]

Amphetaminelike compounds combined with other drugs are frequently employed as bronchodilators for the treatment of asthma and other upper respiratory syndromes.[70] Psychotic reactions have been reported following the use of such preparations, but so too has the phenomenon of alternating psychosis and asthma in a few individuals.

LSD-like Drugs

The discovery of d-lysergic acid diethylamide (LSD) by Hoffman gave the world its most potent known mind-altering substance. Quantities less than 1 mg. of this compound produce a syndrome which may resemble certain stages in the naturally-occurring psychoses. Other related compounds such as psilocybin and dimethyltryptamine produce similar acute behavioral responses. This reaction is characterized by dramatic visual illusions and by a unique destructuring of the usual psychic defenses. Giarman and Freedman's description aptly characterizes this altered state of consciousness:[52]

> Psychotomimetic drugs such as d-lysergic acid diethylamide . . . reliably and consistently produce periods of altered perception and experience without clouded consciousness or marked physiological changes; mental processes that are usually dormant and transient during wakefulness become "locked" into a persistent state. The usual boundaries which structure thought and perception become fluid; awareness becomes vivid while control over input is markedly diminished; customary inputs and modes of thought and perception become novel, illusory, and portentous; and with the loss of customary controlling anchors, dependence on the surroundings, on prior expectations, or on a mystique for structure and support is enhanced. Psychiatrists recognize these primary changes as a background state out of which a number of secondary psychological states can ensue, depending on motive, capacity and circumstance. This is reflected in the terminology that has grown around these drugs; if symptoms ensue, the term psychotomimetic or psychodysleptic is used; and if mystical experience, religious conversion, or a therapeutic change in behavior is stressed, the term psychedelic or mind "manifesting" has been applied.
>
> The drugs and clinical states set up a "search for synthesis," and the motives and capacities of subjects and patients to achieve this are obviously of importance if one is to assess outcomes and compare and contrast these states. [p. 2][52]

The following example of LSD-induced altered state of consciousness exemplifies the kind of experiential destructuring which may attend the use of this and similar compounds. This letter was written by a young college student during the ten hours of an LSD experience. He recovered completely at the end of this period and did not, in retrospect, regard this drug experience as a "bad trip."

> Hi again Marilyn. I think that you hurt me and I haven't had the honesty to admit it so there I have admitted it and you can be happy. . . . It is late and I'm getting very high with a gross and stupidly terrible idea. I must admit Marilyn, yes, that you are so much like my mother. It's like Mom when she used to punish me, she used to hit me and I think you will hit your children a lot like my mother. Yes, in your admonishing role you are

like my mother, with the same kind of disapproval of my behavior it's the same feeling that I used to get when my mother disapproved of my doing something that I get now when Marilyn says I'm irresponsible. It's the same feeling I mean that when I was young I had a kind of feeling of guilt, remorse, anger, and shame—all of the normal little child's feelings. I have the same kind of feeling now when Marilyn my mother admonishes and reprimands me for my irresponsibility and I fear that when she gives me the same feeling I used to get from my mother, then she couldn't be good for my children and my children are very important. . . . I think I have finally figured it out! I'm afraid that I am going to die. If I die and I am not a Christian I will go to hell. God, am I afraid to die! I might commit suicide. My papers are due—my papers are due. . . . Why am I so afraid to lose Marilyn. There is a sense in which my fear of going insane is linked with losing her. . . . I am only now very tired, a bit depressed about my papers and sorry about Marilyn so I am really alright. . . . At least I have enough sense to go to bed now. I fear being crazy and admitting it to myself because then I might commit suicide like my brother. I'm going to bed. If Bill goes to the University Health he might be right and if they found out that I'm crazy I might really be crazy and if I were crazy I might commit suicide. I'm afraid everything is closing in on me, troopers and everything. I'm so tired! I'm going to bed—good night Marilyn.

This excerpt is not presented as a typical LSD experience, but rather as an experiential account suggesting the manner in which this kind of altered consciousness may reactivate certain painful intrapsychic issues and heighten the experience of conflict at certain critical developmental periods. Such an interaction between drug-induced state and intrapsychic conflict and defense may be involved in many "bad trips" or extended psychotic states related to drug use. Bridger's ideas concerning the interaction of stress and psychotomimetic drug effect seem relevant in this context.[23,24] He notes that animal experiments suggest that psychotomimetic drugs facilitate the association of a conditioned and an unconditioned stimulus so long as the animal is still under the stress of a learning paradigm where an aversive unconditioned stimulus is being used. Bridger concludes that such drugs

facilitate the intrapsychic merging of symbol and the object symbolized.

We have noted that conflicts which are depicted in the phenomenology of psychotomimetic drug-induced states can be understood as genuine conflictual issues for the individual which were under control prior to the drug-induced state. The drug experience appeared to have breached an intrapsychic buffer zone between certain kinds of current experience and internal "symbols" of vulnerability, similar to the way an antigen–antibody response might be facilitated. A similar mechanism has been called "catathymic" and proposed by Faergeman as operative in "psychogenic psychoses". The ability of the individual to control, tolerate, or modulate this "anamnestic response" would be expected to vary, as it does in drug-induced states.

That stress or conflict occurring *during* a psychotomimetic episode can lead to further dyscontrol over the content, intensity, and quality of subjective experience has been noted by the adherents of the Peyote ceremonies, "lay pharmacologists" using these drugs, and medical scientists.[48] Blacker[14] speculated that avoidance of aversive stimuli, learned in the drug state (in which the least stressful adaptation is to cease vigilant reaction and "go with" the experience) may characterize some of the passivity and amotivational behavior of chronic drug users. The loss of perceptual constancies, of "barrier" functions from the banal to those regulating reality adaptations, has been noticed,[48] and the inability to ward off or put bounds around intrapsychic or external stimuli has been noted in the so-called "flashback" phenomenon.[88] The model of the traumatic neuroses in which repetitive noxious experience recurs after the mastery of ongoing stimuli was unexpectedly disrupted (or the "stimulus barrier" breached), and the need to synthesize the intensities of experience, has been noted as a possible mechanism in this inconstantly occurring after effect of LSD or mescaline. The phenomena occurs generally briefly, and not as the lay imagination conceives it, as a miniature "re-run" of hours of a particular LSD episode; thresholds for observations of minor alterations of states of consciousness are often enhanced—both by publicity and perhaps by the drug experience—and the interpretation of these effects can lead to panic and excessive focus upon subjective states. In any event, the experience and its mastery during the drug state possibly accounts for the variability of outcomes, and certainly defines the chief characteristics of these states in which the operations of variables such as expectation, group structuring and reinforcement, and individual experience and coping, are strikingly revealed as both crucial and variable. It is nevertheless noteworthy that animals can detect very low and behaviorally inapparent doses of these drugs and distinguish LSD from mescaline, for example.[25] Accordingly, the neural and chemical mechanisms evoking these perceptions are of some interest in understanding brain function and psychoticlike behaviors.

Initial comparisons of the LSD state with naturally occurring psychoses tended to conclude that the two were not related.[62] Later comparisons have shown that some psychotic reactions can be characterized by the "psychedelic" form of experience which may accompany the use of LSD-like drugs.[18] Cumulative-dose experiments performed with LSD-like compounds tend to produce tolerance[1,66,67] unlike the effects in amphetamine experiments (in which psychosis supervenes). Response to and resistance to noxious stimuli after several days of LSD has not been systematically examined in man. In animals on tolerance dosage schedules, such stimuli can enhance or disrupt certain performances and apparently do not show tolerance.[48] The LSD-precipitated psychotic reaction—an extended psychosis following LSD use—tends to be somewhat different from the amphetamine-induced psychoses. The former may be associated with more ecstatic elements and less routinely with psychotic suspiciousness. Drugs in these two classes also tend to produce different EEG effects in animals and these differences have led investigators to propose these drugs as prototypes of two distinct classes of psychotomimetic drugs.[103–105] Whether the effects of cumulative doses of amphetamine (or the immediate as well as

prolonged effects of acute doses of methamphetamine) are linked to persisting effects of intermediate metabolites of the drug is not precisely known.[6] The presence of LSD in the body can be roughly correlated with different phases in the drug response.[3] For example, it is apparent that four to eight hours after the acute LSD effects (which correspond to the half-life of the drug in plasma), suspiciousness and ideas of reference are characteristic when the acute "TV show in the head" is over.[48,87] It would be misleading to suggest, therefore, that the syndromes are distinctively different with the two drugs at the clinical level, as evident from the following example.

The patient was Nancy, a twenty-year-old female in her second year at college. She was basically rather easygoing but was particularly influenced by her father whom she described as a "man of principle," and who was frequently very critical of her. She took a summer trip alone and was given LSD by some travelers she met along the way. The psychosis which resulted was later described by Nancy during her recovery in the following manner:

I had spent the whole summer testing out life styles. So I decided to take a trip out west to see what I could learn from others. That's when I met this fellow Ray. I was fascinated by the life they lived—lots of drugs and sex. I felt this was the opening up of sex for me. You have to understand that this was a complete change in life style for me, a new world completely. Some parts were beautiful. I took several capsules of acid over the two-week period and began to see significance in things. They mentioned a dog and I thought I had become a dog sexually. Maybe, I thought, they were trying to teach me not to be up tight about sex. I began to have the notion that I would have a sex-change operation. Maybe I was a guy trapped in a woman's body. My mind was running like crazy. I thought I was adopted, maybe sterile or suffering from mental retardation. I saw a double rainbow and that made me believe there was hope. Noises were especially loud. Anything I ever had as a problem my mind dug up. Particularly problems with my father and with church. All the books I had ever read in my life seemed to come back to me. I thought I might have a terminal disease, be sterile or pregnant. So much was hitting my head at once. I often had a very strong urge to laugh. My body was supersensitive. I thought my bed would separate and that I would be torn in half, that the top half of me belonged to the devil and I would pay for what I had done. On my way to a hospital I noticed that everything behind me was being burned or destroyed. Again the idea of the atom bomb having been dropped came to me. I thought I would die and be reborn. In the hospital I thought one of the nurses was the devil. That meant I was split in quarters—half of me was a devil and half a woman. Also I was afraid to move for fear that something terrible would happen. I thought there was something registering my movements. I had an idea that I had to save the neighborhood. Sometimes I felt only capable of destruction, other times I thought I could save others.

Of particular significance in this kind of syndrome are the dynamic issues related to guilt and self-debasement. Such concerns have emerged repeatedly in cases we have seen and in reports of psychotic reactions related to LSD ingestion. In some ways the prolonged LSD-psychosis is similar, at least at the level of clinical analysis, to psychotic depression. Conflictual issues of guilt and shame seem uniquely heightened and thrust into awareness by these drugs. Long-term ingestion of LSD-like compounds may result in amotivational states which can be ego-syntonic and associated with atypical belief systems or delusional ideas.[53]

Although the actual mechanism of action of LSD-like drugs is unknown, a remarkably reliable property of psychoactive drugs in this class is their biochemical and physiological effect upon 5-hydroxytryptamine-containing neurons.[2] There is tentative evidence that psychotic reactions following LSD may be associated with decreased formation of 5-hydroxyindoleacetic acid, a metabolite of 5-hydroxytryptamine, in cerebrospinal fluid,[16] a finding consistent with the neurochemical effect of acute administration of LSD-like drugs to animals.[*]

Cannabis

Although there has been some controversy concerning the psychotogenic potential of cannabis-containing compounds, the question, apparently, is primarily one of dose. In countries where strong cannabis preparations are available, psychotic reactions are not uncommon.[†] Although the basic pharmacology is somewhat different, the spectrum of psychotic reactions to cannabis compounds is quite similar to that seen in LSD-related psychoses. Under experimental conditions with human subjects, Jones[69] has shown that higher doses of cannabis produce effects indistinguishable from LSD on many behavioral scales. An unusual study[99] documents the strikingly increased incidence of quasi-schizophrenic psychoses in a group of American servicemen during a period when hashish usage was extensive. With high doses of the active ingredient, Δ9-THC (delta-9-tetrahydrocannabinol) a number of LSD-like psychotomimetic effects occur, but the dysphoric episode is generally terminated by drowsiness—unlike LSD effects.[63] Experienced users are aware of paranoidlike responses after unexpectedly high doses, i.e., a hypervigilance and ideas of reference. There are many features and factors in psychotic reactions to cannabis which require differentiation in future research. These include the role of prior state. Most studies, such as the report of Mayor LaGuardia's Committee on Marihuana in 1944, indicate a small incidence of paranoid reactions although a general harmlessness of the experience for most individuals. Paranoid reactions have been ascribed to the use of prepsychotic or vulnerable subjects. The role of active metabolites in any persisting effects and the role of factors in both cumulative effects of moderately small, frequent dosages and of high dosage of the more potent hashish require further attention and clarification.

L-Dopa

Psychotic reactions following L-Dopa therapy for Parkinsonism occur in a substantial portion of treated patients.[26,27,32,55] Perhaps because this population is an older one and often uses anticholinergic drugs in addition to

[*] See references 47, 50, and 86.

[†] See references 58, 71, 73, 81, 94, 97, and 106.

L-Dopa, a significant number of these reactions are associated with some of the symptoms of delirium. Although actual reports are rare according to Snyder,[91] apparently L-Dopa can induce psychotic symptoms in a clear sensorium in some cases. L-Dopa can induce a manic reaction or exacerbate psychotic symptoms in individuals who have a prior history of manic and schizophrenic behavior. Celesia and Barr[26] emphasize that patients with postencephalitic Parkinsonism appear most susceptible to the spectrum of psychoses induced by L-Dopa. The role of "prior state" (perhaps prior imbalances in neurohumoral storage and release involving receptors and systems reacting to acetylcholine, catecholamines, and indoleamines) recurs as an explanatory factor in individual response. Celesia and Barr describe the unique characteristics of central L-Dopa intoxication; namely, psychosis and various dyskinetic symptoms, particularly facial and lingual dyskinesias. When LSD was given forty-eight hours following reserpine pretreatment, oculogyric crises and dystonia were observed.[50] Interestingly, such dyskinetic and extrapyramidal syndromes have not been a prominent aspect to the amphetamine psychoses, although stimulation of dopamine receptors is thought to play a major role in the mediation of several components of the amphetamine psychoses. Preexisting receptor sensitivity may be a differentiating factor in the clinical manifestations of dopaminergic stimulation.

Drugs Used in the Treatment of Psychological Depression

The monoamine oxidase inhibitors and tricyclic antidepressants, compounds effective in the treatment of certain depressive syndromes, may be associated with acute psychotic reactions even when employed at the usual therapeutic doses,[9] as illustrated by the following case.

EXAMPLE. A 28-year-old man, depressed and seclusive for months, was treated with a monoamine oxidase inhibitor. After two weeks he became more verbal and less depressed. However, he soon began to be hyperactive, agitated, and grandiose as exemplified in the following excerpt from a letter he wrote at that time to a woman whom he had known only a few days and who had been frightened by his intensity:

Dear Jane: I know the reason you have run away from everyone and from me, the man you said you would share everything openly with, who believed in you and who trusted you to keep your word, not to be childish or afraid, is because you had a difficult menstrual period for a week and a very upsetting one which both of us can't take. I pray desperately every night that you will phone me or come back to me for help. Do you think everything we ever said and did together meant *nothing* [his emphasis] or was *false* or *sinful?* Dear God in Heaven, give me strength to face this crisis. If Jane has sinned please let me take her sins as mine so that she may come to me or heaven, serene and unmolested. If Jane or any other girl I've known should need blood or eyes or even a heart, let them be compatible with mine that I may give my organs freely to them, though my worthless, homely self dies. Amen. . . . I started excellent dancing lessons and want you to come. I brought you a six hundred dollar wedding night ceremony present, about a thousand dollars of clothes and apartment furnishings, and I've dusted my hope chest off to share with you alone.

This manialike state with elements of elation and depression subsided over several days following the withdrawal of the drug. Elation or psychotic suspiciousness may be observed in the course of tricyclic antidepressant drug treatment and tends to subside rapidly following drug withdrawal and antipsychotic drug therapy. In such cases one assumes that there is some innate proclivity to psychotic or manic states. These drugs have been shown to exacerbate psychotic symptoms in individuals who have been diagnosed as schizophrenic. Tricyclic compounds, as noted above, also possess significant anticholinergic activity and may be associated with delirium. The clinical distinction between a primary manic or psychotic state versus delirium with psychosis during tricyclic therapy may be difficult, but can usually be made by noting the presence or absence of significant disorientation. It is sometimes possible to achieve useful antidepressant results without the recurrence of delirium by a reduction in dosage.

❲ Treatment

The most important step in the treatment of drug-related psychotic episodes is proper diagnosis and removal of the offending drug when possible. With potent pharmacological substances so readily available, a drug-induced reaction should be part of the differential diagnosis of any acute psychotic syndrome.[98] The role of careful history, of "mismatches" between factors such as current stress and prior adjustment and the current mental status, the presence of amnesia or delirioid features may occasionally help in this, although there are few clear-cut pathognomonic features. Conservative management is always indicated where diagnosis is in doubt. The classical principles involved in the treatment of drug-induced delirium apply here: protection of the individual, general nursing care, and a supportive, simplified environment. Unless a pharmacological addition to therapy is clearly indicated, it is wise to avoid compounding the trouble with yet another drug. Where hyperactive behavior is a problem, acute sedation with barbiturates may be as useful as phenothiazine administration. The important role of setting and psychological support for the treatment of psychotic drug reactions has recently been reemphasized. (It is a curious observation that psychotic reactions clearly related to drug use rarely evoke the same sympathy or therapeutic zeal in treatment personnel as do other psychotic states.) If the psychotic reaction is brief and essentially terminated within twenty-four hours one may be justified in providing acute treatment only. However, if the reaction is prolonged or uniquely disturbing to the individual, responsible treatment should include several follow-up visits to determine whether characteristic defensive forces have been redeployed and to evaluate current life stresses the individual is facing which may have con-

tributed to the dysphoric reaction. Where drug use initiates a psychotic process which seems to gain momentum and continue beyond the known duration of drug action, psychiatric hospitalization may be necessary. Flashbacks or related recurrent phenomena present interesting treatment problems in their own right. In general the therapeutic approach involves an avoidance of undue attention to the phenomena themselves and a focus upon attendant life tasks which are being avoided. Sedative antianxiety drugs or low doses of phenothiazines may be of some benefit as in other nonpsychotic conditions where symptom relief facilitates psychological work.

❲ Bibliography

1. ABRAMSON, H. A. in H. A. Abramson, ed., *Conference on Neuropharmacology*, Trans. 3rd Conf., p. 268. New York: Josiah Macy, Jr., Foundation, 1957.

2. AGHAJANIAN, G. "Influence of Drugs on the Firing of Serotonin-Containing Neurons in Brain," *Fed. Proc.*, 31 (1972), 91–96.

3. AGHAJANIAN, G. and O. BING. "Persistence of Lysergic Acid Diethylamide in the Plasma of Human Subjects," *Clin. Pharmacol. Ther.*, 5 (1964), 611–614.

4. ANDERSON, E. "Propylhexedrine (Benzedrex) Psychosis," *N.Z. Med. J.*, 71 (1970), 302.

5. ANGRIST, A. and S. GERSHON. "The Phenomenology of Experimentally Induced Amphetamine Psychosis-Preliminary Observations," *Biol. Psychiatry*, 2 (1970), 95–107.

6. ANGRIST, B., J. SCHWEITZER, A. FRIEDHOFF et al. "The Clinical Symptomatology of Amphetamine Psychosis and Its Relationship to Amphetamine Levels in Urine," *Int. Pharmacopsychiatry*, 2 (1969), 125–139.

7. ANGRIST, B., J. SCHWEITZER, S. GERSHON et al. "Mephentermine Psychosis: Misuse of the Wyamine Inhaler," *Am. J. Psychiatry*, 126 (1970), 1315–1317.

8. ANGRIST, B., B. SHOPSIN, and S. GERSHON. "Comparative Psychotomimetic Effects of Stereoisomers of Amphetamine," *Nature*, 234 (1971), 152–153.

9. BALDESSARINI, R. and R. WILLMUTH. "Psychotic Reactions During Amitriptyline

Therapy," *Can. Psychiatr. Assoc. J.*, 13 (1968), 571–573.

10. BASS, M. "Sudden Sniffing Death," *JAMA*, 212 (1970), 2075–2079.

11. BELL, D. "A Comparison of Amphetamine Psychosis and Schizophrenia," *Br. J. Psychiatry*, 3 (1965), 701–706.

12. ———. "The Experimental Reproduction of Amphetamine Psychosis," *Arch. Gen. Psychiatry*, 29 (1973), 35–45.

13. BETHELL, M. "Toxic Psychosis Caused by Radioactive Iodine," *Br. J. Psychiatry*, 117 (1970), 473–479.

14. BLACKER, K., R. JONES, G. STONE et al. "Chronic Users of LSD: The 'Acidheads'," *Am. J. Psychiatry*, 125 (1968), 341–351.

15. BLATHERWICK, C. "Understanding Glue Sniffing," *Can. J. Public Health*, 63 (1972), 272–276.

16. BOWERS, M. "Acute Psychosis Induced by Psychotomimetic Drug Abuse," *Arch. Gen. Psychiatry*, 27 (1972), 437–442.

17. BOWERS, M., A. CHIPMAN, A. SCHWARTZ et al. "Dynamics of Psychedelic Drug Abuse," *Arch. Gen. Psychiatry*, 16 (1967), 560–565.

18. BOWERS, M. and D. FREEDMAN. " 'Psychedelic' Experiences in Acute Psychoses," *Arch. Gen. Psychiatry*, 15 (1966), 240–248.

19. BOWERS, M., E. GOODMAN, and V. SIM. "Some Behavioral Changes in Man Following Anticholinesterase Administration," *J. Nerv. Ment. Dis.*, 138 (1964), 383–389.

20. BOWERS, M. and D. SINGER. "Thyrotoxicosis and Psychological State," *Psychosomatics*, 5 (1964), 322–324.

21. BRACELAND, F. "Mental Symptoms following Carbon Disulphide Absorption and Intoxication," *Ann. Intern. Med.*, 16 (1942), 246–261.

22. BRAWLEY, P. and J. DUFFIELD. "The Pharmacology of Hallucinogens," *Pharmacol. Rev.*, 24 (1972), 31–66.

23. BRIDGER, W. "Psychotomimetic Drugs, Animal Behavior, and Human Psychopathology," in J. O. Cole, A. M. Freedman, and A. Friedhoff, eds., *Psychopathology and Psychopharmacology*, pp. 133–142. Baltimore: The Johns Hopkins University Press, 1973.

24. BRIDGER, W. and I. MANDEL. "Excitatory and Inhibitory Effects of Mescaline on Shuttle Avoidance in the Rat," *Biol. Psychiatry*, 3 (1971), 379–385.

25. CAMERON, O. "Stimulus Properties of Drugs: LSD as S^D and UCS," Dissertation, University of Chicago, August 1972.

26. CELESIA, G. and A. BARR. "Psychosis and Other Psychiatric Manifestations of Levodopa Therapy," *Arch. Neurol.*, 23 (1970), 193–200.

27. CELESIA, G. and W. WANAMAKER. "Psychiatric Disturbances in Parkinson's Disease," *Dis. Nerv. Sys.*, 33 (1972), 577–583.

28. CLARK, L., W. BAUER, and S. COBB. "Preliminary Observations on Mental Disturbances Occurring in Patients Under Therapy with Cortisone and ACTH," *N. Engl. J. Med.*, 246 (1952), 205–216.

29. CONNELL, P. *Amphetamine Psychosis.* Maudsley Monogr. no. 5, p. 5. London: Oxford University Press, 1958.

30. CROWELL, E. and J. KETCHUM. "The Treatment of Scopolamine-Induced Delirium with Physostigmine," *Clin. Pharmacol. Ther.*, 8 (1967), 409–414.

31. DALY, R., F. KANE, and J. EWING. "Psychosis Associated with the Use of a Sequential Oral Contraceptive," *Lancet*, 2 (1967), 444–445.

32. DAMÁSIO, A., J. LOBO-ANTUNES, and C. MACEDO. "Psychiatric Aspects in Parkinsonism Treated with L-Dopa," *J. Neurol. Neurosurg., Psychiatry*, 34 (1971), 502–507.

33. DOMINO, E. F. "Neurobiology of Phencyclidine (Sernyl), a Drug with an Unusual Spectrum of Pharmacological Activity," *Int. Rev. Neurobiol.*, 6 (1964), 303–347.

34. DOMINO, E. F. and E. LUBY. "Abnormal Mental States Induced by Phencyclidine as a Model of Schizophrenia," in J. O. Cole, A. M. Freedman, and A. Friedhoff, eds., *Psychopathology and Psychopharmacology*, pp. 37–50. Baltimore: The Johns Hopkins University Press, 1973.

35. DUVOISIN, R. and R. KATZ. "Reversal of Central Anticholinergic Syndrome in Man by Physostigmine," *JAMA*, 206 (1968), 1963–1965.

36. EDISON, G. "Hallucinations Associated with Pentazocine," *N. Engl. J. Med.*, 281 (1969), 447–448.

37. ELKES, J. "Effects of Psychotomimetic Drugs in Animals and Man," in H. A. Abramson, ed., *Conference on Neuropharmacology*, Trans. 3rd. Conf., pp. 205–295. New York: Josiah Macy, Jr., Foundation, 1957.

38. ELLINWOOD, E. "Amphetamine Psychosis 1: Description of the Individuals and Process," *J. Nerv. Ment. Dis.*, 44 (1967), 273–280.

39. ————. "Effect of Chronic Methamphetamine Intoxication in Rhesus Monkeys," *Biol. Psychiatry*, 3 (1971), 25–32.

40. ————. "Assault and Homicide Associated with Amphetamine Abuse," *Am. J. Psychiatry*, 127 (1971), 1170–1175.

41. ELLINWOOD, E. and O. ESCALANTE. "Behavior and Histopathological Findings During Chronic Methedrine Intoxication," *Biol. Psychiatry*, 2 (1970), 27–39.

42. ELLINWOOD, E., A. SUDILOVSKY, and L. NELSON. "Behavioral Analysis of Chronic Amphetamine Intoxication," *Biol. Psychiatry*, 4 (1972), 215–230.

43. ERIKSSEN, J. "Atropine Psychosis," *Lancet*, 1 (1969), 53–54.

44. ESCALANTE, O. and E. ELLINWOOD. "Central Nervous System Cytopathological Changes in Cats with Chronic Methedrine Intoxication," *Brain Res.*, 21 (1970), 151–155.

45. FLOWERS, N. and L. HORAN. "The Electrical Sequelae of Aerosol Inhalation," *Am. Heart J.*, 83 (1972), 644–651.

46. ————. "Nonanoxic Aerosol Arrhythmias," *JAMA*, 219 (1972), 33–37.

47. FREEDMAN, D. "Studies of LSD-25 and Serotonin in the Brain," *Proc. 3rd World Congr. Psychiatry*, 1 (1961), 653–658.

48. ————. "On the Use and Abuse of LSD," *Arch. Gen. Psychiatry*, 18 (1968), 330–347.

49. FREEDMAN, D. and N. GIARMAN. "Brain Amines, Electrical Activity, and Behavior," in G. H. Glaser, ed., *EEG and Behavior*, pp. 198–243. New York: Basic Books, 1963.

50. FREEDMAN, D., R. GOTTLIEB, and R. LOVELL. "Psychotomimetic Drugs and Brain 5-Hydroxytryptamine Metabolism," *Biochem. Pharmacol.*, 19 (1970), 1181–1188.

51. GERSHON, S. and B. ANGRIST. "Drug-Induced Psychoses," *Hosp. Practice*, 2 (1967), 36–39, 50–53.

52. GIARMAN, N. and D. FREEDMAN. "Biochemical Aspects of the Actions of Psychotomimetic Drugs," *Pharmacol. Rev.*, 17 (1965), 1–25.

53. GLASS, G. and M. BOWERS. "Chronic Psychosis Associated with Long-Term Psychotomimetic Drug Abuse," *Arch. Gen. Psychiatry*, 23 (1970), 97–103.

54. GONZALES, E. and J. DOWNEY. "Polyneuropathy in a Glue Sniffer," *Arch. Phys. Med. Rehabil.*, 53 (1972), 333–337.

55. GOODWIN, F. "Psychiatric Side Effects of Levodopa in Man," *JAMA*, 218 (1971), 1915–1920.

56. GORDY, S. and M. TRUMPER. "Carbon Disulfide Poisoning with a Report of Six Cases," *JAMA*, 110 (1938), 1543–1549.

57. GRIFFITH, J., J. CAVANAUGH, J. HELD et al. "Dexroamphetamine-Evaluation of Psychotomimetic Properties in Man," *Arch. Gen. Psychiatry*, 26 (1972), 97–100.

58. GROSSMAN, W. "Adverse Reactions Associated with Cannabis Products in India," *Ann. Intern. Med.*, 70 (1969), 529–533.

59. HEDLEY, A. and P. BEWSHER. "Psychosis and Antithyroid Drug Therapy," *Br. Med. J.*, 3 (1969), 596–597.

60. HOCH, P., J. CATTELL, and H. PENNES. "Effects of Mescaline and LSD," *Am. J. Psychiatry*, 108 (1952), 579–584.

61. HOFF, E. "Brain Syndromes Associated with Drug or Poison Intoxication," in A. Freedman and H. Kaplan, eds., *Comprehensive Textbook of Psychiatry*, pp. 759–775. Baltimore: Williams & Wilkins, 1967.

62. HOLLISTER, L. *Chemical Psychosis*. Springfield, Ill.: Charles C. Thomas, 1968.

63. HOLLISTER, L., R. RICHARDS, and H. GILLESPIE. "Comparison of Tetrahydrocannabinol and Synhexyl in Man," *Clin. Pharmacol. Ther.*, 9 (1969), 783–791.

64. HORN, A. and S. SNYDER. "Chlorpromazine and Dopamine: Conformational Similarities that Correlate with the Antischizophrenic Activity of Phenothiazine Drugs," *Proc. Natl. Acad. Sci. USA*, 68 (1971), 2325–2328.

65. HUSSAIN, M. and J. MURPHY. "Psychosis Induced by Oral Contraception," *Can. Med. Assoc. J.*, 104 (1971), 984–986.

66. ISBELL, H., R. E. BELLEVILLE, and H. F. FRASER. "Studies on Lysergic Acid Diethylamide (LSD-25)," *Arch. Neurol. Psychiatry*, 76 (1956), 468–478.

67. ISBELL, H., A. B. WOLBACH, A. WINKLER et al. "Cross Tolerance Between LSD and Psilocybin," *Psychopharmacologia*, 2 (1961), 147–159.

68. JANOWSKY, D., M. EL-YOUSEF, J. DAVIS et al. "Provocation of Schizophrenic Symptoms by Intravenous Methylphenidate," *Arch. Gen. Psychiatry*, 28 (1973), 185–193.

69. JONES, R. "Drug Models of Schizophrenia—Cannabis," in J. O. Cole, A. M. Freedman, and A. Friedhoff, eds., *Psychopathology and Psychopharmacology*, pp. 71–86. Baltimore: The Johns Hopkins University Press, 1973.

70. KANE, F. and R. FLORENZANO. "Psychosis Accompanying Use of Bronchodilator Compound," *JAMA*, 215 (1971), 2116.

71. KEUP, W. "Psychotic Symptoms Due to Cannabis Abuse," *Dis. Nerv. Syst.*, 31 (1970), 119–126.

72. KIMURA, E., D. EBERT, and P. DODGE. "Acute Toxicity and Limits of Solvent Residue for Sixteen Organic Solvents," *Toxicol. Appl. Pharmacol.*, 19 (1971), 699–704.

73. KLEE, G. "Marihuana Psychosis—a Case Study," *Psychiatr. Q.*, 43 (1969), 719–733.

74. LEVIN, M. "Transitory Schizophrenias Produced by Bromide Intoxication," *Am. J. Psychiatry*, 103 (1946), 229–237.

75. ———. "Bromide Psychosis: Four Varieties," *Am. J. Psychiatry*, 104 (1948), 798–800.

76. LIDDEN, S. and R. SATRAN. "Disulfiram (Antabuse) Psychosis," *Am. J. Psychiatry*, 123 (1967), 1284–1289.

77. LOURIA, D., T. HENSLE, and J. ROSE. "The Major Medical Complications of Heroin Addiction," *Ann. Intern. Med.*, 76 (1967), 1–22.

78. LUBY, E., B. COHEN, G. ROSENBAUM et al. "Study of a New Schizophrenomimetic Drug-Sernyl," *Arch. Neurol. Psychiatry*, 81 (1959), 113–119.

79. MEYER, J., F. GREIFENSTEIN, and M. DE-VAULT. "A New Drug Causing Symptoms of Sensory Deprivation," *J. Nerv. Ment. Dis.*, 129 (1959), 54–61.

80. NEWELL, H. and T. LIDZ. "The Toxicity of Atabrine to the Central Nervous System," *Am. J. Psychiatry*, 102 (1946), 805–818.

81. PERNA, D. "Psychotogenic Effect of Marihuana," *JAMA*, 209 (1969), 1085–1086.

82. QUARTON, G., L. CLARK, S. COBB et al. "Mental Disturbances Associated with ACTH and Cortisone," *Medicine* (Baltimore), 34 (1955), 13–50.

83. REDLICH, F. and D. FREEDMAN. *The Theory and Practice of Psychiatry*, p. 741. New York: Basic Books, 1966.

84. REICH, P. and R. HEPPS. "Homicide During a Psychosis Induced by LSD," *JAMA*, 219 (1972), 869–871.

85. ROME, H. and F. BRACELAND. "Psychological Responses to Corticotropin, Cortisone, and Related Steroid Substances," *JAMA*, 148 (1952), 27–30.

86. ROSECRANS, J., R. LOVELL, and D. FREEDMAN. "Effects of Lysergic Acid Diethylamide on the Metabolism of Brain 5-Hydroxytryptamine," *Biochem. Pharmacol.*, 16 (1967), 2011–2021.

87. SALVATORE, S. and R. HYDE. "Progression of Effects of LSD," *Arch. Neurol. Psychiatry*, 76 (1956), 50–59.

88. SHICK, J. and D. SMITH. "Analysis of the LSD Flashback," *J. Psychedel. Drugs*, 3 (1970), 13–19.

89. SHILLIRO, F., C. DRINKER, and T. SHAUGHNESSY. "The Problem of Nervous and Mental Sequelae in Carbon Monoxide Poisoning," *JAMA*, 106 (1936), 669–674.

90. SMITH, D. "An Analysis of 310 Cases of Acute High-Dose Methamphetamine Toxicity in Haight-Ashbury," *Clin. Toxicity*, 3 (1970), 117–124.

91. SNYDER, S. "Catecholamines in the Brain as Mediators of Amphetamine Psychosis," *Arch. Gen. Psychiatry*, 27 (1972), 169–179.

92. SNYDER, S., K. TAYLOR, J. COYLE et al. "The Role of Brain Dopamine in Behavioral Regulation and the Actions of Psychotropic Drugs," *Am. J. Psychiatry*, 127 (1970), 199–207.

93. SOSKIS, D. and M. BOWERS. "The Schizophrenic Experience—A Follow Up Study of Attitude and Posthospital Adjustment," *J. Nerv. Ment. Dis.*, 149 (1969), 443–449.

94. SPENCER, D. "Cannabis Induced Psychosis," *Br. J. Addict.*, 65 (1970), 369–372.

95. SPENSLEY, J. and D. RICKWELL. "Psychosis during Methylphenidate Abuse," *N. Engl. J. Med.*, 286 (1972), 880–881.

96. STOCKINGS, G. "A Clinical Study of the Mescaline Psychosis, with Special Reference to the Mechanism of the Genesis of Schizophrenic and Other Psychotic States," *J. Ment. Sci.*, 86 (1940), 29–47.

97. TALBOTT, J. and J. TEAGUE. "Marihuana Psychosis," *JAMA*, 210 (1969), 299–302.

98. TAYLOR, R., J. MAURER, and J. TINKLENBERG. "Management of 'Bad Trips' in an Evolving Drug Scene," *JAMA*, 213 (1970), 421–425.

99. TENNANT, F. and C. GROESBECK. "Psychiatric Effects of Hashish," *Arch. Gen. Psychiatry*, 27 (1972), 133–136.

100. THOMAS, D. and D. FREEDMAN. "Treatment of the Alcohol Withdrawal Syndrome," *JAMA*, 188 (1964), 316–318.

101. ULLMAN, K. and R. GROH. "Identification and Treatment of Acute Psychotic States Secondary to the Usage of Over-the-Counter Sleeping Preparations," *Am. J. Psychiatry*, 128 (1972), 1244–1248.

102. VICTOR, M. and R. ADAMS. "The Effect of Alcohol on the Nervous System," *Assoc. Res. Nerv. Ment. Dis. Proc.*, 32 (1953), 526–573.

103. WALLACH, M., B. ANGRIST, and S. GERSHON. "The Comparison of the Stereotyped Behavior-Inducing Effects of d- and l-Amphetamine in Dogs," *Comm. Behav. Biol.*, 6 (1971), 93–96.

104. WALLACH, M., E. FRIEDMAN, and S. GERSHON. "2,5-Dimethoxy-4-Methylamphetamine (DOM), a Neuropharmacological Examination," *J. Pharmacol. Exp. Ther.*, 182 (1972), 145–154.

105. WALLACH, M. and S. GERSHON. "A Neuropsychopharmacological Comparison of D-Amphetamine, L-Dopa, and Cocaine," *Neuropharmacology*, 10 (1971), 743–752.

106. WEIL, A. "Adverse Reactions to Marihuana," *N. Engl. J. Med.*, 282 (1970), 997–1000.

107. WEIL-MALHERBE, H. and S. SZARA. *The Biochemistry of Functional and Experimental Psychoses*. Springfield, Ill.: Charles C. Thomas, 1971.

108. WEINSTEIN, M. and A. FISCHER. "Benztropine Toxicity and Atropine Psychosis," *JAMA*, 220 (1972), 1616–1617.

109. YOST, M. and F. McKEGNEY. "Organic Psychosis Due to Talwin (Pentazocine)," *Conn. Med.*, 34 (1970), 259–260.

110. YOUNG, D. and W. SCOVILLE. "Paranoid Psychosis in Narcolepsy and the Possible Dangers of Benzedrine Treatment," *Med. Clin. North Am.*, 22 (1938), 637–646.

CHAPTER 15

ALCOHOLISM: A BIOBEHAVIORAL DISORDER*

Nancy K. Mello and Jack H. Mendelson

❪ Introduction

THIS CHAPTER presents an overview of our current state of knowledge concerning the actions of alcohol, the disease of alcoholism, and patterns of use and abuse in contemporary American society. The basic pharmacology of alcohol effects is reviewed, and the medical, psychological, and social consequences of prolonged alcohol abuse and alcoholism are described. Comparisons are made between alcohol addiction and drug addiction wherever possible. The limitations in our current understanding of the factors which influence the development and main-

tenance of alcohol abuse and alcoholism are discussed, and the potential efficacy of existing treatment approaches is evaluated. We conclude that significant progress in combating alcohol abuse requires clarification of the basic mechanisms of the addictive process to permit development of effective therapies as well as productive straegies for prevention.

Alcohol: Beverage and Drug

All beverage alcohols, wine, beer and distilled spirits, contain the same primary ingredient, ethyl alcohol or ethanol. Ethanol is a relatively simple organic molecule which is produced in abundance by the fermentation processes of microorganisms. Virtually all unicellular organisms have the capacity to produce ethanol given the availability of sugar,

* Portions of this chapter are taken from an administrative report on Alcohol Use and Alcoholism prepared for the Special Action Office for Drug Abuse Prevention of the Executive Office of the President by the senior author.

water, yeast, oxygen, warmth, and an appropriate acid–base balance. These basic ingredients have been present on earth since paleozoic times.

Beverage alcohols differ primarily in ethanol concentration which usually ranges from less than 4 percent for beer, to over 12 percent for wine, to 40–50 percent for distilled spirits. Under ordinary biological conditions, microorganisms do not produce alcohol concentrations in excess of 12–14 percent. However, man's discovery of distillation processes has permitted production of beverage alcohols with a higher concentration of ethanol. Alcohol boils at a lower temperature than water and therefore can be separated from its vehicle and concentrated. The term brandy derives from a German term for burnt distilled wine.[191]

Beverage alcohols also differ in terms of congener content or nonethanol impurities which include vitamins, organic and amino acids, minerals, salts, sugars, etc., as well as low concentrations of the higher alcohols (known as fusel oils) which are relatively toxic.[82] The nonnutritional congener content of distilled spirits is higher than that of wine or beer and has been shown to increase as a function of aging.[86]

It is well known that the rate of alcohol absorption into the blood varies markedly between beer, wine, and distilled spirits.[52,88] [129,130] Some congeners also affect the rate of alcohol absorption.[81] Generally, the higher the alcohol concentration, the more rapid its absorption, whereas the higher the congener concentration, the slower its absorption.

The nutrient value of alcohol is negligible following distillation. The caloric content of beverage alcohols varies between 100 and 200 calories per ounce. However, the extent to which calories in alcohol are equivalent to calories derived from food remains a subject of controversy. Alcoholics tend to eat poorly while they are drinking and it has often been suggested that this is due to the high caloric yield from alcohol. However, it has recently been observed that alcohol addicts receiving a daily total combined caloric intake from food (about 2000 calories) and alcohol averaging

4000 to 5000 calories did not gain weight over a two-month period.[108] The small effective contribution of calories from alcohol to the total caloric pool may reflect the fact that utilization of calories from vitamin-deficient sources such as alcohol is impaired when food intake is adequate.

Alcohol Use in Historical Perspective

Alcohol was first discovered perhaps 200 million years ago and relics of the earliest civilizations show that alcohol was used in religious ceremonies, medical treatment, and in many aspects of daily life. It has been speculated that paleolithic man learned to ferment honey and that the development of agriculture was paralleled by the improvement of techniques for fermentation of fruits and grains, culminating in the process of distillation during the first century A.D.[36,144] The legendary origins of alcohol are intermixed with the religious beliefs of many cultures, and it was commonly considered to be a gift of the Gods. In ancient Egypt and Greece, Osiris and Dionysos were worshipped as the givers of wine. It was believed that the Gods could use this gift to cause madness or enhance pleasure and awareness in the drinker.[191] Later, alcohol itself was imbued with an autonomous power and a trace of animistic thinking about alcohol still persists.

Although festival drunkenness was condoned, the secular use of alcohol was accompanied by many warnings against excessive drinking throughout history. One of the oldest temperance tracts, entitled The Wisdom of Ani, was written in Egypt about 3000 years ago.[144] Denunciation of excessive drinking can be found throughout ancient writings of Greece, Rome, India, Japan, and China as well as in the Old and New Testaments.[23]

The early temperance movement of the 1830s recommended abstinence only from distilled spirits.[51] Subsequently, there developed an increasing opposition to all alcoholic beverages, which were finally banned by the eighteenth amendment in 1920. National prohibition was repealed in 1933 by the twenty-first amendment in response to a complex series of attitude changes about self-regulation of drinking and the dangers of bootlegging. Legal sanctions* proved ineffective in controlling alcohol abuse and in modifying the fact that many people like to drink. In contemporary American society, most adults consume some alcoholic beverages, and, apparently, most do so in a responsible and healthy way.[8]

Medical Use of Alcohol

There is no current medical use of alcohol. Before the introduction of anesthesia, alcohol was used during surgical procedures in an effort to alleviate pain. However, since the dosage of alcohol required to produce loss of consciousness is close to a lethal dose for normal drinkers, alcohol is impractical as an anesthetic agent.

During the early part of the century, alcohol was occasionally used to counteract the alcohol-withdrawal syndrome. Although alcohol did reduce tremor briefly, its duration of action was too short to be practical. Moreover, prolonged use of alcohol merely reinstated the condition of chronic intoxication which leads to withdrawal symptoms following alcohol termination.

Until recently, alcohol was the drug of choice for the treatment of familial action tremor.[182] This condition is now treated with propranolol (a beta-adrenergic blocking agent used in the clinical management of cardiac arrhythmias).[181] The efficacy of both alcohol and propranolol in reducing symptoms of familial action tremor suggests that both may have a common receptor site in the central nervous system (CNS).

Current Patterns of Alcohol Use and Abuse

According to a recent survey of American drinking practices, an estimated two thirds of all adults use alcohol occasionally.[8] Total abstinence accounted for 32 percent of the 2746

representative persons surveyed. There were considerable regional variations in beverage preference and in the usual amount of alcohol consumed.[23]

Of the alcohol users studied, 12 percent were categorized as "heavy" drinkers; i.e., persons who drank almost daily or once a week and often consumed five or more drinks per occasion.[8] There are several problems associated with a compilation of a meaningful volume-frequency index of alcohol consumption.[8,79] Although people may drink comparable total quantities of alcohol over a particular time interval, the extent to which they space drinking or concentrate drinking within a brief period may reflect distinctly different drinking patterns. In contrast to the "heavy" drinker, an alcohol addict may drink between 24 to 32 oz. per day in increments of 2 or 3 oz. per occasion.[103,124] The length of a drinking spree may vary from a few days to two weeks or more.

A follow-up survey of American drinking practices revealed that there was considerable dynamic change in composition of the "heavy" drinking group and of moderate and infrequent drinking groups. During the three-year interval between two successive surveys, 15 percent of the sample had moved out of or into the heavy drinking group.[7] Even in the abstinent group, one third reported that they once used to drink. This high turnover rate is somewhat encouraging insofar as it indicates that heavy drinking does not invariably progress towards alcohol abuse or alcoholism.

Many interrelated sociological, demographic, economic, and psychological variables affect drinking patterns. The largest proportion of problem drinkers appear to be persons of lower socioeconomic status living in urban areas.[8,122] The highest rates of alcohol-related problems were found in urban men, under 25, single and divorced, who often reported disrupted childhoods and a transition from rural to city living. The proportion of heavy drinkers among white and black males was comparable (22 vs. 19 percent), whereas black women showed a considerably higher rate of heavy drinking (11 percent) than white women (4 percent).[23] However, esti-

---

* Recent reviews of the legal status of intoxication and alcoholism may be found in Chapter 7 of *Alcohol and Health*[23] and in *Legal Issues in Alcoholism and Alcohol Usage.*[5]

mates of alcohol abuse prevalence rates based on arrested or hospitalized alcoholics show a higher rate of severe drinking problems among ghetto-reared black males.[143] American Indians and Eskimos have also been shown to be at high risk for the development of alcoholism.[23]

The commonalities that have emerged from cross-sectional survey studies[7,8] do not permit reliable prediction of the development of problem drinking.[23] Both heavy drinkers and abstainers have been described as more discontented and alienated from society than persons who use alcohol in moderation.[23] Data from longitudinal studies suggest that the same childhood patterns predict drinking problems for ghetto-reared blacks and whites. Among both whites and blacks, adult drinking problems appear to be associated with early school problems, delinquency, drug use, and broken homes.[143] These data have been interpreted to suggest that attention to *early* school problems might avert the subsequent progression of school failure and dropout, early drug exploration, and adolescent delinquency.[143]

It is important to recognize that alcohol problems are not restricted to the disadvantaged, but can develop in anyone who drinks alcohol to excess. Alcoholism is considered to be the major drug-abuse problem in contemporary American society.[65] It has been estimated that perhaps 5 million persons suffer from alcoholism.[23] However, it should be emphasized that accurate case finding in alcoholism has been severely limited by the social stigma associated with this disorder.[136] Consequently, accurate estimates of incidence and prevalence have been difficult to obtain.[74] An additional 4 million persons are thought to abuse alcohol and therefore to be at high risk for the development of alcoholism.[23] If these estimates are valid, perhaps 7 percent of the adult population have drinking problems.

The social costs to the afflicted individual and to his family are incalculable. In its severest form, chronic alcoholism is associated with disruption of normal social and family ties; job loss and diminution of earning capacity; compromised physical and psychological health and decreased life expectancy.[126] A profound and progressive isolation and alienation from self and society may sometimes terminate in violent death or suicide.[42,142,165,174]

There is no simple formula to calculate the cost to society of the loss of a productive individual. The social costs of alcoholism have been estimated at levels of $750 million,[65] $2 billion,[126] and $15 billion[23] dollars annually. Recent estimates suggest that $10 billion may be spent each year as a function of lost work time in every sector of the economy.[23] Health and welfare services for alcoholics and their families cost an estimated $2 billion per year.[23] An estimated 45 percent of all arrests in 1965 were for public intoxication, disorderly conduct, and vagrancy.[126] Estimated medical expenses and property damage associated with alcohol problems bring the yearly cost of alcoholism to a total of $15 billion.[23] These estimates, considered in connection with the human costs of alcohol-related traffic fatalities and disrupted lives, testify to the destructive toll of this poorly understood, complex biobehavioral disorder.

Definitions of Alcoholism and Alcohol Abuse

The terms "alcohol abuse" and "alcoholism" are not synonymous, but rather reflect stages in a continuum of severity from problem drinking to chronic alcohol addiction. Traditionally, there has been relatively poor agreement concerning definitions of alcoholism and alcohol abuse. Although the definition: "repetitive, excessive drinking that results in injury to an individual's health, adequate social function, or both," would be generally accepted, considerable variation continues to exist in the formulation of more precise definitions with concomitant criteria for differential diagnosis and implications for treatment.* Definitions are important since they affect the management of the problem. The lack of an adequate definition has often impeded progress in our understanding of alcohol problems.[74,119]

* See references 7, 9, 66, 74, 119, 125, and 189.

SOCIOCULTURAL DEFINITIONS

Although at first glance it may not appear difficult to arrive at a concensus for definition of an alcohol-related problem, there are many conflicting social, cultural, and religious perceptions which contribute to continuing disagreement. Some attempts have been made to define alcohol abuse on the basis of a volume-frequency index of alcohol consumption. This approach is limited, since a particular drinking pattern will not be uniformly accepted in different regions or across various cultures. The Expert Committee of the World Health Organization defines abnormal drinking as that form of drinking which transgresses the normal social and dietary habits of the community.[189] Therefore, heavy drinking in a society which condones drinking would not constitute alcohol abuse, whereas consumption of any alcohol in a society which has rigorous standards of abstinence would be considered alcohol abuse. Depending on the standards employed, any definition of alcohol abuse results either in over-inclusion or under-inclusion of a large number of cases. Consequently, definitions which involve primarily social criteria are limited by the enormous variation in acceptable drinking habits within and between countries.

PHARMACOLOGICAL DEFINITIONS

One resolution of the difficulties associated with sociocultural definitions is to establish diagnostic criteria for alcoholism based on the pharmacological criteria of addiction: tolerance and physical dependence (see discussion on pp. 379–382). Tolerance for and physical dependence upon alcohol is similar to phenomena which may develop following the abuse of other drugs which affect the central nervous system, such as opiates and barbiturates. Tolerance for alcohol refers to the fact that progressively larger quantities are required to produce changes in feelings or behavior which had previously been attained with smaller doses of alcohol. Physical dependence is demonstrated by the fact that the alcoholic experiences discomfort and physical illness when he stops drinking or decreases his alcohol intake. It is not necessary for an alcoholic to stop drinking completely before he experiences withdrawal symptoms, since a relatively small decrease from high blood-alcohol levels may precipitate the onset of this disorder.[58,108]

The pharmacological definition of alcoholism has the advantage of referring to a series of observable events, i.e., the alcohol withdrawal syndrome. This objective definition permits selection of comparable patients for research and treatment evaluation and thereby increases the generalizability of the results. However, the pharmacological definition is limited in that it applies only to the alcohol addict and does not include the early problem drinker. The skid-row alcoholic is the most visible victim of alcoholism and accounts for an estimated 3–5 percent of Americans with alcohol problems.[23] The extent of physical dependence among the middle and upper socioeconomic classes is unknown.

THE DISEASE CONCEPT OF ALCOHOLISM

Demonstration that alcoholism is a form of addiction has led to a gradual acceptance of the idea that alcoholism is an illness and a medical problem. For many decades, alcoholism was considered primarily within the context of moral transgression and social deviancy, and public drunkenness was dealt with in a punitive, criminal-justice system. It has become increasingly evident that legal sanctions and moral pressures have not provided an adequate remedy for this problem. An unfortunate result of the moralistic view of alcoholism was to limit interest in biomedical research on this condition. Our heritage from these years of scientific neglect is relative ignorance concerning even the basic phenomenology of alcoholism. Now that alcoholism, the disease, is considered an appropriate subject for laboratory and clinical investigation and federal resources are available for research, biomedical research interest has increased fourfold in six years (1966–1972).

The disease concept of alcoholism is sometimes criticized because it is thought to be overly restrictive and to imply a linear physical causality without sufficient attention to social and psychological factors. This criticism is based upon a misunderstanding of the disease model of alcoholism. In fact, the model assumes that expression of the disorder depends on an *interaction* between the individual, the agent of the disease (alcohol) and the environment in which the disease process develops (see Figure 15–1). It is well known that disease processes can rarely be explained on the basis of any specific factor within these three categories, but rather on their interrelationships. Even infectious disease is often more closely related to host-resistance factors and environmental variables than to the presence or even the virulence of any given infectious agent.[112,113,119]

One important advantage of a disease model of alcoholism is to stimulate biomedical research and to redirect the attention of physicians to the medical aspects of this disorder. Traditionally, physicians have shown considerable reluctance to treat alcoholics for a variety of reasons and it has been difficult for alcoholics to gain admission to general hospitals.[126] Insofar as alcoholism is now considered to be within the province of medicine,

there should be an improvement in the quality of care for the medical complications of alcohol abuse. Moreover, as the physician begins to accept responsibility for the alcoholic patients, he may become more interested in and skillful at detecting early warning signals of the illness within the context of general medical practice.

A PRACTICAL SOLUTION
COMPREHENSIVE DIAGNOSTIC CRITERIA

A constructive and direct outgrowth of the general acceptance of the disease model of alcoholism is the development of comprehensive diagnostic guidelines by the National Council on Alcoholism.[125] These criteria specify behavioral and attitudinal changes, as well as medical problems, to aid the physician in the early detection of alcohol problems and to permit differential diagnosis of late-stage alcoholism. There has been an attempt to compare the significance of certain subjective reports and objective signs in diagnosing alcohol problems. Common medical complications of alcoholism are specifically indicated and evaluation of possible concurrent psychiatric problems is urged.

Early detection is probably a critical aspect of prevention. Individuals at high risk for alcoholism characteristically deny the contribution of alcohol to any physical or psychological problems that led them to seek medical advice. By careful description of the types of behavioral and medical problems associated with excessive alcohol use, these diagnostic criteria provide a basis for increased awareness of the danger signs of alcoholism and the possibility of early intervention by the alert physician. The extent to which the availability of these diagnostic criteria may increase physicians' acceptance of the patient with alcohol problems remains to be determined.

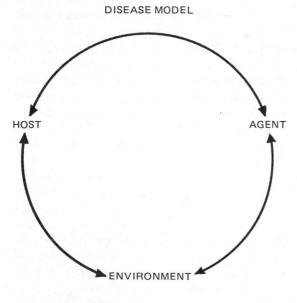

DISEASE MODEL

HOST

AGENT

ENVIRONMENT

Figure 15–1. Schematic diagram of a disease model of alcoholism depicting the interaction between host, agent (alcohol) and the environment.

❲ Pharmacology of Alcohol and Alcohol Abuse

Mechanism of Action of Alcohol

The exact pharmacological mechanisms of the actions of alcohol are unknown. The targets of central and peripheral effects can be specified with some confidence, but the way in which alcohol produces physiological and behavioral changes is not understood. In addition to the effects of alcohol on the central nervous system, which are associated with the subjective and behavioral correlates of intoxication, alcohol ingestion may also result in a sensation of warmth and flushing of the skin (due to dilation of the peripheral blood vessels), muscular relaxation, and stimulation of gastric secretion and peristalsis.[126]

Some of the physiological changes produced by alcohol may be determined by selective and perhaps even genetically controlled factors within an individual. Flushing and peripheral vasodilatation following alcohol consumption has been found to occur with greater frequency and intensity in orientals than in occidentals.[183] Studies of infant responses to alcohol indicate that this phenomenon is not due to cultural, cognitive, or experiential factors.[183] These findings have recently been confirmed and extended to adults.[31] This increased sensitivity of orientals to alcohol may have some influence on their perception of drinking as relatively aversive or pleasurable.

Ethanol is absorbed primarily from the small intestine and its rate of absorption into the blood is influenced by several factors. Rapid drinking produces a higher concentration of alcohol in blood than slowly sipping a comparable amount of alcohol. The rate of absorption increases with increasing concentrations of ethanol (up to a maximum of about 40 percent). However, increasing concentrations of congeners are associated with a slower rate of ethanol absorption. The presence of food in the stomach substantially reduces the rapidity of alcohol absorption, as does a variety of other factors which may slow the emptying time of the stomach. Given the same alcohol intake under the same conditions, a 180-pound man has a lower blood-alcohol level than a 130-pound man. Body weight influences blood alcohol concentrations because alcohol is uniformly distributed throughout the body tissue fluids following absorption. Once alcohol attains equilibrium,

its concentration in body tissues is directly proportional to their water content. Regional concentrations of alcohol are partly dependent on regional differences in water concentration.[70,111]

Because of these interacting variables, it is impossible to accurately predict the blood-alcohol concentration following alcohol ingestion. However, it has been estimated that the usual legal limit of intoxication for operating a motor vehicle (100 mg. alcohol per 100 ml. of blood) is attained after consumption of 6 oz. of distilled spirits on an empty stomach. Three ounces of alcohol may yield a blood-alcohol level of 50 mg./100 ml. whereas 12 oz. yield a level of 200 mg./100 ml. In general, the behavioral effects of alcohol are directly dose related.

Most alcohol is removed by metabolic processes in the liver and only an estimated 2–10 percent is excreted via the kidneys and lungs.[62] The rate of alcohol metabolism is the same in normals and in abstinent alcohol addicts.[110] However, it has been shown that rates of alcohol metabolism may increase as a function of the amount and duration of ethanol ingestion.[56,120] At the present time, there are no pharmacological agents available which significantly enhance rates of ethanol metabolism with a concomitant reduction of acute intoxicating effects of alcohol.

Intoxication: Short-Term Effects of Alcohol

The behavioral level of intoxication is a function of the concentration of alcohol in the blood. It has been shown that low doses of alcohol act as a stimulant whereas higher doses result in central nervous system depression.[48,69,101,111] Increases in intoxication as a function of increased alcohol dosage comprise a continuum from relaxation and mild euphoria to hyperactivity, garrulousness, and aggression to incoordination, confusion, disorientation, stupor, and possibly coma or death. A pleasant tranquility and mild sedation may accompany a blood alcohol level of about 50 mg./100 ml. Motor discoordination may occur at levels of about 100 mg./100 ml.

Above that level, intoxication is obvious and may produce unconsciousness in normal (non-tolerant) drinkers. Concentrations above 500 mg./100 ml. may be fatal.[126] The exact mechanisms by which alcohol effects the brain to produce the behavioral expression of intoxication is unknown.

It was once thought that these sequelae of intoxication reflected a hierarchical disruption of brain centers progressing from structures which control complex cognitive and motor behaviors and critical faculties to structures which control essential life functions such as breathing. It was suggested that the hyperactivity and emotionality associated with intoxication could reflect stimulation of relevant neural structures *or* depression of other neural complexes which normally inhibit the expression of these behaviors. It now appears that alcohol acts on a regulatory system, the reticular activating system, which, in turn, concurrently effects the activity of both the cerebral cortex and subcortical structures.[69,150]

There is no simple relationship between moderate levels of alcohol intoxication and an individual's capacity to perform a variety of cognitive* and motor tasks. In part because of the tranquilizing effects of alcohol, some individuals show improved performance at low doses.[11,176] The behavioral tolerance for alcohol which accompanies alcohol addiction is defined by the lack of impairment of skilled-task performance even at very high blood-alcohol concentrations (150–200 mg./100 ml.).[103,105]

Yet, it has been shown that moderate alcohol doses may impair visual sensory capacities, i.e., specifically brightness discrimination and readjustment after exposure to bright lights. Auditory and tactile sensitivities are not dramatically affected and sensitivity to taste and odor is somewhat impaired.[23,69] It is attention, judgment, and the integration and evaluation of sensory information rather than the quality of sensory information per se that seems to be most affected by alcohol. For example, during intoxication, people tend to

---

* The effects of alcohol intoxication on memory function and sleep will be discussed under Clinical Disorders, pages 382–391.

underestimate object speed and distance as well as the passage of time.[23]

The contribution of alcohol intoxication to accidents is probably a complex combination of sensory-motor impairments, poor judgment, and emotional liability and aggressivity. The effects of alcohol on emotionality and aggressivity are poorly understood. Although alcohol is generally believed to increase emotional liability, considerable evidence suggests that the social context strongly influences both the type and direction of emotional expression during intoxication. Consumption of large amounts of alcohol may facilitate, and perhaps induce, violent and aggressive behavior including homicide, armed robbery with aggravated assault, and other crimes of violence.[165] The possible relationship between alcohol-induced aggressivity and the preponderance of fatal accidents during intoxication remains to be determined.

The role of alcohol intoxication in fatal accidents has been clearly demonstrated. Over half the nonhighway accident fatalities have been shown to involve known alcoholics or alcohol abusers.[23] In the sample studied, work-related fatal injuries occurred far less frequently than accidents in the home.[23] A comparison of the number of positive blood-alcohol levels among accident victims admitted to a hospital emergency ward showed a decrease from highway accidents (30 percent), to home accidents (22 percent) to occupational accidents (16 percent).[178]

The high concordance between automobile accidents and alcohol abuse is well known.[1,174,175] The Injury Control Program of the Public Health Service has estimated that alcohol contributes to or is associated with 50 percent of fatal motor vehicle accidents.[126] An estimated 28,000 highway fatalities were associated with alcohol intoxication during a recent 12 month period.[23] Statistics on drunken-driving fatalities show that a preponderance of the victims had blood-alcohol levels above 150 mg./100 ml.[1,174,175] These high blood-alcohol levels suggest that the single-vehicle casualties studied were not social drinkers, but alcohol addicts with substantial behavioral tolerance for alcohol. The nontolerant individual would show severe motor and cognitive dysfunction at these blood alcohol levels which could interfere with driving altogether.

The effect of alcohol intoxication on sexual function has been the subject of many anecdotes in the nonscientific literature which usually concur with Shakespeare's observation that intoxication provokes desire but impairs sexual performance. Male alcohol addicts are usually described as experiencing diminished heterosexual desire and activity and sexual impotence. Female alcoholics tend to report initiation or increased drinking during the premenstrual period.[2] There are biological data which indicate that chronic alcohol abuse may impair sexual function through a disruption of gonadal function.[114] It is well known that chronic alcoholism in males may be associated with the development of gynecomastia and testicular atrophy, which in turn may be related to a derangement in androgen metabolism. Alcohol intoxication has recently been shown to suppress plasma testosterone levels to well below the normal range in alcohol addicts.[114] Other centrally acting depressant drugs (i.e., heroin, barbiturates, and high dosages of methadone) also suppress plasma-testosterone levels in addicts.[117] Following alcohol, methadone, and heroin withdrawal, plasma-testosterone levels return to predrug baseline or to normal levels.[114–117] The possible endocrine mechanisms which influence the behavioral expression of sexuality (and aggression) are as yet unclear.

Following acute intoxication, a generalized somatic discomfort, commonly called "the hangover," may occur. The physiological determinants of the hangover are not understood. It has not been shown that mixing drinks or the congener content of drinks specifically leads to the development of a hangover. There are no specific treatments for a hangover and little scientific support for the efficacy of the popular remedies.[126]

Alcohol Addiction: Long-Term Effects of Alcohol Abuse

Drug addiction is defined by the pharmacological criteria of tolerance and physical dependence. Some chronic alcohol abusers eventually develop physical dependence upon alcohol. This end stage of alcohol abuse has been clearly shown to be an addictive disorder on the basis of both clinical[170] and experimental observations.[58,109] It was once thought that physical dependence, the alcohol withdrawal syndrome, reflected intercurrent illness or vitamin and nutritional deficiencies. It has now been shown that withdrawal signs and symptoms occur in healthy well-nourished alcoholics solely as a function of cessation of drinking. It has also been possible to induce physical dependence upon alcohol in a variety of experimental animals.*

The crucial determinants of the development of alcohol addiction are unknown, and the nature of the addictive process remains a matter of conjecture.[113] Thus far, no single theory has proved adequate to explain the complex multilevel symptoms which we collectively term alcoholism. Most probably, alcoholism, like any other behavior disorder, derives from many diverse factors in the individual and his environment. The factors which effect a particular individual's susceptibility to alcohol addiction, given a prolonged pattern of heavy drinking, remain to be determined.

TOLERANCE

The process described as "tolerance" occurs as a function of prolonged exposure to a drug. This term refers to the observation that progressively higher doses of a drug are required to produce comparable subjective and behavioral effects. The development of tolerance is far more rapid than that of physical dependence, both for alcohol[71,120] and for narcotics.[71] Tolerance and physical dependence were once believed to be sequential and inseparable aspects of the same underlying addictive process. However, our current understanding of the relationship between tolerance and physical dependence suggests that, although physical dependence is invariably accompanied by the development of tolerance, drug tolerance may occur independently of physical dependence.[19,40,65,152]

* See references 22, 27, 30, 32, 104, 137, 187, and 188.

The alcohol addict shows three types of tolerance which are common to other addictive disorders; i.e., behavioral tolerance, pharmacological tolerance and cross tolerance to other potentially addictive drugs.[149] *Behavioral tolerance* for alcohol is illustrated by the fact that an alcohol addict can drink as much as a quart of bourbon per day without signs of gross intoxication.[103,105,107,108] A number of investigators have found that task performance during sobriety and inebriation may not differ significantly even when blood-alcohol levels are twice 100 mg/ml, the legal limit of intoxication in many states.*

Associated with behavioral tolerance is *pharmacological tolerance* for alcohol. Consistent consumption of as much as a quart of bourbon per day may result in unexpectedly low levels of alcohol in the blood.[107,108] It has been shown that alcohol ingestion does increase the rate of alcohol metabolism in alcoholics and in controls as a function of both amount and duration of alcohol ingestion.[56, 120] However, the ethanol-induced enhancement of the rate of ethanol metabolism appears to be transient and does not persist long after cessation of drinking. A number of studies have shown that the rate of ethanol metabolism in abstinent alcoholics and nonalcoholics is not significantly different.† The dramatic behavioral tolerance for alcohol shown by the alcohol addict cannot be accounted for by a more rapid or effective capacity to metabolize alcohol. This is evidenced by the fact that alcoholics can perform well on difficult tasks even with very high blood-alcohol levels (above 200 mg./100 ml.).[103, 105] These data suggest that the adaptive processes subserving tolerance occur in the central nervous system rather than at a metabolic level.

Cross tolerance refers to the general phenomena of reduced responsivity to drugs other than the primary addicting agent. It has been shown that sober alcoholics metabolize a number of drugs more rapidly than nonalcoholics,[72] and there are reports that alcohol addicts undergoing surgery require far larger doses of anesthetics than nonaddict patients to induce a surgical level of anesthesia.[3,83] Similarly, the alcohol addict may show cross tolerance to other potentially addictive agents such as barbiturates, hypnotics, and sedatives.[149] No cross dependence has been shown between alcohol and opiate narcotics.[40] Finally, the alcoholic shows tolerance for many toxic alcohols and is able to ingest these in quantities that would be fatal for nonalcoholics.[121] It should be emphasized that the phenomena of cross tolerance occurs in the *sober* alcohol addict. Under conditions of intoxication, many drugs contribute to the effects of alcohol, and the alcoholic individual may metabolize these drugs more slowly than normal subjects.[145]

Although alcohol tolerance is striking in the alcoholic, the degree of tolerance, on a comparable dosage basis, is much less for alcohol than for opiates or barbiturates. For example, barbiturate addicts may ingest twenty to thirty times the average hypnotic dose in a twenty-four-hour period. Heroin addicts show similar increases in self-administration over their initial dosage levels. It is well known that some heroin addicts go through withdrawal in order to reduce their tolerance and thereby lower their daily maintenance dosage requirements.[40] The physical limit of tolerance for the alcoholic is more firmly fixed, and even though the alcoholic does develop behavioral tolerance, blood-alcohol levels rarely exceed 450 mg./100 ml. The lethal level of alcohol dosage also remains close to that for normal drinkers, and blood-alcohol concentrations in excess of 500–600 mg./100 ml. result in severe respiratory depression.

PHYSICAL DEPENDENCE

The usual alcohol withdrawal syndrome occurs between twelve and seventy-two hours following cessation of drinking, although the course and severity are quite variable.[168,170] For clinical description see pp. 383–385. Abstinence signs and symptoms may include tremor, profuse sweating, gastrointestinal disorders, nystagmus, hyperreflexia, sleep disturbances, hallucinations, and occasionally, seizures. Remission of major symptoms is usually complete within three to five days. The usual

* See references 11, 25, 103, 105, and 159–161.
† See references 13, 53, 63, 110, 120, and 128.

alcohol withdrawal syndrome is generally similar to mild barbiturate, opiate, and nonbarbiturate sedative withdrawal.[29]

The biological mechanisms underlying alcohol withdrawal and abstinence syndromes generally are unknown. The development of physical dependence is thought to be multiply determined by a complex interaction of neural, endocrine, and metabolic variables.[113] Most attempts to account for the characteristic psychomotor and autonomic hyperactivity associated with drug-withdrawal syndromes have postulated a heightened CNS excitability. The basis for CNS hyperexcitability during withdrawal has often been attributed to a rebound effect following drug-induced depression of neural activity.[65,113] There is considerable neurophysiological evidence consistent with the notion that the CNS becomes more excitable during drug withdrawal.[65,113]

The role of alcohol in facilitating seizure disorders in persons with an underlying epileptic disorder has long been a subject of considerable controversy. It is now thought that alcohol intoxication rather than alcohol withdrawal may increase the probability of seizures in persons with idiopathic or traumatic epilepsy.[169]

Recent data suggest that, following removal of the depressant effect of alcohol, there is an increased sensitivity of the respiratory center to carbon dioxide and hyperventilation.[184,185] It was once thought that alcoholics became acidotic during alcohol withdrawal. However, it has recently been shown that alcoholics develop a significant respiratory alkalosis which correlates both with susceptibility to stroboscopically induced seizures and the occurrence of delirium tremens. These data are of particular interest since several other hyperventilation syndromes, also associated with a respiratory alkalosis, yield clinical syndromes similar to those of alcohol withdrawal.[185] Attempts to treat the alcohol-withdrawal syndrome by administering carbon dioxide to reduce the respiratory alkalosis were rather promising, despite technical difficulties in administering carbon dioxide. The efficacy of pharmacological agents to correct the respiratory alkalosis is currently being evaluated.[184,185]

PSYCHOLOGICAL DEPENDENCE

Definitions of drug dependence are often subdivided into physical dependence and psychological dependence.[190] Psychological dependence is usually inferred when drug use takes priority over other coping mechanisms and assumes a central focus in the organization of daily behavior.[10] The term "psychological dependence" is imprecisely defined and usually used to refer to the motivational factors which underlie drug-seeking behavior *and* to the psychological effects of drug use. This semantic confusion between motivational and drug effect aspects of dependence reflects our current limited understanding of the factors which initiate and maintain drinking episodes. The conditions which initiate and perpetuate heavy drinking behavior are unknown. The resumption of addictive drinking after a period of abstinence probably reflects many psychogenic and stress factors. The possible contribution of the condition of physical dependence upon alcohol to reinitiation of drinking after sobriety is undetermined.[106] It is unlikely that the condition of physical dependence in the sober alcoholic influences drinking behavior in the same way that the presence or absence of food-deprivation affects food seeking behavior.[106] There are no satisfactory explanations for the repetition of excessive drinking and withdrawal sequences, despite the totally predictable adverse medical, social, economic, and often legal consequences. It is the immediate rather than the long-range consequences of alcohol abuse which appear to control drinking behavior.

In trying to account for the persistence of addictive drinking, it is tempting to extrapolate from one's own enjoyment of alcohol and to imagine that the immediate pleasures of drinking negate either the awesome prospect or the concurrent awareness of its many aversive consequences. However, it has been shown repeatedly that alcoholics become progressively more dysphoric, anxious, agitated, and depressed during a chronic drinking sequence.[103] A comparable dysphoria during chronic drug use has been observed in morphine addicts[179] and it has been suggested that increased narcotics intake may be motivated by an effort to regain an initial euphoria. It has also been shown that drinking tends to confirm and aggravate feelings of inadequacy and low self-esteem in alcoholics.[167] Although the voluminous psychiatric literature on alcoholism has tended to present "the alcoholic" as an impulsive hedonist who drinks to dissolve his anxieties and achieve a diffuse sense of omnipotence, direct observations of intoxicated alcoholics reveal a pathetic failure to attain such goals.

The somewhat paradoxical increase in disturbing affect observed in alcoholics during studies of experimentally induced intoxication is difficult to reconcile with information that most alcoholics provide about their drinking experiences during sobriety. It appears that the sober alcoholic does not recall the seemingly aversive aspects of his drinking experience during a subsequent period of sobriety and therefore these aversive consequences cannot effectively modify his future behavior. There are considerable data which converge to suggest that there is a substantial dissociation of experience during drinking, and subsequent recall and expectancy during sobriety.[106] It is possible that psychotherapeutic techniques which involve efforts to integrate experiences during inebriation with awareness during sobriety through the use of videotaped interviews may provide an effective tool for bridging this alcohol-induced dissociation.

A second factor often advanced to account for the perpetuation of drinking is the notion of "craving" which implies that once an alcoholic starts to drink, "he is compelled to continue until he reaches a state of severe intoxication."[96] The circularity inherent in this reasoning is evident, i.e., the concept of "craving" is defined by the behavior that it is evoked to explain. The concept of "craving" with its implication of "loss of control" over drinking has been the source of considerable confusion in the literature on alcoholism and has stimulated continuing debate.[75,106,134] There has been no empirical support for the notion of "craving" on the basis of direct experimental observations of alcoholics given alcohol[108] and clinical material.[103,134] Although this construct appears to be of limited utility, it has long formed the basis for the usual therapeutic goal of total abstinence in the treatment of the alcoholic patient. (See also discussion on Treatment of Alcoholism, pp. 394–395.)

A third factor assumed to be related to the maintenance of addictive drinking is the avoidance of withdrawal signs and symptoms which follow an abrupt reduction in blood-alcohol concentration. If the avoidance of withdrawal signs is the factor which motivates an alcoholic to continue drinking, it would be expected that during a drinking spree, he should drink quite consistently and maintain stable blood-alcohol levels. However, recent data have shown a considerable cyclicity of alcohol self-administration both in primate[187,188] and human alcohol addicts.[108] Despite the attendant discomfort, the alcoholic does not invariably respond to these partial withdrawal signs by increased drinking.[108] This situation may resemble that of the narcotics addict in which it has been suggested that incipient withdrawal signs may add both to the gratification and perpetuation of drug use.[179] The relationship between physical dependence and subsequent drug self-administration is, at best, ambiguous.[104] The assumption that physical dependence is one aspect of an addict's motivation for drug use is a complex and elusive issue to approach experimentally.[64,180] Logically, it is difficult to account for the reinitiation of an addictive drinking sequence, after a prolonged period of sobriety, in terms of physical dependence alone. Presumably, whatever factors first prompted excessive drinking before the development of physical dependence, continue to affect resumption of alcohol abuse.

At the core of the many dynamic formulations concerning the basis of alcohol abuse are two related notions: (1) the alcoholic drinks to achieve a pleasurable subjective state; and (2) the alcoholic drinks to avoid or reduce the impact of current problems. Until progress in behavioral science permits more precise specification of the factors which initiate and perpetuate addictive drinking, the efficacy of attempts to intervene and avert repetition of destructive drinking sequences will be greatly limited. At present, we can only speculate about the possible psychological and social determinants of alcohol dependence.

◖ Clinical Disorders Associated with Alcohol Abuse and Alcoholism

Factors in the Development of Alcoholism

Alcoholism can develop in any man or woman, irrespective of individual personality characteristics, educational, cultural, religious, ethnic, or socioeconomic background. No single psychological, social, or biological variable has yet been shown to predict the development of problem drinking or to uniquely differentiate alcoholics from nonalcoholics. The differences between alcoholic individuals far outweigh the commonalities of repetitive excessive drinking and tolerance for and physical dependence upon alcohol.

Many individuals develop alcohol problems independently of any family history of alcoholism. However, recent evidence suggests the possibility of a genetic component associated with the genesis of alcohol problems.[47,148] Dissociation of familial learning factors from genetic variables is a difficult methodological problem.[41] However, a study of fifty-five adult males, separated during infancy from their biological parents (one of whom had been hospitalized for alcoholism) had a significantly higher incidence of alcoholism than matched adoptee controls.[47] Another study of 164 adoptees showed a significantly greater tendency to develop alcohol problems if the biological parent was an alcoholic than if the adopted parent was alcoholic.[148]

The psychiatric literature on alcoholism contains countless theories which attempt to conceptualize alcoholism in terms of a psychodynamic formulation, a psychosocial developmental model, or as the outgrowth of specific personality characteristics such as depression, dependency, immaturity, hostility, and social isolation. An excellent comprehensive review of psychodynamic and personality factors in alcoholism appears in the first edition of this Handbook.[194] This chapter does not attempt to recapitulate this material, in part because there has been little in the way of novel or substantive revision of the various psychological theories of alcoholism since the Handbook was first published in 1959. Some more recent conceptualizations seem little more than relabeling exercises with terms currently in fashion, e.g., "systems theory" etc. More important, the most plausible and ingenious theories concerning the psychological determinants of alcoholism have contributed little to the development of effective treatment and, for the most part, have been difficult to subject to rigorous experimental scrutiny.

Motivation for drinking varies greatly between individuals as well as within an individual from occasion to occasion. Drinking patterns are idiosyncratic; no consistent behavioral or biological correlates have yet been identified. Anxiety and depression may be far less at the beginning of a drinking episode than during or following prolonged intoxication.[100,103,109,124] Stressful incidents may correlate with either the initiation or the cessation of drinking in alcohol addicts.[103] Alcohol intoxication does not appear to produce any reproducible pattern of social interactions. Often it appears that alcohol may accentuate a person's characteristic mode of coping with his environment and social world. Efforts at objective behavioral analysis of drinking patterns are very new, and the findings are gradually dispelling some basic misconceptions about alcoholism derived from retrospective, self-report data from the sober alcoholic.[103]

The Alcohol-Withdrawal Syndromes

Hippocrates was the first to report an association between alcohol abuse and tremulousness, delirium, and seizure disorders.[193] However, it was not until the late eighteenth and early nineteenth century that the alcohol-abstinence syndrome was accurately described in the medical literature.[156] Despite a long history of clinical observation of the association between cessation of drinking and signs and symptoms characterizing the withdrawal state, the basis of the alcohol-abstinence syndrome was not determined until the mid twentieth century. Studies carried out by Victor and Adams[170] in 1953 provided the first careful clinical documentation of the alcohol-withdrawal states and an accurate classification of the withdrawal syndromes. Based upon these observations three unique, but not mutually exclusive withdrawal states were differentiated: the tremulous syndrome, alcohol-related seizure disorders, and delirium tremens.

The critical determinants of the onset of withdrawal symptoms are unclear, since either a relative decrease in blood-alcohol levels *or* the abrupt cessation of drinking may precipitate the syndrome. The severity and duration of withdrawal symptoms also do not appear to be directly related either to the volume of alcohol consumed or to the duration of a drinking spree. It appears that the pattern of drinking may be more important than the duration of drinking in accounting for the expression of the alcohol-abstinence syndrome.[107] (See also p. 375 and pp. 380–381.)

Tremulousness is the most common withdrawal sign observed following cessation of drinking. Tremulousness may be relatively mild with involvement of only the distal upper extremities, or it may be severe, involving upper and lower extremities as well as tongue and trunk. The onset of tremulousness may occur as early as six hours following cessation of alcohol intake but the peak of intensity of the syndrome usually occurs after 24 to 48 hours of abstinence. Tremor is usually relatively coarse and may be exaggerated or exacerbated when the patient is asked to extend his arms with palms either separated or pronated. Duration of the tremulous state rarely extends beyond seventy-two hours following cessation of drinking but in some cases it may last as long as four or five days.

Tremulousness is often associated with a subjective sensation of moderate to severe anxiety. Hallucinations may also accompany the acute alcohol withdrawal state.[50] Acute alcoholic hallucinosis is usually auditory and there is little support for the notion that these hallucinatory events are related to an underlying schizophrenia.[50] It is also important to emphasize that hallucinosis is not necessarily an index of the severity of the abstinence syndrome. Recent data, obtained under experimental research ward conditions, have shown that hallucinations may occur when alcohol addicts are severely intoxicated as well as following cessation of drinking.[186]

Seizure disorders due to alcohol withdrawal are often associated with antecedent and consequent states of tremulousness, although isolated seizure disorders without tremulousness do occur. Seizure disorders associated with alcohol withdrawal may occur as early as several hours following the last intake of alcohol, but the peak incidence of this syndrome is usually twelve to twenty-four hours following cessation of drinking. Seizures are usually grand mal in nature and are rarely preceded by auras but usually followed by a post-ictal state. Seizures may occur during alcohol withdrawal in patients who have no other evidence of neurological disease and have normal EEG's during sobriety. The occurrence of seizure disorders may herald subsequent development of overt delirium tremens. According to Victor and Adams,[170] approximately one third of all patients who have seizure disorders during alcohol withdrawal eventually develop delirium tremens.

Seizure disorders are not unique to alcohol-withdrawal states and have been observed following withdrawal of many centrally acting drugs. Seizure disorders are commonly seen during barbiturate withdrawal and following cessation of prolonged use of high dosages of meprobamate, chloral hydrate, and paraldehyde. In contrast, the heroin abstinence syndrome is rarely associated with seizure disorders. Although it has been suggested that seizure disorders observed during the alcohol abstinence state represent a latent form of epilepsy which is precipitated either by heavy alcohol use or withdrawal, there is no evidence to support this hypothesis.[169] At present the underlying mechanisms which produce seizure states during alcohol withdrawal are not known.

The term "delirium tremens" is often erroneously used as a generic description of most alcohol-withdrawal states. However, delirium tremens is a distinct and specific disorder which occurs with relative infrequency. In contrast to the common alcohol-withdrawal syndrome, delirium tremens usually occurs late, i.e., seventy-two to ninety-six hours following cessation of drinking. It may be preceded by tremulousness[168,170] and is often preceded by seizure disorders.[170]

Delirium tremens is characterized by profound confusion, disorientation, delusional states, and hallucinatory episodes as well as motor and autonomic dysfunction.[170] Confusional states and delirium are rarely observed in the common tremulousness syndrome of alcohol abstinence. Hallucinations associated with delirium tremens tend to be visual rather than auditory.[33,49] However, there is little empirical support for the popular notion of a "typical" hallucinatory pattern. Although frightening and dysphoric hallucinations may occur, comforting, pleasurable and euphoric hallucinations are also observed, and it is the sensory and perceptual richness of the hallucinatory event that is distinctive.[49] Hallucinations associated with delirium tremens are distinguished from hallucinations of schizophrenia by the intense visual nonideational quality, increased frequency of occurrence at night, and reports of subjective intensification when the patients' eyes are closed.[33,49]

In addition to disorders of the sensorium, patients with delirium tremens frequently show profuse sweating, tachycardia, hyperreflexia, mild to severe tremulousness, hypertension, and fever. Intercurrent illness, particularly pulmonary and gastrointestinal disorders, are also common in these patients. Delirium tremens is a potentially lethal condition in contrast to the relatively benign common tremulous syndrome.[170]

In the process of establishing a differential diagnosis between acute alcoholic tremulousness, seizure disorders, and delirium tremens, it is essential to consider the time course as well as the presence or absence of confusion, disorientation, and autonomic dysfunction. It is also important to remember that alcohol withdrawal is not an all-or-none phenomenon. During the course of chronic drinking, alcohol addicts may experience wide fluctuations in blood alcohol levels as a function of periodicity of alcohol intake plus alterations in the rate of absorption and metabolism of alcohol. A number of clinical and laboratory studies have demonstrated that onset of the withdrawal syndrome, particularly tremulousness, may occur when alcoholics are consuming ethanol, but have a relative decrease in their blood-alcohol levels.[58,107,108] It is impossible to arbitrarily define a critical blood alcohol level for any given individual which either initiates or suppresses the withdrawal state. For example, alcohol addicts who have blood alcohol levels of 300 mg./100 ml. may experience severe abstinence syndromes when their blood alcohol levels fall 100 or only 50 mg./100 ml.[108]

In addition to symptoms which appear to be directly related to alcohol (or partial alcohol) withdrawal, a number of associated disorders may contribute to the severity and duration of the withdrawal syndromes. Alcohol addicts may have disturbances in acid-base, water, and electrolyte balance during alcohol withdrawal.[131] Hyperventilation is frequently observed in the early hours following cessation of drinking and this phenomenon may be associated with induction of respiratory alkalosis and elevated blood pH.[184] Hypomagnecemia may also be found in patients in alcohol withdrawal.[118]

Low serum magnesium levels are probably the result of two factors: poor dietary intake and malabsorption of magnesium associated with heavy drinking, and a shift of magnesium from the intravascular to intracellular fluid compartments.[118,185] Although a state of dehydration may be present in some patients during withdrawal, overhydration may also be a problem.[112,131]

Somatic Disorders

Prolonged alcohol abuse has been shown to have toxic effects on a number of organ systems as well as secondary effects on metabolic processes. Since the liver is the major drug-metabolizing organ in the body, perhaps it is not surprising that *liver damage* is both the earliest and most profound consequence of excessive alcohol use. Alcohol has been shown to induce a transient development of fatty liver in normal drinkers in as little as two days.[146] In chronic alcoholism, there may be a temporal progression from alcohol-induced fatty liver to alcoholic hepatitis or cirrhosis,[85] a potentially fatal condition. The extent to which alcoholic hepatitis, characterized by extensive necrosis and inflammation, may in turn initiate scarring, fibrosis, and finally cirrhosis is unclear. Moreover, although excessive alcohol use almost invariably induces fatty liver, not all alcoholics develop cirrhosis.[85] Recent data suggest that the development of alcohol-induced hyperlipidemia may be related to genetic factors, since alcoholics with primary hypertriglyceridemia develop striking lipid abnormalities during experimentally induced chronic intoxication.[115] Normal drinkers with primary hypertriglyceridemia also develop marked increases in triglyceride levels after acute administration of low doses of alcohol.[39]

Gastrointestinal disorders associated with alcohol abuse are very common. Gastritis and pancreatitis are probably the most frequently encountered gastrointestinal disorders in alcohol abusers. *Gastritis* may progress to gastric or duodenal ulcers which, in turn, may lead to potentially fatal gastrointestinal bleeding. *Pancreatitis* is also a potentially lethal consequence of alcohol ingestion. The mechanism of pancreatitis production in relation to alcoholism is unknown.[20,147] Excessive alcohol use may also intefere with the absorption of essential nutrients and vitamins from the small intestine into the blood stream. The nutritional malabsorption syndrome, so frequently observed secondary to alcoholism, may also contribute to the compromised nutritional status often seen in the alcohol addict.[61,87]

The neurological disorders frequently associated with alcohol addiction are also related to malabsorption of critical nutrients. The most frequently observed disorder of the peripheral nervous system in alcoholics usually involves motor and sensory nerves in the arms and legs. These *peripheral neuropathies* are characterized by pain, impaired movement and coordination, and eventually by muscle wasting. This condition is usually reversible with an adequate diet and cessation of drinking.[97,123]

Disorders of the *central nervous system* may also be associated with chronic alcohol abuse. Until recently, it has not been clear whether these disorders were caused by the direct action of alcohol or a combination of alcohol abuse and poor nutrition. It is now generally believed that nutritional deficiencies are the most important etiological factor in most neurological diseases associated with chronic alcoholism.[26,127,171] The incidence of CNS diseases associated with nutritional deficiency and alcohol abuse is very low.[26] Even in 1953, neurological disease in hospitalized alcoholics ranged only between 1 and 3 percent.[170] There has been a persistent mistaken impression that certain CNS diseases are uniquely associated with alcoholism. Table 15–1 summarizes some other conditions in which CNS diseases traditionally associated with alcoholism are also seen. The clinical neurology and neuropathology associated with amblyopia, cerebellar cortical degeneration, central pontine myelinolysis, myelopathy, Marchiafava-Bignami disease, and Wernicke-Korsakoff syndrome has recently been reviewed by Dreyfus.[26]

The latter two syndromes require some special emphasis because of their historical association with the condition of alcoholism. Marchiafava-Bignami disease is a rare condition of unknown origin, which presents a clinical picture rather similar to delirium tremens, and is characterized by demyelination of the central portion of the corpus collasum.[26] Only about sixty-four cases have been reported in the world literature.[182] The disorder was once thought to occur only in Italian males who drank large amounts of crude red wine.[26,95] This syndrome has subsequently been observed in non-Italian alcoholic patients after abuse of various types of alcohol.[57,59] The pathological changes associated with Marchiafava-Bignami disease have also been found in patients with Wernicke-Korsakoff syndrome.[26]

Wernicke's syndrome is an encephalopathy frequently associated with alcohol abuse. Prolonged alcohol intake, even in the presence of an adequate diet, may result in impairment of

TABLE 15–1. **Disorders of the Central Nervous System Associated with Alcoholism and Other Specific Conditions***

ASSOCIATED CONDITIONS	DISEASES OF THE NERVOUS SYSTEM				
	WERNICKE-KORSAKOFF SYNDROME	AMBLYOPIA	CEREBELLAR CORTICAL DEGENERATION	CENTRAL PONTINE MYELINOLYSIS	MYELOPATHY
Liver Disease					√133, 192
Thyro Toxicosis	√28				
Pernicious Vomiting of Pregnancy	√18				
Strachan's Disease					√35
Nutritional Factors					
Chronic Malnutrition	√35, 76, 153				
Chronic Malnutrition Associated with Disease				√6, 17, 80, 98, 151	
Nutritional Depletion			√94		
Thiamine Deficiencies	√171				
Vitamin B Deficiencies	√171	√54			
Pellagra					√157
Treatment Variables					
Chronic Hemodialysis	√89				
Isonicotinic Acid Hydrazide		√73			

* This material is abstracted from Dreyfus.[26] Numbers refer to bibliographic entries.

eye muscle control due to nerve dysfunction. Although this condition is usually benign and readily reversible following cessation of alcohol intake, it may herald a potentially serious disorder which could lead to a permanent incapacity. This more serious disorder has been termed Wernicke's disease and Korsakoff's psychosis and is characterized by opthalmoplegia, ataxia, weakness, profound disorders of memory and deranged process of thinking.

This syndrome results primarily from vitamin deficiency and, in particular, a deficiency of thiamin.[26,172] Alcohol abusers are at a high risk for the development of vitamin deficiencies because they eat poorly and alcohol may inhibit absorption and transport of vitamins from the GI (gastrointestinal) tract. Remission of opthalmoplegia usually occurs promptly after parenteral administration of vitamin B complex. Ataxia and confusional states clear more slowly. The prolonged derangements of memory (Korsakoff's psychosis) are discussed under Disorders of Memory Function (p. 389).

The possible contribution of alcoholism to *heart* disease is, as yet, unknown. Alcohol is a myocardial depressant[154] and may play some role in the development of cardiomyopathies. A comparison of clinically normal alcoholic patients with cardiomyopathy and normal groups showed abnormalities of cardiac function similar to but quantitatively less than in the cardiomyopathy group.[154]

Less frequent but not uncommon conditions associated with chronic alcohol abuse include disturbances in *blood*-cell formation and anemia, *muscle* disease, and enhanced susceptibility to infection.[123,182] An interaction between poor nutrition and excessive drinking is probably most important in the genesis of these disorders. It is known that alcoholics have a very high incidence of tuberculosis and this infectious disease is most common in individuals who are debilitated and have poor dietary intake.[55]

Affective Disorders and Psychosis

Depression as an antecedent or consequent phenomenon in patients with alcohol-abuse problems has been well documented in the clinical literature.* However, the causation of alcohol problems as unique sequela of affective disorders has never been substantiated. Some individuals with neurotic and psychotic affective disorders may abuse alcohol, but many individuals with these symptoms do not drink heavily and may even abstain from using alcoholic beverages. Although it is tempting to postulate that alcoholics drink to alleviate depression, there is some evidence that chronic drinking enhances depression. A number of studies have shown that depression and dysphoric states are precipitated by or perhaps increased during chronic intoxication.[100,109,124,162] It is therefore important for the physician to recognize that depression is not a necessary "underlying" basis for alcohol abuse and to avoid simplistic formulations for "treatment of the depression" rather than employing a more comprehensive therapeutic approach.

Alcoholism is a common finding in individuals who attempt or commit suicide.[42] It has been estimated that one third of all reported suicides are associated with chronic alcohol abuse.[142,165] However, the available statistics indicate that this figure may be valid only for white middle-aged males.[42] Suicide rates appear to be relatively low for black males over thirty-five, although problem drinking in this group is more likely to occur at an earlier age than for white males.[42] Until more comprehensive data are available, the precise interaction between alcoholism and suicide will remain obscure. On the other hand, there is very good evidence that alcohol consumption frequently occurs prior to suicidal behavior, since

* See references 23, 24, 38, 42, 66, 126, 142, and 177.

about 25 percent of suicide victims have detectable amounts of alcohol in tissue on necropsy examination.[42] It is tempting to postulate that this finding supports the observation that alcohol may enhance dysphoric mood states.[100,109,124,162] Since there are no data available concerning the number of individuals who contemplate suicide, drink, but do not attempt the act, or who are even dissuaded from suicide as a consequence of drinking, the relationship between suicidal behavior and drinking is unclear.

The causal relationship often assumed to exist between alcoholism and a number of psychiatric states is also tenuous at best. The "alcoholic paranoid state" has been listed in the Diagnostic and Statistical Manual (DSM-II), published in 1968 by the American Psychiatric Association. There is no evidence that this behavior disorder is a unique psychosis caused or even aggravated by drinking. An examination of the clinical literature reveals no convincing data which demonstrate either acquisition or remission of a psychiatric disorder as a function of alcohol intake. However, it is not unlikely that patients may initiate drinking or abuse alcohol as one of a series of behaviors associated with recrudescence of a psychotic episode. Assignment of a causal rather than an associational relationship between alcohol abuse and psychotic disorders is naive and impedes development of the basis for a comprehensive differential diagnosis.

"Pathological intoxication" is a term often found in the literature and it is most commonly characterized as uncontrolled and usually violent aggressive behavior and rage following alcohol intake. Rage states have been associated with even very small volume alcohol intake, and a causal basis has been assigned to alcohol in producing the disordered behavior. No such causal basis has been verified in controlled studies, nor has an association between blood alcohol levels, abnormal brain-wave activity, and violence been experimentally validated. As noted previously, some patients may exhibit increased aggressive behavior when intoxicated.[114] However other individuals may become more friendly, while others show no change in behavior. So-called "pathological intoxication" is probably more closely related to host and environmental determinants than to a specific pharmacological effect of alcohol in the CNS.

During recent years, it has been reported that a large number of new admissions to state mental hospitals have alcoholism as a primary diagnosis.[23] Among those patients a significant number have "organic brain dysfunction" which has been linked to alcohol abuse. It should be kept in mind that these patients have a number of similar features in addition to a history of alcohol abuse, e.g., most are poor; most have a past history of marginal nutritional status; most have family backgrounds of low socioeconomic status and poor educational achievement. The apparent increase in the number of admissions of these patients does not necessarily reflect a true increase in prevalence of alcoholism. Rather it may reflect the increased willingness of state institutions to admit these patients as a consequence of decreased duration of hospitalization for other psychiatric patients who are more amenable to psychopharmacological interventions.

The entire category of the organic brain disorders is poorly understood. More rigorous and obsessive relabeling will not provide better insight into the causal determinants of the disorders of cognition, perception, and memory function. Much more knowledge is necessary before the role of alcohol abuse, alone or in combination with other disorders of behavior, can be determined in the genesis and progression of deranged intellectual function and aberrant thought processes.

Disorders-of-Memory Function

Excessive alcohol use has been associated with several types of impaired memory function. These range from a severe persistent amnestic disorder, Wernicke's Korsakoff syndrome,[158] to the transient total memory loss which may accompany heavy intoxication, i.e., the alcoholic "blackout"[43,44] to the fragmentary absence of recall of events during drinking which has been described as a dissociative state.[46,132] The mechanisms which account

for these alcohol-induced memory impairments are unknown.[105]

Wernicke's Korsakoff syndrome is usually associated with pathological changes of the mammillary bodies and the medial thalamus and hypothalamus.[172] The patient presents with anterograde and retrograde amnesia.[158] Although memory of early life experiences is intact, there is usually an inability to recall more recent life circumstances. Patients are unable to acquire new information and often cannot recall, for example, the route to the hospital dining room, the food served at lunch, the name of their doctor, etc. The most comprehensive analysis of the memory deficits associated with the Wernicke's Korsakoff syndrome has been completed by Talland.[158] The extent to which this complex memory disorder is a function of impairment in information storage, or in retrieval of that information is the subject of continuing study.

The alcoholic "blackout" is a general term used to describe a total loss of memory for events during an episode of heavy intoxication. In some instances, intoxicated individuals may drive long distances, fight, be arrested, and subsequently awaken without any recollection of their activities for the past several hours or days. The incidence of "blackouts" is unknown. In a sample of one hundred alcoholics about two-thirds reported experiencing "blackouts".[44] The degree of intoxication does not reliably predict the occurrence of this profound memory loss.[43] Moreover, alcohol-induced periods of amnesia may occur in moderate or heavy drinkers as well as in alcoholics. The frequency of blackout occurrence does appear to correlate with severity of alcoholism, a history of head trauma, malnutrition, and fatigue. It is unlikely that deliberate malingering often accounts for these clinical phenomena.[163] Total loss of memory for significant events is a frightening experience for most patients and "blackouts" do not appear to have any motivational consequences for the maintenance of drinking behavior. The occurrence of blackouts is not necessarily correlated with a history of head trauma. No information is available to rule out the possibility that alcohol-induced blackouts reflect an underlying neuropathological process such as impaired temporal-lobe function which is accentuated by intoxication. Comparable reports of hours or days of amnesia are not a prominent feature of heroin or barbiturate intoxication.

It has been suggested that the "blackout" may be explained in terms of a disruption of "short-term" memory* consolidation by alcohol.[45,163] It is argued that information lost to "short-term" memory would not be available subsequently from "long-term" storage and so could account for a period of global memory loss. The validity of this hypothesis has been the subject of controversy. An alcohol-induced decrement in "short-term" memory function was observed in alcoholics with a clinical history of "blackouts" but not in alcoholics without such a history.[45] However, these findings are inconclusive since no measures of memory function were taken during sobriety and, therefore, it is impossible to establish that memory function did not differ between these two groups before alcohol administration. Another report indicated that alcoholics with a clinical history of blackouts showed "short-term" memory impairment during intoxication but not during sobriety.[163] Since no comparison of the effect of alcohol on memory function in alcoholics *without* a clinical history of blackouts was made, the extent to which blackout history and alcohol may interact uniquely to affect memory function was not determined. A third study compared the performance of alcoholics with and without a clinical history of blackouts, during sobriety, and acute and chronic alcohol intoxication and found no impairment of short-term memory in either group under any condition.[105] It appears that when alcoholic subjects are adequately motivated to perform a task, their

behavioral tolerance for alcohol permits accurate performance, even at very high blood alcohol levels.[105] Visual short-term memory can be disrupted by relatively low doses of alcohol in normal drinkers who lack behavioral tolerance.[12] Data collection on alcoholics with no history of blackouts[159-161] and rhesus monkeys[102] also failed to reveal any direct effect of alcohol on "short-term" memory.

A third form of memory dysfunction associated with alcohol intoxication is the fragmentary absence of recall of some events during a subsequent period of sobriety. In some instances, events during intoxication (e.g., hiding money or alcohol) are only recalled during a subsequent period of intoxication, and therefore fall into the framework of state-dependent effects.[103,132] The observation that behavior learned during a drug state may not occur during a nondrug state, then reoccur during reinstitution of a drug state, has been demonstrated in experimental animals.[132] Simply stated, responses established under specific conditions are most easily elicited once these conditions are re-established. State-dependent dissociation of recall for verbal materials learned during alcohol intoxication has also been shown in normal college students.[46]

Clinically, the dissociative effect of alcohol is most often expressed by a failure to recall aversive consequences of drinking (e.g., depression, anxiety, illness) during a subsequent period of sobriety. Alcohol addicts form positive expectancies about a forthcoming drinking experience, and, following a period of chronic intoxication, they tend to recall their experience in terms of the predrinking expectancy, rather than the events that actually transpired.[99,100,162] The implications of this dissociative phenomena for treatment of the alcoholic were first noted in 1962 by Diethelm and Barr.[24] Patients interviewed under conditions of acute intoxication talked more freely and described emotions, especially guilt and hostility, which they had not discussed during sobriety. Usually these patients forgot the content of these interviews once they became sober again. Traditionally, physicians have

---

* Most concepts of memory function differentiate between a "short-term" registration phase and a "long-term" consolidation phase, with the implication that these are sequential processes required for subsequent information retrieval. A recurrent source of confusion in the short-term memory literature has been the inconsistency in definition of this term. Short-term memory has been variously defined as 1 sec., 5 sec., 1 min., 5 min., and 30 min.

tended to refuse treatment to intoxicated alcoholics. A reevaluation of this principle and an effort to assist patients in integrating feelings expressed during intoxication with self-perception during sobriety could result in more effective psychotherapy for alcoholic individuals.

Sleep Disturbances

There is a prevailing impression that alcohol facilitates sleep. Although this notion is consistent with the usual classification of alcohol as a CNS depressant, it is not supported by electroencephalographic analysis of the effects of alcohol on sleep. It has been generally agreed that "poor sleep" is characterized by a decrease in REM activity and a decrease in stage 4 sleep. It is now well established that acute administration of alcohol does produce a relative suppression of REM activity in normal individuals, alcohol addicts, and experimental animals.[50,67] The effect of alcohol on stage 4 sleep is a controversial issue, but it is agreed that stage 4 is decreased during alcohol withdrawal.[50,67] Sleep of alcoholics is generally light and somewhat fragmented. Such sleep disturbances and insomnia seem to be characteristic symptoms of chronic alcoholism.[67]

There has been considerable interest in the possibility that hallucinations often seen in alcohol addicts during alcohol withdrawal may reflect a REM "overshoot" following a period of alcohol-induced REM suppression. Hughlings Jackson and William James were among the first to suggest the possibility of a neurophysiological continuity between dreaming sleep and waking hallucinatory activity.[34,50] Hallucinosis is sometimes associated with difficulty in discriminating between sleeping and waking states. The idea that REM sleep and dreams are isomorphic is no longer accepted since dreamlike activity has also been reported during non-REM awakenings. However, the hypothesis that REM suppression as a function of chronic alcohol intoxication may facilitate the eruption of hallucinations during withdrawal has received confirmation in several studies of alcohol addicts during a period of *acute* alcohol withdrawal.[50,67] Interpretation of reports of EEG correlates of sleep activity during alcohol withdrawal must be made with caution since it has usually been impossible to obtain adequate baseline sleep measures. Consequently, the high levels of REM activity observed may reflect a combined effect of acute hospitalization and alcohol withdrawal. It is seldom possible to determine the number of hours since the last drink with any degree of accuracy in acute hospital admissions, and this can confuse differential diagnosis of alcoholic hallucinosis versus delirium tremens (see discussion on p. 385).

A recent study of alcohol addicts before, during, and after a period of chronic alcohol consumption did not reveal a consistent REM hyperactivity during alcohol withdrawal.[186] Although hallucinations were frequently associated with an antecedent REM suppression or insomnia, there were no invariant relationships between hallucinosis and REM activity. Also, hallucinations were reported during intoxication as well as during alcohol withdrawal. There were no consistent dose-response relationships between alcohol intake and the subjective intensity of reported dreams or hallucinations.[186] It may be somewhat premature to assume an invariant association between dream-hallucinatory episodes and REM activity, and the drug-suppression-withdrawal overshoot REM hypothesis is currently being reevaluated in several laboratories. Attempts to discern relationships between the presumed physiological accompaniments of the behavioral expressions of intoxication and withdrawal are necessarily restricted by limitations inherent in existing techniques, and the notion of a physiology of dreaming remains a provocative but hypothetical construct.

(Treatment of Acute and Long-Term Alcohol Problems

Treatment for the alcohol-related disorders will be described separately for the acute effects of alcohol intoxication and withdrawal and the chronic phase of the illness. The implications of problems in establishing outcome criteria for current treatment approaches will also be considered in the discussion of treatment evaluation and prevention.

The Treatment Setting

Most physicians treat patients with alcohol-related problems in two clinical situations, each of which involves substantially different problems. In hospital practice, patients are rarely seeking assistance for alcohol problems per se, but are usually under treatment for intercurrent illness associated with alcohol abuse. Therapy is often directed towards solving medical problems of acute illness, with minimal attention to the underlying alcohol problem. Many such patients return to problem drinking once they are discharged from the hospital and then are frequently readmitted with identical or similar disorders.[136,138] This unfortunate recidivism often promotes an attitude of despair in the patient and disdain in the physician and other hospital personnel.

In office practice, despair and disdain are fostered by other factors. Patients seeking aid in this situation generally initiate therapy because of some degree of external coercion. Such coercion may range from threats of an employer to terminate employment to threats of a spouse to end a marriage unless the patient seeks and obtains assistance. In this situation, the patient is usually both frightened and angry and the sum of both conditions is often interpreted by the physician as evidence of lack of motivation to do something about his or her drinking problem. Motivational factors have become so emphasized in diagnosis and therapy that they have frequently been assigned predictive value in determining efficacy of treatment.[16] It is therefore possible for a physician to prematurely assume a poor prognosis for a patient who appears "poorly motivated" and then to employ a "poor-motivation" vs. "good-motivation" dichotomy to account for either success or failure of the treatment provided.[38,78] Since motivational

states are rarely static in patients treated for any disorder, it is obvious that this criterion is not of great value.

Differential Diagnosis

Although there have been significant advances in public perception of alcoholism as a disease rather than evidence of "moral weakness", a severe stigma continues to be associated with this disorder. In most instances, patients with alcohol-related illness recognize this stigma and are reluctant to fully discuss the duration or severity of their drinking problems. Successful case finding and elucidation of past and current problem history taking involve techniques which are common to all psychiatric interviewing procedures. Since these are discussed in other portions of this *Handbook* (see Volume 1, Chapters 53 and 54), they will not be repeated here.

Much attention has been paid to the role of attitudes and values held by physicians in determining their diagnostic approach to patients with alcohol problems.[15] Similar contingencies probably apply to all categories of mental disorders and perpetuation of emphasis on the importance of this issue provides a rationale for accepting or rejecting patients. At the present time, there are no data which specify the optimal qualities, attitudes and approaches in the treating physician as a determinant of treatment outcome.

The process of differential diagnosis for alcohol related problems requires a conceptual approach which has been employed by physicians for many decades in general medicine. In psychiatric practice, this approach often suffers because of lack of basic information about causation and natural history of mental illness. An attempt has recently been made to systematize the diagnostic criteria for alcohol abuse and alcoholism.[125] These criteria include behavioral, physiological, and attitudinal factors, with particular attention to the major illnesses associated with alcoholism and the related patterns of clinical laboratory test abnormalities.[125] Although this system is imperfect, it represents a considerable advance which deserves attention and critical appraisal by physicians.

Treatment of Alcohol Intoxication

There are no effective, readily available means of rapidly reducing the blood-alcohol concentration of a severely intoxicated individual.[176] Although the rate of ethanol metabolism can be increased by fructose administration,[14,90,166] this technique has found little successful clinical application since its discovery thirty-five years ago.[112] Recent explorations of hemodialysis procedures to rapidly reduce blood-alcohol concentrations[173] have limited general applicability because of their expense and potential risk of infection.

Fatal alcohol poisoning is very rare. There are occasional reports of children or adolescents who die of respiratory depression following an overdose of alcohol. However, in view of the many people who drink and the large volumes of alcohol consumed, it must be concluded that alcohol is a relatively safe drug in comparison to the opiate narcotics. It is virtually impossible to drink an acutely toxic amount of alcohol before vomiting or unconsciousness occurs.[126]

The comparative safety of alcohol may also be related to its dual properties as a drug and a food. Alcohol does contain calories and is metabolized like other carbohydrates. The principal enzyme responsible for alcohol metabolism, alcohol dehydrogenase, is ubiquitous in body organs and most highly concentrated in liver.[111] Consequently, the lethal toxic potential of alcohol is counteracted by nature's provision for its rapid degradation.

The recent increase in polydrug abuse requires added caution in treatment of acute intoxication. The concurrent use of several drugs which may act synergistically can result in overdose. Improved techniques for determining the blood concentrations of, e.g., heroin and barbiturates as well as ethanol, can aid the physician in accurate diagnosis. Fast acting pharmacological antagonists are currently available for heroin[64,65] but not for barbiturates or alcohol.

Since acute intoxication in the chronic inebriate is usually complicated by other medical problems (see pp. 385–388) it is essential that the care of afflicted individuals occur in the context of good medical management. Until recently, it has been difficult, especially for impoverished alcoholics, to obtain adequate medical treatment for the acute effects of alcohol. However, it is likely that most of these patients are admitted to hospitals for treatment of acute intoxication under the guise of some other diagnostic criteria.[126,136,138,140]

Following the recent change in the legal status of intoxication and alcoholism in 1966, a number of detoxification centers were established to treat the acute inebriate. While these facilities do provide some resource for patient care, they were seldom established within the mainstream of medical care. Consequently, there is great danger that these centers may become nothing more than a respectable version of the traditional "drying-out" facilities, i.e., the jail or the drunk tank.[9,138]

Treatment of Alcohol Withdrawal

Rather good progress has been made by biomedical scientists in devising new methods for the treatment of the alcohol withdrawal syndrome. Improvements in treatment have occurred primarily because of general advances in medicine which provide more accurate diagnosis and better patient management, i.e., treatment of metabolic disturbances and infections which frequently accompany the abstinence syndrome. Less than twenty years ago, the mortality associated with delirium tremens was reported as about 15 percent in various hospitals and institutions.[170] Today, the incidence of death associated with delirium tremens has fallen to less than 1 percent.[164]

The development of new psychopharmacological agents, particularly the minor tranquilizers, has provided a means of mildly sedating patients and reducing severity of agitation and tremor without compromising the patient's ability to eat well and receive other medical care.[68,168] Chlordiazepoxide (Librium) has been reported to be an effective anti-convulsant in the treatment of withdrawal seizures[68] (see also pp. 383–385).

Treatment of Alcoholism

At present, there is no specific and uniformly efficacious treatment either for the disease of alcoholism or for problem drinking. The treatment techniques that have been used include individual and group psychotherapy, Alcoholics Anonymous, aversive conditioning therapies, Antabuse, vitamin therapies, and LSD treatment, singly or in various combinations. In the few relatively controlled therapy evaluation studies, the rate of improvement or alcohol abstinence following therapy was very low.[177] Since the spontaneous recovery rate for alcoholics has been estimated at about 20 percent,[177] the efficacy of the existing therapies is discouragingly low. These figures compare rather poorly with the improvement rate of heroin addicts treated with methadone, an estimated 70 percent.[37]

The complexities and difficulties involved in treating the chronic alcohol abuser have been thoroughly reviewed by many concerned investigators.* Since all variants of alcoholism are multiply determined, the treatment of alcohol problems presents the challenge of any complex behavioral disorder. The dynamic conceptualizations of an "alcoholic personality" have received no empirical support, and there is considerable heterogeneity on many dimensions, even among the end stage, "skidrow" alcoholics.[103] Although there is no evidence to indicate that alcoholism is invariably associated with a predisposing psychiatric illness, the development of problem drinking rarely occurs in isolation from emotional, interpersonal, and job-related problems. Whatever its origins, alcoholism is characterized by a vast diversity of related difficulties.

The treatment of alcoholism is further complicated by the fact that most people with alcohol problems tend to deny the reality of their illness and to reject treatment. It has been shown that patient acceptance of treatment can be greatly improved if initial hospital contacts are sympathetic and positive.[16] However, physicians have tended to reject alcoholic patients[140] and to avoid diagnosing the problem unless it was glaringly apparent in the terminal phase.[15] Frustration with relapsing patients who deny the significance of their alcohol problems, and limitations of available treatments have contributed to physicians' negative attitudes. The point has often been made that treatment goals for the alcoholic should have limited objectives[15] and a multimodality therapy suited to the needs of the individual and his resources should be offered.[78] The logic of this position is obvious and can be extended to argue for treatment of the alcoholic within the mainstream of medical practice, where the greatest range of medical, psychiatric, and social services is potentially available. However, the question of which treatment will most benefit the patient with alcohol problems remains unanswered. Until there is a better understanding of the disease process of alcoholism, and better treatments available, it is unlikely that the incidence of alcoholism will be greatly reduced, despite the recent improvements in the delivery of health-care services to alcoholics.

The low success rate of current treatment approaches seems to point to the need for an effective pharmacotherapy for alcohol addiction. The recent advances in the treatment of heroin addiction have occurred largely because of the availability of blocking agents or antagonists.[37,64] However, the use of blocking agents for heroin addiction has been criticized because these agents have high addictive potential. An ideal blocking agent for any centrally acting drug of abuse, including alcohol, would have the following characteristics: (1) low addictive potency; (2) little or no synergistic action with other drugs; (3) no central nervous depression or excitatory effects. In essence, the drug of choice for treating alcoholics would be more closely analogous to a narcotic antagonist than a blocking agent. It should be emphasized that the rationale for the use of blocking agents which reduce the subjective effect of a drug is very different from that for the use of Antabuse[64] which produces severe discomfort, and poten-

* See references 4, 9, 38, 91–93, 134, and 177.

tially lethal consequences if taken in combination with alcohol.[93,177]

In view of the wide spectrum of alcohol-related problems, drug therapy alone would not suffice. A variety of other psychological and social interventions would probably be necessary to produce the greatest change in alcoholics with diverse behavioral, biological, and social problems. However, an effective drug therapy would permit other types of therapeutic intervention to occur under conditions where confounding effects of perpetuation of alcohol intake were significantly reduced.

Treatment Evaluation

One of the most important and frequently ignored issues related to the treatment of alcoholism is the problem of evaluation. Unless there are adequate evaluation and follow-up data, it is not possible to demonstrate the efficacy of any treatment approach. One fundamental issue in evaluation is the establishment of valid outcome criteria. The establishment of comprehensive criteria of efficacy which can be uniformly applied to all treatment programs is critical for adequate evaluation. There has been no consensus that the traditional goal of absolute abstinence is the optimal therapeutic goal for the alcoholic.[21,134,135] Indeed, it appears that for many alcohol abusers, giving up drinking completely can also result in severe social and psychological dysfunction.[134,135] There is accumulating evidence that some alcohol addicts may be able to return to social drinking.[21,134,135] The persistent rationale for the treatment criterion of absolute abstinence is based on the erroneous concept of "craving", which is discussed under Psychological Dependence, p. 382.

Once outcome criteria have been formulated, construction of an adequate clinical research design assumes paramount importance. Traditionally, it has been argued that clinical research cannot yield "hard data" because of the complexity of the dependent variables, the difficulties in controlling relevant factors as well as ethical constraints.[91] It is curious that the expectancy for objectivity, sophistication, and accuracy in basic research has not been extended to treatment research. A lack of these qualities in the laboratory would have severe consequences for research development, and it could be argued that casual evaluation of treatment programs could have even more profound consequences for longevity and quality of human life. It does not seem unreasonable to require an even more precise specification of methods and outcome criteria for treatment programs which involve human beings than for isolated physical and chemical studies involving *in vitro* biochemical constituents. Enthusiastic testimonials by proponents of a particular treatment approach are too often substituted for adequate data. Awareness of the difficulties attendant on clinical treatment research should not constitute an excuse for neglecting or evading basic tenets of experimental design.[91] A lucid summary and discussion of basic requirements for the design of clinical research has recently been prepared by Ludwig.[91]

Prevention

There is little question that the best treatment for any disorder is prevention, and significant emphasis has been placed on public education concerning use hazards in virtually all drug-abuse areas. Evaluation of the impact of such public education and prevention efforts is extremely difficult. The problem is complicated by the lack of good data on the incidence and prevalence of alcohol abuse and alcoholism, and the many difficulties associated with adequate case finding (see discussion on pp. 374–376). In the absence of firm incidence data, it is difficult to demonstrate conclusively that public-education programs or attempts to shape attitudes have had a significant impact on alcohol-abuse problems. Some preliminary evidence suggests that naive programs of public education and attitude shaping may sometimes prompt exploration and thereby increase the incidence of drug-abuse-related problems. Unfortunately, problem drinking usually occurs in situations where behavior is not determined by logical thinking, but rather by internal and external stress-contingent factors which are not highly amenable to rational persuasion. People with well-established alcohol related problems may be unresponsive to reminders that a certain pattern of drinking can be dangerous to their health. There is probably no substitute for the early development of responsible attitudes about alcohol use and awareness of the nature of alcohol problems.

Prevention techniques designed to change attitudes are quite distinct from coercive efforts to control distribution of alcohol or to prevent some individuals from drinking through imposition of age limits, etc. Attempts to control alcoholism through prohibition were a dramatic and unequivocal failure.[51] There has been little systematic study of the effects of increased taxation or restricted hours for bars and liquor stores in areas where these techniques have been applied. It is often argued that consumption of low-alcohol-content beverages such as beer may prevent alcoholism. This argument is somewhat misleading in that consumption of large enough quantities of a 6-percent alcohol beverage can yield an alcohol intake equivalent to that of the distilled spirits drinker. Physical dependence upon alcohol has been seen in individuals who consume large quantities of beer and wine.

Until there is a better understanding of the many factors which contribute to the development and maintenance of alcohol abuse, it will be difficult to formulate more effective approaches to the prevention and treatment of alcoholism.

⟪ Bibliography

1. BACON, S. D., ed. "Studies of Drinking and Driving," *Q. J. Stud. Alcohol*, Suppl. no. 4 (1968), 1–10.
2. BELFER, M. L., R. I. SHADER, M. CARROL et al. "Alcoholism in Women," *Arch. Gen. Psychiatry*, 25 (1971), 540–544.
3. BLOOMQUIST, E. R. "Addiction, Addicting Drugs and the Anesthesiologist," *JAMA*, 171 (1959), 518–523.
4. BLUM, E. M. and R. H. BLUM. *Alcoholism: Modern Psychological Approaches to Treatment*. San Francisco: Jossey-Bass, 1967.
5. BOSTON UNIVERSITY LAW-MEDICINE INSTITUTE. *Legal Issues in Alcoholism and Alcohol Usage*. Boston University Law-Medicine Inst. Proc., 1965.
6. CADMAN, T. E. and L. B. RORKE. "Central Pontine Myelinolysis in Childhood and Adolescence," *Arch. Dis. Child.*, 44 (1969), 342–350.
7. CAHALAN, D. *Problem Drinkers*. San Francisco: Jossey-Bass, 1970.
8. CAHALAN, D., I. H. CISIN, and H. M. CROSSLEY. *American Drinking Practices: A National Study of Drinking Behavior and Attitudes*, Monogr. no. 6. New Brunswick, N.J.: Rutgers Center of Alcohol Studies, 1969.
9. CAHN, S. *The Treatment of Alcoholics: An Evaluative Study*. New York: Oxford University Press, 1970.
10. CAMERON, D. C. "Abuse of Alcohol and Drugs: Concepts and Planning," *WHO Chron.*, 25 (1971), 8–16.
11. CARPENTER, J. A. "Effects of Alcohol on Some Psychological Processes," *Q. J. Stud. Alcohol*, 23 (1962), 274–314.
12. CARPENTER, J. A. and B. M. Ross. "Effect of Alcohol on Short-Term Memory," *Q. J. Stud. Alcohol*, 26 (1965), 561–579.
13. CARPENTER, T. M. "The Metabolism of Alcohol: A Review," *Q. J. Stud. Alcohol*, 1 (1940), 201–226.
14. CARPENTER, T. M. and R. C. LEE. "The Effects of Glucose on the Metabolism of Ethyl Alcohol in Man," *J. Pharmacol. Exp. Ther.*, 60 (1937), 264–285.
15. CHAFETZ, M. E. "The Prevention of Alcoholism," *Int. J. Psychiatry*, 9 (1970–71), 329–348.
16. CHAFETZ, M. E., H. T. BLANE, H. S. ABRAM et al. "Establishing Treatment Relations With Alcoholics," *J. Nerv. Ment. Dis.*, 134 (1962), 395–409.
17. CHASON, J. L., R. W. LANDERS, and J. E. GONZALEZ. "Central Pontine Myelinolysis," *J. Neurol. Neurosurg. Psychiatry*, 27 (1964), 317–325.
18. CHATURACHINDA, K. and E. M. McGREGOR. "Wernicke's Encephalopathy and Pregnancy," *J. Obstet. Gynaecol. Br. Commonw.*, 75 (1968), 969–971.
19. COCHIN, J. "The Pharmacology of Addiction to Narcotics," in G. J. Martin and B. Kisch, eds., *Enzymes in Mental Health*, pp. 27–

42. Philadelphia: Lippincott, 1966.

20. COLLINS, J. R. "Major Medical Problems in Alcoholic Patients," in J. H. Mendelson, ed., *Alcoholism*, Vol. 3, pp. 189–214. International Psychiatry Clinics. Boston: Little, Brown, 1966.

21. DAVIS, D. L. "Normal Drinking in Recovered Alcohol Addicts," *Q. J. Stud. Alcohol*, 23 (1962), 94–104.

22. DENEAU, G., T. YANAGITA, and M. H. SEEVERS. "Self Administration of Psychoactive Substances by the Monkey," *Psychopharmacologia*, 16 (1969), 30–48.

23. DEPARTMENT OF HEALTH, EDUCATION, AND WELFARE. *Alcohol and Health*, First Special Report to Congress, Publ. no. DHEW 72-9009. Washington: U.S. Govt. Print. Off., 1971.

24. DIETHELM, O. and R. M. BARR. "Psychotherapeutic Interviews and Alcohol Intoxication," *Q. J. Stud. Alcohol*, 23 (1962), 243–251.

25. DOCTOR, R. G., P. NAITOH, and J. C. SMITH. "Electroencephalographic Changes and Vigilance Behavior during Experimentally Induced Intoxication with Alcoholic Subjects," *Psychosom. Med.*, 28 (1966), 605–615.

26. DREYFUS, P. M. "Diseases of the Nervous System in Chronic Alcoholics," in B. Kissin and H. Begleiter, eds., The Biology of Alcoholism, Vol. 3, pp. 265–290. *Clinical Pathology*. New York: Plenum, 1974.

27. ELLIS, F. W. and J. R. PICK. "Ethanol Intoxication and Dependence in Rhesus Monkeys," in N. K. Mello and J. H. Mendelson, eds., *Recent Advances in Studies of Alcoholism*, Publ. no. (HSM) 71-9045, pp. 401–412. Washington: U.S. Govt. Print. Off.. 1971.

28. ENOCH, B. A. and D. M. WILLIAMS. "An Association Between Wernicke's Encephalopathy and Thyrotoxicosis," *Postgrad. Med. J.*, 44 (1968), 923–930.

29. ESSIG, C. F. "'Alcohol and Related Addicting Drugs," in R. J. Catanzaro, ed., *Alcoholism, the Total Treatment Approach*, pp. 58–69. Springfield, Ill.: Charles C. Thomas, 1968.

30. ESSIG, C. F. and R. C. LAM. "Convulsions and Hallucinatory Behavior Following Alcohol Withdrawal in the Dog," *Arch. Neurol.*, 18 (1968), 626–632.

31. EWING, J. A., B. A. ROUSE, and E. D. PELLIZZARI. "Alcohol Sensitivity and Ethnic Background," *Am. J. Psychiatry*, 131 (1974), 206–210.

32. FALK, J. L. "Behavioral Maintenance of High Blood Ethanol and Physical Dependence in the Rat," *Science*, 177 (1972), 811–813.

33. FEINBERG, I. "Hallucinations, Dreaming and REM Sleep," in W. Keup, ed., *Origins and Mechanisms of Hallucinations*, pp. 125–132. New York: Plenum, (1970).

34. FEINBERG, I. and E. V. EVARTS. "Some Implications of Sleep Research for Psychiatry," in J. Zubin and C. Shagass, eds., *Neurobiological Aspects of Psychopathology*, pp. 334–393. New York: Grune & Stratton, (1969).

35. FISHER, C. M. "Residual Neuropathological Changes in Canadians Held Prisoners of War by the Japanese," *Can. Serv. Med. J.*, 11 (1955), 157–199.

36. FORBES, R. J. *Short History of the Art of Distillation*. Leiden, Netherlands: E. J. Brill, 1948.

37. GEARING, F. R. *Successes and Failures in Methadone Maintenance Treatment of Heroin Addiction in New York City*, Proc. of the 3rd Natl. Conf. on Methadone Treatment, NAPAN-NIMH, PHS Publ. no. 2172. Washington: U.S. Govt. Print. Off., 1970.

38. GERARD, D. L. and G. SAENGER. *Out-Patient Treatment of Alcoholism*, Brookside Monogr. no. 4. Toronto: University of Toronto Press, 1966.

39. GINSBERG, H., J. OLEFSKY, J. W. FARQUHAR et al. "Moderate Ethanol Ingestion and Plasma Triglyceride Levels," *Ann. Intern. Med.*, 80 (1974), 143–149.

40. GOLDSTEIN, A., L. ARANOW, and S. M. KALMAN. *Principles of Drug Action*. New York: Harper & Row, 1968.

41. GOODWIN, D. W. "Is Alcoholism Hereditary? A Review and Critique," *Arch. Gen. Psychiatry*, 25 (1971), 545–549.

42. ———. "Alcohol in Suicide and Homicide," *Q. J. Stud. Alcohol*, 34 (1973), 144–156.

43. GOODWIN, D. W., J. B. CRANE, and S. B. GUZE. "Phenomenological Aspects of the Alcoholic Blackout," *Br. J. Psychiatry*, 115 (1969), 1033–1038.

44. ———. "Alcoholic Blackouts: A Review and Clinical Study of 100 Alcoholics," *Am. J. Psychiatry*, 126 (1969), 191–198.

45. GOODWIN, D. W., E. OTHMER, J. A. HALI-

KAS et al. "Loss of Short Term Memory as a Predictor of the Alcoholic 'Blackout'," *Nature*, 227 (1970), 201–202.

46. GOODWIN, D. W., B. POWELL, D. BREMER et al. "Alcohol and Recall: State-Dependent Effects in Man," *Science*, 163 (1969), 1358–1360.

47. GOODWIN, D. W., F. SCHULSINGER, L. HERMANSEN et al. "Alcohol Problems in Adoptees Raised Apart From Alcoholic Biological Parents," *Arch. Gen. Psychiatry*, 28 (1973), 238–243.

48. GRENELL, R. G. "Alcohols and Activity of Cerebral Neurons," *Q. J. Stud. Alcohol*, 29 (1959), 421–427.

49. GROSS, M. M., E. LEWIS, and J. HASTEY. "Acute Alcohol Withdrawal Syndrome," in B. Kissin and H. Begleiter, eds., The Biology of Alcoholism, Vol. 3, pp. 191–263. *Clinical Pathology*, New York: Plenum, 1974.

50. GROSS, M. M., D. R. GOODENOUGH, J. HASTEY et al. "Sleep Disturbances in Alcohol Intoxication and Withdrawal," in N. K. Mello and J. H. Mendelson, eds., *Recent Advances in Studies of Alcoholism*, Publ. no. (HSM) 71-9045, pp. 317–397. Washington: U.S. Govt. Print. Off., 1971.

51. GUSFIELD, J. R. "Status Conflicts and the Changing Ideologies of the American Temperance Movement," in D. J. Pittman and C. R. Snyder, eds., *Society, Culture and Drinking Patterns*, pp. 101–120. New York: Wiley, 1962.

52. HAGGARD, H. W., L. A. GREENBERG, and G. LOLLI. "The Absorption of Alcohol with Special Reference to Its Influence on the Concentration of Alcohol Appearing in the Blood," *Q. J. Stud. Alcohol*, 1 (1941), 684.

53. HARGER, R. N. and H. R. HULPIEU. "The Pharmacology of Alcohol," in G. N. Thompson, ed., *Alcoholism*, pp. 103–232. Springfield, Ill.: Charles C. Thomas, 1956.

54. HEATON, J. M., A. J. McCORMICK, and A. G. FREEMAN. "Tobacco Amblyopia: A Clinical Manifestation of Vitamin B_{12} Deficiency," *Lancet*, 2 (1958), 286–290.

55. HOWE, L. P. and V. D. PATCH. "Rehabilitating the Tuberculosis Alcoholic," Final Report: Research Study no. RD-2138-P. Washington: Social and Rehabilitative Service, DHEW, 1971.

56. IBER, F., R. M. KATER, and N. CARULI. "Differences in the Rate of Ethanol Metabolism in Recently Drinking Alcoholic and Non-Drinking Subjects," *Am. J. Clin. Nutr.*, 22 (1969), 1608–1617.

57. IRONSIDE, R., F. D. BOSANQUET, and W. H. McMENEMEY. "Central Demyelination of the Corpus Collosum (Marchiafava-Bignami Disease); With a Report of a Second Case in Great Britain," *Brain*, 84 (1961), 212–230.

58. ISBELL, H., H. FRASER, A. WIKLER et al. "An Experimental Study of the Etiology of Rum Fits and Delirium Tremens," *Q. J. Stud. Alcohol*, 16 (1955), 1–33.

59. ISHIZAKI, T., H. CHITANONDH, and U. LAKSANAVICHARN. "Marchiafava-Bignami's Disease: Report of the First Case in an Asian," *Acta Neuropathol.*, 16 (1970), 187–193.

60. ISRAEL, Y. and J. MARDONES, eds., *Biological Basis of Alcoholism*. New York: Wiley-Interscience, 1971.

61. ISSELBACHER, K. J. and E. A. CARTER. "Effect of Alcohol on Liver and Intestinal Function," in N. K. Mello and J. H. Mendelson, eds., *Recent Advances in Studies of Alcoholism*, Publ. no. (HSM) 71-9045, pp. 42–58. Washington: U.S. Govt. Print. Off., 1971.

62. ISSELBACHER, K. J. and N. J .GREENBERGER. "Metabolic Effects of Alcohol on the Liver," *N. Engl. J. Med.*, 270 (1964), 351–356, 402–410.

63. JACOBSEN, E. "The Metabolism of Ethyl Alcohol," *Pharmacol. Rev.*, 4 (1952), 107–135.

64. JAFFE, J. H. "Psychopharmacology and Opiate Dependence," in D. H. Efron, ed., *Psychopharmacology: A Review of Progress 1957–1967*, PHS Publ. no. 1836, pp. 853–864. Washington: U.S. Govt. Print. Off., 1968.

65. ———. "Drug Addiction and Drug Abuse," in L. S. Goodman and A. Gilman, eds., *The Pharmacological Basis of Therapeutics*, pp. 276–313. New York: Macmillan, 1970.

66. JELLINEK, E. M. *The Disease Concept of Alcoholism*. Highland Park, N.J.: Hillhouse Press, 1960.

67. JOHNSON, L. C. "Sleep Patterns in Chronic Alcoholics," in N. K. Mello and J. H. Mendelson, eds., *Recent Advances in Studies of Alcoholism*, Publ. no. (HSM) 71-9045, pp. 288–316. Washington: U.S. Govt. Print. Off., 1971.

68. KAIM, S. "Drug Treatment of the Alcohol Withdrawal Syndrome," in N. K. Mello and

J. H. Mendelson, eds., *Recent Advances in Studies of Alcoholism*, Publ. no. (HSM) 71-9045, pp. 767–780. Washington: U.S. Govt. Print. Off., 1971.

69. KALANT, H. "Effects of Ethanol on the Nervous System," in J. Tremolieres, ed., International Encyclopedia of Pharmacology and Therapy, Sect. 20, Vol. 1. *Alcohols and Derivatives*. New York: Pergamon, 1970.

70. ———. "Absorption Diffusion, Distribution and Elimination of Ethanol: Effects on Biological Membranes," in B. Kissin and H. Begleiter, eds., The Biology of Alcoholism, Vol. 1, pp. 1–62, *Biochemistry*. New York: Plenum, 1971.

71. KALANT, H., A. E. LeBLANC, and R. J. GIBBINS. "Tolerance To, and Dependence On Some Non-Opiate Psychotropic Drugs," *Pharmacol. Rev.*, 23 (1971), 135–191.

72. KATER, R. M. H., D. ZEIVE, F. TOBIN et al. "Heavy Drinking Accelerates Drugs' Breakdown in Liver," *JAMA*, 206 (1968), 1709.

73. KEEPING, J. A. and C. W. A. SEARLE. "Optic Neuritis Following Isonaizid Therapy," *Lancet*, 2 (1955), 278.

74. KELLER, M. "The Definition of Alcoholism and the Estimation of Its Prevalence," in D. J. Pittman and G. R. Snyder, eds., *Society, Culture and Drinking Patterns*, pp. 310–329. New York: Wiley, 1962.

75. ———. "On the Loss-of-Control Phenomenon in Alcoholism," *Br. J. Addict.*, 67 (1972), 153–166.

76. KING, J. H. JR., and J. W. PASSMORE. "Nutritional Amblyopia: A Study of American Prisoners of War in Korea," *Am. J. Opthalmol.*, 39 (1955), 173–186.

77. KISSIN, B. and H. BEGLEITER, eds. The Biology of Alcoholism, Vol. 1. *Biochemistry*, 1971; Vol. 2. *Physiology and Behavior*, 1972. New York: Plenum.

78. KISSIN, B., A. PLATZ, and W. H. SU. "Selective Factors in Treatment Choice and Outcome in Alcoholics," in N. K. Mello and J. H. Mendelson, eds., *Recent Advances in Studies of Alcoholism*, Publ. no. (HSM) 71-9045, pp. 781–802. Washington: U.S. Govt. Print. Off., 1971.

79. KNUPFER, G. "Some Methodological Problems in the Epidemiology of Alcoholic Beverage Usage: Definition of Amount of Intake," *Am. J. Public Health*, 2 (1966), 237–242.

80. LANDERS, J. W., J. L. CHASON, and V. N. SAMUEL. "Central Pontine Myelinolysis: A Pathogenic Hypothesis," *Neurology*, 15 (1965), 968–971.

81. LEAKE, C. D. and M. SILVERMAN. *Alcoholic Beverages in Clinical Medicine*. Chicago: Yearbook Medical Publishers, 1966.

82. ———. "The Chemistry of Alcoholic Beverages," in B. Kissin and H. Begleiter, eds., The Biology of Alcoholism, Vol. 1. *Biochemistry*, pp. 575–612. New York: Plenum, 1971.

83. LEE, T. K., M. H. CHO, and A. B. DOBKIN. "Effects of Alcoholism, Morphinism, and Barbiturate Resistance on Induction and Maintenance of General Anesthesia," *Can. Anaesth. Soc. J.*, 1 (1964), 354–381.

84. LIEBER, C. S. "Alcohol and the Liver," in E. E. Bittar, ed., *The Biological Basis of Medicine*, Vol. 5, pp. 317–344. London: Academic, 1969.

85. LIEBER, C. S., E. RUBIN, and L. M. De-CARLI. "Chronic and Acute Effects of Ethanol on Hepatic Metabolism of Ethanol, Lipids and Drugs: Correlation with Ultrastructural Changes," in N. K. Mello and J. H. Mendelson, eds., *Recent Advances in Studies of Alcoholism*, Publ. no. (HSM) 71-9045, pp. 3–41. Washington: U.S. Govt. Print. Off., 1971.

86. LIEBMANN, A. J. and B. SCHERL. "Changes in Whiskey While Maturing," *Ind. Eng. Chem.*, 41 (1949), 534.

87. LINDENBAUM, J. and C. S. LIEBER, "Effects of Ethanol on the Blood, Bone Marrow, and Small Intestine of Man," in M. K. Roach, W. M. McIsaac, and P. J. Creaven, eds., *Biological Aspects of Alcohol*, pp. 27–53. Austin, Texas: University of Texas Press, 1971.

88. LOLLI, G. and L. MESCHIERI. "Mental and Physical Efficiency After Wine and Ethanol Solutions Ingested on an Empty and on a Full Stomach," *Q. J. Stud. Alcohol.*, 25 (1964), 535–540.

89. LOPEZ, R. I. and G. H. COLLINS. "Wernicke's Encephalopathy. A Complication of Chronic Hemodialysis," *Arch. Neurol.*, 18 (1968), 248–259.

90. LOWENSTEIN, L. M., R. SIMONE, P. BOULTER et al. "The Effect of Fructose on Blood Ethanol Concentrations in Man," *JAMA*, 213 (1970), 1899–1901.

91. LUDWIG, A. M. "The Design of Clinical Studies in Treatment Efficacy," in M. E.

Chafetz, ed., *Proc. 1st Annual Alcoholism Conf. N.I.A.A.A.*, DHEW no. (HSM) 73-9074. Washington: U.S. Govt. Print. Off., 1973.

92. LUDWIG, A. M., J. LEVINE, and L. H. STARK. *LSD and Alcoholism.* Springfield, Ill.: Charles C. Thomas, 1970.

93. LUNDWALL, L. and F. BAEKELAND. "Disulfiram Treatment of Alcoholism," *J. Nerv. Ment. Dis.*, 153 (1971), 381–394.

94. MANCALL, E. L. and W. J. McENTEE. "Alterations of the Cerebellar Cortex in Nutritional Encephalopathy," *Neurology*, 15 (1965), 303–313.

95. MARCHIAFAVA, E. and A. BIGNAMI. "Sopra Un'Alterazione del Corpo Calloso Osservata in Soggetti Alcoolisti," *Riv. Patol. Nerv. Ment.*, 8 (1903), 544–549.

96. MARDONES, J. "The Alcohols," in W. S. Root and F. G. Hofmann, eds., *Physiological Pharmacology.* New York: Academic, 1963.

97. MAYER, R. F. "Peripheral Nerve Conduction in Alcoholics," *Psychosom. Med.*, 28 (1966), 475–483.

98. McCORMICK, W. F. and C. M. DANNEEL. "Central Pontine Myelinolysis," *Arch. Intern. Med.*, 119 (1967), 444–478.

99. McGUIRE, M. T., J. H. MENDELSON, and S. STEIN. "Comparative Psychosocial Studies of Alcoholic and Non-Alcoholic Subjects Undergoing Experimentally-Induced Ethanol Intoxication," *Psychosom. Med.*, 28 (1966), 13–26.

100. McNAMEE, H. B., N. K. MELLO, and J. H. MENDELSON. "Experimental Analysis of Drinking Patterns of Alcoholics: Concurrent Psychiatric Observations," *Am. J. Psychiatry*, 124 (1968), 1063–1069.

101. MELLO, N. K. "Some Aspects of the Behavioral Pharmacology of Alcohol," in D. H. Efron, ed., *Psychopharmacology: A Review of Progress 1957–67*, PHS Publ. no. 1863, pp. 787–809. Washington: U.S. Govt. Print. Off., 1968.

102. ———. "Alcohol Effects on Delayed Matching to Sample Performance by Rhesus Monkey," *Physiol. Behav.*, 7 (1971), 77–101.

103. ———. "Behavioral Studies of Alcoholism," in B. Kissin and H. Begleiter, eds., The Biology of Alcoholism, Vol. 2. *Physiology and Behavior*, pp. 219–291. New York: Plenum, 1972.

104. ———. "A Review of Methods to Induce Alcohol Addiction in Animals," *Pharmacol. Biochem. Behav.*, 1 (1973), 89–101.

105. ———. "Short-Term Memory Function in Alcohol Addicts During Intoxication," in M. M. Gross, ed., *Alcohol Intoxication and Withdrawal: Experimental Studies*, Proc. 30th Int. Congr. on Alcoholism and Drug Dependence pp. 333–344. New York: Plenum, 1973.

106. ———. "A Semantic Aspect of Alcoholism," in H. D. Cappell and A. E. Leblanc, eds., *International Symposium on Alcohol and Drug Research.* Toronto: Addiction Research Foundation, forthcoming.

107. MELLO, N. K. and J. H. MENDELSON. "Experimentally-Induced Intoxication in Alcoholics: A Comparison Between Programmed and Spontaneous Drinking," *J. Pharmacol. Exp. Therap.*, 173 (1970), 101–116.

108. ———. "Drinking Patterns During Work-Contingent and Non-Contingent Alcohol Acquisition," *Psychosom. Med.*, 34 (1972), 139–164.

109. MENDELSON, J. H., ed. "Experimentally-Induced Chronic Intoxication and Withdrawal in Alcoholics," *Q. J. Stud. Alcohol*, Suppl. 2 (1964).

110. ———. "Ethanol-1-C^{14} Metabolism in Alcoholics and Non-Alcoholics," *Science*, 159 (1968), 319–320.

111. ———. "Biochemical Pharmacology of Alcohol," in D. H. Efron, ed., *Psychopharmacology: A Review of Progress 1957–67*, PHS Publ. no. 1836, pp. 769–785. Washington: U.S. Govt. Print. Off., 1968.

112. ———. "Biological Concomitants of Alcoholism," *N. Engl. J. Med.*, 283 (1970), 24–32, 71–81.

113. ———. "Biochemical Mechanisms of Alcohol Addiction," in B. Kissin and H. Begleiter, eds., The Biology of Alcoholism, Vol. 1, *Biochemistry*, pp. 513–544. New York: Plenum, 1971.

114. MENDELSON, J. H. and N. K. MELLO. "Alcohol-Induced Hyperlipidemia and Beta Lipoproteins," *Science*, 180 (1973), 1372–1374.

115. ———. "Alcohol, Aggression and Androgens," *Proc. Assoc. Res. Nerv. Ment. Dis.*, 52 (1974), 225–247.

116. ———. "Plasma Testosterone Levels During Chronic Heroin Use and Protracted Abstinence," *Pharmacologist*, 16 (1974), 193 (Abstract 020).

117. MENDELSON, J. H., J. E. MENDELSON, and V. D. PATCH. "Plasma Testosterone Levels in Heroin Addiction and During Methadone Maintenance," *J. Pharmacol. Exp. Therapeutics*, 192 (1975), 211–217.

118. MENDELSON, J. H., M. OGATA, and N. K. MELLO. "Effects of Alcohol Ingestion and Withdrawal on Magnesium States of Alcoholics: Clinical and Experimental Findings," *Ann. N.Y. Acad. Sci.*, 162 (1969), 918–933.

119. MENDELSON, J. H. and S. STEIN. "The Definition of Alcoholism," in J. H. Mendelson, ed., *Alcoholism*, Vol. 3, pp. 3–16. International Psychiatry Clinics. Boston: Little, Brown, 1966.

120. MENDELSON, J. H., S. STEIN, and N. K. MELLO. "Effects of Experimentally-Induced Intoxication on Metabolism of Ethanol-1-C^{14} in Alcoholic Subjects," *Metabolism*, 14 (1965), 1255–1266.

121. MENDELSON, J., D. WEXLER, P. LEIDERMAN et al. "A Study of Addiction to Nonethyl Alcohols and Other Poisonous Compounds," *Q. J. Stud. Alcohol*, 18 (1957), 561–580.

122. MULFORD, H. A. "Drinking and Deviant Drinking," *Q. J. Stud. Alcohol*, 25 (1964), 634–650.

123. MYERSON, R. M. "Effects of Alcohol on Cardiac and Muscular Function," in Y. Israel and J. Mardones, eds., *Biological Basis of Alcoholism*, pp. 183–208. New New York: Wiley-Interscience, 1971.

124. NATHAN, P. E.. N. A. TITLER, L. M. LOWENSTEIN et al. "Behavioral Analysis of Chronic Alcoholism," *Arch. Gen. Psychiatry*, 22 (1970), 419–430.

125. NATIONAL COUNCIL ON ALCOHOLISM. "Criteria for the Diagnosis of Alcoholism," *Am. J. Psychiatry*, 129 (1972), 127–135.

126. NATIONAL INSTITUTE OF MENTAL HEALTH. *Alcohol and Alcoholism*, PHS Publ. no. 1640. Washington: U.S. Govt. Print. Off., 1968.

127. NEVILLE, J. N., J. A. EAGLES, G. SAMSON et al. "Nutritional Status of Alcoholics," *Am. J. Clin. Nutr.*, 21 (1968), 1329–1340.

128. NEWMAN, H. W. "Acquired Tolerance to Ethyl Alcohol," *Q. J. Stud. Alcohol*, 2 (1941), 453–463.

129. NEWMAN, H. W. and M. ABRAMSON. "Absorption of Various Alcoholic Beverages," *Science*, 96 (1942), 43.

130. ———. "Some Factors Influencing the Intoxicating Effect of Alcoholic Beverages," *Q. J. Stud. Alcohol*, 3 (1942), 351–370.

131. OGATA, M., J. H. MENDELSON, and N. K. MELLO. "Electrolytes and Osmolality in Alcoholics During Experimentally-Induced Intoxication," *Psychosom. Med.*, 30 (1968), 463–488.

132. OVERTON, D. A. "State-Dependent Learning Produced by Alcohol and Its Relevance to Alcoholism," in B. Kissin and H. Begleiter, eds., The Biology of Alcoholism, Vol. 2. *Physiology and Behavior*, pp. 193–217. New York: Plenum, 1972.

133. PANT, S. S., A. N. BHARGAVA, M. M. SINGH et al. "Myelopathy in Hepatic Cirrhosis," *Br. Med. J.*, 5337 (1963), 1064–1065.

134. PATTISON, E. M. "A Critique of Alcoholism Treatment Concepts; With Special Reference to Abstinence," *Q. J. Stud. Alcohol*, 27 (1966), 49–71.

135. PATTISON, E. M., E. B. HEADLEY, G. C. GLESER et al. "Abstinence and Normal Drinking," *Q. J. Stud. Alcohol*, 29 (1968), 610–633.

136. PEARSON, W. S. "The 'Hidden' Alcoholic in the General Hospital. A Study of 'Hidden' Alcoholism in White Male Patients Admitted for Unrelated Complaints," *N.C. Med. J.*, 23 (1960), 6–10.

137. PIEPER, W. A., J. J. SKEEN, H. M. MCCLURE et al. "The Chimpanzee as an Animal Model for Investigating Alcoholism," *Science*, 176 (1972), 71–73.

138. PITTMAN, D. J. and C. W. GORDON. *Revolving Door: A Study of the Chronic Police Case Inebriate*, Monogr. no. 2. New Brunswick, N.J.: Rutgers Center for Alcohol Studies, 1958.

139. PITTMAN, D. J. and C. R. SNYDER. *Society, Culture and Drinking Patterns*. New York: Wiley, 1962.

140. PLAUT, T. F. A. *Alcohol Problems: A Report to the National Cooperative Commission on the Study of Alcoholism*. New York: Oxford University Press, 1967.

141. ROACH, M. K., W. M. MCISAAC, and P. J. CREAVEN. eds., *Biological Aspects of Alcoholism*. Austin, Texas: University of Texas Press, 1971.

142. ROBBINS, E., G. MURPHY, R. WILKENSON et al. "Some Clinical Considerations in the Prevention of Suicide Based on a Study of 134 Successful Suicides," *Am. J. Public Health*, 49 (1959), 888–899.

143. ROBINS, L. N. and S. B. GUZE. "Drinking Practices and Problems in Urban Ghetto Populations," in N. K. Mello and J. H. Mendelson, eds., *Recent Advances in Studies of Alcoholism*, Publ. no. (HSM) 71-9045, pp. 825–842. Washington: U.S. Govt. Print. Off., 1971.

144. ROUECHE, B. *The Neutral Spirit: A Portrait of Alcohol*. Boston: Little, Brown, 1960.

145. RUBIN, E., H. GANG, P. MISRA et al. "Inhibition of Drug Metabolism by Acute Ethanol Intoxication: A Hepatic Microsomal Mechanism," *Am. J. Med.*, 49 (1970), 800–806.

146. RUBIN, E. and C. S. LIEBER. "Alcohol-Induced Hepatic Injury in Nonalcoholic Volunteers," *N. Engl. J. Med.*, 278 (1968), 869–876.

147. SCHAPIRO, H., L. D. WRUBLE, and L. G. BRITT. "The Possible Mechanism of Alcohol in the Production of Acute Pancreatitis," *Surgery*, 60 (1966), 1108–1111.

148. SCHUCKIT, M. A., D. A. GOODWIN, and G. WINOKUR. "A Study of Alcoholism in Half Siblings," *Am. J. Psychiatry*, 128 (1972), 1132–1136.

149. SEEVERS, M. H. and G. A. DENEAU. "Physiological Aspects of Tolerance and Physical Dependence," in W. S. Root and F. G. Hofman, eds., *Physiological Pharmacology*, pp. 565–640. New York: Academic, 1963.

150. SEIXAS, F. A. and S. EGGLESTON, eds. "Alcoholism and the Central Nervous System," *Ann. NY. Acad. Sci.*, 215 (1973).

151. SHURTLIFF, L. F., E. T. AJAX, E. ENGLERT et al. "Central Pontine Myelinolysis and Cirrhosis of the Liver," *Am. J. Clin. Pathol.*, 46 (1966), 239–244.

152. SMITH, A. A. "Inhibitors of Tolerance Development," in D. H. Clouet, ed., *Narcotic Drugs: Biochemical Pharmacology*, pp. 424–431. New York: Plenum, 1971.

153. SMITH, D. A. and M. F. A. WOODRUFF. *Deficiency Diseases in Japanese Prison Camps*, Medical Research Council, Special Report Series, no. 274. London: Her Majesty's Stationery Office, 1951.

154. SPODICK, D. H., V. M. PIGOTT, and R. CHIRIFE. "Preclinical Cardiac Malfunction in Chronic Alcoholism," *N. Eng. J. Med.*, 287 (1972), 677–680.

155. SUNDBY, P. *Alcoholism and Mortality*, Publ. no. 6. Oslo, Norway: The National Institute for Alcohol Research, 1967.

156. SUTTON, T. *Tracts on Delirium Tremens, on Peritonitis and Other Inflammatory Afflictions*. London: Thomas Underwood, 1813.

157. SYDENSTRICKER, V. P. and E. S. ARMSTRONG. "Review of 440 Cases of Pellagra," *Arch. Intern. Med.*, 59 (1937), 883–891.

158. TALLAND, G. A. *Deranged Memory*. New York: Academic, 1965.

159. ———. "Effects of Alcohol on Performance on Continuous Attention Tasks," *Psychosom. Med.*, 28 (1966), 596–604.

160. TALLAND, G. A., J. H. MENDELSON, and P. RYACK. "Experimentally-Induced Chronic Intoxication and Withdrawal in Alcoholics. Pt. 4, Tests of Motor Skills," *Q. J. Stud. Alcohol*, Suppl. 2 (1964), 53–73.

161. ———. "Experimentally-Induced Chronic Intoxication and Withdrawal in Alcoholics. Pt. 5, Tests of Attention," *Q. J. Stud. Alcohol*, Suppl. 2 (1964), 74–86.

162. TAMERIN, J. S., S. WEINER, and J. H. MENDELSON. "Alcoholics' Expectancies and Recall of Experiences during Intoxication," *Am. J. Psychiatry*, 126 (1970), 1697–1704.

163. TAMERIN, J. S., S. WEINER, R. POPPEN et al. "Alcohol and Memory: Amnesia and Short-Term Function during Experimentally Induced Intoxication," *Am. J. Psychiatry*, 127 (1971), 1659–1664.

164. TAVEL, M. E., W. DAVIDSON, and T. D. BATTERTON. "A Clinical Analysis of Mortality Associated with Delirium Tremens; Review of 39 Fatalities in a 9-Year Period," *Am. J. Med. Sci.*, 242 (1961), 18–29.

165. TINKLENBERG, J. R. "Alcohol and Violence," in P. Bourne and R. Fox, eds., *Alcoholism: Progress in Treatment*, pp. 195–210. New York: Academic, 1973.

166. TYGSTRUP, N., K. WINKLER, and F. LUNDQUIST. "The Mechanism of the Fructose Effect on the Ethanol Metabolism of the Human Liver," *J. Clin. Invest.*, 44 (1965), 817–830.

167. VANDERPOOL, J. A. "Alcoholism and the Self-Concept," *Q. J. Stud. Alcohol*, 30 (1969), 59–77.

168. VICTOR, M. "Treatment of Alcoholic Intoxication and the Withdrawal Syndrome. A Critical Analysis of the Use of Drugs and Other Forms of Therapy," *Psychosom. Med.*, 28 (1966), 636–650.

169. ———. "The Pathophysiology of Alcoholic Epilepsy," *Res. Publ. Assoc. Nerv. Ment. Dis.*, 46 (1968), 434–454.

170. VICTOR, M. and R. D. ADAMS. "The Effect

of Alcohol on the Nervous System," in *Res. Publ. Assoc. Nerv. Ment. Dis.*, 32 (1953), 526–573.

171. ———. "On the Etiology of the Alcoholic Neurologic Diseases with Special Reference to the Role of Nutrition," *Am. J. Clin. Nutr.*, 9 (1961), 379–397.

172. VICTOR, M., R. D. ADAMS, and H. G. COLLINS. *The Wernicke-Korsakoff Syndrome.* Philadelphia: Davis, 1971.

173. WALDER, A. I., J. S. REDDING, L. FAILLACE et al. "Rapid Detoxification of the Acute Alcoholic with Hemodialysis," *Surgery*, 66 (1969), 201–207.

174. WALLER, J. A. "Factors Associated with Alcohol and Responsibility for Fatal Highway Crashes," *Q. J. Stud. Alcohol*, 33 (1972), 160–170.

175. WALLER, J. A. and R. G. SMART. "Impaired Driving and Alcoholism: Personality or Pharmacologic Effect?" *J. Safety Res.*, 1 (1969), 174–177.

176. WALLGREN, H. and H. BARRY. *Actions of Alcohol*, Vol. 1. *Biochemical and Physiological Aspects.* Amsterdam: Elsevier, 1970.

177. ———. *Actions of Alcohol*, Vol. 2. Chronic and Clinical Aspects. Amsterdam: Elsevier, 1970.

178. WESCHLER, H., E. H. KASEY, D. THOM et al. "Alcohol Level and Home Accidents," *Public Health Rep.*, 84 (1969), 1043–1050.

179. WIKLER, A. "On the Nature of Addiction and Habituation," *Br. J. Addict.*, 57 (1961), 73–79.

180. ———. "Personality Disorders. III: Sociopathic Type, The Addictions," in A. M. Freedman and H. I. Kaplan, eds., *Comprehensive Textbook of Psychiatry*, pp. 939–1003. Baltimore: Williams & Wilkins, 1967.

181. WINKLER, G. F. and R. R. YOUNG. "The Control of Essential Tremor by Propranolol," *Trans. Am. Neurol. Assoc.*, 96 (1971), 66–68.

182. WINTROBE, M. M., R. D. ADAMS, I. L. BENNETT et al. *Harrison's Principles of Internal Medicine*, 6th ed. New York: McGraw Hill, 1970.

183. WOLFE, P. H. "Ethnic Differences in Alcohol Sensitivity," *Science*, 175 (1972), 449–450.

184. WOLFE, S. M., J. MENDELSON, M. OGATA et al. "Respiratory Alkalosis and Alcohol Withdrawal," *Trans. Assoc. Am. Physicians*, 83 (1969), 344–352.

185. WOLFE, S. M. and M. VICTOR. "The Physiological Basis of the Alcohol Withdrawal Syndrome," in N. K. Mello and J. H. Mendelson, eds., *Recent Advances in Studies of Alcoholism*, Publ. no. (HSM) 71-9045, pp. 188–199. Washington: U.S. Govt. Print. Off., 1971.

186. WOLIN, S. J. and N. K. MELLO. "The Effects of Alcohol on Dreams and Hallucinations in Alcohol Addicts," *Ann. N.Y. Acad Sci.*, 215 (1973), 266–302.

187. WOODS, J. H., F. I. IKONI, and G. WINGER. "The Reinforcing Properties of Ethanol," in M. K. Roach, W. M. McIsaac, and P. J. Creaven, eds., *Biological Aspects of Alcoholism*, pp. 371–388. Austin, Texas: University of Texas Press, 1971.

188. WOODS, J. H. and G. D. WINGER. "A Critique of Methods for Inducing Ethanol Self-Intoxication in Animals," in N. K. Mello and J. H. Mendelson, eds., *Recent Advances in Studies of Alcoholism*, Publ. no. (HSM) 71-9045, pp. 413–436. Washington: U.S. Govt. Print. Off., 1971.

189. WORLD HEALTH ORGANIZATION. Expert Committee on Alcohol, First Report, Technical Report Series, no. 84. Geneva: WHO, 1955.

190. WORLD HEALTH ORGANIZATION. Expert Committee on Drug Dependence, Technical Report Series no. 407:6. Geneva: WHO, 1969.

191. YOUNGER, W. *Gods, Men and Wine*, The Wine and Food Society. Cleveland, Ohio: World Publishing Co., 1966.

192. ZIEVE, L., D. F. MENDELSON, and M. GOEPFERT. "Shunt Encephalomyelopathy. II. Occurrence of Permanent Myelopathy," *Ann. Intern. Med.*, 53 (1960), 53–63.

193. ZILBORG, G. and G. W. HENRY. *A History of Medical Psychology.* New York: Norton, 1941.

194. ZWERLING, I. and M. ROSENBAUM. "Alcoholic Addiction and Personality," in S. Arieti, ed., *American Handbook of Psychiatry*, 1st ed., Vol. 1, pp. 623–644. New York: Basic Books, 1959.

CHAPTER 16

PSYCHOSIS ASSOCIATED WITH HEREDITARY DISORDERS

I. Herbert Scheinberg

⟪ Introduction*

THE EFFECTS of hereditary abnormalities on the central nervous system may be manifested as mental retardation, disturbances of neurological function, or psychiatric disorders. Where the abnormal heredity is confined to a single gene, or gene pair, it is, paradoxically, rather more common for two or three of these phenotypic disturbances to be seen than is true where more numerous and less well-defined genetic abnormalities are present. Thus Huntington's chorea and Wilson's disease generally produce neurological *and* psychiatric dysfunction, though a single dominant gene or a single pair of recessive ones, respectively, is the cause of each disease.

* A section on the genetic terminology used in this chapter appears at the end.

Yet the poorly understood combinations of several genes which predispose to senile psychoses are not generally also associated with impairment of intellectual and neurologic function.[7,8]

Mental retardation is by far the commonest hereditary disorder of the central nervous system associated with genetic abnormalities that are more or less well-defined biochemically. In phenylketonuria, maple syrup urine disease, homocystinuria, histidinemia, and galactosemia—to cite the best known of perhaps fifty nonchromosomal disorders—a specific block in normal amino acid metabolism leads to the accumulation of sufficient amounts of intermediate compounds to be toxic to the brain.[15,21] In other instances of mental retardation, such as the autosomal recessively transmitted Tay-Sachs disease, or the chromosomal abnormality associated with the cri-du-chat syndrome, there is little knowledge of the biochemical mechanisms involved.[15]

Neurological dysfunction—alone or with other manifestations of CNS disorder—is characteristic of Huntington's chorea, Wilson's disease, familial or hereditary tremor, and the genetically heterogeneous group of congenital disorders, of which a number are hereditary, collectively diagnosed as cerebral palsy.

Both psychotic and nonpsychotic psychiatric disturbances may be seen in a number of hereditary disorders which are either well-defined syndromes, such as Huntington's chorea, or are the result of a complex interplay of hereditary endowment and environment, such as the senile psychoses. Both classes can be due, in large measure, to the indirect effects on the ego's functioning of a crippling or life-threatening disease, as discussed below under Wilson's disease. There is little doubt, however, that the specific and direct biochemical effects of a disorder, e.g., the accumulation of large and toxic excesses of copper in the brains of patients with Wilson's disease, can sufficiently derange brain function to produce psychiatric disorders.

(Huntington's Chorea

Huntington's chorea is a widespread hereditary disorder of the CNS which is transmitted as an autosomal dominant and has an incidence of about four per 100,000 in Europe and the United States and about four per 1,000,000 in Japan.[15] Clinical manifestation of the illness is rarely noted in childhood; the onset, generally, occurs between the fourth and sixth decades. Classically, chorea and the existence of the disease in members of previous generations of the patient's family are sufficient criteria for the diagnosis.[18] Frequently, ". . . ataxia, dysarthria, dysphagia, dysphasia . . ." may be present; onset may occur in childhood; there may be, not uncommonly antedating peripheral neurological disturbances, ". . . amnesia, judgment, and/or orientation defects . . . ;" and there are almost always concomitant emotional disturbances including depression, with suicidal impulses, or a clinical picture indistinguishable from schizophrenia.[18]

There is no biochemical knowledge of the disease; there is no chemical, clinical, or pathological test or finding which is diagnostic; and there is no specific treatment known. Except, possibly, for a test based on the administration of L-Dopa,[9] diagnosis is made solely on clinical grounds and the physician is totally unable to tell if a child of a patient carries the dominant abnormal gene which causes the disease or is free of this abnormal allele, and will neither contract nor be able to transmit the disorder. Until diagnostic clinical manifestations are noted, every such child has to be considered to have an even chance of possessing, or not possessing, the abnormal gene. Since signs and symptoms may not occur until the sixth decade, the problem of genetic counselling becomes difficult indeed.[17,20]

Management of patients, once it is clear that Huntington's chorea is present, is limited to nonspecific chemotherapy, for both the neurological and psychiatric disturbances, and to supportive psychotherapy.[19,20] Because of the physician's inability to diagnose the illness before clinical manifestations have appeared, the uncertainties that surround the individual and his relatives are almost as tragic as the effects of the disorder itself on the afflicted individual.[10]

(Wilson's Disease

Wilson's disease, with an incidence of about one in 200,000, is similar to Huntington's chorea in being hereditary (though transmitted in autosomal recessive fashion), in severely affecting the CNS, both neurologically and psychiatrically, and in not manifesting itself clinically early in life. In contrast, however, there is a great deal of biochemical information about the disease, diagnostic chemical tests can be applied, and specific therapy is available.

The etiologic agent causing the pathological

changes which underlie the disease is copper, toxic excesses of which are accumulated in the CNS. Diagnosis is possible in the asymptomatic as well as the ill patient by the demonstration of a deficiency (less than 20 mg./100 ml. of serum) of the plasma copper-protein, ceruloplasmin, *and* an excess (greater than 250 μg./g. dry liver) of hepatic copper. Specific treatment consists of the administration of D-penicillamine, which removes copper from the symptomatic patient, in whom marked clinical improvement generally results, and from the asymptomatic one, in whom manifestations of the disease may be indefinitely prevented.[12,16]

Almost all diets contain 2–5 mg. of copper and this amount is more than sufficient to supply the body's need for this essential element, which is present in a number of proteins such as cytochrome oxidase and tyrosinase. The total body content of copper is about 150 mg., and virtually none is lost in the urine so that the normal individual excretes in his stools, principally from bile, almost precisely the amount absorbed from the diet. In Wilson's disease, a defect in the excretion of the absorbed copper has been inherited so that the metal accumulates slowly, but steadily, in the liver. Eventually destruction of hepatic parenchyma results in the release of relatively large amounts of copper to the blood whence it diffuses into the brain, the corneas (where it produces the diagnostic Kayser-Fleischer rings), the kidneys, and into almost every other tissue and organ. The toxic effects of copper in all these sites constitute Wilson's disease.

From this sequence it is apparent that copper first reaches toxic levels in the liver and, indeed, this organ almost invariably shows pathological changes by the time the diagnosis of Wilson's disease is first made even though the patient may be asymptomatic. Yet in only about 40 percent of patients who become symptomatic is the liver the source of the initial clinical manifestations of the disease. In another 30–40 percent neurological signs are first noted while neurotic, psychotic, or bizarre behavioral disorders herald the onset in perhaps 25 percent.[14] Many patients suffer from significant psychiatric disturbance after an initial hepatic or neurological onset. Thus, in one group of twenty-two patients with Wilson's disease, nine, or 41 percent, had a psychiatric diagnosis of which three appeared to be psychotic.[5] Of forty-nine of our patients with Wilson's disease, thirty, or 61 percent, had significant psychiatric disturbances, of which nine were classified as psychotic.

The emotional disturbances seen in these patients do not appear to be associated with significant mental retardation or impairment. (Emphasis on the intellectual impairment due to hereditary defects has probably tended to obscure the fact that more subtle forms of psychological disease can also be so caused.) Of the group of forty-nine patients just referred to, nineteen were evaluated on the Wechsler Adult Intelligence Scale (or the Wechsler Intelligence Scale for Children): individual IQ scores ranged from 57 to 135, with an average full-scale IQ for the group of 94.[14]

Very few sophisticated psychiatric studies of patients with Wilson's disease have yet been made. Before the introduction of penicillamine, the hepatic and neurological disease, progressive and fatal, overshadowed the psychiatric illness. With the availability of effective chemotherapy, on the other hand, treatment—and prophylaxis—of hepatitis, tremors, and dysarthria have been so dramatically successful that recently attention has been given to investigating the frequent accompanying psychiatric disorder which is usually not life-threatening.

Beard, writing in 1959 before penicillamine was generally available, described a patient with indubitable Wilson's disease who also suffered from schizophrenia.[2] He defined the latter as consisting of delusions of reference, and hallucinations and affective flatness in a setting of clear consciousness without insight. Although he found a number of patients in the literature who were said to suffer from both Wilson's disease and schizophrenia, he considered the latter diagnosis generally to be incorrect, with the patients suffering instead from less well-defined ". . . confusional state(s) or dementia." This conclusion follows from Beard's assumption that schizophrenia is a specific illness developing in a patient with "... a schizoid personality or hereditary disposition . . . ," and he clearly differentiates the latter from the abnormal pair of genes which causes Wilson's disease.

In the relatively superficial psychiatric studies reported since, it is impossible either to describe a particular psychiatric syndrome specific for Wilson's disease or to differentiate the patients' manifestations from the psychiatric disorders seen in general practice. Six representative examples, selected from our patients, follow:

1. A middle-aged man spent the last ten years of his life in a (New York State) mental hospital, which he entered, before the diagnosis of Wilson's disease was made, with a diagnosis of paranoid schizophrenia.

2. A young man, of high intelligence and normal stability, suddenly began to suffer from, and act out, voyeuristic compulsions which soon led to his arrest, and a suicidal attempt while in jail.

3. An adolescent girl manifested neurotic disturbances to such a degree that psychoanalytic treatment was initiated. Within six years mild neurological abnormalities appeared and she became psychotically depressed and withdrawn.

4. An adolescent boy pushed a woman visitor into a swimming pool and chased his father with a shotgun before either neurological or hepatic abnormalities of Wilson's disease had become observable.

5. A married man in his early thirties attacked without warning an elevator operator in the belief that this man was threatening to kill his children.

6. A woman in her thirties had, over a period of about ten years, several alternating episodes of mania and depression which have required hospitalization in a state mental hospital.[13]

Since 1960, the majority of patients with Wilson's disease have received regular therapy with penicillamine with marked clinical improvement which has, obviously, been particularly well documented with respect to hepatic and neurological disease. There is little doubt, however, in the minds of physicians who have treated more than one or two patients with this disease, that the psychiatric disorders also improve to a greater extent than would be expected in a similar group of patients without Wilson's disease.[5,14] Although this is as difficult to document as is the efficacy of any psychiatric therapy, the courses of the six patients described above are of some interest:

1. This man remained hospitalized and, despite intensive treatment to remove the excess copper, worsened progressively and died.

2. Life-long treatment with penicillamine, begun in 1960, was initially accompanied by weekly sessions of therapy with a psychiatrist which later were occasionally reinstituted for several months at a time. Neurological recovery from a state of near-incapacity has been complete. The patient has a wife and three children, effectively manages a moderately large and complex family business, and is active in civic and charitable activities.

3. Psychiatric and penicillamine treatment resulted in disappearance of the patient's mild neurological manifestations. A psychotic episode with depressive and schizophrenic overtones ended her marriage and required almost six months of hospitalization. Following discharge, treatment with penicillamine was accompanied by psychiatric treatment, chiefly involving a variety of tranquilizing and mood-elevating drugs. She married a second time, adopted a child and, despite continued immaturity, has managed to live a reasonably fulfilling life as a housewife in a city 1000 miles from her mother, on whom she remains quite dependent.

4. This boy, whose older untreated brother had died of Wilson's disease, was treated with penicillamine and manifested no further psychiatric abnormalities. Mild neurological disabilities supervened before treatment was begun and these have persisted but produce no significant incapacity.

5. Treatment with penicillamine, and brief psychiatric hospitalization and treatment, have returned this man to a normal neurological and psychiatric state.

6. One further episode of mania and depression required hospitalization after regular treatment with penicillamine was instituted.

In the ensuing twelve years, however, only two episodes, requiring brief hospitalization, have interrupted her normal life.

These results, and the impression that[5] ". . . the incidence of psychiatric disturbances is higher in patients with Wilson's disease than it is in the average neurological patient population . . ." make it difficult to escape the conclusion that the psychiatric abnormalities of Wilson's disease represent more than the reactions of a patient to a crippling and life-threatening disease. Such reactive emotional abnormalities are clearly part of the picture, but the toxic neurological effects which copper deposits can produce, the fact[2] that there is ". . . widespread cortical damage . . . ," and the improvement in psychiatric dysfunction which follows removal of some of the excess copper, strongly suggest that too much of this metal can directly derange the integrative functions of the brain.

(Acute Intermittent Porphyria

The term "porphyria" is used to describe a number of disorders of porphyrin metabolism, some of which are inherited.[21] Acute intermittent porphyria is the best known, the most intensively studied, and the form usually associated with psychiatric findings. The incidence of the disease, which probably occurs in all races, is around one in 5000.[21] It is generally thought to be transmitted as an autosomal dominant.[21] However, incidental and incomplete data which are given in two reports[1,11] not primarily concerned with genetic aspects do not support this. They present no evidence of occurrence in successive generations, and they indicate an incidence in affected families of 22 and 20 percent when the propositus of each sibship is subtracted from its number of patients.[1,11] These characteristics are more consonant with an autosomal recessive mode of inheritance than with a dominant mode, where one expects to find patients in successive generatons and an incidence of 50 percent among sibs of affected families.

Acute intermittent porphyria is character-ized by episodes of severe abdominal pain with nausea and vomiting. There may be accompanying fever and leukocytosis, and paresis or even paralysis of various muscle groups. Attacks may last for hours or days and are followed by long periods of good health. The ingestion of barbiturates—or perhaps other drugs—and acute infections are generally considered to be capable of precipitating attacks.

Biochemically the illness is associated with the excretion of porphobilinogen and its metabolic precursor, δ-aminolevulinic acid, in the urine in amounts which may exceed 100 mg. daily. Because of the nonspecificity of the clinical picture a firm diagnosis should not be made unless these intermediates of heme biosynthesis can be demonstrated.

Acute intermittent porphyria has been considered by many authors to be characterized by psychiatric complications. Most commonly, these are thought to accompany the acute episodes with a ". . . complete return to clarity and reason . . ." when the attack subsides.[11] The description of these manifestations varies from mild irritability or depression to delirium or frank psychosis.[1] In a rather widely publicized paper in the British Medical Journal the episodic madness of King George III has been unequivocally attributed to acute intermittent porphyria. Presumably by referring his aberrant behavior to a genetically caused excess of porphobilinogen and δ-aminolevulinic acid rather than to unknown mechanisms these authors[11] conclude that ". . . this diagnosis clears the House of Hanover of an hereditary taint of madness. . . ."

Unfortunately, the psychiatric investigation of this disease has been relatively naive and confined to conscious manifestations. Investigators have differed widely in their conclusions, as is implicit in a review of previous studies by Ackner, Cooper et al.[1] The psychiatric disorders noted have been considered to be (1) a consequence of the inherited metabolic error, though by unknown pathogenic mechanisms; (2) reactions to a recurrent but solely somatic disorder which the patients generally know to be life-threatening; (3) causative of the acute attack; or (4) coincidental findings. In the study by Ackner et al.

the ". . . importance of emotional disturbances in precipitating acute attacks . . .", and the suggestion that the ". . . porphyric patient has a background of neurotic instability . . ." are not considered to be supported by the evidence in the literature. In their study of thirteen patients they could find no evidence for a psychogenic factor in the etiology of the disorder, nor for a neurotic predisposition. Although ". . . psychiatric symptoms commonly occur during an acute attack of porphyria . . . (they may) be largely psychogenic and unrelated to the underlying metabolic defect."

Clearly, treatment of the psychiatric manifestations which may accompany the acute attacks of porphyria is necessarily nonspecific. As noted, these disturbances subside when the attacks are over.[3]

There are several other disturbances in porphyrin metabolism* which are inherited, but they have little or no association with psychiatric abnormalities.[21]

(**Discussion**

Wilson's disease, Huntington's chorea, and acute intermittent porphyria are similar in that each is caused by the inheritance of only one, or a pair of, abnormal genes. Their dissimilarities are greater than this shared characteristic. Thus, we know nothing of the biochemical defect caused by the abnormal gene of Huntington's chorea and have no chemical or pathological means of confirming the diagnosis, before or after the disease is clinically manifest; there is no effective treatment. There is no doubt that psychiatric disturbance is a major characteristic of the disease, but we do not know if the emotional disorder is a reaction to the somatic, neurological disease or is a direct result of the unknown biochemical defect, or is due to both.

We know at least the probable chemical locus of the biochemical defect which under-

lies acute intermittent porphyria—somewhere in the pathway of the biosynthesis of heme—but we know neither what the primary gene product—enzyme or protein—of the abnormal, or normal, gene is, nor how or if the abnormal amounts of porphobilinogen and δ-aminolevulinic acid produce the somatic symptoms of the acute attack. Unlike what appears to be true of Wilson's disease and perhaps Huntington's chorea, the available data leave quite uncertain whether the psychiatric manifestations which have been observed are in any way specifically related to the biochemical defect, or whether they solely constitute the reactions to a recurrent and life-threatening illness.

Although we also do not know what the primary gene product of the "Wilson's disease gene," or its normal allele is, we have considerably more information about the etiology and pathogenesis of this disorder. The inborn metabolic error results in gradually increasing deposits of copper throughout the body, and the clinical manifestations of the disorder, very probably including to a significant degree the psychiatric disturbances, are the direct result of copper toxicity. In part, of course, the emotional abnormalities also represent reactions to a chronic disease which, untreated, is progressively disabling and ultimately fatal. Freud predicted, in 1920, that deeper molecular knowledge about psychiatric disease would make psychoanalytic techniques of treatment obsolete.[4] His prediction is, to a modest degree, fulfilled by the unquestionable improvement, in the psychiatric disease of a significant number of patients with Wilson's disease, which accompanies the pharmacological removal of a portion of excess copper. Such improvement appears to be accelerated if psychotherapy, or nonspecific chemo-psychotherapy, or both, accompanies the life-long administration of D-penicillamine to remove copper.

These diseases are the only instances of hereditary psychosis about which we have any biochemical genetic knowledge. Unfortunately, they constitute an insignificant proportion of all psychiatric disease. There is little doubt that heredity plays a significant, if not the dominant, role in the etiology of the psychoses,

---

* Porphyria variegata, hereditary coproporphyria, erythropoietic porphyria, and erythropoietic protoporphyria.[21]

and of other psychiatric disturbance,[6–8,15] but those causative effects are probably a summation of at least several synergistic genes. We have little knowledge about the linkages of these genes, the disorders associated with them, and no knowledge of the biochemical consequences of having inherited the normal or abnormal allele. Pick's disease is apparently associated with a dominant gene and, perhaps, Alzheimer's and Jakob-Creutzfeldt's presenile dementias have genetic determinants, but these vague bits of data are of little aid to diagnosis and of none to therapy.[6]

Jervis[6] summarizes our ignorance of these hereditary, emotional disorders: ". . . the precise nature of these genetic factors remains undetermined . . ." This ignorance includes for each such psychiatric disease, the number of genes involved as well as the structure, function, and concentration of their primary gene product and the manner in which the genetic endowment interacts with the individual's physical and emotional environment. At present, we have a significant part of such knowledge for only a few hereditary diseases of the CNS. In these, furthermore, psychosis is not the dominant clinical manifestation, and the primary interaction of the abnormal genes is with physical, not emotional, aspects of the environment. In phenylketonuria, galactosemia, the sphingolipidoses, and Wilson's disease the single-gene defect results in the accumulation of a normal chemical metabolite to concentrations which are toxic to the CNS. Just to speculate on the number of genes possibly involved etiologically in schizophrenia, and how they may interact with the patient's emotional milieu, internal and external, is to make depressingly obvious how far we are from the time predicted by Freud fifty years ago: "the deficiencies in our description (of emotional disorders) would probably vanish if we were already in a position to replace the psychological terms by physiological or chemical ones . . . On the other hand it should be made quite clear that the uncertainty of our speculation has been greatly increased by the necessity for borrowing from the science of biology. Biology is truly a land of unlimited possibilities. We may expect it to give us the most surprising information and we cannot guess what answers it will return in a few dozen years to the questions we have put to it. They may be of a kind which will blow away the whole of our artificial structure of hypotheses." [pp. 82–83][4]

❨ Genetic Terminology

Every inherited characteristic of a living organism is a consequence of a particular gene or of gene interaction. For some organisms, which are called "haploid", each characteristic is governed by unpaired genes; other organisms, including human beings, are termed "diploid" and possess a pair of genes for each characteristic, with one member of the pair derived from the father and the other from the mother. The number of genes in each human individual is unknown, but may approach 1,000,000.

A gene may be "autosomal," in which case it is present on one of the forty-four nonsex determining chromosomes; or it may be sex-linked, in which case it is located on the X chromosome. A gene is linked to other genes when all are present on the same chromosome, and are generally inherited as a unit.

A gene is termed "dominant" if the possession of one gene of a pair is sufficient to produce a specific disease, irrespective of the nature of its paired mate. A gene is "recessive" if both members of the pair must be abnormal for the disease to be produced. There are often two or more forms of a given gene, each of which is called an allele, and only one, or a pair, of which can be present in an individual. Where a disease-associated gene is recessive, the heterozygote, i.e., the individual with one abnormal and one normal allele, is called a "carrier" of the disease and, generally, does not manifest any clinical abnormalities.

All genes function either by determining the structure of a protein, termed the "primary gene product," or by regulating the rate and conditions under which the primary gene product is synthesized.

Inherited diseases may also be the consequence of the possession of more, or less, than the normal complement of forty-six chromosomes, or of abnormal forms of chromosomes. Such diseases are generally much more gross in their clinical effects than single-gene disorders for the obvious reason that a chromosome contains many genes.

⟨ Bibliography

1. ACKNER, B., J. E. COOPER, C. H. GRAY et al. "Acute Porphyria: A Neuropsychiatric and Biochemical Study." *J. Psychosom. Res.*, 6 (1961), 1–24.

2. BEARD, A. W., "The Association of Hepatolenticular Degeneration with Schizophrenia," *Acta Psychiatr. Neurol. Scand.*, 34 (1959), 411–427.

3. CARNEY, M. W. P. "Hepatic Porphyria with Mental Symptoms," *Lancet*, 2 (1972), 100–101.

4. FREUD, S. (1920) "Beyond the Pleasure Principle," in J. Strachey, ed., *Standard Edition*, Vol. 18, pp. 7–64. London: Hogarth, 1950.

5. GOLDSTEIN, N. P., J. C. EWERT, R. V. RANDALL et al. "Psychiatric Aspects of Wilson's Disease (Hepatolenticular Degeneration): Results of Psychometric Tests During Long-Term Therapy," *Am. J. Psychiatry*, 124 (1968), 1555–1561.

6. JERVIS, G. A. "The Presenile Dementias," in *Mental Disorders in Later Life*, 2nd ed., pp. 262–288. Stanford: Stanford University Press, 1956.

7. KALLMAN, F. J. "The Genetics of Psychoses; An Analysis of 1232 Index Families," Congrès International de Psychiatrie, VI. Génétique et Eugénique, pp. 1–40. Paris: Hermann, 1950.

8. KALLMANN, F. J., L. FEINGOLD, and E. BONDY. "Comparative Adaptational, Social, and Psychometric Data on the Life Histories of Senescent Twin Pairs," *Am. J. Human Genet.*, 3 (1951), 65–73.

9. KLAWANS, H. C., G. W. PAULSON, and A. BARBEAU. "Predictive Test for Huntington's Chorea," *Lancet*, 2 (1970), 1185–1186.

10. LYNCH, H. T., W. L. HARLAN, and J. S. DYHRBERG. "Subjective Perspective of a Family with Huntington's Chorea," *Arch. Gen. Psychiatry*, 27 (1972), 67–72.

11. MACALPINE, I. and R. HUNTER. "The 'Insanity' of King George III: A Classic Case of Porphyria," *Br. Med. J.*, 1 (1966), 65–71.

12. SCHEINBERG, I. H. and I. STERNLIEB. "Wilson's Disease," *Ann. Rev. Med.*, 16 (1965), 119–134.

13. ———. "Copper Metabolism and the Central Nervous System," in O. Walaas, ed., *Molecular Basis of Some Aspects of Mental Activity*, Vol. 2, pp. 115–116. New York: Academic, 1967.

14. SCHEINBERG, I. H., I. STERNLIEB, and J. RICHMAN. "Characterization of the Psychiatric Manifestations of Wilson's Disease," in D. Bergsma, I. H. Scheinberg, and I. Sternlieb, eds., *Wilson's Disease*, Birth Defects Original Article Series, Vol. 4, no. 2, pp. 85–87. New York: The National Foundation—March of Dimes, 1968.

15. SLATER, E. and V. COWIE. *The Genetics of Mental Disorders*. London: Oxford University Press, 1971.

16. STERNLIEB, I. and I. H. SCHEINBERG. "Prevention of Wilson's Disease in Asymptomatic Patients," *N. Engl. J. Med.*, 278 (1968), 352–359.

17. WHITTIER, J. R. "Genetics in Psychiatric Practice," *Eugenics Q.*, 5 (1958), 9–15.

18. ———. "Clinical Aspects of Huntington's Disease," in A. Barbeau and J.-R. Brunette, eds., Progress in Neurogenetics. Proc. 2nd Int. Congr. of Neuro-Genetics and Neuro-Ophthalmology, World Fed. Neurol., Montreal, Sept., 1967. Vol. 1. *Huntington's Disease*, pp. 632–644. Amsterdam: Excerpta Medica Foundation, 1969.

19. WHITTIER, J. R., G. HAYDU, and J. CRAWFORD. "Effect of Imipramine (Tofränil) on Depression and Hyperkinesia in Huntington's Disease," *Am. J. Psychiatry*, 118 (1961), 79.

20. WHITTIER, J. R., A. HEIMLER, and C. KORENYI. "The Psychiatrist and Huntington's Disease (Chorea)," *Am. J. Psychiatry*, 128 (1972), 1546–1550.

21. WORLD HEALTH ORGANIZATION SCIENTIFIC GROUP. "Screening for Inborn Errors of Metabolism," WHO Tech. Rep. Ser. no. 401. Geneva: WHO, 1968.

CHAPTER 17

MENTAL DISORDERS WITH HUNTINGTON'S CHOREA

A. Clinical Aspects

John R. Whittier[*]

❰ Introductory Remarks

A BRIEF historical review of events since the first edition of the *American Handbook of Psychiatry* is of interest. The first printing of the *Handbook* was in 1959, and it had run through nine printings by 1967. In that year, by coincidence, a remarkable wave of attention was paid to Huntington's disease (chronic progressive hereditary chorea). This was evidenced by the fact that during the decade ending 1959 there had been approximately 120 publications in the scientific literature on the disease. The number had increased to over 350 during the decade ending 1969. Furthermore, the first international symposium on the disease was held in September of 1967 in Mon-

treal. This symposium brought together a group of investigators which reviewed what was known of the disease to that time, and proceedings were subsequently published by the hosting Congress of Neurogenetics and Neuro-ophthalmology of the World Federation of Neurology.[6] In 1967 there was also created the Committee to Combat Huntington's Disease, spurred by the interest of a single individual, Marjorie Guthrie, whose husband died of Huntington's disease. The Committee grew from a single small group in that year to a national organization with headquarters in New York and more than fifty chapters in the United States and other countries by 1974. This Committee was also responsible for assisting the World Federation of Neurology Research Commission on Huntington's Chorea not only in holding its 1967 symposium but also in holding a centennial sym-

* The author wishes to acknowledge the assistance of Pearl Band and Roslyn Laiterman in preparation of the clinical aspects of this chapter.

posium in 1972 celebrating the description by George Huntington of the disease and resulting in publication of the first book devoted entirely to its present status.[5] The publication is a comprehensive review to which anyone interested in special aspects of the disease, including those of interest to psychiatrists, may refer.

In the relatively short time since 1967, there has been a great increase in the number of investigators devoting a major part of their efforts to clinical and pathological aspects of Huntington's disease (H.D.). New concepts regarding aspects of the underlying pathological physiology have appeared. The effect of L-Dopa, other chemicals, and of neurotransmitters on the disease has been studied. Development of new techniques and the refinement of previous techniques have progressed, including fluorescence microscopy, electron microscopy, and methods of chemical analysis of human brain obtained at autopsy or by biopsy.

The role of the psychiatrist with regard to the disease varies, depending on the orientation of the patient or family member and the nature and setting of the psychiatrist's practice. Useful previous reports dealing with the role of the psychiatrist in summary manner are available.[88,91]

⟪ Nature of the Disease

The disease is unusual by reason of its genetic mechanism. It passes from one generation to another by a Mendelian pattern of autosomal dominant gene with almost complete penetrance. This means that a parent who carries the gene and lives long enough will ultimately develop the disease. If there are offspring, of either sex, the probability for each of acquiring the disease and passing it to their offspring in the same manner is 50 percent. Although the disease has been thought to "skip" generations there is general agreement that this never occurs. "Skipping" is usually the result of inadequate family history, or of death of a gene-carrying parent prior to the appearance of symptoms. The underlying pathology is

that of a slowly progressive atrophy limited to selected sites in the brain only. It is characterized by distinctive neuropathological changes (see section on Neuropathology) in a process usually extending over a period of ten to fifteen years. Onset of more or less blatant symptoms only after the first three decades insures that a pool of individuals "at risk" for the disease is almost always available. In most populations studied to date, a prevalence of six per 100,000 general population is found.[63] Some pockets of exceptionally high prevalence are known, as in Maracaibo, Venezuela, and in the Moray Firth area of Scotland. Knowledge of and attitudes toward the disease by the populations in areas of high prevalence should be of special interest to psychiatrists.

Clinical Picture

The symptoms of the disease may be considered as "usual early patterns" and "usual advanced patterns." The usual early patterns may have an "early onset" form with severe mental retardation, rigidity, and epileptic seizures appearing in the first year of life and rapidly progressing to profound neurological disability and death in three to five years. This early onset form has recently been shown to occur more often when the affected parent of such an offspring was the father.[4,87] The attention of psychiatrists is usually not drawn to such patients.[78] Other patterns of early onset occur in the juvenile and adolescent period.[21,52] Here behavior disorders occur, including asocial, antisocial, and withdrawal disorders, emotional lability, depression, a strong tendency to sexual promiscuity, and abuse of drugs and alcohol. These patients are likely to come to the attention of psychiatrists. Recognizing the symptoms either as reactive to the presence of known disease in the family (even in instances where the offspring eventually can be shown to be gene-free by their subsequent course) or as those generated from early influence by the gene in initial stages of the actual disease presents as a challenging situation.

The symptoms in the usual advanced state are the result of years of the slow progressive selective atrophy of the brain which characterizes the disease. Symptoms and signs appear gradually, and are slowly progressive with onset in the second and third decades. In the fourth and fifth decades they are fully developed. They include psychiatric symptoms such as irritability, hostility, assaultiveness, and depression, and behavioral symptoms including alcoholism, drug abuse, and promiscuity. Neurological symptoms appear, including chorea, incoordination, dysarthria, aphasia, ataxia, pseudo bulbar palsy and bulimia, and defects in memory, orientation and judgment. For psychiatrists it is important to recognize that psychiatric symptoms may long precede the appearance of the neurological symptoms.[20,22,23] A tendency for depression and suicide appears to occur more frequently in females, and for assaultiveness and homicide more frequently in males.[79] Despite the relatively low reported prevalence, there are many investigators who believe it is considerably higher. Psychiatrists should always elicit as complete a family history as possible from any patient coming to their attention because of the serious personal, social, economic and other complications arising from a failure to make early diagnosis. Psychiatric symptoms may be the only ones present for many years before the typical choreic symptoms appear. Conversely, chorea alone, late in onset, may exist with very little dementia.

The chorea is typical in pattern, characterized by the occurrence of abnormal involuntary movements (AIMS), caused by contractions of muscle groups occurring at different sites in irregular sequence. Collaboration of contracting and relaxing muscle groups is preserved, so that movements of body surfaces or segments take place. Contractions may not be of sufficient magnitude or arrangement to cause displacement of a limb or body segment, but they can be detected by careful continuous observation. They do not occur during sleep. Standardized motion picture recording over a period of years has been extremely helpful in distinguishing at risk individuals with abnormal involuntary movements patterned as chorea from at risk individuals with normal involuntary movements (NIMS)

resulting from anxiety. When sufficiently forceful and occurring at appropriate sites, the movements produce a sequence of grotesque posturing and distorted or uncoordinated voluntary movements.

Chorea may occur in any part of the visible, voluntary, muscular apparatus such as face musculature, especially perioral and periorbital, and the chest, including diaphragmatic musculature and resulting in markedly irregular breathing patterns which in themselves contribute to speech abnormalities. Speech abnormalities and very slight movements of axial musculature and of fingers tend to occur during the early stages of the disease. The inability to keep the tongue protruded is almost pathognomonic in advanced cases, and reduction in time of maintained tongue protrusion often occurs early in the adult. A tendency to familial stereotype appears not only in the time of onset of the disease (juvenile or adolescent as compared to adult) but also in the sites of choreic activity. A rigid form without chorea is recognized. A tendency also appears for offspring of patients with Huntington's Disease to display increased frequency of medical disorders unassociated with Huntington's Disease.[56]

A remarkable tendency to promiscuity in both young and old (lack of sexual inhibition, remarked upon in 1872 by Huntington for elderly patients) favors on the one hand illegitimacy with its attendant difficulties in tracing family lines, and, on the other hand, what appears to be a real tendency to high fecundity; families of a parent with the disease tend to be unusually large.[70] This latter observation may very well be related to abnormally high sexual activity by reason of the underlying degeneration of especially caudate and putamen nuclei, whose purpose includes many aspects of inhibition of behavior. The apparently high parental fecundity may also be interpreted, however, as deriving from the denial mechanism which is so common in the disease.

The rate of progression of the disease may vary greatly between individuals. It is much more rapid with early than late onset cases. The influence of stress in some form of other appears unequivocal in causing symptoms to appear for the first time, or in worsening symptoms already present. Pregnancy and head injury have been reported as unusually common stressor events.[54]

Diagnosis

Probably because of the sites of degeneration in the brain and the stress generated even in gene-free at risk individuals with a family history of the disease, an unusually long list of psychiatric and neurological disorders require consideration and exclusion. It must be repeatedly emphasized that only the affirming of a positive family history after energetic tracking of the family line, pursued with such persistence and in such depth as is perhaps done properly only by a geneticist, permits the differentiation of H.D. from other disorders.[64] Psychiatric disorders include anxiety, which is capable of ubiquitous manifestations, and schizophrenic reactions, especially paranoid and catatonic, torticollis, tic (including the syndrome of Gilles de la Tourette), and especially depressions of one or another variety. Perioral, periorbital, and facial choreic movements are occasionally mistaken for schizophrenic grimaces. Among neurological disorders, Huntington's disease is most frequently misdiagnosed as Parkinson's disease or multiple sclerosis. Sydenham's chorea, and chorea occasionally presenting with general medical disorders should provide no diagnostic problem, but the disorders of Creuzfeldt-Jakob and Hallervorden-Spatz, familial paroxysmal choreoathethosis, cerebellar disorders including olivopontocerebellar atrophy, and the diseases of Alzheimer and Pick may present diagnostic problems resolved only by a neurologist.

"Senile chorea" probably is an entity, but can usually be distinguished from Huntington's disease by the pattern of severe AIMS in the presence of relatively mild or absent dementia, and a well-established negative family history. Posthemiplegic chorea is almost invariably unilateral. A recent review listed eighty-five diseases to be considered in differential diagnosis.[11]

Urgent search is underway for a specific test capable of detecting the disease before the onset of symptoms.[35] The effort has been notably unsuccessful, except perhaps for evidence that an L-Dopa challenge may evoke choreic AIMS in at risk subjects (and worsen chorea if present already).[35,36,41,50] The lack of an early sensitive test prior to onset of recognizable early symptoms has been probably the single most troublesome aspect of the management of Huntington's disease, since the stress of knowledge of its presence in the family and the drive to child bearing precede the signs and symptoms required for diagnosis in at risk individuals. Specifically, lumbar puncture and specialized examination of spinal fluid have had no value. The electro-encephalogram has been shown to be without value in early stages of the disease. When disease is advanced, abnormal EEG patterns usually appear as flattening of wave forms. Pneumoencephalography shows dilated lateral ventricles and widened sulci, which characterize the ultimate generalized atrophy of affected brains. Psychological testing offers no diagnostic help. Electromyography has nothing specific to offer. Special applications of tremometry[26] may ultimately be helpful in early diagnosis. Electro-oculography is still in the experimental stage but shows considerable promise.[73] Cineseismography is one of the newer methods for quantifying abnormal involuntary movements of all types, and may be helpful in a battery of tests for secondary phenomena.[54,56] By this method, motion-picture records are made of movements and their detection by the sensitive surface of a metabolic scale. Brain biopsy is now being performed, and the tissue studied by a variety of sophisticated methods, but this is not practical for routine purposes, although some abnormalities in cortical tissue may ultimately be accepted as specific.

(Management

The way in which psychiatrists become drawn into what is best referred to as a management relation to patients (referred to as probands in the case of the first in the family coming to his attention) and their family depends upon many factors, including the psychiatrist's type of practice, his geographic location, the administrative setting in which he may operate, and the special diagnostic resources available to him. Most patients hospitalized for Huntington's disease are in its advanced stages, and are usually found in state hospitals, Veterans Administration hospitals, or nursing homes.

Patients usually appear as troubled family members either from a direct line who are at risk and have not yet developed the disease or who are showing early signs of the disease. In either case, anxiety and depression and combinations of these may be present.[86]

Collateral members of affected families may come to the psychiatrist's attention with symptoms of anxiety and depression arising from their awareness of the disease if it has only recently come to their attention and they have little knowledge of its nature. In any case, psychotherapy is indicated in whatever form the psychiatrist can offer, and this does not exclude patients with the disease suffering from its nonneurological consequences. The first priority of therapy should be to insure that the patient's knowledge of the disease is as complete as he is capable of comprehending, the information being communicated by a therapist who is free of anxiety. This may take preliminary exploration of the area, and instruction over a period of time. Indeed this educational process alone may, if properly handled, alleviate much of the symptomatology. If a definite diagnosis has not been made, there should be no hesitation by the psychiatrist to refer to a neurologist or a medical center. Most experience, contrary to what might be expected, is that a positive diagnosis is less likely to generate symptoms than it is to relieve them. This is apparently because uncertainty by itself creates fear or anxiety. It is always desirable to proceed carefully giving knowledge concerning the disease, and especially in conveying the fact that diagnosis has been made.[71] Many patients stoutly assert that they wish to know whether they have the disease when, in fact, at least for the moment,

they do not. However, if a patient is asked, why he wishes to know, one can be guided by the answer: "I would find the nearest tall building and jump off it." This carries quite different implication than "At least I would know and be able to plan in advance depending on how bad my condition might become."

Psychotherapy should resort to the aid of professional genetic counseling if available, Sometimes it is not; references to detailed reports of management are provided in this chapter.[87,89] In addition, referral may be made to special resources, such as geographical listing of genetics counseling centers regularly updated by the National Foundation-March of Dimes.[7] The Committee to Combat Huntington's Disease now has chapters in almost every state, and the national organization in New York can provide information about a nearby chapter. Contact by patients with these chapters usually provides strong additional support for psychotherapy. In some situations, physical, social and economic assistance may be available, as in the Veterans Administration. Legal referral may occasionally be necessary because individuals may have problems relating to vocational, professional, and economic planning, marital and parental situations, or insurance and driving coverage. With regard to application forms, individuals should usually be informed that if they are truthful concerning the presence of Huntington's disease in the family, they may risk rejection or increased insurance premiums, or be subjected to special tests for a driver's license. If they are not truthful, and difficulties arise they may lose insurance coverage and be subject to heavier penalties for damages incurred in accidents. Problems of this nature often require a psychiatrist, but unfortunately they do not always have the information to offer. Very often the expectation is that somebody else will take care of this responsibility, such as a neurologist or a geneticist. The result is that the patient is never provided with the information he requires in order to advance the psychotherapeutic relation which should always include correct information, appropriately presented. The situation is analogous to many of those arising from over-specialization in medicine, unless provision is made for specifying functions in an organization. Of course, in some rural situations a psychiatrist may be the only individual available to a family either to alert a family to the presence of Huntington's disease or to see that their needs are properly met.

A variety of medications are effective in the psychiatrist's handling of patients, whether they are symptomatic with chorea and non-neurological problems, or at risk. A series of effective antichoreic medications include reserpine in doses increasing from 2 to 12 mg. per day; chlorpromazine in appropriate dosage, usually 50 mg. three times a day or single dose at bedtime, and fluphenazine or haloperidol, either given in dosage from 2 to 15 mg. per day. All these medications usually are increased by steps over a period of several weeks. Benefit to the chorea, anxiety, and delusions or other mental aberrations should be expected before adverse side effects, usually drowsiness or dystonic reactions. The latter can be appropriately managed with benztropine in dosage of 2 mg. or biperiden (2 mg.) 2 mg. twice a day or more. Diazepam is useful during the day and for sleep, as is the newer compound fluorazepam.

Depression, which is so frequent and common, responds to antidepressant medications, which the psychiatrist should choose as he desires.[89] Imipramine in dosage of 50 mg. three times a day or single dose at bedtime is quite reliable. In some instances antidepressants alone may worsen the chorea.

It is more generally recognized that neurosurgical procedures on brain or peripheral nerves is of no benefit, and may damage a tissue already undergoing progressive handicap.

Complications in early stages include depression of suicidal degree which should be handled appropriately; Huntington's disease is no contraindication of electroconvulsive therapy. As the disease advances, the neurological symptoms singly or in combination usually lead to bedfast state, and watch must be kept for the usual complications of pneumonia, skin ulcers, fractures of long bones or skull, urinary tract infections, and the like.

In conclusion, Huntington's disease can be seen as a condition that may be rightfully judged a paradigm for hereditary medical disorders in general and for psychiatric disorders in particular, complicated by neurological symptoms.

B. Neuropathology

Leon Roizin and Mavis A. Kaufman

DUNLAP[24] supplemented the literature review* with a personal detailed neuropathologic study based on seventeen positive† cases of Huntington's chorea, twelve questionable cases, and thirty or more control cases. Many selective destructive lesions in the human striatum had failed to give clear evidence of any definite function of this region. Wilson's[91] experimental work on anthropoid animals "in which the striatum was first electrically stimulated and then in large part destroyed on one side," showed little, if any, difference from normal controls. Therefore Dunlap attempted (in the above mentioned study) to determine whether gross or microscopic changes could be found in the central nervous system "in all cases of Huntington's chorea which would distinguish this disease process from all others."

Grossly, the brains in the "positive" cases of Huntington's chorea were small and of diminished weight. The reduction was chiefly, if not entirely, in the forebrain, with marked general atrophy affecting the convolutions, the deep white matter, and particularly the corpus striatum, which was less than half the normal size. The cerebellum was regarded as essentially normal in all cases except one, and its

average weight equaled that of the controls, but further study would have been desirable. No conclusions were reached regarding the other nuclear constituents of the extrapyramidal system.

Microscopically, the corpus striatum showed a remarkable loss of nerve cells in the putamen, especially in the posterior three fourths; less loss in the anterior fourth and in the head of the caudate nucleus; and probably no loss of nerve cells in the globus pallidus. In the majority of cases, an extensive neuroglial proliferation, most marked where the neurons were fewest, was noted. In the red nucleus no constant or definite neuronal or neuroglial changes were identified. The corpus subthalamicum and the substantia nigra were too little studied to justify a definite opinion.

The nerve cells of the cerebral cortex were nearly always "dark staining, small, and shrunken in appearance."[24] The cytoarchitecture was not obviously disorganized, and as a whole, the neurons were "probably" not reduced in number as compared with the control cases. The neuroglial nuclei of the cortex looked smaller, darker, and more abundant than in the control cases. The neuroglial fibers were usually most abundant in the zone of junction of gray and white matter or in the deepest layers of the gray matter, where many of the glial nuclei were large, pale, and vesicular.

The white matter of the cerebral hemispheres, in general, was thought to be con-

---

* See references 1, 2, 8, 9, 33, 38, 39, 40, 43, 45, 47, 48, 51, 82, and 90.

† Every member of this group had, in addition to the characteristic motor disorders and mental symptoms of Huntington's chorea, a family history of uninterrupted heredity from parent to child, and was considered free from all objections.

siderably more reduced in amount than the gray matter. No abnormality in the gray or white matter of the cerebellum or in the dentate nucleus was observed, with the exception of one case (see further comments on pp. 421–422; electron-microscopic observations on pp. 425–432, and H.C. in children on p. 422).

In conclusion, Dunlap[24] felt that there were constant lesions of a definite type in the corpus striatum and in the gray and white matter of the cerebrum. Several authors* have found changes similar to those described by Dunlap. Some authors, in addition, have described areas of tissue necrosis which doubtless had a vascular origin[29,61,68] but such lesions sometimes appeared distant from the involved blood vessels, being then possibly a sequence to angiospasm.[91] Such findings, however, were not specific or of constant character and were found not to be related to the duration of the disease.

Subsequent studies by Davidson et al.[17] es-

* See references 34, 49, 57, 59, and 60.

sentially confirmed Dunlap's findings, with the exception that these investigators observed more marked changes in the third cortical layer of the cerebral cortex and changes in the cerebellum in two of the three cases studied. In contrast to Dunlap's cases, but in conformity with Jakob's,[44] they found that the rostral portions of the striatum were more involved than the caudal.

In view of the fact that these minor discrepancies could also be attributed to some individual variability of the disease process and possibly some difference in investigative techniques, we (Roizin and Kaufman) reviewed some of Dunlap's[24] original material and added ten selected unquestionable cases of chronic, progressive Huntington's chorea. We shall mention only some of the most outstanding neuropathological findings in our series.

Microscopic examination of the CNS revealed, in general, various degrees of atrophic changes of the cerebrum (Figure 17–1) and loss of weight. The leptomeninges, particu-

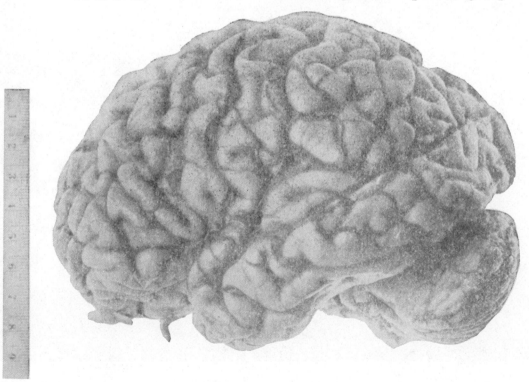

Figure 17–1. Huntington's chorea. Gross appearance of the brain, revealing pronounced atrophic changes.

larly over the atrophic gyri, often appeared thickened. Coronal or horizontal sections of the brain revealed various degrees of narrowing of the cerebral convolutions, deepening and widening of the sulci, thinning of the gray and white matter of the cerebrum and corpus callosum, variable atrophic changes of the caudate nucleus and putamen, and variable degrees of internal hydrocephalus frequently, but not exclusively, of the anterior horns of

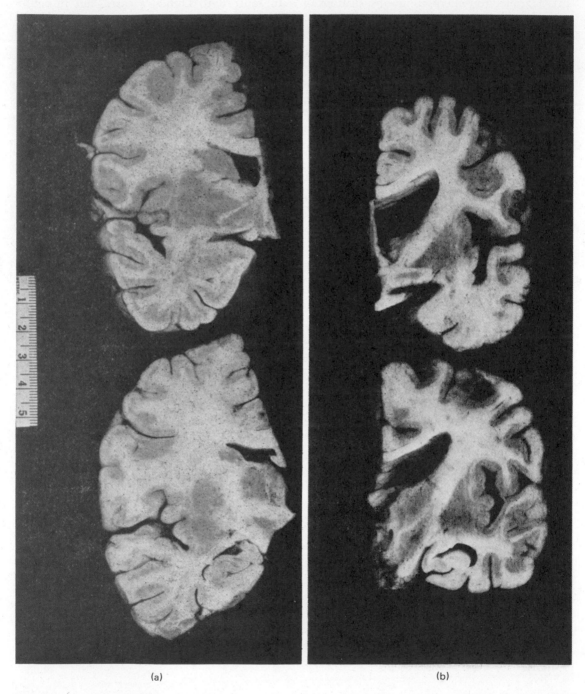

(a)   (b)

Figure 17–2.   (a) Coronal section through a control brain; (b) Huntington's chorea as described in the text.

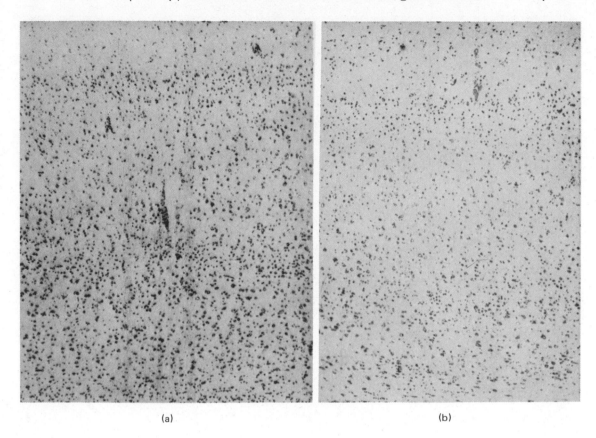

(a)   (b)

Figure 17–3. (a) Section from the frontal lobe of a control case; (b) section from the same region (approx.) of a case of Huntington's chorea, revealing prominent reduction in number of the nerve cells in various cyto-architectural areas. Nissl stain. Low-power magnification.

the lateral ventricles (Figure 17–2). In some cases the brain stem also appeared somewhat smaller than in comparable controls.

Microscopic examination disclosed a degenerative, generally chronic, process of variable intensity and distribution. In some instances the middle layers appeared more prominently involved (Figure 17–3 (b)), in others the deeper layers; in still others, the involvement appeared more diffuse in character (Figure 17–4 (a)). Here and there, circumscribed neuronal rarefraction or small acellular areas were also encountered (Figure 17–4 (b)). Though frequently the smaller neurons appeared severely involved, in some instances the large pyramidal cells showed chromatolysis as well as lipid degeneration. Increased neuroglial density (marginal or subcortical) was observed particularly in association with the more pronounced degrees of atrophy.

Neuronal degeneration and various degrees of numerical reduction were observed in the putamen and the head of the caudate nucleus. Generally, the most marked involvement was of the smaller nerve cells (Figure 17–5 (a)), but the larger neurons Figure 17–5 (b)) in the putamen and caudate nucleus as well as in the globus pallidus were not always spared. As a matter of fact, Sudan III and Sudan black stains, particularly in long-standing chronic cases, revealed the presence of increased intraneuronal lipid material. Similar changes were also encountered, in various degree, in the hypothalamus, in the different nuclear formations of the brain stem and medulla (particularly the inferior olives), and in the Purkinje cells and dentate nucleus of the cerebellum. In some cases the Ammon's horn also appeared to be involved. Increased satellitosis, pseudoneuronophagia, and neuronophagia

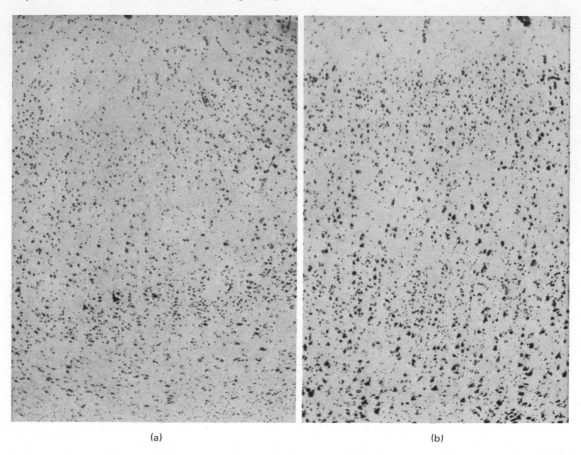

(a)   (b)

Figure 17–4. Huntington's chorea. Cortical regions showing (a) diffuse and (b) small, focal areas with reduction in number of neurons. Nissl stain. Medium-power magnification.

were, at times, prominent in the caudate nucleus and putamen. In the same structures, increased gliosis (Figure 17–6), fibrillary as well as protoplasmic, was frequent. In some instances hypertrophic astrocytes were quite prominent and frequently independent of the blood-vessel walls. There was periaqueductal gliosis in some cases, and in one case marked atrophy and severe gliosis of the inferior olivary nuclei of the medulla were noted. Myelin-sheath stains disclosed in four cases some subcortical pallor and myelin rarefaction as well as poor differentiation of the tangential systems. Almost complete status dysmyelinatus was present in two cases. Moderate arteriosclerotic changes with some lipid deposits and perivascular fibrosis were noticed in five cases. In one instance calcium deposits within the walls and in a perivascular location were ob-

served. Abundant deposits of calcium and amorphous material giving an intense iron reaction, involving particularly the basal ganglia, were found in one case. Now and then, amyloid bodies in a periventricular location, in perivascular areas, or in the white matter were also identified. Senile plaques were detected with silver impregnation in one case.

Clinicopathological studies on Huntington's chorea occurring in the first decade are considered to represent about 1 percent of the total number of patients. The incidence of this disease in the general population is one in 24,000.[46] In addition, typical choreatic movements are often absent in children. Instead they may have hypokinesia, muscular rigidity, epilepsy, cerebellar symptoms, and mental retardation. The cause of death is frequently bronchopneumonia.[13,46,62]

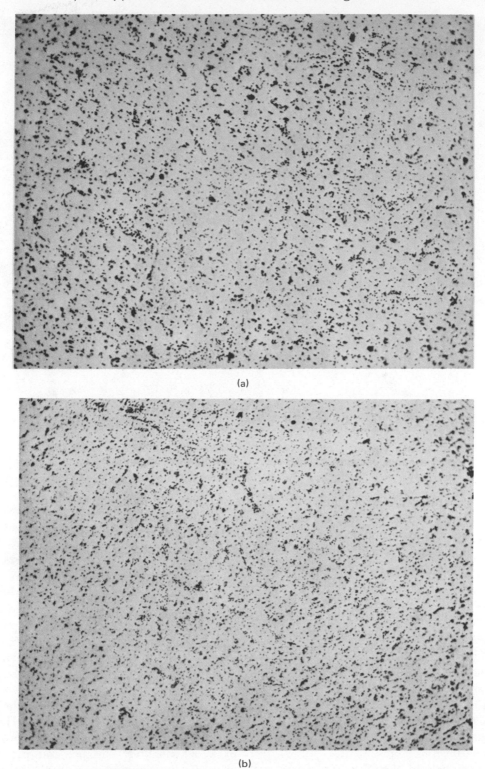

(a)

(b)

Figure 17–5.   Huntington's chorea. Putamen: (a) Various degrees of very pronounced diminution of the neurons (particularly of the small nerve cells) and (b) neuronophagia and increased density of glial nuclei. Nissl stain. Low-power magnification.

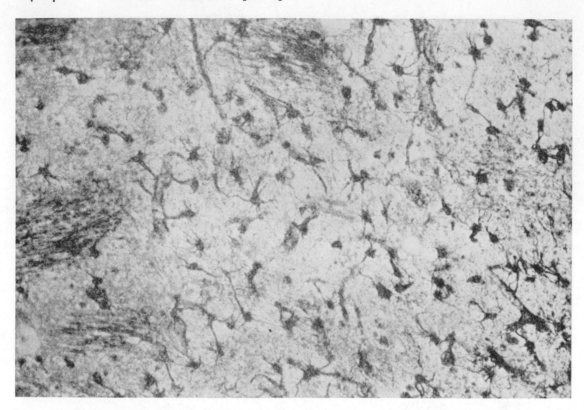

Figure 17–6. Huntington's chorea. Putamen: Astrocytic gliosis as described in the text. Cajal's gold sublimate impregnation. High-power magnification.

Grossly the cerebrum and the cerebellum show various degrees of generally diffuse* atrophy (brain weight 940–980 g.[46]). There is a striking decrease in size of the caudate nucleus, less marked reduction of the putamen and slight of the globus pallidus.

The most common microscopic findings consist of various degrees of decrease in neurons throughout the cerebral cortex. Pronounced to complete loss of neurons in the caudate nucleus is the most frequent feature. In the putamen often only a few large neurons are present with frequent absence of all small ones. The globus pallidus may show some loss of neurons or be well-preserved. Decrease of neurons is also encountered in the subthalamic and red nuclei. The substantia nigra contains less pigment than expected, usually without loss of neurons.

In the cerebellum, the folia are atrophic and the molecular layer reduced in width. The Purkinje cells are particularly depleted. Granular and dentate nuclei neurons are also reduced in number.

In some instances considerable loss of neurons was observed in the inferior olives of the medulla.[46]

Sparse fat-laden cells in the perivascular regions, moderate decrease of myelin in the globus pallidus, very pale or diminished strionigral fibers were prominent in certain cases. Also dense gliosis of globus pallidus, putamen, and Bergmann's layer, as well as increased glial reaction in the molecular layer and dentate nuclei of the cerebellum have been observed in several cases.

It appears from earlier clinicopathological studies that, in the classical type of Huntington's chorea, the neuropathological process is of a degenerative, chronic, and progressive character, involving principally the neurons of the caudate nucleus and putamen, and to a somewhat lesser degree the cerebral cortex. However, in some cases correlated systems

* In some instances particularly fronto-parietal.[46,62]

also are affected, though to a lesser degree and inconsistently.

From an etiopathogenetic point of view, some authors have interpreted the lesions as a primary degeneration of the small cells of the putamen caudate system and of the third and fifth cortical layers. The Vogts[83,84] Jakob,[44] and others assumed that these two sets of structures comprised a "biologically combined organ"[90] subjected to an abiotrophic* process[12,14] As was demonstrated above, however, the lesions in Huntington's chorea are generally diffuse and not specific in character.[15] Other authors regarded the lesions as being due to a "primary progressive gliosis" and the neuronal degeneration as being secondary in character.[16,37] On the other hand, some investigators believed that vasular involution comes first,[27] and that both parenchymatous and glial changes are secondary. The diversity of opinion seems to indicate that, thus far, specific and consistent data are not available for conclusive determination of the pathogenetic mechanisms in Huntington's chorea.† It would appear that the choreic individual is congenitally predisposed to develop, at a certain period of life, the characteristic clinicopathologic syndrome which we have briefly reviewed. Hence, heredity has assumed the role of the principal "etiopathogenetic" factor.

Inborn errors of metabolism in degenerative processes‡ and mental disorders[71] have been suggested as possible factors, based upon the assumption that the morbid changes may be caused by the lack of specific enzymes. Mental abnormalities as by-products of inborn biochemical errors[30] of different degree have been ascribed to phenylketonuria, porphyria, methemoglobinemia, amaurotic idiocies, gargoylism, and other cerebral lipoidoses,[71] as well as to some involutional degenerative processes such as Alzheimer's and Pick's presenile psychoses, although the pathognomonic enzyme abnormality has not been specifically

identified as yet. A similar parallel inborn biochemical abnormality also could be assumed for Huntington's chorea. In support of this suggestion, one should consider that, according to some investigators,[71] hereditary dispositions due to metabolic errors are mainly of two kinds. The first type is almost always genetically homozygous and the affected subject lacks an enzyme because the abnormal genes present in duplicate fail to produce it. These people show signs of a constant abnormality throughout life, or at least from an early age. A carrier with one normal and one abnormal gene is still able to make the necessary enzyme. The second type is less regular in appearance and can have a dominant inheritance. At times, the inborn error gives rise to symptoms only under special circumstances or stress (see below).

During the last two years our combined electron-microscope and histochemical-enzyme studies[74] revealed the following salient findings: (1) The fine structure of the nuclei of cerebral cortical neurons appeared, at times, denser than usual and contained clumps of circumscribed masses of compact osmiophilic granules and/or irregularly dispersed particulate material. The nuclear membranes and their "pores" also show fine structural alterations. Enzyme reaction products of acid phosphatases (AcP) and glucose-6-phosphatase (G-6-P) were usually observed in higher concentrations in the denser regions of the nucleus and at the periphery. (2) Some nucleoli also showed changes and only the pars granulosa and chromosa were differentiated. At times the nucleolus contained dense and light zones composed of granular material. (3) The rough endoplasmic reticulum was scanty and irregularly distributed. Frequently there were abnormal enlargements of the cisternae. In some instances the cisternae showed varying degrees of degranulation. Free ribosomal granules were irregularly dispersed and often reduced in number (Figure 17–7). (4) The Golgi canaliculi formed irregular patterns and frequently the canalicular outlines were blurred and their lumens not discernible (Figure 17–8). The distribution of AcP, G-6-P, and TPP (thiamine pyrophosphatase) reac-

---

* This is a term coined by Gowers[32] to indicate an inherent constitutional weakness or a "defective vital endurance" and "premature decay" of the affected parts of the nervous system.

† See references 27, 28, 58, 65, 67, 75, and 92.

‡ See references 25, 31, 76, 77, and 84.

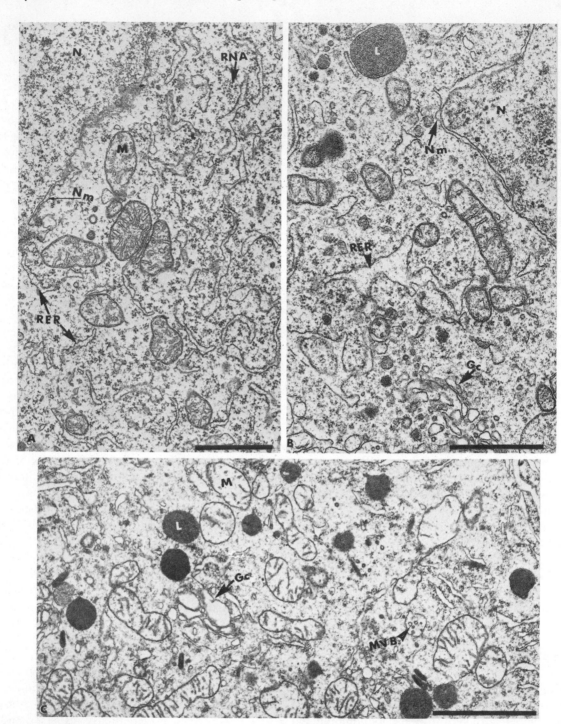

Figure 17–7. Various degrees of fine structural changes of the rough endoplasmic reticulum and RNA distribution in the cytoplasm of some neurons as described in the text. Magnification: (a) ×29,500; (b) ×35,400; (c) ×39,530.

Scale: 1mm. = 1000μ

Explanation of symbols: Gc = Golgi complex or the smooth component of the endoplasmic reticulum; M = mitochondrian; MVB = multivesicular body; Nm = nuclear membrane; N = nucleus; RER = rough component of the endoplasmic reticulum; RNA = ribosomal granules.

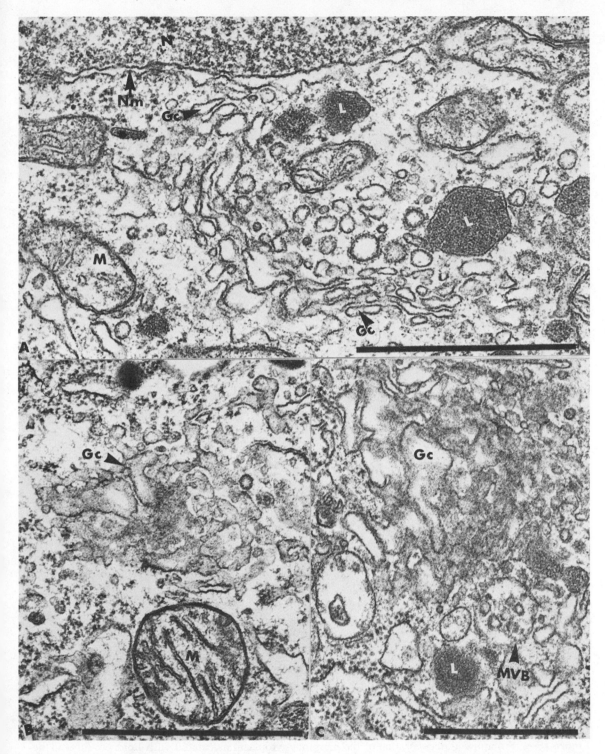

Figure 17–8.   Various stages of fine structural changes and disorganization, especially of the Golgi system as described in the text. Magnification: (a) and (b) ×64,900; (c) ×45,815
Scale: 1mm. = 1000μ
Explanation of symbols: Gc = Golgi caniculi; L = lysosomes;   M = mitochondrian;   MVB = multives-icular body; N = nucleus; Nm = nuclear membrane.

tion products differed and, at times, they had an extracanalicular location. (5) The lysosomes displayed marked variations in number and many were pleomorphic. They showed various stages of metamorphosis particularly in the vicinity of or within areas containing lipid products and lipofuscin bodies (Figure 17–9). AcP, G-6-P, and, to a lesser degree, TPP reaction products were distributed in various concentrations and configurations in lysosomes which were in various stages of auto- and heterophagism. (6) Degenerative

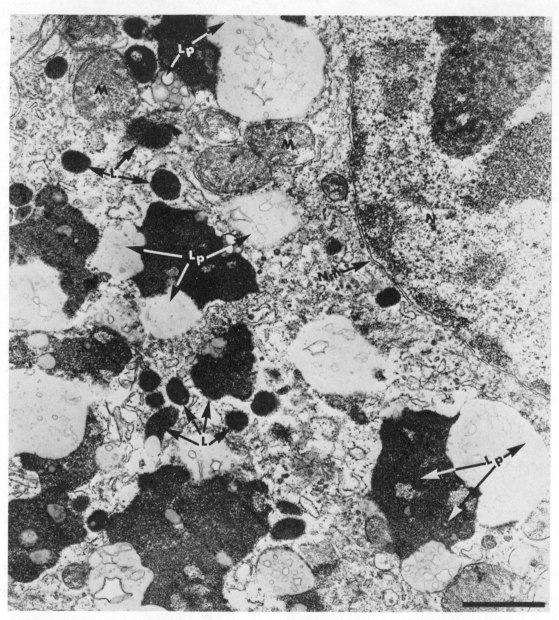

Figure 17–9. Pronounced degeneration of the neuronal cytoplasm associated with lipid products of degeneration and lipofuscin. Lipid products of degeneration intertwined with lipofuscin pigment associated with increase in number of lysosomes. Magnification: ×28,560
Scale: 1mm. = 1000μ
Explanation of symbols: L = lysosomes; Lp = lipofuscin compounds; M = mitochondrian; N = nucleus; Nm = nuclear membrane.

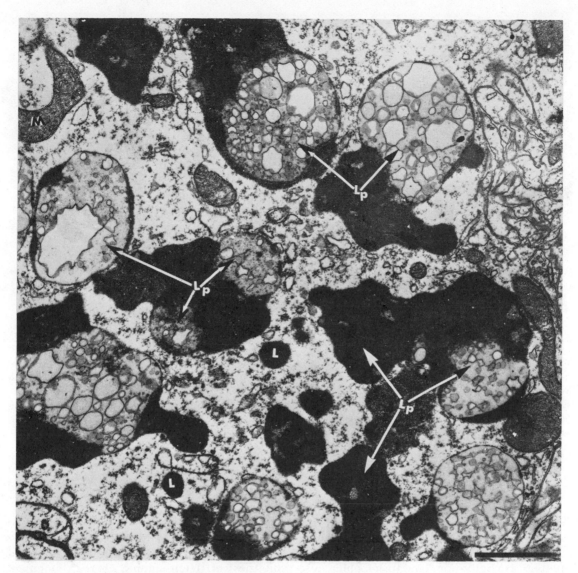

Figure 17–10. Multivacuolated lipofuscin structures intertwined with degenerative lipid material. Magnification: ×25,960
Scale: 1mm. = 1000μ
Explanation of symbols: L = lysosomes; Lp = lipid with lipofuscin vacuolated structures; M = mitochondrion.

products showing variations in osmiophilia were frequently observed in contact with or intertwined with multiforme varieties of lipofuscin bodies (Figure 17–10). The latter were most often observed in the cytoplasm of neurons, particularly in the perinuclear regions. They were also encountered in the glial cells (Figure 17–11), in perivascular regions, and in lesser numbers within the blood-vessel walls. AcP, TPP and G-6-P reaction products were irregularly distributed in differing concentrations, except within vacuolated structures where they were lacking (Figure 17–12). (7) Glycogen granules were found particularly in glial cell processes in the neurophil often in perivascular areas. They were occasionally seen in the axoplasm of neurons or in the presynaptic terminals. (8) Mito-

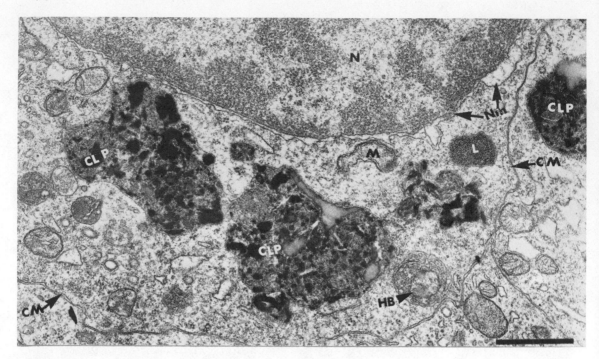

Figure 17–11. Composite lipid products undergoing digestive processes in cytolysomes as described in the text. Magnification: ×26,550.

Scale: 1mm. = 1000μ

Explanation of symbols: CLP = composite lipid products; CM = cellular membrane; HB= heterogeneous body; L = lysosome; M = mitochondria; N = nucleus; Nm = nuclear membrane.

chondria (polymorphometabolosomes) showed variation in number, shape and size. There were also concomitant variations in the configuration of the cristae and osmiophilia of the matrix. Some mitochondria contained AcP reaction products. (9) Multivesicular bodies and heterogeneous bodies which varied in number, configuration, and osmiophilia also contained AcP, TPP, and G-6-P reaction products. Centrioles were sometimes seen in the vicinity of the Golgi system. (10) Of the synaptic complex, the presynaptic terminals often showed reduced numbers of vesicles, which, at times, were associated with variable numbers of organelles some of which were undergoing degenerative changes. Variations in the fine structure and osmiophilic character of the synaptic cleft and subsynaptic web were observed. (11) In several instances the axoplasm contained variable numbers of mitochondria and organelles which gave an appearance resembling axonal dystrophy (Figure 17–13). In addition, AcP and G-6-P

reaction products were found in differing concentrations independent of the presence of organelles (Figure 17–12). (12) Intra- and interlamellar myelin degeneration was observed in some cases. Our control material is still inadequate to make appropriate comparisons. However, these findings in cerebral biopsies of Huntington's chorea[*] augment those reported previously by Tellez-Nagel et al.[80] in that additional histochemical studies were carried out which have enabled us to demonstrate previously undescribed pathological features.[74]

Although our understanding of possible pathogenic mechanisms based on electron-microscope studies is limited, since only the cerebral cortex was examined, similar investigations will be carried out on basal ganglia

[*] This biopsy material is part of a multidisciplinary research investigation on Huntington's chorea carried out in cooperation with S. Stellar, N. Willson, and J. Whittier, supported in part by the St. Barnabas Medical Center Research Foundation for the Neural Sciences.

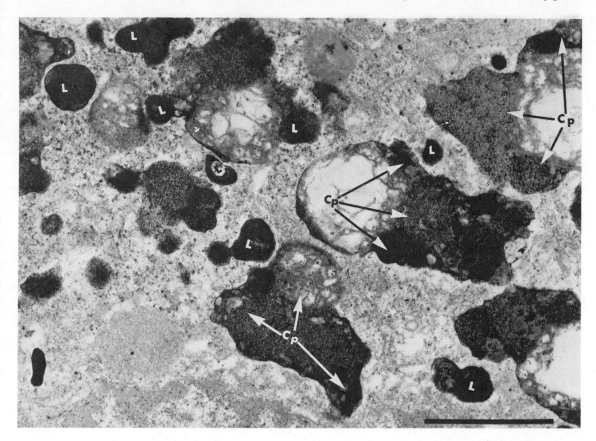

Figure 17–12.   Combined electron-microscope and histochemical reaction for glucose-6-phosphatase showing presence of various amounts of glucose-6-phosphatase reaction products as described in the text. Magnification: ×45,720.
Scale: 1mm. = 1000μ.
Explanation of symbols: L = lysosme;   Cp = composite lipofuscin, glucose-6-phosphatase enzyme reaction products distributed over portions of dense lipofuscin structures.

tissue when it becomes available. With these factors in mind we would like to hypothesize as follows: (1) The ultrastructural alterations in the nucleus and nucleolus, the changes in the endoplasmic reticulum including degranulation, and the irregular distribution and decrease in the number of cytoplasmic ribosomes may be related to disordered protein metabolism. Further studies are needed to determine whether these findings can be correlated with the protein abnormalities recently reported in Huntington's chorea by Igbal et al.[42] (2) Some investigators (Novikoff et al.[66] and Roizin et al.[73]) have suggested that the endoplasmic reticulum is in communication with the nuclear membranes, lysosomes (and correlated structures), and multivesicular bodies

and that it serves as a unitary system concerned with intracellular transport mechanisms. In light of these considerations, it appears possible that the fine structural alterations and irregular distribution of the AcP., G-6P, and TPP reaction products in the Golgi complex and related organelles might be due to a disorder of intracellular transport mechanisms. With respect to the latter it would be of interest to consider its possible significance in lipofuscin body formation in the sense that the degenerative changes of the Golgi canaliculi and its subunits may interfere with or deprive the lysosomes of a continuous supply of the enzyme systems necessary for digestive mechanisms (DeDuve and Wittaux[18,19]). The subsequent accumulation of the lipofuscin

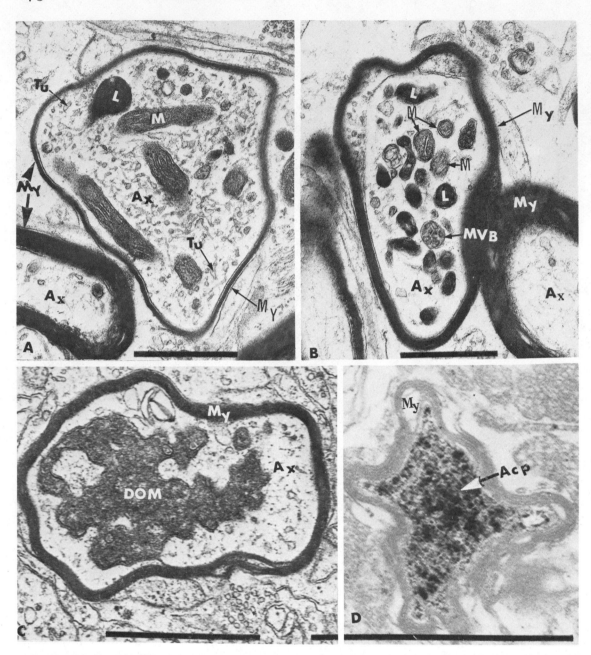

Figure 17–13. (a) Myelinated axon showing pleomorphism of neural tubules and increased number of organelles. Magnification: ×30,480. (b) Myelinated axon with axoplasm containing a large number and variety of organelles undergoing some degenerative changes. Magnification: ×28,650. (c) Myelinated axon revealing dense osmiophilic material as described in text. ×40,650. (d) Axoplasm field with acid phosphatase reaction products. ×77,290.

Scale: 1mm. = 1000μ

Explanation of symbols: Acp = acid phosphatase reaction product; Ax = axon; DOM = dense osmiophilic material; L = lysosomes; M = mitochondrian; MVB = multivesicular body; My = myelin; Tu = neural tubules.

bodies[81] may not only be the result of a failure of cell exocytosis (Brunk and Ericsson[10]), but it may also be due to the fact that the accumulated "residues" were incompletely digested or metabolized as a result of a lack of some lysosomal enzymes. This might result in a molecule which is too large to pass readily through the membranes. (3) The axonal involvement and some of the fine structural alterations of the synapses and their respective subunits may represent some functional and histochemical disorders of the neuronal communication mechanisms.

❨ Bibliography

1. AITKEN, W. "Morbid Appearance in a Case of Chorea. The Connection of This Disease with Imbecility and an Alteration in the Substance of the Brain," *Glasgow Med. J.*, 1 (1853), 92.
2. ALZHEIMER, A. "Über die Anatomische Grundlage der Huntingtonschen Chorea und der Choreatischen Bewegungen Überhaupt," *Z. Ges. Neurol. Psychiatr.*, 3 (1911), 566.
3. ANTON, G. "Über die Beteiligung der Grossen Basalen Gehirnganglien bei Bewegungsstörungen und Insbesondere bei Chorea," *Jahrb. Psychiatr.*, 14 (1896), 141.
4. BARBEAU, A. "Parental Ascent in the Juvenile Form of Huntington's Chorea," *Lancet*, 2 (1970), 937.
5. BARBEAU, A. and J.-R. BRUNETTE, eds., *Progress in Neurogenetics*, Proc. 2nd Int. Congr. Neuro-Genetics and Neuro-Ophthalmology, World Fed. Neurol. Montreal, Sept., 1967, Vol. 1, *Huntingtons's Disease*, pp. 509–694. Amsterdam: Excerpta Medica Foundation, 1969.
6. BARBEAU, A., T. N. CHASE, and G. W. PAULSON, eds. Advances in Neurology, Vol. 1. *Huntington's Chorea, 1872–1972.* New York: Raven, 1973.
7. BERGSMA, D., H. T. LYNCH, and R. J. THOMAS, eds. *International Directory of Genetic Services*, 4th ed. New York: The National Foundation-March of Dimes, 1974.
8. BONHOEFFER, K. "Ein Beitrag zur Localisation der Choreatischen Bewegungen," *Monatsschr. Psychiatr. Neurol.*, 1 (1897), 6.
9. BROADBENT, W. H. "Remarks on the Pathology of Chorea," *Br. Med. J.* (1869), 345; also reported before the London Med. Soc., 1865–66.
10. BRUNK, U. and J. L. E. ERICSSON. "Electron Microscopical Studies on Rat Brain Neurons. Localization of Acid Phosphatase and Mode of Formation of Lipofuscin Bodies," *J. Ultrastruct. Res.*, 38 (1972), 1.
11. BRUYN, G. W. "Clinical Variants and Differential Diagnosis," in A. Barbeau, T. N. Chase, and G. W. Paulson, eds., Advances in Neurology, Vol. 1, *Huntington's Chorea, 1872–1972*, pp. 51–56. New York: Raven, 1973.
12. BUZZARD, E. F. and J. G. GREENFIELD. *Pathology of the Nervous System.* London: Constable, 1921.
13. BYERS, R. K. and J. A. DODGE. "Huntington's Chorea in Children. Report of Four Cases," *Neurology*, 17 (1967), 587.
14. CANFIELD, R. M. and J. J. PUTNAM. "A Case of Hemiplegic Chorea with Autopsy and Remarks," *Boston Med. Surg. J.*, 11 (1884), 220.
15. COURVILLE, C. B. *Pathology of the Central Nervous System.* Mountview, Calif.: Pacific Press Publ. Assoc., 1945.
16. D'ANTONA, S. "Contributo all'Anatomia Patalogica della Corea di Huntington," *Riv. Patol. Nerv. Ment.*, 19 (1914), 321.
17. DAVIDSON, C., S. P. GOODHART, and H. SHLIONSKY. "Chronic Progressive Chorea, The Pathogenesis and Mechanism; A Histopathologic Study," *Arch. Neurol. Psychiatry*, 27 (1932), 906.
18. DE DUVE, C. "General Properties of Lysosomes, The Lysosome Concept," in A.V.S. de Rouck and M. P. Cameron, eds., *Ciba Foundation Symposium on Lysosomes*, pp. 1–31. Boston: Little, Brown, 1963.
19. DE DUVE, C. and R. WATTIAUX. "Functions of Lysosomes," *Ann. Rev. Physiol.*, 28 (1966), 435.
20. DEWHURST, K. "Personality Disorder in Huntington's Disease," *Psychiatr. Clin.*, 3 (1970), 221–229.
21. DEWHURST, K. and J. OLIVER. "Huntington's Disease of Young People," *Eur. Neurol.*, 3 (1970), 278–289.
22. DEWHURST, K., J. E. OLIVER, and A. L. McKNIGHT. "Sociopsychiatric Consequences of Huntington's Disease," *Br. J. Psychiatry*, 116 (1970), 255.
23. DEWHURST, K., J. OLIVER, K. L. K. TRICK et

al. "Neuro-psychiatric Aspects of Hunting-ton's Disease," *Confin. Neurol.*, 31 (1969), 255–258.

24. DUNLAP, C. B. "Pathologic Changes in Huntington's Chorea," *Arch. Neurol. Psychiatry*, 18 (1927), 867.

25. ELLIOT, K. A. C., I. H. PAGE, and J. H. QUASTEL. "Neurochemistry: The Chemical Dynamics of Brain and Nerves," Spring-field, Ill.: Charles C. Thomas, 1955.

26. FALEK, A. "An Ongoing Study in Early Detection as Part of a Comprehensive Program in Huntington's Chorea," in A. Barbeau, T. N. Chase, and G. W. Paulson, eds., Advances in Neurology, Vol. 1. *Huntington's Chorea, 1872–1972*, pp. 325–327. New York: Raven, 1973.

27. FEREMUTSCH, K. "Vascular Disease of Striatum Producing Clinical Picture of Chronic Progressive Chorea in Two Siblings," *Monatsschr. Psychiatr. Neurol.*, 127 (1954), 227.

28. FROMENTY, M. L. "Progressive Chorea with Dementia Due to Murine Typhus," *Presse Méd.*, 59 (1951), 91.

29. FROTSCHER, R. "Ein Beitrag zum Krankheitsbild der Chorea Chronica Progressiva," *Arch. Psychiatr.*, 47 (1910), 790.

30. GARROD, A. E. *Inborn Errors of Metabolism*, 2nd ed. London: Hodder, 1923.

31. GATES, R. R. *Human Genetics*, Vol. 2. New York: Macmillan, 1946.

32. GOWERS, W. R. *Lectures in the Diagnosis of the Disease of the Brain*. London: Churchill, 1885.

33. HAMMOND, W. A. *A Treatise on the Diseases of the Nervous System*, 6th ed., p. 722. New York: Appleton, 1876.

34. HASSIN, G. B. *Histopathology of the Peripheral and Central Nervous System*, p. 433. Chicago: Hamilton, 1948.

35. HEMPHILL, M. "Tests for Presymptomatic Huntington's Chorea," *N. Engl. J. Med.*, 287 (1972), 823–824.

36. ———. "Pretesting for Huntington's Disease," *Hastings Center Rept.*, 3 (1973), 12–13.

37. HOFFMANN, J. "Über Chorea Chronica Progressiva (Huntingtonsche Chorea, Chorea hereditaria)," *Arch. Pathol. Anat.*, 111 (1888), 513.

38. HUGHES, M. "Social Significance of Huntington's Chorea," *Am. J. Psychiatry*, 3 (1925), 537.

39. HUNT, J. R. "Progressive Atrophy of the Globus Pallidus," *Brain*, 40 (1917), 58.

40. HUNTINGTON, G. "On Chorea," *Med. Surg. Reptr.*, 26 (1872), 317.

41. HUSQUINET, H., G. FRANCK, and C. VRANCKX. "Detection of Future Cases of Huntington's Chorea by the L-Dopa Load Test: Experiment with Two Monozygotic Twins," *Adv. Neurol.*, 1 (1973), 301–310.

42. IGBAL, K., I. GRUNDKE-IGBAL, M. L. SHELANSKI et al. "Abnormal Proteins in Huntington's Disease," *J. Neuropathol. Exp. Neurol.*, 33 (1974), 172.

43. JACKSON, J. H. "Observations on the Psychology and Pathology of Hemichorea," *Edinburgh Med. J.*, 14 (1868), 294.

44. JAKOB, A. "Die Extrapyramidalen Erkrankungen im Lichte der Pathologischen Anatomie und Histologie und die Pathophysiologie der Extrapyramidalen Bewegungsstörungen," *Klin. Wochnschr.*, 3 (1924), 865.

45. JELGERSMA, G. "Neue Anatomische Befunde bei Paralysis Agitans und bei Chronische Chorea," *Neurol. Zentralbl.*, 27 (1908), 995.

46. JERVIS, G. A. "Huntington's Chorea in Childhood," *Arch. Neurol.*, 9 (1963), 244.

47. JOSEPHY, H. "Huntingtonsche Krankheit," in O. Bumke, and O. Foerster, eds., *Handbuch der Neurologie*, Vol. 16, p. 729. Berlin: Springer, 1936.

48. KALKHOF, J. and O. RANKE. "Eine Neue Chorea Huntington-Familie," *Z. Ges. Neurol. Psychiatr.*, 17 (1913), 256.

49. KIESSELBACH, G. "Anatomischer Befund eines Falles von Huntingtonscher Chorea," *Monatsschr. Psychiatr. Neurol.*, 35 (1914), 525.

50. KLAWANS, H. L., G. W. PAULSON, S. P. RINGEL et al. "The Use of L-Dopa in the Presymptomatic Detection of Huntington's Chorea," in A. Barbeau, T. N. Chase, and G. W. Paulson, eds., Advances in Neurology, Vol. 1. *Huntington's Chorea, 1872–1972*, pp. 295–310. New York: Raven, 1973.

51. KLEIST, K. "Anatomischer Befund bei Huntingtonschen Chorea," *Z. Ges. Neurol. Psychiatr.*, 6 (1913), 423.

52. KORENYI, C. and J. R. WHITTIER. "The Juvenile Form of Huntington's Chorea: Its Prevalence and Other Observations," in A. Barbeau, T. N. Chase, and G. W.

Paulson, eds., Advances in Neurology, Vol. 1. *Huntington's Chorea, 1872–1972,* pp. 75–77. New York: Raven, 1973.

53. ———. "Dyskinesia Analysis," *Dis. Nerv. Syst.,* 35 (1974), 169–171.

54. KORENYI, C., J. R. WHITTIER, and D. CONCHADO. "Stress in Huntington's Disease (Chorea): Review of the Literature and Personal Observations," *Dis. Nerv. Syst.,* 33 (1972), 339–344.

55. KORENYI, C., J. R. WHITTIER, and G. FISCHBACH. "Cineseismography: A Method for Measuring Abnormal Involuntary Movements of the Human Body," *Dis. Nerv. Syst.,* 35 (1974), 63–65.

56. KORENYI, C. and R. WITTMAN. "Prevalence of Medical Disorders Other than Huntington's Disease in Offspring of Symptomatic and at Risk Parents," *Dis. Nerv. Syst.,* 35 (1974), 17–19.

57. LEWANDOWSKY, M. and E. STADELMANN. "Chorea Apoplectica," *Z. Ges. Neurol. Psychiatr.,* 12 (1912), 530.

58. LEWY, F. H. "Historical Introduction: The Basal Ganglia and Their Diseases," *Assoc. Nerv. Ment. Dis. Proc.,* 21 (1940), 1.

59. LHERMITTE, J. and P. PAGNIEZ. "Anatomie et physiologie pathologiques de la chorée de Sydenham," *Encéphale,* 25 (1930), 24.

60. LICHTENSTEIN, B. W. *A Textbook of Neuropathology,* p. 80. Philadelphia: Saunders, 1949.

61. MARIE, P. and J. LHERMITTE. "Les Lésions de la chorée chronique progressive (chorée d'Huntington). La dégénération atrophique cortico-striée," *Ann. Méd.,* 1 (1914), 18.

62. MARKHAM, C. H. and J. W. KNOX. "Observations on Huntington's Chorea in Childhood," *J. Pediatr.,* 67 (1965), 45.

63. MYRIANTHOPOULOS, N. C. "Review Article: Huntington's Chorea," *J. Med. Genet.,* 3 (1966), 298–314.

64. ———. "Huntington's Chorea: The Genetic Problem Five Years Later," in A. Barbeau, T. N. Chase, and G. W. Paulson, eds., Advances in Neurology, Vol. 1. *Huntington's Chorea, 1872–1972,* pp. 149–159. New York: Raven, 1973.

65. NOTKIN, J. "Convulsive Manifestations in Huntington's Chorea," *J. Nerv. Ment. Dis.,* 74 (1931), 149.

66. NOVIKOFF, A. B. "Lysosomes in Nerve Cells," in H. Hyden, ed., *The Neuron,* p. 319. Amsterdam: Elsevier, 1967.

67. NOYES, A. P. *Modern Clinical Psychiatry,* Philadelphia: Saunders, 1939.

68. OPPENHEIM, H., and H. HOPPE. "Zur Pathologischen Anatomie der Chorea Chronica Progressiva Hereditaria," *Arch. Psychiatr.,* 25 (1893), 617.

69. PALM, J. D. "Longitudinal Study of a Preclinical Test Program for Huntington's Chorea," *Adv. Neurol.,* 1 (1973), 311–324.

70. PEARSON, J. S. "Behavioral Aspects of Huntington's Chorea," *Adv. Neurol.,* 1 (1973), 701–715.

71. PENROSE, L. S. "Inborn Errors of Metabolism in Relation to Mental Pathology," in K. A. C. Elliott, I. H. Page, and J. H. Quastel, eds., *Neurochemistry,* p. 807. Springfield, Ill.: Charles C. Thomas, 1955.

72. PETIT, H. and G. MILBLED. "Anomalies of Conjugate Ocular Movements in Huntington's Chorea: Application to Early Detection," in A. Barbeau, T. N. Chase, and G. W. Paulson, eds., Advances in Neurology, Vol. 1. *Huntington's Chorea, 1872–1972,* pp. 287–294. New York: Raven, 1973.

73. ROIZIN, L., K. NISHIKAWA, J. KOIZUMI et al. "The Fine Structure of the MVB and Their Relationship to the Ultracellular Constituents of the CNS," *J. Neuropathol. Exp. Neurol.,* 26 (1967), 223.

74. ROIZIN, L., S. STELLAR, N. WILLSON et al. "Electron Microscope and Enzyme Studies in Cerebral Biopsies of Huntington's Chorea," *Trans. Am. Neurol. Assoc.,* 99 (1974), in press.

75. ROSENBAUM, D. "Psychosis with Huntington's Chorea," *Psychiatr. Q.,* 15 (1941), 93.

76. SJOGREN, T. "Vererbungsmedizinische Untersuchungen über Huntington's Chorea in einer Schwedischen Bauern Population," *Z. Menschl. Vererb. Konstitutionslehre,* 19 (1935), 131.

77. STERN, C. *Human Genetics.* San Francisco: Freeman, 1949.

78. STEVENS, D. L. "The Classification of Variants of Huntington's Chorea," in A. Barbeau, T. N. Chase, and G. W. Paulson, eds., Advances in Neurology, Vol. 1. *Huntington's Chorea, 1872–1972,* pp. 57–64. New York: Raven, 1973.

79. TAMIR, A., J. WHITTIER, and C. KORENYI. "Huntington's Chorea: A Sex Difference in Psychopathological Symptoms," *Dis. Nerv. Syst.,* 30 (1969), 103.

80. TELLEZ-NAGEL, J., A. B. JOHNSON, and R. D. TERRY. "Studies of Brain Biopsies of Patients with Huntington's Chorea," *J. Neuropathol. Exp. Neurol.*, 33 (1974), 172.

81. TOTH, S. E. "The Origin of Lipofuscin Age Pigments," *Exp. Gerontol.*, 3 (1968), 19.

82. VOGT, C. "Quelques Considérations générales à propos du syndrome du corps strie," *J. Psychol. Neurol.*, Ergh., 4 (1911–12), 479.

83. VOGT, C., and O. VOGT. "Zur Lehre der Erkrankungen des Striären Systems," *J. Psychol. Neurol.*, 25, Ergh., 3 (1920), 631.

84. ———. "Precipitating and Modifying Agents in Chorea," *J. Nerv. Ment. Dis.*, 116 (1952), 601.

85. WAGNER, R. and H. K. MITCHELL. *Genetics and Metabolism*. New York: Wiley, 1955.

86. WERNER, A. and J. J. FOLK. "Manifestations of Neurotic Conflict in Huntington's Chorea," *J. Nerv. Ment. Dis.*, 147 (1968), 141.

87. WHITTIER, J. R. "Management of Hunting-

ton's Chorea: The Disease, Those Affected, and Those Otherwise Involved," in A. Barbeau, T. N. Chase, and G. W. Paulson, eds., Advances in Neurology, Vol. 1. *Huntington's Chorea, 1872–1972*, pp. 743–753. New York: Raven, 1973.

88. WHITTIER, J. R., G. HAYDU, and J. CRAWFORD. "Effect of Imipramine (Tofranil) on Depression and Hyperkinesia in Huntington's Disease," *Am. J. Psychiatry*, 118 (1961), 79.

89. WHITTIER, J. R., A. HEIMLER, and C. KORENYI. "The Psychiatrist and Huntington's Disease (Chorea)," *Am. J. Psychiatry*, 128 (1972), 1546–1550.

90. WILSON, S. A. K. "Progressive Lenticular Degeneration: A Familial Nervous Disease Associated with Cirrhosis of the Liver," *Brain*, 34 (1912), 295.

91. ———. *Modern Problems in Neurology*, Chaps. 7–11. New York: Wood, 1929.

92. ———. *Neurology*, Vol. 2. Baltimore: Williams & Wilkins, 1940.

CHAPTER 18

MENTAL RETARDATION

I. Nature and Manifestations

Sterling D. Garrard and Julius B. Richmond

MENTAL RETARDATION is an arbitrary concept. It is often discussed in a medical and psychiatric context as if it were a homogeneous clinical entity, a disorder, or even a disease. This clinical viewpoint is reinforced somewhat circularly for physicians by the inclusion of the rubric in the classification of diseases in medicine and psychiatry. From a rigorous clinical standpoint, however, mental retardation is an imprecise, lumping term rather than a single, homogeneous entity. Unfortunately, a discussion of the "nature and manifestations" of mental retardation may further reinforce the notion that it is a naturalistic phenomenon.

The individuals who are assigned to the category of "mentally retarded" through clinical processes vary widely with respect to their genotypic, etiologic, anatomic, neurophysiologic, psychometric, cognitive, prognostic, and most other characteristics. For many, if not most, traits the scale of the phenotypic variation within the retarded population approxi-

mates that in the population at large. Since most traits vary continuously rather than discontinuously between the two populations, the retarded and nonretarded groups tend to merge without a sharp line of demarcation. Their separation ultimately depends upon the application of arbitrary criteria. While the differences between the populations are primarily those of degree rather than of kind, there is a group of persons with mentally retarded behavior which represents a separate population. This group is set apart chiefly by its association with genetic mutations, cytogenetic abnormalities, and biomedical disorders of the central nervous system.

The heterogeneity within the category of mental retardation sharply limits the utility of the term for medical-psychiatric, educational, psychological, administrative, and scientific purposes. Because of the large numbers of variables which influence behavior within the total population of retarded individuals, different samples of the population tend to include differing mixtures of subgroups. Even when carefully matched on a selected set of variables, homogeneous comparison groups are difficult to obtain. Over the years, this problem undoubtedly has confounded the interpretation and replication of innumerable studies in the field of mental retardation. The heterogeneity of the population highlights the fact that mental retardation is not a medical, psychological, educational, or sociological entity. For this reason, in part, mental retardation cannot be fully understood from the perspective of any one discipline.

Mental retardation does not stand alone as a field for scientific investigation. Its scientific roots lie within the subdivisions of developmental psychology, e.g., intelligence and cognition, attention and habituation, learning theory and behavior principles, language, and psycholinguistics. The understanding of mental retardation is advanced only as far as investigations in the component fields of developmental psychology. Although particular developmental issues may be studied to advantage within the retarded population, developmental psychology is the mirror within which mental retardation must be viewed for scientific purposes.

⟦ Definition and Classification

An awareness of two constructs is necessary for an understanding of mental retardation. The first construct pertains to intelligence. It is assumed heuristically here that quantities of "intelligence" are normally distributed in the population. Within this framework, psychometric tests have been constructed to yield a normal distribution of test abilities with respect to a reference population. These tests provide an objective basis for measuring and defining low intelligence. Mental retardation is a second construct which is dependent upon the preceding one but is not identical with it. This construct is derived, in part, from the nontest behaviors of individuals at the low end of the distribution of measured intelligence. Within this framework, mental retardation may be attributed to persons with low

measured intelligence whose adaptive behavior is also judged to be impaired or unintelligent. *Accordingly, low measured intelligence is not always synonymous with mental retardation.* From the perspective of learning theory, mental retardation reflects both insufficient and inappropriate learning. In the final analysis, however, "mental retardation" is a clinical term which refers to a reduced velocity and deviant direction of behavioral development.

The formal definitions of mental retardation, which are pertinent to clinical practice in the United States, are discussed in two reference books. These definitions reflect a consensus of prevailing professional views and are subject to periodic revisions as concepts change. The *Manual on Terminology and Classification in Mental Retardation*, 1973 Revision, of the American Association on Mental Deficiency (AAMD) defines mental retardation as follows: "Mental retardation refers to significantly subaverage general intellectual functioning existing concurrently with deficits in adaptive behavior, and manifested during the developmental period."[29] The interrelated *Diagnostic and Statistical Manual of Mental Disorders* (DSM-II, 1968) of the American Psychiatric Association (APA),[1] which adapts the *International Classification of Diseases* (ICD-8, 1968) of the World Health Organization[62] to American usage, defines mental retardation in somewhat similar terms as follows: "Mental retardation refers to subnormal general intellectual functioning which originates during the developmental period and is associated with impairment of either learning and social adjustment, or maturation, or both."

These definitions assign two essential properties to mental retardation, namely, low intellectual functioning and deficient adaptive behavior. In keeping with these definitions, dual criteria are required for an inference of mental retardation at an operational level, namely, measured intelligence at or below a selected level *and* demonstrated deficiencies in adaptive behavior. Strictly speaking, only the combination of a low IQ score plus deficient adaptive behavior equals mental retardation. Any other combination of impairment and nonimpairment in these two areas does not equal mental retardation. "Learning disabilities," many poverty-associated learning "failures," and other forms of intellectual growth deflections are automatically excluded from the clinical category of mental retardation by these criteria, even though causal and functional continuities may exist between them.

The necessity for dual criteria for a "diagnosis" of mental retardation reflects a distrust of either criterion alone as a basis for identification. An exclusive reliance on intelligence test scores would result in the labeling of many individuals whose behavioral adequacy could be demonstrated in a variety of circumstances. In addition, minority-group members would be inappropriately included within the clinical category of mental retardation in appreciable numbers. In a sense, *the adaptive behavioral criterion is intended to provide a double check on the psychometric criterion in the clinical labeling process.* Unfortunately, the relative lack of precision of adaptive behavioral scales in separating retarded from nonretarded behaviors at borderline levels leaves considerable room for subjective judgments in this area. These judgments may ultimately be crucial in the labeling of large numbers of children, especially in minority groups. Because of the subjective latitude which enters into the application of the adaptive behavioral criterion, the category of mental retardation cannot be clearly delineated throughout its entire range. Except for measured intelligence, the available diagnostic tools lack sufficient discriminatory power to be useful for identification in many instances.

The APA manual distinguishes five levels of mental retardation, based entirely upon measured intelligence in this system; adaptive behavior is not considered. Levels are delineated by ranges of IQ scores (test unspecified) as follows: (1) borderline, IQ 68–85; (2) mild, IQ 52–67; (3) moderate, IQ 36–51; (4) severe, IQ 20–35; and (5) profound, IQ less than 20. The borderline level in this classification has been widely criticized because it would result in the potential inclusion of at least 16 percent of the total population within the category of retardation.

The AAMD manual, on the other hand, classifies the severity of mental retardation independently in the areas of measured intelligence (i.e., test behaviors) and adaptive behavior (i.e., nontest behaviors). In each behavioral domain four levels of severity are distinguished. The criterion for mental retardation is fulfilled with respect to measured intelligence by scores which are more than two standard deviations below the mean of a standardized test. In the AAMD system, the controversial borderline category of the APA manual is eliminated. The remaining four levels of severity with respect to intelligence test scores are delineated by standard deviation intervals as shown in Table 18–1.

The adaptive behavioral criterion is fulfilled in the AAMD system when rating scales and observer judgments lead to the conclusion that adaptive behavior is significantly below the population norms for the age group. Adaptive behavior here refers to the behavioral phenomena which contribute most strongly to the social perception of retardation. Areas of in-

TABLE 18–1. **Levels of Severity of Mental Retardation by Measured Intelligence (AAMD)**

DESCRIPTIVE LEVELS	STANDARD DEVIATION RANGES	REPRESENTATIVE IQ SCORES	
		STANFORD-BINET AND CATTELL (S.D. 16)	WECHSLER SCALES (S.D. 15)
Mild	−2.01 to −3.00	68–52	69–55
Moderate	−3.01 to −4.00	51–36	54–40
Severe	−4.01 to −5.00	35–20	39–25*
Profound	Below	19 and below	24 and below*

* Extrapolated.

terest in this context include self-help and personal independence, sensorimotor development, communication, socialization, reasoning, and judgment in meeting societal expectations, academic skills pertinent to community living, self-direction and responsibility, occupational attributes, maladaptive behaviors, and the like. Levels of adaptive behavioral deficiency are labeled mild, moderate, severe, and profound. At its upper limit the mild level of deficiency corresponds to a significant, negative deviation from population norms (analogous to —2 standard deviations for intelligence test scores, but lacking in this degree of precision). At its lower limit the profound level of deficiency corresponds to an almost complete lack of adaptation. The AAMD manual provides descriptive patterns of adaptive behavioral functioning by age and level which may be helpful in estimating severity. It is intended, however, that standardized scales, e.g., the Vineland Social Maturity Scale[17] and the AAMD Adaptive Behavior Scales,[44] will be used in combination with clinical judgment to classify levels of adaptive behavioral deficiency.

(Biomedical "Causation"

In a strictly logical framework, medical diagnoses, diseases, and pathological processes do not define mental retardation; only behavioral criteria do this. Conversely, behaviors which are labeled mentally retarded do not define or signify pathological processes or medical disorders; only biomedical criteria do this.

There are no direct relationships between specific medical diagnoses and specific learning or adaptive behavioral characteristics. Many interacting variables, including innumerable environmental contingencies, are interposed between biomedical phenomena and particular behaviors. From this perspective, a medical diagnosis or disorder can never be viewed as the sole or proximate "cause" of mental retardation. Lately, the behaviorists have been particularly vocal in indicating that

the explanatory power of medical diagnoses for mentally retarded behavior is limited and that the techniques of behavioral intervention are independent of the dictates of medical etiologies.

General associations are noted, however, between mental retardation and various medical diseases, syndromes, disorders, findings, and events. Presumably, these associations are mediated through pathological processes which affect the response capacities for learning and predispose individuals to behaviors which may be labeled abnormal. The correlation between a medical diagnosis and mental retardation approaches unity in the case of Down's syndrome or mongolism. Here, the association is so strong that the recognition of the medical syndrome at birth is considered tantamount to the identification of mental retardation, even though the behavioral criteria may not be fulfilled until some time in the future. A number of additional medical disorders are correlated with retardation in this way at different levels of probability. The AAMD manual includes a separate medical classification for the coding of conditions which are presumed to be etiologically associated with retardation.[29] Similar coding requirements are contained in the APA manual.[1]

When viewed from a medical perspective, the mentally retarded population is roughly separable into the following two groups: Group 1, a small group with abnormal medical findings, and Group 2, a large group without abnormal medical findings. The divisibility of the retarded population into two groups on the basis of medical findings has been noted in the literature for many years. In the past, various terms have been applied to these groups as follows: extrinsic and intrinsic, secondary and primary, exogenous and endogenous, organic and subcultural, pathological and physiological, and the like. Although these terms imply a binary view of causation which is no longer tenable, the separation into two groups is useful for medical diagnostic purposes. The relationships between these two groups and the major etiological categories

TABLE 18–2.   **Relationships between two medically distinguishable groups within the retarded population and postulated etiological categories**

MEDICAL DIAGNOSES (20–25 percent of total retarded population)	MULTIFACTORIAL – POLYGENIC (75–80 percent of total retarded population)	
Single mutant genes (metabolic diseases)		
Malformation syndromes (including cytogenetic)	Complex causation low socioeconomic status learning experiences	Tail of "normal" distribution of intelligence.
Sequelae of prior disease (prenatal, perinatal, postnatal)	disadvantaged or predisposing to retardation	
Miscellaneous progressive neurological diseases	subclinical or undiagnosed prior disease	
Group 1. Abnormal medical findings: includes more than 20–25% of the total retarded population.	Group 2. No abnormal medical findings.	

which are postulated within the retarded population are shown in Table 18–2.

From a practical standpoint, the yield of medical diagnoses will be limited to Group 1. Some individuals in this group will have specific medical diagnoses which can be currently and directly verified; included in this category will be the metabolic diseases, malformation syndromes, and certain progressive neurological diseases, e.g., subacute sclerosing panencephalitis. Other individuals in this group will have medical disorders which cannot be currently or directly verified, because the findings represent sequelae of conditions which were active for a limited time only during the prenatal, perinatal, or postnatal periods. In these instances, the applicable diagnoses must be inferred retrospectively; the validity of these inferences will depend upon the degree of specificity of the residual findings and/or of the available historical data. If neither the findings nor the history justify a specific diagnostic inference, the abnormal findings must be considered to be idiopathic or undiagnosable.[13] Individuals with idiopathic findings

contribute to the size of Group 1 in indeterminate numbers. It is commonly estimated, however, that persons with assignable medical etiologies account for 20–25 percent of the total retarded population. Table 18–2 shows the proportionate representation (estimated) of medical findings and diagnoses within the retarded population. Table 18–3 presents a simplified medical classification which can serve as a framework for the medical diagnostic approach. Representative medical disorders which are included in Table 18–3 for illustrative purposes will not be discussed here.

Group 1 is delineated by five sets of medical findings which provide access to the etiologic categories in Table 18–3. Since these findings are always presumptive of a medical etiology or "cause" for mentally retarded behavior, the medical examination should be directed toward their identification. These findings are not mutually exclusive and may occur in any combination in a single individual. The five sets of findings with a high diagnostic payoff in relation to the etiologic categories in Table

18–3 are the following: (1) a cluster of abnormal neurological signs; (2) neurological deterioration or developmental regression; (3) a malformation cluster; (4) positive laboratory tests for abnormal concentrations of metabolites in body fluids; and (5) a documented neurological disease in the past. These findings and their diagnostic implications will be discussed briefly below.

Positive neurological signs are, perhaps, the most frequent indications of medical abnormality which are associated with Group 1. Significant here are one or more localizing or major signs; two or more nonlocalizing, minor, or "soft" dysfunctional signs; or a developmental or IQ which is three standard deviations or more below the mean of a standardized test (roughly equivalent to a score of 50 or below). Since the latter finding is regularly associated with major pathology of the central nervous system (CNS), a low IQ per se at these levels is usually interpreted as an abnormal neurological sign. Identifiable medical diseases and syndromes are heavily concentrated among individuals at these low IQ levels. If identified, positive neurological signs dictate additional investigations for disorders in the categories of metabolic abnormalities, malformation syndromes, and progressive neurological diseases, as shown in Table 18–3.

Neurological deterioration or developmental regression points to currently active dis-

TABLE 18–3.   **Simplified Classification of Medical Disorders Which May Be Etiologically Associated with Mentally Retarded Behavior**

METABOLIC DISEASES, SINGLE MUTANT GENES	MALFORMATION SYNDROMES AND CLUSTERS, CYTOGENETIC AND NON-CYTOGENETIC	NEUROLOGICAL SEQUELAE OF TIME-LIMITED DISORDERS: PRE-, PERI-, OR POSTNATAL	MISCELLANEOUS PROGRESSIVE NEUROLOGICAL DISEASES

Phenylketonuria	Malformation cluster with a cytogenetic anomaly; pattern of anomalies may or may not be specific	Prenatal
		  Teratogenic agents
		  Maternal phenyl-
		    ketonuria
			Subacute sclerosing panencephalitis

Histidinemia			Lead intoxication

Homocystinuria		Rubella virus
		  Cytomegalovirus
		  Herpesvirus hominis
			Hydrocephaly

Maple syrup urine disease	Down's syndrome
	  E_1-trisomy (47,18+)
	  D_1-trisomy (47,13+)		

Argininosuccinic acidemia	Cat-cry syndrome (46, 5p-)	Perinatal Low birth weight	

Glycosaminoglycans: mucopolysaccharidoses	Malformation cluster without demonstrable cytogenetic abnormality; recognizable pattern of anomalies	prematurity; small for gestational age
		  Malnutrition
		  Asphyxia; acidosis
		  Hypoglucosemia
		  Rh isoimmunization and kernicterus	

Galactosemia			
Gangliosidoses: Tay Sachs, etc.			

	Acrocephalosyndactyly (Apert's syndrome)
	Oral-facial-digital syndrome
	Rubenstein-Taybi syndrome
	Cornelia de Lange syndrome
		Postnatal
		  Child abuse
		  Intracranial trauma
		  Meningitis
		  Encephalitis	

	Malformation cluster; no demonstrable cytogenetic abnormality; no recognizable pattern		

eases. Evidence for deterioration should be obtained from documented, longitudinal observations whenever possible, but lacking this, from the history as provided by family members or other significant nonprofessionals. Rates of regression may be rapid or exceedingly slow and difficult to recognize, either intermittent or continuous. If abnormal neurological signs are identified in a person with mental retardation, active disease of the CNS must be considered. Evidence for progressive neurological deterioration points to the metabolic disorders and active neurological diseases as shown in Table 18–3. Evidence for nonprogressive neurological abnormalities (especially when accomplished by a continuous advance in developmental level) points to the residual effects of prior disease. In these instances, the etiology may or may not be assignable.

Malformation clusters are important contributors to the abnormal medical findings which characterize Group 1. Significant here is the combination of two and, especially, three or more malformations, either of major organs or of minor structures, including dermatoglyphics. In some instances, the cluster of anomalies may be associated with a cytogenetic abnormality. In other instances, the cluster of anomalies may conform to a recognizable syndromic pattern in the absence of a demonstrable cytogenetic abnormality. In still other instances, the cluster of anomalies may be unclassifiable and unassociated with a cytogenetic abnormality. Malformation clusters suggest disordered embryogenesis. If accompanied by mental retardation and abnormal neurological signs, they generate an inference that structural abnormalities of the CNS are also present. Regardless of the specificity of the clinical pattern, malformation clusters provide an indication for cytogenetic studies. Several useful catalogues are now available to aid the physician in the clinical identification of malformation syndromes.[6,35,41,53]

Positive laboratory tests for abnormal concentrations of metabolites in body fluids, or for deficient enzyme activity, point directly to the genetic disorders of metabolism.[2,14,19,50] Pre-determined protocols of qualitative or semiquantitative screening tests for metabolic diseases, especially for the amino acid disorders, are often applied in the medical evaluation of individuals with mental retardation. Positive results from these tests must always be confirmed by specific procedures. Assays for enzyme activity are undertaken selectively in situations in which a specific disease, e.g., a ganglioside storage disease, is suspect on the basis of the family history or clinical findings.

A *documented disease or insult* to the central nervous system in the past may be crucial for the subsequent assignment of etiology in instances of nonprogressive neurological abnormalities. Presumably, abnormalities of this type represent the sequelae of prior time-limited diseases. Precise diagnoses of these diseases must be established during their active phase. Retrospective diagnoses, which are based entirely upon the recall of events, or nonspecific, residual findings, are at best speculative. Prenatal or fetal diseases are presumed to be major contributors to the residual category in Table 18–3. Since intrauterine disorders are exceptionally difficult to identify, either concurrently or retrospectively, the etiology of many nonprogressive neurological abnormalities cannot be assigned.[13] The findings are labeled idiopathic under these circumstances.

These five sets of findings are not the only presumptive indications for a medical etiology or "cause" in individuals with mental retardation. Many other pathological findings (e.g., cutaneous lesions of neuroectodermal disorders, chorioretinitis, microcephaly, intracranial calcifications, and the like) may be identified during the course of medical examinations and contribute to diagnostic or etiologic inferences. In addition to the neurological abnormalities which may be elicited by the medical examinations of physicians, psychologists regularly find evidence for impaired cortical and neurointegrative functions during psychological and psychoeducational testing. In the future, neurophysiological techniques may also be applied clinically and permit the recognition of subtle biological abnormalities which now cannot be identified, e.g., in the areas of evoked potentials, attention and habituation, expectancy patterns, sleep patterns, and the like.[20] Developments of this type may expand the numbers of individuals with retardation in whom biological abnormalities can be demonstrated.

Group 2 of the retarded population is distinguished by an apparent absence of the abnormal medical findings which characterize Group 1. Group 2 includes the majority, perhaps 75–80 percent, of the total retarded population. The severity of the retardation here is limited to the mild level, whereas all levels are included in Group 1. Several etiologic subgroups undoubtedly exist within Group 2 which are not separable through medical technology. The causes of mentally retarded behavior here are believed to be multifactorial and to involve complex interactions between polygenic inheritance factors, experiential factors, and subclinical medical factors.

❲ Polygenic "Causation"

Geneticists estimate that 70 percent of all mental retardation can be encompassed etiologically within the framework of polygenic inheritance of a graded characteristic.[28] In this context, each of the segregating polygenes is assumed to have a small effect on trait variation by comparison with the total variation observed for the trait. Gene effects of this type presumably account for "physiological" trait variations which conform to a normal or continuous distribution. By contrast, major or single mutant gene effects may account for discontinuous or "pathological" traits.

Tests for the measurement of intelligence have been constructed and standardized to yield a normal distribution of test abilities or scores with respect to a reference population. These tests, in turn, generate the assumption that a trait "intelligence" exists which is normally distributed and polygenically determined. If normally distributed, 99.73 percent of intelligence test scores will predictably lie within three standard deviations above or below the mean of a standardized test. On the Stanford-Binet with a standard deviation of 16, scores from 52–148 would be included within this range; on the Wechsler Scales with a standard deviation of 15, scores from 55–145 would be included. These ranges presumably reflect the "physiological" spread of intelligence due to polygenic inheritance.

A normal frequency distribution also predicts that 2.14 percent of intelligence test scores will lie between two and three standard deviations below the mean. Many individuals with scores in this range are labeled mildly retarded. Those who are distinguished by an absence of abnormal medical findings may reflect the low end of the continuum of intelligence due to the segregation of polygenes. The observed frequency of IQ scores in this range, however, exceeds the predicted frequency due, presumably, to medical pathology and other influences which will be examined subsequently.[16]

The concept of polygenic inheritance in relation to measured intelligence has been supported by numerous studies which involve correlational pairings.[21] These studies have indicated that intragroup resemblance in intellectual abilities increases in proportion to the degree of genetic relationship, i.e., the greater the gene overlap the greater the similarity in intelligence, whether or not the paired individuals have shared the same environment. Empiric risk figures for mild mental retardation, as derived from family studies, have also been consistent with a polygenic hypothesis.[45] Finally, the distribution of IQ scores along a social class gradient has been regarded as consistent with the distributional expectations due to polygenic inheritance given conditions of social mobility and assortative mating.[11]

Multiple studies in white populations in more or less uniform environments have estimated that heritability accounts for 60–80 percent of the total variance in intelligence test scores.[49] On the assumption that the variance attributable to heritability is equally high in all groups, it has been reasoned that differences in mean IQ scores between black and white populations or social classes are genetically determined, i.e., are due to differences in the distribution of genotypes for high and low IQ.[36,37] Environmentalists, on the other hand, have argued that statistical estimates of heritability apply only to a particular population in a relatively constant environment. Measures in another population with a different distribution of environmental characteristics do not necessarily show the same proportion of genetic and environmental variances. From this standpoint, it is hypothesized that heritability will account for more of the variance in optimal environments and less of the variance in suboptimal environments. Accordingly, differences in mean IQ scores between racial and social groups are attributed to environmental disadvantage. It is concluded in this framework that a phenotypic distribution of IQ scores neither reflects the distribution of genotypes for intelligence nor is immutable.[40]

Obviously, psychometric instruments influence the phenomena which are measured and the conclusions which are reached concerning polygenic and sociocultural "etiologies." If cognitive capacity is not fully matched by cognitive competence or performance in response to the demands and conditions of a test, an artifact of measurement will occur.[10] In recent years, interest in the concept of general intelligence has yielded somewhat to the study of differentiated intelligence, i.e., of the various subabilities which are hypothesized to affect mental functioning. If not necessarily clarifying the genotypic issues, such studies provide a refined view of the differences in performance between subgroups of the population (or individuals) under specific demand situations.[37] While some abilities may be more resistant to training and experience than others, *psychometric items are always culture-bound.*

◖ Sociocultural "Causation"

As has been noted, the majority of individuals in the retarded category are classified as mildly retarded. Usually, no single etiological or causal influence can be identified in this group. Presumably, mental retardation at this level represents a final symptomatic pattern of IQ and adaptive behavioral effects due to multiple interacting variables. Because correlations with social class and ethnic minority status are high in this group, the terms "cultural-familial" and "sociocultural" are frequently applied to it.

Epidemiological and prevalence studies provide a useful perspective from which to view the social implications of mild mental retardation.[9,22,30,55] It should be noted first that all studies of prevalence have shown that severe mental retardation (i.e., moderate, severe, and profound levels) is distributed across social classes without a significant gradient. Prevalence has been remarkably constant in all studies at approximately three to four per 1000 children between five and eighteen years of age. Virtually all individuals with severe retardation have significant signs of medical pathology. For this reason, biomedical causalities are thought to account for the excess frequency of low IQ scores (below 52–55) beyond the predictions of a normal frequency distribution.[16]

The prevalence of mild mental retardation, on the other hand, has varied between studies according to the criteria, instruments, population characteristics, and sampling techniques employed, and the locale or country studied. Roughly, prevalence ratios by severity are as follows: mild twenty, moderate four, severe one. Aside from actual prevalence rates, however, three important epidemiological characteristics of mild mental retardation emerge from these studies.

The most striking epidemiological feature of mild mental retardation is its disproportionate social distribution, i.e., its social gradient. The discrepancy between the top and the bottom of the social scale is marked enough to suggest that this form of mental retardation is virtually specific to the lowest social classes. A dramatic increase in prevalence occurs particularly at IQ levels equal to or greater than sixty between social classes 3 to 5 (as determined by the occupation of the head of the household). As a generalization, it may be concluded that the prevalence of mild mental retardation increases by a factor of two for each step downward in social class.

The second outstanding epidemiologic

characteristic of mild mental retardation is its disproportionate age distribution. This distribution has been designated as the "schologenic hump."[56] Mild mental retardation has a low prevalence in the preschool years, increases rapidly in frequency during the early school years, peaks dramatically during puberty and adolescence, and declines sharply again thereafter, in part, as a reflection of the role of the schools in identification. In some studies, the prevalence of mild mental retardation reaches twenty to forty per 1000 population in the age group 10–14 years. It is assumed that movement of many individuals into and out of the category of mild mental retardation accounts for these age specific prevalence rates. The importance of the behavioral demands of particular social settings and of the labeling process on the prevalence of mild mental retardation is highlighted by these studies.[43] Since the label of mental retardation is difficult to remove, professionals should be exceedingly wary of stigmatizing anyone at the mild level who might move out of the category.

The third outstanding epidemiological characteristic of mild mental retardation is the frequent absence of abnormal medical findings. This feature was documented most clearly by Birch et al. in a superb epidemiological study of mental retardation in eight-to-ten-year old children in Aberdeen, Scotland.[9] In this homogeneous white population, one third of the children with IQ scores above 50 (up to 75) had abnormal neurological findings as defined by one localizing or two nonlocalizing signs. However, only one fourth of children with IQ scores equal to or greater than 60 (up to 75) had abnormal neurological findings as defined. The numbers of children with neurological abnormalities in the latter group were ten times greater than in a sample of normal children. In other studies, it has been estimated that 20–50 percent of mildly retarded children will present abnormal medical findings.

Medical findings and social class often interact to influence the prevalence of mild mental retardation.[8] This relationship is demonstrated dramatically with respect to low birth weight and severe perinatal stress. Low-birth-weight infants (above 3½ lb.) in upper social-class families reveal minimal IQ effects, while decreasing birth weight is associated with a marked increase in the frequency of low IQ scores in other social classes.[18] Severe perinatal stress also appears to be compensable in good postnatal environments. The interaction between reproductive and environmental hazards produces a cumulative risk which has a profound effect on the IQ levels of lower class children who are exposed to the severest forms of perinatal stress.[61]

Epidemiological evidence suggests that mild mental retardation is not randomly distributed within low social classes. In a study of prevalence in an American slum, for example, Heber demonstrated that mild retardation was concentrated in families of mothers with low IQ scores.[33,34] Although mothers with an IQ less than 80 made up 40 percent of the total surveyed, they accounted for four fifths of the children with IQ scores less than 80. The offspring of these mothers experienced a marked decline in measured intelligence between three to five years which was followed by a further modest decline until the average measured IQ at twelve to fourteen years approximated the maternal average of 68. The probability of children testing between IQ 55–67 on the Wechsler Scales at twelve to fourteen years was fourteen times greater if the IQ scores of their mothers were in this range than if the mothers' scores were at or above IQ 100. The mothers in this study were comparable in economic level, living conditions, educational background, and the like, and varied only on measured intelligence. This study suggested that a threshold level of maternal IQ might be correlated with most instances of mild mental retardation in low social classes.

Other studies have seemingly corroborated the existence of a progressive form of intellectual retardation (and mild mental retardation) which is associated with low social class for some children.* Cross-sectional data have indicated that groups of disadvantaged chil-

* See references 15, 27, 31, 32, and 55.

dren compare unfavorably with children of high socioeconomic status on intelligence test measures at least by four years of age, and differences tend to increase with increasing age. Groups of disadvantaged children also perform below the national average on all measures of school achievement at all grade levels, and the absolute discrepancies in age levels increase with time. Not all children in low socioeconomic circumstances, however, reveal indications of progressive intellectual or mental retardation.

It is commonly hypothesized that progressive retardation in low social classes results from a deprivation of experiences which are necessary for the development of cognitive competencies for academic learning. Untangling the web of class and specific environmental differences which may contribute to differences in intellectual functioning, however, is a complicated process. Child-rearing practices which favor one cognitive style rather than another, specific types of class-related interpersonal communications which result in specific deficits in intellectual functioning, differences in linguistic styles and form which make mainstream English syntax and vocabulary a second language, differences in patterns of reinforcement contingencies, differences in motivation, differences in pregnancy, nutrition, and health factors, and the importance of social "models," all and more have been postulated and explored.

Race and social class contributions to the mildly retarded category also interact. White group mean IQ scores and black group mean IQ scores may differ by as much as one standard deviation or roughly 15 points.[38] Among the blacks, 18 percent may score below IQ 70, while only two percent of whites score in this range. Mercer has shown, however, that low scores for black and Mexican-American children in Riverside, California, were correlated more with sociocultural status than ethnic or racial background.[43] In each group, mean IQ scores converged progressively toward standard norms as sociocultural background characteristics were successively controlled for similarity to the dominant society.

Mercer's study demonstrated the importance of the labeling process in the determination of the category of mild mental retardation. As a result of her findings, she is currently developing differential ethnic norms for adaptive behavior by subculture in order to obviate the labeling of school children who meet social expectations and demands in their own cultural group. In Mercer's view, low IQ scores predict the need for appropriate educational supports, while adequate adaptive behavior in relation to an appropriate (non-school) reference group should predict the capacity to fill an adult role acceptably. From this perspective, the category of mild mental retardation should be reserved for those children who are "comprehensively" retarded in terms of IQ scores and adaptive behavioral criteria as applied within a cultural context. Much of the confusion regarding the category of mild retardation and the prognosis for those assigned to it results from the unavailability of discriminating criteria for adaptive behavioral adequacy.

From a dynamic viewpoint, the test and nontest behaviors which define mental retardation always reflect the interaction of multiple variables, not only at mild levels but at all levels of severity. In this sense, the assignment of the cause of mental retardation to a single variable or etiology represents an oversimplification. At any given time, mentally retarded behavior may be conceptualized as resulting from an interplay between the person's *response potentialities* (i.e., the polygenetic, physiological, and pathological limitations imposed upon his reacting and coordinating systems), his *learned responses* or competencies (i.e., his cumulative or antecedent learning history as acquired through interactions with his personal, cultural, social, and physical environments), and his *current stimulus-response environment* (i.e., the specific circumstances in which his present specific behaviors are arising).

(Mutability of IQ

Logically, an increase in IQ scores above the criterion level for mental retardation should result in a "cure." IQ changes with time occur at all levels of retardation, either upwardly or downwardly and with or without intentional intervention.[55] As noted previously, the progressive downward movement of group mean IQ scores of low socioeconomic status children corresponds with an increasing frequency of mild mental retardation at puberty and adolescence. In an institutional population, Fisher and Zeaman found the growth of mental age (MA) to be roughly linear between the ages of five and sixteen years at all levels of retardation.[23] The IQ scores declined precipitously during this period, however, due to the slow rate of MA increase. Since the mildly retarded group continued to exhibit MA growth through the late thirties, IQ scores in this group subsequently rose after age sixteen years. Non-institutionalized children with culturally associated retardation have also been reported to make IQ gains in early adulthood.[55]

In general, the greatest potential for IQ change is associated with the most unfavorable social and educational origins of a group. The frequency and extent of IQ changes in retarded children from advantaged environments remain moot questions, especially as consequences of training and education. Intelligence test scores, however, place a primary emphasis upon the products of cognition. During the past two decades, numerous investigations have explored the process of learning among the retarded.* These studies have contributed to a growing technology of education which has permitted retarded individuals to learn complex tasks previously thought to be impossible.[52,59] Even without IQ change, remarkable changes in performance can be achieved through strategies derived from discrimination learning, information theory, learning theory, and the like.

Some aspects of an effective educational program for the retarded child may involve the following: (1) the definition of specific objectives for learning in accord with the present stage and learning characteristics of the child; (2) the ordering of the sequential

tasks necessary to achieve a learning objective; (3) the ordering of the physical and spatial environment to direct attention to the relevant stimulus dimensions of tasks; (4) the ordering of tasks in magnitudes of difficulty which insure a high probability of successful achievement; (5) the use of a range of reinforcing techniques which is appropriate to the task and child; (6) the provision of an appropriate response model which the child can also emulate and imitate; and (7) the creation of a social relationship which enhances motivation and encourages movement toward autonomy.

(Mutability of Adaptive Behavior

Logically, an increase in adaptive behavior above the criterion level for mental retardation should also result in a "cure" even without an IQ increase. There are no generalized behaviors, however, which are specific to retardation.[39] At mild levels, adaptive behavioral retardation is often defined in relation to the specific demands of a particular social setting, especially the schools. Rightly or wrongly, the child's responses in coping with the particular environment serve as the basis for the definition of retardation within that environment. Adaptive behavioral change under these circumstances requires a clear delineation of the behaviors which are contributing to the social definition and a specific strategy for intervention, an endeavor which is often questionable from an ethnic and subcultural perspective.

There are behavioral phenomena, however, which distinguish a child as atypical in virtually all social settings. Basic social skills which are appropriate to the chronological age of the child, for example, may be missing from the behavioral repertoire. These missing skills may relate to toileting, feeding, dressing, bathing, ambulation, play, and communication. The complexity of the skills which are lacking may increase at successive ages. These absent behaviors have the effect of depriving the retarded person of independence and movement through the expected range of social settings for age. There are also maladaptive behaviors

* See references 5, 7, 24, 51, 54, and 57.

which distinguish a person as atypical. These behaviors may involve stereotyped or repetitive acts which consist of body rocking, head rolling, hand flapping, bruxism, twirling, pill-rolling, unusual limb posturing, object spinning, vocal sounds, and the like.[4] A closely related group of self-injurious behaviors may also be observed which includes head-banging, face slapping, self-biting, trichotillomania, and eye poking. Tantrums, aggressive and destructive acts, explosive outbursts, hyperkinesis, lack of impulse control, unconcealed masturbation, inappropriate channeling of erotic feelings, compulsions, unusual fears, negativism, and withdrawal, all represent behaviors which are considered to be undesirable in most settings, and hence, maladaptive. Manifestations of these types are generally independent of social class and are closely correlated with IQ levels and abnormal medical findings. A number of scales are available for the assessment of adaptive behavior in these areas which may serve as useful guides for the specification of training objectives (AAMD[44] Fairview,[46] Cain-Levine,[12] Balthazar,[3] and Watson[60]).

A vast experimental and clinical literature now supports the potency of the techniques of behavior modification for changing behaviors of the preceding types.[25,26,58,59] Through these techniques, maladaptive behaviors can become less frequent; likewise, adaptive behaviors which are available to the child, but infrequent, can become more frequent. Developmentally appropriate behaviors which are not in the behavioral repertoire may also be generated through the chaining of separate steps in a complex behavior or through shaping, i.e., the successive approximation of a terminal behavior. Through these techniques, even severely and profoundly retarded children can learn toileting, self-feeding, self-dressing, communication, and other skills. At the present time, therefore, it is probably appropriate to conclude that all retarded children can be helped to become less retarded in the area of adaptive behavior.

The professional framework in which a child is viewed may determine the interpretation or label which is applied to his adaptive behavior. Many of the behaviors which have been described here may be interpreted in a psychiatric context. In this light, several epidemiological studies have shown that mental retardation is associated with a wide range of psychiatric disorders.[47] In general, the frequency of psychiatric diagnoses is inversely correlated with IQ levels. Although psychoses, especially in mentally retarded adults, are frequently noted, the psychiatric disorders of children with retardation are heterogeneous and nonspecific.[42] The traditional psychiatric syndrome of infantile autism is highly correlated with mentally retarded behavior.[47,48]

⟨ Conclusion

Mental retardation can be viewed from at least three perspectives, namely, medical, behavioral, and sociological. The *medical orientation* (including the genetic) tends to assign the causes for the behaviors which are labeled abnormal to deficiencies and pathological processes *within* the individual. In this context, the focus is often directed toward the assignment of etiology to biomedical diseases and events. Mental retardation may be considered to be a unitary condition here and the individual with retardation to be a patient who requires treatment to achieve health or normalcy. The *behavioral orientation* tends to ignore medical and other etiologies and relates the behaviors which are labeled maladaptive to learning experiences and current-stimulus response events within particular environments; in this context, many of the retarded behaviors are considered to be trainable, manipulable, or extinguishable under specified environmental conditions. The person with retardation is considered here to be one who needs environmental modification to permit appropriate learning and behavior. The *sociological orientation* focuses on differences in the distribution of socioeconomic-cultural variables and upon the labeling process per se. In this context, mental retardation is seen as an artifact of society, of social influences and of social organization. Mental retardation here is regarded as essentially non-clinical, and the burden of causation is placed *outside* the individual.

The heterogeneity of the retarded group defies a single, all-inclusive conceptualization. The medical or clinical perspective, however, limits the view of retardation to instances which are categorized through professional activities and clinical procedures. The sociological perspective broadens the scope of interest to include equivalent sets of behavioral phenomena whether or not they are clinically labeled. Although not mutually exclusive, these two orientations generate different views of the nature and manifestations of mental retardation and somewhat different strategies for intervention. Social change rather than individual change represents the primary difference in emphasis.

⟨ Bibliography

1. AMERICAN PSYCHIATRIC ASSOCIATION. *Diagnostic and Statistical Manual of Mental Disorders*, 2nd ed., Washington: American Psychiatric Association, 1968.

2. AMPOLA, M. G. "Phenylketonuria and Other Disorders of Amino Acid Metabolism," *Pediatric Clin. North Am.*, 20 (1973), 507–536.

3. BALTHAZAR, E. E. *Balthazar Scales of Adaptive Behavior*. Champaign, Ill.: Research Press, 1971.

4. BAUMEISTER, A. A. and R. FOREHAND. "Stereotyped Acts," in N. R. Ellis, ed., *International Review of Research in Mental Retardation*, Vol. 6, pp. 55–96. New York: Academic, 1973.

5. BAUMEISTER, A. A. and G. KELLAS. "Process Variables in Paired-Associate Learning of Retardates," in N. R. Ellis, ed., *International Review of Research in Mental Retardation*, Vol. 5, pp. 221–270. New York: Academic, 1971.

6. BERGSMA, D., ed. *Birth Defects: Atlas and Compendium*. Baltimore: Williams & Wilkins, 1973.

7. BERKSON, G. "Behavior," in J. Wortis, ed., *Mental Retardation and Developmental Disabilities: An Annual Review*, Vol. 5, pp. 55–71. New York: Brunner/Mazel, 1973.

8. BIRCH, H. G. and J. D. GUSSOW. *Disadvantaged Children: Health, Nutrition and School Failure*. New York: Grune & Stratton, 1970.

9. BIRCH, H. G., S. A. RICHARDSON, D. BAIRD et al. *Mental Subnormality in the Community: A Clinical and Epidemiological Study*. Baltimore: Williams & Wilkins, 1970.

10. BORTNER, M. and H. G. BIRCH. "Cognitive Capacity and Cognitive Competence," *Am. J. Ment. Defic.*, 74 (1970), 735–744.

11. BURT, C. "Intelligence and Social Mobility," *Br. J. Statist. Psychol.*, 14 (1961), 3–24.

12. CAIN, L. F., S. LEVINE, F. F. ELZEY. *Cain-Levine Social Competency Scale*. Palo Alto: Consulting Psychologist's Press, 1963.

13. CAVANAGH, J. B. *The Brain in Unclassified Mental Retardation*. Baltimore: Williams & Wilkins, 1972.

14. CROME, L. and J. STERN. *The Pathology of Mental Retardation*. London: Churchill, 1967.

15. DAS, J. P. "Cultural Deprivation and Cognitive Competence," in N. R. Ellis, ed., *International Review of Research in Mental Retardation*, Vol. 6, pp. 1–53. New York: Academic, 1973.

16. DINGMAN, H. F. and G. TARJAN. "Mental Retardation and the Normal Distribution Curve," *Am. J. Ment. Defic.*, 64 (1960), 991–994.

17. DOLL, E. A. *Vineland Social Maturity Scale*. Circle Pines, Minn.: American Guidance Service, n.d.

18. DRILLIEN, C. M. *Growth and Development of the Prematurely Born Infant*. Baltimore: Williams & Wilkins, 1964.

19. EASTHAM, R. D. and J. JANCAR. *Clinical Pathology in Mental Retardation*. Baltimore: Williams & Wilkins, 1968.

20. ELLINGSON, R. J. "Neurophysiology," in J. Wortis, ed., *Mental Retardation: An Annual Review*, Vol. 4, pp. 123–139. New York: Grune & Stratton, 1972.

21. ERLENMEYER-KIMBLING, L. and L. F. JARVIK. "Genetics and Intelligence: A Review," *Science*, 142 (1963), 1477–1479.

22. FARBER, B. *Mental Retardation: Its Social Context and Social Consequences*. Boston: Houghton Mifflin, 1968.

23. FISHER, M. and D. ZEAMAN. "Growth and Decline of Retardate Intelligence," in N. R. Ellis, ed., *International Review of Research in Mental Retardation*, Vol. 4, pp. 151–191. New York: Academic, 1970.

24. ————. "An Attention-Retention Theory of Retardate Discrimination Learning," in N. R. Ellis, ed., *International Review of Research in Mental Retardation*, Vol. 6, pp. 169–256. New York: Academic, 1973.

25. FOX, R. M. and N. H. AZRIN. *Toilet Training the Retarded*. Champaign, Ill.: Research Press, 1973.

26. GARDNER, W. I. *Behavior Modification in Mental Retardation*. Chicago: Aldine-Atherton, 1971.

27. GIRARDEAU, F. L. "Cultural-Familial Retardation," in N. R. Ellis, ed., *International Review of Research in Mental Retardation*, Vol. 5, pp. 304–348. New York: Academic, 1971.

28. GOTTESMAN, I. I. "Genetic Aspects of Intelligent Behavior," in N. R. Ellis, ed., *Handbook of Mental Deficiency: Psychological Theory and Research*, pp. 253–296. New York: McGraw-Hill, 1963.

29. GROSSMAN, H. J., ed. *Manual on Terminology and Classification in Mental Retardation*, 1973 Revision. Washington: American Association on Mental Deficiency, 1973.

30. GRUENBERG, E. M. "*Epidemiology*," in H. A. Stevens, and R. Heber, eds., *Mental Retardation: Review of Research*, pp. 259–306. Chicago: University of Chicago Press, 1964.

31. HAYWOOD, H. C., ed. *Socio-Cultural Aspects of Mental Retardation*. New York: Meredith, 1970.

32. HAYWOOD, H. C. and J. T. TAPP. "Experience and the Development of Adaptive Behavior," in N. R. Ellis, ed., *International Review of Research in Mental Deficiency*, Vol. 1, pp. 109–151. New York: Academic, 1966.

33. HEBER, R. F. "Culture and Familial Retardation," in M. Cohen, ed., *International Research Seminar on Vocational Rehabilitation of the Mentally Retarded*, Special Publications Series, no. 1. pp. 313–324. Washington: American Association on Mental Deficiency, 1972.

34. HEBER, R. F. and R. B. DEVER. "Research on Education and Habilitation of the Mentally Retarded," in H. C. Haywood, ed., *Socio-Cultural Aspects of Mental Retardation*, pp. 395–427. New York: Meredith, 1970.

35. HOLMES, L. B., H. W. MOSER, S. HALLDORSSON et al. *Mental Retardation: An Atlas of Diseases with Associated Physical Abnormalities*. New York: Macmillan, 1972.

36. JENSEN, A. R. "How Much Can We Boost I.Q. and Scholastic Achievement?" *Harvard Educ. Rev.*, 39 (1969), 1–123.

37. ————. "A Theory of Primary and Secondary Familial Mental Retardation," in N. R. Ellis, ed., *International Review of Research in Mental Retardation*, Vol. 4, pp. 33–105. New York: Academic, 1970.

38. KENNEDY, W. A., V. VAN DE RIET, and J. C. WHITE, JR. *A Normative Sample of Intelligence and Achievement of Negro Elementary School Children in Southeastern United States*, Monographs of the Society for Research in Child Development, 28 (1963), no. 6.

39. LELAND, H. "Mental Retardation and Adaptive Behavior," *J. Spec. Educ.*, 6 (1972), 71–80.

40. LEWONTIN, R. C. "Race and Intelligence," *Bull. Atomic Scientists*, 26 (1970), 2–8.

41. McKUSICK, V. A. *Mendelian Inheritance in Man: Catalogs of Autosomal Dominant, Autosomal Recessive, and X-Linked Phenotypes*. 3rd ed. Baltimore: The Johns Hopkins University Press, 1971.

42. MENOLASCINO, F. J., ed. *Psychiatric Approaches to Mental Retardation*. New York: Basic Books, 1970.

43. MERCER, J. R. *Labeling the Mentally Retarded: Clinical and Social Systems Perspective on Mental Retardation*. Berkeley: University of California Press, 1973.

44. NIHIRA, K., R. FOSTER, M. SHELLHAAS et al. *Adaptive Behavior Scales*. Washington, D.C.: American Association on Mental Deficiency, 1969.

45. REED, E. W. and S. C. REED. *Mental Retardation: A Family Study*. Philadelphia: Saunders, 1964.

46. ROSS, R. T. *Fairview Self-Help Scale (1970); Fairview Social Skills Scale (1972)*. Costa Mesa, California: Research Department, Fairview State Hospital.

47. RUTTER, M. L. "Psychiatry," in J. WORTIS, ed., *Mental Retardation: An Annual Review*, Vol. 3, pp. 186–221. New York: Grune & Stratton, 1971.

48. RUTTER, M. L., ed. *Infantile Autism: Concepts, Characteristics, and Treatment*. Baltimore: Williams & Wilkins, 1971.

49. SCARR-SALAPATEK, S. "Race, Social Class, and I.Q.," *Science*, 174 (1971), 1285–1295.

50. SCRIVER, C. R. and L. E. ROSENBERG. *Amino-Acid Metabolism and Its Disorders*. Philadelphia: Saunders, 1973.

51. SERSEN, E. A. "Conditioning and Learning," in J. Wortis, ed., *Mental Retardation: An Annual Review*, Vol. 1, pp. 28–41. New York: Grune & Stratton, 1970.

52. SKINNER, B. F. *Technology of Teaching*. New York: Appleton-Century-Crofts, 1968.

53. SMITH, D. W. *Recognizable Patterns of Human Malformation*. Philadelphia: Saunders, 1970.

54. SPITZ, H. H. "Consolidating Facts into Schematized Learning and Memory System of Educable Retardates," in N. R. Ellis, ed., *International Review of Research in Mental Retardation*, Vol. 6, pp. 149–168. New York: Academic, 1973.

55. STEIN, Z. and M. SUSSER. "Mutability of Intelligence and Epidemiology of Mild Mental Retardation," *Rev. Educ. Res.*, 40 (1970), 29–67.

56. STEVENSON, G. S. in *New Directions for Mentally Retarded Children*. New York: Josiah Macy, Jr., Foundation, 1956.

57. STEVENSON, H. W. *Children's Learning*. New York: Meredith, 1972.

58. THARP, R. G. and R. J. WETZEL. *Behavior Modification in the Natural Environment*. New York: Academic, 1969.

59. WATSON, L. S., JR. "Application of Operant Conditioning Techniques to Institutionalized Severely and Profoundly Retarded Children," *Mental Retardation Abstracts*, 4 (1967), 1–18.

60. ———. *How to Use Behavior Modification with Mentally Retarded and Autistic Children: Programs for Administrators, Teachers, Parents, and Nurses*. Columbus, Ohio: Behavior Modification Technology, 1972.

61. WERNER, E., J. M. BIERMAN, F. E. FRENCH et al. "Reproductive and Environmental Casualties: A Report on the 10-year Follow-up of the Children of Kauai Pregnancy Study," *Pediatrics*, 42 (1968), 112–127.

62. WORLD HEALTH ORGANIZATION. *International Classification of Diseases*, 8th Revision. Geneva: WHO, 1968.

CHAPTER 19

MENTAL RETARDATION

II. Care and Management

Sterling D. Garrard and Julius B. Richmond

TODAY, patterns of service in the area of mental retardation are undergoing a progressive change and differentiation which eventually may enable most persons considered handicapped to live in communities throughout most or all of their lives. Under the impact of the normalization principle and strong advocacy for the retarded at many levels, a range of family support services, training and educational options, domiciliary options, and work options is being developed.[30] In many places, traditional residential institutions have redefined their programs, dispersed some of their functions among small specialized facilities in communities, and/or have become the hub of regional programs.[3,20] All services are being ordered along a continuum which will allow progressive movement of the individual toward as much independence in adult life as the degree of normative skill development will permit.

(Services

Two major groups of services may be considered within the emerging service system as follows: (1) those which are directed toward the maximum cognitive competency and adaptive behavioral outcomes of the developmental period; and (2) those which are directed toward the maintenance of functional and productive capacities in adult life.

Developmental Services

Training and education are the one constant feature of programming throughout the developmental period. During this time, all other professional services are titrated for their specificity against the assessed needs of the child and family.

If identification of developmental retardation occurs in early infancy, home-training programs may be instituted in order to provide parents with the knowledge of appropriate developmental and behavioral objectives and to assist them in acquiring effective techniques of support. These programs may be especially important if the infant or young child with mental retardation, cerebral palsy, or multiple disabilities presents unusual cues or stimuli to parents. In these instances, the automatic or untutored parental responses may be inappropriate, may impede effective learning progress, and may even reinforce maladaptive behaviors. During the preschool period, the focus of training and education shifts to extrafamilial, developmental day-care programs, often with the continuation of a parent educational component. It is noteworthy that preschool programs, such as Head Start, are increasingly accepting children with mental retardation and other handicapping conditions into their services.

By school age, preparation begins for the range of social environments which may be open to the person in adult life. At this time, a few profoundly retarded or multiply handicapped children may be placed in medically oriented institutions or nursing-home programs, where they ideally will receive systematic stimulation, behavior shaping, care, and consistent social contacts. Other children, who are severely or moderately retarded, may enter self-contained special educational programs either in regular schools or in a segregated community facility. Children with mild retardation may receive a variety of educational programs in regular schools as follows: self-contained special education, split regular and special education, regular classroom with special resource teachers, regular classroom with tutors and programmed instructional aids, or regular classroom with no special supports. By the teen years, training and education are vocationally and work oriented and may terminally involve work-study experiences.

The family is viewed as the major resource for the care of the child with mental retardation during the developmental period. All necessary medical, allied health, social, coun-

seling, mental health, recreational, transportational, protective, legal, and other services must be available in order to support the continuation of community living in the nuclear family, if feasible and appropriate. Alternate living arrangements should also be available in foster homes or group homes on a short- or long-term basis, as indicated by the capacities of the nuclear family. Generic service agencies should include staff skills in the range of problems which may be associated with mental retardation.

Massive traditional institutions are now viewed as an option of last resort for developmental services for children with mental retardation. Many institutions at present, however, are integrating their activities with the continuum of community services.[20] A range of services may be offered to the population of a region, for example, in support of continued family care. Specialized residential programs may be provided for multiply disabled children, especially for those from non-urban areas. For many profoundly retarded children with continuing medical needs, developmentally oriented nursing-care programs may be provided in residence. Habilitative residential programs may also be offered with the aim of returning the child to the family or community after specific developmental or behavioral objectives have been achieved. In some instances, a reverse flow is affected in which institutional residents receive all or most of their educational programming in the community. New residential facilities are being constructed in many parts of the country which imaginatively exploit architectural possibilities for normalizing institutional environments. Recently, minimum institutional standards have been adopted for the accreditation of residential facilities which ensure a basic quality of professional care and service.[16]

Ideally, the available range of domiciliary options, work options, and guardianship arrangements should permit parental responsibilities for the person with retardation to end when he reaches adult life. Except in a few instances, this ideal is not yet realized.

Adult Services for the Enhancement and Maintenance of Functional and Productive Capacities

The need for special adult services is determined by the amount of social structuring which the individual requires, i.e., whether independent or dependent living is possible. In either case, the usual generic human-service agencies and programs must be available on a need basis. Special consideration must be given to domiciliary arrangements, work provisions, heterosexual (or homosexual) activities, and legal rights. It is axiomatic that living and work arrangements should enable the person to approximate normative experiences as nearly as the behavioral potential permits.

Domiciliary arrangements may involve institutions, half-way houses, hostels, or small group homes for individuals at moderately and mildly retarded levels. Progression toward decreasing supervision within facilities should be possible as competence for work and independence increases. The psychological meaning of useful and remunerative work for the retarded is underscored here.[5] Vocational rehabilitation services and a spectrum of settings for productive employment are necessary if community living is to succeed. Possibilities for heterosexual relationships and marriage are just beginning to be explored systematically in the face of long-standing social biases.[6]

Edgerton has provided a poignant documentation of the quality of life associated with unsupervised community living for a number of individuals with mental retardation.[8]

tion to identify the children who come through medical channels. Presumptive identification may be achieved in medical office settings if sensorimotor, language, or social development deviates markedly from the norms of screening instruments such as the Denver Developmental Screening Test.[9] Other infants and young children who do not receive care in physicians' offices may be identified in well-child clinics or in their own homes by public health nurses who are trained in developmental surveillance. Many other children are identified first in relation to the demands of day-care, nursery, or preschool programs. The importance of the schools as a source of identification of mild forms of retardation has been previously emphasized. Finally, developmental delay or mental retardation may be suspected first by parents, especially in high socioeconomic families, although even sophisticated parents occasionally overlook signs of difficulty for long periods of time.

Except for school identification, these activities serve chiefly to identify children with the most obvious manifestations of mental retardation. Other agencies, including physicians, may be somewhat less effective in identifying mildly retarded children, especially in the absence of neurological or somatic abnormalities. Unless the objectives of identification are related to specific forms of intervention which can be immediately activated, however, *early labeling is a sterile exercise which may have harmful consequences for some children.* The state of the art in the area of screening and assessment of young children at developmental risk has been recently reviewed by Meier.[23]

❰ Identification

The responsibility for the identification of children with mental retardation is shared by all persons who are concerned with the development of the child, including the parents.[11] Physicians are in a particularly strategic posi-

❰ Evaluation

The "diagnosis" of mental retardation may have different connotations in different settings. It may refer to the formal labeling of a child through professional studies which identify the psychometric and adaptive behavioral criteria. It may refer to a medical evaluation for the identification of etiologies or remediable disorders which may be compounding the developmental and behavioral issues. In still other settings, it may refer to a comprehensive, interdisciplinary study of the child's functional characteristics for the purpose of identifying appropriate objectives for intervention, assigning professional responsibilities, or designating appropriate service resources. None of these "diagnostic" activities is necessarily confined to one location or a single discipline.

Medical Evaluation

The physician follows a definite agenda in the medical evaluation of children with mental retardation. He must identify associated medical disorders which are heritable, thereby permitting genetic counseling for the parents, amniocentesis for intrauterine diagnosis in subsequent pregnancies (where possible), or early recognition in subsequent offspring. In rare instances, a specific treatment may be available which will permit the amelioration or interruption of an underlying genetic disease. As noted in the preceding chapter, the clues which are presumptive of a specific medical disease, including those which are heritable, are the following: (1) positive neurological signs; (2) neurological deterioration; (3) malformation clusters; (4) positive biochemical screening tests; (5) other physical signs, including macular degeneration, ectodermal lesions, and the like; and (6) prior family history of a heritable disorder. The physician must also identify remediable medical disorders which are actively inhibiting development through the restriction of response capabilities. Areas of concern here may include visual acuity, auditory function, convulsive activity, neuromuscular impairment, otologic, orthopedic, cardiac, or similar disorders. The physician may be assisted in this endeavor by a variety of medical specialists and allied health professionals. Many children with mental retardation will have additional disabilities which require treatment. The physician may also be assisted by social workers and psychologists in recognizing potentially remediable psychosocial factors which are actively interfering with cognitive growth and adaptive behavioral development.

Functional Evaluation

Present-day management of mental retardation during childhood is directed toward the production of specified changes in a child's competencies and adaptive behavior.[11] Intervention of this type requires a definition of specific learning and behavioral objectives. A functional analysis of the child's current, observable behaviors is the necessary first step in defining these objectives. Measures of intelligence which compare a child with a standardization group for the primary purpose of categorization have limited usefulness for this purpose; likewise, etiologic diagnoses are meaningless in this context.

A functional analysis of the child's behavior may involve any or all of the following: (1) a determination of his current developmental locus (i.e., his learned behaviors); (2) observation of his learning behaviors or processes; (3) observation and specification of his maladaptive behaviors; (4) observation of the environmental consequences (and possibly antecedents) of his maladaptive behaviors; and (5) delineation of the limitations which are imposed by medical findings on his response capabilities under specific demand situations.

The identification of the child's present locus in a known developmental sequence automatically defines his next developmental steps and delineates appropriate objectives for intervention. In recent years, studies in cognitive psychology, psycholinguistics, and social adaptive behavior (among children with mental retardation) have refined our knowledge of the hierarchical sequences of development, and, in some instances, have contributed to the construction of ordinal or other scales for the purpose of assessment.* It is now possible to specify a child's locus in any of several developmental streams with considerable preci-

---

* See references 21, 22, 25, 26, 28, and 29.

sion. Likewise, a child's educational locus and learning behaviors can be analyzed through psychoeducational instruments and educational observations. Again, the child's locus and functional characteristics delineate the appropriate educational objectives and approaches.

Maladaptive behaviors and those which are inappropriate and unacceptable in particular settings may also be observed and specified. When defined with sufficient precision, maladaptive behaviors can be rank-ordered in terms of importance, counted, and specified as potential targets for modification. The target behaviors which are selected for modification are usually determined in consultation with parents or other involved persons. The attempt to change adaptive behavior requires an analysis of the environmental consequences of the child's behavior as well. Consequent parental behavior and that of other significant persons with whom the child interacts must be specified in this context as simultaneous targets for modification.

(Prescriptive Programming

From the preceding discussion, it is apparent that a new model has evolved in community and residential facilities for professional intervention with children with mental retardation. Prescriptive programming is the keystone of intervention within this model. A prescription is based upon the results of the analysis of a child's current, observable, functional characteristics. When all objectives have been identified and clearly specified, appropriate techniques for intervention can be prescribed, either in the area of training and adaptive behavior, or education. Behavior principles and modern educational concepts supply the technology for intervention of this type. Some features of behavior modification and effective educational programming were noted briefly in the preceding chapter.

A pragmatic test is an essential ingredient of prescriptive intervention. The program which is prescribed must finally be shown to be feasible for implementation within the home, the community facility, or the school, and to have demonstrable efficacy in the production of movement toward the specified objectives. If neither feasible nor effective, the objectives or the techniques of intervention, or both, must be modified.

(Interdisciplinary Model

The interdisciplinary model is an organizational structure through which professional services are delivered to persons with mental retardation.[11,19] The model is based upon the assumption that the complexities of the problems of the individual with mental retardation exceed the resolving power of any single discipline. The professional composition of the interdisciplinary group varies according to the forms and severity of the problems and the age of the person. The professional group at one time or another and in different circumstances may include some combination of the following: psychologists, educators, audiologists and speech pathologists, social workers, vocational counselors and rehabilitationists, allied health professionals, physicians from any of several specialties, including psychiatry, and care staff members. The contributions of each discipline are determined by the match between its specific skills, the functional characteristics of the person, and the priorities for intervention which are established through the interdisciplinary group process. Except for the continuing importance of education during childhood, the contributions of other disciplines may vary from person to person and at different points in the life of the same person.

The interdisciplinary model ensures the availability of appropriate professional skills for the person. In addition, it minimizes professional redundancy by requiring each discipline to define clearly its special expertise vis-à-vis other disciplines. Through the interdisciplinary group process, the disciplines frequently generate a multifaceted view of the person, his problems, and the objectives for intervention which can rarely be duplicated by professionals who work independently.

(Parental Involvement

Many early-infant educational projects have included a subsidiary parent-educational component, and several have worked primarily with parents in the home.[14,17,18] These programs have demonstrated that specific direction of the maternal transactions with an infant or young child can influence developmental outcome under the conditions of the studies. In addition, the growing literature in the field of behavior modification has indicated that parents can be effective agents for intervention in relation to a wide spectrum of behavioral phenomena if provided with knowledge of appropriate objectives and techniques.[4,7,15] It has now been recognized that parents can be taught to be effective teachers, that they can profit from formal specific child-rearing education, and that they can modify their behavior to some degree if they are reinforcing maladaptive behavior.

Present approaches to the education of parents of children with mental retardation often emphasize instruction in the techniques of behavior modification.[4,15] Although few studies have been designed to date with sufficient rigor to permit an objective evaluation of this approach, the education of parents in specific techniques to support the development of their own children has a strong intrinsic appeal. When the education of parents involves the use of the techniques of behavior modification, the parent becomes a contributing and participating member of the professional team concerned with intervention. The parent may then be regarded as a manpower resource for the conduct of the child's program in the natural setting of the home. In the process of generating a prescription for intervention in conjunction with professionals, parents can learn appropriate developmental objectives, participate in the delineation of maladaptive behaviors, and acquire techniques and behaviors through which to fulfill a supportive and effec-

tive role with the child. Under these circumstances, the parental role acquires direction and specificity, and the parent assumes an active rather than a passive stance in relation to the child's problems.

Obviously, the educational approach to parents need not be limited to indoctrination in the techniques of behavior modification. The latter may lead at times to the delineation of objectives which are too narrowly defined from a comprehensive perspective. Any additional combination of the following techniques may be employed in working with parents: individual educational discussions, informational classes, group work, modeling experiences, feedback experiences—possibly with immediate cueing or delayed videotape viewing—and insight counseling.[31]

(Family Support

It is easy to overgeneralize concerning the psychological adaptations of parents, siblings, and the retarded child or adult. Often discussions concerning these adaptations are based upon stereotypes derived from experiences limited to high socioeconomic-status parents who have a severely retarded child. Obviously, the psychological adaptations of parents may vary according to multiple idiosyncratic factors as follows: the severity of mental retardation and the extent of the child's deviancy in behavior and appearance; age of the child; sex of the child and of the parent; age of the parent; sociocultural background; investment in the child for achieving unfulfilled parental ambitions; duration of the marriage and its mutuality and stability; presence or absence of other normal children in the family; religious orientation; orientation toward achievement; past experiences in dealing with adversity; previous attitudes toward handicaps and minority groups; need for social approval; need for utilization of the child in neurotic patterns which may defeat professional efforts for change or improvement.

In general, the adaptational problems of parents reflect anticipated psychological responses to the degree of realistic stress which the child poses. If the child is severely impaired, parents may exhibit a predictable sequence of reactions leading eventually to adjustment in accord with crisis theory.[12,13] A phase of initial stress, shock, grief, and disorganization may be followed by a prolonged phase of reintegration in which feelings of denial and guilt may be associated with the observed behavioral patterns. Eventually, an adaptation is reached which will permit internal comfort and constructive action by most parents. The passage of time and a prolonged expenditure of effort in behalf of the child may be necessary before the latter stage of resolution is reached. During the interim period, specific instruction and concrete assistance for increasing parental effectiveness with the child may be at least as important for psychological movement as the gaining of psychological insight.

Within the broad phases of adaptation, points may occur at which psychological stresses are intensified for parents in association with the maturation of the child. After initial recognition, these points may include: (1) the period at which the child's chronological age ordinarily would permit school attendance; (2) the period of pubescence with increased physical growth, sexual maturity, and sexual or erotic interests; and (3) the period of entry into adult life with the necessity for decisions concerning provisions for living and supervision.

Although the psychological reactions of parents may be homeostatic for them, the overt behavioral correlates of these reactions may be maladaptive for the support of the cognitive and adaptive growth of the child. Management goals are required for parents and the child, therefore, which are both separate and interrelated. In general, the dual objectives can be met most effectively in the context of the child's program setting. Under these circumstances, it is least likely that the professional focus upon the child will be subordinated to an interest in the psychodynamic reactions of the parents. The experienced professional will observe the course of parental adaptations with time, however, as indications of denial, guilt, dependency, and projection are revealed. Individual psychotherapeutic efforts for parents, when indicated, should occur in facilities appropriate for them.

It is inevitable that some of the difficulties associated with the presence of a retarded child in the family, especially at severe levels, will impinge upon the normal siblings and create adjustment problems for them.[1] Again, their problems may be seen as anticipated responses to stress which can usually be assimilated without major disruptive effects. Professional counseling for the parents or the normal siblings may be helpful at times in support of the adaptational processes. The fact that an affected child was born into the family may raise doubts for teenagers regarding their own capacity for parenthood. The provision of accurate information in clear, objective terms will be helpful in dispelling these apprehensions.

The management of erotic feelings and sexual behavior generates more uncertainty and concerns in relation to the child or adult with mental retardation than any other aspect of behavior.[6] Many individuals with retardation reach puberty and adult life without adequate information, understanding, or opportunities to learn appropriate mechanisms for coping with sexual feelings. Parents and professionals alike may systematically avoid specific preparatory efforts in these areas. Parental concerns at adolescence often focus upon unconcealed masturbation, sexual exploitation (either heterosexually or homosexually), pregnancy, and lack of control of sexual impulses. The recent emphasis upon normalization and the increased movement of individuals with retardation in society has highlighted the potential sexual risks. At least at an academic level, attention is now being directed toward the necessity for instituting curricula and training programs for the preparation of children to fill adult social (including sexual) roles. Parental instruction is almost universally needed as a means of enabling them to provide appropriate support for developmental growth in this area.

Professional Decorum

The overt behavior which the professional person manifests in fulfilling his specific responsibilities for the child may have powerful, nonspecific side effects for families.[11] In utilizing himself as an instrument for parental support, the professional person should demonstrate technical competence, provide an appropriate behavioral model with the child, and demonstrate a constancy of interest in the child and family. He should also maintain an expectation of developmental movement in the child in line with the prevailing optimism surrounding present-day approaches to intervention and in recognition of the shaping effect of expectations. Finally, he should respond positively to appropriate parental behaviors and neutrally to inappropriate behaviors as a means of reinforcing parental strengths and attenuating weaknesses. The professional person should be aware, however, of the emotional turmoil which parents may feel and the range of behavioral responses which they may exhibit in relation to a child with severe mental retardation. He may then provide an important, nonspecific source of comfort, if needed, through his listening skills.

Drug Treatment

The physician may be an instrument for increasing the effectiveness of learning and behavioral intervention for some children by prescribing neuropharmacological agents which may modify distracted behavior or control seizures.[10,27] In these instances, the choice of an appropriate agent and dosage requires the joint participation of educators and other disciplines as objective observers of behavioral effects through the use of rating scales and other quantitative measures. Drug therapy, however, cannot substitute for appropriate educational or intervention programs. At times, the behaviors, which a physician is asked to modify through drug treatment, represent behavioral responses to inappropriate or nonindividualized programs or to maladaptive parental behavior. Appropriate program prescriptions should always precede medicinal prescriptions. Neuropharmacological agents do not have the potentiality for modifying basic behavioral patterns or learning characteristics. Only appropriate behavioral programming can accomplish the objective of basic behavioral change.

When prescribing neuropharmacological agents, the physician may be advised to follow the format of a behavior-modification prescription. Thus, the behavior(s) to be modified should be clearly defined and specified in concrete terms. The frequency of the target behavior should be counted with and without medication in the child's home and/or school setting. Measurable changes in school-learning behavior should likewise be demonstrated if academic objectives are the defined targets. *Since neuropharmacological agents are potent drugs with significant potential side effects, treatment should be discontinued if it fails to produce quantitative evidence for the intended behavioral effects.*

Ethical, Moral, and Legal Issues

Mental retardation pinpoints sharply many ethical, moral, and legal dilemmas for the professions and society at large. Judgments concerning the withholding of life-saving medical treatments in individuals who are demonstrably retarded; human experimentation in retarded populations with attendant issues concerning risks and consent; sterilization procedures on the indication of retardation alone; marital prohibitions; institutional commitment procedures; denial of rights and unequal treatment before the law; all and many more discriminatory practices are currently being questioned and sharply attacked.[2] The values and fabric of our society are threatened as long as these inequities are permitted to exist. Strong advocacy for individuals with mental retardation has become a major responsibility for all who are concerned with human life, dignity, and pluralism.

Conclusion

Within the recent past, major changes have occurred, and are continuing to occur, in concepts and practices related to intervention with children and adults with mental retardation. These changes have generated an expectation that the developmental velocity and adaptive behaviors of all children can be modified through specified forms of environmental intervention. During the developmental period, community services in support of family care have supplanted the large institution as a major resource for service and care. In adult life, the thrust toward normalization has led to a variety of living and work options which have contributed to a clarification of the ultimate objectives for developmental interventions. To an important extent, social changes have occurred which have increased the options for a retarded person even when the possibilities for individual change are sharply limited. But communities must be conscious of the extent of the commitment which is required to build a spectrum of community-based services (integrated with institutional services) in order to make these options realistic.[24] Without the commitment of adequate resources, community programs risk the same disenchantment which historically overtook residential institutions.

Bibliography

1. ADAMS, M. E. "Siblings of the Retarded: Their Problems and Treatment," *Child Welfare*, 46 (1967), 310–316.

2. ———. "Science, Technology, and Some Dilemmas of Advocacy," *Science*, 180 (1973), 840–842.

3. BAUMEISTER, A. A., E. C. BUTTERFIELD, eds. *Residential Facilities for the Mentally Retarded*. Chicago: Aldine-Atherton, 1970.

4. BERKOWITZ, B. P., and A. M. GRAZIANO. "Training Parents as Behavior Therapists: A Review," *Behav. Res. Ther.*, 10 (1972), 297–317.

5. COHEN, M., ed. *International Research Seminar on Vocational Rehabilitation of the Mentally Retarded*, Special Publication Series, no. 1, pp. iii–vii. Washington: American Association on Mental Deficiency, 1972.

6. DE LA CRUZ, F. F. and G. D. LA VECK. *Human Sexuality and the Mentally Retarded*. New York: Brunner/Mazel, 1973.

7. DOERNBERG, N. L. "Parents as Teachers of Their Own Children," in J. Wortis, ed., *Mental Retardation: An Annual Review*, Vol. 4, pp. 33–43. New York: Grune & Stratton, 1972.

8. EDGERTON, R. B. *The Cloak of Competence*. Berkeley: University of California Press, 1967.

9. FRANKENBERG, W. K., J. B. DODDS, and W. FANDAL. *Denver Developmental Screening Test*. 1970 Rev. ed. Denver: University of Colorado Medical Center, 1970.

10. FREEMAN, R. D. "Psychopharmacology and the Retarded Child," in F. J. Menolascino, ed., *Psychiatric Approaches to Mental Retardation*, pp. 294–368. New York: Basic Books, 1970.

11. GARRARD, S. D. "Role of the Pediatrician in the Management of Learning Disorders," *Pediatric Clin. North Am.*, 20 (1973), 737–754.

12. GARRARD, S. D. and J. B. RICHMOND. "Psychological Aspects of the Management of Chronic Diseases and Handicapping Conditions in Childhood," in H. I. Lief, V. F. Lief, and N. R. Lief, eds., *The Psychological Basis of Medical Practice*, pp. 370–403. New York: Harper & Row, 1963.

13. HALLENBECK, P. "A Note on a 'New' Method of Studying Change," *Rehabil. Lit.*, 34 (1973), 138–139.

14. HEBER, R. Unpublished study.

15. JOHNSON, C. A. and R. C. KATZ. "Using Parents as Change Agents for Their Children: A Review," *J. Child Psychol. Psychiatry*, 14 (1973), 181–200.

16. JOINT COMMISSION ON ACCREDITATION OF HOSPITALS. *Standards for Residential Facilities for the Mentally Retarded*. Chicago: Joint Commission on Accreditation of Hospitals, 1971.

17. KARNES, M. B., I. A. TESKA, A. S. HODGINS et al. "Educational Intervention at Home by Mothers of Disadvantaged Infants," *Child Dev.*, 41 (1970), 925–935.

18. KLAUS, R. A. and S. W. GRAY. *The Early Training Project for Disadvantaged Chil-*

dren: A Report After Five Years," Monographs of the Society for Research in Child Development, 33 (1968), no. 4.

19. KOCH, R. and J. C. DOBSON. *The Mentally Retarded Child and His Family: A Multidisciplinary Handbook.* New York: Brunner/Mazel, 1971.

20. KUGEL, R. B. and W. WOLFENSBERGER. *Changing Patterns in Residential Services for the Mentally Retarded.* Washington: The President's Committee on Mental Retardation, 1969.

21. LAURENDEAU, M. and A. PINARD. *Causal Thinking in the Child.* New York: International Universities Press, 1962.

22. ———. *The Development of the Concept of Space in the Child.* New York: International Universities Press, 1970.

23. MEIER, J. *Screening and Assessment of Young Children at Developmental Risk.* DHEW Publication no. (OS) 73–90. Washington: The President's Committee on Mental Retardation, 1973.

24. RICHMOND, J. B., G. E. TARJAN, and R. S. MENDELSOHN. eds. *Mental Retardation: An AMA Handbook for the Primary Physician,* 2nd ed. Chicago: American Medical Association, 1974.

25. SAILOR, W., D. GUESS, and D. M. BAER. "Functional Language for Verbally Deficient Children," *Ment. Retard.,* 11 (1973), 27–35.

26. SCHIEFELBUSCH, R. L., ed. *Language of the Mentally Retarded.* Baltimore: University Park Press, 1972.

27. SROUFE, L. A. and M. A. STEWART. "Treating Problem Children with Stimulant Drugs," *N. Engl. J. Med.,* 289 (1973), 407–413.

28. UZGIRIS, I. C. and J. McV. HUNT. *An Instrument for Assessing Infant Psychological Development.* (Unpublished study.) Champaign, Ill.: Psychological Development Laboratory, University of Illinois, 1966.

29. WATSON, L. S., JR. *How to Use Behavior Modification with Mentally Retarded and Autistic Children: Programs for Administrators, Teachers, Parents, and Nurses.* Columbus, Ohio: Behavior Modification Technology, 1972.

30. WOLFENSBERGER, W. *The Principle of Normalization in Human Services.* Toronto: National Institute on Mental Retardation, 1972.

31. WOLFENSBERGER, W. and R. A. KURTZ, eds. *Management of the Family of the Mentally Retarded.* Chicago: Follett Educational Corporation, 1969.

CHAPTER 20

BIOMEDICAL TYPES OF MENTAL DEFICIENCY

George A. Jervis

THE FIRST attempts to isolate specific types of mental retardation in the large population of defectives dates from the last century when cretinism, mongolism, and tuberosclerosis were identified. These attempts have continued with increased success and at present a few hundred biomedical types are on record.

The purpose of this chapter is to describe briefly some of these types. They can be classified into two large categories according to the etiology, i.e., the genetically determined and the environmentally determined. A third category may be added to include types of mental defect of unknown etiology.

The genetically determined types are usually classified into three groups: due to (1) mental defect associated with chromosomal abnormalities; (2) recessive genes, and (3) dominant genes.

❨ Chromosomal Abnormalities

Downs Syndrome, Mongolism

Frequency is estimated at about 1 in 600 births and increases some ten-fold in children born of women over forty years of age. The symptomatology consists of a conglomeration of abnormal physical traits: stunted growth, brachycephalic small skull, round flat face, almond-shaped palpebral fissures which slant inward and downward, epicanthus folds, large tongue, and small chin. The extremities are small, the fifth finger is usually curved and the palm of the hands shows a marked transverse line. There is general muscular hypotonicity. Congenital defects of heart or other organs are common. Mental retardation varies from severe to mild but the majority show a moderate degree of it. See Figure 20–1.

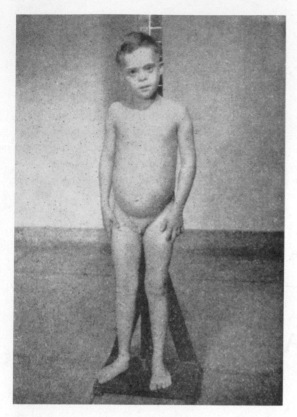

Figure 20–1.   Down's syndrome.

In about 90 percent of the cases, the abnormality of chromosomes consists in an extra chromosome in the twenty-one chromosomes of group G. There are, therefore, forty-seven chromosomes instead of the normal complement of forty-six. In a small percentage of patients there is a different chromosomal arrangement, the extra chromosome is not free but is attached (translocated) to a large chromosome, usually of D group. The total complement is therefore apparently the normal forty-six chromosomes. In a situation of this type the mother may have also a similar translocation, the total amount of her chromosomes being forty-five. The mother, then, has a theoretical chance of one out of three of having other affected children.

Edwards Syndrome, Trisomy E

Frequency is about 1 in 3500 births. Clinical manifestations consist of hypertelorism, palpebral ptosis, small chin, low-set malformed ears, macrognathia, shield chest, flexion deformity of finger, short neck, and congenital heart disease. Mental retardation is severe. Early death is common. The diagnosis rests on the demonstration of extra chromosome eighteen in the E group.

Patau Syndrome, Trisomy D

This is rarer than Trisomy E, the incidence being about 1 in 6000. Clinically, there is microcephaly, microthalmia, cleft lip, cleft palate, malformed ears, polydactily or syndactily, and other malformations. Mental retardation is profound and life expectancy short, from a few months to a few years. The extra chromosome in the D group is number thirteen.

Cat-Cry Syndrome

This syndrome—deletion of short arm of chromosome 5—is characterized by microcephaly, round face, hypertelorism, micrognathia and severe mental retardation. The voice in infancy has a characteristic catlike quality. Numerous other abnormalities in number or structure of autosomal chromosomes resulting in mental deficiency are documented. They are, however, rarer than the ones mentioned.

Several aberration of sex chromosomes in mentally defective individuals are known. The major categories are the following:

Klinefelter disease is clinically manifested by tall stature, underdeveloped secondary sexual characteristics, small and firm testes, clinodactily, cubitus valgus, and often obesity. Mental retardation when present is mild. The karyotype is XXY. The number of chromosome thirty-seven.

In the same group of excessive number of sex chromosomes are cases with *karyotype of XXXY and XXYY*, clinically similar to *XXY* male. Patients with the karyotype XXXXY (thirty-nine chromosome) show, in addition, more severe mental retardation. The hypogenitalism is more evident and several skeletal abnormalities are present.

In the female, the major categories of aberrations of sex chromosomes associated with mental retardation are the *multiple X types.* In patients with three X (instead of two) there is no distinct phenotype and mental retardation is not always observed and, when present, is mild. Cases with four or five X have been occasionally reported. These women are usually mentally defective. The syndrome of multiple X may be promptly diagnosed by examining a buccal smear. The epithelial cells of the mouth mucosa have one less Barr bodies than the number of X's.

Mental Deficiency Due to Recessive Genes

Numerous uncommon types of mental defect may be grouped under this heading. In each condition the family data of the patients are consistent with the hypothesis of a recessive gene being associated with the disease. Therefore, in a group of affected families, when the sibships are examined with proper statistical methods, the ratio of affected to normal sibs is 1 to 3 and the rate of consanguinity among parents of affected children is significantly higher than in the general population. A number of recessive types, in addition, are characterized by the defect of a specific enzyme. However, the causal relationship between the biochemical abnormality and mental defect is not always clear.

Among this group, the following may be briefly described.

PHENYLKETONURIA

The incidence is of the order of 1 in 15,000 children, the highest in these metabolic types. The degree of mental retardation varies but it is usually severe. Physical development is little impaired and life expectancy is not much shorter than normal. Seizures are often present and minor neurological abnormalities can be demonstrated in most patients. The diagnosis is based on the finding of phenylpyruvic acid in the urine. In addition, phenylalanine (an essential amino acid) is present in abnormal quantity in the blood. The demonstration of excess phenylalanine in the blood is diagnostic in the newborn infant when phenylpyruvic acid is not yet present. Early diagnosis is crucial for a successful treatment of the disease. The metabolic abnormality consists in the absence of a specific liver enzyme which metabolizes phenylalanine. The unmetabolized phenylalanine or some of its derivatives are apparently toxic, interfering with normal postnatal development of the brain. Treatment consists of special diets poor in phenylalanine.

HOMOCYSTINURIA

The main clinical manifestations are arachnodactyly, stiff joints, high stature, long limbs, and dislocation of the lenses. The presence of peculiar malar flush may be of help in the diagnosis. Glaucoma and cataracts may be present. Arterial and venous thromboses are frequent. Mental retardation, when present, varies from very mild to moderate. The metabolic abnormality consists of the absence of cystothionine synthetase, the enzyme of sulfur amino acid metabolism catalyzing the conversion of homocystine to cystothionine. The unmetabolized excess of homocystine is excreted in the urine and is easily recognized by a simple test. Low methionine diet may help in the treatment and in a certain number of cases the administration of Vitamin B6 is useful.

MAPLE SUGAR URINE DISEASE

The first clinical manifestations occur in early infancy. There are feeding difficulties, vomiting, spasticity, generalized seizures and unresponsiveness. Hair is coarse, sparse, and kinky (hence the term of kinky hair disease). The urine has a strong odor similar to maple sugar. The metabolic abnormality is in the branched amino acid metabolism. Leucine, valine, isoleucine, and their corresponding keto acids accumulate in blood and urine because of a lack of their proper enzymes. Ketoaciduria results which is diagnostic of the disease. Unless controlled with very difficult dietary measures, the disease is fatal.

HISTIDINEMIA

There are no distinct clinical manifestations aside from mild mental deficiency which is present only in about 50 percent of the cases. Speech defect is noted in some 60 percent.

The metabolic abnormality consists of a missing enzyme (histidase) in the catabolism of histidine. The absence of histidase results in the presence of an abnormal amount of histidine and of its ketoacid (imidazole pyruvic acid) in the blood and urine of patients. A few other rare amino aciduriae with mental defect have been reported.

NEUROLIPIDOSES

The term is used to denote a group of diseases of the central nervous system characterized by the storage of lipid in the brain and other organs. Mental retardation is always present and the conditions are fatal.

Tay-Sachs Disease, the onset of this disease (infantile amaurotic idiocy) is during the first years of life and leads to death in a few years. Neurological deterioration, blindness, and convulsions are major symptoms. Pathologically, the nerve cells are ubiquitously distended and repleted with gangliosides, a complex lipid, small amounts of which are normally present in the brain (see Figure 20–2). The disease is prevalent among Ashkenazi Jews. Prenatal diagnosis may be made by demonstrating the defect of a specific enzyme, hexoseaminidase A, in the cells of the amniotic fluid.

Batten Disease, this disease, neuronal ceroidlipofuscinosis, is a widely investigated lipidosis causing progressive mental retardation and blindness. There are several varieties which are classified according to age of onset and duration. Their common trait is the storage of a complex lipid (lipofuscin) in the brain cells. The nature of the defective enzyme (if any) is not known.

Nieman-Pick disease, in its infantile form, is characterized by a severe progressive mental retardation, blindness, and hepatospenomegaly. The substance accumulating in brain, liver, and spleen is sphingomylin, a lipid normally present in the brain but in smaller quantity. The missing enzyme is sphingomyelinase

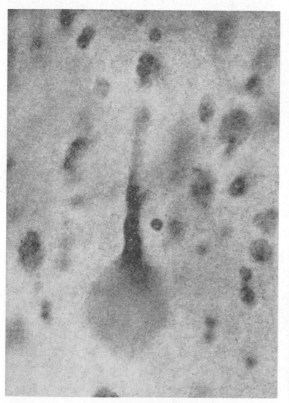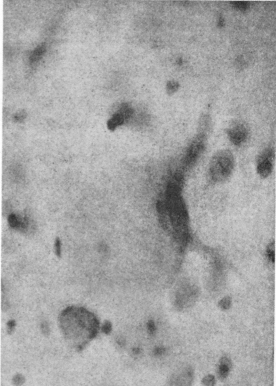

Figure 20–2.   Swollen "ballonlike" nerve cells characteristic of amaurotic idiocy.

which normally breaks down sphingomyelin.

Gaucher disease, in the acute infantile cerebral types, with severe mental deterioration is usually fatal. Spleen and liver are enlarged because of the accumulation of a glycolipid (glucocerebroside) which cannot be metabolized because of the congenital lack of its specific enzyme.

MUCOPOLYSACCHARIDOSES

This is a group of diseases characterized by accumulation of mucopolysaccharides in the cells of various organs, including the brain. With few exceptions the children are mentally defective. Several varieties have been recognized showing minor clinical differences but distinct enzymatic characteristics. The most common are:

Type I, *Hurler Syndrome*, characterized by stunted growth, large head, distorted coarse facial features, clouding of the corneas, large nose, thick tongue, abnormalities of osseous system, short neck, gibbus, and hirsutism (see Figure 20–3). Mental retardation is usually severe and slowly progressive. Mucopolysaccharides in the form of dermatan sulfate and heparan sulfate are present in the urine and the tissues of the body. The enzyme which is missing is alpha-L-Iduzonidase.

Type II, *Hunter Syndrome*, has clinical features similar to Type I but cornea clouding is lacking, mental retardation is less severe, and life expectancy longer. The disease is recessive but sex-linked, so that the patients are only boys. The biochemical characteristics are also similar to Type I, but the missing enzyme is different (sulfoiduromate sulfatase).

Type III, *Sanfilippo syndrome*, has physical features similar to Type II and I in the other varieties of the disease but mental retardation is usually much more marked. In the urine, blood, and tissues mostly heparan sulfate is present. The specific missing enzyme is heparan sulfate sulfatase.

GALACTOSEMIA

The main symptoms of this disease are mental deficiency, hepatosplenomegaly, and cataracts. In newborn, jaundice is usually present. Biochemically, large amounts of galactose and

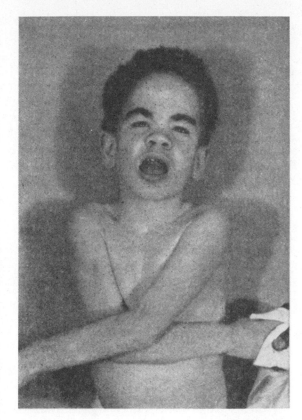

Figure 20–3. Hurler syndrome.

its phosphate are found in the urine and body fluids. The enzymatic defect is in the metabolic pathway from galactose to glucose where a block exists after the galactose phosphate step, due to the missing enzyme which converts galactose phosphate to uridine-galactose. This disease is rare, about 1 in 60,000–70,000 births and can be treated by eliminating milk and milk products from the diet of the infant.

WILSON DISEASE

This disease, hepato lenticular degeneration, is a recessive condition, characterized clinically by progressive extrapyramidal syndrome with intellectual deterioration, and pathologically by cirrhosis of the liver and degeneration of the basal ganglia of the brain. Biochemical alterations consist of very low blood copper, increased excretion of copper in the urine and deposit of copper in the brain, liver, and other organs. Normally, blood copper is closely bound to ceruloplasmin, a blood protein. In

Wilson disease, ceruloplasmin cannot bind copper because of a genetically determined structural alteration (for further review see Chapter 16). Free copper, then, is deposited in the brain, liver, and other organs causing degenerative change. Treatment by chelating agents such as penicillamine is of benefit.

HYPERUCEMIA

In this disease, Lesch-Nyhan, mental and motor retardation are accompanied by athetoid movements and spasms. Peculiar self-mutilating behavior, such as lip-biting and finger-chewing are characteristic. Biochemically, there is an increased production of uric acid, due to a defect of inhibitory enzyme in the uric acid metabolism.

In a second group of recessive conditions associated with mental deficiency, no biochemical abnormalities have been detected thus far.

PRIMARY MICROCEPHALY

Patients are of small stature and the head is particularly small (see Figure 20–4). There are no neurological manifestations but mental deficiency is usually serious. The condition should be differentiated from secondary microcephaly which is more common and is caused by various environmental factors.

ATAXIA TELANGIECTASIA

In this disease, Louis-Barr syndrome, mental defect is accompanied by progressive cerebellar dysfunction and by characteristic telangiectasiae of the bulbar conjunctiva. There is in addition immune incompetence due to the deficiency of immune globuline A.

LAURENCE-MOON SYNDROME

This disease is easily recognized by a cluster of abnormalities, such as pigmentary degeneration of the retina, mental retardation, polydactyly, obesity, and hypogenitalism.

SJÖGREN-LARSON SYNDROME

This disease consists of congenital generalized ichtyosis, pigmentary degeneration of the retina, slowly progressive spastic extensor

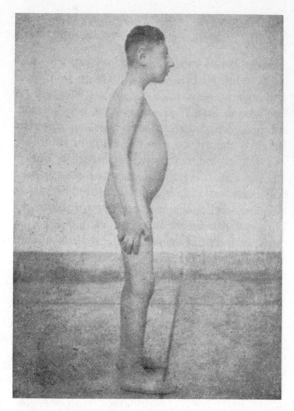

Figure 20–4.   Microcephaly. Chronological age fifteen, mental age three.

plantar response, and mental defect. Epileptic seizures are not uncommon.

COCKAYNE SYNDROME

Mental defect is usually severe and associated with dwarfism, microcephaly, pigmentary degeneration of the retina, hypogenitalism, and malnutrition. The condition is often progressive.

LOWE SYNDROME

Cataract is present early, often at birth, and is frequently accompanied by glaucoma. Metabolic acidosis, rickets, and organic aciduria of renal origin are usually present. Life expectancy is reduced. Mental deficiency is usually severe. The condition is X-linked recessive affecting only boys.

SMITH-LEMLI-OPITZ SYNDROME

The features consist of microcephaly, epicanthus with ptosis, strabismus, small upturned nose with broad bridge, micrognathia, lowset upturned ears, syndactyly or polydactyly, and various deformities of the lower extremities. Mental defect is usually severe and patients fail to thrive.

Mental Deficiency Associated with Dominant Genes

In this group are a few types of genetically determined instances of mental deficiency which are transmitted directly from affected parent to half of the offspring. The occurrence of sporadic forms is explained by assuming that the isolated instance is caused by a mutation in the parental gene. The mutated gene is then transmitted to the offspring. If there are no offspring the instance remains unique. Incomplete symptomatology is often noted in dominant conditions thus adding difficulties to the recognition of the disease.

TUBEROSCLEROSIS

This disease is characterized by the triad mental deficiency, adenoma sebaceous, and epilepsy. Other skin lesions are common, such as areas of discoloration, cutaneous fibroma, and shagreen patches. Retinal nodules and intracranial calcifications are often present (see Figure 20–5). Mental retardation varies from profound to mild. Occasionally, patients with normal intelligence have been on record. Incomplete forms ("formes' frustes") are not rare.

ACHONDROPLASIA

Shortening of the limbs, particularly of the proximal segments, large head with prominent

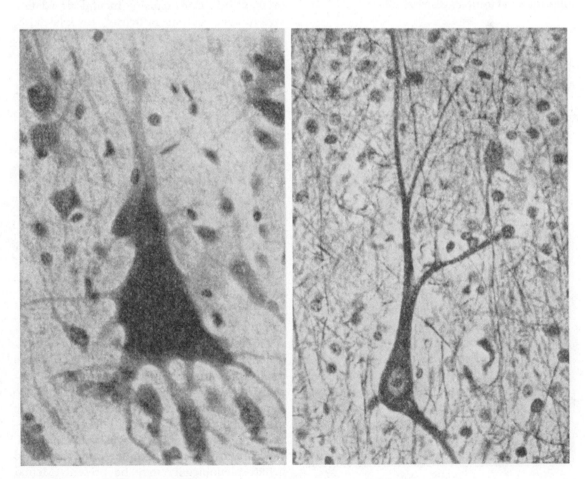

Figure 20–5. Tuberosclerosis.

forehead, and short broad hands are the main physical features of this disease. Mental retardation, usually mild, is present in no more than a third of the patients.

CRANIOFACIAL DYSOSTOSIS

In this disease (Crouzon), distorted shape of head, exopthalmos strabismus, and hypertelorism are characteristic. The orbits are poorly developed. Mental deficiency is mild or moderate, increased intracranial pressure may develop.

ACROCEPHALOSYNDACTYLIA

In this disease (Apert), the head is misshaped, resembling that of Crouzon disease. There is, in addition, fusion of fingers and toes (see Figure 20–6). Several varieties have been described. Mental defect is usually less mild than in Crouzon disease.

ARACHNODACTYLY

In this disease (Marfan), long limbs, spidery fingers and toes, dislocation of lenses, and cardiac defects are the main physical fea-

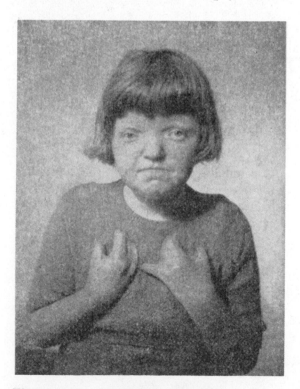

Figure 20–6.   Acrocephalosyndactilia.

tures. Mental deficiency, when present, is mild.

❨ Mental Deficiency Caused by Environmental Factors

Known types of mental deficiency caused by exogenous factors are not as many as those genetically determined, but include a higher incidence in each category.

Mental Defect Due to Infection

Infection may damage the nervous system during intrauterine life, or during infancy and childhood. Damage varies according to the type of infectious agent, the age of subject, and the severity of the acute infection. Among prenatal infections causing mental retardation are rubella, cytomegalovirus, toxoplasmosis, and syphilis.

RUBELLA

Infection of the mother during the first trimester of pregnancy may be transmitted transplacentally to the developing fetus, and damage various organs and systems, including the developing central nervous system. Clinical manifestations in the child are microcephaly, cataract, retinopathy, hepatitis thrombocytopenia, heart defect, and other malformation. Anamnestic data and the clinical picture make possible a prompt diagnosis. Rubella virus can be isolated at birth or shortly after. The widespread vaccination of girls against rubella has considerably reduced the incidence of this condition.

CYTOMEGALOVIRUS INFECTION

This is increasingly recognized as a significant cause of mental retardation. Usually the disease develops during intrauterine life. Apparently nonimmune women who acquire the infection during pregnancy are the most likely to transmit the disease to the fetus. Mild microcephaly is the major clinical manifestation. Chorioretinitis, intracranial calcification, and hepatosplenomegaly may be present. Mental deficiency varies from mild to severe. Excretion of the virus may persist for months after birth. Treatment is of little avail but preventive vaccination has been attempted.

Toxoplasmosis

Transplacental intrauterine transmission of toxoplasmosis is well known although its frequency has not been established. Clinical manifestations in the child consist of microcephaly or, at times, hydrocephaly, with intracranial calcifications. Chorioretinitis is common, cataract, glaucoma, or micropthalmia may be present. Mental retardation is often severe. There is no satisfactory treatment of the disease although the toxoplasm responds to certain sulfa drugs.

Syphilis

Congenital syphilis is the classical example of prenatal infection causing mental deficiency—but its symptoms and signs—saddle nose, notched teeth, interstitial keratosis, deafness, bone lesions and others—are rarely seen among mentally retarded. On the other hand, positive serology in a mentally defective is no evidence that the intellectual impairment is due to syphilis. A peculiar, but today rare, type of congenital syphilis is "juvenile paralysis." This serious deteriorating disease, due to multiplication of the syphilic agent in the brain, shows progressive mental defect, motor paralyses, and often epilepsy.

Encephalitis in Infancy or Childhood

Encephalitis is not rare in children and the accompanying brain damage may result in various degrees of mental retardation. The clinical history of the acute phase is usually characteristic and dramatic. Upon recovery from the acute episode, mental retardation becomes apparent. It is rarely progressive and, in fact, is often regressive. A first group of encephalitides is caused by neurotropic viruses of which many are known.

A particularly severe form is the herpes encephalitis in newborn, probably acquired during delivery from the infected genitalia of the mother.

A second group of encephalitis is due to bacteria and is usually associated with meningitis. The increasing use of antibiotic treatment during the acute phase of bacterial meningo-encephalitis has resulted in a dramatic decrease of the death rate but in a noticeable increase of the number of partially recovered, and often defective, children.

A third group of encephalitides follows common diseases of childhood such as measles, scarlet fever, or chickenpox. Brain involvement usually develops after the original disease has subsided. An allergic mechanism is apparently responsible for this encephalitic reaction.

The clinical picture of the postencephalitic retardate shows a few distinct features indicative of the type of the original disease. Evidence of brain damage often present includes paresis, spasticity, speech defect, disturbance in eye movements, and behavior alterations. The degree of mental retardation varies considerably from case to case and usually cannot be correlated with the type of encephalitis.

(Mental Retardation Clinical Syndromes

In numerous clinically characteristic types of mental deficiency, the data are not sufficient to establish the genetic or environmental nature of the condition.

DeLange Syndrome

Moderate microcephaly and small stature are usually present. Facies is characterized by bushy eyebrows with synophrys, small upturned nose, wide philtrum, low set ears, small mouth, and small chin. There is inability to extend the elbow completely. Syndactily, micromelia oligodactily, actodactily, and clinodactily are often present. Characteristic is a shortening and proximal placement of the thumb. Hirsuitism is common. Mental deficiency is usually severe.

Rubinstein-Taybi Syndrome

Mild microcephaly, hypertelorism, strabismus, antimongoloid slant of the eyes, beak nose, and high palate are common features. The most characteristic trait consists of broad terminal phalanx of the thumb or first toe. At times duplication of the first toe is noted. Laxity of joint ligament, hyperactive reflexes, stiff gait, and unfrequent seizures are other signs. Mental retardation is always present.

Sturge-Weber Syndrome

This is easily recognized because of the presence of angioma covering unilaterally a usually large area of the face. This is accompanied by a calcified angioma of the meninges in the occipital region on the same side as the facial angioma. Associated angioma of the choroid with glaucoma is not rare. Epilepsy is common and hemiplegia often develops. The disease is slowly progressive. Mental retardation is generally present but its severity varies considerably.

Prader's Syndrome

This consists of small stature, striking obesity, particularly in the lower parts of the body where characteristic cuffs around the ankles usually develop. Feet and hands are very small. Secondary sex characteristics are underdeveloped. There is characteristic muscular hypotonia, particularly in infancy. Mental retardation is usually moderate. Diabetes has often been observed in adult patients.

Sotos Syndrome

This is characterized in infancy by the very large proportions of height and weight which are above the 90 percentile. Therefore the term "cerebral gigantism." The head is also large and often dolicocephalic in shape. There are, in addition, hypertelorism, antimongoloid slant of the eyes, drooping eyelids, large ears, and prognathism. Various degrees of mental retardation are noted. The adult patient may have normal height and weight.

Beckwith-Wiederman Syndrome

Large tongue, omphalocele, large kidneys, and a large liver in a large body are distinct features. Hypoglycemia at birth and polycythamia are often seen. A common finding is hyperplasia of endocrine glands. Mental retardation is not always observed and when present is not severe.

Angelman Syndrome

This curious condition (happy puppet syndrome) is recognized by peculiar paroxysms of unjustified laughter and severe mental retardation. Other signs are microcephaly with flat occiput, hypertelorism, prognathism, muscular hypotonia with hyperreflexia, and incoordinated, jerky movements. Epileptic seizures are usually present. A curious trait is the tendency of the child to protrude the tongue for long periods of time.

Williams-Beuren Syndrome

A so-called "elfin face" is characteristic of the syndrome with hypertelorism, epicanthus, upturned small nose, wide mouth, full cheeks, low-set ears, and small chin. Hypercalcemia and supravalvular aortic stenosis are features of the syndrome. Mental retardation, which is not always present, is usually moderate.

❨ Bibliography

1. CROME, L. *Pathology of Mental Retardation.* Baltimore: Williams & Wilkins, 1971.
2. GELLIS, S. S. and M. FEINGOLD. *Atlas of Mental Retardation Syndromes.* Washington: U.S. Department of Health, Education, and Welfare, 1968.
3. HOLMES, L. B., H. W. MOSER, S. HALDORSSON et al. *Mental Retardation: An Atlas of Disease with Associated Physical Abnormalities.* New York: Macmillan, 1972.
4. McKUSICK, V. A. *Mendelian Inheritance in Man,* 3rd ed. Baltimore: The Johns Hopkins University Press, 1964.
5. MOSER, H. W. and P. A. WOLF. *The Nosology of Mental Retardation.* Baltimore: Williams & Wilkins, 1971.
6. PENROSE, L. S. *The Biology of Mental Defect,*

3rd ed. New York: Grune & Stratton, 1963.

7. STANBURY, J. B., J. B. WYNGAARDEN, and D. S. FREDRICKSON. *The Metabolic Basis of Inherited Disease*, 3rd ed. New York: McGraw-Hill, 1973.

8. STEVENS, H. A. and R. HEBER. *Mental Retardation*. Chicago: University of Chicago Press, 1964.

9. VINKEN, P. J. and G. W. BRUYN, eds. *Handbook of Clinical Neurology*, Vols. 10, 13, and 14. New York: American Elsevier, 1973.

PART TWO

Psychosomatic Medicine

CHAPTER 21

CHANGING THEORETICAL CONCEPTS IN PSYCHOSOMATIC MEDICINE[*]

Morton F. Reiser

⟮ Introduction

EVER SINCE man first experienced a sense
of self-awareness, he has been intrigued
with the challenge of understanding
the relationship of mind to body, and has
worked diligently toward developing empirically based conceptual solutions to the mysti-
fying problems it presents. To this day, the
problem eludes solution. The early history of
these efforts has been reviewed elsewhere[6,46]
and this account will pick up the thread of

[*] This Chapter introduces the second part of the
Volume and refers extensively to material covered in
chapters that follow, particularly Chapters 22, 23,
24, 25, and 26. To avoid unnecessary duplication,
many of the bibliographic references listed in those
Chapters have not been repeated. Readers interested
in a thorough follow-up of literature sources, therefore,
are advised to consult those Chapters and their bibliographies as well as the bibliography of this one.

the story toward the end of World War II
when experiences in military psychiatry were
generating considerable serious interest in dynamic psychiatry and in exploring the interrelationships between mind and body in the
etiology and pathogenesis of physical as well
as mental disorders. This chapter takes an historical perspective and is presented in three
parts. It begins with a review of earlier theories and the empirical context from which
they emerged. It emphasizes the important
clinical psychiatric observations and attempts
to define some of their limitations for theory,
while underlining those aspects of earlier data
and theory that seem still to be relevant and
cogent. Part 2 reviews findings that for the
most part followed the main portion of earlier
theory construction, though in fact the time
periods overlap, Part 1 roughly covering
1940–1960 and Part 2, 1955–1972. The work of

this second period immensely widened our data bases and added important new dimensions to available information about the interrelationship between physiological and psychological aspects of bodily function both in health and in disease. Accordingly, it forces reconsideration of earlier theoretical ideas and calls for drastically modified, if not entirely new, formulations. Part 3 begins with the conclusion that it is not possible at this time to construct a satisfactory and empirically sound general theory of etiology and pathogenesis. Rather, attempts are made in the last part of the chapter to extract a general conceptual scheme for approaching the problem of understanding man in health and disease. Throughout the chapter an effort is made to offer some suggestions as to possible shapes and directions for future work and theory construction, and, wherever possible, to bring older ideas into perspective in regard to present thinking.

(Part 1: Earlier Theories

In the first part of the epoch bounded roughly by the years 1940–1960, work proceeded mainly along two lines. First there was combined medical and psychological investigation of selected medical patients. This work aimed at identification and elucidation of the role of psychological conflict (and emotional arousal) in etiology and pathogenesis of medical illness, and in influencing the course of disease, for example, as in inducing remissions or exacerbations or in affecting the rate of progression. Meticulous and detailed combined clinical studies by internists and psychiatrists (Weiss,[89] Engel,[18] Ferris,[21] Wolff,[91] Wolf,[90] Grace,[27] Mirsky,[53] Romano,[20] Levine,[41] Rosenbaum,[65] Saslow,[69] Lidz,[44] and Binger,[8] to name just a few) demonstrated beyond a doubt that many medical diseases first became clinically manifest during periods of psychosocial crisis and that the course of disease can indeed be profoundly influenced by psychological factors. Complications were observed to occur in conjunction with serious psycho-

logical stress, disease processes were observed to accelerate during periods of sustained psychosocial turmoil, and remissions were observed in conjunction with periods of relative psychological tranquility. Further it become clear that the doctor–patient relationship by modulating and ameliorating psychological distress of patients could exert beneficial effects on the symptoms and progression of illness, and could at times augment desired pharmacologic effects of drugs (converse effects were observable as well, albeit with some reluctance on the part of clinicians.)[61,74] Relationships of this nature are regularly observed in hospitals and clinics when healthcare personnel are interested and when they have been trained to observe and to listen. The limited implications of such observed relationships for theories of etiology and pathogenesis will be discussed below.

The second major line of investigation was more experimental and involved the study of patients at first, and "healthy" subjects later, in the clinical psychophysiological laboratory. Although many variations were developed, the basic experimental design consisted of continuous, or repeated, measurements of (relevant) physiological functions during periods of "base line" or "rest" and during periods when attempts were made to manipulate the patient's or subject's emotional state by discussing conflictual topics and/or by exposing him to stimuli designed to elicit specific affects, e.g., anger, anxiety, etc. In this way virtually every tissue and organ of the body innervated by the autonomic nervous system and available for observation or intubation, or accessible to electronic recording from surface or depth electrodes in unanesthetized humans, was shown to be capable of considerable functional variability in reaction to a wide variety of provocative experimental manipulations. The ultimate goal of such experiments was to produce measurable functional changes experimentally in target organs that would mimic or reproduce pathological-physiological patterns of function associated with specific disease states, e.g., gastric hyperacidity and hypermotility, tachycardia, elevated blood pressure, changes in measures of external respiratory dynamics, etc. In fact, it has been possible to demonstrate repeatedly that a wide variety of impressive physiological changes may be so induced but not with the degree of regularity, predictability, and experimental control required for rigorous support of specific etiologic and/or pathogenic hypotheses. As our experience and sophistication have increased, innumerable technical, methodological, and experimental variations on the basic theme have evolved, but a myriad of highly complex problems (control, instrumentation, data reduction, statistical evaluation, and interpretation) connected with such experiments remain, and their limitations for contributing to the solution of problems of etiology and pathogenesis are indeed still considerable.[31,64,79,87]

The central theoretical issue of the epoch (1940–1960) was specificity. What determines whether a patient falls ill of one disease rather than another (why peptic ulcer instead of rheumatoid arthritis, for example)? More to the point in the context of psychosomatic medicine, do specific psychological factors constitute necessary and/or sufficient factors in determining choice of organ system and disease? Specificity in this sense refers to a different phenomenon from that observed in individual patients whereby a repetitive theme may be repeatedly activated at critical points in the history of the disease, making it a repetitive "core issue" for the particular patient, but not generalizable to others. In retrospect it is clear that the clinical and laboratory findings of the period under discussion implicated both specific and nonspecific mechanisms, but more attention and interest was directed to the search for specificity.

Before undertaking a review of the major theories that represented this point of view, it might be well to mention first some of the more general conceptual issues and problems that complicate the field and frustrate attempts to build and evaluate theory. Regardless of our ultimate conviction that mind and body constitute a true functional unity, the fact remains that as observers, investigators, and theorists, we are obliged (whether we like it or not) to deal with data from two separate realms, one pertaining to mind and the other to body. The science of the mind and the science of the body utilize different languages, different concepts (with differing levels of abstraction and complexity), and different sets of tools and techniques. Simultaneous and parallel psychological and physiological study of a patient in an intense anxiety state produces of necessity two separate and distinct sets of descriptive data, measurements, and formulations. There is no way to unify the two by translation into a common language, or by reference to a shared conceptual framework, nor are there as yet bridging concepts that could serve, as Bertalanffy suggests, as intermediate templates, isomorphic with both realms.[82] For all practical purposes, then, we deal with mind and body as separate realms; virtually all of our psychophysiological and psychosomatic data consist in essence of covariance data, demonstrating coincidence of events occurring in the two realms within specified time intervals at a frequency beyond chance. Such findings—our very best ones— tell us nothing in and of themselves about time sequences or causality as ordinarily understood in a linear sequential model. Confronted, then, by covariance findings of this nature, for example an association between a specified dysphoric affect or mood state and the development of a bodily lesion, such as a duodenal ulcer, there are essentially four conceptual schemes that can be evoked to relate the physical to the mental findings (see Figure 21–1). First we might say that there is no more than a coincidental relationship between the psychological and somatic spheres (Figure 21–1 (a)); in essence the duodenum represents a constitutional "weak link in the chain," hence that part of the body is expected to break down in response to stress of any type. A second model would postulate a somatopsychic sequence stating that the dysphoric state represents a psychological response to the organic lesion (Figure 21–1 (b)). A third model would postulate a psychosomatic sequence stating that the physiological changes accompanying the dysphoric mood are pathogenic and, if sustained, lead to peptic ulceration of the duodenal mucosa (Figure 21–1

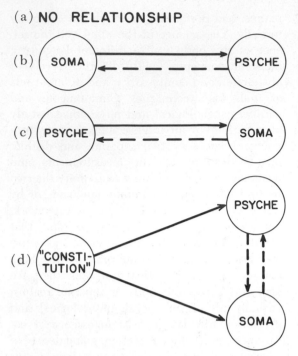

(a) **NO RELATIONSHIP**

(b) SOMA — — — PSYCHE

(c) PSYCHE — — — SOMA

(d) "CONSTI- TUTION" → PSYCHE ⇅ SOMA

Figure 21–1. Conceptual schemes for relating covariant physical and psychological findings in psychosomatic research. (For explanation see text.)

(c)). (Both of the preceding models would also allow for secondary reactive sequences in opposite directions, allowing for feedback from psyche to soma in the first instance, or soma to psyche in the second, thus explaining cyclic (escalating) feedback reactions such as pain, anxiety, spasm, increased pain, etc.) Finally there is a fourth conceptual model which states that the coincident psychic and somatic phenomena in fact represent separate and parallel reflections of a common underlying constitutional factor(s) usually postulated to be related to genetic and early experiential factors (Figure 21–1 (d)). Such a model also allows for secondary reciprocal interplay between the psychic and somatic spheres, as in the preceding two schemes. In essence this is a somatopsychosomatic model.

Another source of theoretical confusion can arise from overlooking the fact that there are at least three phases or epochs in the natural history of any disease. These are probably best considered separately when attempts are made to reconstruct pathogenesis. First is the period preceding manifest clinical appearance of the disease. During this period interest centers on predisposing causes, i.e., the various possible combinations of constitutional (genetic and experiential developmental) factors that may be thought of as programming a *capacity for a specific disease* into the organism. The second phase is that of the actual onset or precipitation. Here interest centers on the forces and mechanisms that precipitate the illness. These ordinarily need be in force only for relatively short periods of time, and need not be (and usually probably are not) the same as those involved in generating predispositions; of course the physiological mechanisms involved in different diseases must be quite different from one another. Third is the last epoch, i.e., the period following the establishment of the disease process. Here interest is on those factors and mechanisms influencing the course of the disease, such as remissions, exacerbations, accelerations, and so on, and these again may be expected to be different from those involved in the two preceding phases. For example, once a disease has become established and the individual has become aware of it, knowledge of the lesion and sensations related to it become incorporated into the self-image and are then subject to symbolic elaboration and incorporation into preexistent conflictual psychological structures. In the somatic realm, as a disease progresses, the role and importance of a variety of influencing factors may change profoundly. For example, the potential of salt to aggravate or accelerate the course of long-standing established essential hypertension in a patient with considerable loss of renal reserve, is very much greater than it is in a patient much earlier in the course of essential hypertension whose renal reserve is still within normal limits. Likewise, in essential hypertension the relative and proportional contributions of neurogenic and humoral factors in maintaining increased peripheral resistance change with time. In duodenal ulcer scarring, pyloric sphincter hypertrophy, sclerosis of blood vessels, etc., all change markedly with time, and play increasingly important roles late in the course of the disease, whereas they may well have been negligible factors earlier in the course. The main point is that both the psychological and the physiological medical data differ in fundamental and important ways, depending upon the phase of the natural history of the disease that is under study, and it clearly may be misleading, and probably quite incorrect, to assume that analysis of the circumstances and mechanisms involved in precipitation of an illness, or in influencing its course (no matter how thoroughly studied and formulated), would necessarily bear any direct relevance for understanding the mechanisms that had been involved in establishing predisposition. A priori, one might very well expect that in considering predisposing factors, disease-specific influences might very well overshadow nonspecific mechanisms in importance, whereas it is entirely plausible that mechanisms involved in precipitating the onset of disease, and in influencing the course of disease once established, might involve nonspecific mechanisms more importantly. These matters will be discussed further at the end of the chapter.

Turning now to a review of the major theories of the 1940s and 1950s, as noted above, the issue of specificity captured the imagination and attention of the major workers of that period. Generally speaking, the observations of experienced clinicians working at that time strongly suggested that it would indeed be both rational and worthwhile to search for specific elements in the personality structure and psychological life of patients that might participate in etiologic and pathogenic processes and contribute to the choice of symptoms and illness. Not only general clinical experience, but systematic profiles of personality (obtained either by structured interview, or projective and inventory-type psychological tests), led to the inescapable conclusion that patients with certain medical disorders, for example, duodenal ulcer, do in fact resemble one another psychologically more than they do members of the general patient population, or homogeneous groups of patients with other specified diseases. George Engel described the situation very aptly by stating that, if one tells an experienced clinician that he has a patient

with ulcerative colitis, the clinician might very well give a surprisingly accurate thumbnail personality sketch of that patient without ever having seen him. The converse, however, Engel is quick to point out, does not hold, that is, given even a detailed account of the patient's personality, it is by no means possible to predict with any degree of confidence what disease, if any, the patient might have.[18] A major question, of course, is whether the psychological personality features, shared by patients with the same disease, may not be shared because they, in fact, arise in reaction to the disease and hence would be expected to be shared. A more subtle but nonetheless cogent question is whether such shared somatic-psychic features may arise in response to an implicit perception or awareness of vulnerability or predisposition even before the disease becomes clinically manifest. This question is posed in beginning the review of the early specificity theories, since it is of central importance in a discussion of linear sequential cause-effect models, as in fact all of these early theories are. It is now generally appreciated that this critical question is unanswerable in retrospective studies, and probably only partially answerable in most longitudinal prospective studies that are feasible of execution in clinical investigations with human subjects. As will be clear later, with respect to more recent field theories, such as currently obtain generally in human biology, this question is much less important, at least in this particular form.

One of the first and most detailed attempts to relate personality to specific illness was the "personality profile" proposed by Flanders Dunbar.[16] While its extensive clinical observations were quite accurate, its clinical and theoretical utility turned out to be very limited, and it is now generally regarded as having mainly historical interest and importance.

A second important theoretical framework emerged from the extensive research program headed by Harold Wolff and his collaborators. The full scope of his investigations can only be appreciated by consulting some of the major original publications such as *Human Gastric Function*, the classic study of a patient with a gastric fistula by Harold Wolff and Stewart Wolff.[91] In essence Wolff postulated that stress diseases arise as part of the human physiological reaction to stress, i.e., "forces or individuals that jeopardize the life or love of a human being . . . which interfere with the realization of his aspirations and needs or block the exercise of his potential. These threats are reacted to by mobilization of an individual's defenses." [p. 1059][92] Thus, the bodily reactions were regarded as having been set in motion as adaptive, protective, or defensive or offensive responses, depending upon the subject's nature, his past experience, and the situation. "They are more or less effective and more or less costly to the individual, depending on these and other factors, such as the nature and integrity of the structures participating in the protective reaction." [p. 1060][92] Wolff and his co-workers postulated patterns of defensive reactions which, they felt, were specifically associated with defensive responses, in particular organ systems, and affecting specified functions such as eating, ejection-riddance, etc. The psychological formulations were based upon personality features and behaviors that were directly observable with minimal or no inference, and that pertained primarily to conscious layers of the patient's personality function and life experiences. Further focus was on psychological observations that could be carried out simultaneously with detailed study and observation of the patient's clinical status, and with measurement of the function of affected organ systems in the physiological laboratory. Naturally, the formulations looked and sounded quite different from those of contemporary psychoanalytic investigators (as will be noted below) but in retrospect, it can be seen that the specificity formulations of Wolff and of Franz Alexander, in particular, are in fact quite compatible in regard to the central themes, though they differ considerably in respect to the level of mental functions emphasized, in the amount of inference involved in constructing theory from observation, and in the dynamic richness and scope of the formulations, as well as the ease with which such formulations could be apposed to (or fitted

with) concurrent measures of clinical status and organ function. For example, the following statement by Harold Wolff regarding "protective patterns of defense involving eating: the stomach and the duodenum," can be compared to Alexander's formulations (quoted later) concerning the specific psychological contributions to disorders of the same organs. Wolff states:

One of the earliest aggressive patterns to manifest itself in the infant is that associated with hunger and eating. In later life, this pattern may reassert itself in certain individuals when they feel threatened; at such times of danger, feelings of anger and deprivation, of longing for emotional support, or of need for being "cared for," may be repressed by the equally insistent assertion that the individual is strong, independent, capable of doing alone, or standing 'on his own feet,' either through actual deprivation of emotional support or an unwillingness to accept it. This feeling state shows itself in the stomach as one of readiness for eating; hypersalivation may also occur. The gastric hyperfunction associated with these feelings is manifested by increased blood flow, motility, and acid secretion. Under such circumstances the mucous membrane was found to be unusually fragile. The hyperdynamic state of the stomach was found to be associated with symptoms, namely heartburn and localized epigastric pain, relieved by food and soda whether or not ulceration was present. [p. 1064][92]

Later, two of Wolff's students, Grace[27] and Graham,[28] formulated a derivative hypothesis which they named "specificity of attitude" hypothesis. This hypothesis states that there is associated with each psychosomatic disease a specific attitude toward the life events that precipitate the first appearance or later exacerbations of the disease. Attitude was defined as: "(1) How a person perceives his own position in a situation—what he feels is happening to him, and (2) What action, if any, he wishes to take." [p. 159][28] It was postulated that attitudes are different for different diseases but that all persons with a given disease would have the same attitude. For comparison with the Wolff and Alexander formulations, the attitude leading to duodenal ulcer was described by Graham as "felt deprived of what was due him and wanted to get even (didn't get what he should, what was owed or promised, and wanted to get back at, get revenge, do to him what he did to me)."[29] Thus, Graham and his co-workers extracted from a broader formulation a distilled statement about attitude which then could be tested quite explicitly by a variety of techniques, including induction of attitudes under hypnosis, while measuring appropriate bodily system responses, as well as by postdiction from interview material by blind raters— postdiction which would match patients with diseases by detecting evidences of "specific attitudes" in the interview material.

Franz Alexander and his associates in 1932 began a series of psychoanalytic studies of patients suffering from chronic organic ailments in which emotional conflicts were thought possibly to play an etiologic role either as primary or contributing factors. Alexander's studies utilized mainly the investigative method of psychoanalysis and proceeded on the basis of a fundamental distinction between "visceral neurosis" and conversion hysteria which he first articulated in 1939. Freud, in his studies on hysteria with Breuer in 1895, had demonstrated that specific unconscious contents could be symbolically expressed in the body language of somatic symptoms through the mechanism of conversion.[9] In 1910, Freud also noted that there could be mechanisms other than conversion whereby unconscious attitudes might alter physiological functions without symbolizing any definite psychic meaning, but did not further specify their possible nature.[22] Alexander formalized the distinction between hysteria and the "visceral neuroses," a term he used in referring to those disorders which were identified with the field of psychosomatic medicine. He pointed out that whereas in conversion hysteria symptom formation acts to resolve unconscious conflict, in the visceral neuroses, the basic conflict remains unresolved; he postulated that the chronic affect associated with unresolved conflict, even though repressed or suppressed, would nonetheless be accompanied by its (appropriate) physiologic concomitants.[3] Alexander theorized that the physiological changes accompanying the chronic emotions

associated with unresolved conflict were the physiological changes then that would give rise, first to altered function in the appropriate organ systems and, if long enough sustained, to alterations in structure and disease. Thus, for each of the seven diseases that he and his colleagues studied, a formulation of specific conflict was derived from the clinical data produced in the course of psychoanalytic treatment and/or investigation. For comparison with the preceding formulations, Alexander's formulation regarding duodenal ulcer is quoted below:

The central dynamic feature in duodenal peptic ulcers is the frustration of dependent desires originally oral in character. The craving to be fed appears later as a wish to be loved, to be given support, money, and advice. This fixation on early dependent situations of infancy comes in conflict with the adult ego and results in hurt pride, since the infantile craving for help is contrary to the standards of the adult, to his wish for independence and self-assertion. Because of this conflict, the oral craving must be repressed. Oral receptiveness when frustrated often changes into oral aggressiveness, and this also becomes repressed because of guilt feelings it provokes. Both oral dependent and oral aggressive impulses may then be frustrated by internal factors—shame and guilt.

The most common defense against both oral dependent and oral acquisitive impulses is overcompensation. The latently dependent or acquisitive person overtly appears as an independent, hard-working individual who likes responsibility and taking care of others. He responds to challenges with increased activity and ambition, works hard and assumes greater and greater responsibilities. This in turn increases his secret longing to lean on others. To be loved, to be helped is associated from the beginning of life with the wish to be fed. When this help-seeking attitude is denied its normal expression in a give-and-take relationship with others, a psychological regression takes place to the original form of a wish to ingest food. *This regressive desire seems to be specifically correlated with increased gastric secretion.* (Italics mine.)

Not all patients suffering from duodenal ulcer overcompensate for their dependent desires with an outward show of 'gogetting' activity. Many of them are overtly dependent, demanding, or disgruntled persons. In such individuals, the dependent tendencies are frustrated not by internal repudiation, but by external circumstances. But even in these overtly demanding patients, a definite conflict about dependent cravings can be discovered. The crucial psychological finding in all ulcer patients is the frustration (external or internal) of passive, dependent, and love-demanding desires that cannot be gratified in normal relationships.

Onset of illness occurs when the intensity of the patient's unsatisfied dependent cravings increases either because of external deprivation or because the patient defends against his cravings by assuming increased responsibilities. The external deprivation often consists in the loss of a person upon whom the patient has been dependent, in leaving home, or in losing money or a position that had given the patient a sense of security. The increased responsibility may take the form of marriage or the birth of a child or the assumption of a more responsible job. [Pp. 15–16][5]

The other six diseases studied by the Chicago psychoanalytic group of Alexander, were bronchial asthma, rheumatoid arthritis, ulcerative colitis, essential hypertension, neurodermatitis, and thyrotoxicosis. For each specific psychodynamic constellation, there was postulated also a specific related "onset situation" i.e., the life conditions preceding illness that affected patients emotionally at the time of onset (by reactivating old conflicts); and a third factor which Alexander designated an X factor by which he meant a constitutional vulnerability of a specific tissue, organ, or system. This then was a multiple factor model in which each of the three factors was considered a necessary but not sufficient cause, with the development of manifest disease depending upon presence and activation of all three in appropriate combination. In Alexander's words, the operational hypothesis of this work could be reduced as follows: "A patient with vulnerability of a specific organ or somatic system and a characteristic psychodynamic constellation develops the corresponding disease when the turn of events in his life is suited to mobilize his earlier established central conflict and break down his primary defenses against it. In other words, if the precipitating external situation never occurs, a patient may, in spite of the presence of the predisposing emotional patterns and of organ

vulnerability, never develop the disease." [p. 77][5]

This then was a linear psychosomatic theory (Figure 21–1(c)). A central feature to note is the postulation that the pathogenic physiological changes involved were conceived of as physiological concomitants of emotion, such as are encountered in mature adult organisms and patterned on the fight-flight physiology of Cannon, namely sympatho-adrenal and/or parasympathetic activation. For example, essential hypertension was seen as resulting from chronically suppressed and repressed rage with concomitant sympatho-adrenal activation and elevation of blood pressure, such as might be seen in acute rage attacks; gastric hypermotility and hypersecretion of acid were seen as the physiological concomitants of vagal stimulation accompanying repressed and suppressed longing for love (equated with longing to be fed).[4] These psychophysiological characteristics of the theory appear as well in the formulations of Harold Wolff and his co-workers.

In retrospect, these early specificity formulations appear rather narrow and oversimplified; to a large degree this may be the result of preoccupation with what we now realize to be a relatively narrow and limited sector of the field. While giving little more than lip service to multiple-factor concepts, these early writers limited their attention to predominantly intrapsychic issues and proximate interpersonal transactions in the psychological realm, and to peripheral autonomic effector mechanisms and end-organ systems in the physiological realm, while relatively little attention was paid to external social systems, to central nervous system mechanisms, or to cellular and molecular biological phenomena. In other words, the formulations may have been premature in the sense that they will have turned out to be incomplete and overinclusive rather than intrinsically incorrect.

Other psychoanalytic investigators of the same time period, particularly Grinker, Schur, and Deutsch, were impressed not only with the ubiquity in "psychosomatic" patients of core conflicts around pregenital issues (as Alexander had been) but also with the extensive and impressive evidence of regression and primitivization of ego functions in these patients, particularly at the time of the life crises associated with precipitation and/or aggravation of the disease and during periods of prolonged active illness. Impressed by the resemblance of pathological physiological function in "visceral neurosis" to the labile relatively unmodulated patterning of physiological responses in infancy and very early childhood, they speculated about its possible significance. Their (essentially epigenetic developmental) theories regard the pathological physiology of psychosomatic diseases as being patterned according to the physiology of infancy and early childhood and postulate the physiological anlagen (X factors) to be constitutional (genetic and early experiential), possibly or probably fixed or programmed into the organism by coincidence (conditioning), and later reinforced in the mother-infant and child-family interactive relationships during development. Two of the investigators of that era, Margolin[47] and Szasz,[81] also were impressed with the primitive "regressive" nature of the physiology, and Szasz spoke of "regressive innervation." These theories stand in sharp contrast to Alexander's theory in two ways: (1) they utilize transactional field rather than linear models, and (2) they postulate the physiological components to be more primitive and less well regulated than the adult patterns evoked in Alexander's theory. Grinker[30] postulated an infinite series of progressive stages of differentiation of body systems from psychosomatic unity at birth to the highly complex differentiated and integrated adult organism. He saw a breakdown in adaptation involving progressive dedifferentiation of varying degrees regressively back through stages of psychosis and various psychosomatic disorders all the way to primitive disorganized and overwhelming panic states (roughly equivalent to the neonatal conditions of total response). Schur[72,73] conceptualized the progressive maturation from infantile "psychosomatic unity" as occurring in two spheres: (1) progressive desomatization of reactions to danger in the physiological sphere (a gradual refinement from general chaotic uncontrolled

total-body responses to the finely modulated, discrete and homeostatically balanced responses of the adult, such as "signal anxiety"), and (2) progressive refinement from primary process thinking to secondary process-controlled thinking (mediated and modulated by small discrete quantities of "delibidinized and deaggressivized" energy) in the psychologic sphere. He emphasized that the ego reacts simultaneously to danger in two ways: evaluating danger and responding to danger. If failure of defensive ego functions under stress and reactivation of unconscious conflict occur, he postulates that danger signals are increasingly evaluated along progressively more (primitive symbolic) primary-process modes and also that there is a concomitant (but not necessarily entirely synchronous) "resomatization" of the response. As the resomatization proceeds to primitive levels, old infantile patterns of bodily response can be reactivated and result finally in disease (the specific organs and processes involved having been predetermined by constitutional factors). He considered that alterations in "ego state" in reaction to stress were of utmost importance in permitting and/or promoting emergence of primitive pathophysiological patterns of function that could then lead to disease. Deutsch[13] also emphasized return to infantile, or primitive developmental points of physiological "fixation" and was, at the same time, quite impressed with the primitive body language (symbolism) encountered in psychosomatic patients and included important elements of pregenital conversion as well as conditioning and genetic endowment in his thinking about specificity of organ and symptom choice. Needless to say, none of these theoretical systems is amenable to empirical testing (given the present "state of the art") but they do bear an interesting conceptual compatibility with many of the newer biological findings to be reviewed later.

A few psychoanalytic clinical investigators, such as Garma[26] and Sperling[75–78] have continued the conceptual tradition begun with Groddeck[32] that considers psychosomatic visceral disorders to arise mainly on the basis of symbolic conversion mechanisms. The observations and rich clinical data about symbolic significance of bodily symptoms and changes are not in question; they are prominent in the data whenever clinicians work at psychological depth with medical patients. But these theories regarding pathogenesis are neither empirically testable at present, nor are they readily reconciled conceptually with recent developments in the biology of disease, nor as noted earlier is it possible in a retrospective historical study to distinguish whether such psychological meanings occur as reactions to the presence and knowledge of illness or whether they antedated illness and may have contributed to its genesis.

The work and the theories of several investigators of this epoch have been reviewed in considerable detail not only because they are considered to be important and representative (and responsible for stimulating a highly productive era of psychophysiological research); but also because many of the main ideas contained in them should ultimately be brought into proper perspective and reconciled with more recent findings and theoretical models. This period produced an enormously rich yield of carefully detailed and documented observations, and of derivative formulations. Many of the *clinical observations themselves* have been confirmed and replicated many times over and by this time have been incorporated into the general body of information about clinical medicine. Many of the psychodynamic formulations, particularly Alexander's work, have been supported as valid *psychological* findings and formulations by other investigators (Mirsky,[50] Weiner,[88] Dongier, Wittkower et al.,[15] Wallerstein et al.,[83] see below). On the other hand, original *psychosomatic* formulations regarding the direct role of specific psychodynamic factors in etiology and pathogenesis of disease have not fared as well in attempts to validate them in careful and often highly sophisticated and elaborate clinical research. Yet at the same time there has been enough partial empirical support to preclude their being summarily dismissed.[5,29] It seems certain that future theories will have to account for the observations,

and it is also likely that the general shape of the major hypotheses may still be discernible in future formulations albeit with different emphases and perspectives, when information from broader data bases and newer systems and transactional theoretical models are taken into account.

❨ Part 2: Modern Developments, 1955–1972

As noted earlier, the work of the first part of the epoch 1940–1960 concentrated mainly on intrapsychic mechanisms, peripheral autonomic and humoral mechanisms in control of target organs and organ systems, and phenomena that seem to bear directly on the issue of specificity, with less attention being paid to broader interpersonal and social ecological factors, to the role of the *central nervous system* (CNS) in mediating between cognitive emotional and peripheral neurovegetative effector mechanisms, to cellular and molecular biologic processes, and to mechanisms of genetic transmission. And there were relatively few studies concerned with dissecting mechanisms and relative contributions of genetic transmission, neonatal, early infant, and child development in determining "constitutional" predisposition, and with the role of nonspecific bodily responses in medical pathogenesis. All of this has changed radically with the tremendous expansion of information that has occurred in the human life sciences and neurobiology since the mid 1950s. Technical breakthroughs in electronics and instrumentation, along with the rapid develoment of computer science, have now made it possible to investigate biological processes that previously had been inaccessible to experimental analysis, and to obtain answers to questions that were previously out of reach. Currently there is a much fuller appreciation of the fact that understanding states of health and disease requires understanding of biological, psychological, and social parameters to be complete. More investigators and theoreticians are appreciative of the obligation to address the complexity of interacting factors and mechanisms in these three spheres as they contribute to the development of an actual phenotype from a genotypic blueprint. This broadened understanding has made it clearer than ever that mind and body cannot be regarded, or dealt with, as separate much longer despite our bondage to Cartesian dualism. Corollary to this is the recognition that subclassification or distinction of psychosomatic from other disorders is rapidly losing (perhaps has already lost) its meaning and utility. The next section will review selected sectors of clinical and related neurobiological research that have contributed to newer perspectives in the field. It is not intended to be a fully comprehensive review, but rather to concentrate on selected fields of study and data that have had major impact on our perspectives regarding relations between mind, brain, and body. Important new work and perspectives in the social, epidemiologic, and transcultural aspects is not included here. For this the reader is referred to Chapter 25.

Longitudinal "Predictive" Studies of Persons at Risk

This section deals with studies of predisposing (physical and psychological) factors and of precipitating (psychosocial) factors in longitudinal studies of populations identified as being at risk for a particular disease by virtue of possessing known biological markers. The best known of such studies are those of Mirsky and co-workers[50,88] on duodenal ulcer which further refined the Alexander concept. Mirsky identified the physiological (genetically-determined) condition necessary, but not sufficient, for the development of duodenal ulcer; that is, the hypersecretion of pepsinogen into the blood.[50–52] He postulated that this inborn trait, through its influence on the mother-infant relationship, would also play a central role in personality development and in determining the type of social-conflict situation that would later be pathogenic for the individual in adult life. This, then, is a circular rather

than linear theory, i.e., it suggests somatopsychosomatic sequences rather than linear psychosomatic ones. It is supported by empirical data gathered in a study on duodenal ulcer by Weiner, Thaler, Reiser, and Mirsky in which independently studied psychological data were used to predict (using Alexander's formulations of core conflict specific for peptic-ulcer) which, of a large number of potential ulcer patients (as determined by pepsinogen level), would actually develop the disease under the psychosocial stress of basic military training.[88] These data, as noted earlier, lend validity to the psychodynamic formulations that Alexander and his colleagues derived from psychoanalytic studies of patients with duodenal ulcer. At the same time it should be emphasized that these studies by Mirsky et al. do not address the question of what the physiological mechanisms may be that lead to actual ulcer formation in the duodenum, and thus do not bear directly at all on the psychophysiological psychosomatic hypotheses advanced by Alexander et al. Similarly, partial support of Alexander's psychodynamic formulations about thyrotoxicosis is provided by the work of Dongier and Wittkower,[15] and of Wallerstein et al.,[83] which demonstrates an association in euthyroid subjects between a high propensity of the thyroid to incorporate I^{131} and the psychological personality characteristics described by Alexander et al. in patients with thyrotoxicosis. The relationship, if any, of this physiological trait and thyroid disease is not clear, and as Weiner[84] has pointed out, the psychological traits may be linked with a tendency toward involvement of the thyroid gland in diseases affecting its secretory function (in either an upward or a downward direction).

In an unfinished statement written shortly before his death, Alexander took into account the findings of Mirsky and others on these newer demonstrated interrelationships of biological, psychological, and social factors in etiology and pathogenesis and indicated some readiness to modify his theoretical model:

These three variables—inherited or early acquired organ or system vulnerability, psychological patterns of conflict and defense formed in early life, and the precipitating life situations—are not necessarily independent factors. It is possible that constitution at least partially determines both the organ vulnerability and the characteristic psychological patterns. At present little is known about the interdependence of these two variables. There is strong indication, however, that the correlation between constitution and characteristic psychiatric patterns is not a simple one. Constitution alone without certain emotional experiences of early life, particularly the early mother-child relation, may not produce a consistent pattern. [P. 17][5]

The power of such risk studies (which are possible only when biological "anlagen" such as pepsinogen are known) can be further amplified when applied to studies of *discordant disease incidence in monozygotic and dizygotic twins.*[56,57] Katz and Weiner point out that risk strategy could be applied in gout (utilizing hyperuricemia to identify subjects at risk);[37] it might also be applicable for the study of rheumatoid arthritis, utilizing certain immune proteins as indicators of risk. Another appropriate application might be in coronary artery disease where there are multiple factors (such as obesity, cigarette smoking, exercise habits, heredity, hypertension, blood lipids, etc.) that are known to affect the risk of myocardial infarction in additive and combined ways (see Chapter 26). In longitudinal risk studies of coronary disease, it would seem worthwhile to study in detail both the nature of the precipitating circumstances, and the psychological personality characteristics of subjects. Such data might then be useful in helping to clarify: (1) the relative roles of specific vs. nonspecific ubiquitous psychosocial stress situations (like bereavement,[55] see below) in precipitation of myocardial infarction; and (2) the relation of "predisposing" psychological characteristics, such as the Type A personality of Friedman and Rosenman,[23,66] to incidence of myocardial infarction. Does "Type A personality" lead to disease by making the person's life stressful, or is it rather a parallel psychological manifestation of an underlying predisposing constitutional factor that also leads to coronary artery disease? (Figure 21–1(d).)

Mortality and Morbidity of Bereavement

Studies on the mortality and morbidity of bereavement exemplify the emergence of data emphasizing *the importance of nonspecific effects of psychosocial stress on physical health.* Rees and Lutkins[60] reported in 1967 on the study of a small community in Wales in which a cohort of 903 close relatives of patients who had recently died were identified as experimental subjects. A group of 878 control subjects from the same community matched for age, sex, and marital status were also identified. The health of the experimental and control subjects was followed for one year following death of the relative or selection as a control subject. During the year of bereavement the death rate in the bereaved subjects was *seven times* that of the controls! A related, and perhaps even more impressive finding was that the risk of death was twice as high if the relatives had died outside the home (including in the hospital) than when they had died in the home. A study of widowers in Britain by Parkes, Benjamin and Fitzgerald[55] yielded similar results and showed that the majority of deaths in the first six months of widowerhood could be accounted for by coronary artery disease in subjects of the appropriate age group. A controlled study by Bennet[7] following the Bristol flood (July 1968) in Britain demonstrated in the twelve months following the flood an increase in morbidity and a 50 percent increase in mortality in subjects whose homes had been flooded compared to those whose homes had not been so affected! The earlier findings of Engel[19] and Schmale,[70,71] demonstrating the high frequency with which real, threatened, or symbolic object loss and separation precede development of illness of any type, are quite consistent with the findings of these British investigators. Taken altogether, the data convincingly demonstrate that bereavement, object loss, and the associated reactive affective states may have profound reverberations in the physical sphere, affecting even the capacity to sustain life itself. The affective and psychological characteristics of these states span a wide spectrum: natural bereavement, aggravated or serious bereavement, depression of various types, and include states that Engel and Schmale feel deserve special designation as "helplessness and hopelessness" associated with attitudes of "giving up" and "given up."[19] Engel postulates that there may be a fundamental biological stress or danger response state in addition to "fight-flight" which he has named "conservation withdrawal." He points out that the metabolic changes associated with such a response would be anabolic, as opposed to the catabolic activation responses of the "fight or flight" reaction described by Cannon, which was used as the exclusive physiological referent for earlier psychosomatic theories. Engel considers that the physiological changes he postulates to occur in "conservation withdrawal" would act in an entirely nonspecific manner by rendering the organism less resistive to *a variety* of pathogenic factors. While the physiology of conservation withdrawal as such has not been documented, there is much evidence that psychoendocrine phenomena may well play an important role in clinical events of this kind (see below).

Psychoneuroendocrinology

Psychoneuroendocrinology constitutes the third major section for discussion here. This field of study serves as a major link between clinical and basic research endeavors. While its main relevance pertains to nonspecific mechanisms in pathogenesis and precipitation of a wide variety of illnesses, it may also have some interesting and provocative indirect implications for the issue of specificity as well. Studies in the psychoneuroendocrine sector probably more than any other single sector have (1) contributed to our growing recognition of the overwhelming importance of nonspecific mechanisms in development of disease; and (2) provided a beginning of vitally important insights into the fascinating and intricate (still incompletely understood) mechanisms by which the CNS is able to mediate between higher mental functions (and psychological responses to psychosocial events)

on one hand, and maintenance of metabolic processes and integrity in body tissues and systems on the other hand. It has, in fact, provided us with an overwhelming sense (incomplete in fine detail) of the highly complex integrated linkages between the limbic forebrain system and (1) the autonomic nervous system (which extends outward to innervate peripheral tissue); and (2) the pituitary (via the hypothalamus) and through it, the entire endocrine system, thus making it possible for the hormones to act as circulating extensions of the nervous system. These relationships and linkages are summarized and discussed fully in Chapters 22, 23, and 24 by Weiner, Hofer, and Mason, respectively. The discussion here will highlight only some issues that are of interest in the context of this particular chapter.

First is the fact that alterations in endocrine function occurring in experimental animals in response to psychosocial stresses have been shown to influence host resistance to a variety of pathogenic organisms and to affect the viability and rate of growth of implanted neoplastic tissue.[1,40] In this connection it should be noted that there is also considerable evidence that central neurophysiological mechanisms may participate more directly in these psychosocial stress effects on host resistance by influencing immunological reactions, including tissue sensitivity to histamine and levels of circulating antibodies[59,80] (see Chapter 29 by Schiavi and Stein). It appears then that the hormones, separately and in combination as described by Mason[48] (see Chapter 21), may play a role not only in stress and hormone-dependent diseases, but also in infectious and neoplastic processes as well.

A second important feature is the phenomenon of *reciprocity between the effectiveness of ego defenses and the level of activation of stress hormone systems* (mainly the sympathoadrenal system and the pituitary-adrenal axis). This was first demonstrated in man in a classic study by Sachar et al. in patients with acute schizophrenic excitement.[68] Subsequently it has been shown to operate in a wide variety of both acute *and* chronic conditions (as noted in several of the chapters that follow). The demonstration of this phenomenon has proved to be of fundamental theoretical significance and brings us a giant step closer to understanding the way in which *intrapsychic phenomena may be interposed between psychosocial vectors on the one hand and alterations in body physiology on the other*. Ego defenses may protect against excessively brisk endocrine activation by functioning effectively; conversely vigorous endocrine activation may take place when ego-defense functions in the psychological sphere are inefficient or totally inadequate. The clinical significance of these findings is further enhanced when it is realized that the pathogenic effects of the adrenal steroids may be mediated not only by their influence on peripheral tissue metabolism, but also in less obvious but nonetheless highly important ways by *their effects on CNS function*[86,43] (to be discussed below).

Third, the endocrine system, like the autonomic nervous system, shows evidence of a waxing and waning of its level of activity in association with regular biologic rhythms— principally the circadian diurnal rhythms, but also longer seasonal rhythms, the menstrual ovulation cycle in females, and certain ultradian rhythms such as the 90-min. REM cycle in sleep. Ordinarily these multiple rhythms, each with different periods, are considered to be in some way synchronized or accommodated to each other. Curtis has reminded us that the potential for psychopathological and pathophysiological effects, when desynchronization between these multiple biologic rhythms takes place, is just beginning to be appreciated and studied.[12] A number of investigators, including Sachar, Roffwarg, Hellman, and their associates, have demonstrated important differences in patterns of endocrine function during different stages of sleep. They have also shown that there are alterations in these patterned relationships in patients in active episodes of psychotic depression.[67] Of related interest are the observations described in this volume by Hofer (Chapter 23), and by Williams and Karacan (Chapter 35), to the effect that autonomic-nervous-system function varies dramatically in different stages of sleep, e.g., the marked increase in variability of some autonomic func-

tions during REM periods has led to considerable interest in possible pathogenic effects, e.g., in certain cardiovascular conditions such as coronary insufficiency with nocturnal angina. Friedman and Fisher[24] and Kripke[39] have adduced evidence that an ultradian ninety-minute rhythm persists throughout a twenty-four-hour period and is not just confined to sleep although its (behavioral) manifestations are different during waking hours. The fact that these sleep and related waking ninety-minute rhythms are, or may be, linked with fluctuations in levels of consciousness (and possibly with changes in patterns of homostatic physiologic regulation) is especially provocative when recalling Schur's formulations[72,73] regarding the significance for medical pathogenesis of "altered ego states"—a psychological term that refers at least partially to altered states of consciousness. It should be recalled also that Breuer and Freud,[9] in their original "Studies on Hysteria," postulated an altered "hypnoidal state" of consciousness as providing the biologic substrate for actual symptom formation.

This sector of work has been (and bears promise of continuing to be) an especially fruitful area for collaboration between psychiatric clinicians and clinical physiologists. Stressful periods of life provide opportunities for *intensive parallel and simultaneous application of depth psychological techniques with neuroendocrine techniques*, and for attempts to arrive at integrated formulations concerning the biological significance of the changes observed. The psychoanalytic technique is particularly well suited for elucidating critical and important details of the psychological aspects, since it provides opportunity for repetitive finely detailed studies at those very times when major changes in balance of intrapsychic forces and in levels of consciousness and ego state are occurring. Since earlier theories, for the most part, took physiological "mechanisms" for granted, it would be desirable to conduct new studies now (such as those carried out by Knapp et al.[38]) in which psychological observations are made in conjunction with observations of these complex biological mechanisms. This will be required before empirically sound improvements can be made in the realm of theory.

Finally it should be noted that Henry, Axelrod, and collaborators[35] have demonstrated increases in adrenal weight and marked increases in adrenal tissue content of the biosynthetic enzymes of norepinephrine in response to an intense psychosocial stress in mice (the same stress that simultaneously leads to development of sustained hypertension and renal pathology in the experimental animals). The enzymes involved in synthesis and metabolism of catecholemines in the CNS have also been shown to be influenced by the hormones of the adrenal cortex (see Weiner, Chapter 22), and it even seems possible that psychoneuroendocrine stress responses may in some way be involved in CNS regulation of biogenic amine metabolism, and thus participate in development of those major affective disorders that are considered possibly *to reflect disturbances in biogenic amine systems.*[45]

Autonomic Conditioning

The fourth section, instrumental conditioning of autonomic responses, is reviewed in Hofer's chapter on the autonomic nervous system. These studies, pioneered by DiCara and Miller and associates, hold major and fundamental significance in regard to etiology and pathogenesis of medical illness.[14,49] Older specificity theories evoking early life "conditioning" as a factor in constitutional predisposition were limited in the scope of possible visceral changes that could be conditioned to those that could be evoked by an unconditioned stimulus as long as the Pavlovian paradigm of classical conditioning was considered the only form applicable to the autonomic nervous system. The demonstration that instrumental conditioning of the autonomic nervous system can occur means that virtually any change in the functional repertoire of the viscera bears the potential for "shaping" and augmentation by instrumental learning. Hofer discusses how this might operate during development, to influence later predisposition to disease. These findings also make it evident that there are, in fact, important functioning

afferent pathways to the brain from autonomically innervated structures, and that feedback effects on the brain from the viscera via the autonomic nervous system pathways are far more important than was previously thought. Study of these pathways and mechanisms should clarify and elucidate many of the previously somewhat mysterious somatopsychic effects encountered in clinical medicine, and, as Hofer points out, may have far-reaching fundamental implications for understanding the interrelationships of the CNS and the autonomic-nervous-system function in integrating behavior and bodily function.

Developmental Psychophysiology

A fifth section deals with research in developmental psychophysiology, which is of course highly cogent to the questions regarding the role that early-life experiences may play, along with conditioning and genetic endowment, in determining "constitution." The most important findings in this field derive from experimental studies on laboratory animals that reach maturity in a short period of time, thus permitting later adult effects of early-life experimental behavioral manipulations to be observed within convenient time periods. For example, Levine and collaborators have developed extensive data on the effects of subtle early manipulations such as "handling" on important parameters of adult behavioral (e.g., excitability) and physiological responses to novel stimulation and stress (responsiveness of the pituitary adrenal system).[42] Levine has also studied long term behavioral influences of sex hormones administered during critical periods of infantile development, elucidating some important developmental aspects of hormonal effects on complex adult patterns of sexual and aggressive behavior.[54,33] Ader and Friedman, in extensive programmatic studies, have developed several animal models of disease susceptibility in which experimental manipulation of infantile experience (such as solitary vs. crowded conditions of raising) has been shown to influence subsequent adult susceptibility or resistance to a number of pathogenic challenges, including various pathogenic microorganisms and viruses, as well as a number of behavioral manipulations known to be stressful.[1,2,25] Their data clearly demonstrate marked effects on "host resistance" in both directions—augmentation or decrease of resistance depending upon the nature of the early-life experimental manipulations, and upon the pathogens and/or stresses employed. Hofer and collaborators have studied maturation of physiological mechanisms regulating heart rate and rhythm in rats, and have demonstrated asynchrony of maturation of sympathetic and vagal systems, and have identified developmental epochs of possible significance as "critical periods" (perhaps even as anlagen of adult pathological response patterns, such as the fatal bradycardia known to occur in certain adult rodents under threat of severe attack).[36] By combining longitudinal developmental studies with techniques of selective breeding, the distinct possibility exists for elucidating the interaction of genetic and experiential factors in determining predispositions or specific susceptibilities of organ systems to specified types of disorders, and even to differential responsiveness to specific pharmacologic agents as Corson has shown in hyperkinetic dogs.[11] A highly important aspect of the work of Henry et al.,[35] mentioned above, consists of the fact that it clearly demonstrates the influence of differential conditions of early rearing and experience upon later susceptibility to developing hypertension and associated adrenal changes in mice exposed to the psychosocial stress he employs. This work is truly noteworthy in that it addresses the entire span of the biological, psychological and social aspects of the experimental disease model; it provides important details of the social stress employed, of behavior, of pathological physiology, of organ pathology, of changes in endocrine and metabolic enzyme systems, and of early developmental parameters as well!

In summary, psychosomatic research has gradually evolved from early case and clinical psychophysiological experiments, to include extensive basic and clinical research that addresses issues ranging from discrete cellular functions at one extreme to transcultural comparisons at the other. Whereas the earliest contributions came mainly from medical psychiatric and psychoanalytic clinicians and from experimental psychophysiologists, an extremely wide range of neurobiological and behavioral scientists are now actively engaged in work related to the field of medicine. A great deal of research is increasingly directed to a study of the mechanisms whereby the brain subserves, regulates and coordinates higher mental and social functions on the one hand, and widespread physiological functions throughout the body on the other. These have become possible because of the technical and methodological breakthroughs that have occurred in the life sciences, in neurophysiology, in endocrinology, in computer science, and in the social and behavioral sciences as well.

⟮ Part 3: Toward a Theory

Considering the findings reviewed in the preceding section, it seems reasonable to think of man as existing in a "bio-psycho-social" field as illustrated in Figure 21–2. This depicts an open transactional system that allows uninterrupted bidirectional flow of information and energy transactions extending from the deepest and most minute recesses of the body (intracellular metabolic processes) to the social field, encompassing cultural forces, even historical forces that contributed to shaping the culture. In the center is the brain which both subserves mental functions and influences (and is influenced by) body function. On the one hand, the higher mental functions, which include mechanisms for regulating interpersonal relations, mediate the individual's transactions with his social environment including family, social groups, and society at large. On the other hand, the brain also in some fashion (mysteriously) "transduces"[85] nonphysical immaterial aspects of the social field (that is, symbolic meanings) into physical-physiological events within the CNS, and these in turn initiate physiological changes throughout the body. At the same time brain function itself is, in turn, influenced by physiological changes

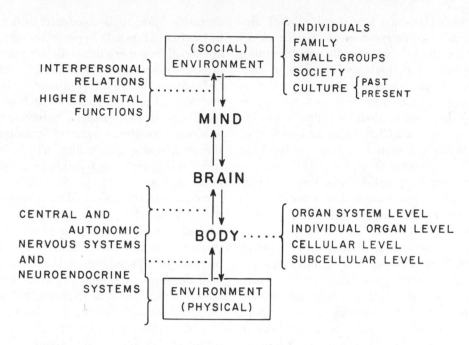

Figure 21–2. The Bio-psycho-social field. (For explanation see text.)

occurring in the periphery of the body. These two-way interchanges of information and energy between the central nervous system (brain) and the periphery (body) are negotiated by the central and autonomic nervous systems and the neuroendocrine systems. This transactional continuity extending from subcellular metabolic processes throughout the body via the brain to the social environment makes it understandable that major life experiences, such as bereavement, can influence even the capacity to sustain the life process itself. A *unique* feature, not explicitly depicted in the diagram, is that the brain, which occupies this interface position between mind and body, *is at the same time itself an organ of the body,* subject to influence by the very same alterations in the body's internal environment that it, in fact, helps to generate. Viewed in this way, the brain can be thought of as a possible "target organ" in sustained and profound stressful reactions. It may not be entirely fanciful to speculate that some forms of functional psychosis may in fact represent "stress diseases" in which the brain is the "target organ."

Considering the apparent complexity of re-

lationships and the incompleteness of our knowledge concerning the mechanisms involved, we do not yet seem to be in a position to construct a satisfactory general theory of etiology and pathogenesis that would account in a parsimonious fashion (as a good theory should) for the variety of ways in which psychosocial forces may be involved in the development of bodily illness. All the same, some implications for the general shape and character, and for some components, of a future theory can be drawn. If etiology and pathogenesis are conceived of as stepwise processes, and the natural history of disease is considered in respect to the separate phases (the phase preceding manifest disease, the phase of precipitation, and the phase of established disease), it appears that varying admixtures of specific and nonspecific mechanisms are involved, the relative proportions depending upon the stage of pathogenesis and phase of the disease process.

In *phase 1*, the period preceding the development of manifest disease, the important issue to be understood is if—and if so, how—a predisposition to a specific disease may be programmed into an individual who is later to be affected. Here we face a complex of elements ordinarily referred to as "constitution." It appears likely that specific programming could involve (1) peripheral tissues in patterns or characteristics of organ function or tissue response, e.g., rate of pepsinogen secretion; (2) the CNS in modular central-nervous-system circuits (see Chapter 19 for a review of central-nervous-system circuits influencing various organ systems); and (3) both peripheral and central: parallel tissue-response pattern *and* central-nervous-system circuits, with appropriate autonomic and endocrine effector linkages.

For many diseases it is clear that necessary but not sufficient programming information is transmitted in the genes; but since the transmission pattern seems to be one of incomplete penetrance, other factors, such as early experience very probably interact and contribute in fundamental ways to determination of "constitutional" predispositions, and it appears that this could occur in several ways.

Developmental physiology suggests that there may be "critical periods" representing crucial stages in maturation when neurovegetative systems responsible for regulation of important visceral functions (such as heart rate and rhythm, peripheral resistance, etc.) may be particularly amenable to sensitizing or conditioning, and sensitive or open to influences by experiential events. Particularly intriguing is the possibility of autonomic conditioning (visceral learning) occurring during such "critical periods," and eventually shaping a predisposition stored in central-nervous-system circuits for highly specific (pathogenic) visceral innervative patterns that could become activated (and pathogenic) under appropriate conditions later in life. The credibility or face validity of such an idea is enhanced by considering the possibilites for continuing reinforcement and further shaping provided by the continuing transactions between infant and mother, and later between child and family, that take place throughout development. Mirsky in his formulations about duodenal ulcer, has described how a basically genic constitutional predisposition in an organ, if expressed in behavior (e.g., as an excessive need to be nurtured and nourished in the case of gastric hypersecretion), may influence the mother's behavior in response to the infant. This in turn would modify subsequent behavior in the infant (perhaps by frustration and intensification of need) which would then feed back to the mother's behavior etc., etc., gradually creating a nidus of "core conflict" in the developing personality which would be specifically and inextricably related to the genic constitutional predisposition. At the same time in the course of development, reactive or protective ego defenses would develop around this vulnerable part of the personality system, and the nature and potential imperfections in this defensive matrix might very well determine the kind of psychosocial stress situation that could be expected to overwhelm the defenses and activate the conflict. Regardless of whether a constitutional predisposition originated in genic transmission and/or autonomic conditioning and/or classical conditioning (by repetitive fortuitous coincidence of stressful events with periods of illness), an epigenetic developmental sequence similar to this might well be expected to take place and eventuate in an individual with specifically patterned interrelated biological, psychological, and social vulnerabilities. Thus the emphasis in regard to this preillness phase of disease seems to weigh heavily in favor of specific preprogramming, with the evidence suggesting that both genetic *and* early developmental factors are involved and in complex interrelated ways. But the data do not permit us to do more than speculate about the possible nature of the interrelationships and the specific mechanisms whereby such effects might actually be induced.

A rather different set of questions arise in considering the phase of precipitation of active disease. Here the problem is one of understanding how psychosocial stress is to be related to activation of illness. In approaching these questions, primary emphasis shifts to the nonspecific factors reviewed in Part 2, i.e., the nonspecific effects of the psychoneuroendocrine stress responses on "host resistance" through effects on immune mechanisms, and through interfering with synchronization of circadian, ultradian and seasonal rhythms, etc. As noted earlier, the nature of the psychosocial stress situations that might be expected to overwhelm psychological defenses and allow for reactivation of conflict in any given individual would be related to his history, and to his personality organization, more precisely to the nature of whatever unresolved core conflicts remain active in him, and require continuing defensive activity. If under stress his defenses fail and his adrenal cortical and other endocrine activity is affected, he might, for example, be less resistant to infection, and develop a clinical infection more readily on exposure to an infective challenge that he would resist under more favorable circumstances. Such nonspecific reactions affect all people and their effects seem to be ubiquitous in medical practice.

But what about that relatively small group of persons supposed to be preprogrammed or predisposed as described above? *In such individuals the proximal pathogenic vector is not thought to be external (as in the case of pathogenic organisms) but rather internal, i.e., a predisposition, albeit previously latent and inactive.* In what way, if any, could the

intrinsically nonspecific changes attendant to psychoneuroendocrine stress response be related to activation of such a process? Or to put the question differently: in what way, if any, could the changes ultimately induced in the body by the endocrine response be favorable or permissive to actual expression of the previously inactive but potential pathogenic mode of function? The findings suggest that this could happen in a number of ways. Neurovegetative and endocrine changes in response to psychosocial stress have been shown to affect higher mental processes such as cognition,[10,58] and could in this way influence perception and evaluation of danger signals and anxiety proneness.[86,43] It could be hypothesized then that sustained pressure from active psychological conflict, with weakening of defenses, might set into motion a cyclic reaction whereby psychological processes involved in evaluation of danger would become increasingly more primitive and symbolic (regressive) as a consequence of the physiological responses they evoke, and that the physiological responses would become increasingly more vigorous as danger signals were evaluated with increasing alarm (Figure 21–3, step

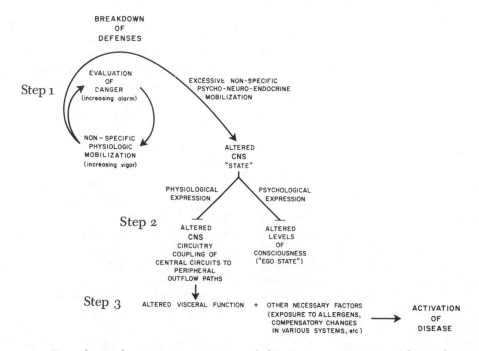

Figure 21–3. Hypothesized steps in precipitation of disease in conjunction with psycho-social stress.

1). One could speculate further that exposure of the brain to vigorous and continuous changes in circulating hormones (changes in the amounts and rates of rise and fall of individual hormones, in profiles among various hormones, in rhythms, etc.) could so affect patterns of central-neurophysiologic regulation that preprogrammed but inactive pathogenic circuits would become active and make connection with appropriate efferent fibers to the viscera, and thereby induce altered visceral function (Figure 21–3, step 2). I have speculated previously[62,63] that such hypothesized altered CNS conditions might be manifested behaviorally in the form of subtly altered states of consciousness (altered "ego states" in psychoanalytic terms as described by Schur;[72,73] or "hypnoidal" states as hypothesized by Breuer and Freud).[9] Such a notion is fully compatible with clinical observations of patients with high levels of free anxiety, and with a number of experimental observations: (1) at least one known state of consciousness (REM sleep) is well known to be associated with markedly altered (less well regulated, more "primitive") patterns of autonomic function; (2) some serious illness episodes (e.g., myocardial infarction, status asthmaticus, hemorrhage from duodenal ulcer, etc.) are known to be precipitated or exacerbated in sleep; and (3) it has been shown that the ultradian ninety-minute rhythm seen in sleep (REM cycle) may continue throughout the twenty-four-hour period and be manifest in behavior (e.g., increased eating behavior) during waking hours.[24]

Finally, in order to activate the specific pathological physiology involved in pathogenesis of a particular disease state (Figure 21–3, step 3) the altered visceral function produced in step 2 (as outlined above) would need to be combined with other factors essential to the particular disease (such as exposure to allergens, pathogens, compensatory and secondary changes in the same and other systems, e.g., circulatory adjustments, etc.) Of course these would be entirely different for each disease, depending upon the nature of its pathological physiology and pathology.

This conceptual schematization of *phase 2*

(precipitation) of disease emphasizes a series of *nonspecific* psychoneuroendocrine changes that may operate to aid in inducing illnesses of all sorts in all people, but which also might facilitate or induce in a smaller group of people so predisposed an altered state of CNS function permissive for activation of specific preprogrammed pathogenic patterns of visceral innervation. In other words, a nonspecific response would prepare the way for emergence of a more specific pathogenic process, with the specific predisposition having been laid down by interaction of psychologically meaningful early experiences with genic endowment in a series of epigenetic somato-psycho-somatic transactions throughout development.

In *phase 3* of disease, i.e., that in which the disease has already been established, it is likely that both nonspecific and specific mechanisms as described above would operate separately or in combination to influence the course and induce exacerbations or complications. But two modifications should be added. First, with increasing progression of disease and diminution in organ reserve, it is entirely possible and plausible that nonspecific changes might very well play an increasingly significant role with time, since less and less functional reserve in organs and resilience in homostatic mechanisms would be available to moderate the disruptive effects of nonspecific stress responses. Second, with time, perception of the disease and its meaning become increasingly elaborated within the individual's self-image and increasingly incorporated into ongoing mental life, particularly in the conflict sphere (Hartmann[34]). Accordingly, symbolically meaningful ideas would with increasing frequency and importance be associated with periods of activated or aggravated pathogenic physiologic responses. It would be expected then that idiosyncratic symbolic meanings connected with the disease would, with increasing frequency, become enmeshed in important issues in the patient's psychosocial field, and in ongoing intrapsychic conflicts as well. This would result in heavy emphasis on symbolic meanings associated with the disease, its signs and symptoms, in the patient's

associations in psychoanalysis or psychotherapy, thereby creating the (probably false)
impression that the disease had originated as a
symbolic conversion mechanism.

In presenting these admittedly fanciful
speculations in the final part of this Chapter, I
have attempted mainly to have them reflect
back to earlier theories while remaining consistent with the ever increasing wave of new
empirical data, and to offer them as guides to
possibly fruitful areas for research and as
rough forecasts or previews of the nature and
shape of (components of) future theory
which is yet to be developed on a sound empirical basis. In any event, it seems reasonably
clear to me that understanding the brain and
its relation to the body on one hand, and to
the mind and social environment on the other,
will probably ultimately provide the key to
the riddle; i.e., full understanding will come
from discovering how the brain orchestrates,
integrates, and at points transduces across the
biological, the psychological, and the social
realms. In keeping with this view, Part Two of
this volume begins with central regulation of
autonomic-nervous-system function, followed
by discussion of the autonomic nervous system
itself, and then by reviews of psychoendocrinology and the data pertaining to the psychosocial parameters of illness in man. Finally
come the separate chapters dealing with specific organ systems and diseases.

❨ Bibliography

1. ADER, R. "The Influences of Psychological
   Factors on Disease Susceptibility in Animals," in M. L. Conalty, ed., *Husbandry
   of Laboratory Animals*, pp. 219–238. London: Academic, 1967.
2. ADER, R. and S. M. PLAUT. "Effects of Prenatal Maternal Handling and Differential
   Housing in Offspring Emotionality, Plasma
   Corticosterone Levels and Susceptibility to
   Gastric Erosions," *Psychosom. Med.*, 30
   (1968), 277–286.
3. ALEXANDER, F. "Fundamental Concepts of
   Psychosomatic Research: Psychogenesis,
   Conversion, Specificity," *Psychosom. Med.*,
   5 (1943), 205–210.
4. ———. *Psychosomatic Medicine*, pp. 104–
   106. New York: Norton, 1950.
5. ALEXANDER, F., T. M. FRENCH, and G. H.
   POLLOCK. *Psychosomatic Specificity*. Chicago: University of Chicago Press, 1968.
6. ALEXANDER, F. and S. SELESNICK. *The History of Psychiatry*. New York: Harper &
   Row, 1966.
7. BENNET, G. "Bristol Floods 1968; Controlled
   Survey of Effects on Health of Local Community Disaster," *Br. Med. J.*, 3 (1970),
   454–458.
8. BINGER, C. A. L., N. W. ACKERMAN, A. E.
   COHN et al. "Personality in Arterial Hypertension," in F. Dunbar, ed., *Psychosomatic
   Medicine Monographs*, pp. 1–228. New
   York: Hoeber, 1945.
9. BREUER, J. and S. FREUD. (1895) "Studies on
   Hysteria," in J. Strachey, ed., *Standard
   Edition*, Vol. 2, pp. 183–252. London:
   Hogarth, 1955.
10. CALLAWAY, E. and S. V. THOMPSON. "Sympathetic Activity and Perception," *Psychosom. Med.*, 15 (1953), 433–455.
11. CORSON, S. A., E. CORSON, V. KIRILCUK et al.
   "Differential Effects of Amphetamines on
   Clinically Relevant Dog Models of Hyperkinesis and Stereotypy: Relevance to
   Huntington's Disease," in A. Barbeau et al.,
   eds., Advances in Neurology, Vol. 1.
   Huntington's Chorea, 1872–1973. New
   York: Raven, 1973.
12. CURTIS, G. C. "Psychosomatics and Chronobiology: Possible Implications of Neuroendocrine Rhythms," *Psychosom. Med.*, 34
   (1972), 235–250.
13. DEUTSCH, F. *The Psychosomatic Concept in
   Psychoanalysis*, pp. 158–161. New York:
   International University Press, 1953.
14. DICARA, L. "Learning of Cardiovascular Responses: A Review and a Description of
   Physiological and Biochemical Consequences," *Trans. N.Y. Acad. Sci.*, 33 (1971),
   411–422.
15. DONGIER, M., E. D. WITTKOWER, L. STE-
   PHENS-NEWSHAM et al. "Psychophysiological Studies in Thyroid Function," *Psychosom. Med.*, 18 (1956), 310–323.
16. DUNBAR, H. F. *Psychosomatic Diagnosis*.
   New York: Hoeber, 1943.
17. ENGEL, G. L. "Studies of Ulcerative Colitis,"
   Am. J. Med., 16 (1954), 416–433.
18. ———. "Studies of Ulcerative Colitis III;
   The Nature of the Psychologic Processes,"
   Am. J. Med., 19 (1955), 231–256.

19. ———. "A Psychological Setting of Somatic Disease: The 'Giving Up—Given Up' Complex," *Proc. Roy. Soc. Med.*, 60 (1967), 553–555.

20. Engel, G. L. and J. Romano. "Studies of Syncope; Biologic Interpretation of Vasodepressor Syncope," *Psychosom. Med.*, 9 (1947), 288.

21. Ferris, E. B., M. F. Reiser, W. W. Stead et al. "Clinical and Physiological Observations of Interrelated Mechanisms in Arterial Hypertension," *Trans. Assoc. Am. Physicians*, 61 (1948), 97–107.

22. Freud, S. (1910) "The Psychoanalytic View of Psychogenic Visual Disturbance," in J. Strachey, ed., *Standard Edition*, Vol. 11, pp. 209–218. London: Hogarth, 1957.

23. Friedman, M., R. H. Rosenman, R. Straus et al. "The Relationship of Behavior Pattern 'A' to the State of the Coronary Vasculature," *Am. J. Med.*, 44 (1968), 525–537.

24. Friedman, S. and C. Fisher. "On the Presence of a Rhythmic, Diurnal, Oral Instinctual Drive Cycle in Man: A Preliminary Report," *J. Am. Psychoanal. Assoc.*, 15 (1967), 317–343.

25. Friedman, S., L. B. Glasgow, and R. Ader. "Psychosocial Factors Modifying Host Resistance to Experimental Infections," *Ann. N.Y. Acad. Sci.*, 164 (1969), 381–393.

26. Garma, A. *Peptic Ulcer and Psychoanalysis*. Baltimore: Williams & Wilkins, 1958.

27. Grace, W. J. "Life Situations, Emotions and Chronic Ulcerative Colitis," in H. Wolff, S. Wolf, Jr. and C. Hare, eds., *Life Stress and Bodily Disease*, pp. 679–692. Baltimore: Williams & Wilkins, 1950.

28. Graham, D. T., J. D. Kabler, and F. K. Graham. "Physiological Response to the Suggestion of Attitudes Specific for Hives and Hypertension," *Psychosom. Med.*, 24 (1962), 159–169.

29. Graham, D. T., R. M. Lundy, L. S. Benjamin et al. "Specific Attitudes in Initial Interviews with Patients Having Different 'Psychosomatic' Diseases," *Psychosom. Med.*, 24 (1962), 257–266.

30. Grinker, R., Sr. *Psychosomatic Research*. New York: Norton, 1953.

31. ———. "Psychoanalytic Theory and Psychosomatic Research," in J. Marmoston and E. Stainbrook, eds., *Psychoanalysis and the Human Situation*, pp. 194–226. New York: Vantage, 1964.

32. Groddeck, G. W. (1926) *The Book of the It; Psychoanalytic Letters to a Friend*. New York: Random House, 1961.

33. Harris, G. W. and S. Levine. "Sexual Differentiation of the Brain and Its Experimental Control," *J. Physiol.* (London), 181 (1965), 379–400.

34. Hartmann, H. *Ego Psychology and the Problem of Adaptation*. New York: International Universities Press, 1958.

35. Henry, J. P., P. M. Stevens, J. Axelrod et al. "Effect of Psychosocial Stimulation on the Enzymes Involved in the Biosynthesis and Metabolism of Noradrenaline and Adrenaline," *Psychosom. Med.*, 33 (1971), 227–237.

36. Hofer, M. A. and M. F. Reiser. "The Development of Cardiac Rate Regulation in Preweanling Rats," *Psychosom. Med.*, 31 (1969), 372–388.

37. Katz, J. L. and H. Weiner. "Psychosomatic Considerations in Hyperuricemia and Gout," *Psychosom. Med.*, 34 (1972), 165–179.

38. Knapp, P. H., C. Mushatt, J. S. Nemetz et al. "The Context of Reported Asthma during Psychoanalysis," *Psychosom. Med.*, 32 (1970), 167–188.

39. Kripke, D. F. "An Ultradian Biologic Rhythm Associated with Perceptual Deprivation and REM Sleep," *Psychosom. Med.*, 34 (1972), 221–233.

40. LaBarba, R. C. "Experiential and Environmental Factors in Cancer; A Review of Research with Animals," *Psychosom. Med.*, 32 (1970), 259–274.

41. Levine, M. *Psychotherapy in Medical Practice*. New York: Macmillan, 1942.

42. Levine, S. and V. H. Denenberg. "Early Stimulation; Effects and Mechanisms; Stimulation in Early Infancy," in A. Ambrose, ed., *Stimulation in Early Infancy*, pp. 3–72. Proceedings of the Study Group on the Functions of Stimulation in Early Post-Natal Development, London, 1967. New York: Academic, 1969.

43. Levitt, E. E., H. Persky, J. P. Brody et al. "The Effect of Hydrocortisone Infusion in Hypnotically Induced Anxiety," *Psychosom. Med.*, 25 (1963), 158–161.

44. Lidz, T. and J. Whitehorn. "Life Situations, Emotions and Graves Disease," in H. Wolff, S. Wolf, Jr., and C. Hare, eds., *Life Stress and Bodily Disease*. Baltimore: Williams & Wilkins, 1950.

45. Maas, J. W. "Adrenocortical Steroid Hor-

mones, Electrolytes, and the Disposition of the Catecholamines with Particular Reference to Depressive States," *J. Psychiatr. Res.*, 9 (1972), 227–241.

46. MARGETTS, E. L. "Historical Notes on Psychosomatic Medicine," in E. D. Wittkower and R. A. Cleghorn, eds., *Recent Developments in Psychosomatic Medicine*, pp. 41–68. Philadelphia: Lippincott, 1954.

47. MARGOLIN, S. G. "Genetic and Dynamic Psychophysiological Determinants of Pathophysiological Processes," in F. Deutsch, ed., *The Psychosomatic Concept in Psychoanalysis*, pp. 3–36. New York: International University Press, 1953.

48. MASON, J. W. " 'Over-All' Hormonal Balance as a Key to Endocrine Organization," *Psychosom. Med.*, 30 (1968), 791–808.

49. MILLER, N. "Learning of Visceral and Glandular Responses," *Science*, 163 (1967), 439–445.

50. MIRSKY, I. A. "Physiologic, Psychologic, and Social Determinants in the Etiology of Duodenal Ulcer," *Am. J. Dig. Dis.*, 3 (1958), 285–314.

51. MIRSKY, I. A., P. FUTTERMAN, and S. KAPLAN. "Blood Plasma Pepsinogen II; the Activity of the Plasma from 'Normal' Subjects, Patients with Duodenal Ulcer, and Patients with Pernicious Anemia," *J. Lab. Clin. Med.*, 40 (1952), 188–199.

52. MIRSKY, I. A., D. FUTTERMAN, S. KAPLAN et al. "Blood Plasma Pepsinogen 1, The Source, Properties, and Assay of the Proteolytic Activity of Plasma at Acid Reactions," *J. Lab. Clin. Med.*, 40 (1952), 17–26.

53. MIRSKY, I. A., S. KAPLAN, and R. H. BROH-KAHN. "Pepsinogen Excretion (Uropepsin) as an Index of the Influence of Various Life Situations on Gastric Secretion" in H. Wolff, S. Wolf, Jr., and C. Hare, eds., *Life Stress and Bodily Disease*, pp. 628–646. Baltimore: Williams & Wilkins, 1950.

54. MULLINS, R. F. and S. LEVINE. "Hormonal Determinants during Infancy of Adult Sexual Behavior in the Rat," *Physiol. Behav.*, 3 (1968), 333–338.

55. PARKES, C. M., B. BENJAMIN, and R. G. FITZGERALD. "Broken Heart: A Statistical Study of Increased Mortality among Widowers," *Br. Med. J.*, 1 (1969), 740–743.

56. PILOT, M. L., E. PRELINGER, R. SCHAFER et al. "Use of a Twin Pool in Developing Interdisciplinary Research," (Abstract), *Psychosom. Med.*, 23 (1961), 443–451.

57. PILOT, M. L., J. RUBIN, R. SCHAFER et al. "Duodenal Ulcer in One of Identical Twins," *Psychosom. Med.*, 5 (1963), 285–290.

58. POLLIN, W. and S. GOLDIN. "The Physiological and Psychological Effects of Intravenously Administered Epinephrine and Its Metabolism in Normal and Schizophrenic Men, II," *J. Psychiatr. Res.*, 1 (1961), 50–67.

59. PRZBYLSKI, A. "Effect of Stimulation and Coagulation of the Midbrain Reticular Formation on the Bronchial Musculature; A Modification of Histamine Susceptibility," *J. Neuro-Visc. Rel.*, 31 (1969), 171–188.

60. REES, W. D. and S. G. LUTKINS. "Mortality of Bereavement," *Br. Med. J.*, 4 (1967), 13–16.

61. REISER, M. F. "Research Findings on the Influence of Countertransference Attitudes on the Course of Patients with Hypertension in Medical Treatment," Round Table on Hypertension, Mid-Winter Meeting; American Psychoanalytic Association, New York; December, 1952. Abstracted in Report of Round Table. *J. Am. Psychoanal. Assoc.*, 1 (1953), 562–574.

62. ———. "Reflections on Interpretation of Psychophysiological Experiments," *Psychosom. Med.*, 23 (1961), 430–439.

63. ———. "Toward an Integrated Psychoanalytic-Physiological Theory of Psychosomatic Disorders," in R. M. Lowenstein, M. Newman, M. Schur et al., eds., *Psychoanalysis —A General Psychology*, pp. 570–582. New York: International Universities Press, 1966.

64. ———. "Models and Techniques in Psychosomatic Research," *Compr. Psychiatry*, 9 (1968), 403–413.

65. ROSENBAUM, M. "Psychosomatic Aspects of Patients with Peptic Ulcer," in E. D. Wittkower and R. A. Cleghorn, eds., *Recent Developments in Psychosomatic Medicine*, pp. 326–344. Philadelphia: Lippincott, 1954.

66. ROSENMAN, R. H., M. FRIEDMAN, R. STRAUS et al. "A Predictive Study of Coronary Heart Disease," *JAMA*, 189 (1964), 15–22.

67. SACHAR, E. J., L. HELLMAN, H. P. ROFFWARG et al. "Disrupted 24-Hour Patterns of Cortisol Secretion in Psychotic Depression," *Arch. Gen. Psychiatry*, 28 (1973), 19–24.

68. SACHAR, E. J., J. MASON, H. S. KOLMER et al. "Psychoendocrine Aspects of Acute Schizophrenic Reactions" *Psychosom. Med.*, 25 (1963), 510–537.

69. SASLOW, G., G. GRESSEL, F. SHOBE et al. "The Possible Etiological Relevance of Personality Factors in Arterial Hypertension," in H. Wolff, S. Wolf, Jr., and C. Hare, eds., *Life Stress and Bodily Disease*, pp. 881–899. Baltimore: Williams & Wilkins, 1950.

70. SCHMALE, A. H., JR. "A Relationship of Separation and Depression to Disease," *Psychosom. Med.*, 20 (1958), 259–277.

71. SCHMALE, A. H., JR. and G. L. ENGEL. "The 'Giving Up—Given Up' Complex Illustrated on Film," *Arch. Gen. Psychiatry*, 17 (1967), 135–145.

72. SCHUR, M. "The Ego in Anxiety," in R. M. Loewenstein, ed., *Drives, Affects, Behavior*, Vol. 1, pp. 67–103. New York: International Universities Press, 1953.

73. ———. "Comments on the Metapsychology of Somatization," in *The Psychoanalytic Study of the Child*, Vol. 10, pp. 110–164. New York: International Universities Press, 1955.

74. SHAPIRO, A. "Influence of Emotional Variables in the Evaluation of Hypotensive Agents," *Psychosom. Med.*, 17 (1955), 291–305.

75. SPERLING, M. "Psychoanalytic Study of Ulcerative Colitis in Children," *Psychoanal. Q.*, 15 (1946), 302–329.

76. ———. "The Psycho-analytic Treatment of Ulcerative Colitis," *Int. J. Psycho-Anal.*, 38 (1957), 341–349.

77. ———. "A Psychoanalytic Study of Bronchial Asthma in Children," in H. I. Schneer, ed., *The Asthmatic Child*, pp. 138–165. New York: Hoeber, 1963.

78. ———. "A Further Contribution to the Psycho-Analytic Study of Migraine and Psychogenic Headaches," *Int. J. Psycho-Anal.*, 45 (1964), 549–557.

79. STEIN, M. "The What, How, and Why of Psychosomatic Medicine," in D. Offer and D. X. Freedman, eds., *Modern Psychiatry and Clinical Research*, pp. 44–58. New York: Basic Books, 1971.

80. STEIN, M., R. C. SCHIAVI, and T. J. LUPARELLO. "The Hypothalamus and Immune Process," *Ann. N.Y. Acad. Sci.*, 164 (1969), 464–472.

81. SZASZ, T. S. "Psychoanalysis and the Autonomic Nervous System," *Psychoanal. Rev.*, 39 (1952), 115–151.

82. VON BERTALANFFY, L. "The Mind-Body Problem," *Psychosom. Med.*, 26 (1964), 29–45.

83. WALLERSTEIN, R. S., P. S. HOLZMAN, H. M. VOTH et al. "Thyroid 'Hot Spots': A Psychophysiological Study," *Psychosom. Med.*, 27 (1965), 508–523.

84. WEINER, H. "The Specificity Hypothesis Revisited," *Psychosom. Med.*, 32 (1970), 543.

85. ———. "Presidential Address: Some Comments on the Transduction of Experience by the Brain; Implications for Our Understanding of the Relationship of Mind to Body," *Psychosom. Med.*, 34 (1972), 355–375.

86. WEINER, S., D. DORMAN, H. PERSKY et al. "Effects on Anxiety of Increasing the Plasma by Hydrocortisive Level," *Psychosom. Med.*, 25 (1963), 69–77.

87. WEINER, H. and M. F. REISER. "Methodological Issues in Psychosomatic Research on Cardiovascular Problems; Retrospect and Prospect," in *Proc. 4th World Congr. Psychiatry*, pp. 2746–2748. Excerpta Medica International Congress Ser. no. 150. Amsterdam: Excerpta Medica Foundation, 1966.

88. WEINER, H., M. THALER, M. F. REISER et al. "Etiology of Duodenal Ulcer I," *Psychosom. Med.*, 19 (1957), 1–10.

89. WEISS, E. and O. ENGLISH. *Psychosomatic Medicine*. Philadelphia: Saunders, 1957.

90. WOLF, S. and E. M. SHEPARD. "An Appraisal of Factors that Evoke and Modify the Hypertensive Reaction Pattern," in H. Wolff, S. Wolf, Jr., and C. Hare, eds., *Life Stress and Bodily Disease*, pp. 976–984. Baltimore: Williams & Wilkins, 1950.

91. WOLF, S. and H. G. WOLFF. *Human Gastric Function*, 2nd ed. London: Oxford University Press, 1947.

92. WOLFF, H. G. "Life Stress and Bodily Disease—A Formulation," in H. Wolff, S. Wolf, Jr., and C. Hare, eds., *Life Stress and Bodily Disease*, pp. 1059–1094. Baltimore: Williams & Wilkins, 1950.

CHAPTER 22

AUTONOMIC PSYCHOPHYSIOLOGY: PERIPHERAL AUTONOMIC MECHANISMS AND THEIR CENTRAL CONTROL

Herbert Weiner

❰ Introduction

SOCIAL AND PSYCHOLOGICAL STIMULI, tasks and constraints and the physiological responses they engender in human and animal subjects, are mediated by hormonal, autonomic, and neuromuscular mechanisms. For this reason, some data and concepts about the organization and function of the autonomic nervous system (ANS) in particular will be presented here in order to add meaning to the psychophysiological relationship which will be outlined in Chapter 23. Little discussion of the control of the neuromuscular system will take place in this Chapter because there is only limited information available about the control of electromyographically recorded activity from muscle. In addition, a full discussion of the neuromuscular transmission would lead the reader too far afield from the main interests of the clinical psychophysiologist.

By definition, the psychophysiologists attempt to record physiological changes after social and psychological stimulation in the intact subject with an absolute minimum of interferences such as the taking of blood samples and intubating blood vessels. At the same time, it behooves the investigator to make absolutely certain that his measurements, which are indirect, validly reflect changes in the functioning of the system or organ under study. Once having made certain of the change he is measuring, he must ascertain that the change occurred from a steady-state baseline. This steady-state probably reflects the product of a number of different physiological parameters: the intrinsic activity of the organ (the denervated heart beats regularly and slowly); the tonic innervation of the organ through the autonomic nervous system which solely modifies the intrinsic rhythm; the effect of neurotransmitter release into the circulation from autonomic nerve endings and the adrenal medulla; the rate of reuptake and metabolism of the free transmitter; the regulation of neurotransmitter biosynthesis, release, and metabolism by the adrenal gland which is under combined hormonal and neural control; and the nature and state of the receptor mechanism for the neurotransmitter at the end organ.

Once the steady-state is disturbed by environmental and psychological variables, dynamic physiological changes begin to occur. The change in physiological function—for instance, an increase in the heart rate from a steady-state level—may be the combination of a large variety of physiological factors, such as a change in cardiac filling, and phasic adrenergic discharge affecting, for example, the sino-auricular node, and increasing atrioventricular conduction velocity, etc. This phasic discharge may, in turn, be regulated by complex central-nervous circuits which lie in all parts of the brain, but particularly in the midbrain, hypothalamus, brain stem, and spinal cord.

Among the important *psychological* parameters affecting acute physiological changes are: the novelty of the stimulus; the expectations of the investigator and the subject; anticipation by the subject of the task ahead; individual response tendencies which, in part, are determined by earlier experiences of the subject; the length of time the subject is given before engaging in a specific task; and the nature and duration of the task or stress.

The kinds of physiological responses which prolonged stresses elicit are different, and are mediated by different mechanisms, than those which are elicited by acute psychological stresses.

With the exception of the EEG,* evoked and other potentials, and electromyographic responses studied by psychophysiologists, all the physiological functions which psychophysiologists record depend primarily on autonomic regulation and control. For example, changes in pupillary size, salivary flow, heart rate, blood pressure, respiratory rate and volume, blood flow through the skin, sweating, gastric motility and secretion, urinary flow, or uterine contraction are to a large extent under autonomic control, although the hormonal regulation of a function also plays a role. Uterine contractility, for example, depends on the stage of the menstrual cycle and the amounts of circulating estrogen and progesterone, etc., while the contractile responses of the pregnant uterus to neural stimuli differs from the non-pregnant one.

This Chapter also attempts to review new information about the autonomic nervous system which has changed our concepts about its functioning.

It used to be said that the sympathetic-adrenergic system mainly discharged as a unit, especially in situations in which the organism responded with the emotions of fright or rage. It used to be believed that the parasympathetic-cholinergic nervous system was mainly organized for discrete and localized discharge and not for mass responses; from a teleonomic point of view, it was considered that it subserves conservative and restorative processes.[13]

These generalizations, however, do not hold in the light of new evidence. Discrete sympathetically mediated responses can be elic-

---

* Even the EEG may be influenced by changes in cardiovascular dynamics.[6]

ited by operant conditioning.[27] Therefore, only under some circumstances does mass discharge of the sympathetic nervous system occur.

Secondly, it is now quite clear that the autonomic nervous system is not only "involuntary." In fact, it can be manipulated by operant techniques which a subject may learn. Furthermore, some "involuntary" functions (such as the alpha rhythm of the EEG) cannot only be recognized but also controlled by their owner. Subjects can also be "taught" to lower their blood pressure. In other words, voluntary control can be achieved over "involuntary" function.

Another new discovery indicates that, in some instances, the transmitter substance of the postganglionic sympathetic nervous system is not norepinephrine but acetylcholine. Therefore, it cannot be correctly assumed that the sympathetic nervous system is exclusively "adrenergic." For example, vasodilatation in skeletal muscle is, in part, brought about by a sympathetic cholinergic system.

In addition, the effects of the norepinephrine release at postganglionic synapses and of epinephrine are, in part, determined by the nature of the receptor.[1] Norepinephrine and epinephrine can cause either excitation or inhibition of smooth muscle, depending on the site and to some extent on its amount. For example, sympathetic discharge produces contraction of the radial muscle of the iris, constriction of the blood vessels of the skin mucosa and lungs, contraction of pilomotor muscles in the skin and the intestinal sphincters, but it also brings about relaxation of the ciliary muscle of the eye, of the bronchial muscles of the lung, and detrusor muscles of the bladder. Where contraction is produced, physiologists classify the receptor as belonging to the α-type, where relaxation occurs they call it the β-type. Some catecholamines mainly affect one type of receptor to produce excitation and others to produce inhibition. Thus, norepinephrine is the most powerful, excitatory catecholamine and mainly affects α-receptors, whereas isoproterenol exhibits the opposite effect. Epinephrine has both excitatory

and inhibitory properties. The majority of adrenergic blocking agents act selectively on the excitatory or inhibitory effects of the catecholamines, and can thus be classified as α- (e.g., phenoxybenzamine) or β- (e.g., 3,4-dichloroisoproterenol) blocking agents.

Cardiac nodes and muscles respond to an increase in sympathetic discharge or the catecholamines, by an increase in rate of discharge and contractile vigor respectively, but have the properties (as defined by their responses to pharmacological agents, i.e., isoproterenol) of the β-receptors.

⟨ The Autonomic Nervous System: Anatomy and Physiology

The more we know about the functioning of the ANS, the better are we able to grasp the meaning of psychophysiological correlations. This leading statement has often been contradicted by psychophysiologists, many of whom tend to be concerned only with demonstrating empirical relationships, or to use psychophysiological techniques to study "covert" behaviors. They argue, with some conviction, that it is not absolutely necessary to understand mechanisms, if it can be demonstrated that training techniques affect physiological function which has been disturbed in disease states, e.g., to lower blood pressure in a patient with essential hypertension by operant techniques.

It is our conviction that such a pragmatic approach evades the basic question of why the blood pressure became elevated in essential hypertension. Although we cannot give an answer to this question, it is fairly widely accepted that an elevated diastolic pressure is but a symptom of essential hypertension, not the disease itself, and represents the end product and an adjustment to altered functions in several different systems—e.g., the brain, adrenal gland, kidney, arteriolar tree, etc.

Therefore, it would seem to be an omission not to be aware of the role of the ANS in a wide variety of bodily functions, including important metabolic and behavioral ones.[3,44]

Anatomy of the Autonomic Nervous System

All structures within and on the surface of the body are innervated by the autonomic nervous system. Obviously, the main motor nerves to skeletal muscle belong to the "voluntary" nervous system, but blood flow within such muscle is autonomically regulated.

One major difference between the motor nerves of the autonomic and the neuromuscular systems is that synaptic connections between the preganglionic and postganglionic fibers of the autonomic system are made outside the neuraxis in a system of ganglia. Emerging from these ganglia, the postganglionic "motor" nerves are further organized into a system of peripheral plexuses, the constituent fibers of which are largely unmyelinated and, therefore, have much slower conduction velocities. They reveal other characteristics than the motor neurones of the neuromuscular system. Denervation of autonomically innervated structures does not preclude their function in the same manner that the function of striated (noncardiac) muscle does.

The two divisions of autonomic efferent fibers—the sympathetic and parasympathetic—innervate the heart, and the same glandular and other structures which are composed of smooth muscle. Traditionally, this arrangement has led to the concept, very popular in psychophysiology, that their functions are antagonistic. Actually, the level of activity in an effector organ at any one moment is the algebraic sum of many influences, i.e., a decrease in adrenergic excitation, while keeping cholinergic excitation steady, may appear as if cholinergic excitation had increased. In fact, recent advances have forced a modification of the old view. For instance, vasodilatation in muscle is mediated by a *sympathetic*, postganglionic cholinergic mechanism. The algebraic sum is also influenced by circulating neurohumors.

The efferent cells of preganglionic sympathetic fibers lie in the intermediolateral columns of the spinal cord from the level of the eight cervical to the second or third lumbar vertebra. Their axons pass with the anterior nerve roots to a series of twenty-two interconnected, paravertebral ganglia where they form synaptic connections with postganglionic sympathetic fibers. Among the most important of these fibers are the ones passing from the superior cervical ganglion to the eye, the lacrimal, submaxillary, and parotid glands, and the heart. The heart also receives postganglionic sympathetic innervation from the middle and inferior cervical ganglia. The superior cervical ganglion also sends postganglionic fibers up the carotid canal to innervate the pineal gland. The biosynthesis of melatonin in that gland is regulated by the light-stimulated release of norepinephrine from the terminals of these sympathetic fibers.[3,43,45]

The receptors of the radial muscle of the iris are of the a-type; an increase in sympathetic activity produces contraction. β-receptors obtain in the ciliary muscle of the eye, sinoatrial and atrioventricular nodes, cardiac atria, ventricles, and conduction system of the heart. Excitation therefore produces relaxation of the ciliary muscle, an increase in heart rate and conduction velocity, in the force of contraction of the heart and in the rate of its intrinsic pacemaker.

The stellate ganglion receives its input mainly from T_1 (first thoracic vertebral level) and sends postganglionic fibers to the heart, lungs, and bronchi whose muscles contain mainly β-receptors which are relaxed by an increase in sympathetic activity. However, the musculature of the lungs also contains a-receptors and is, therefore, subject to constriction by sympathetic excitation.

The celiac ganglion receives sympathetic input from T_{5-9} through the greater splanchnic nerve which also directly innervates the adrenal medulla. Other ganglionic input comes from the lesser splanchnic (T_{10-11}) and the least splanchnic nerves (T_{11-12}). Postganglionic fibers from the celiac ganglion innervate the liver, bile ducts, gall bladder, splenic capsule, stomach, small bowel, proximal colon, kidney, and ureter. Sympathetic excitation is mediated by β-receptors in the stomach and intestine to decrease motility and tone, and by a-receptors to contract its sphincters. The capsule of the spleen is contracted by the mediation of *a*-receptors. Sympathetic discharge induces the biosynthetic enzymes of norepinephrine and epinephrine, so that adrenal-gland levels of these enzymes are raised. On the other hand, dopamine blood levels are raised by an increase in biosynthesis in sympathetic fibers, and not by its liberation from the adrenal medulla.

From the levels of T12–13 preganglionic fibers pass to the superior and inferior mesenteric ganglia. The former innervate the distal colon and rectum to decrease motility and increase the contraction of the anal sphincters; the latter supplies the urinary bladder whose *β*-receptors relax the detrusor muscle while *a*-receptors of the trigone and sphincter are made to contract. Ejaculation of semen is produced by sympathetic activity. The type of receptor in the appropriate muscle is not known.

Fibers from the lower thoracic and the first three lumbar segments also supply the sacral ganglia which send postganglionic fibers to blood vessels, hair follicles, and sweat glands of the legs.

Their postganglionic fibers ("gray rami") are carried in spinal nerves for distribution to blood vessels of the skin, sweat glands, hair follicles and the vessels in skeletal muscle. Except for a double system of receptors in the skeletal muscles of the legs, all of these structures contain *a*-receptors. Thus, constriction of blood vessels and slight local secretion of sweat glands are produced when these receptors are stimulated.

Anatomy of the Parasympathetic Nervous System

The cells of origin of the parasympathetic nervous system[22] reside in nuclei of the third, seventh, ninth, and tenth cranial nerves, and in the gray matter of the second, third, and fourth segments of the sacral spinal cord. The axons of these cells pass to ganglia which lie close to the organs which they innervate. From the Edinger-Westphal nucleus of the oculomotor nerve, cells pass to the ciliary ganglion whose postganglionic fibers inner-

vate the sphincter muscle of the iris and ciliary muscle, both of which contract on nerve or ganglionic stimulation.[22]

Excitation of fibers from the nucleus of the facial nerve pass to the sphenopalatine ganglion and thence to the lacrimal gland to cause tears to flow. Parasympathetic excitation produces salivation and vasodilation in the nasal and oral cavity by virtue of outflow from the same nerve via the chorda tympani and ganglia which innervate the sublingual and submaxillary gland. The glossopharyngeal nerve sends preganglionic fibers to the otic ganglion from which postganglionic fibers pass to the parotid gland. The motor nucleus of the vagus nerve sends very long preganglionic fibers to all the viscera except the distal colon, bladder, ureter, and genitalia which receive innervation from cell bodies in S2-4, spinal cord segments via the pelvic nerves. The parasympathetic ganglia lie on or in the organs they innervate. Short postganglionic fibers pass to the receptor sites in them. In the wall of the gastrointestinal tract, vagal preganglionic fibers synapse around the ganglion cells of the plexuses of Auerbach and Meissner. Parasympathetic excitation produces dilatation of blood vessels in most organs; other muscles such as those in the bronchial tree, stomach, intestine, gall bladder, and the detrusor muscle of the bladder are made to contract, or their tone and motility is increased by parasympathetic discharge. A decrease in heart rate to the point of atrioventricular (AV) block is produced by vagal discharge which also reduces conduction velocity in, and the contractile force of the heart. Secretion of all exocrine glands is increased by parasympathetic discharge. Penile erection is produced by it.

In other words, most organs are doubly innervated, except for the adrenal medulla, pilomotor muscles, many vascular beds in skin, and muscle and the sweat glands of the skin.

Neurotransmission in the Autonomic Nervous System

Central to our understanding of the function of the autonomic nervous system is the concept of neurotransmission.[8] Autonomic nerve impulses elicit responses in smooth and cardiac muscle, exocrine and some endocrine glands, and postsynaptic neurones by the liberation of specific, identified chemical substances. Great strides have been made in our understanding of the storage, release, biosynthesis, and removal of these substances. But our understanding of the receptor mechanisms by which these substances exert their effect postsynaptically is just barely beginning.

Acetylcholine is the neurotransmitter of all *postganglionic parasympathetic fibers* and a few *postganglionic sympathetic fibers*, such as those leading to the sweat glands and the sympathetic vasodilator fibers. *Preganglionic sympathetic* and *parasympathetic fibers* release acetylcholine. A branch of the greater splanchnic nerve which innervates the adrenal medulla also releases acetylcholine, and may influence the biosynthesis of norepinephrine and epinephrine in this gland by the induction of the enzyme, tyrosine hydroxylase (TH).*

Norepinephrine is the principal sympathomimetic substance in *postganglionic sympathetic nerves*.[4] (It may also play a role as an inhibitory neurotransmitter in clearly defined tracts in the brain such as the median forebrain bundle and a tract from the locus coeruleus to Purkinje cells in the cerebellum. Other amines such as histamine, serotonin, and certain amino acids, γ-aminobutryic acid and glycine—may also play unidentified roles in central neurotransmission.)

The effect of the neurotransmitter substances on end organs and postsynaptic fibers is in part a function of whether they produce excitation or inhibition; the intrinsic activity of the innervated structure; the state of the receptor of that structure; and the rates of synthesis, release, reuptake and enzymatic destruction or diffusion of the neurotransmitter. All these factors determine the ultimate response of the end organ whose activity the psychophysiologist wishes to measure.

There are, of course, fundamental differences between the responses of autonomically

innervated structures and those innervated by striated muscle. Seeing that psychophysiologists are interested in responses from both types of structures, these differences might be worth dwelling upon. Preganglionic autonomic fibers are typically myelinated and have the properties of B-fibers, whereas motoneurons (A-fibers) have a larger diameter and thus a much greater conduction rate and shorter spike duration and absolute refractory period. Postganglionic sympathetic axons are unmyelinated (sC-fibers), have smaller fiber diameters, the slowest conduction velocity (in comparison to A and B fibers) and a relatively long spike-potential and absolute refractory period.

The responses of the effector organ is, in part, also the product of relatively slower destruction and thus more prolonged action of the transmitter.

Skeletal muscle responds to a single stimulus to its motor nerve by a brief solitary event —the action potential of the muscle, measured by EMG (electromyogram), followed by the muscle twitch which can be recorded as a smooth increase and then decrease in muscle tension. When a sympathetic axon is stimulated, a muscle action potential shows an initial deflection followed by a series of asynchronous deflections which continue for several seconds after repolarization of the nerve fiber has occurred. The tension record of the smooth muscle shows a gradual and prolonged buildup associated with each muscle action potential change. The transmitter agent remains and continues active long after nerve action has ceased.

Synaptic Transmission

The same mechanism of axonal transmission applies in postganglionic adrenergic and cholinergic fibers. The nerve-action potential consists of a self-propagated reversal of negativity of the axonal membrane (seen from the point of view of the internal potential of the axon) as a result of the admission of sodium and egress of potassium ions.[19] When the action potential arrives at the presynaptic terminal either excitatory or inhibitory transmitter is re-

* Acetylcholine is, of course, the transmitter substance at all neuromuscular junctions involving skeletal muscle and may play a role in neurotransmission in the CNS.

leased by a mechanism that is not wholly understood.

In all probability, and based on the model of neuromuscular transmission, there is a continuous quantal release of transmitter during the resting state which does not, however, produce enough depolarization of the postsynaptic membrane to reach the "firing level."[19] When the "firing level" is reached, a postsynaptic action potential is generated.

When the excitatory transmitter combines with postsynaptic receptors, a localized depolarization occurs which can be recorded by means of an intracellular electrode, as an excitatory postsynaptic potential (EPSP)—that is, a decrease in negativity of the direct current (DC) potential by virtue of an increase in permeability of all ions, particularly those of sodium and potassium. Inhibitory transmitters produce the opposite effect—that is, hyperpolarization with an increase in negativity of the DC (the inhibitory postsynaptic or IPS) potential due to an increase in permeability to potassium and chloride ions.

When the "firing level" has been reached, a propagated action potential is produced in the nerve, and a muscle action potential in most skeletal and cardiac muscle. In certain types of tonic skeletal muscle and in smooth muscle in which propagated impulses do not occur, an EPSP initiates a local contraction, while in gland cells it initiates secretion, probably by means of the induction of enzymes.

Acetylcholine

The excitatory transmitter in autonomic ganglia is acetylcholine. It is probably synthesized by choline acetylase in the region of axon terminals and stored in highly concentrated, ionic form in synaptic vesicles. Acetylcholine is rapidly removed presumably by a specific and specialized enzyme, acetylcholinesterase,[31] which splits the molecule into choline and acetic acid, once acetylcholine is liberated into the synaptic cleft. Acetylcholinesterase, on the other hand, is located at the surface in the infoldings of the postjunctional membrane, and in the subneural apparatus of the motor end plate of most skeletal muscle. In the superior cervical ganglion of the cat, the enzyme is located external to the presynaptic membrane.

Modification of synaptic transmission at ganglia is produced by epinephrine and norepinephrine. They can depress transmission in low doses, and in even lower concentrations enhance it. Thus, it has been proposed that the regulation of transmission may occur by an interaction of acetylcholine and these two catecholamines.

In sympathetic postganglionic fibers, Burn[7] has suggested that acetylcholine is released on stimulation which, in turn, causes the release of norepinephrine to act on effector organs. However, this hypothesis which would explain many diverse observations is not generally accepted. If confirmed, it would give acetylcholine a role additional to that of a neurotransmitter.

In fact, such a role is suggested by the fact that acetylcholine, choline acetylase and acetylcholinesterase are present at a variety of nonsynaptic sites. It has also been suggested that it plays a role in axonal conduction, in the regulation of membrane transport and permeability, and as a local hormone.

PHYSIOLOGICAL EFFECTS OF ACETYLCHOLINE

All of the physiological effects of acetylcholine are very brief because of the speed with which it is hydrolysed by acetylcholinesterase. The effects noted are mainly those that might be expected after stimulation of postganglionic parasympathetic nerve fibers.

In the cardiovascular system, it may produce vasodilatation, a decrease in blood pressure, bradycardia, arrhythmias, including partial or complete atrioventricular block, and ventricular standstill, etc. But most of these effects are counteracted because of the simultaneous release of catecholamines by the adrenal medulla. In fact, in man, the drug has to be given in large doses and rapidly, to produce these and other effects such as lacrimation, salivation, sweating, cough, and vomiting which are due to increase in tone, amplitude, and peristaltic activity of the stomach.

CATECHOLAMINES AND ADRENERGIC TRANSMISSION

We owe to Elliot[9] the concept of adrenergic transmission, to von Euler[38] the identification of norepinephrine as the adrenergic transmitter, and to Axelrod[4] the explanation of the metabolic disposition and some of the steps in the biosynthesis of norepinephrine and epinephrine. From the point of view of integrative behavioral biology and psychophysiology in particular, recent advances in understanding the role of the catecholamines in the brain and periphery have wide-ranging significance.

Epinephrine is synthesized in five steps from the amino acid phenylalanine:

rine is thought largely to be localized in chromaffin cells, particularly of the adrenal medulla. Both are stored as catecholamine-adenosine triphosphonucleotide salts in storage granules. During their synthesis, the biosynthetic step from dopa to dopamine takes place in the cytoplasm of nerve terminals. Dopamine enters the granules of postganglionic nerves and the adrenal medulla, and is then converted into norepinephrine. In the adrenal medulla, norepinephrine leaves the granules, is converted to epinephrine in the cytoplasm and reenters another set of granules where it is stored. After nerve stimulation and when norepinephrine appears in the blood stream, about half is taken up again and

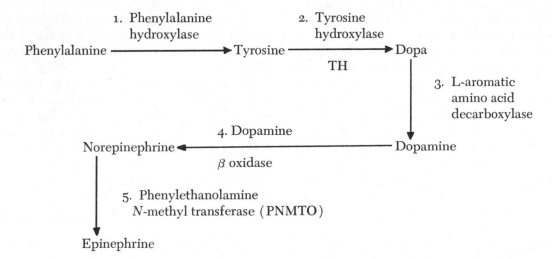

The enzymes involved in this biosynthetic pathway are not specific and it may be that other biosynthetic steps to epinephrine are possible. Furthermore, the enzyme L-aromatic aminoacid decarboxylase also participates in the synthesis of important biogenic amines such as histamine, tyramine and serotonin.

Also of interest is that epinephrine, the end product of biosynthesis, inhibits tyrosine hydroxylase (TH) while TH is induced transsynaptically and by cortisol. In the same manner PNMT is induced, while dopamine is liberated into the blood stream by adrenergic nerve endings.

Once synthesis has occurred norepinephrine is stored in the terminals of postganglionic sympathetic fibers and brain, while epineph-

stored intracellularly in neurons, and the other half is rapidly degraded by two enzymes, monoamine oxidase (MAO) and catecholamine-O-methyl transferase (COMT), to produce 3,4-dihydroxymandelic acid (by MAO), 3-methoxy-4-hydroxymandelic acid (by COMT), and normetanephrine (by COMT). Normetanephrine is further degraded into 3-methoxy-4-hydroxyphenylglycol by MAO, and conjugated with sulfate or glucoronide.

The mechanism of release of norepinephrine by the nerve action potential is as yet unknown (see above). In the adrenal medulla, preganglionic fibers release acetylcholine which may combine with receptor sites at the surface of the chromaffin cells, following which calcium ions may enter these cells to mobilize stored catecholamines.

The fate of released epinephrine is similar to that of norepinephrine according to the following scheme:

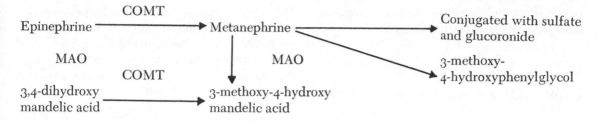

Physiological Effects of Adrenergic Transmitter Substances

Catecholamines can produce powerful excitation and inhibition of smooth muscle, depending on which muscle it acts and in which dosage. As mentioned in the introduction, norepinephrine's action is chiefly excitatory and isoproterenol's chiefly inhibitory; epinephrine has equivalent excitatory and inhibitory effects. In the CNS norepinephrine is postulated to be an inhibitory transmitter.

Physiological Effects of Epinephrine

Epinephrine and norepinephrine have different effects on heart rate, epinephrine being more likely to increase it. Both increase the reflex vagal tone through stimulation of mechanoreceptors in the carotid sinus and aortic arch; but the vagal afferent activity after epinephrine is less than after norepinephrine. Furthermore, epinephrine has a more potent effect in stimulating the β-receptors of the heart to keep the blood pressure comparatively low. Epinephrine also reduces peripheral resistance when compared to norepinephrine. The net effect is that norepinephrine tends to increase heart rate less, but to increase diastolic and systolic blood pressure and peripheral resistance more. In fact, the main effect of epinephrine is to raise the systolic blood pressure, the mean pulmonary-artery pressure, stroke volume, cardiac output, and coronary blood flow. It is well known that it may cause cardiac arrythmias (especially

premature ventricular contractions). Muscle blood flow is greatly increased to the detriment of the blood flow in the skin which is much reduced. Splanchnic blood flow (especially hepatic flow) is increased by it, as are oxygen consumption, blood sugar, lactic acid levels, free fatty acids, plasma cholesterol, phospholipids, and some lipoproteins.

The chief effect of epinephrine is to constrict arterioles, thereby raising the blood pressure. But the action of epinephrine on other smooth muscle depends on the type of epinephrine receptor involved. Bronchial smooth muscle is dilated by it and gastrointestinal muscle relaxed or inhibited. On the other hand, the splenic capsule is contracted by epinephrine, partly accounting for the increase in circulating red blood cells following stress, or hemorrhage.

The behavioral effects of epinephrine injected into human subjects are headache, apprehension, restlessness, and tremor. Such effects are, however, not always produced in all subjects. Much depends on the prevailing mood of the subject, the circumstances under which the drug is given, and what kinds of previous experiences are aroused in the subject.

Physiological Action of Norepinephrine

In contrast to epinephrine, norepinephrine acts mainly on α-receptors except for its action on the β-receptors of the heart. It has much fewer metabolic effects than epinephrine, although in some cells it stimulates the induction of adenylcyclase and thus cyclic AMP in the same manner as epinephrine does.[34] Hyperglycemia is produced by norepinephrine. As mentioned earlier, its cardiac effects are mainly to increase diastolic blood pressure, although systolic blood pressure is also increased; cardiac output remains unchanged or is decreased. Blood flow is reduced through the brain, kidney, liver, and skeletal muscle by virtue of its vasoconstrictor action, while coronary blood flow is increased. Bradycardia is produced reflexly, by norepinephrine; it may cause cardiac arrhythmias.

(Integrative Autonomic Mechanisms

Afferent Fibers of the Autonomic Nervous System

A very rich system of visceral afferent fibers, about which still relatively little is known, passes from most organs by means of non-myelinated fibers into the nervous system via the pelvic, splanchnic, vagus, and other nerves. Visceral afferent fibers make up a major proportion of the total fiber content of these nerves. About one-half of the splanchnic nerve and even more of the vagus are afferent. Other autonomic afferent fibers from skin structures and blood vessels in striated muscle run centripetally in somatic nerves. The cell bodies of most visceral afferent fibers are located in the dorsal root ganglia of spinal nerves, and in the equivalent sensory ganglia of cranial nerves, e.g., the nodose ganglion of the vagus and the petrosal ganglion of the ninth nerve. Visceral afferent impulses then pass into the dorsal horns of the spinal cord and make synaptic connections with cells in the intermediolateral columns of the spinal cord and in respective cranial nerve nuclei. These cells give rise to afferent fibers which pass to the autonomic ganglia outside the spinal cord.

Autonomic afferent fibers mediate visceral sensation (including pain originating in organs, and are, in part, responsible for "referred" pain). They regulate visceral and hormonal interrelationships and a number of very important respiratory, visceromotor, vasomotor, bladder, and cardiac reflexes. The mechanoreceptors of the carotid sinus and aorta, and the chemoreceptors of the carotid and aortic bodies play a crucial role in the regulation of respiration, heart rate, and blood pressure. These receptors are also involved in the regulation of aldosterone production. Stimulation of the mechanoreceptors at the junction of the thyroid and carotid arteries in the dog inhibits aldosterone* production, while a fall in blood pressure increases the output of this steroid. Cutting the thyrocarotid branch of the vagus nerve or occluding the inferior vena cava also increases the production of aldosterone. In addition, an increase in carotid sinus activity reflexly reduces adrenal catecholamines and antidiuretic hormone output.

The principal arterial baroreceptors are in the aortic arch and carotid sinus. Sudden increases in pressure at the carotid sinus produce a marked increase in frequency of discharge in baroreceptor afferent units, which adapt slowly during continued elevation of pressure. When the pressure is pulsatile rather than constant, the firing rate is greater and in concert with the ascending limb of the pressure change. Afferent activity in the mesenteric nerves may also be increased by perfusion of the duodenum with various food stuffs.

Pulmonary artery baroreceptors are active at normal pulmonary artery pressures and seem to respond mainly to the rate of pressure change with each pulse. Pressure receptors within the atrium and ventricle of the heart also produce two types of afferent neuronal activity. A burst of activity occurs with each atrial contraction and is proportional to its amplitude. Another burst of activity occurs at the time of ventricular systole; in other words, these neuronal units fire proportional to the amount of filling of the pulmonary and systemic venous system. Ventricular receptors provide inputs proportional to changes in systolic ventricular tension.

The arterial chemoreceptors adapt slowly and are mainly influenced by variations in arterial pO_2, pCO_2, and pH. In the steady-state, there is a continuous discharge which is markedly enhanced by changes in the partial pressure of oxygen in arterial blood, an increase in

* Aldosterone is the principal steroid, produced by the adrenal cortex, regulating body salt.

arterial CO_2 tension, or a fall in blood pressure.

The largest group of vagal afferents comes from the lungs. Stretching of lung inflation receptors in bronchioles and bronchi increases the firing rate of these afferent units; some adapt rapidly, others slowly. Those receptors which are slowly adapting are probably involved in cardiovascular reflexes.

Sensory inputs which travel in somatic, not sympathetic afferent nerves, arise from muscle, the skin of the face, and from viscera and are involved in reflex cardiovascular adjustments which occur with exercise, with facial stimulation, or stimulation of the vibrissae in mammals, during the diving reflex, or visceral irritation and inflammation. Other sources of input, probably mediated by autonomic afferents, arise from the gut, kidney, and bladder.

From the viscera, sympathetic afferents travel either by an extraspinal pathway by way of the sympathetic chain which finally enters the spinal cord, or by way of the ipsilateral spinal fasciculus gracilis, or by a bilateral pathway in the anterolateral region of the white matter of the cord. Some of the pathways of splanchnic origin reach the cerebral cortex via the thalamus, others pass to the posterior hypothalamus.

In other words, a wide variety of physiological stimuli may influence afferent activity in autonomic nerves, and therefore act as input to the CNS. This input, in turn, interacts with ongoing central activity, so that regulation of a wide variety of peripheral physiological processes occurs. Probably the regulation of blood pressure is the best understood process. A review of the integration and regulation of blood pressure by the nervous system allows one to conclude that only some afferent impulses from mechanoreceptors and chemoreceptors in the heart and major blood vessels, and from the peripheral vascular tree, ascend higher in the nervous system than the medulla and pons. Yet, the vasomotor system of the brain stem is also in turn under the control of two major circuits, one of which—the sympathetic vasodilator system—has in all probability important implications for psychophysiology, as the following account will show.

Organization of Autonomic Reflexes

There is some evidence that autonomic reflex activity may be mediated by autonomic ganglia without the participation of the spinal cord. Preganglionic fibers may give off collaterals to ganglia other than the ones they innervate, so that stimulation of the distal part of a preganglionic fiber isolated from the spinal cord may activate ganglia lying proximally. Although such evoked activity is known as an "axon" reflex, it is not a reflex in the true sense. Axon reflexes play a part in man in the vasodilatation produced in muscle after contraction. Postganglionic "axon" reflexes have also been invoked to explain local sweat responses to electrical stimulation of the skin, but this response may be due to branching postganglionic fibers; branching occurs near the innervated area so that fibers are sent in all directions. To explain the local sweat response one would have to postulate that stimuli pass antidromically up one fiber and orthodromically down another to cause sweating. Other vasomotor responses of the skin are truly reflex. The afferent arc of the reflex may either be sensory or autonomic.

Visceral autonomic afferents may also produce reflex striped muscle contraction. The abdominal muscles contract when the gut or peritoneum are irritated.

Two main kinds of regulatory mechanisms determine activity in preganglionic autonomic neurones which are maintained in a continuous but variable state of neuronal activity. There are segmental sensory and autonomic inputs through dorsal roots, inputs from pontomedullary neurons, and finally from neural circuits which descend from structures which lie rostral to the brain stem.

In animals whose spinal cords have been cut above the thoracic level, a state of spinal shock is present and all autonomic reflexes are depressed: Blood pressure and peripheral resistance are low, the urinary bladder is paralyzed, there is no regulation of body temperature and no sweating. But after several weeks, blood pressure levels rise; further rises occur when the skin of the body is touched or pinched below the level of transection. After the "spinal shock" passes off, some body-temperature control and sweating is then re-established. For example, profuse sweating can be provoked by stimulation of the skin of the body. Urination, defecation, and sexual reflexes reappear and can also be stimulated by stroking the appropriate segments of the body. Chronic decerebrate preparations demonstrate many of the characteristics of the spinal animal with regard to autonomic reflexes, except that arterial pressure is well-maintained, and none of the profound blood-pressure changes, which are precipitated by changes in posture and seen in spinal animals, occur.

Decorticate animals do not show any of the changes in autonomic reflexes seen when more extensive amounts of the nervous system are removed. But these animals do respond to pinching of the skin by "sham" rage behavioral responses and a coordinated massive autonomic (sympathetic) discharge.

Spinal reflexes may be monosynaptic or multisynaptic. Their segmental arrangement is as follows:

Head and neck	T1-5
Pupillodilatation	C8-T1
Arms	T2-9
Lacrimal gland	T1-3 (sympathetic)
Cardiac acceleration	T2-6
Vasomotor responses, sweating:	
Upper trunk	T4-9
Lower trunk	T9-L2
Lower extremities	T12-L2
Abdominal viscera	T4-L2
Genitourinary and anorectal (sympathetic) reflexes	L1-2

Central (Supramedullary) Control of Autonomic Functions

We have seen that autonomic reflexes can either be local or spinal. And it is characteristic of the reflexes in spinal man that they are massive and can be set off by trivial cutaneous stimulation or by temperature alterations. Generally speaking, these very marked re-sponses are attenuated by a complex series of neuronal circuits that course throughout the nervous system. As mentioned earlier, amongst the most important regulatory devices are those to be found in the hypothalamus. At least, and in the case of the body-temperature control system, these mechanisms are arranged in such a reciprocal manner that negative feedback characterizes their interactions. The posterior and lateral nuclei of the hypothalamus are concerned with the regulation of food intake and temperature; their stimulation leads to massive sympathetic discharge including norepinephrine release.

In the hypothalamus, parasympathetic functions are regulated by midline nuclei in the region of the tuber cinereum and nuclei lying closer to the anterior section. Inputs from the limbic system, cortex, thalamus, and striatum probably modulate the activity of these hypothalamic centers. Stimulation of the perifornical hypothalamus can alone elicit complex emotional behaviors in cats as well as marked sympathetically mediated changes in blood pressure and heart rate, and produce piloerection, etc.[11]

Regulation of Blood Pressure

CENTRAL (BRAIN-STEM) MECHANISMS

Before going on to speak about the neurogenic control of blood pressure and peripheral resistance, some general remarks seem in order.

Concepts about the neurogenic control of blood pressure are, in part, limited by the fact that so much of our knowledge of cardiovascular regulation, and the control of blood pressure in particular, derives from observations made on excised organs and anesthetized animals while varying a single input. Only with the development of new recording methods has it been feasible to make observations on intact unanesthetized animals.

These new techniques eliminate various kinds of artifacts caused, for example, by exposing the heart and lungs in acute experiments, and by anesthesia. In addition, behavioral observations can be made in unanesthetized animals while studying cardiovascular function during exercise or while the animal is interacting with its environment, or during brain stimulation, etc.

Chronic brain stimulation may be used to induce elevations of blood pressure while the animal's behavior is observed. Finally, the hope would be to develop in the future, knowledge of the complete neural and neuronal pathways and the activity in them during such manipulations.

The rapid cardiovascular adjustments which precede and accompany exercise demonstrate a case in point.[33] Whereas these adjustments were once considered to be instigated purely by peripheral mechanisms, it is now believed that the onset of vasodilation and increased flow in muscle, heart rate, and output, etc., at the start of exercise, emanate from the nervous system as an autonomic concomitant to the muscular activity which is under volitional control. These cardiovascular changes at the start of exercise can be abolished by lesions in the fields of Forel, and can be replicated by stimulation in this area.

In other words, there exist integrated patterns of cardiovascular and motor activities, exemplified by the changes with exercise. Furthermore, these cardiovascular adjustments seem quite specific to a given behavioral activity; other adjustments probably occur with other activities.

In this way one might expect that our ignorance about the neuronal activity which must underlie volitional activity, its correlated affect, and circulatory changes would gradually be dispelled. At present, we know little about the pathways which subserve the emotions of anger, fear, resentment, or the adjustments with exercise.

We also know little about how these emotional states influence homeostatic cardiovascular mechanisms. It is not unlikely that they do so by biasing tonic neuronal activity in complex circuits which run between the mechanoreceptors, the medulla, the midbrain, the hypothalamus, and limbic and cerebral cortices. If different cardiovascular adjustments accompany different behavioral activities, then it is likely that central excitatory influences on the brain stem and hence vaso-

constrictor outflow may be quite selective. For example, the sympathetic vasodilator discharge pattern emanating from the hypothalamus is characterized by adrenergic discharge to almost the entire vascular bed, with the exception of skeletal muscle. The same differential effects occur in vasoconstrictor fibers when activated by cortical stimulation.

The foregoing statements must have some validity in the light of Miller's work[27] and from studies on the organismic response known as the "defense" reaction which was first described by Hess.[16] Sympathetic vasodilation in muscle, increased heart rate, vasoconstriction in vascular beds other than muscle, and increased secretion of catecholamines occur during the defense reaction. Analogous vascular changes are found in man during states of fear, and mental arithmetic, and may occur during anticipatory states.

The behavior of cats when the defense reaction is elicited consists of growling, hissing, running, pupillary dilation, and piloerection. The defense reaction occurs not only when the hypothalamus near the entrance of the fornix is stimulated, but also with stimulation of the dorsomedial amygdala and striae terminalis. The axonal connections between these nuclear regions and others are still not certain. That other connections must exist is suggested by the fact that it is known that the cerebral cortex attenuates the violence of the defense reaction.

The defense reaction is mentioned as an example of a selective vasomotor and behavioral response, and because Folkow and Rubinstein[11] have been able to produce sustained hypertension by mild and intermittent, daily stimulation for several months in the area of the hypothalamus known to elicit the defense reaction.

Different affective states in man can be accompanied by other and different cardiovascular changes. For example, when a man is hostile or resentful the blood vessels of the gastrointestinal mucosa dilate.

PERIPHERAL RESISTANCE BY THE CNS

Central to current notions about CNS regulation of blood pressure[21,39] is that vasomotor regulation is brought about through variations in vasoconstrictor tone. Decreased vasoconstrictor discharge leads to vasodilation, increased discharge to constriction.

Afferent impulses pass from the carotid sinus and aortic arch mechanoreceptors responsive to stretch, and from chemoreceptors which are sensitive to increases in arterial pCO_2. Stimulation of the mechanoreceptors leads to vasodilation by inhibition of tonic vasoconstrictor outflow, while stimulation of the chemoreceptors causes vasoconstriction. From the carotid mechanoreceptors, afferent impulses pass via the sinus nerve to the medullary vasomotor centers. At high blood pressures neural discharge is sustained, not phasic, and adaptation may occur to such pressures. However, different firing patterns in the sinus nerve occur and depend on fiber size, because the sinus nerve contains fibers of varying diameters. In view of the fact that cutting the sinus nerve increases blood pressure, tonic discharge from the mechanoreceptors must also be present.

Afferent impulses also arise from the atrial walls of the heart and ventricles, and from the walls of the great veins. Sensory, especially pain receptors, influence vasomotor tone, possibly via the agency of the medullary center. In addition to input to the vasomotor center from mechano- and chemoreceptors, etc., input may travel in sympathetic afferent fibers to enter the cord.

We owe to Ranson[32] and Alexander[2] most of our knowledge about the vasomotor center. The pressor area lies in the lateral reticular formation of the rostral two-thirds of the medulla, while the depressor center lies medially in the reticular formation and more caudally in the medulla. Tonic inhibition of spinal cardiovascular mechanisms largely emanates from the depressor zone. The neurons of both of these medullary areas are continually active. Tonic excitatory influences from the pressor area impinge on the same spinal neurons. But the synaptic events at spinal vasomotor neurons and the patterns of interactions of the two descending influences on them largely remain unknown. The intensity of the discharge in preganglionic vasocon-

strictor neurons must be the resultant of the two descending tonic influences. The frequency of tonic discharge in the thoracic sympathetic outflow is relatively low, and discharge occurs in rhythmic bursts, in concert with the pulse beat and respiration. Thus, the afferent discharge is probably driven by input to the medullary center from mechanoreceptors in the great vessels and its branches.

The fall in arterial pressure on activation of mechanoreceptors is probably largely accomplished by peripheral vasodilation in muscle, the splanchnic bed, and the skin through inhibition of vasoconstrictor tone.

The mechanisms subserving vasomotor tone have been reviewed above because of the role that mechanoreceptor activity has played in the hypotheses about the maintenance of elevated blood pressure.

Acute and chronic elevations in arterial pressure result from denervation of the sino-aortic region. But, in animals, at least, the resulting hypertension is labile and accompanied by tachycardia. The elevated blood pressure could be lowered in dogs by exercise and hypotensive drugs with considerably more ease than essential hypertension can be in man.

The effects of denervating mechanoreceptors, though instructive in their own right, do not necessarily prove or disprove their role in naturally occurring essential hypertension. There is considerable evidence to suggest that the carotid sinus reflex remains active and functioning in essential hypertension but that the mechanoreceptors adapt to high levels of blood pressure and, therefore, no longer act maximally to reduce pressure levels. This adaptation occurs in dogs within one to two days after a renal artery is clamped, and is characterized by an increase both in threshold and the range of response of the mechanoreceptors. Recordings from the sinus nerve show a decrease in discharge frequency with changes in pressure in these hypertensive animals.[26] It is not as yet clear what the nature of this adaptation to higher blood pressure is. It is likely to be due to the direct effect of a high systemic pressure rather than to a chemical substance. Such an adaptation to an elevated mean blood pressure would act to sustain it; the decrease in afferent discharge would lead to decreased inhibition of vasomotor tone and therefore further vasoconstriction. These data have led to therapeutic measures designed to counteract the adaptation of the mechanoreceptors. Electrical stimulation of the sinus nerve lowers blood pressure in hypertensive patients.

Stretching of the mechanoreceptors has effects on the CNS in addition to lowering the blood pressure. Bonvallet et al.[6] have distended the carotid sinus while maintaining blood pressure at a constant level, to produce cortical synchronization. They believe that an increase in afferent activity occluded the tonic, corticopetal, desynchronizing influences of the midbrain reticular activating formation. Therefore, one might postulate that if mechanoreceptor adaptation occurs in hypertension, there would be a tendency in the opposite direction, i.e., for cortical desynchronization and behavioral arousal.

An elevated blood pressure may affect the CNS directly and in addition to the effects mediated by mechanoreceptors. Thus Baust et al.[5] reported that raising the blood pressure may directly cause desynchronization of the EEG in the *encéphale isolé* cat, by virtue of its effect on the mesencephalic reticular formation. The mechanical effect of a rise in blood pressure may cause the firing rate of single posterior hypothalamic and mesencephalic reticular neurons to increase. One might well ask, therefore, if this mechanical stimulus also causes the release of humoral substances (for example, vasopressin).

Central Control of the Vasomotor Center

In the cerebral cortex, for example, there are widely distributed points which, on stimulation, modify the blood pressure and which may be way stations in complex circuits of which the medullary and spinal centers are a part.

Stimulation of the gyrus poreus and the sigmoid gyrus in cats and the motor strip in monkeys increases the blood pressure. In addition, when the sensorimotor cortex of the cat is stimulated changes in renal volume occurred without blood-pressure changes, while chronic stimulation of the anterior sigmoid gyrus in cats produced renal vasoconstriction and renal cortical ischemia.

Presumably, these cortical stimuli facilitate vasomotor discharge by pathways and synaptic connections which largely remain unknown. One of the known outflow tracts from the sigmoid gyrus and the pericruciate cortex is the pyramidal tract. In fact, there is evidence that this tract is involved in the regulation of vasomotor activity, possibly by means of collaterals to the pons and medulla or by influencing spinal autonomic mechanisms directly.

Other cortical areas may produce their effects by other pathways, presumably to the hypothalamus. Lesions of the hypothalamus yielded vasomotor responses to stimulation of the surfaces of the posterior orbital gyrus.

On stimulation of frontal, and temporal cortical structures, pressor and depressor effects occur in many mammals including man. The corticofugal pathways mediating such effects are largely unknown; they are believed not to synapse in the hypothalamus.

On the other hand, the effects of rhinencephalic stimulation are most probably transmitted via the hypothalamus. Several rhinencephalic areas (the anterior limbic cortex, anterior insula, and the hippocampal gyrus) on stimulation produce changes in blood pressure. The cingulate gyrus, both in man and apes, is involved in blood-pressure regulation. Amygdala stimulation reduces blood pressure. When a number of midline structures—the nonspecific thalamic nuclei and the midbrain reticular system—are subjected to high-frequency stimulation, marked elevations of blood pressure occur. The effects of such stimulation persist after stimulation stops. Pressor and depressor reflexes may be inhibited by stimulation of the vermis of the cerebellum, presumably by modifying ongoing activity in bulbopontine vasomotor and hypothalamic centers.

The synaptic interactions of these various regions of the brain have not been worked out by intracellular methods. Interactions of the foregoing areas with hypothalamic neurons and with inputs from the mechanoreceptors to the medullary centers may be particularly important in the regulation of blood pressure.

Not only does high-frequency stimulation of the hypothalamus produce acute phasic increases in blood pressure, but the rate of hypothalamic stimulation is linearly related to the impulse frequency in single fibers of the inferior cardiac and the cervical sympathetic nerves. An occlusive interaction between activity produced by baroreceptor activation and hypothalamic stimulation has also been found, while blood-pressure increments produced by stimulation of a peripheral sensory nerve are facilitated by hypothalamic stimulation.

Following the end of simple hypothalamic stimulation, the blood pressure continues to stay elevated for some minutes, possibly due to the release of vasopressin, and perhaps norepinephrine. Furthermore, varying the frequency of stimulation of a particular hypothalamic site may change a pressor to a depressor response by causing tonic vasoconstrictor discharge to cease. Effects on local changes in blood vessels have also been noted upon stimulating the hypothalamus. In unanesthetized animals blood-pressure increases may be accompanied by expressions of rage when the hypothalamus is stimulated.

From the hypothalamus pathways involved in vasomotor regulation may pass to, or through the mesencephalon. Axons may then travel directly to the spinal cord, or synapse in the tegmentum of the midbrain and the periaqueductal gray matter, or they may travel via the median longitudinal fasiculus to end on medullary neurons. Other descending brainstem pathways, such as the ventrolateral reticulospinal pathway, have also been implicated in vasomotor regulation. Therefore, it seems likely that midbrain reticular formation contributes to cardiac control.

In summary, there is still considerable controversy about the detailed anatomy of supramedullary and suprasegmental outflow from the brain responsible for vasomotor control. From the medulla, excitatory impulses pass to spinal vasomotor neurons in the ventrolateral portion of the spinal cord, while inhibitory influences travel in crossed pathways in the dorsolateral columns.

Spinal and Peripheral Vasomotor Regulation

Stimulation in the medullary pressor area causes bilateral increase in the tonic discharge frequency in the inferior cardiac nerve, and an ipsilateral increment of discharge in cervical sympathetic neurons. Presumably, the inputs from higher centers modify spinal vasomotor reflexes which are released when the spinal cord is cut. Tonic vasoconstrictor discharge still occurs in spinal animals, or in animals in whom the buffer nerves have been cut. Spinal vasomotor neurons continue to be responsive to afferent inputs even after cord transection. Sympathetic pathways extend from the lateral horn of the spinal gray matter to sympathetic paravertebral ganglia. Vasoconstrictor fibers to blood vessels and skin emanate from the thoracolumbar outflow. Their effects are transmitted by postganglionic nerve terminals.

Single unit recordings of pre- and postganglionic sympathetic fibers yield data as to a low rate of transmission and frequency of discharge. The degree of regional vasoconstriction is proportional to the rate of stimulation of the cervical sympathetic trunk. Most significantly, a small change in the rate of stimulation may bring about a marked change in resistance to flow, so that there is a hyperbolic relationship between frequency of stimulation and peripheral resistance.

In most vascular compartments, the narrow range of sympathetic vasomotor discharge exerts virtually full control over the smooth muscle effector cells. Folkow and Uvnäs[12] have suggested that there are regional differences in vasoconstrictor discharge. It is plausible that central autonomic neuronal pools regulating tonic discharge to different vascular regions, may exhibit different excitability levels. Some, while remaining active, may not increase sympathetic discharge in one vascular region but may do so in another. If excitatory drive increases or release from inhibition occurs in neuronal circuits, sudden phasic enhancement of vasoconstrictor discharge may occur in one region and not another.

Neural mechanisms probably exist for massive, phasic increase of vasomotor discharge in appropriate circumstances but also for finely graded differential activity of automatic control over vasoconstrictor tone, due to quantitative differences in excitability levels of neuronal discharge to different parts of the vascular tree.

In addition to the regulation of vasomotor tone by mechanisms outlined above, there are other sympathetic vasodilator mechanisms. Such vasodilator nerves to skeletal muscles of mammals may be regulated by pathways from the motor cortex via the hypothalamus, tectum of the midbrain, and the ventrolateral medulla oblongata, from where they travel to the spinal cord. When stimulated, vasodilation in skeletal muscle is accompanied by constriction in the splanchnic bed and skin. As far as is known this second system is tonically active. Its outflow runs peripherally to muscle in cats and dogs and possibly to the skin. Little is, as yet, known about the nature of the transmitter substance, or the more intimate neurophysiological properties of this system.

The blood-pressure changes that occur with stimulation of various areas of the brain are, therefore, in part, mediated by the medullary vasomotor center and, in part, by spinal mechanisms to bring about changes in peripheral resistance. Unfortunately, neurophysiologists interested in using blood pressure as their dependent variable do not usually measure changes in cardiac output or resistance to account for the changes in blood pressure. They then fall into the same mistake as many psychophysiologists, which is to measure only a single dependent variable.

Regulation of Respiration: Central Mechanisms

The regulation of rhythmic respiration depends on the alternation of activity of neurons lying in two parts of the pontomedullary respiratory center. The inspiratory center lies in the ventral reticular formation of the upper medulla. Its neurons are driven by the CO_2 tension of arterial blood and by input from chemoreceptors to produce an increase in depth of inspiration finally leading to active expiration. The expiratory center lies lateral, dorsal, and rostral to the inspiratory center in the medulla, and has a tonic inhibitory function on the inspiratory center.

These two centers are the minimal mechanism for the regulation and maintenance of respiratory rhythm. They are profoundly influenced in the intact organism by neural influences coming from more rostral levels.

In the rostral part of the pons lies an inhibitory center, while in the middle and caudal part of the pons a center is found which tonically controls the inspiratory center to prevent respiratory arrest in inspiration with maximal inflation of the lungs.

Several midbrain centers control the lower ones; e.g., stimulation of the posterior hypothalamus produces a paroxysmal increase in respiratory rate. The lateral thalamus reduces the rate of respiration on stimulation. As one would expect, the main cortical sites in mammals from which changes of respiratory rate, depth, and rhythm can be obtained are the temporal, inferior, and superior precentral and orbito-frontal (inhibitory) cortices. This expectation is based on the fact that respiratory patterns can be altered "at will," or in coordination with speaking, singing, laughter, and breath-holding.

From a physiological point of view, normal respiration is regulated by rhythmic periods of inhibition of the tonically active, medullary inspiratory center. This inspiratory tonus is modulated not only by the medullary expiratory center which is progressively excited during inspiration; it begins to discharge during inspiration to inhibit activity in the inspiratory center. Further control on inspiration is exerted by inhibition of the medullary inspiratory center by the pontine centers so that inspiratory tonus, mediated by the phrenic nerve, is transformed into rhythmic respiration by a series of reciprocally inhibiting interactions amongst brain-stem neurons which regulate respiration.

Of particular interest to psychophysiologists

is that the respiration can be markedly influenced by intellectual work which increases its frequency and reduces its amplitude. The type and frequency of respiration may also be changed by exercise and emotional states, such as anticipation, excitement (sexual or otherwise), anxiety, and depressive mood. These states are accompanied by changes in respiratory rhythm. In the hyperventilation syndrome, both the depth and frequency of respiration are enhanced.

Because of the close interaction of psychological factors and respiration, and of respiration and circulation, it becomes incumbent on the psychophysiologist to monitor respiration when measuring cardiovascular variables.

Interaction of Cardiac and Respiratory Function

Rhythmic fluctuations of blood pressure and heart rate are seen in the steady-state in concert with inspiration and expiration. Integration of cardiac and respiratory function is achieved centrally. The receptor sites are: (1) The pulmonary artery baroreceptors which are particularly sensitive to changes in the rate of pressure with each pulse mainly to adjust respiratory ventilation to changes in venous return; (2) The arterial chemoreceptors which respond to a fall in arterial oxygen tension and/or a rise in the partial pressure of arterial CO_2. When stimulated, there is a marked increase in respiration, a reflex fall in heart rate, and a rise in blood pressure, due to an increase in peripheral resistance. There is also vasoconstriction in muscle, skin, viscera, and the kidney, and increased catecholamine production. These responses are mediated, in part, by the hypothalamus; and (3) The lung inflation receptors which respond to stretching of smooth muscle in the lung with inflation to produce a cessation of inspiration. These receptors are also responsible for most of the cardiovascular changes seen during the normal respiratory cycle. Vagal afferent pathways mediate the responses to stretch. Increased pulmonary stretching suppresses the reflex inhibitory effects on the heart when arterial chemoreceptors are stimulated. The central

pathways mediating stretching pass both to the bulbar respiratory center and to the hypothalamus and cerebral cortex.

Central Regulation of the Galvanic Skin Resistance

One of the most frequent tools used by psychophysiologists is galvanic skin resistance, or conductance (the reciprocal of resistance). The local factors which are responsible for conductance or resistance changes most likely have to do with sweating and blood flow through the skin. The more general factors influencing it are psychological stimuli and states.

Removal of the telencephalon, forebrain, and thalamus in cats causes a marked increase in the galvanic skin response, while diencephalic destruction causes it to decline and finally to disappear, suggesting that the telencephalon exerts inhibitory control on the diencephalon in the regulation of the reflex. Yet there is additional evidence that another set of inhibitory influences on the reflex stem from the ventromedial portion of the medullary reticular formation which, when released from facilitatory diencephalic inputs, causes the reflex to disappear. When this caudal set of neurons is cooled or blocked by anesthesia, the reflex is very active. Spinal transection at the level of the first cervical vertebra abolishes the GSR (galvanic skin response).

There is further evidence that there are neuronal mechanisms modulating the bulbar mechanism for GSR regulation in the caudate nucelus and anterior cerebellar lobe.

Central Regulation of Body Temperature

Two important psychophysiological variables—the moisture of the skin, and respiration—are also involved in heat loss and conservation. Perspiration and panting are processes which cause the body to lose heat.

The hypothalamus is involved in the control of these functions when environmental temperature changes.

Animals, including man, with lesions of the

anterolateral hypothalamus cannot regulate their temperature in a warm environment. Body temperature will then rise. When placed in a cold environment, body temperature is maintained because the physiological changes for heat loss fail. In man, heat loss is usually achieved by vasodilatation of the skin, perspiration, and increased respiration.

If lesions are placed in the dorsolateral portion of the posterior hypothalamus, the animal cannot make the necessary physiological adaptations, either to a cold or a hot environment. Why should both forms of adaptation be lost? In all probability, fibers from the anterior (heat loss) hypothalamic nuclei are interrupted by the lesion which also destroys the posterior (heat conservation) mechanisms. The heat conservation mechanisms of the body include epinephrine secretion and shivering to increase heat production, and cutaneous vasoconstriction and piloerection to conserve heat within the body.

Stimulation or local heating of the anterior hypothalamic centers produces sweating, panting, and cutaneous vasodilation and causes core temperature to drop, especially if the environmental temperature is low. Cold-induced shivering is prevented by anterior hypothalamic stimulation. Yet, when the animal is exposed to cold, the threshold to stimulation is increased.

The two hypothalamic centers seem, therefore, to regulate each other reciprocally. The input to these centers is probably a dual one—one for cold and the other for heat—from cutaneous thermoreceptors, and from thermoreceptors within the body (especially within the cranial cavity) sensitive to internal changes in temperature.

It follows from this review that it is essential to maintain a constant environmental temperature if one is measuring skin resistance or conductance in psychophysiological experiments.

Central Control of Gastric Secretion

There is evidence to suggest that intracerebral stimulation and lesions of various parts of the nervous system may stimulate or inhibit the secretion of acid and pepsin, or change the production and quality of gastric mucus. For example, low intensity (but long-term) stimulation of the anterior hypothalamus in cats has produced hyperplasia of the gastric mucosa. In dogs, a lesion of the anterior hypothalamus increased the basal acidity of the gastric contents, but did not change the secretory response to maximal histamine stimulation. It may be that the cerebral cortex tonically inhibits gastric secretion. Both in dogs and in man, decortication raised the basal secretion of acid in the stomach.

These findings are difficult to interpret. Obviously, species differ in their responses to brain stimulation. In addition, the effects of stimulation on the nervous system are always difficult to interpret; partly because different stimulus strengths and frequencies produce different results.

Presumably, the excitatory effects of brain stimulation are mediated by the vagus nerve. But we do not know how these excitatory effects interact with known central inhibitory influences on vagal discharge. An increase in neural activity in the vagus nerve causes an increase in gastric motility and secretion. But the vagus is not purely excitatory; it also mediates inhibitory influences on the physiological activities of the stomach. We still do not now very much about just how these two opposing influences affect the stomach, for example, we do not know how increased vagal discharge can cause a dissociation of acid from pepsin secretion. The kind of information that is needed to resolve this problem is exemplified by the work of Iggo and Leek,[18] who have recorded the action potential from single axons of the vagus nerve of sheep, and related the pattern of discharge from some of these to contractile movements of the stomach.

A dual mechanism for the regulation of gastric acid secretion also seems to be present in the hypothalamus. Acute increases in gastric acid secretion, as evidenced by a decrease in the pH of gastric juices, can be induced by anterior hypothalamic stimulation. Vagotomy abolishes this response. Stimulation of the posterior hypothalamus produces a delayed increase in gastric acid secretion which reaches its peak after three hours; this response is not mediated by the vagus nerve, but may be mediated by adrenal cortical hormones because bilateral adrenalectomy abolishes it.

Chronic posterior hypothalamic stimulation can produce gastric and duodenal hemorrhage due to ulceration. The increase in gastric acid secretion produced by insulin also seems to act by the medium of the hypothalamus and vagal afferent outflow.

All the mechanisms which produce acid secretion in the stomach are still not known. Vagal afferents to the stomach may control gastrin and pepsinogen secretion. Gastrin is a polypeptide which regulates acid secretion in the stomach, and is, in turn, regulated both by the vagus and by a negative feedback mechanism by increases in the acid content of gastric juice.

The Hypothalamus and Other Psychophysiological Relationships

SEXUAL BEHAVIOR

The autonomic nervous system is clearly involved in the sexual act, both erection and ejaculation are under its control. In addition, during sexual intercourse changes in heart rate, blood pressure, respiratory rate and depth, vasomotor changes, and sweating have been recorded.[26] Psychological factors are presumed to play a considerable role in determining the range and extent of such changes, and the responsiveness of the subject during sexual intercourse.

Very much less is known about the role of the autonomic nervous system in sexual behavior other than sexual reproduction. However, it is known that in mammals the posterior hypothalamus plays a part in sexual behavior and oestrus.

In fact, most of the work on sexual behavior has focused on its hormonal control. The hypothalamus is also involved in patterned emotional behaviors—such as the "defense reaction"—which always has very marked concomitants of autonomic arousal. Involved in these patterns is the complex relationship between the limbic input to hypothalamic activity.

The hypothalamus also plays a role in behavioral states such as sleep and wakefulness, in immune responses, in stress reactions, in the prevention of pulmonary edema, in eating behavior, in aggressive behavior, and in the control of the secretion of pituitary trophic hormones. The implication of the autonomic nervous system in these responses remains to be elucidated.

⟨ Other Psychophysiological Phenomena

Psychophysiologists also measure electrical phenomena, such as the electroencephalogram (EEG), "evoked" potentials (EP), the "contingent negative variation" potential (CNV), and the electromyogram (EMG).

Despite the fact that it is over forty years since the EEG was first described, we still do not know what aspects of neuronal or other neural functioning it reflects. It is used to measure differences of activity in behavioral steady-states such as sleep and quiet wakefulness, delirium and coma. It is affected in its activity by drugs, mental activity, sensory input, and by changes in the blood pressure, etc.

Evoked potentials (EP) can be recorded from the scalp following stimulation of receptors—such as in the eye, ear, or skin—by means of special computer techniques which accumulate time-locked signals. Much controversy has surrounded the EP, because in the intact subject time-locked scalp muscle potentials must be differentiated from a signal of cerebral origin. EP's reflect the activity of sensory receiving areas to incoming impulses in specific sensory tracts produced by the stimulus. The early waves of the EP are believed to consist of activity in thalamocortical projections, the arrival of impulses in cortical neurons and their responses to them. No one knows what central processes the later waves represent. In fact, the mechanism of EP wave forms has resisted analysis to date.

A special form of EP is the CNV, a slow negative D.C. wave recorded from the forehead which is produced when a subject attends to a task. It again must be differentiated from muscle EMG activity such as produced by blinking of the eyes.

General speaking, EP and CNV are influenced mainly by central states—such as variations in attention, sleep, drugs, etc. However, it should be noted that in animals, at least, the early components of the EP are largest in deep barbiturate narcosis.

The EMG's are usually recorded from the skin surface by means of special electrodes, and reflect tonic and phasic changes in tension in large numbers of muscle fibers. They are particularly useful in demonstrating changes in eye, neck, or submental muscle tone during sleep stages. Eye movements are present and tonic submental activity is minimal during REM period sleep. Muscle tension is increased during apprehensive or alerted states.

The regulation of muscle tone is not fully understood. It is reflexly maintained by segmental mechanisms, and regulated by two sets of afferent input. Inhibitory and excitatory influences play upon the alpha-motoneuron through the mediation of the inhibitory Renshaw cell of the cord, and by descending pyramidal, vestibulospinal, rubrospinal, reticulospinal, and other pathways.

Further Integrative Mechanisms

The Relationship Between the Autonomic and Endocrine System

Many of the problems in inference and interpretation about the results of psychophysiological experiments would be simplified if multiple rather than single physiological variables were measured. This would allow the psychophysiologist to obtain a broader view of the biology of responses to the independent variables which he has chosen for his experiment.

For it is increasingly apparent that there are very important interactions between central and peripheral autonomically mediated responses and the endocrine system, and, there-

fore, metabolic processes. What is more, the interactions between these systems occur in both directions. We have seen that ACTH (adrenocorticotrophic hormone) by increasing cortisol production in the adrenal cortex, induces PNMT which, in turn, catalyzes the biosynthesis of epinephrine from norepinephrine. Epinephrine, in turn, mobilizes liver glycogen, through the medium of cyclic AMP (adenosine monophosphate) to increase blood sugar. Insulin increases gastric secretion reflexly through the vagus nerve. Mechanoreceptors in the great blood vessels reflexly and, in part, regulate the release of the mineralocorticoid, aldosterone, which plays a central role in the control of electrolyte metabolism and hence body water, and at the same time regulate catecholamine and ADH release. Sympathetic discharge can bring about renin release from the kidney, hence angiotensin production, and thereby influence the blood pressure. Angiotensin II may increase the firing rate of supraoptic neurons, and hence increase the release of antidiuretic hormone, thereby diminishing urine production. Angiotensin II may also influence CNS mechanisms directly to increase the blood pressure. The sympathetic nervous system mediates the light-induced regulation of melatonin which, in turn, at least, and in some mammals, influences oestrus behavior.

The central integration of autonomic outflow, as well as many metabolic processes, occurs in the hypothalamus. The control and regulation of the pituitary trophic hormones is carried out by hypothalamic cells. These are believed to "transduce" electrical impulses into chemical substances, by the release of biogenic amine neurotransmitters which, in turn, control the release of corticotrophin, follicle-stimulating and thyrotrophin releasing and other factors. Posterior pituitary hormones such as ADH are particularly sensitive to environmental and other (such as painful) stimuli through the medium of the anterior hypothalamus and the hypothalamico-neurohypophysial tract.

Generally speaking, responses to rapid and short-term environmental changes are mediated neurally by the autonomic nervous system by means of ganglionic relays and postganglionic terminals to release neurotransmitter substances at local sites. Physiological adaptations to slowly changing or long-term environmental stimuli or situations are carried out both by neuronal and hormonal agents. These hormones act "at a distance" and often at widespread sites. The release of each hormone has its own time course as discussed in Chapter 24. Intermittent and repeated environmental changes may bring about eventual physiological adaptation. When repeated or continuous environmental factors are imposed on young animals, their physiological responses later in life are determined by the earlier experience,[14,15] thus providing a basis for our understanding of a critical problem in all psychophysiological research, i.e., that of individual differences in response tendencies.

A special and very interesting interaction between the autonomic nervous system, behavior, and hormones has been worked out in the pineal gland.

Fiske et al.[10] had shown that the weight of the pineal gland decreases when rats are kept in continuous light. Under such lighting conditions female rats remain in continuous vaginal oestrus. These, and the observation that extracts of the pineal gland of cattle inhibits oestrus, led to the observation that melatonin reduces the incidence of oestrus in the rat.

We owe to Axelrod and his group,* the elucidation of the biosynthetic pathway of melatonin from tryptophane:

release of melatonin, and this would explain why continuous light produces persistent oestrus.

Axelrod and his associates have worked out the rather complex and indirect pathway from retina to pineal and the manner in which the biosynthetic machinery of the gland is influenced:

Environmental light in the mammal passes via the retina → inferior accessory optic tract → medial forebrain bundle to the medial terminal nucleus of the accessory optic system → preganglionic sympathetic fibers of the spinal cord → the superior cervical ganglion from which postganglionic fibers pass upward to the parenchymal cells of the pineal gland whose terminal release norepinephrine.[28]

At the same time light clearly also stimulates the retina to entrain impulses which pass via the classical visual pathways to the visual cortex, and in an as yet mysterious way to produce the experience of discriminated light.

The release of noradrenaline in the pineal gland influences the formation of melatonin from tryptophane by inducing the enzyme, N-acetyltransferase[20] (which converts serotonin into N-acetylserotonin).

Two further points about the regulation in the pineal gland need, however, to be made. One highlights the importance of taking into account the time during a biological rhythm, and, the second, the importance of the age of the animal, at which an experiment is done.

The first case is illustrated by the fact that

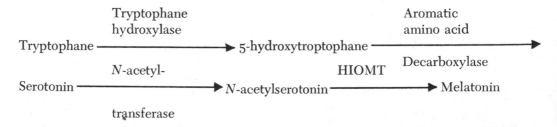

Wurtman, Axelrod, and Phillips[45] showed that levels of hydroxyindole-O-methyltransferase (HIOMT) in the pineal gland are elevated when rats are kept in continuous light. Therefore, light reduces the synthesis and

* See references 3, 28, 35, 43, and 44.

there is a biological rhythm for the content of serotonin in the pineal[44]—one of the important precursors of melatonin—and for norepinephrine in the pineal gland. The content is high during the day under normal lighting conditions, and low at 11:00 P.M. This rhythm is endogenous, although its driving oscillator is unknown. Despite its endogenous nature, the oscillator can be entrained by light, e.g., when day and night are reversed experimentally.[35]

Norepinephrine content, on the other hand, which reaches its highest levels at night is not controlled by an endogenous oscillator but is under the direct environmental control of light. Thus, its high nocturnal content corresponds to the high nocturnal content of HIOMT, and, therefore, of melatonin synthesis.

It is, however, of great interest that the oscillator for serotonin is not operative until the rat is six days old.[28] Furthermore, in young rats before they are twenty-seven days old, light affects the serotonin level in the pineal gland by an extraretinal pathway; after this age this earlier pathway is no longer operative.

(Integrative Function of the Autonomic Nervous System

Certain generalizations about the overall function of the ANS in maintaining homeostasis have beclouded the fact that sympathectomized animals do survive and lead quite a normal existence. They eat, grow, sleep, and reproduce in the laboratory. They may not be able to suckle their young, and may be unduly cold-sensitive. Only under conditions of stress do responses fail but even then stresses must be quite severe (such as asphyxia stress) to reveal the absence of sympathetic regulatory devices. In other words, there seem to be adaptations to the absence of the sympathetic nervous system, in which otherwise redundant mechanisms take over its function.

(Modern Concepts

Modern concepts about the autonomic nervous system no longer tend to focus as much on its role in maintaining the "constancy of the internal environment." Rather, its role is seen as one of the three main mediators of the organism's responses to his natural or social environment.

This view is implicit in Walter Cannon's work but in retrospect it is a point of view that has been underplayed. Rather, the field of psychophysiology has moved in the direction of the study of controllable psychological and sociological variables in the laboratory while measuring single physiological ones. Furthermore, such studies deal only with responses in the acute experimental situation. We know very much less about the autonomically mediated responses to chronic "stresses."

The study of organismic responses, that is, the integrated psychological and a broad range of physiological responses, to everyday, naturally occurring situations requires different methodologies. The responses obtained by new techniques may require further analysis in the laboratory.

However, a giant step has been taken in this direction by the research performed in the laboratories of Axelrod,[4] Henry,[14] and Kopin.[24] They have combined a number of techniques, taken from such diverse fields as ethology, experimental psychology, biochemical pharmacology, and enzymology, to demonstrate the effects on animals of short-term and long-term exposure to stress and how such exposure affects mediating autonomic mechanisms.

Very acute stresses, preparation for activity and novel experiences, are now known to be divided into anticipatory and reactive phases, and are associated with increases in systolic blood pressure, heart rate, and catecholamine and steroid excretion, etc. In all likelihood these changes are largely mediated neuronally. The mechanism underlying the increase in catecholamines, especially norepinephrine secretion, appears to be due to a sharp increase in norepinephrine synthesis from tyrosine but not dopa, when an increase in sympathetic nerve activity occurs. However, no increase in tyrosine hydroxylase activity occurs, so that either no new enzyme is formed or formation is inhibited by norepinephrine.

The absence of change in tyrosine hydroxylase content of tissue during acute stresses or stimulation stands in contrast to the change that is produced by sustained stress or sympathetic nerve activity.

Thoenen, Mueller, and Axelrod[29,30,36] have shown that a reflex increase in sympathetic nerve activity over several days produced a marked increase in TH activity in the adrenal gland and in the superior cervical ganglion of the rat, and in the brain stem of the rabbit. The activity of PNMT is also increased. By a number of experimental procedures Axelrod and his co-workers have shown that the changes in content of these enzymes in the adrenal gland and in the superior cervical ganglion are not only neuronally mediated but depend on the formation of new protein.[30] In other words, they have shown that the increase in TH activity is transsynaptically induced.

The increase of PNMT produced by neuronal activity is, however, also under the control of ACTH.[4,42] It depends on new protein (enzyme) synthesis and occurs even in hypophysectomy and the administration of ACTH. To a much lesser degree, the two other biosynthetic enzymes, TH and dopamine hydroxylase, are similarly controlled.

That these changes in enzyme activity with sustained neuronal activity are not only the product of the laboratory is attested to by the exquisite work of Henry and his co-workers.[14,15] It confirms the fact that chronic stress produces marked changes in the biosynthetic enzymes of norepinephrine, but, in addition, it produces correlated changes in blood pressure and renal pathology.

The results of this research have been confirmed by the use of the restraint technique. Further evidence for the dually mediated changes in adrenal enzyme content has been obtained. Other work, using this method, provides insight into some of the possible brain mechanisms mediating these changes.

Restraint-immobilization has potent effects on the peripheral and central content of biogenic amines. Kvetnansky and Mikulaj[23] have shown that in rats immobilization for ninety minutes produces an increased excretion level of norepinephrine and epinephrine, associated with a decrease in adrenal epinephrine (but not norepinephrine) content which persisted for twenty-four hours after its conclusion. With persistent immobilization, adrenal epinephrine content was unaffected, but norepinephrine content increased, while the urinary excretion of epinephrine remained increased. These results suggest that the adrenal medulla enhances its ability to replace released epinephrine with repeated immobilization stress. This "adaptation" to stress appears to be due to a neuronally dependent elevation of TH and PNMT in the adrenal medulla.[24] When immobilization is stopped, TH levels diminish with a half-life of about three days.

Following the end of immobilization there is a latency period of about six hours for levels of TH and PNMT to become elevated. Further elevations of levels occur in the next seven days of immobilization, but after six weeks of daily immobilization, no further increases occur.

The long-term increase in catecholamine levels in the adrenal medulla produced by immobilization are not only neuronally dependent but are *also* under the control of ACTH. After hypophysectomy, depletion levels with restraint are greater than in control animals, and levels of TH and PNMT fall. On repeated immobilization, TH levels but not PNMT in hypophysectomized rats do, however, rise but never to control levels. The use of TH levels in operated rats is neuronally dependent in the main, whilst the rise in PNMT, and some of the rise in TH levels, depends almost entirely on ACTH administered prior to the stress.

On the other hand, serum dopamine-β-hydroxylase (which transforms dopamine into norepinephrine) was increased after one thirty-minute immobilization of rats, and continues to increase with daily immobilization for a week. The source of this increase is not, however, the adrenal gland but sympathetic nerves.

Immobilization stress of three hours also significantly accelerates the disappearance of radioactive norepinephrine from heart and kidney. The question of how immobilization stress is centrally translated into these neuronally and hormonally dependent peripheral changes is unanswered except for some very interesting work by the Welches.[41] They showed that restraint stress can cause a greater elevation of *brain* norepinephrine and serotonin in mice who previously had spent eight to twelve weeks in isolation, when compared to littermates housed in groups.

This elevation of brain amines occurs despite the fact that the isolated mice have slower baseline turnover of brain biogenic amines than those housed with others.

This work has several important implications. The isolated mice were behaviorally more hyperexcitable than the housed controls. In other words, previous experience affected behavioral response tendencies, while the finding of different turnover rates and greater elevations with immobilization clearly indicates that previous experience may lead to individual differences in brain biogenic amines as well as behavior.

This work further points up the contention brought forth in this chapter that autonomic and endocrine mechanisms are closely interrelated and interacting. The full range of these interactions and mutually regulating mechanisms is still to be worked out.

Finally, psychophysiology brings us face to face with a major scientific and philosophic issue. Which are the means by which psychological responses—thoughts, feelings, their awareness, etc.—are translated, if indeed they directly are, into autonomically mediated responses?[40] In other words—the mind–body problem. There is no answer to this question, and therefore, much of the meaning of psychophysiological correlations and concomitances remains obscure, meaningless, or without significance.

(Technical Aspects

In addition to having mastered a number of skills, psychophysiologists must have considerable expertise in instrumentation. Special attention must be given to make their instruments reliable and valid: For example, special instruments have been devised for measuring blood pressure in intact subjects.

All the techniques which have been devised require some knowledge of electronic recording devices. For the technical aspects of psychophysiology, the reader is referred to the *Manual of Psychophysiological Methods.*[37]

(Concluding Remarks

The data and concepts reviewed in this chapter are mainly derived from acute experiments performed on anesthetized animals. In addition, these experiments tend to have as their purpose the study of a single dependent autonomic variable, while varying an independent other variable. Such analytic experiments tend to obscure the complex, integrated adjustments that occur in autonomic function in intact, free-ranging animals, and to obscure patterns of autonomic change brought about by changes in the animal's environment. There is some evidence that patterned autonomic changes (and behavioral changes) may be quite specific to particular situations. They may be different in an animal anticipating avoidance conditioning than they are in anticipation of muscular exercise. Or, they may be different in an animal anticipating a fight with another, than during the actual engagement.

Yet, any understanding of autonomic functioning must be based on knowledge of the intrinsic mechanisms which underlie them. For this reason these mechanisms have been reviewed. In Chapter 23, Hofer will review the principles which govern autonomic psychophysiological relationships in the natural life of man and animals. These relationships have been studied in the laboratory or field in intact animals. The data derived from these studies reveal a different level of organization of autonomic functioning than an analytic experiment can do.

(Bibliography

1. AHLQUIST, R. P. "A Study of the Adrenotropic Receptors," *Am. J. Physiol.*, 153 (1948), 586–600.

2. ALEXANDER, R. S. "Tonic and Reflex Functions of Medullary Sympathetic Cardiovascular Centers," *J. Neurophysiol.*, 9 (1946), 205–217.

3. AXELROD, J. "The Pineal Gland," *Endeavor*, 29 (1970), 144–148.

4. ———. "Noradrenaline: Fate and Control of Its Biosynthesis," *Science*, 173 (1971), 598–606.

5. BAUST, W., H. NIEMCZYK, and J. VIETH. "The Action of Blood Pressure on the Ascending Reticular Activating System with Special Reference to Adrenaline-Induced EEG Arousal," *Electroencephalogr. Clin. Neurophysiol.*, 15 (1963), 63–72.

6. BONVALLET, M., A. HUGELIN, and P. DELL. "The Interior Environment and Automatic Activities of the Reticular Cells of the Mesencephalon," *J. Physiol. (Paris)*, 48 (1956), 403–406.

7. BURN, J. N. and M. J. RAND. "Sympathetic Postganglionic Mechanism," *Nature*, 184 (1959), 163–165.

8. ECCLES, J. C. *The Physiology of Synapses.* Berlin: Springer, 1964.

9. ELLIOT, T. R. "The Action of Adrenaline," *J. Physiol.*, 32 (1905), 401–467.

10. FISKE, V. M., G. K. BRYANT, and J. PUTNAM. "Effect of Light on the Weight of the Pineal in the Rat," *Endocrinology*, 66 (1960), 489–491.

11. FOLKOW, B. and E. H. RUBINSTEIN. "Cardiovascular Effects of Acute and Chronic Stimulation of the Hypothalamic Defence Area in the Rat," *Acta Physiol. Scand.*, 68 (1966), 48–57.

12. FOLKOW, B. and B. UVNÄS. "Do Adrenergic Vasodilator Nerves Exist?" *Acta Physiol. Scand.*, 30 (1950), 329–337.

13. GOODMAN, L. S. and A. GILMAN. *The Pharmacological Basis of Therapeutics*, 3rd ed. New York: Macmillan, 1965.

14. HENRY, J. P., D. L. ELY, and P. M. STEPHENS. "Role of the Autonomic System in Social Adaptation and Stress," *Proc. Int. Union Physiol. Sci.*, 8 (1971), 50–51.

15. HENRY, J. P., P. M. STEPHENS, J. AXELROD et al. "Effect of Psychosocial Stimulation on the Enzymes Involved in the Biosynthesis and Metabolism of Noradrenaline and Adrenaline," *Psychosom. Med.*, 33 (1971), 227–237.

16. HESS, W. R. *Das Zwischenhirn.* Basel: Schwabe, 1949.

17. HODGKIN, A. L. *The Conduction of the Nervous Impulse.* Springfield: Charles C. Thomas, 1964.

18. IGGO, A. and B. F. LEEK. "An Electrophysiological Study of Single Vagal Efferent Units Associated with Gastric Movements in Sheep," *J. Physiol.*, 191 (1967), 177–204.

19. KATZ, B. "Quantal Mechanism of Neural Transmitter Release," *Science*, 173 (1971), 123–126.

20. KLEIN, D. C. and J. WELLER. "Serotonin N-Acetyl Transferase Activity is Stimulated by Norepinephrine and Dibutyryl Cyclic Adenosine Monophosphate," *Fed. Proc.*, 29 (1970), 615.

21. KORNER, P. I. "Integrative Neural Cardiovascular Control," *Physiol. Rev.*, 51 (1971), 312–367.

22. KUNTZ, A. *The Autonomic Nervous System.* Philadelphia: Lea & Febiger, 1953.

23. KVETNANSKY, R. and L. MIKULAJ. "Adrenal and Urinary Catecholamines in Rats during Adaptation to Repeated Immobilization Stress," *Endocrinology*, 87 (1970), 738–743.

24. KVETNANSKY, R., V. K. WEISE, and I. J. KOPIN. "Elevation of Adrenal Tyrosine Hydroxylase and Phenylethanolamine-N-Methyl Transferase by Repeated Immobilization of Rats," *Endocrinology*, 87 (1970), 744–749.

25. McCUBBIN, J. W., J. H. GREEN, and I. H. PAGE. "Baroreceptor Functions in Chronic Renal Hypertension," *Circ. Res.*, 4 (1956), 205–210.

26. MASTERS, W. H. and V. E. JOHNSON. *Human Sexual Response.* Boston: Little, Brown, 1966.

27. MILLER, N. E. "Learning of Visceral and Glandular Responses," *Science*, 163 (1969), 434–445.

28. MOORE, R. Y., A. HELLER, R. J. WURTMAN et al. "Visual Pathway Mediating Pineal Response to Environmental Light," *Science*, 155 (1967), 220–223.

29. MUELLER, R. A., H. THOENEN, and J. AXELROD. "Increase in Tyrosine Hydroxylase Activity after Reserpine Administration," *J. Pharmacol. Exp. Ther.*, 169 (1969), 74–79.

30. ———. "Inhibition of Transsynaptically Increased Tyrosine Hydroxylase Activity by Cycloheximide and Actinomycin D," *Mol. Pharmacol.*, 5 (1969), 463–469.

31. NACHMAHNSON, D. *Chemical and Molecular*

Basis of Nerve Activity. New York: Academic, 1959.

32. RANSON, S. W. "New Evidence in Favor of a Chief Vasoconstrictor Center in the Brain," *Am. J. Physiol.*, 42 (1916), 1–8.

33. RUSHMER, R. F. *Cardiovascular Dynamics.* Philadelphia: Saunders, 1970.

34. SEEDS, N. W. and A. G. GILMAN. "Norepinephrine Stimulated Increase of Cyclic AMP Levels in Developing Mouse Brain Cultures," *Science*, 174 (1971), 292.

35. SNYDER, S. H., J. AXELROD, and M. ZWEIG. "Circadian Rhythm in the Serotonin Content of the Rat Pineal Gland: Regulating Factors," *J. Pharmacol. Exp. Ther.*, 158 (1967), 206–213.

36. THOENEN, H., R. A. MUELLER, and J. AXELROD. "Increased Tyrosine Hydroxylase Activity after Drug-Induced Alteration of Sympathetic Transmission," *Nature*, 221 (1969), 1264.

37. VENABLES, P. H. and I. MARTIN, eds. *A Manual of Psychophysiological Methods.* New York: Wiley, 1967.

38. VON EULER, U. S. "Adrenergic Neurotransmitter Functions," *Science*, 173 (1971), 202–206.

39. WEINER, H. "Psychosomatic Research in Essential Hypertension," *Bibl. Psychiatr.*, 144 (1970), 58–116.

40. ———. "Some Comments on the Transduction of Experience by the Brain," *Psychosom. Med.*, 34 (1972), in press.

41. WELCH, B. L. and A. S. WELCH. "Differential Activation by Restraint Stress of a Mechanism to Conserve Brain Catecholamines and Serotonin in Mice Differing in Excitability," *Nature*, 218 (1968), 575–577.

42. WURTMAN, R. J. and J. AXELROD. "Control of Enzymatic Synthesis of Adrenaline in the Adrenal Medulla by Adrenal Cortical Steroids," *J. Biol. Chem.*, 241 (1966), 2301–2305.

43. WURTMAN, R. J., J. AXELROD, and E. W. CHU. "Melatonin, A Pineal Substance: Effect on Rat Ovary," *Science*, 141 (1963), 277–278.

44. WURTMAN, R. J., J. AXELROD, and D. E. KELLY. *The Pineal.* New York: Academic, 1968.

45. WURTMAN, R. J., J. AXELROD, and L. S. PHILLIPS. "Melatonin Synthesis in the Pineal Gland: Control by Light," *Science*, 142 (1963), 1071–1072.

CHAPTER 23

THE PRINCIPLES OF AUTONOMIC FUNCTION IN THE LIFE OF MAN AND ANIMALS

Myron A. Hofer

⟮ Introduction

WHEN GALEN[30] described the anatomy of the visceral neural network 1800 years ago, he was led to conclude that this structure functioned to promote "sympathy" or communication and harmony between internal organs. Although the use of the word "autonomic" nervous system dates from a mere seventy-five years ago,[58] parts of Galen's hypothesis regarding its function have survived, and the word "sympathetic" is used to denote the thoracolumbar portion of the system.

The modern literature on autonomic psychophysiology is immense and I will not attempt to survey the field; the reader is referred to recent books and review articles for this purpose.* Rather this chapter will deal with a few studies selected to illustrate the *principles* which appear to govern autonomic-nervous-system (ANS) functions in the organism during its natural life. The concepts which arise from new data will be emphasized, and will be related to disease processes. Emphasis will be placed on interpretation, on clinical implications, and on future directions, in this way hoping to represent the current state of our understanding of the field.

The previous chapter has dealt with the or-

* See references 6, 9, 23, 31, 33, 52, 53, 75, 83, 88, 94, 97, 102, 110, and 113.

ganization of the ANS at the level of its peripheral and central mechanisms, and reviewed the contribution of laboratory studies to our understanding. This chapter will consider the properties of the ANS as it functions while the organism interacts with its environment. What are the characteristics of its functioning while the subject is at rest, in response to changes in the environment and as a part of emotional and behavioral responses to signals processed by the central nervous system (CNS)? Is the system organized differently at different developmental stages? Is it primarily an effector system or are there major roles for its afferent pathways? Does activity of the autonomic system show effects of learning as does the musculo-skeletal system, and to what extent do the systems differ? Finally, what processes may account for the appearance of the unusually intense or poorly coordinated responses which can produce lasting damage or even death?

Our understanding of the role of the ANS in the economy of the organism was greatly advanced by Claude Bernard[8] and W. B. Cannon,[20] whose elegant experiments led them to an understanding of the negative feedback properties of autonomic function which served to maintain relative constancy of the "milieu interieur," or "homeostasis," in the face of constantly varying environmental conditions. It has since been recognized that such control systems are a general property of biological organization and are present in endocrine, metabolic, and cellular systems in the human.[99] They are also thought to be a characteristic of central neural functioning, mediating conscious experience.[11] Since the time of Cannon, accumulating data has forced modification in our concept of homeostasis to account for the fact that hierarchies are established in the organization of central integration, so that certain functional levels may be maintained at the expense of homeostasis in another area or system. An example of this is the maintenance of temperature regulation at the expense of water and electrolyte balance during extreme heat. Observations such as these have led to the concept of variable set points and a servomechanism model. That is, the central nervous system, under certain conditions, can raise or lower the level of function in a given system toward which adjustments are made. It is in this way that central neural states may act to modify autonomic regulation.

The complex interplay of neural, endocrine, and cellular metabolic processes outlined in the previous chapter illuminates the multiple determinants of level of autonomic function and has important consequences for further understanding. The first is that any given function controlled by the ANS, for example, heart rate, can only approximate a steady state and in reality is subject to a constantly fluctuating interplay of feedback from numerous other systems such as carotid baroreceptors, pulmonary tension receptors, gastric mechanoreceptors, etc., as well as being affected by many systems outside the ANS. The second consequence is that a given change in level of any one autonomic effector system can be produced by one of several different mechanisms. A rise in heart rate, for example, may be produced by a decrease in vagal tone secondary to subsidence of a gastric contraction, or by an increase in sympathetic tone following baroreceptor stimulation, occasioned by a fall in blood pressure due to pooling of extracellular fluid in the legs while sitting down after walking; the list can go on and on. The third consequence of this multiple servocontrol organization is that the response (to a standard environmental stimulus) in any given ANS effector function is greatly affected in degree and even in direction by the current status of continuing and reverberating homeostatic adjustments in other parts of the system as they play back upon the given response system.

These consequences create an extraordinary range of possible variability in autonomic effector function under natural conditions. There is a considerable degree of unpredictability even between observations of steady states and in response to even the most discrete and definable stimulation. The variability is large both within the individual from one point in time to the next and between individuals at any given time.

Some of the sources of variability can be

minimized by the controls which are possible in clinical laboratory investigation. However, very few studies have been done with the highly desirable control, for example, of extra-cellular fluid volume, which so affects cardiovascular regulation and then indirectly many other functions. Diet, temperature, humidity, and the activity of human experimental subjects, are arduous controls when they must be maintained for days prior to an experiment.

If this were the extent of the interactions at work in the functional control of the ANS, this section of the chapter would be shorter but less interesting. There are, in addition to the homeostatic feedback characteristics of the system, two major forms of servomechanism "override" exerted by the CNS. The first of these are the regular, time-related processes of circadian rhythms and of developmental changes. The second involve the irregularly occurring events in response to which the balanced homeostatic organization is overridden by central neural activity, apparently of higher priority, for example, by responding to symbolic environmental stimuli, such as a signal that an athletic contest is about to begin, before the physiological demands of the event itself.

❲ Man at Rest

No studies have been performed in which all or most of the interconnected systems of the ANS described above have been measured simultaneously in man even under basal conditions. Therefore, no complete picture is available of the patterned functioning of the ANS. A few investigators have been aware of the necessity of studying the *pattern* of levels of functioning and have emphasized the importance of the relationship of the level of activity in one function to that in another.

Sargent and Weinman,[86] in an intensive study of army recruits, simultaneously measured more than thirty physiological variables, half of them directly reflecting autonomic neural activity and the others involving water, electrolyte, and nutritional metabolic systems.

Repeated measurements were made at intervals over several-week periods and repeated at a different season of the year. Because the subjects were in the Army, they were under unusual control by the experimenters, so that such factors as diet and activity could be strictly prescribed throughout the experiments. The most striking finding in the observations made at rest was the great individuality of the patterns exhibited by each subject. Like fingerprints, the relationship of one autonomic effector system to another was very different in one individual than in another. There seemed to be no one characteristic pattern for the group. In the observations made on the same individuals at a different season of the year (six months later), the individual patterns had changed. Moreover, there did not seem to be any regularity in the kinds of changes in the individual patterns.

The complex nature of the interrelationships between component parts of the ANS, the extreme individuality of the patterns of ANS activity observed between individuals in the resting state at one point in time, and the inconstancy of a given pattern in the same individual with time (despite rigorous efforts to reproduce an identical resting state) are all fundamental characteristics of ANS organization.

These and other data are consistent with the conceptual scheme outlined in the Introduction, in which multiple feedback relationships between the widespread organ systems innervated determine a complex pattern of balance, subject to a host of environmental factors as well as to individual differences in relative set points. How certain environmental, internal biological, and psychological processes come to exert predictable control over this organization will be the focus of this chapter.

❲ Circadian and Other Rhythms

So far we have examined the functioning of the ANS only in the resting state and only at a single point in time. Repeated observations in man over a period of days disclose pronounced regular, rhythmic fluctuations in all autonomic functions studied.[27,62,66] The previous chapter has described some of the transduction mechanisms for altered neurotransmitter and enzyme levels. Although individuals show slight differences in the timing and scope of these fluctuations, everyone has daily high and low points in levels of functions, many of these independent of environmental lighting, activity, posture, and even of sleep. The low points generally occur during the time of darkness, and the high points soon after dawn and awakening, although there are many exceptions to this generalization.

Although these rhythms can be synchronized by such natural rhythmic environmental events as light and temperature change, and can be caused to cycle at slightly more or less than an exact twenty-four-hour period, they retain their rhythmic behavior in the absence of external cues, thus indicating the existence of an internal "clock" with rhythmic oscillations in set points of ANS function.[82] After prolonged deprivation of all usual daily cues (e.g., isolation in a cave)[66] circadian rhythms become desynchronized, each running at its own period, either slightly more or slightly less than twenty-four hours in length, creating a steadily changing pattern of relationships between individual functions.

Cyclic fluctuations of a shorter period, often approximating ninety minutes in duration, have also been described for some functions and are termed ultradian.[62] More familiar are the annual, seasonal, and monthly rhythms. Autonomic balance has been shown to alter in a rhythmic fashion in time with the human menstrual cycle.[107]

(Developmental Changes

Circadian rhythms in autonomic function are not present at birth in the human, with the exception of skin resistance. Most physiological functions studied show an ultradian rhythm throughout the first postnatal months.[39] Heart rate becomes circadian in rhythmicity at four to twenty weeks but body temperature requires twenty to forty weeks. The factors affecting the rate and regularity of development of these rhythms in early life is an area of current study. Both the inanimate and the social environment of the baby during this early period have been shown to affect maturation of rhythmic behavior.[1,85]

In addition to the ultradian, circadian, and seasonal rhythms, the span of an individual's life exerts its own temporal patterning on ANS functioning. Such levels of ANS functioning as heart rate and blood pressure are known to vary systematically with age in man.[4,59] Blood pressure rises with each decade from birth onward. Resting-heart rate increases after birth during the first few months, is maintained at relatively high rates in childhood, then shows a pronounced decline, reaching a low plateau in adolescence, and rising again slightly throughout adulthood. The pattern is very similar for at least one animal species, the rat, in which it is possible to determine some of the factors involved, Adolph[2] has shown that the rat heart responds to neurotransmitters from late stages in fetal life, and that developmental changes are neurally mediated and not due to maturational changes in the myocardium itself. Hofer's work[41,43] has demonstrated that the high rates during late infancy are the result of high sympathetic tone and that this is, in turn, supported by the mother through her milk which appears to act via a neural mechanism involving the CNS. The subsequent decline of heart rate in late childhood in both rat and man is the result of increasing vagal tone, which had not been present earlier.

The existence of distinctly different patterns of autonomic organization at different developmental stages and the interactions of environmental and social factors in the development of adult patterns are areas with much promise for future study (see below).

(Autonomic Responses

We have developed a picture of the ANS in man at rest under basal conditions as a dynamic system organized to maintain certain levels of function by an elaborate network of checks and balances. These levels of function, in turn, vary in a highly systematic rhythmic fashion around each twenty-four-hour period, programmed by an internal clock which is synchronized ("entrained") by certain daily recurring environmental events. The multiple interconnected feedback relationships described above and in the preceding chapter may alter the intensity and even the direction of a response to a given stimulus, depending on the status of these systems at the time of stimulation. Partly as a result of these interactions, the resting or prestimulus level in a single autonomic effector system can only be a rough predictor of response according to the "initial value" effect.[37,46,105] (By this empirical rule, response magnitude should be inversely related to initial resting level.)

As indicated above, in evaluating autonomic responses in man we must distinguish between (1) nonspecific or spontaneous activity bursts; (2) the final level of function attained during the response; and (3) the magnitude of change in level as a result of the response. Lacey[54] has emphasized that these parameters must be considered independently. He has also shown that responses in different autonomic functions (e.g., heart rate, skin resistance or blood pressure) to the same stimulus have a low correlation. As a result, *patterns* of responses will be more meaningfully related to stimuli than single variables. Nevertheless it is worth pointing out that a *general* relationship can be demonstrated to exist between measures of intensity of physical stimulation (e.g., touch or noise) and magnitude of response in autonomic variables (e.g., skin conductance, heart rate, or finger volume).[21] This simple quantitative principle operates in addition to a number of more complex qualitative determinants of direction and intensity of response which will be discussed later in the chapter.

The autonomic system is organized to respond to a large variety of environmental events in which the organism participates. These will be discussed below, beginning with the simplest and leading to the complexity of elicited emotional states.

Orienting Responses

A fairly uniform pattern of altered ANS activity follows a novel and unexpected change in the environment. For example, a sudden sound, even a weak one, or a sudden reduction in an ongoing level of sound, elicits cortical alerting with characteristic EEG and evoked potential changes, accompanied by a sudden increase in skin conductance, a fall in heart rate and in both systolic and diastolic blood pressure, vasoconstriction in the extremities and vasodilation in external cerebral vessels.[20,91] This response pattern becomes progressively less intense and finally disappears if the same stimulus is repeated several times (habituation), but may at any time be elicited again by a qualitatively different stimulus, for example, a tone of a different pitch.

If the stimulus which initially elicits an orienting response is repeatedly followed by a task which the subject is motivated to perform, it continues to elicit the same ANS pattern and fails to habituate. The stimulus now has "signal properties," continues to arouse attention, and may also arouse some ANS preparatory adjustments appropriate to the task which is about to be performed, e.g., tachycardia before exercise. The ANS pattern thus becomes modified through a process of conditioning (see below, under Autonomic Learning).

The Laceys[57] have studied the relationship between the heart-rate deceleration observed in response to a signal for a reaction-time test and the subject's performance on the test. They have found data to support the hypothesis that the ANS adjustments of the orienting response serve the purpose of increasing cortical vigilance via ANS afferent feedback to the CNS (see below under Afferent Influences.)

It is apparent that even such a relatively simple psychophysiological human response is in fact a pattern of great complexity. Real understanding of its nature is a formidable analytic task. At present the barest descriptive outline of the full pattern is possible.

Defense Responses

With more intense stimuli, the orienting response is discernible only during the initial portion of the subject's response to the first such stimulus presented, and is rapidly overtaken by another pattern, the defense response.[91] Some of the physiological characteristics of the orienting response are retained, (e.g., EEG activation, increased skin conductance and peripheral vasoconstriction) in a prolonged and intensified form. Other autonomic functions change in the opposite direction: heart rate and blood pressure are generally increased and external cerebral blood vessels are constricted. Muscle tone and respiratory frequency and amplitude are usually increased in the moments following stimulation at near painful intensity. These patterns and appropriate behavior have been elicited by brain-stimulation studies as described in the preceding chapter. Another characteristic of defense responses is that they do not cease to occur after the first one or two repetitions of the stimulus (habituation) as do orienting responses. They do undergo a complex series of changes in patterning with repetition, although little systematic data are available on this point.

It is worth noting that the behavior of the organism is quite different in response to weak as compared to strong stimuli (provided these stimuli have not acquired special signal properties). Weak stimuli generally elicit a turning of gaze and posture toward the stimulus and often result in approach of the organism to the stimulus, associated with conscious experience which may be described as curiosity or attention. Strong stimuli generally elicit withdrawal or even generalized escape movements, movement away from the stimulus and the experience of pain and fear.

There is evidence that some of the autonomic correlates of the defense response (e.g., increases in heart rate and blood pressure) may activate afferent ANS pathways serving to reduce cortical excitability and diminish or attenuate the impact of the stimulus upon the CNS[57] (see below under Afferent Influences).

The autonomic responses cited may also be viewed as preparatory mobilization of some of the characteristic physiological changes of physical exertion, preparing the animal for fight or flight. Increased survival capability of animals so prepared has presumably resulted in a selective process favoring this form of ANS organization during evolution.

Exertion

We move now to a consideration of the functional organization of the ANS during physical and mental activity which is sustained and organized over a period of time. For many years, the alterations in cardiovascular dynamics during exercise were explained as proceeding from increased venous return due to the pumping action of active skeletal and respiratory muscles and to vasodilation in muscle beds produced by the local accumulation of metabolites. Hemodynamic principles discovered in isolated heart-lung preparation were freely applied in unchanged form to the intact, unanesthetized animal. The role of the ANS was thought to be entirely reflexive, as in the Bainbridge reflex, whereby the increased cardiac rate during exercise, although mediated by sympathetic nerves, was thought to be reflexively dependent on increased venous filling.

Rushmer and Smith[84] have summarized the large body of evidence which reinstates the CNS and its autonomic cardiovascular connections as prime movers in the cardiovascular as well as the behavioral patterns of exercise. Some aspects of their work have been described in the previous chapter. Central to this chapter is their finding that the cardiovascular changes characteristic of physical exercise in the dog could be elicited either by anticipation of treadmill exercise or by brain stimulation under anesthesia, despite the fact that in these two situations no exercise occurred. Thus, although the behavior and the characteristic ANS cardiovascular adjustment pattern ordinarily occurred together and appeared to share common central neural pathways, either could occur without the other. This demonstration of the dissociability of behavioral and physiological events in the simple situation of treadmill exercise illustrates a fundamental principle of ANS function and of how it is organized in relation to behavior (and conscious experience) which I will return to repeatedly in the subsequent sections.

The autonomic control of regional vascular tone, and of cardiac rate and force of contraction during physical exertion, is brought into play with almost exactly the same pattern of changes during the performance of *mental* tasks such as mental arithmetic. Brod's now classic studies[15] show that the most frequent pattern during serial subtractions was one of increased cardiac rate and output, with a fall in total vascular resistance despite vasoconstriction in skin and renal vascular beds. Muscle beds, such as the forearm, showed increased flow and thus decreased vascular resistance. Blood pressure, both systolic and diastolic, rose slightly.

These studies by Brod and Rushmer and Smith, and others[15,84] employing simultaneous measures of cardiac output and regional blood flow, permit calculations of changes in vascular resistance by regions, and give a far more complete understanding of ANS functioning than the usual psychophysiological studies. For example, as Brod's studies show, two subjects with similar increases in blood pressure may nevertheless differ remarkably in the balance between cardiac output and total peripheral resistance. He was able to define a second pattern, occurring in a minority of subjects in whom cardiac output actually fell during mental arithmetic. In these people (four of eighteen studied), total peripheral resistance consistently increased and this could be attributed to increases in extrarenal vascular resistance exclusive of the muscular (forearm) vascular bed. All subjects showed increases in blood pressure, so that Brod's differentiation of subjects into "output" and "resistance" types would have been impossible without the multiple simultaneous measures.

Brod states that the test provoked "emotional stress," and gives as evidence that "subjects blushed, became tense and nervous and made frequent mistakes which caused them

great embarrassment." Thus, even in this very standardized task situation the subjects' emotional response became a major (uncontrolled) variable. One wonders whether the "output" and "resistance" types of ANS pattern could have been differentiated in terms of the emotions present while performing the task. The work of Funkenstein[29] and Wolf et al.[109] in the 1950s suggests, on the basis of the very indirect cardiovascular measures then available, that those who suppress hostility and do not express their anger at the experimenters directly, give rise to the "resistance" type of pattern. The vital importance of the relationship of the subject to the experimenter will be considered further below.

Appetitive Behavior

Since the process of digestion is complex and the autonomic physiology involved is adequately covered in standard physiology texts I will only mention that a highly reproducible pattern of changes in motility, secretion, and blood flow are set in motion by the ANS in response to digested food. The degree of higher neural control over this process is illustrated by the anticipatory changes in salivary secretion, gastric motility, and heart rate,[74] occasioned by signals prior to the appearance of the food itself and mediated by ANS activity.

Sexual behavior is characterized by many responses organized through the ANS, the central neural pathways which have been described in the previous chapter. Some of these are similar to those occurring with any exertion (greatly increased pulse and blood pressure) but many are quite specific. There appears to be a shift of blood flow to the skin rather than away from it as in ordinary exercise, and local vascular engorgement (e.g., lips, ear lobes, nipples, and genitalia) is pronounced and unique to this form of stimulation. Profound alteration in sweat and specialized glandular secretion, and patterned changes in respiratory depth and rate, are also mediated over autonomic pathways. The regular course of development of these changes throughout an episode of sexual intercourse for both male and female has been described by Masters and Johnson,[63] as well as the variations in timing and stages which occur. Despite the lack of sophisticated physiological instrumentation, their observations have made clear the general outlines of these patterned responses and opened up an area which had previously never been studied systematically.

Special Situations

There are a number of additional life situations, less commonly encountered than those previously described, which evoke pronounced autonomic changes. These have been amply reviewed.[27,104] Many of them may be considered to be primarily physical stressors, such as heat, cold, and centrifugal acceleration, but also arouse emotional responses and other psychological processes which participate in the final autonomic response patterns. Since many of the responses are quite similar to the defense and exertional responses already described, I will deal with others which exemplify a different sort of autonomic pattern, one in which marked *decreases* in cardiac output and other adjustments occur which appear to serve the function of conserving rather than mobilizing the resources of the individual. Brain sites have been identified which give rise to behavioral and autonomic patterns on stimulation which bear some resemblance to this class of responses.[61]

The most clear-cut example of this kind of response is the dive reflex. Present in most mammals, this sudden and profound cardiovascular adaptation occurs most clearly in sea mammals such as the seal, but also in diving birds such as the duck. It has recently been studied in man and in dogs by Elsner.[25] When a man immerses his face in water, while holding his breath, an immediate and profound vagal bradycardia occurs. Elsner recorded one healthy young man who sustained an eighteen-second period of asystole. This cardiac rate change is part of a complex pattern of readjustments. There is massive peripheral vasoconstriction which shunts blood away from all areas capable of anaerobic metabolism, such as muscle and the splanch-

nic area, thus preserving blood oxygen stores for brain and myocardium. The cardiac output accomodates to a much smaller functioning vascular bed by decreasing markedly. Sensory stimuli capable of eliciting this response include both tactile activation in the distribution of the trigeminal nerve, and the pulmonary afferent stimulation involved in sudden breath holding.[73] Anoxia does not develop in time to play a role in these immediate responses. Metabolic adjustments taking place during prolonged dives have been reviewed by Andersen.[5]

Forced—as contrasted with spontaneous—dives in seals have been reported to elicit episodes of atrial fibrillation and ventricular tachycardia[68] and Wolf[108] has suggested that some cases of unexplained sudden death in adult and infant humans may involve the mechanism of the dive reflex.

A response which is less consistent among individuals, but which can be elicited by a variety of stimuli is fainting or "vasovagal syncope."[26] Typically, the early phases of this response are characterized by piloerection, dilation of the pupils, cardiac acceleration, and decreased blood flow to the skin and viscera. However, blood flow to the muscles is increased greatly. (This vascular response is a critical element and can be largely blocked by intraarterial atropine, indicating the role played by cholinergic sympathetic vasodilator fibers.) A fall in systemic vascular resistance occurs, accompanied by a decrease in cardiac output rather than a compensatory increase. Blood pressure falls, systolic before diastolic, and finally a vagal bradycardia occurs. If the subject is erect, brain blood flow is seriously compromised and he loses consciousness. The slowing of the heart is not a necessary part of the phenomenon and syncope can occur without it. Muscular inaction may play a necessary role in the development of the condition, since the fall in cardiac output is partially due to lack of venous return from the muscular venous pump.

A lack of ANS support for cardiac output in the face of decreased peripheral resistance and muscle-bed vasodilation is the basic pattern of ANS organization in this form of syncope. The stimulus situation which most regularly provokes this ANS response is blood loss, and occurs in experienced blood donors after 15–20 percent of blood volume is removed. Pooling of blood and loss of effective blood volume by filtration of plasma into dependent limbs during prolonged maintenance of the standing position can lead to syncope, as it may occur on the parade ground. Cutaneous vasodilation in a hot environment is an ANS response which predisposes to the development of this more complex ANS response. Most interestingly, syncope may be provoked by apparently trivial stimuli which have signal properties (e.g., the sight of blood), or sometimes in association with physical pain.

The response appears to be one in which musculoskeletal inaction is superimposed upon peripheral ANS responses appropriate to vigorous exertion. This in itself does not explain the fall in cardiac output or the bradycardia. Graham[35] emphasizes a sudden cessation of the hyperdynamic state, and has found a subjective sense of relief just before syncope as, for example, when an injection has been completed and the needle is withdrawn. Engel[26] has evidence from other situations which point to a cognitive and emotional state of helplessness and "giving up" which immediately precedes the syncopal episode.

(Altered Central States

The relationship of central neural states to the functional organization of the ANS is poorly understood. Only emotional states have received much study, although they are vastly more difficult to reproduce and subject to numerous methodological complications. As a result, they will be considered in a separate section. Recent work on the state of sleep has made it clear that the ANS is organized very differently during sleep and even according to the subdivisions (stages) of the state of sleep. The fact that ANS response characteristics can differ substantially according to changes in central neural state has clear implications for our understanding of how the ANS operates in the complex situations developing in natural life when emotions, physical activity, sleep, mental tasks, cognitive processes, and psychological defenses are all operating together.

Sleep

Rapid "flurries" of changes in respiratory rate, blood pressure, finger blood flow and heart rate occur in close association with rapid eye movements during stage "REM sleep."[89] In addition, it has recently been shown that flurries of spontaneous fluctuations in skin resistance—"GSR (galvanic skin response) storms," occur predominantly in Stage 4, slow-wave sleep.[16] Heart-rate responses to an auditory stimulus (see Orienting Responses, p. 532) are found to be *more* pronounced and to have markedly different shape and latency during Stage 2 and Stage REM than when the subject was awake or in Stage 3–4 of sleep.[48] Furthermore, there was no habituation of the heart-rate response as long as the subject remained asleep! Another important difference involves the thresholds for activation of responses in relation to the threshold of arousal. In Stage 2, the EEG response (k-complex) first appeared to tones 30 decibels (db.) below that required for arousal from sleep. The finger-pulse response occurred 15 db. below arousal threshold, the heart-rate response at 5 db., and the electrodermal response did not occur until the subject was aroused from sleep sufficiently to show an awake EEG and made a motor response.[48]

These findings argue definitively against any concept of ANS function as operating on a simple arousal continuum from low levels of function during basal states in sleep to the highest levels during the heights of arousal in response to maximal stimulation. Rather, the functional organization seems to be reprogrammed during shifts in central neural state, so that specific response characteristics, spontaneous activity levels, and thresholds are all altered in a highly complex manner. Even such fundamental a characteristic as habituation can be suspended during certain stages of sleep.

During the flurries of autonomic activity

and inhibition in REM sleep, patients with borderline cardiovascular adjustment may enter frank pulmonary edema or life-threatening cardiac arrhythmia. It is out of slow-wave sleep that classic night terrors arise.[17] In these, profuse sweating and violent tachycardia have been noted, indicating intense autonomic activation. Mental content is usually fragmentary and indistinct, although intense anxiety is usually described. In contrast, ordinary anxiety dreams occurring during REM sleep may involve exceedingly vivid and specific hallucinatory experiences, also with intense affects aroused, but this intense emotional activation may occur *without* any alteration in autonomic variables recorded at the time of the dream.[80] Autonomic flurries are more regularly associated with periodic REM than with dream content.[4]

These observations raise an extremely important point to be kept in mind throughout the remainder of this section. The ANS is not organized so that there is any *necessary* relationship between feeling state and levels of autonomic activation. Emotions, or indeed any consciously recognized states, are not causally related to changes in the ANS and indeed the two are not necessarily associated. Both conscious state and autonomic activity can vary independently. It is this generally unrecognized fact which helps to explain why efforts to use the measurement of autonomic variables as indicators of mental state have generally been unsatisfactory or difficult to reproduce. In the example given, the state of sleep appears to act to dissociate the emotions from the autonomic responses. Our knowledge of how this is accomplished is fragmentary but we know that other conditions may have the same effect during other states.[87,93] Research needs to be redirected toward analysis of the processes responsible for full or partial dissociation between feeling state and ANS activity.

Transcendental Meditation

Wallace and co-workers have obtained data on ANS function during a relatively simple form of focused attention (transcendental meditation) and have revealed a hypometabolic state with markedly decreased oxygen consumption, decline in blood lactate, respiratory rate, and heart rate while skin resistance markedly increased.[100] Blood pressure remained unchanged. The EEG showed increased quantity and amplitude of slow alpha rhythm at 8–9 hz. These changes were compared with changes in a few subjects who were hypnotized or asleep; the oxygen consumption, in particular, was reduced far more swiftly and more dramatically during meditation than during either of the other altered CNS states.

Little systematic work has been done on ANS organization during induced alterations of consciousness and this appears to be a fertile area for future work.

Emotion

I have reviewed in some detail the organization of ANS function in a variety of relatively well-defined conditions and in response to relatively simple stimuli, in order to provide a base from which to move on to the welter of data which has been collected on ANS function in emotional states. If we view emotions as consisting of altered central states which interact with numerous other processes (described in other sections of this chapter) in determining autonomic response patterns, we will avoid much of the difficulty which has beset the area of the autonomic nervous system and emotion.

One of the major difficulties experienced by investigators in this area has been in collecting and adequately describing the psychological data with which they sought to correlate their physiological measurements. In fact, for a time, some seemed to be attempting to describe and even quantify emotional states *in terms of* measurements of ANS function. Other investigators, convinced by the results of such attempts that this was the wrong approach, adopted the position that qualitative differences in emotional state were of little importance, but that degree of arousal determined the intensity of a general ANS activation pattern consisting of heightened sympathetic activity in all portions of the system. This position is still held by many workers despite the considerable body of evidence which has accumulated against a simple arousal model,[56,77] some of it described above. Finally, much of the data collected in experimental situations fails to take into account such facts as the importance of the subject's preconceived ideas about the experiment and his relationship with the experimenters themselves. These variables have repeatedly been shown to have a determining effect on the degree, direction, and patterning of ANS response to the supposedly "standardized" emotional experience under study. For example, Weiner et al.[102] demonstrated that maximal physiological responses often occur on the first exposure to the laboratory and before the procedure for inducing emotional states was begun. Then, when the subject made up a story in response to a thematic apperception test (TAT) card but did not have to tell it to the experimenter, the autonomic responses were a fraction of those observed during the verbal report of similar mental content. Thus, the subject's autonomic responses were determined as much by his relationship with the experimenter as by the psychological stimulus being studied (TAT cards).

Studies in animals are leading to an appreciation of the highly specific autonomic patterning which is present during emotional states, and to an understanding of the processes which determine these patterns. Zanchetti[114] has shown, for example, that whereas cats show a diffuse, prolonged, bilateral cholinergic vasodilation during immobile alerting caused by the sight of a dog, a localized, discrete cholinergic vasodilation occurs with attack movement, limited to the moving limb only. Rats subjected to brief electric shock show decreased blood pressure immediately afterwards when shocked in pairs but increases after being shocked alone.[106]

The old view that autonomic nervous regulation is governed simply by homeostatic principles is no more erroneous than the more recent view that autonomic responses in man are determined by emotions and can be simply correlated with affects. To be sure, situations designed to arouse one particular affect tend in general to arouse a pattern of autonomic response which can be statistically differentiated from that occurring when a different affect is provoked.[54,72] However, simple tracking, tapping, or reaction-time tasks with minimal affective arousal, evoke similar autonomic patterns which likewise show a similar "situational stereotypy" as Lacey[56] termed it. Also there are the converse findings that some subjects show minimal or no response in the autonomic systems monitored, despite the presence of affective arousal.[54] From this evidence we must conclude that the relationship between emotional states and autonomic response patterns is far from simple. In fact, there is new evidence that the two may be predictably dissociated by manipulating the contingencies of the situation. Associations between emotional behavior and the ANS may be the result of frequent concomitance, rather than of a necessary functional relationship.

Brady[13] studied monkeys which were anticipating electric shock during a three-minute auditory signal immediately preceding the shock. The emotional behavior studied was inhibition of a stable, previously conditioned, lever-pressing response for food reward. The physiological variables recorded were systolic and diastolic blood pressure and heart rate. Each of a series of monkeys was followed through a long series of repetitions of this basic paradigm, with variations being periodically introduced only in the contingencies between signal and electric shock. These studies provide many examples of clear-cut alterations in autonomic patterning without concomitant detectable changes in emotional behavior. Likewise, changes in emotional behavior were observed to occur without alteration in the associated autonomic patterns. Furthermore, these experiments demonstrate how environmental contingencies affect both autonomic pattern and emotional behavior and suggest that the processes by which responses are evoked in the two systems may be functionally independent.

We thus confront again one of the central unanswered questions in ANS psychophysiology: what are the factors responsible for the maintenance and disruption of correlated functioning of emotional experience, behavior, and physiology by the CNS during life experience? Although other sections of this chapter describe functional characteristics of the ANS which bear on this question, there are several approaches dealing particularly with emotional states which should be mentioned in this section.

Psychological defenses and general coping mechanisms involving cognitive and behavioral processes intervene between stimulus and response in the human, and have been shown to modify the relationship between the situation and the affective and physiological responses.[72,112] Although more work has been done on this subject in the psychoendocrine than the autonomic areas, there is ample evidence that classical intrapsychic defenses as well as cognitive styles ("leveling–sharpening," "field independence–dependence") may modify autonomic responses as well as mental experience.[38,47,102] These findings generally describe an interaction by which intensity of affect and of autonomic reactivity are concurrently reduced by psychological processes which tend to ward off, transform, avoid, or blunt the impact of the potentially painful experience.

Another view, based primarily on clinical observations, describes the converse relationship: the repression of affects (particularly anger) is held to result in greater autonomic responses to a situation whereas affect expression reduces the autonomic disturbance. This theory is sometimes used as a hypothesis for the etiology of some psychosomatic illness.[3] Oken[71] has specifically tested this notion and found little general support for it. In fact, his data slightly suggest a contrary result. Systolic blood pressure, heart rate, respiratory rate, skin resistance, and muscle-blood flow were all somewhat *more* responsive in those subjects in the high extremes of affective range and lability. The low affect group did, however, show a statistically insignificant tendency toward greater responsiveness in three measures of peripheral vasoconstriction.

The foregoing study used healthy volunteers and it has been shown that patients with an illness involving the ANS (Raynaud's Disease) were physiologically more responsive in the organ system of their illness than healthy people.[67] In yet another study, Weiner[102] found that young patients with labile essential hypertension showed relatively reduced cardiovascular responses to an emotionally arousing laboratory situation. They showed reduced affective response and failed to show increased physiological responses. A few individuals were notable exceptions to this generalization. Until we can understand these and other contradictory findings, we must remain aware that there is still a great deal to be learned about the relationship between psychological functioning, affects, and autonomic responses.

For example, we generally think of the autonomic system as an effector system working on the internal environment, much as the musculoskeletal system works on the external world. Autonomic responses are thus viewed as regulatory, adaptive, or even pathogenic for *viscera*. And yet there is mounting evidence that autonomic responses may play a role in regulating *central* psychological processes and emotional states through afferent feedback. This new role for the ANS may force modification of many of our concepts regarding the role of autonomic responses and the emotions. Autonomic responses may serve to temper, modulate, and shape central emotional states.

(Afferent Influences

Perhaps the most exciting and least appreciated aspect of how the ANS works involves its function in conveying information from the internal organs to the CNS. This topic has been surprisingly neglected during years of research on the ANS and it is commonplace to find autonomic pathways represented in textbooks as one-way effector pathways. It is almost as if the collapse of the James-Lange theory of emotions (that they were *caused* by visceral sensations) took with it all study of ANS afferent function. The previous chapter has outlined the anatomy and neurophysiology of these afferent pathways.

Russian work on classical conditioning involving "interoceptive signaling" has continued over the years, however, and has demonstrated that humans can make very fine discriminations among visceral sensations previously thought to be diffuse and global.[79] For example, a water jet at one location along the small bowel mucosa can be distinguished from another several inches away, after appropriate training. Recent experience with biofeedback training suggests that information about internal states is available to the CNS, but is ordinarily appreciated only in the most vague and poorly differentiated manner. Training improves the clarity and discrimination of the internal perceptions and may provide the basis for some voluntary control over internal processes (see below under Autonomic Learning.)

A second area which has exciting potential significance for our understanding of ANS function, involves the role of afferents from cardiovascular organs in controlling central neural functions, such as attention, and perhaps in modulating affective states. The evidence for this concept has been reviewed recently by the Laceys.[57] Neurophysiological and neuroanatomical studies have been reviewed in the previous chapter. The most impressive direct behavioral evidence for the central effects of this afferent feedack has been provided by Zanchetti and co-workers,[7] who have shown that the behavioral syndrome of "sham" rage in the decorticate cat can be instantaneously halted by stimulating pressoreceptive afferent fibers from aortic arch or carotid sinus.

Lacey[57] has evidence from studies with humans, using reaction-time measurements, that decreases in heart rate immediately before a task may function to improve performance. This effect is presumed to be mediated through cortical alerting via autonomic afferent pathways, the converse of the inhibitory effects observed with increases in blood pressure. Obrist[70] has subsequently shown, however, that the decreases in chin electromyogram (EMG) and respiratory rate are equally

or even more closely related to performance. His data suggest a more generalized and complex pattern of preparatory adjustments capable of altering afferent feedback to the CNS over a number of different pathways. These short-term effects, mediated over afferent neural pathways, complement and/or counterbalance long-term effects of ANS activation operating over hormonal pathways.

These findings suggest how autonomic responses, such as increases in blood pressure, by stimulating baroreceptor nerves, may act to damp or even block central neural responses to environmental stimulation. This suggestion is a particularly interesting one because of the implications it has for psychophysiological theory. The ANS response is no longer viewed as simply deriving from or reflecting a central state but as having the function of feedback control over the central neural state. Here is more evidence that emotional behavior and autonomic responses may have to be studied as organizationally distinct subunits capable of having important interactions, rather than as components of a single integrated response pattern.

⟨ Individual Differences

In the preceding section I have described some of the organized patterns of autonomic regulation which are characteristically found during certain states, activities, and behaviors occurring in the course of natural life. The complexity of the patterns possible, the interrelationships of the various effector pathways, and their afferent feedback have already been introduced as contributing to remarkable differences between individuals in the actual ANS patterns shown under these conditions. Fortunately, we have some fundamental data to answer the following questions: To what extent are individual differences important? Is there consistency in these differences when the individual is repeatedly observed in the same situation? To what extent is a given individual consistent in his autonomic patterning in response to different situations?

Lacey[54,56] has found that the mean skin conductance and heart-rate changes of a group of college-age, male subjects during a cold pressor test can be reliably differentiated from the pattern of the group during a reaction-time test or during attention to a tape-recorded story. Differences in mean direction of heart-rate response, as well as differences in degree, characterize each situation. However, if the individual data are examined, many deviations from the mean group pattern can be found. Such individual patterns are not simply the result of random variability with time due to the action of interrelated variables such as temperature or fluid intake which may influence ANS function. Lacey has shown that individual patterns are maintained to a significant degree over intervals as long as four years and are thus consistent modes of functioning.[54] Here again, there are exceptions, approximately one third of the subjects showing correlations between test and retest below $r = 0.30$. Finally, if test situations are not too dissimilar, correlation can be found in individual patterns across different situations, although there are notable individual exceptions. In general, individuals show a significant tendency to respond consistently in a pattern which is characteristic for them. For example, one autonomic variable may be found to be minimally reactive to a wide variety of situations and another, maximally reactive. Interestingly there is some evidence that subjects with complaints in a given system tend to be most responsive in that system,[67] a fact with some implication for pathological mechanism (see below). In addition, subjects who are variable instead of consistent in their individual response patterns have been studied and found to differ, for example, in cognitive style.[54]

Thus we are faced with the fact that the ANS pattern is determined to a significant degree both by the situation and by the characteristics of the individual, as well as by uncontrolled factors productive of more random-appearing variability. The attention to individual differences has been far greater in psychophysiology than in other areas of biological study, where they are obscured by

analysis which emphasizes the cental tendency of large groups of subjects. The factors which correlate with these individual differences appear to be almost limitless, and yet we have only fragmentary information on the most obvious, the genetic determinants.

Most of the available genetic studies on autonomic function involve blood-pressure regulation, reviewed by Pickering.[76] Identical twins show extremely high correlation in blood pressures from normal to hypertensive range, fraternal twins less so. Rats can be bred to be hypertensive and so, apparently, can humans, although there is disagreement as to the mode of inheritance. No studies have been done on the *extent* of interindividual variability in blood pressure which can be accounted for by genetic determinants, for example by studying identical twins raised in separate environments. Other aspects of autonomic functioning have been more neglected, and no detailed study of autonomic response patterning in identical and fraternal twins has been done, to my knowledge. Despite this lack of real information, there is a strong tendency for genetic factors to be taken for granted as important determinants of autonomic functional organization.

Numerous investigators have attempted to understand the differences between individuals in ANS response pattern to a given situation as a function of their psychological response to the situation.[2,54] Others have found that enduring characterological or cognitive differences between individuals are associated with ANS pattern differences.[29,35] A focus on the transaction between the subject and the experimenter[101] or the patient and the therapist[54] is preferred by others, and here again significant associations can be demonstrated between these interchanges and the pattern of ANS responses.

All this evidence leaves no doubt that the regulation of ANS function is influenced by a range of neural systems serving a wide variety of affective and cognitive functions. We lack any unifying hypothesis through which these myriad influences can be logically arranged and we have no clear idea how any of these influences may become so prepotent as to cause alterations of pathological intensity which are not compensated by homeostatic regulation. Some processes by which ANS organization can be altered or molded during life experience will be discussed below.

⟨ Plasticity of Function

Throughout the discussion thus far, individual differences in ANS functional organization have been repeatedly encountered. For the most part, these individual characteristics are relatively stable, and are thought to be an expression of the interaction between genetic and environmental determinants in the previous life history of the subject.

In recent years, two kinds of research have begun to explore the environmental contribution to the development of individual differences in ANS response, the role of autonomic learning and the effects of early experience on physiological development. Both of these kinds of environmental interactions have already been shown to have the capacity to alter psychophysiological function in consistent and systematic ways. Knowledge of these processes may help us to understand the origin of psychosomatic illness, to treat such conditions more effectively, and even to prevent their occurrence.

Autonomic Learning

The ANS, in most of its effector systems, demonstrates the three basic forms of short-term adaptation characteristic of the musculo-skeletal nervous system: (1) learning not to respond (habituation); (2) learning by association (classical conditioning); and (3) learning by effect (instrumental conditioning).

The simplest and, paradoxically, the least thoroughly studied form of short-term adaptation is the phenomenon of habituation, the progressive waning of response to a repeated stimulus. I have touched on this phenomenon earlier when discussing the orienting response.

It must be distinguished from simple metabolic fatigue or adaptation of peripheral sense organs, and this is done operationally by demonstrating that after habituation, the effector system can be readily utilized for another response or the response can be elicited by a *qualitative* change in the stimulus used. Thus, habituation is a specific form of learning of immense adaptive usefulness in coping, physiologically, with a situation of unavoidable, repeated, or prolonged stimulation. This form of learning has been demonstrated in most aspects of autonomic regulation and has been reviewed at the behavioral, neurophysiological (autonomic), and cellular levels.[32,49,50,91]

An intriguing and poorly understood aspect of habituation is its duration. Obviously, if habituation were permanent, adult organisms would be almost unresponsive except to stimuli never previously encountered. Some responses, particularly to weak stimuli, return within minutes or hours after the last stimulus presentation; others remain inhibited for days. If habituation is carried out over a number of days, the specific effect can last for weeks. Months later, after apparent recovery, some responses will rehabituate in one or two trials, indicating prolonged residual effect.[32] Very painful and emotion-arousing stimuli or those related to the drives of hunger and sex show little or no long-term habituation.

There is evidence that habituation of autonomic responses involves central inhibitory systems and its rapidity is correlated with the rate of extinction of classically conditioned responses.

The second form of autonomic learning, the "conditional reflex" of Ivan P. Pavlov,[74] has received more research attention than any other aspect of autonomic functioning. In this form of plasticity, the kinds of autonomic patterned responses described above (e.g., in exercise or digestion) come, at least partially, under the control of previously neutral signal stimuli because of repeated temporal association. The sign heralds the event and subsequently comes to elicit the response which could previously be elicited only by the event itself. The signal is generally termed the conditioned stimulus and the event, the unconditioned stimulus. This simple learning paradigm has served as a useful model for the study of psychophysiological processes and even for the etiology of psychosomatic illness, wherein an organism responds in accordance with past experience in preference to current physical realities. To give a clinical example, classical conditioning may be involved when the asthmatic child in the city begins to wheeze at the sight of the car which usually takes him to the country, well before any rural allergens have reached his respiratory system.

Unfortunately, it has rarely been possible to study classical conditioning under the natural conditions of everyday life. The phenomenon remains a laboratory model and there are no data to tell us the extent to which this form of learning actually moulds specific autonomic responses in the individual throughout his development.

The range and variety of classical conditioning phenomena involving the ANS is truly impressive.[19,78,79] Almost any stimulus which reaches the CNS, including visceral sensation ("interoceptive" stimuli) can acquire the capacity to activate almost any autonomic effector system, provided an unconditioned stimulus can be found which acts through the CNS to produce a response in the desired autonomic effector system. The signal (conditioned) stimulus must precede the physiological (unconditioned) by an interval ranging from less than half a second to as long as a minute for adequate conditioning to take place. Centrally acting drugs serve as well as physical stimuli, such as electric shock, and with interoceptive stimuli much longer pairing intervals are effective. Generally, conditioned responses are small relative to the unconditioned responses, may fluctuate in amplitude after being established, and can even disappear after repeated elicitation. The timing of the conditioned response (whether "anticipatory" to the unconditional stimulus or coincident with it) and its magnitude are affected by: (1) the time interval between the signal and the physiological stimulus; (2) the intensity and nature of the physiological stimulus; (3) the central state of the organism; and (4)

the frequency, timing, and number of previous associative pairings. Repeated stimulation by a strong physiological stimulus may alter thresholds of response to mild signal stimuli, irrespective of associative pairing. This is often called "pseudoconditioning" and can be differentiated by the use of appropriate experimental controls.

This form of physiological learning can be conceptualized as a sophisticated extension of adaptive physiological organization. By this means the organism can prepare in advance for an environmental demand, such as a sudden burst of exertion, thus reducing the latency of appropriate physiological alterations, e.g., increased blood flow to the muscles. Indeed, some of the most elegant and complete descriptions of widespread classically conditioned cardiovascular responses come from the work of Rushmer and Smith[84] on dogs repeatedly studied before treadmill-exercise tasks. Such studies approximate natural conditions in which the signal stimuli are complex, often involving a whole environment including other people, and activate many sensory pathways. Likewise the unconditioned stimulus may also involve all aspects of ANS regulation in an organized pattern. These situations are very different from the excessively discrete stimuli used in the laboratory and a great deal less is known about the properties of classical conditioning under such circumstances. For instance, Hofer has shown[41] that in people who are currently undergoing classical conditioning experience, naturally occurring life situations interact with the conditioned state to release the specific conditioned physiological response well in advance of its usual time of onset.

In the course of the exhaustive research conducted by Russian scientists on classical conditioning, a phenomenon began to emerge which has greatly extended the implications of learning for an understanding of ANS function in health and disease. For example, Lisina (cited by Razran)[79] noted that although the usual classically conditioned vascular response to electrical shock was vasoconstriction, occasional vasodilatory responses took place. If the shock was made to terminate early whenever vasodilation occurred, there was little effect. However, if the subject was allowed to watch his own plethysmogram, he soon learned to vasodilate in response to the shock pairings and thus escape some of the electric shock. This suggested that the ANS response could be modified by an awareness of the consequences of the response, not simply by previous association of stimuli.

For many years it was believed that autonomically mediated behavior could be modified by classical but not by instrumental training methods.[51] In the last few years new data have appeared to demonstrate that the ANS may also participate in the kind of learning which depends upon the consequences of a given response.

In an impressive series of experiments, Miller, DiCara, and others[24,64] have demonstrated that salivation, heart rate, blood pressure, peripheral vasomotor activity, intestinal motility, renal and gastric blood flow can be either increased or decreased by a procedure of rewarding spontaneous fluctuations in the desired direction. The desired autonomic response can be progressively "shaped" to increasing magnitude by progressively altering the criterion level for reward by either brain stimulation or shock avoidance.

These experiments were carried out under curare with controlled positive pressure respiration as a control to rule out possible mediation of autonomic changes via reflex responses to a primary musculo-skeletal maneuver, such as breath holding, carried out by the voluntary motor system. Initially conceived as a necessary control, it was found that the learning effect was much more readily obtained under curare than under natural conditions and this has raised problems of interpretation of their results. Does the explanation lie in the enormously simplified afferent feedback available to the curarized animal, resulting in a relative amplification of visceral information necessary for instrumental learning? Or is it that curare and positive pressure respiration alter the central neural state so as to produce a unique functional organization not available to the animal under normal conditions? If the ANS *is* capable of instrumental

learning during the natural state, why are the changes produced in both animals and man so small in magnitude and require so much training to achieve by present methods? These questions are currently under intensive investigation.

Answers to these problems bear directly on the implications this form of autonomic learning may have for the behavior of the ANS in health and disease. If environmental rewards occur following an autonomic response and if this "reinforcement" increases the likelihood and magnitude of the ANS response when the situation recurs, this may be the way in which specific autonomic responses, such as syncope or bronchoconstriction, become unusually frequent and severe in some people. This idea will be enlarged upon in the next section but it is clearly of considerable importance to understand the conditions controlling the ease and rapidity of instrumental learning in the ANS.

A major issue in our knowledge of how the ANS functions involves its specificity. In the same way that the ANS was thought to be capable only of classical conditioning, it was also, until recently, thought to be capable only of diffuse discharge. We have noted the tendency for patterns of integrated activity involving all effector systems to be a common mode of operation. By differential reinforcement, again under curare, DiCara and Miller showed that it was possible for the ANS to dilate blood vessels in one ear and not in the other. Likewise, heart-rate increases could be produced without altering blood pressure and, vice versa, the same with heart rate and intestinal contraction. Clearly, discrete and specific alterations of ANS activity can be predictably demonstrated.

DiCara[24] and Goesling and Brener[34] present evidence that a *pattern* of musculo-skeletal, respiratory, and cardiac activity is in fact conditioned under curare, although the first two are not evident until the animal recovers from the curare. Rats previously trained for high heart rates under curare are more active, more emotional by various criteria,[24] and have much higher respiratory rates[23] than those trained for low heart rates when the animals are replaced in the training situation without curare. What is actually learned is a pattern involving musculo-skeletal, respiratory, and autonomic cardiac pathways. Further training without curare can separate the cardiac from the other physiological and behavioral changes, but no further increase in cardiac rate change is accomplished. Brener[34] has shown in another way that musculo-skeletal and cardiac changes are functionally interrelated and even centrally interdependent. Animals trained to be active to avoid electric shock, when subsequently trained to alter heart rate under curare, showed increased heart rate regardless of which direction of change they were being trained for under curare. Those trained to inactivity before heart-rate training showed decreased heart rate, regardless of reinforcement contingencies under curare. Thus, the direction of heart-rate change under curare was more powerfully determined by their previous behavioral training than by the more immediate autonomic training under curare. These experiments suggest that there are important interactions between somatomotor and autonomic learning experience. An understanding of these interactions may take us a long way toward learning how these processes may determine autonomic responses to environmental events in natural life situations.

The role of this form of plasticity in the *internal* economy of the organism is also of considerable theoretical importance. For instance, to what extent are homeostatic regulatory processes acquired through learning rather than developed according to genetic plan? Miller et al.[64] have shown that an excess of extracellular water or salt can function as a drive and that a return to normal water and electrolyte balance, accomplished by visceral hormonal and autonomic responses, can function as a reward in an experimental situation. The implication is that homeostatic autonomic responses may be acquired and shaped by the action of reward in the form of a return of the internal milieu to normal. Moreover, the imbalances caused by disease processes are countered by autonomic readjustments which may be learned in the same way through the effect of tending to return the internal state toward status quo. This important new hypothesis on the origin and maintenance of homeostatic functioning in health and disease urgently needs experimental testing.

A parallel development accompanying the growth of interest in autonomic reward learning has been the attempt to apply these training techniques to the treatment of disturbed autonomic function, such as arrhythmias of neural origin and hypertension. These techniques will be reviewed in subsequent chapters on these disease states.

To return for a moment to the experiments described above[79] the subjects did not change their autonomic response when rewarded by shock escape until they were provided with additional feedback over exteroceptive pathways by being allowed to watch the plethysmograph write-out. Brener[14] gave subjects an opportunity to hear their heart beat amplified and they were eventually trained to be able to press a button every time they felt their heart beat, in the absence of sound amplification. After this training in visceral awareness, the subjects were able to increase or decrease heart rate "voluntarily" to a significantly greater extent than control subjects.

By what strategies do subjects accomplish this "voluntary" control? Some use respiratory or musculo-skeletal intermediary behavior, others attempt to create certain mental states, and still others cannot describe how it is done. Contrived strategies are not always the most effective. In applying biofeedback to the therapeutic situation, no other reward is necessary to the patient than return of his biofeedback signal toward normal levels.[103]

This work is in its infancy and requires a great deal more carefully controlled investigation, but it promises to open up new links between conscious experience and the autonomic nervous system.

Early Experience Effects

Mounting evidence over the past ten years has made it clear that behavior, visceral responses, and even survival of the adult under stress can be predictably influenced by alterations in early experience during development of the organism.[69],[97] Of the visceral alterations produced in this way, the pituitary adrenocortical system is the only one which has been extensively studied. There is enough direct evidence however, to conclude that autonomic responses can also be shaped by these long-term developmental interactions.[10],[12,28] If autonomic neural regulation and response patterning can be influenced by early experience, then knowledge about these processes may help us to understand how a particular adult can have acquired psychosomatic vulnerabilities.

In 1961, during John P. Scott's classic studies on socialization in dogs, his co-workers[28] observed that if puppies were left in the company of other dogs without human contact for the first twelve weeks of life, they showed heart-rate responses to electric shock at fourteen weeks of age which were significantly different from dogs which had had as little as one week "socialization" experience with people when they were seven-week-old puppies. If the week of socialization experience occurred either earlier or later than seven weeks it was less effective in altering both cardiac response and behavior. This age was thus described as a "critical" period for the effect of socialization in the dog. The influence of restricted as opposed to increased locomotor, sensory, and social experience on the development of heart-rate regulation has been further documented by two independent studies.[10,12] They both showed higher heart rates in response to a variety of stimuli in adult rats which had been raised in early environments with increased stimulation. Restricted or isolated early living conditions, in contrast, predisposed to bradycardia in response to stimulation by noise. Handling of neonatal rat pups, known to produce an altered adrenocortical response to stress during adulthood, has been shown to increase the level of heart rate and decrease its variability during a period of stimulation of the adult rat by white noise. These demonstrations make the importance of early experience in the development of autonomic response tendencies clear but do not tell us *how* the experience comes to affect autonomic regulation in later life. As yet we cannot even say whether early handling works primarily by a direct stimulating effect on the pups or through altering maternal behavior toward those pups. Recent studies have shown that handling the mother can affect adrenocortical reactivity of her offspring in later life[98] and that separation of rat pups from their mother, at two weeks of age, produces a marked alteration in autonomic cardiac balance.[44]

Studies have shown that the influence of early experience is not confined to small differences in autonomic response pattern but can reliably affect mortality rates from starvation, surgery, and metabolic derangement as well as modify susceptibility to experimental gastric-ulcer formation.[69] In all these conditions, the ANS is known to play an important regulatory role and it is reasonable to suppose that altered ANS function may mediate these early experience effects.

Knowledge of the development of autonomic neural integration is just beginning to accumulate and our understanding of how early experience and its timing may shape the course of development is rudimentary. This is an area of active research interest which should contribute significantly in the next years to our understanding of the origin of psychosomatic illness.

⟮ Pathophysiological Mechanisms

Having outlined the functional characteristics of the ANS in relation to both the internal and the external environment, I will conclude and summarize by attempting to sketch how these characteristics may operate in the exacerbation or production of disease states during interaction of the organism with its environment. I would like to emphasize how tenuous the links are between what we know of autonomic functioning and the production of illness in the organism. The natural history of man is characterized by repeated adaptive challenges posed by his social and physical environment. The predominant function of the ANS is not only to respond to the envi ronment but to return to baseline, not only to react but to repair. As Richards has so elegantly described,[81] medical illness can be characterized as disordered homeostatic balance. Yet little is known of the factors which sustain imbalance or cause prolonged over- and underresponse. New data suggest that homeostatic organization may be acquired through physiological learning, rather than be dictated by genetic mechanisms alone. If this is so, some individuals may acquire the potential for prolonged disorders of homeostatic balance and thus a proclivity toward illness. We do not yet have any clear idea of how or when such characteristics might be acquired.

The ANS, through its central neural integration, is one of the prime organizers of homeostasis, and we may justifiably examine its functional properties in search for the mechanisms of disordered function and look to the relationship of the organism with its environment as an important contributor to the etiology of illness. But in our present state of knowledge we must do so with the intent of generating testable ideas rather than outlining established principles.

Although homeostatic regulation is organized to return function within the ANS to a set level, priorities appear to exist so that homeostasis in one area of the system may be maintained at the expense of severe disequilibrium in another. The example was given of temperature homeostasis being maintained at the expense of water and electrolyte balance during heat stress, in order to illustrate the role of the ANS in determining the form of physiological disruption following environmental stress. Since there appear to be highly individual patterns of autonomic neural balance and integration among the effector systems, certain individuals may be more susceptible and others relatively resistant to disruption by an identical environmental stress. These individual patterns may be predominantly determined by genetic mechanisms or by previous environmental adaptations such as a high-salt diet. Furthermore, autonomic functions fluctuate in regular rhythms leading to a period during the twenty-four-hour cycle when susceptibility to under-

or overresponse to a given stressor is relatively increased. During the course of development, autonomic balance changes markedly so that different life stages are associated with a greater likelihood of certain pathological responses. For example, clinicians are aware that autonomic responses to manipulation of the upper gastrointestinal (GI) tract, such as salivation, retching, and bradycardia are more intense during childhood and adolescence than in later life.

Autonomic responses to environmental stimulation and to mental and physical tasks appear to have some immediate adaptive function in preparing the organism internally to function more effectively in its environment. However, the repeated, frequent elicitation of defensive, alerting, and exertional responses has been demonstrated to produce sustained hypertension, vascular and renal lesions, and increased mortality in animal colonies under specified conditions.[40] Alterations of ANS function during altered states of consciousness, such as REM sleep, may precipitate episodes of congestive failure, arrhythmia or angina pectoris in cardiac patients because of the "flurries" of tachycardia, and bradycardia and vasoconstriction characteristic of the autonomic function during that state of sleep. Likewise, transient emotional states are associated with a wide variety of autonomic patterns and responses which may precipitate decompensation of chronic disease states. Stroebel[95] has found evidence that certain emotional states cause a prolonged disruption of the organized patterns of circadian rhythmicity. The resulting autonomic disorganization may increase disease susceptibility. Avoidance learning contingencies may serve to perpetuate such disorders of central neural homeostatic control.

None of these interactions account for the clinically observed fact that some people are unusually prone to *highly specific* kinds of autonomic responses of extreme intensity, for example asthma, in the absence of allergenic stimulation. The facts on autonomic learning and early experience effects allow us to build a theoretical model for the acquisition of such highly specific autonomic pathophysiologic response tendencies. It seems possible that a certain early experience occurring at a sensitive period may alter the genetically programmed development of reactivity in autonomic function, either through shifting baseline set point, variability, or the capacity to habituate. Such early experience may at the same time elicit a characteristic primitive emotional state. Then, through associative learning, a particular physiological response may become conditioned to signal stimuli which, at this development stage, characteristically precede physiological stimulation. The response is thus more frequently elicited and by ordinarily trivial stimuli. In addition, if the response tends to be followed by reward or by the avoidance of unpleasant events, instrumental conditioning may gradually strengthen and shape the autonomic response until a highly specific and intense physiological response is produced in that particular individual.

One may exemplify such a series of processes in the hypothetical development of bronchial asthma. A tendency toward respiratory hyperactivity may be set in motion by an early experience, such as maternal separation, which provokes repeated and prolonged crying, and a concomitant emotional state which may be termed "separation anxiety." Subsequently, exposure to heavy concentrations of pollen precipitates asthma in association with environmental cues which thereafter acquire the capacity to elicit mild bronchoconstriction over autonomic pathways. The parents respond to the mild wheezing elicited by these conditioned cues with exaggerated attention, gifts, and permission to avoid unpleasant duties. They may even cancel an intended departure from home. These rewards or "reinforcement," which may depend upon the emotional state generated by threatened separation, increase the likelihood and intensity of asthmatic episodes in the future. The child learns, perhaps without conscious awareness, that he can get what he wants by asthmatic breathing.

At this point, the emotional state elicited in this person by threatened separation has become associated (through classical and instrumental learning processes) with a highly specific autonomic response pattern: intense bronchospasm, mucous secretion, etc., that is, clinical asthma. Inborn autonomic correlates of an emotional state thus may become specifically modified by particular developmental experiences. The emotional state, however, is subject to further modification by a number of other psychological processes and experiences which may even disassemble this organization and "cure the disease."

The emotional states deriving from the early separation experience, and the human relationships built upon them, thus may become interwoven with the specific physiological effects of the experience on the development of the child's respiratory system. Both associative and instrumental learning may function to stamp in and intensify what might otherwise be a mild and transient period of childhood wheezing. Further learning and emotionally trying human relationships may finally generate the severe reactive asthma which has earned the term "psychosomatic."

❲ Bibliography

1. ADER, R. "Early Experiences Accelerate Maturation of the 24-hr. Adrenocortical Rhythm," *Science*, 163 (1969), 1225–1226.

2. ADOLPH, E. R. "Ranges of Heart Rates and Their Regulations at Various Ages (Rat)," *Am. J. Physiol.*, 212 (1967), 595–602.

3. ALEXANDER, R., T. M. FRENCH, and G. H. POLLOCK, eds., Psychosomatic Specificity, Vol. 1. *Experimental Study and Results.* Chicago: University of Chicago Press, 1968.

4. ALTMAN, P. L. and D. S. DITTMER. *Biological Handbooks: Respiration and Circulation.* Bethesda, Md.: Fed. of Am. Soc. for Exptl. Biol., 1971.

5. ANDERSON, H. T. "Physiological Adaptations in Diving Vertebrates," *Physiol. Rev.*, 46 (1966), 212–243.

6. APPLEY, M. and R. TRUMBULL, eds., *Psychological Stress—Issues in Research*. New York: Appleton-Century-Crofts, 1967.

7. BACCELLI, G., M. GUAZZI, A. LIBRETTI, and A. ZANCHETTI. "Pressoreceptive and

Chemoreceptive Aortic Reflexes in Decorticate and in Decerebrate Cats," *Am. J. Physiol.*, 208 (1965), 708–714.

8. BERNARD, C. In J. Fulton, ed., *Selected Readings in the History of Physiology*, p. 307. Springfield, Ill.: Charles C. Thomas, 1930.

9. BLACK, P., ed. *Physiological Correlates of Emotion*. New York: Academic, 1970.

10. BLIZARD, D. A. "Individual Differences in Autonomic Responsivity in the Adult Rat— Neonatal Influences," *Psychosom. Med.*, 33 (1971), 445–457.

11. BOWLBY, J. *Attachment and Loss*, Vol. 1, Attachment. New York: Basic Books, 1969.

12. BOYLES, W. R., R. W. BLACK, and E. FURCHTGOTT. "Early Experience and Cardiac Responsivity in the Female Rat," *J. Comp. Physiol. Psychol.*, 59 (1965), 446–447.

13. BRADY, J. V., D. KELLY, and L. PLUMLEE. "Autonomic and Behavioral Responses of the Rhesus Monkey to Emotional Conditioning," *Ann. N.Y. Acad. Sci.*, 159 (1969), 959–975.

14. BRENER, J., R. A. KLEINMAN, and W. J. GOESLING. "The Effects of Different Exposures to Augmented Sensory Feedback on the Control of Heart Rate," *Psychophysiology*, 5 (1969), 510–516.

15. BROD, J., V. FENCL, Z. HEJL et al. "Circulatory Changes Underlying Blood Pressure Elevation during Acute Emotional Stress (Mental Arithmetic) in Normotensive and Hypertensive Subjects," *Clin. Sci.*, 18 (1959), 269–278.

16. BROUGHTON, R., R. POIRE, and C. TASSARINI. "The Electroderm (Tarchanoff Effect) during Sleep," *EEG Clin. Neurophysiol.*, 18 (1965), 691–708.

17. ———. "Sleep Disorders: Disorders of Arousal?" *Science*, 159 (1968), 1070–1074.

18. BROWN, C. C. "The Parotid Puzzle: A Review of the Literature on Human Salivation and Its Application to Psychophysiology," *Psychophysiology*, 7 (1970), 66–85.

19. BYKOV, K. M. and W. H. GANTT. *The Cerebral Cortex and the Internal Organs*. New York: Chemical Publishing, 1957.

20. CANNON, W. B. *Bodily Changes in Pain, Hunger, Fear and Rage*, 2nd ed. New York: Appleton, 1929.

21. DAVIS, R. C. and A. M. BUCHWALD. "An Exploration of Somatic Response Patterns: Stimulus and Sex Differences," *J. Comp. Physiol. Psychol.*, 50 (1957), 44–52.

22. DAVIS, R. C., A. M. BUCHWALD, and R. W. FRANKMANN. "Autonomic and Muscular Responses and Their Relation to Simple Stimuli," *Psychol. Monogr.*, Vol. 69, no. 20, 1955.

23. DICARA, L. "Heart Rate Learning in the Non-Curarized State, Transfer to the Curarized State and Subsequent Retraining in the Non-Curarized State," *Physiol. Behav.*, 4 (1969), 621–624.

24. ———. "Learning of Cardiovascular Responses: A Review and a Description of Physiological and Biochemical Consequences," *Trans. N.Y. Acad. Sci.*, (1971), 411–422.

25. ELSNER, R., D. L. FRANKLIN, R. L. VAN CITTERS et al. "Cardiovascular Defense Against Asphyxia," *Science*, 153 (1966), 941–949.

26. ENGEL, G. L. *Fainting-Physiological and Psychological Considerations*, 2nd ed. Springfield, Ill.: Charles C. Thomas, 1962.

27. FOLK, G. E. *Introduction to Environmental Physiology-Environmental Extremes and Mammalian Survival*. Philadelphia: Lea & Febiger, 1966.

28. FREEDMAN, D. G., J. A. KING, and O. ELLIOT. "Critical Period in the Social Development of Dogs," *Science*, 133 (1961), 1016–1017.

29. FUNKENSTEIN, D. H., S. H. KING, and M. E. DROLETTE. *Mastery of Stress*. Cambridge, Mass.: Harvard University Press, 1957.

30. GALEN, C. *De Usu Partium Corporis Humani*, cited by D. Sheehan in "The Discovery of the Autonomic Nervous System," *Arch. Neurol. Psychiatry*, 35 (1936), 1081.

31. GELLHORN, E. *Emotions and Emotional Disorders—A Neurophysiological Study*. New York: Hoeber, 1963.

32. GLASER, E. M. *The Physiological Basis of Habituation*. London: Oxford University Press, 1966.

33. GLASS, D. C., ed. *Neurophysiology and Emotion*. New York: Rockefeller University Press, 1967.

34. GOESLING, W. J. and J. BRENER. "Effects of Activity and Immobility Conditioning Upon Subsequent Heart Rate Conditioning in Curarized Rats," *J. Comp. Physiol. Psychol.*, 81 (1972), 311–317.

35. GRAHAM, D. T., J. D. KABLER, and L. LUNSFORD. "The Course of Vasovagal Fainting.

A Diphasic Response," *Psychosom. Med.*, 23 (1961).

36. HALBERG, F. "Chronobiology," *Ann. Rev. Physiol.*, 31 (1969), 675–725.

37. HEATH, H. A. and D. OKEN. "Change Scores as Related to Initial and Final Levels," *Ann. N.Y. Acad. Sci.*, 98 (1962), 1242–1256.

38. HEIN, D. L., S. I. COHEN, and B. M. SHMAVONIAN. "Perceptual Mode and Cardiac Conditioning," *Psychophysiology*, 3 (1966), 101–107.

39. HELLBRUGGE, T., J. LANGE, J. RUTENFRANZ et al. "Circadian Periodicity of Physiological Functions in Different Stages of Infancy and Childhood," *Ann. N.Y. Acad. Sci.*, 117 (1964), 361–373.

40. HENRY, J. D., J. P. MEEHAN, and P. M. STEPHENS. "The Use of Psychosocial Stimuli to Induce Prolonged Systolic Hypertension in Mice," *Psychosom. Med.*, 29 (1967), 408–432.

41. HOFER, M. A. "Regulation of Heart Rate by Nutritional Factor in Young Rats," *Science*, 172 (1971), 1039–1041.

42. HOFER, M. A. and L. E. HINKLE. "Conditioned Diuresis in Man: Effects of Altered Environment, Subjective State and Conditioning Experience," *Psychosom. Med.*, 26 (1964), 653–660.

43. HOFER, M. A. and M. F. REISER. "The Development of Cardiac Rate Regulation in Preweanling Rats," *Psychosom. Med.*, 31 (1969), 372–388.

44. HOFER, M. A. and H. WEINER. "The Development and Mechanisms of Cardiorespiratory Response to Maternal Deprivation in Rat Pups," *Psychosom. Med.*, 33 (1971), 353–362.

45. HORD, D. J., L. C. JOHNSON, and A. LUBIN. "Differential Effect of the Law of Initial Value on Autonomic Variables," *Psychophysiology*, 1 (1964), 79–87.

46. HUTT, C. and S. J. HUTT. "The Neonatal Evoked Heart Rate Response and the Law of Initial Value," *Psychophysiology*, 6 (1970), 661–668.

47. ISRAEL, N. R. "Leveling-Sharpening and Anticipatory Cardiac Response," *Psychosom. Med.*, 31 (1969), 499–509.

48. JOHNSON, L. C. "A Psychophysiology for All States," *Psychophysiology*, 6 (1970), 501–516.

49. KANDEL, E. R. and W. A. SPENCER. "Cellular Neurophysiological Approaches in the Study of Learning," *Physiol. Rev.*, 48 (1968), 65–134.

50. KATIN, E. S. and R. J. McCUBBIN. "Habituation of the Orienting Response as a Function of Individual Differences in Anxiety and Autonomic Lability," *J. Abnorm. Psychol.*, 74 (1969), 54–60.

51. KIMBLE, G. A. *Hilgard and Marquis, Conditioning and Learning*, 2nd ed., p. 100. New York: Appleton-Century-Crofts, 1961.

52. KNAPP, P. H. *Expression of the Emotions in Man*. New York: International Universities Press, 1963.

53. KUNTZ, A. *The Autonomic Nervous System*. Philadelphia: Lea & Febiger, 1953.

54. LACEY, J. I. "Psychophysiological Approaches to Evaluation of Psychotherapeutic Process and Outcome," in E. A. Rubenstein et al., eds., *Research in Psychotherapy*, pp. 160–208. Washington, D.C.: Am. Psychol. Assoc., 1959.

55. ———. "Somatic Response Patterning and Stress: Some Revisions of Activation Theory," in M. Appley and R. Trumbull, eds., *Psychological Stress*, pp. 14–37. New York: Appleton-Century-Crofts, 1967.

56. LACEY, J. I. and B. C. LACEY. "The Law of Initial Value in the Longitudinal Study of Autonomic Constitution: Reproducibility of Autonomic Response and Response Patterns over a Four-Year Interval," *Ann. N.Y. Acad. Sci.*, 98 (1962), 1257–1290.

57. ———. "Some Autonomic-Central Nervous System Interrelationships," in P. Black, ed., *Physiological Correlates of Emotion*, pp. 205–207. New York: Academic, 1970.

58. LANGLEY, J. N. "On the Union of Cranial Autonomic (Visceral) Fibers with the Nerve Cells in the Superior Cervical Ganglion," *J. Physiol.*, 23 (1898), 240–270.

59. LIPTON, E. L., A. STEINSCHNEIDER, and J. B. RICHMOND. "The Autonomic Nervous System in Early Life," *N. Engl. J. Med.*, 273 (1965), 147–154, 201–208.

60. ———. "Autonomic Function in the Neonate: VII-Maturational Changes in Cardiac Control," *Child Dev.*, 37 (1966), 1–16.

61. LÖFVING, A. "Cardiovascular Adjustments Induced from the Rostral Cingulate GYRUS with Special Reference to Sympatho-Inhibitory Mechanisms," *Acta. Physiol. Scand.*, 53, Suppl. 184 (1961), 1–79.

62. LUCE, G. *Biological Rhythms in Psychiatry*

and Medicine. Washington: U.S. Govt. Print. Off., 1970.

63. MASTERS, W. H. and V. E. JOHNSON. *Human Sexual Response*. Boston: Little, Brown, 1966.

64. MILLER, N. "Learning of Visceral and Glandular Response," *Science*, 163 (1969), 439–445.

65. MILLER, N., L. V. DICARA, and G. WOLF. "Homeostasis and Reward: T-Maze Learning Induced by Manipulating Antidiuretic Hormone," *Am. J. Physiol.*, 215 (1968), 684–686.

66. MILLS, J. N. "Circadian Rhythms during and after Three Months in Solitude Underground," *J. Physiol.*, 174 (1964), 217–231.

67. MITTELMAN, B. and H. G. WOLFF. "Affective States and Skin Temperature: Experimental Study of Subjects with 'Cold Hands' and Raynaud's Syndrome," *Psychosom. Med.*, 4 (1942), 5–61.

68. MURDAUGH, H. V., J. C. SEABURY, and W. L. MITCHELL. "Electrocardiogram of the Diving Seal," *Circ. Res.*, 9 (1961), 358–361.

69. NEWTON, G. and S. LEVINE. *Early Experience and Behavior*. Springfield, Ill.: Charles C. Thomas, 1968.

70. OBRIST, P. A., R. A. WEBB, and J. R. SUTTERER. "Heart Rate and Somatic Changes during Aversive Conditioning and Simple Reaction Time Task," *Psychophysiology*, 5 (1969), 696–723.

71. OKEN, D. "Relation of Physiological Response to Affect Expression," *Arch. Gen. Psychiatry*, 6 (1962), 336–351.

72. ———. "The Role of Defense in Psychological Stress," in R. Roessler and N. Greenfield, eds., *Physiological Correlates of Psychological Disorders*, pp. 193–210. Madison: University of Wisconsin Press, 1962.

73. PAULEV, P. "Cardiac Rhythm during Breath Holding and Water Immersion in Man," *Acta. Physiol. Scand.*, 73 (1968), 139–150.

74. PAVLOV, I. P. (1927) *Conditioned Reflexes: An Investigation of the Physiological Activity of the Cerebral Cortex*. New York: Dover, 1960.

75. PICK, J. *The Autonomic Nervous System— Morphological Comparative, Clinical and Surgical Aspects*. Philadelphia: Lippincott, 1970.

76. PICKERING, G. *The Inheritance of Arterial Pressure in High Blood Pressure*. New York: Grune & Stratton, 1968.

77. PRIBRAM, K. H. "Emotion: Steps toward a Neuropsychological Theory," in D. C. Glass, ed., *Neurophysiology and Emotion*, pp. 3–40. New York: Rockefeller University Press, 1967.

78. PROKASKY, W. F. *Classical Conditioning*. New York: Appleton-Century-Crofts, 1965.

79. RAZRAN, G. "The Observable Unconscious and the Inferable Conscious, in Current Soviet Psychophysiology: Interoceptive Conditioning, Semantic Conditioning and the Orienting Reflex," *Psychol. Rev.*, 68 (1961), 81–147.

80. REISER, M. F. "Reflections on Interpretations of Psychophysiologic Experiments," *Psychosom. Med.*, 23 (1961), 430–439.

81. RICHARDS, D. W. "Homeostasis: Its Dislocations and Perturbations," *Perspect. Biol. Med.*, 3 (1960), 238–251.

82. RICHTER, C. P. *Biological Clocks in Medicine and Psychiatry*. Springfield, Ill.: Charles C. Thomas, 1965.

83. ROESSLER, R. and N. GREENFIELD, eds. *Physiological Correlates of Psychological Disorder*. Madison: University of Wisconsin Press, 1962.

84. RUSHMER, R. F. and O. A. SMITH. "Cardiac Control," *Physiol. Rev.*, 39 (1959), 41–69.

85. SANDER, L., G. STECHLER, H. JULIA et al. "Continuous 24 Hour Interactional Monitoring in Infants in Two Caretaking Environments," *Psychosom. Med.*, 34 (1972), 270–282.

86. SARGENT, F. and K. P. WEINMAN. "Physiological Individuality," *Ann. N.Y. Acad. Sci.*, 134 (1966), 696–719.

87. SCHACTER, S. and J. SINGER. "Cognitive, Social and Physiological Determinants of Emotional State," *Psychol. Rev.*, 69 (1962), 379–399.

88. SHAPIRO, D. and G. E. SCHWARTZ. "Psychophysiological Contributions to Social Psychology," *Ann. Rev. Psychol.*, 21 (1970), 87–112.

89. SNOWDON, C. T., D. D. BELL, and N. D. HENDERSON. "Relationship between Heart Rate and Open Field Behavior," *J. Comp. Physiol. Psychol.*, 58 (1964), 423–430.

90. SNYDER, F., D. R. MORRISON, and F. GOLDFRANK. "Changes in Respiration, Heart Rate and Systolic Blood Pressure in Human Sleep," *J. Appl. Physiol.*, 19 (1964), 417–422.

91. SOKOLOV, Y. N. *Perception and the Condi-*

tioned Reflex. New York: Macmillian, 1963.

92. SOLLBERGER, A. *Biological Rhythm Research.* New York: Elsevier, 1965.

93. STEIN, M. "Some Psychophysiological Considerations of the Relationship between the Autonomic Nervous System and Behavior," in D. C. Glass, ed., *Neurophysiology and Emotion,* pp. 145–154. New York: Rockefeller University Press, 1967.

94. STELLAR, E. and J. SPRAGUE, eds. *Progress in Physiological Psychology,* Vols. 1, 2, and 3. New York: Academic, 1967–1970.

95. STROEBEL, C. F. "The Importance of Biological Clocks in Mental Health," in E. A. Rubinstein, and G. V. Coelho, eds., *Behavioral Sciences and Mental Health,* pp. 286–314. Public Health Service Publication 2064, Washington: Govt. Print. Off., 1971.

96. THOMAN, E. B. and S. LEVINE. "The Role of Maternal Disturbance and Temperature Change in Early Experience Studies," *Physiol. Behav.,* 4 (1969), 143–145.

97. TOBACH, E., ed. "Experimental Approaches to the Study of Emotional Behavior," *Ann. N.Y. Acad. Sci.,* 159 (1969), 621–1121.

98. TOBACH, E., L. R. ARONSON, and E. SHAW. *The Biopsychology of Development.* New York: Academic, 1971.

99. VON BERTALANFFY, L. *General System Theory.* New York: George Braziller, 1968.

100. WALLACE, R. K., H. BENSON, and A. F. WILSON. "A Wakeful Hypometabolic Physiologic State," *Am. J. Physiol.,* 221 (1971), 795–799.

101. WEINER, H. "Current Status and Future Prospects for Research in Psychosomatic Medicine," *J. Psychiatr. Res.,* 8 (1971), 479–498.

102. WEINER, H., M. T. SINGER, and M. F. REISER. "Cardiovascular Responses and Their Psychological Correlates. I: A Study of Healthy Young Adults and Patients with Peptic Ulcer and Hypertension," *Psychosom. Med.,* 24 (1962), 477–488.

103. WEISS, T. and B. T. ENGEL. "Operant Conditioning of Heart Rate in Patients with Premature Ventricular Contractions," *Psychosom. Med.,* 33 (1971), 301–322.

104. WEYBREW, B. B. "Patterns of Psychophysiological Response to Military Stress," in M. Appley and R. Trumbull, eds., *Psychological Stress,* pp. 324–353. New York: Appleton-Century-Crofts, 1967.

105. WILDER, J. "Modern Psychophysiology and the Law of Initial Value," *Am. J. Psychotherapy,* 12 (1958), 199–221.

106. WILLIAMS, R. B. and B. EICHELMAN. "Social Setting: Influence on the Physiological Response to Electric Shock in the Rat," *Science,* 174 (1971), 613–614.

107. WINEMAN, E. W. "Autonomic Balance Changes during the Human Menstrual Cycle," *Psychophysiology,* 8 (1971), 1–6.

108. WOLF, S. "The Bradycardia of the Dive Reflex—A Possible Mechanism of Sudden Death," *Trans. Am. Clin. Climatol. Assoc.,* 76 (1964), 192–200.

109. WOLF, S., P. CARDON, E. SHEPARD et al. *Life Stress and Essential Hypertension.* Baltimore: Williams & Wilkins, 1955.

110. WOLF, S. and H. GOODELL, eds. *Harold G. Wolff's Stress and Disease.* Springfield, Ill.: Charles C. Thomas, 1967.

111. WOLF, W. "Rhythmic Functions in the Living System," *Ann. N.Y. Acad. Sci.,* 98 (1962), 753–1326.

112. WOLFF, C. T., M. A. HOFER, S. FRIEDMAN et al. "Relationship between Psychological Defenses and Mean Urinary 17—Hydroxycorticosteroid Excretion Rates, Parts I and II," *Psychosom. Med.,* 26 (1964), 576–609.

113. WOLSTENHOLME, G. E. W. and J. KNIGHT, eds., *Physiology, Emotions and Psychosomatic Illness,* CIBA Foundation Symposium. Amsterdam: Elsevier, 1972.

114. ZANCHETTI, A. "Emotion and the Cardiovascular System of the Cat," in G. E. W. Wolstenholme and J. Knight, eds., *Physiology, Emotions and Psychosomatic Illness,* pp. 201–219. CIBA Foundation Symposium. Amsterdam: Elsevier, 1972.

CHAPTER 24

CLINICAL

PSYCHOPHYSIOLOGY

Psychoendocrine Mechanisms

John W. Mason

❮ Some Theoretical Implications of Psychoendocrinology

THE RECOGNITION that endocrine systems are remarkably sensitive to both acute and enduring psychological influences is a relatively recent and notable historical development. Only since the 1950s have biochemical methods for hormone measurement become sufficiently specific, sensitive, and precise to permit reliable experimental exploration of the scope and significance of psychoendocrine relationships. As a result, it has now become clear that, in viewing central nervous system organization, the endocrine systems are properly regarded as representing a *third effector* or *motor system* of the brain, along with the autonomic and skeletal-muscular systems. The far-reaching implications

of this new insight for biology, in general, and for psychophysiology and psychosomatic medicine, in particular, are still only beginning to be recognized and put to creative use.

Perhaps the broadest of these implications lies in the new and strategically important leverage that recent knowledge of neuroendocrine systems provides in gaining an understanding of the organization of central mechanisms which *integrate the internal environment*. While the innervation of smooth and cardiac muscle and exocrine glands by the autonomic nervous system has been long recognized as a mediating link between the brain and selected visceral structures, the discovery of neuroendocrine systems extends the scope of central nervous system (CNS) coordination of the *internal* environment to the level of virtually every body tissue and cell via the circulatory distribution of hormones.[54] In a historical perspective, then, it is clear that lack of knowledge of this major mediating link between the brain and peripheral bodily processes severely impeded earlier efforts to deal with the important problem of how the many separate unit functions of the body are integrated or coordinated in the overall fashion necessary to maintain the exquisite homeostatic equilibrium of the organism as a whole. This problem has long been regarded by biological theoreticians as one of the most fundamental and crucial issues in biology.[3,95,53]

In general, the implications of neuroendocrine linkages for psychosomatic medicine may be viewed in two closely interrelated perspectives. First, hormonal responses may be viewed, from principally a psychiatric orientation, as *reflecting intrapsychic processes* and as providing a relatively objective approach to the qualitative and quantitative study of psychological mechanisms. As knowledge develops that particular psychological processes are determinants or correlates of particular endocrine reactions, then the psychoendocrine approach can become a very useful tool for the testing and development of psychiatric theory, particularly in the elusive area of emotional and related intrapsychic processes. Secondly, psychoendocrine reactions may be viewed, from principally a medical orientation, in terms of their possible significance in the *mediation* of the effects of psychopathological processes upon bodily tissues in the pathogenesis of psychosomatic disorders. It may be possible from a strategic standpoint, for example, to initiate an endocrinological search for abnormal hormonal profiles or altered response patterns in patients with psychosomatic illnesses, independently of psychological collaboration, if necessary, in order to test the hypothesis that characteristic endocrine abnormalities, reflecting integrative disorders, are regularly present in such illnesses. If such endocrine imbalances can be demonstrated, then the second phase, involving the more complicated and laborious work of defining the relevant psychological concomitants, of evaluating the role of nonpsy-

chological factors, and of establishing criteria for evaluating the pathogenetic significance of hormonal changes, could be undertaken with greater confidence that this conceptual approach warrants such a large investment of effort.

In the relatively brief span of two decades, there have been only a few preliminary ventures in psychoendocrine research into the study of psychosomatic patients, but psychoendocrinologists have been mainly preoccupied with the basic psychophysiological exploration of the significance of hormonal responses as reflections of intrapsychic processes. To put it simply, the principal orientation has been, "what may be learned about psychological processes by the measurement of blood and urinary hormone levels"? As is often the case following the introduction of revolutionary new methods, developments in the psychoendocrine field have been rapid and wide ranging, with many probing attempts to test the relative power and usefulness of new tools and to define the scope of their application. While the total body of accumulated facts is already quite substantial, the distribution of effort in psychoendocrine research has been rather uneven, with a few areas receiving much attention, while other important issues and approaches have barely been explored. Much necessary attention has also been given to practical obstacles in research technique. Particularly encouraging progress has been made in the developing and refining of difficult new methods, the devising of effective, often novel, strategic and tactical research approaches, and in beginning to solve some of the formidable human and organizational problems hindering efforts to achieve the interdisciplinary cooperation which is so essential to progress.[54]

In summarizing the status of psychoendocrinology, therefore, the general picture might be described as that of a young science emerging from an initial period of considerable flux and preliminary exploration, but now tending to move into a more stable period of consolidation and sharper focussing of effort. A number of reviews provide detailed summaries of research findings and dogma in the field, but also tend to present a somewhat incomplete view of the scope of issues and approaches, because of the disproportionate emphasis on a few selected research objectives and endocrine systems in most early research efforts.* Some principal aims in this chapter, therefore, are not only to outline highlights of present knowledge in psychoendocrinology, but also to point out gaps in knowledge, to present a more balanced theoretical perspective of the evolution of issues and approaches in the field, and, hopefully, to convey something of the historical sense of scientific adventure and breakthrough which has pervaded psychoendocrine research in its infancy. In doing so, the personal bias of the author will undoubtedly be evident, both in the conceptual approach and in a predilection often to cite firsthand experimental observations in preference to equally, or more, relevant observations of other workers. It is hoped, however, that the sense of historical and conceptual continuity and the broad overview of issues provided by this frankly personal approach may compensate, in some measure, for the lack of a more eclectic review of the field.

(Basic Scientific Foundations of Clinical Psychoendocrinology

While this chapter is oriented primarily in terms of clinical aspects of psychoendocrinology, it is important to recognize that interdisciplinary cooperation between many basic neurosciences has established a solid experimental foundation for the clinical field. Psychoendocrine research may, indeed, be viewed as beginning with the pioneering experimental observations reported in 1911 by Cannon and de la Paz that the adrenal medulla releases hormone in the cat during the emotional arousal associated with confrontation by a barking dog.[12] The apparent utility of the

* See references 8, 45, 49–51, and 83.

multiple physiological consequences of sympathetic-adrenal medullary response, in terms of visceral preparation for the strenuous muscular exertion required for flight or struggle or in preparation for injury, was brilliantly elaborated by Walter Cannon.[11] In 1936, Selye provided preliminary evidence that a second endocrine system, the pituitary-adrenal cortical axis, also with extensive influences on many metabolic functions, responded to "mere emotional stimuli" in rats.[89] It was not until about 1952, however, that the major breakthroughs in hormone assay methodology, such as the chromatographic Nelson-Samuel's method for the determination of 17-hydroxy-corticosteroid (17-OHCS) levels in plasma, ushered in the modern era of psychoendocrine research which has led to the realization that the scope of endocrine systems involved in psychoendocrine relationships is extremely broad. In the 1970s, in fact, we reach a point where it is difficult to exclude any endocrine system as being entirely independent of psychological or neural influences.[60]

Fortunately, the development of new hormone-assay methods during the 1950s coincided with availability of a number of important new methods and developments in the basic brain and behavioral sciences. The extensive work of Harris and others in neuroendocrinology demonstrated the functional significance of the hypothalamo-hypophyseal portal capillary system as a neuro-humoral link between the hypothalamus and the anterior pituitary gland.[28,29] This finding greatly increased the scope of neuroendocrinology, from concern with only the few hormones of the posterior pituitary, sympathetic-adrenal medullary system, and, perhaps, the vago-insulin system, to the inclusion of the many additional hormones of the anterior pituitary gland and of the target endocrine glands of the pituitary trophic hormones. Recognition of the hypothalamic-anterior pituitary linkage as a major point of neuroendocrine articulation, thus, provided an anatomical basis for exploring brain influences on secretion of growth hormone, prolactin, adrenocorticotropin (ACTH) thyrotropin (TSH), luteinizing hormone (LH), follicle-stimulating hormone (FSH), and, consequently, cortisol, thyroxine, testosterone, estrogens, progesterone, and related adrenal cortical, thyroid, and gonadal hormones, in addition to the hormones representing previously recognized neuroendocrine linkages, such as epinephrine, norepinephrine, vasopressin, oxytocin, and insulin.[48]

A substantial science of neuroendocrinology has consequently developed since the 1950s with the demonstration, by such neurophysiological techniques as electrical stimulation or ablation of local brain areas in laboratory animals, including primates, that not only the hypothalamus but also such distant brain regions as the amygdaloid complex, hippocampus, and midbrain exert modulating influences on hormone secretion.[62] Much of the work done so far on localization or mapping of neural influences on hormone secretion, however, has been limited to intrahypothalamic studies and to only a few hormones, particularly those of the pituitary-adrenal cortical system. Modern neuroanatomical knowledge of limbic system-midbrain circuitry and of direct and indirect projection pathways to the hypothalamus presents a most inviting opportunity for future systematic studies of the neural substratum for psychoendocrine processes, which is still a largely unexplored area, particularly in relation to such hormones as testosterone, thyroxine, insulin, and others for which excellent assay methods have recently become available.

Another important series of experiments has been concerned with the demonstration and characterization of neurosecretory releasing hormones in the hypothalamus, which appear to be the specific humoral links between the hypothalamus and anterior pituitary cells. Included are the corticotropin-releasing hormone (CRH), thyrotropin-releasing hormone (TRH), luteinizing-hormone releasing factor (LHRF), follicle-stimulating hormone-releasing factor (FSHRF), growth hormone releasing factor (GHRF), and prolactin-inhibiting factor (PIF).[68,77] These hormones and factors are presumably secreted by final common pathway neurones in the hypothalamus and

then via the hypothalamo-hypophyseal portal system act selectively to bring about changes in the secretion rate of the various anterior pituitary hormones. The hypothalamic final common pathway neurones, incidentally, not only represent an anatomical boundary line, but appear also to define a boundary line between scientific disciplines as well. In general, research at the hypothalamic level and below has been largely in the field of endocrinology, while research on higher brain influences on endocrine regulation has been pursued largely in the central-nervous-system sciences.

The field of experimental psychology has also made important contributions to the development of a basic science foundation for psychoendocrinology. While naturalistic approaches to eliciting emotional arousal in animals, such as by immobilization, crowding, etc., have been fruitful, the use of behavioral conditioning methods has provided a considerably more sophisticated and systematic approach to psychoendocrine studies in animals. As an example, in a "conditioned avoidance" procedure, during which a monkey must press a hand lever in the presence of a red light in order to avoid an electric shock to the foot, an organized and reproducible pattern of multiple psychoendocrine responses has been observed.[52] The contingencies of such conditioning procedures may be arranged in a great variety of ways in order to vary the quality or intensity of the emotional disturbance which is elicited.[46,47,49]

While it is beyond the scope of this chapter to elaborate further on how the basic brain disciplines may be useful, particularly in various interdisciplinary combinations in the study of psychoendocrine mechanisms, it is important for the clinician to keep in mind that a growing body of knowledge, developing from neuroanatomical, electrophysiological, experimental psychological, neurochemical, and neuropharmacological approaches, is building a substantial basic science foundation which complements, supplements, and illuminates related research in clinical psychoendocrinology.

⟨ The Development of Issues and Approaches in Clinical Psychoendocrinology

The Sensitivity of the Pituitary-Adrenal Cortical System to Psychological Influences

While W. B. Cannon had laid the groundwork for psychoendocrinology almost forty years earlier with his work on the sympathetic-adrenal medullary system, it is a curious historical fact that modern psychoendocrine research evolved largely out of a period of intensive, popular interest in the pituitary-adrenal cortical system, following the publication of Selye's sweeping and provocative "stress" concepts in 1950. Selye's "stress" formulations, ascribing special importance to the apparent "non-specificity" of the pituitary-adrenal cortical response to "nocuous" stimuli,[90,55] had a considerable impact not only on endocrinological research, but also intrigued many behavioral scientists because of the implication of psychological stimuli among the various "stressors" capable of eliciting ACTH release. The findings of Selye and other workers prior to the early 1950s were based on relatively indirect and crude indices of adrenal cortical activity, however, so that a foremost objective in the psychoendocrine field, when the reliable, chromatographic, microanalytical methods for 17-OHCS measurements in blood and urine became available after 1952, was simply to see if the earlier observations of corticosteroid responses to psychological stimuli could be confirmed by more refined endocrinological and psychological methods. Many endocrinologists were initially rather skeptical that psychological factors would be found to play a significant role in pituitary-adrenal cortical regulation in comparison with such drastic physical stimuli as trauma, exercise, cold, fasting, hemorrhage, and so on. Considerable attention was, therefore, devoted in early psychoendocrine experiments to the elimination or control of physical stimuli as independent variables. The burden

of proof, in a sense, was on the psychoendocrinologist to rule out, in rigorous fashion, any remote possibility that concomitant physical stimuli, particularly muscular activity, might be causing corticosteroid changes attributed to psychological influences.

Within several years, substantial and convincing evidence emerged from many laboratories, using a variety of experimental approaches, which established beyond any reasonable doubt the reality of pituitary-adrenal cortical responsiveness to psychological influences. Particularly influential among these early experiments were the rather captivating observations of Thorn, Fox, and their co-workers, on Harvard oarsmen in relation to the annual Harvard-Yale crew race. Indications of increased adrenal cortical activity on the race day were observed, not only in the crew members, but in the coach and coxswain as well.[93] In 1956, a report of later extensions of these studies indicated that psychological factors associated with competition or with time-trial sessions were far more potent determinants of urinary 17-OHCS elevations than muscular work alone.[31] Also capitalizing on natural stressful life situations, Bliss and his co-workers reported in 1956 that plasma or urinary 17-OHCS increases were prevalent in medical students taking final college examinations, in relatives of emergency room patients, and in subjects exposed to a variety of other natural and contrived situations associated with emotional reactions.[5] Board et al. reported marked plasma 17-OHCS elevations in acutely disturbed psychiatric patients, and correlations were observed between the intensity of endocrine and psychological disturbances.[6] The demonstration by Mason et al. of consistent plasma 17-OHCS elevations in rhesus monkeys during conditioned emotional disturbances permitted systematic separation of psychological from physical factors as experimental determinants of hormone release. Chair-restrained monkeys pressing a hand lever to avoid an aversive stimulus during "conditioned avoidance" sessions, as one example, showed marked plasma 17-OHCS responses, while the same monkeys, pressing the lever at an equal or greater rate in order to obtain food, showed no 17-OHCS elevations, thus militating against the variable of muscular activity associated with lever pressing as a determinant of 17-OHCS release in the "avoidance" situation.[57] A host of other psychoendocrine studies involving stressful life situations such as aircraft flight, anticipation of surgery, military combat, hospital admission, etc., compiled overwhelming and consistent evidence of pituitary-adrenal cortical response to emotional stimuli in human subjects.[49]

By the late 1950s, then, it was generally recognized not only that psychoendocrinology rested on a solid experimental foundation, but that psychological stimuli were, in fact, among the most potent of all natural stimuli to the pituitary-adrenal cortical system. The potency of psychological stimuli in ACTH regulation was evident not only in the marked 17-OHCS elevations observed in severely stressful life situations in normal subjects and in the even greater increases seen during some acute psychiatric disturbances, but was perhaps most impressively demonstrated in the striking sensitivity with which relatively subtle environmental or psychological influences were often reflected in 17-OHCS levels. In the rhesus monkey, for example, urinary 17-OHCS levels reflected the day-to-day level of activity in the laboratory in which animals were housed, being highest on Monday, fairly stable from Tuesday to Friday, and decreasing by 30 percent during the weekend when people were absent.[46] When the same monkeys were transferred from a busy, active laboratory setting to a quiet, private room, and screened visually from each other, their chronic, mean basal 17-OHCS level consistently ran 50 percent lower than in the original setting.[56] Many workers were impressed by the sensitivity of 17-OHCS levels to such factors as the "first experience" or novelty effect, population density, and various, often seemingly minor, social influences.[13,49,56] Studies of plasma 17-OHCS levels in normal young adults viewing commercial motion pictures provided one particularly striking demonstration of the sensitivity of this psychoendocrine system. In the

same group of subjects, 17-OHCS levels were observed to rise during a distressing war movie, and then to decrease sharply on two other occasions during the observation of Disney nature films, as shown in Figure 24–1.[96]

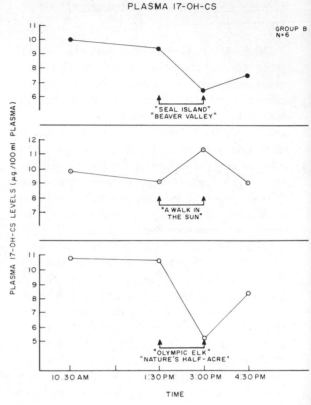

Figure 24–1. Elevation and suppression of plasma 17-OHCS levels in group of normal young adults viewing commercial movies.[95] (U.S. Army photograph.)

These and many other observations indicated not only great sensitivity of hormonal response to psychosocial stimuli, but also suggested that the concept of "tonicity," similar to that in the autonomic and skeletal-muscular effector systems, applies to the neuroendocrine systems as well. Rather than to use the concept of a "normal," absolute hormonal level, it may be more valid to think in terms of an ongoing "basal" or "tonic" 17-OHCS level in any given individual which may be either raised or lowered on an acute or chronic basis, depending upon environmental, psychological, or other factors.

The unequivocal and repeated demonstration of the sensitivity of the pituitary-adrenal cortical system to psychological stimuli, isolated from attendant physical stimuli by various experimental approaches, may be viewed, then, as representing a historically important and decisive first phase of psychoendocrine research which established the field as a viable science and opened the way for future development. If there has been experimental overemphasis in any phase of psychoendocrine research, it was probably in these initial studies directed at the question "Does the pituitary-adrenal cortical system respond to psychological stimuli or not"? For some time after it was settled beyond any reasonable doubt that psychological stimuli elicited ACTH release, there was a tendency for workers to continue to devote considerable research effort to adding still more stressful situations to the list of those in which ACTH-cortisol release occurs. It appears, in fact, that this question was viewed by many as the principal, if not the sole, issue in the field and that much general interest and participation was withdrawn at the conclusion of this phase of psychoendocrine research.

As a smaller group of workers persisted in psychoendocrine research, however, it became increasingly clear that many important issues and approaches remained to be explored. A survey of some of these less well recognized issues and approaches is a special objective of this chapter. It should be borne in mind that, in the discussion of psychiatric theory, the vantage point of the author is not that of a clinical psychiatrist, but rather of a physiologist who has worked in close collaboration with research psychiatrists for many years. It should also be emphasized that the major part of the work on the development of concepts in psychoendocrinology up to the present time is based upon research on the pituitary-adrenal cortical and sympathetic-adrenal medullary systems. The resultant emphasis on these systems in this chapter should not be construed necessarily as implying that they have a preeminent role in the psychoendocrine apparatus as a whole. Only similarly intensive future study of the pituitary-thyroid, pituitary-gonadal, and other neuroendocrine systems can eventually provide a proper perspective concerning the relative significance of individual systems in psychoendocrinology.

Psychoendocrine Reflections of Emotional States

In the initial phase of psychoendrocrine research when primary emphasis was largely on isolating psychological stimuli in "pure" form from physical stimuli, and on evaluating the relative sensitivity of hormone levels to psychological versus "physical" stimuli, only rather scattered and preliminary efforts were made to define the *nature* of the psychological mechanisms which were reflected in hormonal responses. The general and plausible assumption was that hormonal levels were probably a rather direct index of emotional state, particularly of the level of anxiety. Many early studies simply employed situational criteria of threat, with the assumption that a given situation would be anxiety-provoking to the subjects, but without validating this assumption by objective psychological assessment of actual emotional reactions in relation to hormonal responses in individual subjects.

A number of laboratories, however, began to deal with this difficult issue directly and to develop or evaluate psychological methods which would permit correlational studies, comparing hormonal levels with specific emotional states. A principal approach was the development of relatively objective and reproducible methods for clinical assessment of the levels of anxiety, depression, and anger on a roughly quantitative rating scale. Special care was taken to evaluate and develop intraobserver and interobserver reliability in these methods. As was expected, such ratings did show significant correlations with 17-OHCS levels under certain conditions. Persky et al., for example, found that objective ratings of increase in anxiety, depression, and anger were proportional to changes in plasma 17-OHCS levels in anxious patients during stressful interviews.[71]

Another approach was the use by Price et al. of projective tests to evaluate affective state and 17-OHCS correlations in patients on the day before elective cardiac surgery.[74] In this study, significant correlations were not observed between 17-OHCS levels and any specific affective state, such as anxiety or anger, but rather with several measures such as the neutral content, introversive tendencies, extended F+ percent and unpleasant content, all of which may be regarded as reflecting emotionality in a more general sense. As additional experience accumulated in the human, with such techniques as estimates or ratings of affect based on psychiatric interview and observation, clinical psychological testing, and self-reporting by subjects, it was generally found that, while these techniques were useful in establishing rather rough, general correlations between emotional reactions and 17-OHCS levels, this hormonal system did not appear to be related to any one specific affect, such as anxiety. Together with studies in experimental animals, the clinical studies suggested the general conclusion, rather, that 17-OHCS levels reflect a rather undifferentiated psychological state, for which such terms as arousal, hyperalerting, involvement, or anticipation of coping activity might be appropriate. In other words, while 17-OHCS levels may be a useful index of the *occurrence, intensity* and perhaps *duration* of emotional arousal, the pituitary-adrenal cortical system alone did not appear to provide leverage in the study of the *qualitative differentiation* of affective states. It should be emphasized, however, that more intensive, in-depth, psychodynamic studies remain to be undertaken, particularly with regard to such questions, for example, as the 17-OHCS reflections of anger and the various ways anger is handled or expressed, or with regard to pleasant states of arousal. The work of Levi and his co-workers has indicated that certain pleasant states, such as sexual arousal, are associated with catecholamine elevations and suggests the need for further systematic study of pleasant stimuli in psychoendocrine research.[43,45]

A rather promising approach to the issue of whether endocrine indices may be used to differentiate emotional states, however, has emerged from other studies of the sympathetic-adrenal medullary system. Although chromatographic methods for measurement of plasma and urinary catecholamines were available during the 1950s, considerably less attention was devoted to the catecholamines than to the corticosteroids in psychoendocrine research. One of the practical reasons for this, no doubt, was the greater difficulty of the fluorimetric methods used for catecholamine analysis, particularly in the plasma. Earlier psychophysiological studies by Ax[1] and by Funkenstein et al.,[26] based upon cardiovascular indices, had suggested that epinephrine and norepinephrine might be differentially related to fear and anger reactions. Funkenstein et al., for example, postulated that anger directed "outwardly" is associated with norepinephrine predominance, while anger direct "inwardly" is reflected in epinephrine predominance. Curiously, these intriguing early leads have not yet been thoroughly evaluated with modern psychoendocrine techniques, although a few more or less incidental observations have been made in clinical studies of urinary catecholamine levels which appear consistent with Funkenstein's hypothesis. Some studies of plasma corticosteroid and catecholamine patterns during acute emotional disturbances in the monkey have also provided encouragement for further exploration of the psychoendocrine differentiation of emotional states. In a study of six different psychologically stressful situations, all associated with plasma 17-OHCS and norepinephrine elevations in the monkey, significant plasma epinephrine elevations were observed in only three of the situations. Thus, two psychoendocrine reaction patterns were defined, pattern 1 with 17-OHCS and norepinephrine, but not epinephrine, elevation and pattern 2 with elevation of all three hormones. In general, the most striking distinction between the situations associated with the two different hormonal response patterns was apparently the presence of a high degree of unpredictability, uncertainty, or ambiguity in the pattern-2 situations. Unpleasant elements were present in all situations, but in the pattern-1 situations the animal knew exactly what to expect, while in the pattern-2 situations the animal knew threatening events were likely, but did not know exactly what they would be or when to expect them.[58,61] When one also considers that such hormones as thyroxine, testosterone, insulin, growth hormone, and estrone can now be determined quantitatively by reliable assays and have been shown to respond to psychological stimuli,[52] it is clear that the issue of psychoendocrine differentiation of both acute and sustained emotional states remains largely an open question, and there is a need for further resourceful and systematic research along these lines, particularly in longitudinal studies of human subjects.

Psychoendocrine Reflections of Psychological Defenses

One of the most fascinating and illuminating approaches in psychoendocrinology has developed from recurrent observations of the marked individual variations in psychoendocrine reactions between different people exposed to the same stressful situation. In the face of a real, life-threatening event, such as cardiac surgery, for example, some subjects showed marked anticipatory 17-OHCS responses, while others showed little or no 17-OHCS change.[74] Although such observations were at first often regarded with annoyance, since they diminished the significance of group-mean levels in data analysis, it soon became clear that a fundamental and intriguing question was raised concerning the psychological correlates of these individual differences in endocrine response to a seriously threatening event. The simple logic which emerged as this issue was faced, was that if 17-OHCS levels provide a sensitive index of general emotional arousal, as had already been established, by the same token they should provide a means of studying the opposing psychological forces which prevent, minimize, or counteract emotional arousal in the face of threat.

While a number of early workers recognized this issue,[74,21,70] the emergence of this approach is particularly well illustrated in the psychoendocrine studies by Friedman et al.,[25] and Wolff et al.,[98,99] of "chronic psychological stress" in the parents of children with leu-

kemia. One of the most striking findings in these parents was the persistence of characteristic individual differences between subjects in chronic mean basal urinary 17-OHCS levels over periods of months or years. Figure 24–2 summarizes the mean 17-OHCS levels and the range of fluctuation, representing repeated sampling over many months, in a group of mothers during the course of their child's leukemic illness. While a few subjects showed a substantial range of fluctuation, most of the mothers maintained stable levels with a remarkably constricted range and could be characterized with some confidence as individually falling into "high" (above 6 mg./day), "middle" (between 4–6 mg./day), and "low" (below 4mg./day) subgroups on the basis of chronic mean basal urinary 17-OHCS levels. Considering the tragic and disruptive circumstances, the presence of average or low mean 17-OHCS values in most subjects suggested the operation of remarkably effective defensive psychological mechanisms. Injection of ACTH and other observations indicated that adrenal exhaustion was not the explanation.[25] The fact that some individual subjects with the lowest chronic mean 17-OHCS levels tended to suppress their levels *even lower* on days when stressful or unpleasant events occurred, in contrast to "high" subjects whose levels usually rose still higher on stressful occasions, as shown in Figure 24–3, especially drew attention to the possibility of *suppressive* or *overcompensatory* defensive psychological mechanisms as being reflected in 17-OHCS levels in the "low" group. An exploratory survey of defensive organization revealed that several of the subjects with the lowest mean 17-OHCS levels characteristically employed denial to a marked degree in coping with the implications of their child's illness. These and other preliminary observations were sufficiently suggestive of the reflection of defensive styles in chronic 17-OHCS levels that a predictive psychiatric study was done, in which correlations between mean 17-OHCS level, as predicted by the psychiatric assessment of the effectiveness of psychological defenses, and the actual chronic mean basal level were examined and found to be significant both for

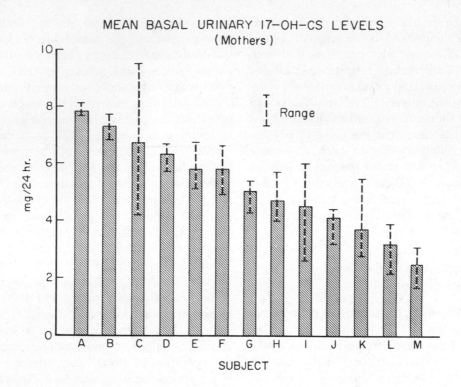

Figure 24–2. Individual differences in chronic mean urinary 17-OHCS levels between mothers of fatally ill children.[97] (U.S. Army photograph.)

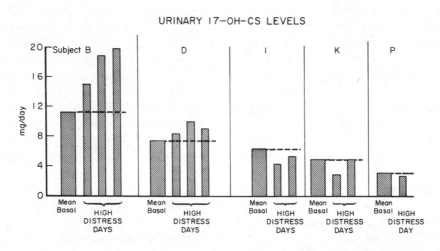

Figure 24–3. Difference in direction of 17-OHCS response to superimposed acute disturbance in some "high" versus "low" 17-OHCS excretors included in Figure 24–2.[47] (U.S. Army photograph.)

the fathers ($r = 0.80$) and the mothers ($r = 0.59$).[98]

There were some particularly illuminating anecdotal observations in certain parents in whom temporary relinquishment or ineffectiveness of habitual defenses were associated

with prompt and dramatic 17-OHCS changes. Figure 24–4, for example, presents the case of a mother in whom the predictive psychiatric interviews were associated inadvertently with the undermining of her usual defenses of detachment and rationalization. During the in-

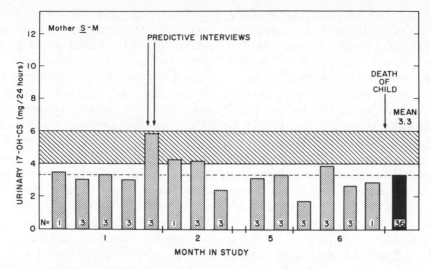

Figure 24–4. Longitudinal study showing 17-OHCS response to relinquishment of psychological defenses during psychiatric interviews.[98] (U.S. Army photograph.)

terviews, which represented her first experience with a psychiatrist, there was an outpouring of suppressed, painful thoughts concerning personal problems which she "had not talked to anyone about in years." During and immediately following this period, her urinary 17-OHCS level rose from the "low" into the "middle" (shaded) range, but with the reestablishment of her usual defenses, her 17-OHCS level declined and never again rose into this range, even during the final days before the death of her child.[98]

A second case presents an impressive example of the pitfalls of assessing affect unilaterally without considering defensive organization in psychoendocrine studies. This mother was by all overt appearances almost constantly upset, as judged by the content and style of her speech, the associated facial expressions, the tremulous actions, and so on. Accordingly, the ward staff initially regarded her as among the most distressed parents in the entire study. Figure 24–5, however, shows that her urinary 17-OHCS levels were gener-

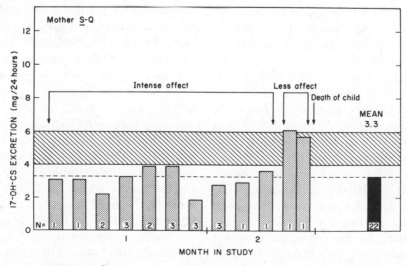

Figure 24–5. Longitudinal study in which 17-OHCS levels reflect use of affective display as a defensive style.[98] (U.S. Army photograph.)

ally quite stable and low, ranging between only 2 to 4 mg./day during a two-month period when such overt signs of intense affective distress were shown. Two days before her child's death, observers were struck with a sudden decrease in outward signs of affective distress, as she attended quietly to her child's needs, during which period her 17-OHCS levels rose to nearly 6 mg./day. This type of dissociation between overt affect ratings and 17-OHCS levels has since been observed in other subjects and appears to reflect a defensive style in which the display of signs of affective distress or frailty serves an effective coping function, perhaps from both an intrapsychic and manipulative standpoint, i.e., in which affect display or expression is employed as a "defense."[99] Psychiatric assessment involving conventional affect ratings alone would, of course, have been misleading in such cases and it is only in the deeper psychodynamic context of defensive organization that the significance of the psychoendocrine data appear to be clarified. The same general conclusion is suggested by other cases in which the reverse relationship of marked 17-OHCS elevations, occurring in the absence of overt evidence of affective distress, was observed in persons who "suffer in silence," or who subjectively are oblivious of inner distress.

Confirmation of a relationship between chronic 17-OHCS levels and defense effectiveness was reported by Rose et al., in a predictive study of Army recruits during basic training patterned after the parent study.[82] This study, in addition, drew attention to some further methodological and theoretical issues involved in this psychoendocrine approach. In assessing effectiveness of defenses in individuals during basic training, it became especially clear that a particular defensive style is not inevitably associated with a particular characteristic 17-OHCS picture in all situations. The specific demands of the current environmental or social setting must clearly be taken into account in relation to the individual's coping style. A defensive style which might be quite effective in maintaining psychoendocrine sta-

bility during basic training, for example, might be relatively ineffective in another life setting where the environmental realities and demands are quite different. An often overlooked methodological corollary of this conclusion, then, is that one cannot expect a consistent correlation between any specific behavioral trait or test score and hormone level to occur in all situations, but must always view psychological-endocrine correlations in the context of the specific social setting, and make accordingly careful observations and assessment of the relevant social variables. This study made also clear that certain nonpsychological variables, such as body weight, environmental variables such as temperature, and historic variables such as early parental death may relate to chronic 17-OHCS level.[73] These findings emphasize the necessity to avoid simplistic methodological approaches and to deal with an increasing range of interacting psychological, social, and nonpsychological factors as multiple codeterminants of chronic 17-OHCS levels.

Still another issue in the psychoendocrine study of defensive organization is illustrated by the work of Mattson et al., who made long-term studies of 17-OHCS levels in hemophilic boys.[65] In judging *psychosocial* adaptation to the illness, he found that those patients regarded by the staff as "good" adapters, being generally cooperative, controlled, and pleasant showed high 17-OHCS levels, while the "poor" adapters, being often uncooperative, irritable, and complaining tended to have low 17-OHCS levels. A deeper psychodynamic analysis of the two subgroups, however, tended to suggest that the organization of ego defenses in the "poor" adapters, although associated with poor social adjustment, was more effective from an intrapsychic standpoint in minimizing affective distress and maintaining low 17-OHCS levels than that in the socially "good" adapters. These observations indicate the need to recognize that effectiveness of defenses, as viewed in terms of social adaptation, may present quite a different picture than when viewed in terms of internal or physiological homeostatic adaptation.

Finally, the psychodynamic implications of experimental observations suggesting that common mental or psychomotor activities are reflected in 17-OHCS levels should also perhaps be considered in the context of defensive styles. The acute suppression of 17-OHCS levels during the viewing of Disney nature movies, for example, raises the question of the likelihood that many comparable everyday activities may be similarly reflected in psychoendocrine adjustments.[96,47] Levi has shown similar suppression of urinary catecholamine levels in subjects viewing natural-scenery films.[45] These findings suggest the possibility that such seemingly similar everyday tension-relieving activities as reading, television viewing, knitting, card games, hobbies, or other self-selected recreational or diverting activities may also be reflected sensitively in hormonal adjustments. This is still a largely undeveloped area in psychoendocrine research, but even the limited information available suggests that it is necessary to bear the role of tension-relieving activities in mind as another variable to be considered in the assessment of the balance between the arousal and antiarousal forces which operate as multiple determinants of psychoendocrine reactions.

One may view the development of psychoendocrine research, then, as providing a succession of insights into the nature and scope of the relevant psychological factors which are codeterminants of hormonal levels. As indicated previously, a broad basic generalization emerging from 17-OHCS studies is that psychoendocrine state at any given point is a resultant of a balance between two sets of opposing forces, those promoting arousal and those defending against arousal. It is increasingly clear that the organization of defensive or antiarousal mechanisms must be considered in a very broad sense, as involving not only the classical intrapsychic defenses, but the full range of mental processes and psychomotor activities which may counteract the mechanisms promoting emotional arousal or involvement.

The practical implications of these generalizations for psychoendocrine methodology relate to the necessity in future studies to assess an increasing array of psychosocial factors concurrently, including quality and intensity of *affect*, *defensive* or coping mechanisms in the broadest sense, and *social* setting, all in the perspective of the dynamic factors operating in each individual subject. This is a tall methodological order, to be sure, and represents a major obstacle to future progress in psychoendocrinology. On the other hand, there is already evidence that the feedback from psychoendocrine experiments can facilitate the development of suitable methods for psychiatric assessment of the above psychosocial factors, by providing leverage and economy in several ways, particularly by virtue of the highly objective indices hormone measurements afford in helping dissect out of the maze of psychological and social variables those which bear the greatest *relevance* to the psychoendocrine processes.

Once given the premise that 17-OHCS measurements provide an objective index of the balance between arousal and antiarousal mechanisms, it follows that the research psychiatrist is given a tool which may be applied to the study of many issues in psychiatric theory, such as those concerned with neurotic, psychotic, psychosomatic, social, and developmental processes, insofar as these relate to emotional and defensive mechanisms. The remainder of this chapter will deal mainly with illustrations of such psychoendocrine approaches in diverse and overlapping areas of psychiatric research.

Psychoendocrine Reflections of Neurotic Processes

One of the most striking paradoxes in this field, so far, is the very limited degree to which psychoendocrine approaches have been applied to the study of neurotic processes. Few, if any, studies have been expressly designed to deal systematically with the testing of theoretical concepts of neurosis or even with the descriptive psychoendocrine study of severely neurotic patients. Most of the few available data suggesting the usefulness of this approach have been incidentally derived from anecdotal observations of individual neurotic patients encountered in "normal" groups or in groups of patients with medical or psychosomatic illnesses.

One such example from the study of parents of leukemic children involved a father with a long-standing neurotic hypersensitivity to rejection by others. Normally, his urinary 17-OHCS level was about 10 mg./day, but one weekend a remarkable elevation to 30 mg./day was noted. This elevation was not attended by any readily evident outward signs or verbal expression of distress, although the ward staff was well-trained and experienced in the clinical rating of emotional behavior. Only a careful reconstruction of the events of the weekend in the psychodynamic context of the patient's neurotic style appeared to clarify the psychoendocrine findings. During this weekend, the subject had been forced by circumstances for the first time to spend many hours in close contact with his ill child, a teen-age boy with whom the father felt rejected and uncomfortable. Normally, the father on each weekend visit would spend a few minutes with his son and then would busy himself with other activities on the ward or elsewhere so as to avoid all but minimal contact with the child, while the mother stayed in attendance. On the weekend of the father's marked 17-OHCS elevation, however, the mother was absent from the hospital because of a family emergency at home, and the father was unable to avoid involvement in the interpersonal situation which apparently activated a strong neurotic reaction.[99]

Another case history was that of a young man who volunteered as a normal "control" subject and lived for many weeks in a hospital-ward setting with other young healthy adults. This subject showed evidence of an exaggerated, neurotic need for approval, low self-esteem, and fear of rejection, and was constantly actively seeking out personal contacts with other subjects and the ward staff. His chronic mean basal urinary 17-OHCS level, established over a period of many weeks, was about 11 mg./day. Following his success in

becoming engaged to a young woman, also participating in the project as a subject, his 17-OHCS levels sharply fell to a new, stable plateau of about 5 mg./day for the period of several weeks that the engagement lasted.[47] While some mild behavioral changes appeared to coincide with the changes in hormone level adjustment, they did not appear commensurate in intensity with the degree of hormonal change.

A number of other similar observations have been made suggesting that marked, psychologically induced 17-OHCS changes can occur in the absence of *overt* clinical signs of associated emotional disturbance and with virtually *no subjective awareness* of the person of any feelings of affective distress or arousal. Since it is characteristic of many neurotic subjects, in the process of self-alienation, to have unconsciously learned to lose or repress awareness of certain unacceptable feelings, and since such repression of self-awareness can be a major obstacle to rehabilitative efforts during therapy, the possibility that psychoendocrine changes may objectively reflect intrapsychic processes of the neurotic patient seems well worth further exploration. The discrepancy between the striking magnitude of the somatic or psychoendocrine reaction and the minimal clinical or subjective manifestation of intrapsychic disturbance is the particularly impressive feature of the preliminary observations suggesting this approach. Are neurotic defenses, strategies, or conflicts particularly prone to lead to psychoendocrine or somatic reactions or disorders? Are different patterns of neurotic trends or conflicts reflected in characteristic psychoendocrine reaction patterns? Is there a characteristic psychoendocrine reflection of neurotically repressed anger, as compared to that for anger handled in other manners? These are random examples of many similar questions which have not yet been approached directly and systematically, although it now appears feasible to do so with the tools of modern psychoendocrine research.

Initially, perhaps the most appropriate tactical approach for the exploration of such questions would be the intensive, longitudinal, in-depth psychodynamic study of individual neurotic patients during psychoanalysis, with emphasis on the *post hoc* qualitative study of intrapsychic processes in the light of recurrent psychoendocrine reaction patterns. Eventually, as this approach yields pilot information and working hypotheses, more objective and predictive methods could be introduced to test the validity of such hypotheses in a more rigorous manner. Finally, because of the relatively high incidence of neuroticism in patients with psychosomatic disorders, the psychoendocrine reflections of neurotic processes in such patients may provide not only objective indices of intrapsychic disorders but offer the possibility of a three-way correlational study of psychological, endocrine and somatic processes. Knapp and his co-workers have performed some valuable pioneering work in the development of methodological guidelines for this approach in their long-term studies of asthmatic patients.[40,64] While the usefulness of psychoendocrine approaches to the study of neurotic processes is still largely speculative and unproven, there are compelling reasons to regard it as one of the most potentially fruitful and powerful of all psychoendocrine approaches to the testing of psychiatric theory, and certainly so far one of the most unexplored and neglected.

Psychoendocrine Reflections of Psychotic Processes

Early psychoendocrine studies of schizophrenic patients between about 1945 and 1955 led to considerable confusion, largely because of methodological limitations from biochemical, physiological, and psychiatric standpoints.[49] An early hypothesis that chronic schizophrenia was associated with hypoadrenalism[72] was not subsequently confirmed as methodological approaches became more refined during the 1950s.[4,49] It should be emphasized that the conceptual approach in early psychoendocrine research on psychosis evolved from the quest for a biochemical abnormality or deficiency which might have pathogenetic significance in schizophrenia. In this respect, the orientation is quite different from the mainstream of recent psychoendocrine research, which has largely viewed hormonal responses as reflections, rather than as determinants, of intrapsychic reactions, although both views are valid and their relative importance remains to be elucidated, as will be discussed later.

The classical study of acute schizophrenic patients by Sachar represents one of the finest models of the application of psychoendocrine approaches to the testing of psychiatric theory.[88] Using a conceptual view of the natural course of acute schizophrenic reactions as being divided into several clearly defined phases of illness from initial breakdown to eventual recovery, he studied endocrine correlates of such clinical phases. Figure 24–6 presents an example of a case illustrating how closely such clinical phases correlate with equally well-defined phases of endocrine change. During the initial turmoil phase, when the patient's characteristic defense mechanisms have been overwhelmed, emotional distress and 17-OHCS and catecholamine levels are very high. With the subsequent formation of a consoling psychotic delusional system, becoming well established by about the eleventh day, hormone values subside to a lower, more stable level. During this period of psychotic equilibrium, the patient's picture of himself and his style of interaction with others is completely narcissistic, and affective distress is minimal. Then, as the doctor and ward staff begin to challenge and undermine the patient's psychotic defenses during the 4th week, the patient reveals his true devalued self-image, and the affective distress of anxiety and depression reappears with associated increases in hormone levels. As the patient eventually arrives at a more mature, clinically improved "equilibrium," with minimal affective distress, hormone levels stabilize in a range very close to that observed during the earlier psychotic "equilibrium" phase. Similar correlations between hormonal and psychological phases were observed in longitudinal studies of additional patients of the same type.[88]

These findings suggest that the psychotic system operates defensively to minimize both emotional distress and associated endocrine disturbance. Sachar's observations were among the first to call attention to the important role of psychological defenses in the maintenance of physiological as well as psychological homeostasis. This work also points

tion for the earlier confusion and conflicting findings in psychoendocrine studies, when clinical phases were often not evaluated in close relation to the period of hormone sampling. Thus, it is not surprising that "contrast" studies of groups of normal subjects versus patients in chronic psychotic equilibrium may show no differences in group mean 17-OHCS

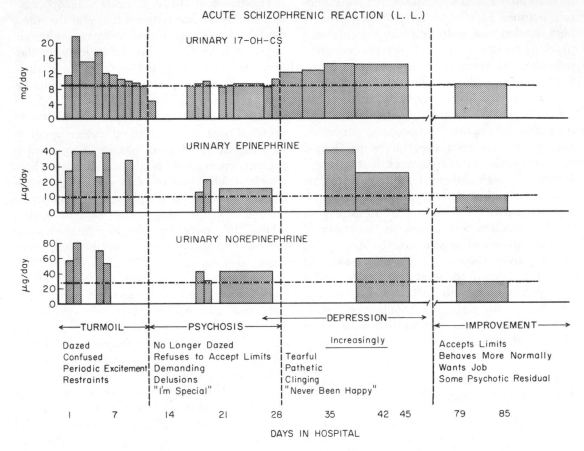

Figure 24–6. Longitudinal study showing correlations between clinical and endocrine phases during course of acute schizophrenic reaction.[84] (U.S. Army photograph.)

out that it is essentially the *effectiveness* of defenses, whether they be normal, neurotic or psychotic in character, which is reflected in 17-OHCS levels, thus setting a pattern for later psychoendocrine studies of defensive organization. It is also particularly noteworthy that at the time the patient is the most severely psychotic and withdrawn, emotional distress is often minimal, and 17-OHCS levels are similar to those following eventual clinical recovery. This observation provides a plausible explana-

levels. Only when the dynamic factors involved in defensive organization are viewed in relation to the life setting does the significance of the psychoendocrine picture begin to become clarified. Finally, Sachar suggests that endocrine measures may not only provide a form of validation of theoretical classification of key phases in the course of a type of psychosis, but may also provide helpful guidelines to the psychotherapist, as he supports or challenges the patient's psychological defenses.[88]

Another example of psychoendocrine evaluation of psychodynamic issues is provided by studies of the manic state, which clinically has been regarded by some observers as involving considerable intrapsychic distress, and by others as a more comfortable, restitutive state. Longitudinal studies of corticosteroid levels in manic patients have been reported by a number of workers.[9,21,76] Generally it has been found that pituitary-adrenal cortical activity is relatively low during manic phases, in contrast to the higher levels during depressed phases. These findings may be interpreted as providing physiological support for the clinical hypothesis that mania, with its elements of euphoria and denial, represents a counteracting, protective defense against the painful distress associated with depression.

Psychoendocrine Reflections of Depressive Processes

Although a discussion of depressive syndromes obviously overlaps with that in the previous sections on neurotic and psychotic processes, the considerable emphasis on studies of depression in psychoendocrine research merits special mention. In 1956, Board et al., reported marked plasma 17-OHCS elevations in acutely depressed patients shortly after hospital admission.[7] While others confirmed these findings, it was subsequently found in longitudinal studies which extended well beyond the hospital admission period that 17-OHCS levels did not invariably correlate significantly with the severity of depressive symptoms.[49]

In a study by Bunney et al., for example, two general subgroups of depressed patients could be distinguished on the basis of chronic urinary 17-OHCS levels.[10] One group, characterized by high and labile 17-OHCS levels, appeared to be more aware of, and involved in, the struggle with their illness. The second group, although also having high ratings on the depression scale, had relatively low and stable 17-OHCS levels and appeared to have differently organized defenses, often employing denial of their illness or related problems.

This study indicated that the symptoms of depression alone are not necessarily associated with 17-OHCS elevations, but that, again, a more holistic, psychodynamic view of defensive organization must be taken, particularly in view of the considerable heterogeneity of clinical depressive syndromes.

The incisive studies of Sachar and his co-workers have, in particular, contributed greatly to the clarification of psychoendocrine research on depression. In a study designed to test the psychiatric hypothesis that certain depressive reactions serve a defensive function against acknowledgment of painful feelings of disappointment or anger, dynamic factors were carefully assessed throughout the period of psychotherapy in a relatively homogeneous group of patients with reactive depression. Elevated 17-OHCS levels were generally not observed in those patients except during episodic "confrontation" periods, when the painful losses which precipitated their depressive reactions were being dealt with during therapy. Emphasis was placed on distinguishing the affects associated with loss and mourning from the organized syndrome of melancholia.[85,86] Sachar also has presented a penetrating critique of early psychoendocrine research on depression which should be an important guide to future work in this field. The failure of many studies to consider important control issues, such as the psychoendocrine response to hospital admission, the social milieu throughout hospitalization, the interference of certain central-acting medications, the criteria for control data to be compared with illness data, as well as the failure to take psychodynamic factors into account, are implicated as probable reasons for inconsistencies and confusion in early psychoendocrine research on depression.[84]

At present, then, it appears that outward signs of depression are not necessarily associated with 17-OHCS elevations, and that the intrapsychic processes which are associated with the marked 17-OHCS changes often seen in depressed patients remain to be qualitatively characterized in future studies, which take into account dynamic factors as a basis for distinguishing the many different syndromes in which signs of depression are a prominent feature.

Psychoendocrine Approaches to the Study of Developmental Processes

It logically follows that insofar as endocrine measures reflect intrapsychic processes, then such measures may be used to study experiential and genetic influences on the development of those same intrapsychic processes. The marked individual differences in psychoendocrine responses observed between different subjects exposed to the same stressful situation provides one point of departure for research along such developmental lines. Under relatively highly standardized conditions, for example, six adult rhesus monkeys were exposed to two-week sessions of a conditioned emotional disturbance, conditioned "avoidance," during which they were required to press a hand lever at times in order to avoid an aversive stimulus. Of the six monkeys exposed to this procedure, two showed marked 17-OHCS elevations, two showed mild 17-OHCS elevations, and two animals actually showed *suppression* of 17-OHCS levels, which was not, incidentally, associated with elevated preexperimental 17-OHCS baselines. While no genetic or early developmental data were available on these animals acquired as adults, it was noteworthy that there appeared to be a close correlation between *direction* of 17-OHCS response and the extent of their prior laboratory experience and handling. The monkeys showing marked 17-OHCS elevations were laboratory-naive, while the monkeys showing suppression of 17-OHCS levels were veterans of many laboratory experiments.[47] While these studies of adult monkeys may not be viewed as developmental in the usual sense, they did, along with other observations in animals,[49,79] suggest the possible importance of even short-term experiential factors in the determination of psychoendocrine reaction patterns and raised the issue of the need for systematic developmental studies.

Some findings perhaps more directly related to this approach emerged from studies by Poe et al. of childhood history in relation to indi-vidual differences in chronic mean 17-OHCS levels in ninety-one Army recruits studied during basic training. Of the fourteen men in this group who had lost a parent by death, twelve had 17-OHCS levels in the upper or lower quartiles. In the "high" 17-OHCS quartile, five of the six subjects had lost their mother, while five of the six subjects in the "low" 17-OHCS quartile had lost their father.[73] So far, no subsequent attempts have apparently been made to pursue this finding further or to search for possible psychological correlates of endocrine differences in subjects who experienced parental deaths during childhood.

More broadly, it appears that psychoendocrine reflections of emotional and defensive mechanisms may provide useful adjuncts to the psychological study of the early development of these intrapsychic mechanisms and represent an objective basis for testing theories of developmental stages based entirely on psychological observations. In addition to the well-established usefulness of corticosteroid and catecholamine levels in defining individual characterological differences, the recent availability of improved methods for determination of testosterone and other sex hormones adds even further interest to developmental approaches. At present, however, there is a dearth of psychoendocrine data on virtually all phases of early development, from the first year through adolescence and this approach awaits further exploration.

Psychoendocrine Approaches to the Study of Social Processes

The social setting of psychoendocrine studies has already been emphasized as an important variable to assess in relation to psychodynamic factors and hormonal reaction patterns. Some of the specific examples of the ways in which social influences may be reflected in hormonal levels suggest in addition that psychoendocrine approaches may be useful to social scientists in the systematic study of social interactions, particularly those occurring in small groups.

One of the social phenomena apparently reflected in psychoendocrine studies is what might be called the "emotional contagion effect." An early observation suggesting this interpretation was the close similarity of 17-OHCS levels in crewmen of a B-52 bomber during a nonstop flight to Argentina under unusually stressful conditions. The pilot had extremely high urinary 17-OHCS levels of about 20 mg./day (compared with a mean normal of about 7 mg./day in men). The other three crewmen, who were back in the plane working closely together, all ran very similar elevated levels of about 13 mg./day.[46] The rarity of 17-OHCS levels of 13 mg./day, even in large groups of human subjects in stressful situations, suggested the possibility that a socially communicated "13 mg./day atmosphere" prevailed in this aircraft on the flight day.

Similar conclusions were suggested in the studies of other small, closely-knit groups of five to six human subjects. In each of three different groups of young men anticipating ninety-six-hour sleep-deprivation sessions, mean plasma 17-OHCS levels differed appreciably from one group to the next. Yet, within each group, the individual 17-OHCS values clustered very closely around the particular group mean at the end of the control week during which the men had been continuously in close social communication.[56] The tendency for 17-OHCS levels in most individual members of a group anticipating a stressful experience to cluster around an "equilibrium level" was also observed in normal young adults anticipating movie-viewing experiences.[56] In studies of normal young adults during hospitalization, however, it was found that, while some groups had a very narrow range of intragroup corticosteroid levels after the individuals lived together for a while, other groups showed a much wider range of intragroup individual variation in a similar setting.[56] These observations suggest that certain group dynamics may be reflected in psychoendocrine parameters, particularly when the group is relatively small and the members have been together for some time in a relatively intimate and stressful setting.

Many observations in animals have also indicated that such parameters as population density and social hierarchy are reflected in endocrine activity.[13,49] Of particular interest are the elegant studies by Rose and his co-workers of plasma testosterone levels in monkeys living in social groups. These studies have shown correlations between plasma testosterone levels, dominance rank, and various levels of agonistic behavior. Testosterone fluctuations in individual male monkeys have also been observed in relation to such social or sexual stimuli as defeat in combat or introduction to a colony of females.[79,80]

Similarly creative psychoendocrine approaches would appear to be feasible in human groups, for example, in relation to various group-therapy approaches, yet little has been done so far along these lines. The naturalistic character of group interactions, as contrasted to the contrived laboratory investigator-subject settings, seems rather promising as an experimental approach for psychoendocrine studies in human subjects. Again, both the potential and the limitations of this approach are defined by the rationale that to the extent that hormonal reactions reflect emotional and defensive organization, and to the extent which such intrapsychic processes are related to social interactions, then psychoendocrine approaches should be useful to the investigator of social processes.

Psychoendocrine Approaches to the Study of Occupational Activities

The sensitivity of corticosteroid and catecholamine levels to such everyday activities as viewing motion pictures has already been mentioned. It has been shown by Wadeson et al.,[96] and Levi[45] that hormonal levels may rise during the viewing of certain movies and fall during the viewing of other movies. These experiments convey a rather dynamic sense of hormonal levels shifting up or down from one short time segment to another during the day in reaction to an experience not unlike many other common activities of everyday life. The question naturally arises as to whether or not similar hormonal reactions do occur in association with a much larger range of everyday activities, including occupational as well as recreational pursuits, even though we do not normally think of many of these activities as being associated with appreciable changes in affective state.

In a series of resourceful studies, Levi and his co-workers have indeed demonstrated that certain occupational tasks have psychoendocrine reflections in the activity of the sympathetic-adrenal medullary system. He found urinary catecholamine increases and hyperlipoproteinemia, for example, in persons performing an exacting industrial task of sorting out four slightly different sizes of steel balls in the presence of distracting noise and lights.[45] In another study, Levi found that conditions of everyday work, such as whether it is performed on a piecework or salaried basis, were reflected in urinary epinephrine and norepinephrine levels in young women who were invoicing clerks.[44] Frankenhaeuser et al., have also reported urinary catecholamine changes in association with psychological tests involving arithmetic and inductive tasks.[22] In another study, it was found that individual psychoendocrine differences associated with performance of mental activities or tasks may, in turn, be correlated with individual differences in the effectiveness of performance. Subjects showing the greatest improvement in performance of proofreading or coding tasks in a stressful setting were also those who showed the largest increase in norepinephrine excretion in association with the task.[23]

While we have as yet minimal data with which to evaluate this general approach, it is certainly a provocative notion to consider that our daily routines are composed of a sequence of episodic segments in which hormonal increases and decreases reflect associated shifts in mental and psychomotor activities, which may perhaps be divided into general classes, such as tension-building or tension-relieving, on a psychological basis. The dynamic factors involved in emotional and defensive organization of individual subjects would, of course, have to be taken carefully into account in the interpretation of findings emerging from this approach. Recent research with plasma cortisol measurements at frequent intervals has shown some striking periodic increases and decreases in hormonal levels over the course of the day.[30] One of the issues raised by these findings is whether such "ultradian" fluctuations represent simply an "on and off" physiological mechanism of glandular release of hormone in periodic bursts, or if the fluctuations are largely a reflection of shifting inputs into the neuroendocrine machinery, particularly perhaps a reflection of shifting intrapsychic functioning in relation to moment-to-moment events, thoughts, and activities. While this is certainly a technically difficult issue to approach experimentally, its practical and theoretical implications for occupational stress research and psychosomatic medicine provide a compelling basis for its further exploration.

(Psychological Reflections of Endocrine State

While recent psychoendocrine research has been oriented primarily in terms of the influence of psychological factors upon hormone secretion, the important fact should be kept in mind, of course, that interactions between the brain and the endocrine glands operate in both directions. It is known that many hormones exert influences on neural and psychological processes, although our knowledge of such effects is still very limited, largely because of the unusually difficult methodological problems involved in assessing the affected CNS processes. The early work of Reiss and his associates in England was directed at this "other side of the coin" in psychoendocrinology, i.e., the possible clinical importance of the effects of abnormal hormone levels upon the brain as a pathogenetic factor in various psychiatric disorders.[75] The psychiatric symptoms which often accompany certain clinical endocrinopathies have long been recognized.[92] The hypothesis that a deficiency of gonadal hormone secretion, leading to an immature level of psychosexual functioning, might be a pathogenetic factor in certain schizophrenic patients was formulated many years ago,[32] but could not, at that time, be rigorously tested because of the lack of specific and reliable methods for gonadal hormone measurement in blood and urine. Such methods, however, are now available. The striking and regular fluctuations in mood state associated with the menstrual cycle in many women provide another example of observations which strongly suggest hormonal influences upon intrapsychic processes and probably presents one of the best natural opportunities for the experimental study of such correlations. The recent development of radioimmunoassay methods for the measurement of the gonadotropins and of the individual gonadal steroids now makes possible a highly refined endocrinological approach to this clinical problem. The research of Rose and his co-workers, involving the study of correlations between plasma testosterone and agonistic behavior, presents another excellent model of how the general problem of viewing psychoendocrine relationships in both directions may be approached experimentally.[41,78] It is clear that the study of hormonal feedback upon the brain is another aspect of psychoendocrinology which is worthy of greater attention in the future, particularly because of the recent availability of many long-awaited, refined methods of hormone assay.

It should also be mentioned that there is a considerable body of neurochemical and psychopharmacological research which indicates that biogenic amines in the brain may be involved in the development of affective disorders such as depression and mania. The possible role of various hormones upon the metabolism and balance of the biogenic amines within the CNS has, therefore, become yet another area of current interest in psychoendocrine research. Some caution is probably well-advised in this area, however, for several reasons, perhaps particularly with regard to the pitfall of placing overemphasis prematurely on a single hormone before a broader survey for possible multiple, interacting hormonal influences on the biogenic amines is completed.

(Psychoendocrine Approaches to the Study of Psychosomatic Disorders

Most of the psychoendocrine approaches discussed up to this point have been oriented in terms of the study of hormonal changes as reflections of psychological processes. The central issues have revolved around the use of hormone measurements as sensitive, objective, roughly quantitative reflections of the intrapsychic processes involved in emotional and defensive organization. It has also been emphasized that the great bulk of psychoendocrine research since the 1950s, furthermore, has been focused on the pituitary-adrenal cortical and the sympathetic-adrenal medullary systems.

In turning, finally, to the question of the implications of psychoendocrine approaches for psychosomatic medicine, it is necessary to broaden our conceptual approach to consider some fundamental facts of endocrine physiology. The basic question now becomes, "Can psychologically determined hormonal changes play a mediating, pathogenic role, along with concurrent autonomic changes, in the development of somatic illnesses?" In approaching this question, the modus operandi of hormones at the cellular level becomes a highly relevant issue. A particularly crucial fact is that hormones are now known to exert their effects upon metabolic or cellular processes in a complex, *interdependent* way. In general, a given metabolic process is regulated by numerous hormones which are aligned into a balance of opposing and cooperating forces, with antagonistic, synergistic, additive, and permissive relationships present between the hormones in relation to the regulation of any particular cellular process. As a result, no single hormone controls any single metabolic process, but there is always a *balance between interdependent forces*. Thus, in considering the regulation of lipid metabolism, for example, a substantial number of hormones must be taken into account, including norepinephrine, insulin, cortisol, epinephrine, growth hormone, thyroxine, and estrogens.[53] Carried to its logical conclusion, then, this basic feature of endocrine physiology dictates the conclusion that an understanding of the regulation of the functional state of any given cellular process at any given time can only be achieved by viewing the current *overall hormonal balance* as the final, key determinant of the cellular activity in question.[53] In practical terms, this means that little success is to be expected in approaches which attempt to relate psychological processes and somatic illnesses through a view of any *single* mediating psychoendocrine system in isolation. It means that an increasing number of concurrent hormonal measurements, involving as many endocrine systems as possible, should be incorporated into psychoendocrine studies of psychosomatic disorders.

Another body of evidence supports this conceptual approach in addition to the reasoning based on cellular aspects of endocrine physiology. With the recent, revolutionary advances in hormone-assay methodology, it has become feasible to measure a large number of hormones concurrently and to test the hypothesis that the many endocrine systems, which have anatomical contacts with the brain, are responsive to psychological influences. Figure 24–7 shows the pattern of multiple hormonal responses to a seventy-two-hour conditioned emotional disturbance in a series of "conditioned avoidance" experiments in monkeys.[52] First of all, it is evident that every hormone measured changed in reaction to this stressful situation, although the dynamics of change differ considerably from one hormone to the next, particularly with regard to temporal features. Two general hormone-response subgroups may be distinguished on the basis of initial direction of change. The levels of the corticosteroids, epinephrine, norepinephrine, thyroxine or butanol-extractive iodine (BEI), and growth hormone all rise initially, while the levels of insulin, androgens, and estrogens drop initially. Following the session, the latter hormones tend to rebound above baseline levels. The possibility that the organization of this acute psychoendocrine response pattern represents a "catabolic-anabolic" sequence of coordinated responses in preparation for muscular exertion, according to Cannon's formula-

tion,[11] fits well with our present knowledge of the role of each of these hormones in relation to energy metabolism. The critical interpretation of these experiments has been discussed

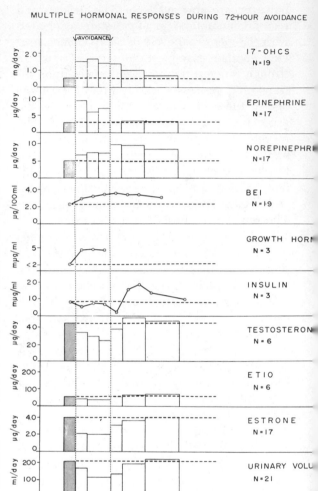

Figure 24–7. Organization of multiple hormonal responses to sustained conditioned emotional disturbance (conditioned avoidance) in rhesus monkeys.[52] (U.S. Army photograph.)

at length elsewhere,[52] but their general relevance to psychosomatic studies seems clear. While this stereotyped pattern of acute psychoendocrine response is demonstrable under certain conditions in the monkey, how might the pattern of hormonal balance be variously altered on an acute and chronic basis by the complex psychological machinery which has already been demonstrated in corticosteroid and catecholamine studies to exert such profound and varying effects on endocrine function from one individual to the next? Are particular characterological patterns of psychological organization reflected broadly in the pattern of overall hormonal balance? If we view psychosomatic illnesses as fundamentally *integrative disorders*, does the pattern of organization of overall hormonal balance distinctively reflect the particular integrative disorder involving emotional and defensive processes? If so, does the altered pattern of hormone balance appear to constitute a pathogenetic link to the associated somatic disorder? These questions represent the general lines along which working hypotheses can be perhaps most logically developed in the light of current psychoendocrine data and theory.

As yet, however, only the most preliminary efforts have been made to test the usefulness of this broadly based, holistic psychoendocrine approach to the study of psychosomatic disorders. Such efforts, while quite limited so far, have provided some useful guidelines and leads for future work in this area. In a study of hormonal patterns of recruits during basic training, for example, several hormonal abnormalities were noted during the week prior to onset of acute adenovirus respiratory illnesses. A gradual decline in thyroid hormone levels, spiking corticosteroid and catecholamine elevations several days before the onset of illness, and a high percentage of extremely high or extremely low corticosteroid, thyroid hormone, or androgen levels appeared to characterize the period preceding respiratory infections.[59] These findings suggest that it may be worthwhile to evaluate further the working hypothesis that stress-related, *preillness, multiple* changes in overall hormonal balance may play a pathogenetic role in altering host resistance to infectious illnesses.

In a preliminary study of obese patients, Troyer et al.[94] have observed that two general classes of endocrine abnormalities should be considered. First, the *mean chronic profile* of hormonal balance appears to be altered, with the levels of certain hormones chronically higher or lower than those in normal groups or other patient populations. Secondly, the pattern of *acute responsiveness* reflected in changes in hormonal balance with psychological or other stimuli may be distinctively altered in patients with psychosomatic illnesses. A number of acute episodes were observed in obese patients, for example, in which the anabolic hormones rose at the same time that the catabolic hormones rose, a pattern quite different from that observed during acute arousal in the normal monkey. It is also especially interesting, incidentally, that these marked acute hormone responses apparently occurred in the patients generally without overt expression or subjective awareness of emotional distress.[94] In two obese subjects studied earlier, however, details of life events and some knowledge of dynamic factors in the individual patient suggested that neurotic processes were suddenly activated at the time of the hormonal changes. These pilot observations require considerable further evaluation, but are mentioned here primarily to indicate the kinds of methodological and theoretical issues which bear consideration in the design of psychoendocrine studies of medical patients. Endocrine sampling in long-term longitudinal studies of patients should yield both a chronic mean hormonal profile and an acute psychoendocrine response pattern so that both of these parameters, in turn, can be studied for possible relationships to psychological and somatic parameters.

While the technical and organizational problems which make this multidisciplinary approach difficult are substantial and require resourceful and energetic efforts for their solution, historically it now appears within our grasp. It is not often that a generation has suddenly new experimental methods at its disposal which make possible the testing of a promising but unproven concept of disease. While much of medicine, with the ever-increasing trend towards specialization, continues to pursue the course of viewing disease as a local or regional phenomenon, the opportunity is now open to pursue, at a new level of sophistication, a view of many *diseases as disorders of integration*. We have long thought of endocrine systems as largely governed by relatively simple, humoral, nearly infallible self-regulatory mechanisms. The new knowledge that highly complicated psychological influences are superimposed upon the humoral machinery for endocrine regulation raises the possibility that disorders of bodily function may result when the more complex, and probably more fallible, psychological machinery preempts, disrupts, or otherwise works at odds against the simpler, lower-level, humoral machinery of endocrine regulation. Certainly, there are few, if any, conceptual approaches to the genesis of disease presently envisioned in medicine which are potentially more far-reaching, logically appealing, and challenging.

⟨ Appendix: Some Control Issues and Experimental Tactics in Psychoendocrine Research

While it is beyond the scope of this chapter to discuss in detail such relevant research issues as nonpsychological determinants of endocrine activity which may act as interfering independent variables in psychoendocrine studies, control measures in experimental design, selection and validation of hormone assay procedures, etc., it may be useful to review briefly several of the problems which have most commonly proven pitfalls in past psychoendocrine research.

Quality-Control Check System for Hormone-Assay Methods

Since hormone assay methods are generally quite delicate microanalytical procedures, in which such subtle factors as minor variations in day-to-day laboratory technique, fluctuations in environmental temperature, variability in reagent batches, instrument malfunction, glassware contamination, etc., can cause major errors in the accuracy of results, it is *essential* that quality-control checks which are as rigorous and comprehensive as possible be incorporated into every analytical run. Even in the most experienced laboratories, such methods may suddenly give unreliable results and days or even weeks of trouble-shooting may be required in order to locate the source of error. A sound quality-control check system cannot, of course, prevent such breakdowns of methods, nor the associated loss of samples or time, but it has the all-important advantages of providing the investigator with a highly reliable and objective basis for accepting or rejecting biochemical results in each analytical run, and of greatly reducing the chance of accepting erroneous results as valid. These advantages apply equally whether the biochemical determinations are made by the investigator himself, by a close colleague, or by a distant commercial laboratory. The following system, outlined in a general way, can be applied to most blood or urinary hormone-assay procedures with appropriate modifications.

First, a large pool of plasma or urine should be obtained so as to provide about 100 or more aliquots of the same volume as will be normally collected for individual routine analyses of unknown samples from experimental subjects. The number of aliquots is arbitrary and mainly decided by convenience, in terms of providing a supply to last several months for the method in question. If, for example, the method requires a 1–ml. aliquot for each determination, if two control samples are included in each analytical run, and if three analytical runs are made each week, then 102 aliquots would provide a seventeen-week supply of control samples. The concentration of hormone in the original pool should be reasonably close to the concentration range present in the samples from the subject population to be studied. The original raw pool should be divided into three equal subpools, designated C_1, C_2, and C_3. Subpool C_1 should remain untreated, as it was collected. To subpool C_2, a quantity of crystalline or highly purified hormone should be added so as to increase the hormone concentration in each aliquot by an amount just slightly greater than the standard deviation of the method. The principle involved here is that C_2 should be clearly distinguishable from C_1 by the analytical method, but just barely so. In other words, if aliquots from C_1 and C_2 are repeatedly analyzed in twenty or thirty successive runs, the highest values obtained for C_1 aliquots should only very rarely exceed the lowest values obtained on C_2 aliquots. If too much hormone is added to C_2 and the concentration difference is too great between C_1 and C_2 so that they are too easily distinguishable, then in some methods this may lead to conscious or unconscious bias on the part of the technician. To subpool C_3, then, an amount of purified hormone, twice as great as that added to C_2, should be added so that C_2 and C_3 aliquots will be just comfortably distinguishable by the method and values from the two subpools rarely overlap.

Once the three subpools are thus prepared, and the added hormone in subpools C_2 and C_3 well-mixed by shaking, each subpool should then be divided into the small individual aliquots for individual analyses. Next comes the important matter of coding the bottles with numbers in such a way as to give no indication to the technician of which subpool is represented. A code sheet is prepared listing numbers from 1 to 100, or whatever total number of aliquots there may be, and samples are then numbered in order after they are drawn at random from the three subpool groups. The code sheet might read, for example, 1 (the only number actually on the tube) = C_2, 2 = C_1, 3 = C_2, 4 = C_3, 5 = C_3, 6 = C_1, etc. The biochemist receives only the tubes with the numbers 1, 2, 3, 4, 5, 6, etc. The responsible investigator should maintain custody of the code sheet in such a way as to keep the procedure blind, but to supply immediate feedback to the chemist or technician after each run is completed. The control samples should be stored frozen, with a substantial number of aliquots kept in the same freezer as the unknown samples from experimental subjects. If the freezer should ever malfunction, the control samples may provide some valuable indication as to whether serious damage to hormone concentrations has resulted from high temperatures or not. For most methods, at least two control samples

should be included in each run, preferably one at the beginning and one at the end of the series of tubes being analyzed. Immediately after the control samples are initially prepared, six to ten samples should be analyzed from each subpool so as to establish an approximate mean value and standard deviation for each subpool before proceeding with the analysis of unknown samples.

While this system provides a reliable check against the great majority of sources of analytical error, it is not infallible and will not detect, for example, an occasional random error caused by the contamination of a single tube. In such an instance, the investigator can only ask for several replicate determinations of any sample giving a value far away from the expected range. In the main, however, the system is extremely valuable in monitoring day-to-day accuracy and in providing reassurance to the investigator, particularly when in search of psychological correlates, that the hormone values are valid.

Choice of Blood- and Urine-Sample Collection Schedules

There are several guidelines for the design of hormone-sampling schedules which have proven useful in promoting the interpretability of psychoendocrine experiments. The first principle, perhaps, is that the sample-collection times should be closely attuned to the dynamics of the endocrine response and the stimulus under study. It is known, of course, that the levels of some hormones such as epinephrine, norepinephrine, and growth hormone are very labile, showing marked elevations or decreases within a matter of minutes. Other hormones, such as cortisol, thyroxine, or testosterone, apparently change more slowly. While some general guesses about optimal sampling intervals can be made from previous work on various hormones, it is desirable in any particular study, whenever possible, to carry out a few pilot experiments with frequent enough samples so as to define roughly the temporal configuration of hormonal-response curves. Once this is established, a more economical collection design with fewer samples can be devised with greater assurance that response peaks will not be missed because of inappropriate sampling intervals.

Another extremely important practice is the obtaining of *multiple* control or base-line samples *before* the onset of any experimental manipulations on either an acute or prolonged basis. Because of the well-known potency of anticipatory reactions, especially those involving novelty or uncertainty, as stimuli to many endocrine systems, at least two, and preferably more, preexperimental samples should always be obtained in order to establish the slope of hormonal change against which experimental stimuli are superimposed. It is probable that few factors have led to greater confusion and error in the interpretation of experiments on endocrine regulation than failure to obtain multiple base-line samples.

A number of other control and methodological issues, such as the advantages of long-term "longitudinal" studies of individual patients over "contrast" studies of large groups in the exploratory phases of psychoendocrine research, the importance of social milieu during hospitalization, the selection and validation of psychological methods, the need to consider circadian and ultradian hormonal rhythms in experimental design, and the role of nonpsychological determinants, such as age, sex, medications, smoking, posture, bed rest, muscular activity, environmental temperature, nutrition, etc., have all emerged as important considerations in psychoendocrine research and are discussed in greater detail elsewhere.[35,36,45,49,84]

(Bibliography

1. Ax, A. "The Physiological Differentiation between Fear and Anger in Humans," *Psychosom. Med.*, 15 (1953), 433–442.

2. Berkeley, A. W. "Level of Aspiration in Relation to Adrenal Cortical Activity and the Concept of Stress," *J. Comp. Physiol. Psychol.*, 45 (1952), 443–449.

3. Bernard, C. In A. Pi-Suner, ed., *The Whole and the Parts: Classics of Biology*, p. 313. New York: Philosophical Library, 1955.

4. Bliss, E. L., C. J. Migeon, C. H. Branch et al. "Adrenocortical Function in Schizophrenia," *Am. J. Physiol.*, 112 (1955), 358–365.

5. ———. "Reaction of the Adrenal Cortex to Emotional Stress," *Psychosom. Med.*, 18 (1956), 56–76.

6. Board, F., H. Persky, and D. A. Hamburg. "Psychological Stress and Endocrine Functions. Blood Levels of Adrenocortical and Thyroid Hormones in Acutely Disturbed Patients," *Psychosom. Med.*, 18 (1956), 324–333.

7. ———. "Psychological Stress and Endocrine Functions. Blood Levels of Adrenocortical and Thyroid Hormones in Patients Suffering from Depressive Reactions," *Arch. Neurol. Psychiatry*, 78 (1957), 612–620.

8. Brown, G. M. and S. Reichlin. "Psychologic and Neural Regulations of Growth Hormone," *Psychosom. Med.*, 34 (1972), 45–60.

9. Bunney, W. E., Jr., E. L. Hartmann, and J. W. Mason. "Study of a Patient with 48-Hour Manic-Depressive Cycles: II. Strong Positive Correlation between Endocrine Factors and Manic Defense Patterns," *Arch. Gen. Psychiatry*, 12 (1965), 619–625.

10. Bunney, W. E., Jr., J. W. Mason, and D. A. Hamburg. "Correlations between Behavioral Variables and Urinary 17-Hydroxycorticosteroids in Depressed Patients," *Psychosom. Med.*, 27 (1965), 299–308.

11. Cannon, W. B. *Bodily Changes in Pain, Hunger, Fear, and Rage*. Boston: Branford, 1929.

12. Cannon, W. B. and D. de la Paz. "Emotional Stimulation of Adrenal Secretion," *Am. J. Physiol.*, 27 (1911), 64–70.

13. Christian, J. J. "Phenomena Associated with Population Density," *Proc. Natl. Acad. Sci.*, 47 (1961), 428–449.

14. Elmadjian, F., J. M. Hope, and E. T. Lamson. "Excretion of Epinephrine and Norepinephrine Under Stress," *Recent Prog. Horm. Res.*, 14 (1958), 513–553.

15. Euler, U. S., V. *Noradrenaline*. Springfield, Ill.: Charles C. Thomas, 1956.

16. ———. "Quantitation of Stress by Catecholamine Analysis," *Clin. Pharmacol. Ther.*, 5 (1964), 398–404.

17. Euler, U. S., V., C. A. Gemzell, L. Levi et al. "Cortical and Medullary Adrenal

Activity in Emotional Stress," *Acta Endocrinol. (Kbh.)*, 30 (1959), 567–573.

18. Fox, H. M. "Effects of Psychophysiological Research on the Transference," *J. Am. Psychoanal. Assoc.*, 6 (1958), 413–432.

19. Fox, H. M., S. Gifford, A. F. Valenstein et al. "Psychophysiological Correlation of 17-Ketosteroids and 17-Hydroxycorticosteroids in 21 Pairs of Monozygotic Twins," *J. Psychosom. Res.*, 14 (1970), 71–79.

20. Fox, H. M., B. J. Murawski, A. F. Bartholoway et al. "Adrenal Steroid Excretion Patterns in Eighteen Healthy Subjects," *Psychosom. Med.*, 23 (1961), 33–40.

21. Fox, H. M., B. J. Murawski, G. W. Thorn et al. "Urinary 17-Hydroxycorticosteroid and Uropepsin Levels with Psychological Data: A Three-Year Study of One Subject," *Arch. Intern. Med.*, 10 (1958), 859–871.

22. Frankenhaeuser, M. and S. Kareby. "The Effect of Meprobamate on Catecholamine Excretion during Mental Stress," *Percept. Mot. Skills*, 15 (1962), 571–577.

23. Frankenhaeuser, M. and P. Patkai. "Catecholamine Excretion and Performance during Stress," *Percept. Mot. Skills*, 19 (1964), 13–14.

24. Frankenhaeuser, M. and B. Post. "Catecholamine Excretion during Mental Work as Modified by Centrally Acting Drugs," *Acta. Physiol. Scand.*, 55 (1962), 74–81.

25. Friedman, S. B., J. W. Mason, and D. A. Hamburg. "Urinary 17-Hydroxycorticosteroid Levels in Parents of Children with Neoplastic Disease," *Psychosom. Med.*, 25 (1963), 364–376.

26. Funkenstein, D. H., S. H. King, and M. E. Drolette. *Mastery of Stress.* Cambridge: Harvard University Press, 1957.

27. Hamburg, D. A. "Plasma and Urinary Corticosteroid Levels in Normally Occurring Psychological Stresses," in S. Korey, ed., *Ultrastructure and Metabolism of the Nervous System*, pp. 426–452. Baltimore: Williams & Wilkins, 1962.

28. Harris, G. W. *Neural Control of the Pituitary Gland.* London: Arnold, 1955.

29. ——. "Hypothalamic Control of the Anterior Lobe of the Hypophysis," in W. S. Fields, B. Guillemin, and C. A. Carton, eds., *Hypothalamic-Hypophyseal Interrelationships*, pp. 31–45. Springfield, Ill.: Charles C. Thomas, 1956.

30. Hellman, L., F. Nakada, J. Curti et al. "Cortisol Is Secreted Episodically by Normal Man," *J. Clin. Endocrinol. Metab.*, 30 (1970), 411–422.

31. Hill, S. R., Jr., F. C. Goetz, H. M. Fox et al. "Studies on Adrenocortical and Psychological Response to Stress in Man," *Arch. Intern. Med.*, 97 (1956), 269–298.

32. Hoskins, R. G. *The Biology of Schizophrenia.* New York: Norton, 1946.

33. Hubble, D. "The Endocrine Orchestra," *Br. Med. J.*, 1 (1961), 523–528.

34. ——. "The Psyche and the Endocrine System," *Lancet*, 2 (1963), 209–214.

35. Ingle, D. J. "Parameters of Metabolic Problems," *Recent Prog. Horm. Res.*, 6 (1951), 159–194.

36. ——. *Principles of Research in Biology and Medicine.* Philadelphia: Lippincott, 1958.

37. Johansson, S., L. Levi, and S. Lindstedt. *Stress and the Thyroid Gland: A Review of Clinical and Experimental Studies, and a Report of Own Data on Experimentally Induced PBI Reactions in Man.* Reports from the Laboratory for Clinical Stress Research, no. 17. Stockholm, Nov. 1970.

38. Johns, M. W., T. J. A. Gay, J. P. Masterton et al. "Relationship between Sleep Habits, Adrenocortical Activity, and Personality," *Psychosom. Med.*, 33 (1971), 499–503.

39. Katz, J. L., P. Ackman, Y. Rothwax et al. "Psychoendocrine Aspects of Cancer of the Breast," *Psychosom. Med.*, 32 (1970), 1–18.

40. Knapp, P. H., C. Mushatt, S. J. Nemetz et al. "The Context of Reported Asthma during Psychoanalysis," *Psychosom. Med.*, 32 (1970), 167–188.

41. Kreuz, L. E. and R. M. Rose. "Assessment of Aggressive Behavior and Plasma Testosterone in a Young Criminal Population," *Psychosom. Med.*, 34 (1972), 321–332.

42. Kreuz, L. E., R. M. Rose, and J. R. Jennings. "Suppression of Plasma Testosterone Levels and Psychological Stress: A Longitudinal Study of Young Men in Officer Candidate School," *Arch. Gen. Psychiatry*, 26 (1972), 479–482.

43. Levi, L. "The Urinary Output of Adrenaline and Noradrenaline during Different Experimentally Induced Pleasant and Unpleasant Emotional States: A Summary," *J. Psychosom. Res.*, 8 (1964), 197–198.

44. ——. "The Stress of Every Day Work as Reflected in Productiveness, Subjective

Feelings, and Urinary Output of Adrenaline and Noradrenaline Under Salaried and Piece-work Conditions," *J. Psychosom. Res.*, 8 (1964), 199–202.

45. LEVI, L., ed. "Stress and Distress in Response to Psychological Stimuli," *Acta. Med. Scand.*, 191, *Suppl.* 528 (1972).

46. MASON, J. W. "Psychological Influences on the Pituitary-Adrenal Cortical System," *Recent Prog. Horm. Res.*, 15 (1959), 345–389.

47. ———. "Psychoendocrine Approaches in Stress Research," in *Symposium on Medical Aspects of Stress in the Military Climate*, pp. 375–419. Washington: Walter Reed Army Institute of Research, 1964.

48. ———. "The Scope of Psychoendocrine Research," *Psychosom. Med.*, 30 (1968), 565–575.

49. ———. "A Review of Psychoendocrine Research on the Pituitary-Adrenal Cortical System," *Psychosom. Med.*, 30 (1968), 576–607.

50. ———. "A Review of Psychoendocrine Research on the Sympathetic-Adrenal Medullary System," *Psychosom. Med.*, 30 (1968), 631–653.

51. ———. "A Review of Psychoendocrine Research on the Pituitary-Thyroid System," *Psychosom. Med.*, 30 (1968), 666–681.

52. ———. "Organization of the Multiple Endocrine Responses to Avoidance in the Monkey," *Psychosom. Med.*, 30 (1968), 774–790.

53. ———. " 'Over-all' Hormonal Balance as a Key to Endocrine Organization," *Psychosom. Med.*, 30 (1968), 791–808.

54. ———. "Strategy in Psychosomatic Research," *Psychosom. Med.*, 32 (1970), 427–439.

55. ———. "A Re-evaluation of the Concept of 'Non-Specificity' in Stress Theory," *J. Psychiatr. Res.*, 8 (1971), 323–333.

56. MASON, J. W. and J. V. BRADY. "The Sensitivity of Psychoendocrine Systems to Social and Physical Environment," in P. H. Liederman and D. Shapiro, eds., *Psychobiological Approaches to Social Behavior*, pp. 4–23. Stanford: Stanford University Press, 1964.

57. MASON, J. W., J. V. BRADY, and M. SIDMAN. "Plasma 17-Hydroxycorticosteroid Levels and Conditioned Behavior in the Rhesus Monkey," *Endocrinology*, 60 (1957), 741–752.

58. MASON, J. W., J. V. BRADY, and W. W. TOLSON. "Behavioral Adaptations and Endocrine Activity—Psychoendocrine Differentiation of Emotional States," in R. Levine, ed., *Endocrines and the Central Nervous System*, pp. 227–250. Baltimore: Williams & Wilkins, 1966.

59. MASON, J. W., E. D. BUESCHER, M. L. BELFER et al. "Pre-illness Hormonal Changes in Army Recruits with Acute Respiratory Infections," (Abstract) *Psychosom. Med.*, 29 (1967), 545.

60. MASON, J. W., C. C. KENION, D. R. COLLINS et al. "Urinary Testosterone Responses to 72-Hour Avoidance Sessions in the Monkey," *Psychosom. Med.*, 30 (1968), 721–732.

61. MASON, J. W., G. F. MANGAN, JR., J. V. BRADY et al. "Concurrent Plasma Epinephrine, Norepinephrine, and 17-Hydroxycorticosteroid Levels during Conditioned Emotional Disturbances in Monkeys," *Psychosom. Med.*, 23 (1961), 344–353.

62. MASON, J. W., W. J. H. NAUTA, J. V. BRADY et al. "The Role of Limbic System Structures in the Regulation of ACTH Secretion," *Acta. Neuroveget.*, 23 (1961), 4–14.

63. MASON, J. W., E. J. SACHAR, J. R. FISHMAN et al. "Corticosteroid Responses to Hospital Admission," *Arch. Gen. Psychiatry*, 13 (1965), 1–8.

64. MATHE, A. A. and P. H. KNAPP. "Emotional and Adrenal Reactions to Stress in Bronchial Asthma," *Psychosom. Med.*, 33 (1971), 323–340.

65. MATTSON, A., S. GROSS, and T. W. HALL. "Psychoendocrine Study of Adaptation in Young Hemophiliacs," *Psychosom. Med.*, 33 (1971), 215–225.

66. MICHAEL, R. P. and J. L. GIBBONS. "Interrelationships between the Endocrine System and Neuropsychiatry," *Int. Rev. Neurobiol.*, 5 (1963), 243–292.

67. MILLER, R. G., R. T. RUBIN, B. R. CLARK et al. "The Stress of Aircraft Carrier Landings. 1. Corticosteroid Responses in Naval Aviators," *Psychosom. Med.*, 32 (1970), 581–588.

68. NALBANDOV, A. V., ed. *Advances in Neuroendocrinology*. Urbana: University of Illinois Press, 1963.

69. NAUTA, W. J. H. "Central Nervous Organization and the Endocrine Motor System," in A. V. Nalbandov, ed., *Advances in Neuroendocrinology*, pp. 5–21. Urbana:

University of Illinois Press, 1963.

70. OKEN, D. "The Role of Defense in Psychological Stress," in R. Roessler, ed., *Physiological Correlates of Psychological Disorder*, pp. 193–210. Madison: University of Wisconsin Press, 1962.

71. PERSKY, H., D. A. HAMBURG, H. BASOWITZ et al. "Relation of Emotional Responses and Changes in Plasma Hydrocortisone Level after Stressful Interview," *Arch. Neurol. Physiol.*, 79 (1958), 434–447.

72. PINCUS, G., H. HOAGLAND, H. FREEMAN et al. "A Study of Pituitary-Adrenocortical Function in Normal and Psychotic Men," *Psychosom. Med.*, 11 (1949), 74–101.

73. POE, R. O., R. M. ROSE, and J. W. MASON. "Multiple Determinants of 17-Hydroxycorticosteroid Excretion in Recruits during Basic Training," *Psychosom. Med.*, 32 (1970), 369–378.

74. PRICE, D. B., M. THALER, and J. W. MASON. "Preoperative Emotional States and Adrenal Cortical Activity: Studies on Cardiac and Pulmonary Surgery Patients," *Arch. Neurol. Psychiatry*, 77 (1957), 646–656.

75. REISS, M., ed. *Psychoendocrinology*. New York: Grune & Stratton, 1958.

76. RIZZO, N. D., H. M. FOX, J. C. LAIDLAW et al. "Concurrent Observations of Behavior Changes and of Adrenocortical Variations in a Cyclothymic Patient during a Period of 12 Months," *Ann. Intern. Med.*, 41 (1954), 798–815.

77. ROSE, R. M. "Androgen Responses to Stress: I. Psychoendocrine Relationships and Assessment of Androgen Activity," *Psychosom. Med.*, 31 (1969), 405–417.

78. ———. "The Psychological Effects of Androgens and Estrogens—A Review," in R. I. Shader, ed., *Psychiatric Complications of Medical Drugs*, pp. 251–293. New York: Raven Press, 1972.

79. ROSE, R. M., T. P. GORDON, and I. S. BERNSTEIN. "Sexual and Social Influences on Testosterone Secretion in the Rhesus," (Abstract) *Psychosom. Med.*, 34 (1972), 473.

80. ROSE. R. M., J. W. HOLADAY, and I. S. BERNSTEIN. "Plasma Testosterone, Dominance Rank, and Aggressive Behavior in Male Rhesus Monkeys," *Nature*, 231 (1971), 366–368.

81. ROSE, R. M., J. W. MASON, and J. V. BRADY. "Adrenal Responses to Maternal Separation and Chair Adaptation in Experimentally Raised Rhesus Monkeys (Macaca mulatta)," in C. R. Carpenter, ed., *Proc. 2nd. Int. Congr. Primates*, Vol. 1, pp. 211–218. New York: Karger, 1969.

82. ROSE, R. M., R. O. POE, and J. W. MASON. "Psychological State and Body Size as Determinants of 17-OHCS Excretion," *Arch. Intern. Med.*, 121 (1968), 406–413.

83. RUBIN, R. T. and A. J. MANDELL. "Adrenal Cortical Activity in Pathological Emotional States. A Review." *Am. J. Psychiatry*, 123 (1966), 387–400.

84. SACHAR, E. J. "Corticosteroids in Depressive Illness: A Re-evaluation of Control Issues and the Literature," *Arch. Gen. Psychiatry*, 17 (1967), 544–553.

85. SACHAR, E. J., J. M. MACKENZIE, and W. A. BINSTOCK. "Corticosteroid Responses to Psychotherapy of Depressions: I. Evaluations during Confrontation of Loss," *Arch. Gen. Psychiatry*, 16 (1967), 461–470.

86. SACHAR, E. J., J. M. MACKENZIE, W. A. BINSTOCK et al. "Corticosteroid Responses to Psychotherapy of Depressions: II. Further Clinical and Physiological Implications," *Psychosom. Med.*, 30 (1968), 23–44.

87. SACHAR, E. J., J. W. MASON, J. R. FISHMAN et al. "Corticosteroid Excretion in Normal Young Adults Living under 'Basal' Conditions," *Psychosom. Med.*, 27 (1965), 435–445.

88. SACHAR, E. J., J. W. MASON, H. S. KOLMER, JR. et al. "Psychoendocrine Aspects of Acute Schizophrenic Reactions," *Psychosom. Med.*, 25 (1963), 510–537.

89. SELYE, H. "A Syndrome Produced by Diverse Nocuous Agents," *Nature*, 138 (1936), 32.

90. ———. *Stress*. Montreal: Acta, 1950.

91. SILVERMAN, A. J., S. I. COHEN, B. M. SHMAVONIAN et al. "Catecholamines in Psychophysiologic Studies," *Recent Adv. Biol. Psychiatry*, 3 (1961), 104–117.

92. SMITH, C. K., J. BARISH, J. CORREA et al. "Psychiatric Disturbances in Endocrinologic Disease," *Psychosom. Med.*, 34 (1972), 69–86.

93. THORN, G. W., D. JENKINS, J. C. LAIDLAW et al. "Response of the Adrenal Cortex to Stress in Man," *Trans. Assoc. Am. Physicians*, 66 (1953), 48–64.

94. TROYER, W., J. MASON, and J. HIRSCH. "A Preliminary Psychoendocrine Study of

Obese Patients," unpublished observations.

95. VON BERTALANFFY, L. *Modern Theories of Development*. London: Oxford University Press, 1933.

96. WADESON, R. W., J. W. MASON, D. A. HAMBURG et al. "Plasma and Urinary 17-OHCS Responses to Motion Pictures," *Arch. Gen. Psychiatry*, 9 (1963), 146–156.

97. WILLCOX, D. R. "The Serial Study of Adrenal Steroid Excretion," *J. Psychosom. Res.*, 4 (1959), 106–116.

98. WOLFF, C. T., S. B. FRIEDMAN, M. A. HOFER et al. "Relationship between Psychological Defenses and Mean Urinary 17-OHCS Excretion Rates. I. A Predictive Study of Parents of Fatally Ill Children," *Psychosom. Med.*, 26 (1964), 576–591.

99. WOLFF, C. T., M. A. HOFER, and J. W. MASON. "Relationship between Psychological Defenses and Mean Urinary 17-OHCS Excretion Rates: II. Methodological and Theoretical Considerations," *Psychosom. Med.*, 26 (1964), 592–609.

100. YATES, F. E. and J. W. MARAN. "Stimulation and Inhibition of Adrenocorticotropic (ACTH) Release," in W. Sawyer and E. Knobil, eds., *Handbook of Physiology, Section on Endocrinology*. Washington: American Physiological Society, forthcoming.

CHAPTER 25

PSYCHOSOCIAL AND EPIDEMIOLOGICAL CONCEPTS IN MEDICINE

John J. Schwab

THIS CHAPTER will present some of the concepts of psychosocial medicine as they relate to psychosomatic disorders, particularly in groups. This will involve an examination of the epidemiology of psychosomatic disorders, their frequency and distribution, the demographic characteristics of the afflicted, and changing patterns of susceptibility and illness. Then we will look at some of the ideas about relationships between sociocultural processes and health or illness. In this chapter, the term "psychosocial medicine" refers to the health and illness of groups.

In any discussion of psychosocial medicine, we should be aware of certain unanswerable questions. Can we attribute psychosomatic illnesses and behavioral disorders to sociocultural processes? When a sufficient number of individuals within a group becomes ill, should the entire group be labeled a "sick society"?[35] Can an entire group react, analogous to an individual, in such a way that it becomes ill? Although we cannot find definitive answers to these questions, we know that numbers of persons, groups, can display similar reactions, that they may be predisposed to mental and psychosomatic illnesses, possibly by learning and conditioning, and that certain illnesses may become epidemic as a result of that predisposition, perhaps by conditions leading to shared "definitions of the situation,"[127] or even by contagion.

In his introduction to *Psychosocial Medicine: A Study of the Sick Society*, Halliday states that:

A group, like an individual, may be viewed both physically and psychologically. . . . If [the physical] needs are not satisfied its "physical health" declines and the group becomes a *sick population* characterized by high rates of sickness and death due to reasons such as malnutrition, infectious diseases, infestations, and so on. In its psychological aspects a group appears as a society with psychological or social needs. If these needs are not satisfied, its "psychological health," which is also its "social health" declines and the group becomes socially sick, that is, a *sick society*. The medical approach to the study of the sick society is called "psychosocial medicine." [p. 10][35]

Our concepts of psychosocial medicine extend back to Hippocrates'[44] *Airs, Waters, and Places* which deals specifically with the influence of the environment on the organism—not only physical factors such as climate and the character of the terrain, but also socioenvironmental factors such as the habits and the child-rearing practices of various peoples as they relate to health and disease. His treatise, therefore, may be considered as the first essay on ecologic medicine.

Hippocrates described some specific psychosomatic afflictions and associated their frequency with certain sociodemographic characteristics. For example, in comparison to other peoples, the nomadic Scythians were an infertile group. He attributed their infertility to their constitutions: "They are stout and fleshy in appearance; they have ill-marked joints, and are flabby and lacking in tone; their lower alimentary canals are moist beyond the ordinary."[11] He related both their constitutional deficiencies and their infertility to their habits and customs. Wealthy Scythians spent almost all of their lives on horseback. The men developed edema and severe varicosities of their lower extremities while the fat, indolent women had menstrual difficulties: "The monthly cleansing process does not take place in proper fashion, but is scanty and of short duration."[11] But the impotence and the menstrual difficulties, Hippocrates noted, were diseases only of the wealthy who could afford horses. The poor, who walked or ran while the tribes moved from place to place, did not have these afflictions. Hippocrates stated that the wealthier Scythians' manner of life was one factor responsible for their infertility. As further etiological evidence, he noted that: "an

important proof of this is furnished by their female servants; for no sooner do they have intercourse with a man than they become pregnant, this being due to their lives of hard toil and to the sparseness of their frames."[11]

In this classic, Hippocrates supplied us with an explanatory model for examining populations and their illnesses in a psychosocial context. Life styles, which were directly related to social class (in conjunction with constitutional factors), affected both the men and the women in ways which resulted in infertility in the upper classes. In addition to pointing out that the frequency of infertility varied with social class, he noted that the child-rearing practices were influential. In contrast to other peoples, the wealthy Scythians did not swaddle their children, but instead, just allowed them to ride in wagons. Although Hippocrates does not state explicitly that the children were neglected by not being swaddled, he intimates that their life style was conducive to the development of their constitutional deficiencies and thus their infertility.

This ancient description of the relationship between sociocultural processes and psychosomatic illness furnishes a background for looking at the psychosocial aspects of psychosomatic disorders. A rationale for this approach is provided by the studies which have shown repeatedly that psychosomatic disorders are unequally distributed within and between populations. Also, at times certain psychosomatic afflictions have been epidemic; some examples are tarantism in the Middle Ages, fainting in the Victorian Era, and coronary heart disease today.

In an editorial in *Science*, Stallones[121] quotes Andrija Stampar: "No matter what the number of physicians may be, they will never improve people's health by individual therapy." Stallones does not minimize the importance of direct medical care but he does assert that the major health benefits of the last century ". . . have resulted from the operation of undirected, nonspecific influences. Advances in medical knowledge and the decline of disease are simultaneous results of a general improvement in the quality of life." He maintains that: "To define, explain, and gain control of the various and extremely effective determinants of disease requires a deep appreciation of the ecological systems of which they are a part." He concludes that different environmental experiences are responsible for differences in the frequency of illness between different populations and that substantial improvements are possible if ". . . we are able to understand and control the general environmental factors contributing to disease."[121]

Both the unequal distribution of illnesses within a given population and the significance of the social environment have been shown by Hinkle and Wolff's prospective studies of health and disease over a period of more than twenty years. Working initially with a healthy, homogeneous population, they found that episodes of illness were not randomly distributed; instead, the most frequently ill 10 percent of the subjects experienced 34 percent of the total sickness disability in contrast to the healthiest 10 percent who experienced only 1 percent of the total sickness disability.[41] The ill group was also found to be accident prone. A positive correlation was discovered between what was characterized as a "good attitude and the ability to get along with people" and a low frequency of illness. No differences in the childhoods of the two groups were found but the group with the highest frequency of illness was characterized as "unhappy, insecure, discontented, and with a large number of interpersonal problems."[41] The difference in the rates of absence from work was hypothetically explained by the correlation between the frequency of illness and both unfulfilled expectations and perceptions of a stressful life.

The results from their extended work with five different populations (100 Chinese immigrants, 76 Hungarian refugees, 1527 skilled workmen, 1700 semiskilled women workers in New York City, and 132 recent college graduates) were remarkably similar to their earlier findings.[43] Episodes of illness were not randomly distributed among the members of any of the groups; in each of the groups, during twenty years of adult life, 25 percent of the members experienced approximately 50 percent of all the episodes of illness. The healthiest 25 percent in each group experienced less than 10 percent of the total number of illness episodes. Furthermore, differences in susceptibility to illness were not limited to any specific syndromes:[43]

In every group the members displayed a difference in their susceptibility to illness in general, regardless of its type, or of the causal agents apparently involved. Thus, as the number of episodes experienced by an individual increased, the number of different types of disease syndromes that he exhibited increased also. Although a great many of these syndromes might involve one or two organ systems, episodes of illness were not limited to a few systems; instead, as the number of episodes of illness experienced by an individual increased, the number of his organ systems involved in disease increased also. Likewise, as the number of episodes he experienced increased, he exhibited illnesses of an increasing variety of etiologies. He was likely to have more "major," irreversible and life-endangering illnesses, as well as more "minor," reversible and transient illnesses. Finally, as the number of his "bodily" illnesses increased, the number of his "emotional disturbances" and "psychoneurotic" and psychotic manifestations (here categorized as "disturbances of mood, thought, and behavior") usually increased also.

These findings have been obtained consistently in each of these five groups, regardless of the sex, race, culture, economic or social background, environment or life experiences of the people studied.

Then Hinkle and Wolff found that their subjects had peak periods in which the number of illness episodes appeared as clusters of different syndromes, of varying degrees of severity, and from several etiological sources. They concluded that "efforts to adapt to the social environment are to some degree involved in the majority of all of the illness episodes that occur among the adult population."[43] They emphasize that the state of the host is only one determinant of illness, that a man's susceptibility to illness is influenced by "his relation to the society in which he lives and the people in it."[43] Their studies yielded no evidence for labeling any special category of disease as psychosomatic; instead, they think that all forms of illness are influenced by reactions to life situations and the patient's relation to his environment.

TABLE 25–1.   **Frequency and Distribution of Psychosomatic Illness**

AUTHOR	YEAR	PERCENT OF SAMPLE WITH PSYCHOPHYSIOLOGICAL SYMPTOMS
General Populations		
Hollingshead and Redlich[45]	1958	7–13
Leighton et al.[47,62,65] (Stirling County Study)	1959	59
Srole et al.[61,120] (Midtown Manhattan Study)	1962	60
Pasamanick[87]	1962	3.65
Surveys of Medical Practice		
Watts[132]	1962	26.5 (Great Britain)
Crombie[19]	1963	40
Kessel and Munro[56]	1964	1.68 (Scottish town)
Finn and Huston[29]	1966	20
Mazer[73]	1967	30
African and Aboriginal Societies		
Leighton et al.[63]	1963	84 (Yoruba)
Kidson and Jones[57]	1968	1.4 (Australian aborigines)

Hinkle and Wolff found, therefore, that illnesses were unequally distributed within the five homogeneous groups they studied. A look at the epidemiology of psychosomatic disorders and psychophysiological symptoms in a number of different populations in various parts of the world reveals varying frequencies in different populations.

(**Frequency and Distribution**

It appears that the frequency of psychosomatic illness, and particularly psychophysiological symptomatology, has been rising since World War II. As shown in Table 25–1, both epidemiological studies and surveys of physicians' practices have shown that psychophysiological illness is a common affliction.* In the Stirling County Study,[62] the psychophysiological symptom pattern turned out to be the most common, present in 59 percent of the total sample. Of the respondents in the Midtown Manhattan Study,[61,120] 60 percent had so-

* See references 19, 29, 45, 47, 56, 57, 61–63, 65, 73, 87, 120, and 132.

matic complaints. In their study of psychiatric treatment patterns in New Haven, Hollingshead and Redlich[45] reported psychosomatic reactions in 7–13 percent of patients in various social classes. In a survey of Baltimore households, conducted in 1961, Pasamanick[87] found a prevalence rate of 3.65 percent for psychophysiological disorders.

In our epidemiological study of a southeastern county which is in the throes of social change, we are finding that large numbers of people are ill with various types of diseases. In a preliminary random community sample of 322 adults, 31 percent were rated as impaired according to our criteria of social psychiatric impairment; 42 percent reported psychophysiological illnesses; and 42 percent were rated as having some degree of physical illness (27 percent mild and 15 percent moderate or severe).[105,112]

Of the more than 1600 respondents in our major community sample, 7 percent reported that they had had peptic ulcers, 3 percent asthma, and 8.6 percent reported having had hypertension at some time in their lives. About 6 percent reported having a "nervous stomach," 8 percent symptoms of indigestion, and almost 10 percent headaches at the present time.

Physicians' surveys also attest to the high frequency of psychosomatic illnesses and psychophysiological symptoms. Finn and Huston's[29] analysis of medical practices in Iowa disclosed that about 20 percent of the adults consulting physicians had psychosomatic illnesses. In a study of psychiatric conditions in general practice, Mazer[73] reports that 30 percent of the medical patients were diagnosed as psychophysiologic. Kessel and Munro's[56] summary of surveys from Scotland, Australia, and London, and Watts'[132] study of general practitioners in Britain report a great variability in one-year-period prevalence rates in various communities, ranging from 1.68 percent in a small Scottish town to 26.5 percent in Britain. Maintaining that a strict enumeration of psychosomatic disorders in medical practice is misleading, Crombie[19] concludes that 40 percent of patients going to practitioners had mixed organic-emotional illnesses.

These findings, notwithstanding variations in methodology and results, illustrate that the prevalence of psychophysiological illnesses is a health problem of substantial magnitude. Furthermore, evidence of the increasing frequency of psychosomatic disorders, e.g., peptic ulcer,[21] diabetes,[12] and especially coronary heart disease,[49,52,72] indicates that these illnesses can be regarded as epidemic, at least in Western societies.

It may be argued that this increase is more apparent than real because the population at risk is larger for a number of reasons; e.g., many would have formerly died early deaths from infectious diseases before antibiotics were discovered. Spain,[119] however, concludes from an analysis of vital statistics that there is considerably increased morbidity and mortality from psychosomatic illness, and that the base has moved toward younger age groups.

Early investigators believed that psychophysiological illnesses were unevenly distributed throughout the world, prevalent in industrialized societies, but relatively rare among primitives.[35] Studies by Kidson and Jones,[57] Leighton, et al.,[63] and Seguin,[116] for example, found great variability in primitive societies, ranging from 1.4 percent in Australian aborigines[57] to 84 percent in the Yoruba in Nigeria.[63]

With increasing industrialization throughout the world, parity may be reached in terms of distribution of psychosomatic illnesses.[97,99] However, data concerning this distribution and particularly transcultural comparisons, are difficult to evaluate and are obviously subject to erroneous interpretations because the epidemiological task is complex and social psychiatry is in its infancy.[35]

(Demographic Characteristics of the Afflicted

Age

Table 25–2 summarizes the findings of major epidemiological studies with reference to age and psychosomatic disorders. Although psychosomatic disorders do occur in children, they are generally considered to be afflictions of adult life. The authors of the Midtown Manhattan Study found that psychosomatic symptoms increase with age. However, they did not sample subjects aged sixty and older. In our preliminary community study, we also found a linear relationship up to the age of sixty; psychophysiological illness was present in 37 percent of those under the age of thirty, 41 percent in those between thirty and forty-four years old, and 51 percent in the forty-five-to-fifty-nine age group. But in those over the age of sixty, the percentage with psychophysiological illnesses dropped to 43 percent. It should be noted, however, that most of our respondents over the age of sixty, about 80 percent, had physical illnesses of some type; as the percentage with psychophysiological illnesses among the elderly diminished, the percentage with physical illnesses increased. The elderly, as a group, are more and more plagued by ill health. Harrington,[37] in discussing "the golden years," paraphrases Yeats, "(This) is no country for old men."

Earlier, Halliday[35] suggested that a rising frequency of psychophysiological symptomatology in younger age groups was evidence of

TABLE 25–2.   Relationship of Age and Psychosomatic Disorders

AUTHOR	YEAR	AGE GROUP	RESULTS
Leighton et al.[47,62,65] (Stirling County Study)	1959	30–70	Increase with age
Srole et al.[120] (Midtown Manhattan Study)	1962	All ages	Increase with age
Finn and Huston[29]	1966	15–64 − 15, 65 +	Increase with age Prevalence diminished
Pasamanick[87]	1957	− 15, 65 +	Prevalence diminished
U.S. National Health Survey[21]	1960	35–54	Highest incidence of peptic ulcer in men
Mazer[73]	1967	45 +	Fewer psychophysiological disorders in men

greater incidence of psychosomatic illness. He found that peptic ulcer affected increasingly larger numbers of young people in Britain in the 1930s. He contended that these age shifts were due to the accumulation of persons who were predisposed to psychosomatic illness because of changes of conditioning during childhood. Studies found somewhat lower psychophysiological illness rates for the adolescent–young adult group and the elderly group.[29,87] This may indicate an inverse relationship between psychosomatic illness and depressive illness, since the latter appears to be increasing in these groups.[106,107]

Sex

The male–female ratio for psychophysiological symptoms in recent times has been reported by various investigators as 1 to 1,[47,62,65] 1 to 3,[87] and 2 to 3.[132] In our research with medical patients we found that women expressed significantly greater dissatisfaction with their bodily parts and functions than men.[108] Although we were not attempting to delineate psychosomatic entities, we concluded that women tended to somatize while the men were more stoical.[111] In our recent community study, 47 percent of the women were found to have psychophysiological illness in contrast to 32 percent of the men. Certain illnesses such as peptic ulcer and asthma were more common in the men than in the women, while hypertension, for example, was reported almost twice as often in the women than in the men.

Marked shifts in the sex ratio were described by Halliday[35] as being characteristic of psychosomatic disorders. Surveying this point historically, he notes that there was a reversal of the sex ratio for both diabetes and peptic ulcer from the nineteenth to the twentieth century. In the nineteenth century, peptic ulcer, which Dragstedt[25] has called "the wound stripe of civilization," was a woman's disease, but it became primarily an affliction of men in the present century.[35] Halliday notes that "the official *Medical History of the (First) Great War* did not even mention the term 'duodenal ulcer'."[35] In the United States, although more men than women suffer from peptic ulcer, the ratio has changed in the last few decades from at least 4 to 1 to 2.5 to 1.[21]

In our community study, 10.3 percent of the white men and 5.6 percent of the white women reported having had peptic ulcer at some time in their lives, but in the blacks this large sex differential was not present, i.e., 5.7 percent of the men reported having had peptic ulcers, as compared to 4.5 percent of the women. Coronary heart disease is much more frequent in men than in women, at least 2 to 1,[49] but the sex difference diminishes with increasing age.

Data concerning the disproportionate sex ratios of various psychosomatic diseases have been given sociocultural interpretations by Halliday,[35] Jennings,[51] and others. Fluctuations in sex ratio probably reflect the fact that social change does not exert a uniform influence on both sexes simultaneously. On the contemporary social scene, as women move out of their traditional roles to participate more actively in the occupational and social fields previously dominated by men, they are exposed to added stresses.[132] During this transition, there is greater role conflict and ambiguity, particularly for women. In fact, the "identity crisis," which is being conceptualized as a discrete illness entity for youth, may also have to be applied to many women, at least to the career women and working mothers. As they are subjected to role strain, susceptibility to both well-known and newer forms of psychosomatic illness is likely to increase. Perhaps we will see some convergence of differential psychosomatic sex ratios. But genetic and endocrine, as well as social factors, are influential in determining different reactions; even with comparable social stresses on both men and women, it is likely that some disorders will continue to be more frequent in one sex than in the other.

Social Class

Although Karl Marx once said that: "It is not the consciousness of men that determines their being, but, on the contrary, their social being that determines their consciousness,"[71] and novelists from Dickens to Steinbeck have described the misery of lower-class status, Hollingshead and Redlich's[45] work called our attention to the inverse relationship between social class and the prevalence of psychiatric illness, including the psychosomatic. Their lower-class patients somatized complaints to a greater extent than did the upper-class patients. Crandell and Dohrenwend,[18] reviewing both the Midtown Manhattan and Stirling County Studies, concluded that there is "a distinct tendency for lower-class groups to express psychological distress in physiological terms." Table 25-3 summarizes the findings regarding social class from a number of studies.

Most observers of our social scene have found[34,63,95] that the lower class is afflicted with a greater frequency of illness of almost

TABLE 25–3.   **Relationship of Social Class to Psychosomatic Illness**

AUTHOR	YEAR	RESULTS
Hollingshead and Redlich[45]	1958	Frequency of psychophysiological reactions inversely related to social class
Leighton et al.[47,62,65]	1959	Psychophysiological disorders more common in poorly integrated communities
Stamler et al.[122]	1960	High frequency of coronary heart disease in males in all socioeconomic groups

Srole et al.[120]	1962	Inversely related to class
		    Arthritis
		    Hypertension
		    Neuralgia
		Positively related to class
		    Colitis
		    Hives
		    Hay fever
		Other illnesses showed only erratic relationships with class
		Bell-shaped curve for hypertension

Pasamanick[87]	1963	U-shaped curve for hypertension

all types. We found that psychophysiological illness was much more prevalent in lower-income groups, i.e., present in 52 percent of those with annual family incomes of less than $3000 per year, and in 66 percent of those with incomes between $3000–5999 per year; but the figure dropped to 25–30 percent in the higher-income groups. A larger percentage of our lower-income respondents than those with higher annual family incomes had physical illness and also more lower- than higher-income respondents were rated as having social psychiatric impairment. For example, 67 percent of those with annual incomes under $3000 and 45 percent of those with annual incomes of $3000–5999 per year had physical illnesses, in contrast to 21–30 percent of those with annual incomes above $10,000. And 49 percent of those with annual incomes of less than $3000 and 42 percent of those with incomes from $3000–5999 were rated as having some degree of social psychiatric impairment, but impairment rates declined to about 15 percent in higher-income groups.

Just a few years ago, Coles[17] reported that the physical health of migrant laborers "deteriorates early in life." Comparisons of certain illness rates in families with incomes under $2000 and those over $7000[96] reveal that heart disease, arthritis, mental and nervous conditions, hypertension, and some physical impairments are two to four times more common in the lower-income group.

Race

Prior to World War II psychosomatic illnesses were believed to be relatively infrequent in Negroes. However, Rowntree's[98] evaluation of 13 million selective-service registrants in World War II showed a "marked increase in incidence of psychosomatic disease in the Negro, who in peacetime appeared relatively immune." Halliday,[35] in 1948, astutely recognized that the Negroes have always been a "second nation" within the United States and he also noted that the incidence of psychochosomatic disorders in Negroes was rising abruptly. Death from hypertension is seven

times more common in nonwhites than in whites.[122] This variation may be due to genetic differences but, as Stamler[122] has indicated: "The patterns of discrimination and segregation which Negroes experience in the United States may induce psychologic stresses, strains, frustrations, etc. These primary central nervous system effects may be responsible for the greater occurrence of hypertension in this racial group."

We found that fewer blacks than whites reported a history of peptic ulcer, but more blacks, especially the women, reported hypertension. Certain symptoms such as headaches and no appetite, were reported more frequently by the blacks, complaints of headache were particularly common in the younger black women.[113]

The work of M. Schwab[114] on hallucinations points to the difficulty in evaluating certain symptoms in black groups. Our preliminary community study showed that hallucinations were reported about twice as frequently by blacks than whites. In a small, southern, black community, she found that reports of hallucinations among the blacks were limited primarily to elderly men and young women. The elderly men's hallucinations could be interpreted as coping mechanisms since the themes centered on peaceful, religious topics; in contrast, the young women's hallucinations, usually filled with terrifying themes, were regarded as evidence of psychopathology and personal distress.

The facts showing that there are greater amounts of illness of all types in the lower class point to the plight of the nonwhites in the United States today who comprise the overwhelming majority of the low-income families.[9,37,96] In our countywide study, we found that the higher rates of social psychiatric impairment and poor physical health in the blacks were correlated with poverty and little education. This correlation between lower social status and illness has been found consistently in other studies.

Although the physical and cultural deprivation associated with being poor and uneducated is apparent to observers of our social scene, we found that social structural factors, such as low incomes, did not account completely for the high rates of social psychiatric impairment in the young blacks.[110] Strikingly, 52 percent of the younger blacks were found to be impaired, as compared to 33 percent of the whites. Comparative analyses for sex, age, education, and income revealed that the high impairment rate in the younger blacks was not as strongly related to low income as was true for the older group.

We suggest that the young black adults have been exposed, during their formative years, to the sociocultural change that has taken place in the last two decades. In their youth they witnessed the turbulence of America in the 1960s, and participated in the struggles accompanying desegregation. But their opportunities were limited for sharing in the life styles and material benefits of the wider society displayed by the media. At the same time the protective traditional cultural patterns of the Southern blacks were being assailed on two fronts, i.e., subordinated and exploited by the dominant white society on one hand and challenged and repudiated on the other by groups stressing African heritage and black power and scorning the former accommodations to the caste system.

Some of the blacks, e.g., the younger age group, can be seen as experiencing a conflict between competing sets of conditioned responses, such as parental restraints on assertion and aggression versus growing emphasis on pride in individuality and ethnicity. Such a situation produces cognitive dissonance and the dilemmas of the "marginal man." Marginality, a concept developed by Park[84] and elaborated by Stonequist,[123] describes persons caught between two different and often antagonistic cultures. Spiritual instability, intensified self-consciousness, restlessness, and malaise were noted by Stonequist as characteristic of the "marginal man."

But some changes in the social position and the health of the blacks can be expected as the nonwhites follow various paths to alleviate their distress. Within the decade of the 1960s, the nonwhite social scene changed rapidly.

This group, once sociologically perceived as a homogeneous subcultural entity, is composed now of diversified groups, socially stratifying within themselves as they develop new ideologies and allegiances. We now see four different patterns in the black population: (1) the militant separatists; (2) the nonviolent protestors; (3) those moving toward middle-class status; and (4) the poor, apathetic group. The Negro who is attempting to obtain a share of the goods of middle-class America by adopting the dominant white value system frequently becomes psychosomatically ill in following this path.[55] The apathetic group, analogous to Marx's "Lumpenproletariat," will probably continue to have at least as much illness as always, unless the caretaking functions of the government intervene. What will happen to those who are expressing their current discontent—both the aggressive separatists and the nonviolent protestors—remains to be seen.

The "second nation,"[35] the nonwhites, therefore, is rapidly becoming one composed of groups. We would expect, then, to begin to see differential manifestations of psychosomatic disorders within these groups as they become increasingly heterogeneous.

(Changing Patterns of Susceptibility and Illness

Many observers of our medical scene* have repeatedly maintained that there are continuing changes in both individual and group susceptibility to psychosomatic as well as to other diseases. These may be attributed in part to sociocultural transformations. Many changes in types of disease have occurred within our lifetime. For example, tuberculosis, once a scourge, has declined drastically throughout the Western world. This decline paralleled higher living standards. However, a rise in tuberculosis has been noted in the ghetto population of New York in the last few years.[7]

Some other infectious diseases, considered

* See references 5, 10, 35, 88, 91, and 125.

to be under control a few years ago, are reappearing as public-health menaces. Recent outbreaks of diphtheria, typhoid fever, and poliomyelitis can be traced to deteriorating public-health standards and facilities relative to the increased population, crowding, and migration, and to apathy resulting from overconfidence in the belief that immunizations and other precautions are no longer necessary. But the sharp rise in VD rates is probably one of the clearer examples of psychosocial influences. The massive movement of young men to and from Southeast Asia for a decade and the emergence of penicillin-resistant strains of gonococci are only in part responsible for the increasing frequency of gonorrhea in the United States today.[131] Numerous complex social and cultural processes have been converging to facilitate the spread of this disease. One of the most noticeable is the change to freer sexual mores. But this is only one aspect of a vast mosaic which includes the intergenerational conflict, with protesting youth living in communes and at times openly practicing polygamy, or even androgyny, as they reject the establishment's values. Moreover, promiscuity among adolescents and the large numbers of divorces even among the middle-aged reflect the changing social structure. The technological triumph represented by *the pill* may be the significant factor underlying the changes on the social scene which are linked to the spread of venereal disease.

Although changes in the incidence of carcinoma are still enigmatic, they may be related to dietary and smoking habits. Carcinoma of the stomach is now rare,[92] while carcinoma of the lung has become prevalent. Quisenberry[92] believes that ethnic variations in distribution and types of carcinoma in Hawaii are due to sociocultural forces, as well as genetic factors, but that with increased intermarriage and integration, the epidemiological picture will become more uniform.

Increased susceptibility to psychosomatic disease is taken for granted as a hazard of urban and suburban living.[33] Cities, of course, have been regarded historically as sources of illness as well as social evil. In *The Prelude*,[134]

Wordsworth described urban distress with the words: "Among the close and overcrowded haunts/Of cities where the human heart is sick. . . ."

Today, psychosomatic illness may be considered one of the American "crowd diseases," particularly among the mobile population. Stamler[122] points out that hypertension is much more common in Negroes who have moved to urban centers. In their epidemiological studies of hypertension, Geiger and Scotch[31] note a tendency toward high blood pressure in urban groups.

In many respects most of the world is being westernized, at least in terms of urbanization[20] and technological change.[27] In Nigeria, for example, Leighton et al.[63] found a higher incidence of psychophysiological illness in towns than in villages. Scotch's[115] comparative study of Zulus in rural and urban settings confirms these findings. Seguin[116] has described a marked increase in psychosomatic illness among Peruvians who migrate from the Sierra to the cities of the plain; according to him, they are undergoing "psychosomatic disadaptation."

Malzberg found that mental illness was more common among Negroes who migrated from the South to the North, than among those born there.[70] In our preliminary county study in the Southeast, we found the highest rates of social psychiatric impairment (including psychophysiological illnesses) among the "hypermobile," i.e., those who had moved nine or more times in the last ten years. The lowest rates were found in those who had moved only four to eight times during the last ten years.[109]

More than a century ago, De Toqueville[130] remarked that the Americans were restless in the midst of their prosperity: "A man builds a house in which to spend his old age, and he sells it before the roof is on . . . he settles in a place, which he soon afterwards leaves *to carry his changeable longings* elsewhere." (Italics ours.) That restlessness may be an American trait, but if so, it appears to be intensifying with contemporary social change. We found that mobility was associated with low rates of social psychiatric impairment when it was not carried to the extreme of hypermobility. Geographic mobility demands changing life styles affecting interactions with relatives and friends; especially for whites, it involves minimizing if not severing reliance on kinship networks. For our mobile, low-impairment group, it appears that the social interaction necessary to maintain adequate mental health is provided by the rapid acquisition of new friends whose life styles are similar or compatible.

Our initial findings on mobility are in keeping with Kantor's[54] conclusion that there is no simple, direct relationship between migration and mental illness. Adjustment to migration, she found, varies with: (1) the individual's social characteristics, attitudes toward moving, and preparedness; (2) with the sociopsychological aspects of the situation; and (3) with the characteristics of the sending and receiving communities. With the "National Incorporation of the South,"[69] the new elite is at home in Suburbia, U.S.A., in the North, South, East, or West.

Not only are patterns of illness changing but new forms are emerging and others are disappearing.[26] Syncope, once an appropriate social response, now occurs rarely. Of 1628 respondents in our community study, only eighty stated that they had ever fainted and only seven men and one woman reported that they had fainted during the preceding year. Schulte[104] maintains that fainting is not an adequate form of emotional discharge in our more complex society in which a wide variety of psychophysiological cardiovascular disorders occurs. With the widespread prevalence of coronary heart disease, complaints of chest pain communicate distress and ensure that the sufferer will receive sympathy and medical attention. We could view syncope as a conditioned social response in the nineteenth century, particularly in Victorian Britain, and chest pain as its equivalent in our current era.

Accident proneness is an everyday phrase, understood by laymen as well as professionals. Smart and Schmidt's[118] finding that ulcer patients had more traffic accidents per capita

than the general driving population supports Halliday's[35] thesis regarding the association of psychosomatic affections. Also, a rising frequency of posttraumatic neurosis, in Modlin's[77] terms, the postaccident syndrome, appears to be directly related to our rapid social and technological expansion. Modlin described the patients exhibiting this syndrome in both social and medical terms; they are integrated into society before the trauma but, in reality, they cannot adapt to the rate of technological change. After the accident they cannot cope because of limited "intrapsychic capacities which, in a crowded world of swift mobility, precipitant crises, and incredibly intricate technological innovations, render them disablingly vulnerable to the inevitable hazards of *living* in such a world."

The most common type of psychophysiological reaction that we see in our Psychiatric Consultation Service at the University of Florida does not have a label, indeed it is difficult to define as an entity. These are the "garden variety" medical patients equivalent to those whom Von Mering and Earley[74,75] call the "problem patients" in medical practice. A typical patient complains of numerous conventional and occasionally bizarre somatic complaints; his diagnostic workup may reveal minor or borderline abnormalities; he appears both anxious and depressed; and when questioned, he tells of interpersonal difficulties, discontent, frustration, and despair. The patient's personal problems are often compounded by the effects of medications, drugs, and alcohol which he has taken in an attempt to alleviate his distress with life and enable him to cope with the complexities of everyday living. Such patients, who, in von Mering and Earley's words, display "undifferentiated health aberrations," are becoming more and more numerous throughout the Western world.

Exotic diseases such as those produced by voodoo and hex, formerly treated only in isolated areas by root workers and witch doctors, are now seen in Negro migrants to ghetto areas.[129] Ellul,[27] in *The Technological Society*, tells of a new disease, "brought on by modern city life . . . which might be called urbanities." During the 1960s, a number of reports of epidemic hysteria appeared.[30,60]

Relationships

The psychosocial relationship of social factors, such as income levels, or cultural habits and customs, to health or illness is, of course, debatable. But certain relationships between the social environment and either health or illness have been established. In their review of more than forty different studies, Dohrenwend and Dohrenwend[23] conclude that "low socioeconomic status within a community is consistently found to be associated with relatively high overall rates of (psychological) disorder."

Whether the high rate of illness in low-income groups is due mainly to genetic factors, "drift" down the social scale, or causative social processes, is a major unanswered question. But the climate of poverty does include crowding, contact with the noxious and the infirm, nutritional deficiencies, physical and cultural deprivations, and often a quality of despair, if not desperation.

Sociocultural deprivation, as well as physical deprivation, appears to influence health and illness. Thoroughman and Pascal[128] showed by both retrospective and prospective studies that ulcer patients with intractable symptoms who scored high on a scale for environmental deprivation responded poorly to surgical treatment. In East European countries, deprivation is also a concern for research. For example, Mester and Mester[76] reported from Budapest that surgical success for the treatment of biliary disease is less frequent in patients who come from large poor families. Chertok et al.[15] and Destounis[22] concluded that economic difficulties were possibly responsible for vomiting in pregnancy.

The frequency of object loss preceding many illnesses has been related to socioeconomic changes.* Mutter and Schleifer[79] found that object loss frequently preceded the onset of physical illnesses in children and that in many, family disorganization was rampant.

* See references 3, 28, 58, 66, 79, 83, 100, and 101.

They concluded, ". . . changes in the psychosocial setting interacting with the psychological and social organization of the child and his family are relevant to the onset of somatic illness in children."

Animal studies show clear-cut relationships between the social environment and various types of illness and disorder. Rats separated from their mothers early in life were found by Ader and Friedman[4] to have a higher mortality rate from inoculated carcinosarcoma cells than did controls. Henry et al.[40] found that mice socially stressed by aggregating and mixing responded with hypertension. Calhoun's[13] classic study of the overpopulation of rats in a confined area demonstrated that crowding is associated with higher mortality rates, prematurity, and massive disorganization.

Principles of psychosocial medicine hold that man and his environment (which is now almost exclusively a social, man-made environment) are inseparable, interacting, and mutually influential. Thus, sociocultural processes, role functions and expectations, the personality and the self, with its instinctual and social needs, comprise a mutable, complex system. From this point of view, it is difficult to speak about exact etiological factors, especially as constants over extended periods of time, since the entire system is an interacting one, and we are always in the midst of social change and culture lag. Moreover, the epidemiology of psychosomatic and mental disorders is still in an embryonic, but developing, phase. In view of the lack of sound, descriptive epidemiology, inferences about etiology may be premature. Psychosocial medicine does consider that health and illness are relative conditions on a continuum, that they reflect the social-self system and that groups, as well as individuals, exist in varying states of health and illness.

Halliday developed the concept of a psychosomatic affection as an illness produced by multiple etiological factors and also as one which is characterized by "a *synergy* of causes"[35] (italics ours). He proposed an ontogenetic theory of psychosomatic affections which was grounded on the "progressive unfolding of a 'life' in historical time in accordance with the orderly mode of development characteristic of its species."[35] Particularly during the stages of infancy both the physical and emotional development of the child depend upon approval and disapproval by others, freedoms and frustrations, adaptations, and defenses, which are eventually woven into patterns of psychobiological reactivity that relate to health and illness.

In his *Concept of a Sick Society*, Ollendorff asserts that: "Society as a whole is fundamentally responsible for the phenomena which are reproduced in every human being."[82] He emphasizes, in Reichian terms, that character formation occurring in infancy and childhood results from ". . . the endless process of structuring as promoted by the impact of society as a whole."[82] Thus, the influence of society is seen fundamentally as being much greater than that of the immediate family, which can be viewed as just a more or less faithful transmitter of the prevailing social forces. Ollendorff also notes that character formation too frequently involves the development of character armor as a result of the prolonged series of incessant bombardments to which the infant and the child are exposed.

Brody[12] notes that in Western cultures there is an oversocialization of middle-class and undersocialization of lower-class children, particularly in terms of expression of feelings, training for identity, and communication. He thinks that the underprivileged group should be evaluated in terms of "multiple impairment" and "cultural exclusion," referring to those who do not have the "opportunity to share fully in the symbolic experience of the society."

The child-rearing practices employed by groups may be the vital determinants of psychosocial health or illness. Hippocrates' observations on the manner in which the Scythian children were reared and its relationship to the sexual and menstrual disorders in adult life, therefore, presage the tenets of modern social psychology and social psychiatry.

Halliday related the changes "in the worlds of the child and of the adult that took place between the 1870s and the 1930s in Britain"[35] to changes in the incidence of various ill-

nesses. Hysteria, common in Victorian England and frequent among enlisted men in the British Army in World War I, was seen much less often during World War II. Halliday describes the physical environment of the infant in the 1870s as appallingly bad; lack of sanitation, overcrowding, poverty, etc., led to high rates of bodily impairment and infant mortality. But viewed psychologically, he emphasizes that infants and young children were allowed a great deal of freedom; babies were breast fed, carried in the arms or swaddled (the perambulator first appeared only in the 1880s and was owned only by the wealthy); toilet training took place "in its own good time."[35] The "vital drives"[35] of early childhood were not inhibited; Halliday associates these child-rearing practices with fewer physiological dysfunctions. But he also notes that the frustrations imposed on the older child during the Oedipal period, and the problems with the patriarchal father were probably responsible for the high incidence of hysteria.

In contrast, the infants reared in the 1930s were fed from bottles according to schedule; "the 'infant in arms' had become the 'kid in the carriage' ";[35] bowel training was instituted early and thoroughly. Since there were fewer children, they were more noticeable and thus more closely watched and controlled. The family was based on the parental dyad. Physically, the environment had improved so that the infant mortality rate had fallen drastically. But psychologically, Halliday thinks that the imposed system of conditioning in child-rearing practices was conducive to physiological dysfunctions which became psychophysiological illnesses in later life. Furthermore, he notes that the stern father of the 1870s became the "daddy" in the 1930s, and that this also may be in part responsible for the decline in the incidence of hysteria.

Presciently, Halliday pointed out that certain changes in the world of the adults between the 1870s and the 1930s were also conducive to the development of the obsessive character type who was afflicted with numerous tensions and physiological dysfunctions. Many of these changes, which Halliday described in the 1940s, became the cries of alarm heard in the late 1960s. He described them as: (1) increasing separation from the outward roots in Mother Earth; (2) increasing disregard of cosmic and biological rhythms; (3) increasing frustration of manipulative creativity; (4) increasing pace of change in the structure of society; (5) increasing standardization and repression of individual expression; and (6) increasing absence of aim and direction.[35]

Halliday compared the indices of communal physical health (general death rate, infant-mortality rate, and certain infectious disease rates), which declined between 1900 and 1939, with indices of communal, psychological, or social health (infertility rate, suicide rate, certain psychosomatic-illness rates), which rose sharply between 1900 and 1939, and concluded that Great Britain was a "sick society."[35] He attributed the psychosocial illness which afflicted Great Britain and which was present elsewhere in Western societies to the "failure of the integration of the social group (which) is attended by failure of integration of the 'psychoneuro-endocrine system' of its members."[35] He stated that "the 'causes' of the weakening of those 'psychological bonds that enable the members of a community to live and work together' are therefore to be sought in the 'causes' that disintegrate social patterns in such a manner and to such a degree that the social equilibrium of the community cannot be restored."[35] He regarded social disequilibrium as the first stage of functional breakdown which is succeeded by social disintegration with a further weakening of the psychological bonds necessary for health.

As theorists of social change maintain, the causes of social disintegration may be produced by external forces, e.g., defeat in war, or from inner tensions, e.g., class conflict, or from decay as a natural phase of its life cycle. Halliday believed that the accelerated changes concomitant with the industrialization of Great Britain in the nineteenth century brought about rapid changes in family, religious, cultural, occupational, and economic patterns so that the "total social system became changed at an ever-accelerating rate, until a point was

reached when the national equilibrium was so seriously upset that disintegration set in."[35]

How social disintegration affects individuals or groups to produce illness, of course, has never been precisely determined. The Leightons[47,62,65] correlated increased psychiatric illness with community disintegration in the Stirling County Study. They postulate that sentiments are a bridging concept for analyzing relationships between the sociocultural environment and mental health or illness. Of particular importance are the "essential striving sentiments" which concern physical security, sexual expression, giving and receiving love, spontaneity, a sense of orientation in relation to society, of belonging to a moral order, etc.[62] Thus, "sociocultural situations can be said to *foster* psychiatric illness if they *interfere* with the development and functioning of these (striving) sentiments, since the latter, in turn, affect the essential psychical condition."[62] Therefore, an individual reacts to a disturbance in the essential psychical condition ". . . by seeking to remove the disturbance. When the process of this removal is inadequate (maladaptive to the personality), this fact is manifest in symptoms and impairment. . . . Symptom formation, however, is not the inevitable outcome."[65]

A number of models have been developed, but not tested, which relate sociocultural processes to the self. As evidenced by the work of Parsons,[86] Goodenough,[32] and Thomas and Bergen,[126] these models emphasize the importance of role theory and focus on the influence of role expectations, role participation, and role strain as determinants of behavior which have implications for psychosocial health and illness.

In *Toward a General Theory of Action*, Parsons[86] proposes an overarching series of constructs which embrace personality and society. He emphasizes that the personality and society are systems and that role participation is at the boundary, linking the individual personality and society: "One particular crucial aspect of the articulation of personality with the social system is the organized system of interaction between ego and 'alter' based upon role expectations."[86] Parsons refers explicitly to the degree of integration or disintegration being, in effect, located at the points of articulation of the personality and social systems. Thus, role expectations and role participation are subject to strain when there are sufficient dislocations in the social systems or disturbances within the personality. Parsons' concepts have implications for health and illness, indeed, for societal conflicts. He states that: "The group of problems centering around conformity, alienation, and creativity are among the most crucial in the whole theory of action because of their relevance to problems of social stability and change."[86]

In *Rethinking Status and Role*, Goodenough[32] distinguishes between personal identity and social identity. He insists upon flexible and dynamic concepts of status and role which emphasize the importance of boundaries and identities for the health of individuals and groups. In her book, *Purity and Danger*, Mary Douglas[24] describes, from an anthropological perspective, the significance which certain groups have placed on boundaries as necessities for ensuring societal integration and cohesion.

Thomas and Bergen[126] propose a model which relates social change to psychological malfunctioning. Social processes define roles and role expectations; personality organization at several levels mediates between role expectations and the instinctual and social needs of the self. Social roles, particularly expectations, embody approval and disapproval in our interpersonal relationships, and elaborated rewards and strains. Tensions and strains become particularly visible when roles and barriers diffuse, when values shift, and when the rate of social and culture change accelerates. Furthermore, Thomas and Bergen maintain that social and culture change affect the way an individual expresses the needs of the self, either by approving or by limiting the number and the modes by which the needs of the self are expressed. Either way, sociocultural processes require flexibility and changes within the personality organization in order to reduce tension within the group, within the social-self system, and/or within the individual.

At least implicitly, these schemata which attempt to explain how the social environment influences health or illness equate illness with maladaptation or see it as the result of stress. Equating illness with maladaptation, basically a Darwinian concept applicable to evolution, runs the risk of being tautological. Furthermore, we should be aware of Kluckhohn's[59] appraisal of adaptation as applied to social man: "We require a way of thinking that takes account of the pull of expectancies as well as the push of tensions, that recognizes that growth and creativity come as much or more from instability as from stability, and that emphasizes culturally created values as well as the immediately observable external environment."

The stress-strain model of illness, which uses a metaphor from a simpler mechanistic era, suggests an essentially mechanical relationship between man and the environment. As explained by Langner and Michael in *The Midtown Manhattan Study*,[61] noxious, or potentially noxious, factors constitute stress, and the reaction to the *stress* is termed "strain." They compare to a situation in engineering, in which a structure is tested by subjecting it to induced stress (e.g., tension, compression, etc.). The object may become deformed under such stress. This reaction—the deformation—is strain. Then, in reference to humans, they say: "We know that personality, the sum of a person's relatively reliable ways of acting and reacting, can become deformed because of stress."

Langner and Michael recognize the limitations of this model: "People are not wooden beams or iron bars."[61] Instead, humans are unpredictable; they symbolize, attach meanings to objects, situations, etc., and react to those meanings or ideas. "It is primarily this capacity of man to symbolize that turns a similar event into a catastrophe for one and a blessing for the other. If 'one man's meat is another man's poison,' how can we define stress in terms of the stimulus rather than the reaction? We can make some generalizations about what stress is because there are cultural and societal uniformities of 'meat' and 'poison' that are somewhat broader than the individual variations."[61] Some factors, constitutional, physical, and emotional, mediate between stress and strain to determine whether the outcome for a given individual will be health or illness. Socioeconomic status, for example, can be viewed either as a factor which is potentially stressful (e.g., poverty) or as one which mediates between other types of stress and strain (e.g., affluence).[61]

In terms of the stress-strain model, illness, or simply symptoms, are seen as reactions to noxious environmental forces. This is a useful frame of reference, especially for the study of fairly large populations, i.e., symptoms would be most common in the groups which are under the most stress, subject, of course, to elaborate mediating factors.

During the last few years, scales have been developed which evaluate the number, kinds, and significance of life events which are associated with the onset of disease. These scales are based primarily on the work of Schmale and others in the Rochester group which related object loss to the onset of physical and/or mental illness.[100,101] The theoretical construct is based on the assumption that certain life events, usually considered to be adverse, are stressful and thus require psychological and social readjustments.

The most widely used is The Social Readjustment Rating Scale of Holmes and Rahe[46] which contains forty-three items "indicative of the life style or of the kinds of events occurring in the individual's life . . . [which] involve an adaptive response on the part of the person affected."[36] The forty-three events range from death of spouse, divorce, and marital separation to a change in eating habits, vacation, and minor violations of the law. Each item is weighted in numerical Life Crisis Units (LCU)—death of spouse receives 100 LCU, while a minor violation of the law receives eleven LCU. Thus the subject receives a total score; higher scores ostensibly reflect greater stress and have been found to be associated with illness and presumably "high risk."

Paykel and his colleagues at Yale[89,90] have also developed a life-events scale which contains thirty-three items which are comparable to those in The Social Readjustment Rating Scale. In a controlled study, they found that depressed patients had a general excess of life events before the onset of depression.[89] Moreover, the depressed patients had significantly more losses or exits from the social field than the control group, who, in contrast, reported more entrances into the social field.

Both of these scales are being standardized with minority groups and used in cross-cultural epidemiological investigations. Their simplicity and ease of scoring are attractive features. But, an event that is defined by one individual as adverse, or even catastrophic, may be regarded by another as a relatively minor, meaningless, or even fortunate occurrence, depending on his "definition of the situation." The common use of these scales, however, yields precise information about the relationships of life events to illness and thus adds to our knowledge about the stress-strain model and, particularly, the significance of the social environment in health and disease.

The various models which relate psychosocial processes to illness in the individual and the group can be criticized for the risk of being tautological, because they are so all-inclusive that they cannot be adequately tested, or because they ultimately fall back on Thomas' definition of the situation. He asserted that: "Preliminary to any self-determined act of behavior there is always a . . . *definition of the situation* . . . gradually a whole life-policy and the personality of the individual himself follow from a series of such definitions."[126] This is a fundamental tenet of social psychology and how the situation is defined accounts for individual variation. Moreover, Thomas emphasized that there is "always a rivalry" between the individual's spontaneous definitions and the definitions of situations furnished him by society.

When carried to its logical extreme, this thesis, with its emphasis on the individual, appears to contradict concepts of psychosocial medicine which emphasize group reactivity in response to socioenvironmental stresses. Moreover, the thesis cannot explain such undisputed facts as epidemics. But we should not dismiss Thomas' insights so quickly; particularly in our contemporary era when we are witnessing sociopolitical polarization and group coalescence, subject to the impact of instant visual communication, we can postulate that shared definitions of a situation account for collective behavior, epidemics, etc.

The studies of Hinkle and his colleagues of relatively large populations demonstrate that the "reaction of a man to his life situation has an influence on all forms of illness."[43]

Other studies have shown that even a *single* adverse event such as real, threatened, or symbolic object loss, as presented by Schmale,[101] Adamson,[3] and others, or bereavement as shown by the work of Parkes,[85] is followed by illness of various types and severity. Furthermore, in a theme that reminds us of Halliday's[35] concept of a psychosomatic affection as one having *multiple* etiological factors and one which is characterized by a synergy of causes, Christenson and Hinkle[16] state that the interactions between man and his world are so complex ". . . that it is a gross oversimplification to attempt to explain 1 or 2 of their categories of illness simply on the basis of the way that they ate, how much they smoked, what happened to them in their childhood, or the way that they react to their present occupations." This point of view about etiology is emphasized by Stallones[121] in his editorial on community health. He deplores a reductionist approach, advocates a "synthetic systems-oriented approach" to the study of illness, and exhorts us to be concerned with "clusters of causes and combinations of effects."

A general systems approach, expressive of the metaphors of our technological era, has become a fashionable way to view man and the universe, to try to comprehend man and his ecosystems. Such an approach states explicitly that the systems, biological, social, and even cosmic, are open ones.[8] But Abelson, in an editorial in *Science*[1] commenting on D. H. Meadows et al., *The Limits to Growth*, reminds us that to some extent, "the concept of earth as a closed system is an appealing one, and in some respects it is valid."

In addition to considering the evidence which indicates that we are dealing with closed systems, e.g., the quantities of oxygen are limited, among certain animals overpopulation leads to social disorganization or death, and our cities decay after reaching a certain size, we should keep in mind Hinkle's statement about taking "a unitary view of the man-environment relationship" and abandoning "the needless dichotomy of a 'physical' and a 'social' environment."[41] Moreover, in discussing the relationship between the internal and external environments, he compares biological and social organizations. Just as individual cells or organs are sacrificed to maintain the organism, "the lives of individual men are subordinated to the requirements of the societies of which they are members."[41] He points out that social groups behave "as if the primary duty of the individual is to fulfill the various social roles in which he finds himself."[41] Thus, Hinkle stresses the importance of role functions and expectations in our modern society and he foretells that: "In the future we can expect that no small part of human illness will be determined by the interaction of men with other men, and by their adaptations to the social roles that are thrust upon them."[41] This unitary concept of man and his environment, the reaffirmation of Spencer and Durkheim's view of society as a living organism, and the focus on social roles as determinants of health and illness, make a strong case for the increasing relevance of psychosocial medicine in our contemporary era. Our epoch has already been described by Allen Wheelis[133] as *The End of the Modern Age*; with the discoveries in theoretical science, dating from Niels Bohr's work on the structure of the atom in 1917, it appears that the principle of uncertainty is just as applicable to the movement of an electron as it is to the vicissitudes of ordinary existence for human beings. The dire conclusions drawn in *The Limits to Growth* indicate that we are, indeed, creatures whose biological, social, and other systems are not only closed ones but may be finite. This acknowledgment is implicit to the concepts of psychosocial medicine.

This discussion of the relationships between social processes and psychosomatic illnesses from a psychosocial point of view has centered on many aspects of current social-science theories, particularly role functions and expectations, and the stress-strain model of illness, as well as the concept of adaptation. However, the presence of new epidemics such as coronary heart disease and the recurrences of epidemic hysteria compel us to consider contagion as a possible mechanism for transmitting psychosocial illnesses.

Contagion and Epidemics

In his classic work, *The Epidemics of the Middle Ages*,[39] Hecker described behavioral and psychosomatic disorders as well as diseases such as the black death. He tells that the dancing mania "was propagated by the sight of the sufferers, like a demoniacal epidemic over the whole of Germany and the neighboring countries to the northwest, which were already prepared for its reception by the prevailing opinions of the times."[39] This strange affliction, characterized by wild dancing, screaming, bodily distortions, mental aberrations, abdominal pain, and even convulsions, affected entire communities between 1374 and the beginning of the seventeenth century. Hecker reports that at one time it affected 500 inhabitants in Cologne and that once the streets of Metz were filled with 1100 dancers. In discussing the causes of this "mental plague," he mentions that the wretched and oppressed populace had been subjected to great natural disasters, famines, and the "incessant feuds of the barons"[39] which resulted in miserable conditions, club law, and the corruption of morals. Furthermore, Hecker maintains that the disposition of mind, peculiar to the Middle Ages, accounted for the long duration of this "extraordinary mental disorder."

In Italy, tarantism prevailed as a great epidemic in the fifteenth and sixteenth centuries. The predominant symptoms were melancholia, weeping, death resulting from paroxysms of laughter or tears, diarrhea, and a sensitivity to music. In fact, dancing to the tarantella relieved the symptoms. Hecker believed that these strange disorders, as well as the mass outbreaks of hysteria which he described, spread by "morbid sympathy"[39] until

they became real epidemics. He states that "imitation—compassion—sympathy, are imperfect designations for a common bond of union among human beings—for an instinct which connects individuals with the general body."[39] Thus, in the midst of societal disintegration, these strange diseases were spread "on the beams of light—on the wings of thought."[39]

Although we would like to explain psychosocial illness by scientific theories, we cannot entirely dismiss the part played by sympathy and contagion. There is some evidence that psychosomatic illnesses spread by interpersonal contagion. Winkelstein, as cited by Spain,[119] investigated the household aggregates of hypertensive patients, composed of both blood-related and nonrelated persons. The blood pressures of the nonrelated persons in these "hypertensive" households were higher than those of controls.

In 1955 an epidemic occurred at the Royal Free Hospital in London. Over 300 staff members became ill with severe malaise, slight fever, the subjective features of hyperventilation, and both evanescent and bizarre neurological symptoms which often followed a glove and stocking distribution.[67] The term "benign myalgic encephalomyelitis" has been applied as a diagnosis to about fifteen such outbreaks.[2,68] McEvedy and Beard[67] have reviewed these epidemics and conclude that they are psychosocial phenomena which should be termed "myalgia nervosa."

In 1943 Schuler and Parenton,[103] in reporting on an epidemic of hysteria in a Louisiana high school, noted that descriptions of such phenomena were abundant in the medical literature in the nineteenth century but that publications on the subject had become rare; in fact, they could not find "a single publication in the United States for over 40 years."[103] They concluded that the "phenomenon of the 'mental epidemic' is not exclusively historical, nor is it confined necessarily to ignorant and backward populations."[103] In 1958, Taylor and Hunter[124] described an epidemic of hysteria which occurred on an open hospital ward among female patients who suffered mainly neurotic and psychosomatic symptoms. Since then, mass hysteria associated with fears of having been bitten by insects was reported among the workers in a textile plant in South Carolina in 1963.[14] This is reminiscent of the epidemics of tarantism in Italy during the late Middle Ages, when the victims imagined they had been bitten by tarantulas.

During the 1960s a number of outbreaks of epidemic hysteria were reported in the United States and Britain, particularly among high school students.[30,60,78] Comparable epidemics have also been reported in nonwestern nations such as Taipei[48] and East Africa.[53] In discussing these mass outbreaks, Jacobs emphasizes that the "social and cultural contexts are most important in defining why they take place when they do and where they do . . . ."[48] Other authors such as Kagwa[53] refer to the basic similarity of such affections, "in man at different psychosocial developmental levels regardless of race or locale."

Redl[93] has indicated that an occurrence of contagion does not occur unless there are restraints to be reduced. This insight helps to explain that epidemics occur not only at times when unfavorable social conditions are conducive to the outbreaks, but also at times when repression is manifest. From this point of view, the epidemics of hysteria in the Victorian Era can be seen as miscarried revolts against the sexual repression of that time. We are concerned about the increasing sociopolitical repression in the United States today which may lead psychosocially to mass outbreaks of various mental and behavioral phenomena.

Drawing on the works of these writers[48,53, 93] since Hecker's day, we can also note that, in addition to social restraints and repressive forces, adverse conditions of life and a certain disposition of the mind are conducive to epidemics. Taylor and Hunter[124] explain that, "It often requires the adoption of a particular idea by a pluralistically stirred group before the accumulated emotions can be freely expressed. This idea will then appear to have been 'infectious' and to have aroused 'collective' emotions."

The high acceptability ratings given by various study groups to illnesses such as ulcer, arthritis, asthma, diabetes, and heart disease, relative to the low acceptability ratings for tuberculosis, alcoholism, and mental illness in Tringo's study[131] can be interpreted as evidence that we are a psychosomatically oriented society. Moreover, it was explained that the psychosomatic illnesses were acceptable because of their high frequency and "lessened shock value."[131]

The increasing incidence of coronary heart disease indicates that it has now become an epidemic of immense proportions. Mathers and Eliot[72] point out that 500,000 Americans die every year from ischemic heart disease and the latest figures indicate that 675,000 persons will die from coronary heart disease in 1974. Harris states that: "We are again in the age of the great pandemics. Our plague is cardiovascular."[38]

The shift of the age base to younger groups is further evidence that this disease is now epidemic; for men between the ages of twenty-five and forty-four, the death rate from coronary heart disease has risen from forty-six to fifty-two per 100,000 between 1950 and 1972.[80]

Ironically, Hinkle[41] notes that this disease appears to be "the outgrowth of several features of our society that we regard as most desirable."[41] These include a high standard of living with an abundant diet which is rich in fat and protein, a highly developed technology which reduces the demand for physical labor, a longer life expectancy with continued exposure to the abundant diet and lack of exercise, social mobility with its demands for alertness, and cigarette smoking to relieve consequent anxieties and tensions.

In a comprehensive review of over 160 papers dealing with the psychological and social precursors of coronary heart disease, Jenkins has come to the following conclusions: Seven general categories of social psychological factors can probably be considered as correlates of this illness. Although no consistent relationship has been observed between a single social-status index and coronary heart disease, status incongruity or inconsistency (discrepant levels of occupation, education, and income for an individual) appears to be associated prospectively with the disease. Although the evidence about social mobility is not definite, a positive relationship has been found between coronary heart disease and intergenerational mobility, and for migration. Higher levels of anxiety and neuroticism seem to precede coronary heart disease although the relationship between manifest anxiety and denial may complicate these conclusions. Life dissatisfactions and environmental stress are reported frequently by coronary heart disease patients. The coronary-prone behavior pattern (Type A) is related to increased risk. This pattern consists of the following traits: competitiveness, striving for achievement, impatience, and other characteristics—"consistent with the 'Protestant Ethic,' with urbanized Western civilization. . . ."[50]

The frequency and acceptability of diseases such as ulcer and coronary heart disease, the prevalence of psychophysiological symptoms, and the mass outbreaks of hysteriform illnesses with various somatic manifestations reflect the social environment. Our contemporary scene is: "Swept with confused alarms of struggle and flight/Where ignorant armies clash by night."[6] The rampant aggression, internal as well as external, which is now a part of everyday life, the lowered morale, and the national loss of confidence (expressed by political leaders, liberal and conservative, Democrats and Republicans) and the turbulent intergenerational conflict can occur only when a society is undergoing disintegration or at a juncture in history when an era is drawing to a close—when its forms are outworn and rejected, when its ethic is obsolete.

Concepts of psychosocial medicine hold that societies or groups exist in varying states of psychological health and illness; that sociocultural processes determine the state of a society's health; that the availability of the material necessities of life is a requisite for health; that shared sentiments both promote and reflect the health of the group; that through child-rearing practices and learning, societal patterns are reproduced in individuals, and that groups react like individuals. These concepts are extensions of Aristotle's statement that, "Man is by nature a social animal. . . . Society is something in nature that precedes the individual. Anyone who either cannot lead the common life or is so self-sufficient as not to need to, and therefore does not partake of society, is either a beast or he is a god."[117]

Basic concepts of psychosocial medicine also affirm that man's environment, now almost exclusively a social and a man-made one, can be pathogenic. Many of the indices of a society's psychological or social health, which Halliday used to characterize Great Britain as a "sick society" in the 1930s, are applicable to the United States in the late 1960s and early 1970s. Particularly, the increasing incidence of coronary heart disease and the rising suicide rate among the young show that our social environment can be lethal as well as pathogenic.

Once a society has been diagnosed psychosocially as "sick," Halliday states the methodology for investigating the nature and the etiology of the social sickness then calls for studying the three following questions:[35]

1. What kind of social group is this, that is, what group characteristics are relevant and causal?
2. Why did the community become sick when it did, that is, what are the causal and environmental factors?
3. Why did the community take ill in the manner it did?

When we find answers to these questions, then we can develop "social therapeutics—whose aim would be to alter etiologically relevant group characteristics and etiologically relevant factors so that reintegration could be secured and a sick society restored to health."[35]

(Bibliography

1. ABELSON, P. H. "The Limits to Growth," *Science*, 175 (1972), 1197.
2. ACHESON, E. D. "The Clinical Syndrome Variously Called Benign Myalgic Encephalomyelitis, Iceland Disease and Epidemic Neuromyasthenia," *Am. J. Med.*, 26 (1959), 569–595.

3. ADAMSON, J. D. and A. H. SCHMALE. "Object Loss, Giving Up, and the Onset of Psychiatric Disease," *Psychosom. Med.*, 27 (1965), 557–576.

4. ADER, R. and S. B. FRIEDMAN. "Social Factors Affecting Emotionality and Resistance to Disease in Animals. V. Early Separation from the Mother and Response to a Transplanted Tumor in the Rat," *Psychosom. Med.*, 27 (1965), 119–122.

5. ANGRIST, A. "Progress and Paradox in Pathology and Medicine," *Pharos*, 32 (1969), 48–53.

6. ARNOLD, M. "Dover Beach," in R. Aldington, ed., *The Viking Book of Poetry of the English Speaking World*, Vol. 2, p. 972. New York: Viking, 1958.

7. BENNETT, C. G. "Mayor's Panel Finds TB on Rise Here," *New York Times*, Dec. 18 (1968), 95.

8. BERTALANFFY, L., VON. "General System Theory and Psychiatry," in S. Arieti, ed., *American Handbook of Psychiatry*, 1st ed., Vol. 3, pp. 705–721, New York: Basic Books, 1966.

9. BLEIBTRAU, H. K. "The Impact of Urbanization on Human Evolution," unpublished paper.

10. BOYD, W. *A Text-Book of Pathology*, Chap. 1. Philadelphia: Lee & Febiger, 1953.

11. BROCK, A. J. *Greek Medicine*. New York: Dutton, 1929.

12. BRODY, E. B. "Transcultural Psychiatry, Human Similarities, and Socioeconomic Evolution," *Am. J. Psychiatry*, 124 (1967), 616–622.

13. CALHOUN, J. B. "Population Density and Social Pathology," in L. Duhl, ed., *The Urban Condition*, pp. 33–43. New York: Basic Books, 1963.

14. CHAMPION, F. P. and R. TAYLOR. "Mass Hysteria Associated with Insect Bites," *J. So. Carolina Med. Assoc.*, 59 (1963), 351–353.

15. CHERTOK, L., M. L. MONDAZAIN, and M. BONNAND. "Psychological, Social, and Cultural Aspects of Sickness during Pregnancy," *Activitas Nervosa Superior* (Praha), 4 (1962), 394–401.

16. CHRISTENSON, W. N. and L. E. HINKLE. "Differences in Illness and Prognostic Signs in Two Groups of Young Men," *JAMA*, 177 (1961), 247–253.

17. COLES, R. "The Lives of Migrant Farmers," *Am. J. Psychiatry*, 122 (1966), 271–285.

18. CRANDELL, D. L. and B. P. DOHRENWEND. "Some Relations Among Psychiatric Symptoms, Organic Illness, and Social Class," *Am. J. Psychiatry*, 123 (1967), 1527–1538.

19. CROMBIE, D. L. "The Procrustean Bed of Medical Nomenclature," *Lancet*, 1 (1963), 1205–1206.

20. DAVIS, K. "The Origin and Growth of Urbanization in the World," *Am. J. Sociol.*, 60 (1955), 429–437.

21. DEPARTMENT OF HEALTH, EDUCATION, AND WELFARE. *Health Statistics from the U.S. National Health Survey*, Series B, no. 17. Washington: U.S. Govt. Print. Off., 1960.

22. DESTOUNIS, N. "Les Facteurs economiques, culturels, sociaux ayant retenti sur secteur donné sur les complications de la grossesse —Une étude psychosomatique," *Bull. Off. Soc. Int. Psycho-Prophylax. Obstetr.*, 6 (1964), 23–30.

23. DOHRENWEND, B. P. and B. S. DOHRENWEND. *Social Status and Psychological Disorder: A Causal Inquiry*. New York: Wiley, 1969.

24. DOUGLAS, M. *Purity and Danger*. New York: Praeger, 1966.

25. DRAGSTEDT, L. R. "The Role of the Nervous System in the Pathogenesis of Duodenal Ulcer," *Surgery*, 34 (1953), 902–903.

26. DUBOS, R. *Man Adapting*. New Haven, Conn.: Yale University Press, 1965.

27. ELLUL, J. *The Technological Society*. New York: Random House, 1967.

28. ENGEL, G. L. "The Concept of Psychosomatic Disorders," *J. Psychosom. Res.*, 11 (1967), 3–9.

29. FINN, R. and P. HUSTON. "Emotional and Mental Symptoms in Private Medical Practice," *J. Iowa St. Med. Soc.*, 56 (1966), 138–143.

30. FRIEDMAN, I. T. "Methodological Considerations and Research Needs in the Study of Epidemic Hysteria," *Am. J. Public Health*, 57 (1967), 2009–2011.

31. GEIGER, H. J. and N. A. SCOTCH. "The Epidemiology of Essential Hypertension," *J. Chronic Dis.*, 16 (1963), 1151–1182.

32. GOODENOUGH, W. H. "Rethinking 'Status' and 'Role,'" in S. A. Tyler, ed., *Cognitive Anthropology*, pp. 311–330. New York: Holt, Rinehart, & Winston, 1969.

33. GORDON, R. and K. K. GORDON. "Psychosomatic Problems in a Rapidly Growing Suburb," *JAMA*, 170 (1959), 1757–1764.

34. GRAHAM, S. "Socio-Economic Status, Illness,

and the Use of Medical Services," in E. J. Jaco, ed., *Patients, Physicians, and Illness*, pp. 129–134. Glencoe, Ill.: Free Press, 1958.

35. HALLIDAY, J. L. *Psychosocial Medicine: A Study of the Sick Society*. New York: Norton, 1948.

36. HARMON, D. K., M. MASUDA, and T. H. HOLMES. "The Social Readjustment Rating Scale: A Cross-Cultural Study of Western Europeans and Americans," *J. Psychosom. Res.*, 14 (1970), 391–400.

37. HARRINGTON, M. *The Other America*. Baltimore: Penguin, 1963.

38. HARRIS, T. G. "Affluence, the Fifth Horseman of the Apocalypse: A Conversation with Jean Mayer," *Psychol. Today*, 3 (1970), 43.

39. HECKER, J. F. C. *Epidemics of the Middle Ages*. Translated by B. G. Babington. London: Woodfall, 1844.

40. HENRY, J. P., J. P. MEEHAN, and P. M. STEPHENS. "The Use of Psychosocial Stimuli to Induce Prolonged Systolic Hypertension in Mice," *Psychosom. Med.*, 29 (1967), 408–432.

41. HINKLE, L. E. "Relating Biochemical, Physiological, and Psychological Disorders to the Social Environment," *Arch. Environ. Health*, 16 (1968), 77–82.

42. HINKLE, L. E., R. H. PINSKY, I. D. J. BROSS et al. "The Distribution of Sickness Disability in a Homogeneous Group of 'Healthy Adult Men,'" *Am. J. Hygiene*, 64 (1956), 220–242.

43. HINKLE, L. E. and H. G. WOLFF. "Ecological Investigations of the Relationship between Illness, Life Experiences, and the Social Environment," *Ann. Intern. Med.*, 49 (1958), 1373–1388.

44. HIPPOCRATES. *The Medical Works of Hippocrates*. Translated by J. Chadwick and W. N. Mann. Oxford: Blackwell Scientific Publications, 1950.

45. HOLLINGSHEAD, A. B. and F. C. REDLICH. *Social Class and Mental Illness*. New York: Wiley, 1958.

46. HOLMES, T. H. and R. H. RAHE. "The Social Readjustment Rating Scale," *J. Psychosom. Res.*, 11 (1967), 213–218.

47. HUGHES, C. C., M. TREMBLAY, R. N. RAPOPORT et al. The Stirling County Study of Psychiatric Disorder and Sociocultural Environment. Vol. 2. *The People of Cove and Woodlot*. New York: Basic Books, 1960.

48. JACOBS, N. "The Phantom Slasher of Taipei: Mass Hysteria in a Non-Western Society," *Soc. Problems*, 12 (1965), 318–328.

49. JENKINS, C. D. "Psychologic and Social Precursors of Coronary Disease (Part I)," *N. Engl. J. Med.*, 284 (1971), 244–255.

50. ———. "Psychologic and Social Precursors of Coronary Disease (Part II)," *N. Engl. J. Med.*, 284 (1971), 307–317.

51. JENNINGS, D. "Perforated Peptic Ulcer: Changes on Age, Incidence, and Sex-Distribution in the Last 150 Years," *Lancet*, 1 (1940), 395–398.

52. KAGAN, A., W. KANNEL, T. DAWBER et al. "The Coronary Profile," *Ann. N.Y. Acad. Sci.*, 97 (1963), 883–894.

53. KAGWA, B. H. "The Problem of Mass Hysteria in East Africa," *East Afr. Med. J.*, 41 (1964), 560–566.

54. KANTOR, M. B. "Internal Migration and Mental Illness," in S. Plog and R. B. Edgerton, eds., *Changing Perspectives in Mental Illness*. New York: Holt, Rinehart, & Winston, 1969.

55. KARDINER, A. and L. OVESEY. *The Mark of Oppression*. New York: World Publishing, 1951.

56. KESSEL, N. and A. MUNRO. "Epidemiological Studies in Psychosomatic Medicine," *J. Psychosom. Res.*, 8 (1964), 67–81.

57. KIDSON, M. and T. JONES. "Psychiatric Disorders among Aborigines of the Australian Western Desert," *Arch. Gen. Psychiatry*, 19 (1968), 413–417.

58. KISSEN, D. "Psychosocial Factors, Personality, and Lung Cancer in Men Aged 55–64," *Br. J. Med. Psychol.*, 40 (1967), 29–43.

59. KLUCKHOHN, C. *Culture and Behavior*. New York: Free Press, 1962.

60. KNIGHT, J. A., J. I. FRIEDMAN, and J. SULIANTI. "Epidemic Hysteria: A Field Study," *Am. J. Public Health*, 55 (1965), 858–865.

61. LANGNER, T. S. and S. T. MICHAEL. The Midtown Manhattan Study. Vol. 2. *Life, Stress and Mental Health*. New York: McGraw-Hill, 1963.

62. LEIGHTON, A. H. The Stirling County Study of Psychiatric Disorder and Sociocultural Environment. Vol. 1. *My Name Is Legion: Foundations for a Theory of Man in Relation to Culture*. New York: Basic Books, 1959.

63. LEIGHTON, A. H., T. A. LAMBO, C. C.

HUGHES et al. "Psychiatric Disorder in West Africa," *Am. J. Psychiatry*, 120 (1963), 521–527.

64. LEIGHTON, D. C. Personal communication, 1969.

65. LEIGHTON, D. C., J. S. HARDING, D. B. MACKLIN et al. The Stirling County Study of Psychiatric Disorder and Sociocultural Environment. Vol. 3. *The Character of Danger*. New York: Basic Books, 1963.

66. LESHAN, L. "Cancer Mortality Rate: Some Statistical Evidence of the Effect of Psychological Factors," *Arch. Gen. Psychiatry*, 6 (1962), 333–335.

67. MCEVEDY, C. P. and A. W. BEARD. "Royal Free Epidemic of 1955: A Reconsideration," *Br. Med. J.*, 1 (1970), 7–11.

68. ———. "Concept of Benign Myalgic Encephalomyelitis," *Br. Med. J.*, 1 (1970), 11–15.

69. MCKINNEY, J. C. and L. B. BOURQUE. "The Changing South: National Incorporation of a Region," *Am. Sociol. Rev.*, 36 (1971), 399–412.

70. MALZBERG, B. "Mental Disease among American Negroes: A Statistical Analysis," in O. Klineberg, ed., *Characteristics of the American Negro*, pp. 371–400. New York: Harper, 1944.

71. MARX, K. and F. ENGELS. "On Class," in C. W. Mills, ed., *Images of Man*, pp. 101–120. New York: Braziller, 1960.

72. MATHERS, D. H. and R. S. ELIOT. "Predicting and Preventing Sudden Death," in R. S. Eliot, ed., *Acute Cardiac Emergency*, pp. 281–286. Mt. Kisca, New York: Futura Publishing, 1972.

73. MAZER, M. "Psychiatric Disorders in General Practice: The Experience of an Island Community," *Am. J. Psychiatry*, 124 (1967), 609–615.

74. MERING, O. VON. "The Diagnosis of Problem Patients," *Human Organ*, 25 (1966), 20–23.

75. MERING, O., VON and L. W. EARLEY. "Major Changes in the Western Medical Environment," *Arch. Gen. Psychiatry*, 13 (1965), 195–201.

76. MESTER, B. F. and Z. MESTER. "Psychological Analysis of the Biographical Data of 83 Patients with Biliary Disease," *Am. Med. Psychol.*, 119 (1961), 447.

77. MODLIN, H. "The Postaccident Anxiety Syndrome: Psychological Aspects," *Am. J. Psychiatry*, 123 (1967), 1008–1012.

78. MOSS, P. D. and C. P. MCEVEDY. "An Epidemic of Overbreathing Among Schoolgirls," *Br. Med. J.*, 2 (1966), 1295–1300.

79. MUTTER, A. and M. SCHLEIFER. "The Role of Psychological and Social Factors in the Onset of Somatic Illness in Children," *Psychosom. Med.*, 28 (1966), 333–343.

80. NEWSWEEK. "Heart Attack: Curbing the Killer," 79 (May 1, 1972), 73–74.

81. NEWSWEEK. "VD: The Epidemic," 79 (Jan. 24, 1972), 46–50.

82. OLLENDORFF, R. H. V. "Concept of the Sick Society," unpublished work.

83. PARENS, H., B. J. MCCONVILLE, and S. M. KAPLAN. "The Prediction of Frequency of Illness from the Response to Separation," *Psychosom. Med.*, 28 (1966), 162–176.

84. PARK, R. E. "Human Migration and the Marginal Man," *Am. J. Sociol.*, 33 (1928), 881–893.

85. PARKES, C. M. "The Psychosomatic Effects of Bereavement," in O. W. Hill, ed., *Modern Trends in Psychosomatic Medicine*, Vol. 2. New York: Appleton-Century-Crofts, 1970.

86. PARSONS, T. and E. A. SHILS, eds. *Toward a General Theory of Action*. Cambridge, Mass.: Harvard University Press, 1962.

87. PASAMANICK, B. "A Survey of Mental Disease in the Urban Population: An Approach to Total Prevalence by Diagnosis and Sex," *J. Nerv. Ment. Dis.*, 133 (1961), 519–523.

88. PAUL, J. R. *Clinical Epidemiology*. Chicago: University of Chicago Press, 1966.

89. PAYKEL, E. S., J. K. MEYERS, M. N. DIENELT et al. "Life Events and Depression, a Controlled Study," *Arch. Gen. Psychiatry*, 21 (1969), 753–760.

90. PAYKEL, E. S. and E. H. UHLENHUTH. "Rating the Magnitude of Life Stress," *Can. Psychiatr. Assoc. J.*, 17, Suppl. 2 (1972), SS93–100.

91. PELLER, S. *Quantitative Research in Human Biology and Medicine*. Bristol, England: Wright, 1967.

92. QUISENBERRY, W. B. "Sociocultural Factors in Cancer in Hawaii," *Ann. N.Y. Acad. Sci.*, 84 (1960), 795–806.

93. REDL, R. "The Phenomenon of Contagion and 'Shock Effect' in Group Therapy," in K. R. Eissler, ed., *Searchlights on Delinquency*, pp. 315–328. New York: International Universities Press, 1949.

94. RENNIE, T. A. C. and L. SROLE. "Social

Class Prevalence and Distribution of Psychosomatic Conditions in an Urban Population," *Psychosom. Med.*, 18 (1956), 449–456.

95. RICHARDSON, W. C. *Dimensions of Economic Dependency*, Health Administration Perspectives, no. A4. Washington: U.S. Govt. Print. Off., 1967.

96. RICHMOND, J. B. "Toward a Developmental Psychosomatic Medicine," *Psychosom. Med.*, 25 (1963), 567–573.

97. ROSEN, G. "The Evolution of Social Medicine," in H. E. Freeman, S. Levine, and L. G. Reeder, eds., *Handbook of Medical Sociology*. Englewood Cliffs, N.J.: Prentice-Hall, 1963.

98. ROWNTREE, L. G. "Psychosomatic Disorders as Revealed by Thirteen Million Examinations of Selective Service Registrants," *Psychosom. Med.*, 7 (1945), 27–30.

99. SARVOTHAM, T. G. and J. N. BERRY. "Prevalence of Coronary Heart Disease in an Urban Population in Northern India," *Circulation*, 37 (1968), 939–953.

100. SCHMALE, A. H. "Relationship of Separation and Depression to Disease: A Report on a Hospitalized Medical Population," *Psychosom. Med.*, 20 (1958), 259–277.

101. ———. *Object Loss, "Giving Up," and Disease Onset: An Overview of Research in Progress*. Washington: Walter Reed Army Institute of Research, 1964.

102. SCHMALE, A. H., S. MEYEROWITZ, and D. C. TILLING. "Current Concepts of Psychosomatic Medicine," in O. W. Hill, ed., *Modern Trends in Psychosomatic Medicine*, Vol. 2, pp. 1–25. New York: Appleton-Century-Crofts, 1970.

103. SCHULER, E. A. and V. J. PARENTON. "A Recent Epidemic of Hysteria in a Louisiana High School," *J. Soc. Psychol.*, 17 (1943), 221–235.

104. SCHULTE, W. "Syncopal Attacks and Cardiac Phobias as Models of Psychosomatic Diseases, with a Discussion of the Biographical and Sociological Correlations," *Klin. Wochenschr.*, 40 (1962), 1088–1093.

105. SCHWAB, J. J. "Psychosomatics and Consultation," *Psychosom.*, 13 (1972), 9–12.

106. SCHWAB, J. J., M. R. BIALOW, J. M. BROWN et al. "Sociocultural Aspects of Depression in Medical Inpatients: II. Symptomatology and Class," *Arch. Gen. Psychiatry*, 17 (1967), 539–543.

107. SCHWAB, J. J., M. R. BIALOW, C. E. HOLZER et al. "Sociocultural Aspects of Depression in Medical Inpatients: I. Frequency and Social Variables," *Arch. Gen. Psychiatry*, 17 (1967), 533–538.

108. SCHWAB, J. J. and J. D. HARMELING. "Body Image and Medical Illness," *Psychosom. Med.*, 30 (1968), 51–61.

109. SCHWAB, J. J. and N. H. McGINNIS. "Social Change, Cultural Change and Mental Health," in *Proc. 5th World Congr. Psychiatry*. Excerpta Medica International Congress Ser., no. 274, Part 1, *Psychiatry*, pp. 703–709. Amsterdam: Excerpta Medica Foundation, 1973.

110. ———. "Social Psychiatric Impairment: Racial Comparisons," *Am. J. Psychiatry*, 130 (1973), 183–187.

111. SCHWAB, J. J., N. H. McGINNIS, and J. D. HARMELING. "Anxiety, Self-Concept, and Body Image: Psychosomatic Correlations," in J. J. Lopez-Ibor, ed., *Proc. 4th World Congr. Psychiatry*. Excerpta Medica International Congress Series, no. 150, Part 4, *Free Communications*, pp. 2715–2717. Amsterdam: Excerpta Medica Foundation, 1968.

112. SCHWAB, J. J. and G. J. WARHEIT. "Evaluating Southern Mental Health Needs and Services: A Preliminary Report," *J. Fla. Med. Assoc.*, 59 (1972), 17–20.

113. SCHWAB, J. J., G. J. WARHEIT, G. SPENCER et al. "Concurrent Psychiatric and Medical Illness," in J. Bierer, V. Hudolin, and J. Masserman, eds., *Proc. 3rd Int. Congr. Soc. Psychiatry*, Vol. 4, pp. 157–163. Zagreb: Amali, 1970.

114. SCHWAB, M. "Hallucinatory Behavior in a Southern Negro Community," in P. Adams, ed., *Humane Social Psychiatry*, pp. 125–133. Gainesville, Fla.: Tree of Life Press.

115. SCOTCH, N. A. "A Preliminary Report on the Relation of Sociocultural Factors to Hypertension Among the Zulu," *Ann. N.Y. Acad. Sci.*, 84 (1960), 1000–1009.

116. SEGUIN, C. A. "Migration and Psychosomatic Disadaptation," *Psychosom. Med.*, 18 (1956), 404–409.

117. SELDES, G. *The Great Quotations*, p. 67. New York: Lyle Stuart, 1960.

118. SMART, R. G. and W. S. SCHMIDT. "Psychosomatic Disorders and Traffic Accidents," *J. Psychosom. Res.*, 6 (1962), 191–197.

119. SPAIN, D. M. "Discussion: Sociocultural Factors in Chronic Organic Disease," *Ann. N.Y. Acad. Sci.*, 84 (1960), 1031.

120. SROLE, L., T. S. LANGNER, S. T. MICHAEL et al. The Midtown Manhattan Study, Vol. 1. *Mental Health in the Metropolis.* New York: McGraw-Hill, 1962.

121. STALLONES, R. A. "Community Health," *Science,* 175 (1972), 839.

122. STAMLER, J., M. KJELSBERG, and Y. HALL. "Epidemiologic Studies on Cardiovascular-Renal Diseases: I. Analysis of Mortality by Age-Race-Sex-Occupation," *J. Chronic Dis.,* 12 (1960), 440–455.

123. STONEQUIST, E. V. *The Marginal Man,* pp. 139–158. New York: Scribners, 1937.

124. TAYLOR, F. K. and R. C. A. HUNTER. "Observation of a Hysterical Epidemic in a Hospital Ward: Thoughts on the Dynamics of Mental Epidemics," *Psychiatr. Q.,* 32 (1958), 821–829.

125. TAYLOR, I. and J. KNOWELDEN. *Principles of Epidemiology,* 2nd ed. Boston: Little, Brown, 1964.

126. THOMAS, C. S. and B. J. BERGEN. "Social Psychiatric View of Psychological Malfunction and Role of Psychiatry in Social Change," *Arch. Gen. Psychiatry,* 12 (1965), 539–544.

127. THOMAS, W. I. In H. Blumer, ed., *An Appraisal of Thomas and Zanecki's "The Polish Peasant in Europe and America."* New York: Social Science Research Council, 1939.

128. THOROUGHMAN, J. C., G. R. PASCAL, W. O. JENKINS et al. "Psychological Factors Predictive of Surgical Success in Patients with Intractable Duodenal Ulcer," *Psychosom. Med.,* 26 (1964), 618–624.

129. TINLING, D. C. "Voodoo, Root Work, and Medicine," *Psychosom. Med.,* 29 (1967), 483–490.

130. TOQUEVILLE, A., DE. *Democracy in America,* Vol. 2. New York: Knopf, 1945.

131. TRINGO, J. L. "The Hierarchy of Preference toward Disability Groups, *J. Spec. Educ.,* 4 (1970), 295–306.

132. WATTS, C. A. H. "Psychiatric Disorders," *Stud. Med. Popul. Subj.,* 14 (1962), 35–52.

133. WHEELIS, A. *The End of the Modern Age.* New York: Basic Books, 1971.

134. WORDSWORTH, W. *The Prelude, or Growth of a Poet's Mind,* E. de Selincourt, ed. London: Oxford University Press, 1960.

CHAPTER 26

PSYCHOLOGICAL ASPECTS OF CARDIOVASCULAR DISEASE*

Chase Patterson Kimball

❨ Introduction

IN CONSIDERING the psychological aspects of cardiovascular disease four areas are discussed: (1) coronary artery disease; (2) congestive heart failure; (3) hypertension; and (4) special aspects of diagnosis and treatment. Although the reader will note psychological variables common to each of these processes, the emphasis is different in each situation. In coronary artery disease, attention is given to the precursant behavioral factors and concurrent social events. In congestive heart failure, emphasis is placed upon the interrelationship of sociological, psychological,

and physiological stress factors in precipitating failure in the presence of structural myocardial or valvular changes. In hypertension, the progressive nature of the disease is considered in terms of effecting different psychosocial relationships for each stage. The section on the psychological aspects of special procedures in diagnosis and treatment discusses cardiac catheterization, cardiac pacemakers, intensive care units, cardiovascular surgery, and the new operant conditioning techniques.

The psychological aspects are discussed in terms of three phases: (1) preillness behavior patterns and personality; (2) the psychological state of the individual at the time of onset; and (3) the emotional and psychological reaction to illness. In each of these phases, the reader will find that it is difficult to separate strictly psychological phenomenon from the

---

* This chapter has a subsection on Psychophysiological and Psychodynamic Problems of the Patient with Structural Heart Disease by Morton F. Reiser and Hyman Bakst on pages 618–624.

physioanatomic on one hand or from the socioenvironmental on the other. Wherever possible, the interaction of these variables with one another is stressed, rather than an implied linear or causal relationship between them. The literature is identified in considerable detail not only to provide current and historical reference sources for the interested student, but also to convey the complex interrelationships that prevail. At the same time, the significance of the findings presented are discussed in terms of their relevance and applicability to clinical problems. For example, the section on Psychological Aspects of Diagnosis and Treatment identifies the increasing attention that investigators have given to the adaptational responses of patients with catastrophic illness and the significance of these in their care.

(Coronary Artery Disease

Epidemiological Precursors

A discussion of psychosocial factors, precursant, concurrent, or consequent to the development and onset of cardiovascular and coronary artery disease begins with the work of epidemiologists.[222] Specific factors implicated by epidemiological study are diet— including caffeine—serum lipids, elevated blood pressure, smoking, diabetes, obesity, and cultural and genetic traits.[57,115] To date, almost all of these studies have been of men. The Framingham studies conducted during the 1960s correlated cholesterol levels, elevated blood pressure and smoking with atherosclerosis.[44] Heavy cigarette smokers experienced a three-fold increase in incidence of myocardial infarction and death from any cause over noncigarette, i.e., pipe and cigar, and former smokers. Although the study failed to demonstrate a relationship with angina pectoris, it did show a correlation of the latter with weight gain after the age of twenty-five.[50,107] Other investigators have verified these relationships and suggested that smoking may act both as an independent factor and in association with other risk factors.[72,221,231]

Paffenbarger and his colleagues have reviewed the college health records of individuals who subsequently developed cardiovascular disease, identifying eight precursors for victims of coronary disease: heavy cigarette smoking, higher blood pressure levels, excess body weight, shortness of stature, nonparticipation in athletics, early parental death, only-child status and "sociopsychological exhaustion".[161-163] Thomas, in a prospective study of medical students has found similar correlations.[229,230,235,237] More recently the lower incidence of atherosclerotic heart disease in some areas of the United States has been related to the increased Lithium content in the water supply.[245] A similar correlation has been suggested for mental illness, which is made more interesting by at least one study which suggests that patients with cardiovascular disease often have cyclothymic personalities.[243] In a study of young men with coronary artery disease, Hatch et al. have found that overnutrition and heavy smoking may interact with hereditary factors to accelerate the progress of coronary atherosclerosis.[86] Among the genetic factors cited are short stature, vascular defects, and abnormalities in the intermediary metabolism of lipoproteins and carbohydrates.

Psychosocial Precursors

In a review of the psychosocial precursors of coronary artery disease, Jenkins cites and evaluates 162 studies.[103,104] He sees the need for larger prospective studies to examine the psychosocial variables: behavior patterns, crisis-related disease-onset situations, and social incongruity. He suggests that these studies address themselves to four patterns of coronary artery disease: (1) survivors vs. (2) nonsurvivors of myocardial infarctions; (3) individuals with silent infarctions; and (4) patients with angina pectoris. Such studies, he anticipates, will identify relative importance for each of the psychosocial variables as related to different disease patterns. The following discussion identifies some of the correlations between psychosocial variables and coronary artery disease.

SOCIAL

Hinkle, on the basis of an earlier review of the social and biological correlates of coronary artery disease, hypothesized that diet, activity patterns, increased latitude for social mobility, and striving behavior foster, via neuronal and hormonal mechanisms, a biochemical environment in the blood stream that accelerates atherosclerosis, facilitating occlusion of coronary arteries, impairing blood supply to the heart muscle, and making arrhythmias and death more likely.[96] He believes that social and behavioral variables cannot be dealt with in broad general categories such as "stress" and "mobility" but must be studied as discrete, carefully limited, vigorously defined concepts or entities. Coronary artery disease is the outcome of a complex interaction of many variables in which no single one predominates. In an examination of the variables occupation and education, Hinkle and his colleagues executed a five-year survey of 270,000 Bell System employees establishing that: (1) men attaining the highest levels of management do not have a higher risk of coronary artery disease than men at the lowest levels; (2) there was no added risk for men elevated quickly or transferred; (3) men who had college degrees on entering the company had a lower attack rate, lower death rate, and lower disability rate at every age, in every part of the country, and in all departments; (4) the difference in risks exists at the time of employment; and (5) may be the result of biological differences in noncollege as opposed to college men related to social and economic background and resulting habits, e.g., smoking, diet, childhood health care.[97]

Other investigators have studied the relationship of social class to the incidence of coronary artery disease. Friedman and Hellerstein examined this incidence in four groups of lawyers presumably divided on the basis of economic and ethnic background.[63] Lawyers in the highest and lowest groups had a lower incidence than those falling in the middle groups. Bruhn et al. related a lower incidence of death from myocardial infarction with the stability of the community in the comparison of a mixed ethnic town with one composed primarily of lower socioeconomic Italians.[26] In a study of major significance, Shekelle et al., on the basis of a prospective study of 1472 middle-aged male Caucasians free of coronary heart disease, concluded that the incongruities in social status are associated with the risk of coronary heart disease.[214] They demonstrated that the incidence increased as the number of incongruities per subject increased. Men with four to five incongruities had six times the risk compared to men with no incongruities. This finding was not explained by correlations with serum cholesterol, arterial pressure, blood glucose, age, educational status, weight, or cigarette smoking. An interesting relationship was observed between level of education and manifestation of cardiac symptoms with men in the highest and lowest strata manifesting angina pectoris as opposed to the middle strata where symptoms and signs of myocardial infarction prevailed.

Caffrey, in a retrospective study of monks with myocardial infarctions, emphasized that a profile of scores relative to a number of factors is of greater significance in ascribing possible etiogenicity than single factors.[30] For monks, he suggests that such a profile including behavior pattern type A, i.e., a moderately high level of responsibility, a family background of lower socioeconomic status, a fairly sedentary occupation in one who has previously enjoyed a good deal of exercise, related to a greater likelihood of myocardial infarction. Cassel et al. comparing a prevalence vs. an incidence study among rural Georgians concluded that the previous high association of coronary artery disease in higher social class white men as opposed to lower rates for lower-class blacks was gradually disappearing presumably because of the increasing behavioral similarities in the two groups, especially among the younger men.[31]

BEHAVIORAL

Since 1958, Friedman and Rosenman and their associates have published extensive retrospective and prospective surveys relating a behavior pattern, identified as type A, to coronary artery disease.[64–67,194–196] In their initial studies, they correlated behavioral factors including intense ambition, competitiveness, constant preoccupation, the stress of occupational deadlines, and a sense of urgency with elevated serum cholesterol, increased blood clotting, *arcus senilis* and clinical coronary artery disease. Subsequently, they have measured the physiological reactions of subjects listening to a specially designed tape recording of two monologues, noting that individuals designated as type A manifested greater respiratory excursions, more frequent clenching of fists and body movement on listening to a dull, hesitant, monotonous, repetitive monologue as compared to individuals identified as having a type-B behavior pattern.[66] In a later, retrospective analysis of prospectively obtained data, 80 of 113 men who developed coronary heart disease or higher serum alpha lipoproteins had been rated as exhibiting behavior pattern type A. In a two year follow-up study, 70 of 3524 employees developed coronary heart disease as demonstrated by infarction or angina. All of these had initially shown an abnormal lipoprotein pattern, hypertension and/or type-A behavior pattern. Of the three, the latter was the single most constant factor. In contrast to the high risk of coronary artery disease identified for type-A behavior, they established a substantially lower risk for a type-B behavior pattern, presumably the converse of type A.[196] A man with type B was considered to be essentially immune to the development of clinical coronary heart disease if he exhibited a serum cholesterol level less than 226 μg./100 ml., a serum triglyceride level less than 126 μg./100 ml. or a serum B/∞ lipoprotein ratio less than 2.01 singly or in combination. On a study of the vasculature of type A and type B succumbing to death for whatever cause, they identified that the former exhibited severe coronary atherosclerosis six times more frequently than the latter.[64] In a recent review article[194] of their findings, a more graphic description for the individual with type-A behavior is suggested as a coat of arms showing a clenched fist wearing a stop-watch. The association of coronary artery disease and type-A behavior is associated with parental coronary artery disease, elevated cholesterol, cigarette smoking, and elevated diastolic blood pressure. The possible role of the hypothalamus is suggested.[194] Electrical stimulation of the diencephalon and lesions in the fornix, medial portion of the lateral hypothalamus and either ventromedial or dorsomedial nucleus have produced transient and persistent elevations in plasma cholesterol levels in rats. These elevations have also been associated with more active behavior patterns. Pursuing their search for a more objective identification of individuals with behavior pattern type A, the Friedman group has developed a twenty-item questionnaire and a voice analysis method of taped interviews which, they report, have achieved this objective.[106] Jenkins, in a computerized analysis of the questionnaire reports an astounding 73 percent correlation with interview assessment of type-A pattern.[105]

Bahnson has suggested another personality type for men with coronary artery disease in which passive and dependent traits rather than assertive and dominant ones are manifested.[10] This more "passive" pattern is hypothesized as developing from unresolved attachments to mothers as opposed to fathers which is suggested for type A.

The work of Friedman and Rosenman is in some ways a refinement of that pioneered by Flanders Dunbar in the 1930s and 1940s.[54] Based on an extensive review of the literature until that time and the intensive examination of 1600 hospital admissions, she identified personality profiles for patients with a variety of illnesses, including coronary occlusion, hypertensive cardiovascular disease, angina, rheumatic heart disease, and arrhythmias. Her profiles included not only obsessive-compulsive personality traits, but also passive-aggressive defenses for the expression of hostility and anger, rigid middle-class social patterns, and involved symbiotic family relationships. For each of these illnesses she delineated one or more features in several areas of the individual's psychosocial field that was characteristic for the group as a whole. These early identifications have spurred other investigators toward more specific examinations using more sophisticated methodologies.[113,156,227]

More thorough studies, such as those of Storment, have failed to confirm an overall personality type for cardiovascular illness, although accord sometimes has been reached for selected traits, such as stability of mood in patients with coronary occlusion and over-criticalness in hypertensives.[226] Other studies continued to investigate the possible correlations between personality and cardiovascular disease. More often than not, it seems that what is considered as personality is poorly defined and refers rather to one or several specific traits. Besides this difficulty, as several critics suggest, many of the studies have been retrospective and as such are more suggestive of types of responses to coronary disease rather than of common psychological precursors. Studies have included highly selected survivors, ignoring the 30 percent who died before inclusion, as well as those with "silent" infarctions who are rarely identified. Prospective studies, focusing on more objective measurements and larger numbers may overcome some of these deficits. The few prospective studies that have been executed have attempted to answer some of these criticisms. Lebovits et al. noted that individuals who died of coronary artery disease had higher Minnesota Multiphase Personality Inventory (MMPI) scores on several testings as compared with those who survived.[132] Among survivors there had been a worsening of MMPI scores between the first and second examinations prior to infarction as compared to individuals who did not subsequently develop heart disease. Brozek followed 258 business and professional men between the ages of forty-five and fifty-five, over fourteen years, subsequently comparing thirty-one who developed coronary disease with 138 who did not.[25] The former showed higher hypochondriasis scores on the MMPI, were more "aggressive" in their interests, and had higher scores on the Activity Drive Scale of the Thurstone Temperament Schedule.

Of studies that have been retrospective, Ibrahim et al. have suggested that the similarities in characteristics that they and others have identified probably are related to the reaction of patients to the disease.[99] They studied hypertension and elevated serum cholesterol in a coronary group and compared it with two at-risk groups, noting that two-thirds of the coronary group as opposed to one-fifth of the noncoronary group showed low-level manifest hostility and elevated levels of anxiety and regression. However, Shekelle et al., based on cross-sectional and longitudinal observations of middle-aged men, conclude that a psychological pattern is not related to either the risk of coronary heart disease nor is its occurrence related to the loss or acquisition of psychological patterns.[213]

Other retrospective studies have contrasted victims of cardiac disease with other populations. Bendian and Groen found patients with myocardial infarctions to be extroverts and suggested a cyclothymic personality for coronary patients.[13] Minc et al., found cardiac patients to show a greater degree of rational control.[154] Their patients showed greater inhibition both in behavior as measured by standard psychological tests and in cerebral cortical functioning as measured by alpha-wave frequency, critical frequency flicker, and reaction time. Cohen and Parsons contributed a negative correlation showing that there was no difference in time perception in coronary patients as opposed to others, and hypothesized that what previous investigators had identified in this regard related to socioeconomic variables.[38] Dreyfuss et al., observed that victims of myocardial infarction viewed the environment as more conflict-laden, the outcome of their actions as more unclear and with less certainty of success.[52] They felt their study supported Cleveland's and Johnson's hypothesis of weak ego boundaries based on the identification of chronic restlessness, underlying passivity, suppressed hostility, and sexual conflicts.[37] Subsequently Dreyfuss noted that infarction frequently occurred in depressed patients.[51] Wolff described compulsivity, repressed hostility, strong repressive superegos, and unfulfilled oral needs for psychiatric patients with angina pectoris.[269] Bruhn et al., contrasted survivors with non-survivors noting greater depression as determined by the MMPI for the latter.[27]

In summary of the psychosocial aspects of

coronary artery disease during the past decade on the basis of carefully constructed hypotheses and methods, several conceptual approaches to the study of the precursors of coronary artery disease have emerged. Paffenbarger, Thomas, and the Framingham group have noted the association of such risk factors as smoking, hypertension, cholesterol levels, early parental death, and activity patterns with the subsequent development of coronary artery disease.

Hinkle[96,97] has produced striking evidence suggesting that higher education at the time of employment is the signal variable correlating with a lower incidence of coronary artery disease. He suggests that this may be related to social and economic factors. Shekelle et al.[214] have introduced the intriguing observation that social incongruity is related to increasing risk for coronary artery disease. Friedman, Rosenman, and their associates[64–67,194–196] have repeatedly identified the type-A behavior pattern as the single most frequent variable correlating with the development of coronary artery disease. Jenkins[103,104] through a computerized analysis of interview and questionnaire data has verified this. The social, behavioral, and physiological interrelationships remain to be elucidated. To what extent these are mutually independent or dependent, genetically or epigenetically determined or cumulative remain for present and future investigators to unravel.

Stress and Illness Onset Precursors

In recent years, attention of investigators has turned increasingly to the environmental situation in which cardiovascular disease is first experienced. The stress researchers, while not ignoring the importance of genetic and previous behavior patterns, identify catastrophic events occurring in temporal proximity to the first symptoms and signs of cardiac disease.[143] Harold Wolff, a father of modern stress research, in a number of carefully designed and executed studies demonstrated a relationship between stressful situations and such physical factors as circulatory efficiency, faulty exercise tolerance, hemodynamic re-

sponse, cardiac arrhythmias, renal blood flow, electrocardiogram, and blood-pressure changes in patients with and without structural heart disease.[268] He identified that stress occurring concurrently with physical activity delayed return of cardiovascular factors to the resting state following cessation of activity. Noting that individuals responded cardiovascularly to stressful situations either hyper- or hypodynamically, he offered as an explanation that the type of response depended on the symbolic significance (often learned) of the stress to the perceiver. Only in this way and for the individual was stress specific for a specific cardiovascular response. Fisher noted that patients with cardiovascular disease frequently presented a history of working excessively under self-imposed and environmental pressure, and reported a gradual increase in the number and intensity of stressful situations prior to the onset of manifest heart disease.[59] Van der Valk and Groen emphasized the occurrence of myocardial infarction in a work situation as a result of interpersonal conflict precipitating an exaggeration of aggressive behavior.[243] Liljefors and Rahe, in a study of identical twins correlated life dissatisfactions as the single most consistent factor with the severity of coronary heart disease, as distinguished from smoking, obesity, hypercholesterolemia, the medical history and the physical examination.[137] Raab reviewing 305 studies relating stress factors to coronary artery disease suggested that emotional and sensory stresses resulted in central nervous system arousal of the pituitary-adrenal and sympathoadrenomedullary systems resulting in the overproduction of adrenocortical steroids and sympathomimetic catecholamines leading to a depletion of myocardial potassium, elevation of blood pressure, and local myocardial hypoxia.[180] He included fear, anxiety, anger, frustration, and optical, accoustical, and thermal percepts among precipitating stimuli.[178] Wolf, studying sudden death from myocardial infarction and cardiac arrhythmias attributed these to undampened autonomic discharges in response to either afferent information from below or impulses resulting from integrative processes in the brain involved in adaptation to stressful life experiences or both.[263] He suggested that triggering stimuli were effective in situations of weary dissatisfaction, frustration, feelings of abandonment and dejection, especially at times when emotional reactions were not forthcoming from others. Engel emphasized both inhibitory and excitatory parasympathetic responses in association with stressful situations as leading to sudden death, the determinants of the response depending upon individual psychobiologic perception and reaction to stress.[56] Paul identified the epidemiologic and prodromal causes of sudden death relating these to arrhythmias and abnormal free fatty acid metabolism.[165] Rees and Lutkins found a six-fold increase over the expected mortality in deaths from myocardial infarction in London widowers within a six-month period following the death of their spouses.[181] Critics such as Horvath view present research as imprecise because of the failure to carefully identify and measure stress.[98] Minc sees coronary artery disease as a disease of civilization, and as a consequence of an attempt at intellectual control over feeling and subsequent behavior conditioned by a social environment that disallows emotional response to stress, resulting in an arousal of the autonomic nervous system.[153] Werko suggests that attention to the changing social structure in the community may be of the greatest importance in the prevention of ischemic heart disease.[255] These speculations lead into metaphysical contemplations regarding the relationship of the disease and civilizations which go beyond our present knowledge and our methods of research.

In summary, the situation in which myocardial infarction, physiological decompensation, or sudden death occurs has been the subject of several investigations. The illness onset situation, whether of the initial process or a recurrence, is seen as a stressful one leading to psychological and physiological changes. Stressful situations are frequently associated with loss and bereavement which in the vulnerable or sensitized individual may lead to psychological and physiological decompensation. The particular stress eliciting a reaction may be nonspecific and is dependent on other factors predilecting the individual to a vulnerable physiological state. The reaction of individuals are variable, both psychologically and physiologically. Since different individuals may react hyper- or hypodynamically to the same stressful situation, it is not possible to universally associate specific stresses with specific patterns of response. Individual variation of response depends on how the individual perceives the stress symbolically, and on innate or learned patterns of physiological response associated with that percept.

Reactions to Coronary Artery Disease

Perhaps of more immediate application and reward in the field of the psychological aspects of cardiac disease are the investigations of the individual's reactions to the symptoms, signs, and diagnosis of cardiovascular disease, for it is at these points that specific and often life-threatening emotions and the defenses against these may be precipitated. Examples are the studies of Hackett and Cassem and Olin, who identified denial in subjects with chest pain at the time of myocardial infarctions as causing delay in seeking medical attention.[81,159] Their subjects, many of whom were sophisticated in the various meanings of chest pain, attributed their discomfort to more benign conditions than myocardial infarction. Although some subjects had previous infarctions, these too tended to use the expression, "I thought it couldn't happen to me," in describing their reaction to substernal pain. If this occurs in survivors and repeat victims, the question may be asked how often this or a similar response occurs in subjects who die before seeking medical help. If this pattern occurs in as many individuals as some epidemiologists believe, then a study of this reaction may be a crucial consideration for psychiatrists and other workers in preventive cardiology. Although most subjects studied have been observed to use denial at one or more points in their reaction to cardiac disease, observers have noted that, whereas in the early phase of illness it is simply a denial of the symptoms as a way of contending with anxiety over the possibility of death, this early denial is a fragile and brittle defense which subsequently is replaced by more characterological mechanisms in which the denial of illness and of its significance may become manifest by inappropriate behavior, also threatening to the recovery of the individual. Arlow has noted that the manifestation of anxiety in anginal patients depends upon the defenses the individual erects to cope with this anxiety which, in turn, are determined by the individual's previous experience as well as his current emotional state.[8] He sees overwhelming panic leading to the use of repression and denial. Ideation encountered in these patients includes fear of dying, fantasied loss of love, abandonment, and at times aggressive and homosexual impulses as means of coping with this fear. Croog et al., identified greater denial in postinfarction patients of Jewish or Italian background than in those patients of British or Irish descent.[41] They demonstrated the persistence of denial in 20 percent of their subjects over a year's time. Bakker, contrasting individuals with arteriosclerotic heart disease with anginal patients, identified more emotional lability, tenseness, conflict, and compulsivity in the latter.[11] Cleveland and Johnson compared postcoronary with presurgical patients, noting chronic restlessness, underlying passivity, and suppressed hostility in the former.[37] Rosen and Bibring related behavioral reaction to myocardial infarction to age and social status.[192] Depression and scrupulous cooperation were greater in older patients, whereas cheerfulness and active defiance were seen in younger ones. Anxiety was more prevalent in white-collar workers, while casualness prevailed in blue-collar workers. Croog and Levine, studying reactions of patients between the age of thirty and sixty to myocardial infarction, found that higher-status individuals showed a greater awareness of emotional stress as an etiological factor than lower-status patients who were less inclined to talk about their reaction to illness.[40] Rodda et al., also identified greater anxiety in younger patients, and depression in older patients.[191] Druss and Kornfeld following survivors of cardiac arrest described the defense mechanisms invoked to control anxiety precipitated by this

experience.[53] Subjects reported violent and frightening dreams, and identified various theories and explanations in order to integrate the experience of having been dead and reborn. Residual problems included insomnia, irritability, and restriction of activities beyond what was medically appropriate.

Treatment and Management

The recognition of chronic anxiety and persistent depressive states in patients with coronary artery disease has led a number of investigators toward examining models of therapeutic intervention. Pelser emphasizes that many patients experience myocardial infarction at a time when they are already under emotional strain and that in the course of treatment they should be given permission to ventilate and discuss their frustration about the broader emotional field.[167] Noting that these patients frequently manifest behavior pattern type A and do poorly in passive situations, he stresses the need for the physician to seek the active cooperation of the patient in his recovery. He suggests that the patient who has usually repressed hostile feelings be encouraged to complain and make demands on his environment, now that he is ill as a means of giving expression to his pent-up frustrations. Bilodeau and Hackett investigated the reaction of postmyocardial infarction patients meeting together with a psychiatric nurse over a three-month period.[15] Subjects that came under discussion in this group process included: current and future states of health, effects of illness on one's life, the role of the patient and its effect on the family, the history of the illness, and medical care following discharge. Adsett and Bruhn have written about the advantages of short-term group psychotherapy for postmyocardial infarction patients and their wives.[3] Hellerstein and Friedman finding unnecessarily limited sexual activity among patients with arteriosclerotic heart disease emphasized the need for counselling patients and their spouses about this important function.[91] Wishnie et al., describing the anxiety and depression in infarction patients after returning home emphasized the need to prepare the patient for the weak, fearful, uncertain feelings he may experience.[261] Among the recommendations they make to the medical team caring for these patients are: regular telephone contact during early convalescence, establishment of a program of mental and physical activity, avoidance of vague advice, prescription of drugs for sleep and of tranquilizers for anxiety, and assisting the patient in altering his lifetime habits in order to adapt to coronary disease. Walter et al., describe the effect that arrhythmias have on patients with coronary disease, leading to symptoms of cerebral ischemia including dizziness, giddiness and syncope.[247] These reactions may be both a cause of and a reaction to anxiety and may be allayed by working with the patient's chronic anxiety.[146] Patients with symptoms of angina pectoris frequently experience this distress at times of stressful environmental situations leading to emotional conflict. At other times, some of these patients are subject to conversion reactions imitative of their anginal disease.[71,256] Conversion reactions frequently occur in patients with underlying anxiety and covert depression relating to their illness. These patients may become increasingly hypochondriacal and develop what has been called a cardiac neurosis superimposed on their cardiac disease. Psychiatric intervention in the form of relaxation techniques has been employed in these situations by Rifkin.[189] Wincott and Caird identify two phases of concern regarding the return of cardiac patients to work.[260] In the first phase, the individual is concerned with employment and finances. Later, after returning to work, he is concerned about increased dependence, invalidism, and performance. Williamson et al., followed seventy-four patients admitted with congestive heart failure to a coronary care unit finding that only two were asymptomatic and functioning normally after a year.[259] Twenty-four had returned to work but were symptomatic. Another nineteen, although ambulatory, were unable to assume life activity. Seven remained bed-ridden and twenty-two had died. Concerned about the staggering morbidity and mortality, they saw this as a critical area for further research. Wells finds physi-

cians and employers partly responsible for patient failures to return to work and sees the need to educate employers and insurance companies and for employee retraining programs.[252] Perlman et al., contrasted 105 patients with congestive heart failure with fifty controls, finding long-standing emotional problems, difficulty in accepting illness, overt denial, and major problems concerning living arrangements.[169] Rosenberg found that patients with congestive heart failure showed improved function and a lower hospital-readmission rate after participation in a group-education program.[193]

Finally Riseman suggesting that few of the injunctions about activity, food, blood pressure, smoking, alcohol, anticoagulants, and vasodilators are proven, believes that the best course for the patient to follow is moderation in all things, gradually returning to normal activity and moderate exercise.[190] He should reduce weight, limit intake of saturated fats, control blood pressure, and eliminate or reduce cigarette smoking. Psychotherapy may be necessary to achieve moderation for the coronary patient with type A behavior.

❲ Conclusions

A summary of the studies that have been cited herein suggests that coronary artery disease is more likely to occur in the individual who: (1) has a family history of cardiovascular disease; (2) lives in a family or social structure in which genetic determination and/or sociocultural values foster a particular behavior pattern; (3) lives in a physical environment in which cardiotoxic factors are present; (4) engages in an aggressive, competitive, upward-mobile culture without resolving internal conflicts about dependency, passivity, and sexuality; (5) becomes involved in nonspecific stressful situations in which these unresolved conflicts are aggravated, leading to a psychobiological decompensation elaborated through the stimulation of the hypothalamus from above and below with an excitation of both autonomic and adrenal cortical activity; and

(6) develops, in the face of morphological change and physical decompensation, behavioral patterns that are predicted by the direct effect of those changes on the central nervous system and the psychological defenses erected to contend with vulnerability and chronic illness. The elaboration and identification of all of these factors in a particular patient will lead the physician to an identification of those for which help can be sought, as well as to a greater awareness of and empathy for the affected individual.

A review of the psychological aspects of cardiovascular disease as presented above commences with the limited genetic and environmental factors that are known. Genetic factors may include either a single genetic substrata that determines predisposition to both a behavior pattern such as Type A and coronary artery disease, or the two independent factors closely linked may be inherited separately but usually together. On the other hand, the association between cardiovascular disease and particular psychological patterns may result from the occurrence of heart disease such as rheumatic fever at a vulnerable time in development, resulting in psychological fixation at that stage and subsequent distorted development.[58,138] In the case of the individual with congenital heart disease, the structuring of personality and behavior patterns may also result from the effects of the disease on the intellectual development and/or the limitations imposed by parents and society on the individual with heart disease.[2,36] Other patterns are identified in terms of the reactions of individuals to acquired heart disease, their emotional responses, and the defenses erected to contain these. An interesting theoretical consideration is that the early association of cardiovascular response to environmental events with repetition becomes conditioned and reinforced. In time the environmental stimulus triggering the cardiovascular response may be replaced and internalized as a symbolic stimulus which no longer needs the same external event for activation. With constant repetition and under the appropriate environmental milieu (internal or external) secondary changes such as atherosclerosis and cardiomyopathies develop. An extensive review of the literature suggests that the relationship is not a linear and unidirectional one between two variables but is more likely a cyclical process including multiple variables that may be stimulated at various points in the cycle. Hence, personality variables may lead to behavior which is cardiotoxic, but cardiovascular disease may also lead to behavior or reactions that are neurotogenic.[203] For either of these reactions to take place, the simultaneous occurrence of other variables including genetic, psychosocial and environmental may need to be present. For the individual patient, an examination of the individual's psychological and physical development, the psychosocial field in which the illness is exacerbated or precipitated, and the reaction of the patient, his family, and society to his illness is necessary in order to assist the patient and his family in the very arduous and circuitous road to maximum rehabilitation.

Psychophysiological and Psychodynamic Problems of the Patient with Structural Heart Disease*

Morton F. Reiser and Hyman Bakst

(Congestive Heart Failure

Physiological Considerations

The basic physiological problems involved in structural heart disease that leads to congestive failure can be understood as one of supply and demand. With the progressive decrease in cardiac reserve that results from the heart lesion, there ensues progressive difficulty in maintaining adequate cardiac output in response to varying functional demands.

Congestive heart failure will develop whenever myocardial capacity is inadequate to meet the metabolic demands of the body. Certain events then occur which lead to the classical picture of congestive failure, and chief among them is the impairment of normal renal mechanisms with the resultant retention of salt and water.[170] The ultimate responsibil-

* This section through p. 624 is modified from the corresponding section in Chapter 33, Psychology of Cardiovascular Disorders by Morton F. Reiser and Hyman Bakst, appearing in the 1st ed. of the *American Handbook of Psychiatry*, Vol. 1, New York: Basic Books, 1959.

ity for this fluid and electrolyte imbalance must be assigned to circulatory inadequacy, but the immediate and crucial mechanism is altered renal function.[173] Consideration of congestive failure must therefore be concerned not only with disordered circulatory dynamics but with the physiological factors controlling the disposition of sodium chloride and water by the kidney.[129]

The balance between tissue needs and the ability of the heart muscle to meet them may be disrupted by increasing the demand or by reducing the functional cardiac reserve. Infection, exertion, increase in blood volume, certain paroxysmal arrhythmias, and emotional stress are all factors which may lead to a relatively abrupt increase in the demand for cardiac work. Diminution in coronary blood supply, inflammation (myocarditis, myocardosis),[172] arrhythmias which reduce efficiency of cardiac function and emotional stress are factors which may lead to relatively rapid decrease in the heart's capacity to perform work. Increased demand and decreased capacity may occur in combination, and as reserve decreases with time and advancing disease, progressively smaller loads determine the limits of compensation.

There is a direct relationship between cardiac output and effective renal-plasma flow; diminished cardiac output lowers the glomerular filtration rate, thereby producing a decrease in salt and water excretion.[111,147] This is not the sole regulating mechanism however, and it has been established that the renal tubule may operate independently of the glomerulus in this respect. The renal tubule is the second discrete regulator of sodium chloride and water balance. For purposes of simplification, the glomerulus may be considered to be affected primarily by hemodynamic changes. Tubular function, on the other hand, is modified chiefly by humoral agents.[129]

The humoral agents which affect tubular function include the antidiuretic hormone (ADH) of the neurohypophysis, which promotes water reabsorption, and the adrenal corticosteroids, which promote sodium retention. Of the latter, the most potent is aldosterone, but other steroids (hydrocortisone, corticosterone) also exert an appreciable effect.[135] Norepinephrine can also cause marked change in sodium excretion. Both adrenal activity and altered circulatory dynamics are necessary for the development of edema, the prime feature of congestive failure. There are many factors which evoke increased aldosterone activity in congestive failure, including dietary restriction of sodium, impaired hormone degradation due to hepatic congestion, and elevated serum potassium levels. In addition, those adrenal steroids which are under ACTH (adrenocorticotrophic hormone) control all have sodium-retaining activity and can, at times, tip the balance in the direction of failure. The role of emotional stress in increasing adrenal cortical activity is well known and will be referred to more fully in the following section when the emotional factors in congestive failure are discussed.

In attempting to clarify the mechanisms underlying the clinical phenomena which concern us, it is pertinent to consider the ways in which psychological stress may affect circulatory equilibrium, either by increasing current demand or by decreasing available supply, and/or by altering renal function.

Psychophysiological Changes Leading to Increased Cardiac Work Demand

It has been repeatedly demonstrated that "emotional stress" may be accompanied by measurable changes in arterial blood pressure, heart rate, stroke volume, cardiac output, and peripheral resistance.* Perhaps the most carefully and extensively documented study from a physiological point of view is that of Hickam and co-workers[95] who utilized a spontaneous, nonspecific stress situation—an important academic exam—in order to demonstrate differences in measurements reflecting circulatory dynamics obtained during "emotional tension" from measurements obtained during relative relaxation. The subjects were twenty-three healthy medical students. Each student was examined just before the critical exam and then again a day or two later, after having been informed that he had passed. The average cardiac index (volume output of the heart l./min per m.² body-surface area) before the exam was 2 l./min. per m.² greater than that measured during relative relaxation. When this figure was converted to "work load," it corresponded to a load which would be demanded by increasing oxygen consumption by an amount equal to the basal metabolism.

In Hickam's work, as well as in that of other authors cited in the footnote on this page, the meaning of the psychological stress and the nature of the reaction to it were not specifically studied in the individual subjects. Hickam noted that the pattern of mobilization varied in his subjects, and described three patterns. For the largest part of the group, anxiety was accompanied by an increase in cardiac index, decrease in peripheral resistance, and relatively small rise in mean arterial pressure. In a smaller second group, the "anxious state" was associated with a slight to moderate rise in peripheral resistance, with a rise in mean

* See references 6, 9, 68, 80, 95, 126, 127, 184, 186, 202, 215, 223, 224, 242, 262, and 265.

blood pressure and no change or a slight decrease in the cardiac index. In three subjects there were rises in cardiac index but large moment-to-moment fluctuations in stroke volume and heart rate.

Much research has been done in an effort to determine whether specific differences in pattern of circulatory response may be related to specific differences in the concomitant emotion involved. The investigative group headed by H. Wolff at Cornell, through the use of structured stimuli (introduction of conflictual topics during interview), have described relationships between different directly observed (and subjectively reported) affects and different patterns of circulatory mobilization.[262,264–266,268] Funkenstein et al.,[68] working with groups of healthy subjects under a specified stressful task, have described three patterns of emotional response which they designate: "anger-in," "anger-out," and "anxiety." On the basis of ballistocardiographic, heart-rate, and blood-pressure recordings taken simultaneously, they reported that subjects showing the "anger-out" pattern developed circulatory changes similar to changes produced by the administration of noradrenalin. (This resembles the second pattern described by Hickam, see above.) Subjects showing "anxiety" and "anger-in" reactions demonstrated changes similar to those that would be produced by injection of adrenalin (resembling the first pattern described by Hickam). Ax[9] and Schachter,[202] working on subjects who were exposed to laboratory situations deliberately staged to evoke either anxiety or hostility, reported differences in pattern of circulatory changes similar to those described by Funkenstein.

The implication of this is that outwardly displayed anger is accompanied by a release of norepinephrine, whereas anxiety and anger directed inward are accompanied by the release of epinephrine. It should be noted that these implications have been drawn by indirect inference from measurement of circulatory functions, and the studies did not include assays of the hormone levels in the blood. The inferences drawn are also open to criticism, since they were based upon quantitative amplitude measurements of ballistocardiographic tracings obtained by the use of direct-body pickup instruments which cannot be satisfactorily calibrated. The issue may be more complicated than this, since Lacey and co-workers have advanced definite evidence to show that individual differences in pattern of response may be largely reflections of constitutional differences, and only partly reflect specific connections between specific affects and particular patterns of response.[126,127] Reiser, Weiner, and Thaler,[186,187] in recording circulatory functions during projective psychological testing, observed the first two patterns reported by Hickam, as well as an intermediate group which, like Hickam's, seemed too variable from moment to moment for adequate qualitative classification. In all subjects, brisk responses (of the same magnitude as those reported by Hickam and others) occurred in association with little directly observable or subjectively reportable evidence of affect. The amount of affect which could be identified in this way was not sufficient for classification. Differential patterning of the circulatory responses appeared to be related more to differential attitudes toward the examiner, but the experiment did not allow for adequate exploration of the unconscious aspects of this relationship. Although the question of specific relationships between affects and physiological patterns of circulatory response is left open, these studies singly and collectively demonstrate that emotion is accompanied by circulatory changes which may greatly increase the amount of work required of the heart. Stevenson et al., have demonstrated that the circulation recovers from the effects of exercise slowly and inefficiently during states of emotional tension, thus prolonging the strain upon the heart.[224]

Most of the studies referred to above deal with changes in healthy subjects whose circulatory systems were presumably normal. The studies of Hickam, Wolff, and others were extended to patients with valvular disease and limited cardiac reserve, with similar results. Striking is Hickam's demonstration in a patient with severely limited cardiac reserve that the effects of exercise and anxiety were similar and were in the direction of developing con-gestive failure. Cardiac index and pulmonary arterial pressure were determined by cardiac catheterization. With anxiety as well as with exercise, there was a failure of the cardiac index to rise, accompanied by an increase in pulmonary arterial pressure.[95]

Psychophysiological Changes Leading to Decreased Myocardial Capacity

Diminution in functional cardiac reserve during tension may occur as a result of inter-ference with intrinsic cardiac mechanisms governing heart rate and rhythm. Changes in the electrocardiogram reflecting such inter-ference with cardiac mechanisms have been repeatedly demonstrated by numerous work-ers, including Katz et al.,[112] Mainzer and Krause,[144] and Wendkos.[253,254] This litera-ture has been reviewed by Weiss.[250]

Psychophysiological Changes Altering Renal Function

There have been only a few studies which bear directly on the role of emotional factors as they affect renal function. Diuresis has been reported in both animals and man following emotional stress, and investigations have been conducted on the effect of specific emotions on fluid and electrolyte balance. Schottstaedt and his co-workers have reported a series of such studies, and indicated a direct correlation of certain emotional response patterns with spe-cific types of alteration of water and sodium excretion. They found that feelings of anger, uneasiness, and apprehension produced in-creased rates of water and sodium excretion, whereas feelings of depression were associated with decreased rates.[12,205]

Confirmation of these findings by other in-vestigators has not been reported and further research on these psychophysiological rela-tionships is needed. Other evidence bears di-rectly on the relationship between emotions and adrenal cortical activity[60,61,208] and be-tween adrenal cortical activity and renal tubu-lar function.[129,173] Thus, by inferential rea-soning, one may hypothesize a sequential

psycho-adreno-renal pathway as an important factor in the clinical manifestations of conges-tive failure.

Clinical Observations

In view of the psychophysiological findings summarized above, it is not surprising to find that stressful events often precede the devel-opment of episodes of congestive failure in patients with established cardiac disease and limited reserve. This expectation can be affirmed readily on the medical wards of any hospital. Chambers and Reiser interviewed twenty-five consecutive patients who were admitted to the wards of the Cincinnati Gen-eral Hospital because of congestive heart failure.[36] An acute emotionally stressful ex-perience had immediately preceded the de-velopment of congestive failure in 76 percent. In each instance these events seemed to have highly specific meaning for the patient in rela-tion to his previous life experiences and con-flicts, and in most they were superimposed upon a chronic state of sustained emotional tension. An important aspect of these findings lies in the fact that most of these patients had been through similar conflictual crises previ-ously without having developed congestive heart failure, that is, similarly stressful experi-ences occurring before the critical limitation of cardiac reserve had developed, had not re-sulted in clinical disturbance of the patients' circulatory equilibrium. It was only after the underlying progressive heart disease had re-sulted in serious loss of cardiac reserve that the stressful events assumed clinical impor-tance in respect to circulation. All of the pa-tients in this series were seriously ill and ex-hibited advanced forms of heart disease and serious degrees of cardiac decompensation. They were the type of patient in whom the extent of underlying cardiac pathology might so impress the physician that he might well not feel it necessary to search for a specific precipitating factor. It is important to recog-nize that the extent of the underlying heart damage does not ordinarily account for the nature of the forces immediately responsible for the abrupt onset or worsening of congestive failure. In the same study it was noted that marked improvement in clinical status coincided with providing the patient an opportunity to share and discuss his difficult life with the physician. It was further observed that a continuing supportive relationship with the physician aided in avoiding further unresolved emotional crises and stabilized the clinical course to a great extent (without, of course, effecting any change in the extent of the underlying heart damage).

In summary, the tenuous balance between work load and cardiac reserve in patients with structural heart disease and diminished cardiac reserve may be seriously disturbed by the various circulatory responses that accompany psychological stress. In this fashion, serious episodes of congestive heart failure may be precipitated and sustained by emotionally stressful situations.

Somatopsychic Problems

In a discussion of the somatopsychic problems in patients with structural heart disease, it is useful to identify those factors intrinsic to cardiac disease which may operate as stressful agents in the psychological sphere, and thus demand attempts at adjustment on the part of the patient. The clinical effects of each of them stem from the fact that they act as sources of anxiety. The end results may come about in two ways, either as the result of untoward effects of free anxiety and other affects upon the tenuous circulatory balance, or as the result of indirect consequences of anxiety, namely behavior which stems from maladaptive use of ego defenses against anxiety. These maladaptive behavioral phenomena, in turn, may complicate or aggravate the circulatory problem. They may lead to behavior which interferes with the patient's ability to utilize a prescribed medical regimen, for example, refusal to take digitalis. They may also be reflected in more general aspects of the patient's personality adjustment and lead to psychiatric problems (e.g., depression) which may not immediately affect circulation but may require therapeutic attention in their own right. The complexity of these direct and indirect conse-

quences, and the manner in which they may in themselves lead to mobilization of additional anxiety (thus completing feedback cycles), is schematically illustrated in Figure 26–1.

The psychological burden imposed by the onset and/or diagnosis of heart disease may stem from any or all of three general sources. The first source is constituted by the symptoms themselves. The abrupt onset of sensations, such as breathlessness, severe precordial pain, palpitation, dizziness, etc., is anxiety provoking. The initial anxiety generated at the onset of an acute episode may impose considerable additional burden upon the already compromised circulation.

The second source is the threat inherent in the diagnosis of heart disease. Any illness may cause anxiety because of actual or threatened damage to bodily integrity. In the case of the heart anxiety is exquisitely exaggerated. The reasons for this are general and universal. The central indispensable role of the heart in maintaining life provides an appropriate background for the use of its mental representation as a symbolic object of awesome unconscious fears. Ample reinforcement comes from folklore, symbolic language conventions, and a vast popular literature. It is probable that the diagnosis of heart disease activates fears of sudden, unexpected, and catastrophic death. The danger implied by the diagnosis is not to be minimized here, but it should be pointed out that fears may exaggerate and amplify it out of proportion. For example, the unconscious threat may be no less intense to the patient who is informed of the discovery of a functional cardiac murmur than it is to the patient confronted by a diagnosis of serious advanced rheumatic heart disease. In addition to these fears stemming from the diagnosis, there may be specific additional factors causing conflict. For example, a patient who has had a highly charged ambivalent relationship with a relative or close friend who died of heart disease may have unresolved problems of identification and guilt.

The third source of anxiety stems from the fact that the patient experiences (or can anticipate) a real limitation of his physical capac-

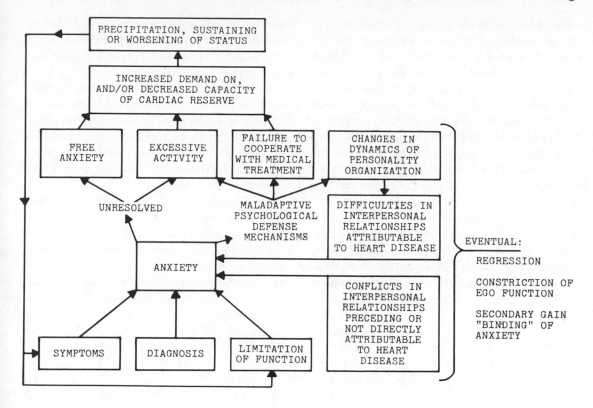

Figure 26-1. Psychophysiological relationships in patients with structural heart disease.

ity, and knows that this will be progressive. The adaptive task imposed upon the patient cannot be underestimated. Successful or ideal adjustment necessitates realistic acceptance of the loss and the attendant limitations which it imposes. It also necessitates rearrangement of living patterns which take these limitations into account and at the same time make maximal utilization of residual capacities. Many factors influence the degree to which the patient succeeds in meeting this challenge. The most important are: (1) the severity of the specific emotional impact of heart disease; (2) the strength of his personality; (3) reactions and attitudes of medical personnel, particularly his doctor; and (4) the reactions of people close to him. The psychological trauma inherent in the development of a cardiac disorder may severely aggravate a preexistent psychiatric problem. In some instances it serves as a precipitant for the development of major psychiatric difficulties in a previously satisfactorily integrated personality.

There are a number of ways in which the handling of anxiety may lead to unsatisfactory responses. Inadequately resolved anxiety may worsen the medical condition, as described above. In addition, psychological mechanisms, which ordinarily have the function of defending against anxiety, may be inappropriately and maladaptively mobilized in the patient's attempt to defend against the threat. For example, specific ego defenses such as denial (for example, of illness) and reaction-formation (for example, against dependent wishes) may lead to open, unrealistic, and rebellious unwillingness to adhere to a prescribed medical regimen. This is a problem frequently encountered in middle-aged men with coronary disease, and such behavior may unwittingly be self-destructive. So far as it contributes to progression and aggravation of symptoms and further actual constriction of the patient's physical capacity, it creates new anxiety, and in this indirect way another type of vicious cycle is established.

Disturbances in the sphere of behavior may not be restricted to issues centering on the physical disorder and its care. Profound changes may develop in the basic functional organization of the personality. Extensive reliance upon defenses, such as projection and displacement, may lead to drastic changes in the patient's view of the world and his reactions to specific people. Unconsciously determined changes in significant and important relationships may result—for example, dissolution of business associations, divorce, etc. These too may represent fresh sources of tension and conflict which lead to still another type of feedback cycle. Even without this, symptomatic behavior of this magnitude represents major psychopathological development and demands therapeutic attention in its own right.

As the situation progresses, more far-reaching long-term changes may become evident. As in any major illness, strong regressive tendencies develop, and when these are added to and combined with the kinds of developments described above, a process is instituted which may eventuate in serious constriction of all aspects of ego-function in general, and, in particular, in restriction of the defensive operations of the ego to relatively few mechanisms that are for the most part maladaptively utilized. The cardiac status becomes part of the self-image, and the personality becomes constricted, rigid, brittle, and fragile. The cardiac status may become a nuclear part of the patient's style of conducting interpersonal relationships, and this is most often manifested by behavior which exploits the physical condition in the service of secondary gains which may acquire considerable value.

One additional mechanism should be mentioned, which can be described as a form of "binding of anxiety." Whenever serious physical disease (or a physical condition which can be treated as "serious") develops during a period when the patient is grappling with a serious unconscious psychological conflict, the physical disease may be seized upon as a way of resolving the conflict. For example, the illness may provide a way of avoiding the issue by precluding the conflictual activity and may thus reduce the importance of the conflict to a state where it is of academic interest only. Two typical and frequently seen examples of this mechanism can be cited. The first is the example of the patient in early adolescence who has not yet reached a satisfactory resolution of problems centering on issues of sexuality and independence; chronic invalidism for such a patient may provide a very convenient way out. The second example is that of the overtly aggressive and ambitious man who harbors unresolved problems about success. Here again, even early manifestations of cardiac disease may offer a face-saving occasion for retrenchment and retreat from vocational growth. In other words, the status of illness may acquire a powerful psychic value because it offers opportunity for "acceptable" avoidance of serious conflicts that would be activated in a fuller life sphere.

(Essential Hypertension

Introduction

The concept of essential hypertension remains variable and imprecise despite increasingly sophisticated techniques for correlating physiological and biochemical processes with elevated blood pressure. An etiological and physiological explanation for more than 90 percent of hypertension remains undeveloped.[171]

Essential hypertension is generally identified by blood-pressure readings of greater than 140/90 mm. Hg. for which an etiology has not been identified. Its incidence is usually higher for each advancing decade. Its prevalence is greater in some geographical areas and sociocultural groups than in others. The readings themselves may be associated with progressive symptoms and signs. The former includes "top-of-head" headaches, dizziness, ringing in the ears, and irritability. Signs include epistaxis, elevated blood-pressure readings, and retinal changes. Secondary symptoms and signs are associated with pathophysio-anatomic changes occurring in organ systems, especially the heart, kidneys, and brain.

The course of the disease may be benign or malignant. Recent statistics suggest that even in benign situations, the course is relentlessly progressive despite a slower development of secondary organ involvement.[21] What governs the differences between a benign and a malignant course remains essentially unknown, although a recent study has suggested different renin and aldosterone patterns in patients with hypertension which seem to have prognostic value in terms of myocardial infarcts and cerebrovascular accidents.[29] Nevertheless, we are left with a poorly defined phenomenon which undoubtedly groups together symptoms, signs, and secondary pathophysioanatomic manifestations for which future research may establish one or more precise etiological factors.

Epidemiological Considerations

Before considering the psychological aspects of essential hypertension, some attention needs to be given to epidemiological findings. Similar to coronary artery disease, epidemiological considerations are fragmentary and for the most part supply only limited impressions upon which derivative formulations are based. The picture is further complicated by the seemingly conflicting findings often reported from the epidemiological field. Studies in the United States have demonstrated that hypertension is higher among urban than among rural dwellers, among lower than upper classes, among blacks than whites, and in men than women.[22] It is also noted that the development of hypertension is more frequently observed and of greater severity in the rural dweller who moves to the city than in the individual who has always lived in the city.[74]

Donaldson, studying changes in disease incidence and prevalence among rural Africans undergoing acculturation, noted that hypertension was greater in the more acculturated urban groups.[49] Obvious correlates of acculturation are changes in life style which include food, housing, work, and interpersonal relations. The changes in disease patterns are probably more complex than the apparent associations suggest. For example, the changes observed may be related to an unmasking of a latent genetic predisposition in a population that rarely became manifest in the less sophisticated and more socially supporting tribal state where infectious disease and starvation frequently lead to early death. Other relative factors may be considered, although supporting data are lacking. Blood-pressure levels identified as falling in the hypertensive range in one geographical area and biocultural population are not necessarily equivalent to identical values for another area and group. These studies suggest that both genetic and environmental factors are related in the pathogenesis of essential hypertension.

PSYCHOBIOLOGICAL VARIABLES

The ensuing discussion examines genetic and environmental variables in terms of their interrelationships with psychological ones in individuals developing hypertension. In considering these interactions, several hypotheses are entertained: (1) the psychological and social aspects of behavior related to hypertension may be independent derivatives of the same or a different (though inherited together) genetic factor as the physiological component; (2) the psychological and physiological components may become associated during the course of development; and (3) the psychological component may be a reaction to the disease process.

LONGITUDINAL STUDIES

Thomas is the most prominent among recent investigators of hypertension.[229-237] For more than twenty years, she has studied prospectively the development of hypertension and associated diseases in medical students. In the course of her investigations, she has made the following correlations: (1) the proportion of students in graduating classes manifesting clinical hypertension was three times that in younger classes; the proportion showing transitory hypertension was double; (2) in the former group, 62.5 percent gave a history of parental hypertension compared with 36.0 percent in the latter; (3) the "at-risk" groups also tended initially to manifest higher resting blood pressures, elevated cholesterol levels, and more intense reactions to stress behaviorally; (4) psychologically, she noted apparent submissiveness of the predisposed individual under the domination of a parent; and (5) the onset of hypertension occurring as an anniversary reaction or in the setting of an unrealistic marriage. She suggested that the observed hypercholesterolemia represented an inborn metabolic defect; that the inheritance of the deficit might be governed by a single locus, although modifying genes and environmental factors were important in determining clinical expression; and that the total behavioral pattern developing under stress might also reflect an inborn predisposition.

Paffenbarger and his associates have also made correlations between characteristics observed in college students and subsequent disease.[161] Undergraduate patterns of cigarette smoking, elevated blood pressure, increased body weight, shorter body stature, early parental death, heart consciousness, and nonparticipation in varsity sports were associated with the occurrence of subarachnoid hemorrhage and occlusive stroke, pathology frequently resulting from chronic hypertension. Associated with heart consciousness and cigarette smoking, Paffenbarger noted emotional distress in terms of anxiety and irritability.

SOME BIOLOGICAL CORRELATES WITH BEHAVIOR

Specific biological variables have been identified in patients with hypertension. Similar to some of the psychological variables discussed below, these are as likely to be secondary to the development of hypertension as they are to be precursors. Renin, angiotensin I and II, and aldosterone may also be considered in this light. Through the accumulation of data via longitudinal studies such as those cited above it may be possible for an eventual distinction to be made.

Schneider and Zangari noted an association of anxiety, tension, fear, anger, and hostility with decreased clotting time, increased viscosity, and elevated blood pressure.[204] With feelings of depression, dejection, and of being overwhelmed, they noted prolonged clotting time, normal viscosity, and normal blood pressure. Hypertensive as opposed to normotensive subjects demonstrated decreased clotting time to the stress of the pressor test.

Testosterone and estrogen have been cited as affecting blood-pressure levels in addition to hormones of the pituitary-adrenal axis.[92] Susceptible male mice developed marked hypertension and aggressive behavior when subjected to social stress, whereas susceptible castrated male mice under the same circumstances remained normotensive and nonaggressive. However, when the latter mice were given testosterone, blood pressures rose and aggressive behavior developed. In some lower sociocultural groups, premenopausal women tend to manifest higher blood pressure than men; the reverse pattern prevails following menopause.[207] Among upper sociocultural groups, the reverse pattern has been observed. These findings suggest that age, sex, and other variables are more than biological but interact with sociocultural roles and the personalities and life situations involved with these. Women who have family histories of hypertension and personal histories of toxemia of pregnancy appear more sensitive to the hypertensive effects of estrogen preparations.[119,128,248] They also appear more likely to experience a depressive response to these preparations.

Von Eiff suggests that hereditary factors prime the pressor center of the hypothalamus to respond hyperactively to environmental stresses leading to increased blood pressure.[244] Yamori et al., have found lower concentrations of norepinephrine in the lower brain stem and hypothalamus of spontaneously hypertensive rats as compared to normotensive ones.[271] This was associated with a lower concentration of L-amino acid decarboxylase, but not of tyrosine hydrogenase, suggesting that abnormal metabolism of ergotrophic hormones may be related to hypertension. Sjoerdsma has noted that monoamine oxidase inhibitors lead to a decarboxylation of alpha dopamine, resulting in what is in effect a medical sympathectomy.[218] This is of interest, inasmuch as clinical observations have frequently suggested a correlation between depression and hypertension, and that the latter tends to improve with the treatment of the former with antidepressants. These fragmentary findings are identified in order to suggest the direction of neurophysiological research in seeking a central mechanism affecting blood pressure.[55] These and others have yet to be woven into an integrated formulation. The actual regulation of blood pressure is a highly complex phenomenon and, as Penaz has noted, depends also on the mechanical parts of the system such as the heart as well as central nervous control.[168]

PSYCHIATRIC RELATIONSHIPS

As long ago as 1902, Alexander noted that blood pressure was frequently elevated in patients suffering from acute melancholia, as opposed to chronic melancholia or mania.[6] Altschule corroborated this observation, finding that elevation of blood pressure was the rule in patients with involutional depression whereas patients with schizophrenic states more often showed blood pressure readings below the normal range.[7] Readings in patients displaying manic behavior were only occasionally elevated. Vanderhoof et al., demonstrated a lower blood flow in patients with schizophrenic states as opposed to those with affective psychoses.[241] Heine et al., studying hypertension in severely depressed patients, observed a decrease in blood pressure for the agitated patients following improvement in their mental status.[89] However, those patients manifesting less agitation and having a history of more frequent depressive episodes were less likely to demonstrate a change in blood pressure following treatment. They suggest that chronicity of emotional stress correlates with irreversible changes in the regulation of blood pressure.

OVERVIEW OF PSYCHOPHYSIOLOGICAL RELATIONSHIPS

Several reviews are first briefly identified and discussed to serve as reference for the student interested in further pursuit of this subject.

Alexander was one of the first investigators to consider hypertension as a progressive sequence of psychopathophysiological changes.[5] Not ruling out the possibility of a constitutional instability of the vasomotor system, he observed that the specific neurotic handling of excessive and inhibited hostile impulses precipitated by a conflictual situation was associated with extreme fluctuations of the blood pressure. In time, with repetition of the conflictual episode, he suggested that these patterns tended to become fixed leading to chronic neurotic states associated with elevated blood pressure and still later to the organic consequences of this condition. Much of the work of subsequent investigators has elaborated on data that have been interpreted as supporting this hypothesis. However, Binger in 1951, reviewing more than 200 articles, suggested that no one had "hit the mark" in establishing a relationship between psychological influences in the etiology of hypertension.[16] Despite the enormous growth of the literature in the intervening decades, it is still possible to make a similar assessment. Nevertheless, many of the variables that have been identified have assisted the clinician in approaching and attempting to understand the patient with hypertension.

Brod conceptualizes hypertension as an intensified and extended normal hemodynamic response to an acute emotional stress, consisting of a redistribution of cardiac output, with blood shifted from the viscera and skin to the skeletal muscles, myocardium, and brain, advantageous for the performance of strenuous muscle work.[23] The increased blood supply to the muscles is in part secondary to the release of epinephrine and is partly related to a reflex involving cholinergic fibers. This pattern is analogous to the circulatory response produced in animals by electrical stimulation of the hypothalamus, which is accompanied by apprehensive and rage behavior identified as "defense system." Brod hypothesizes that this is an old phylogenetic reaction which has been transferred from a threatening external situation to a symbolic internalized stimulus. Whereas, phylogenetically, the reaction would cease with the removal of the provoking stimulus, in the human situation the internalized symbol remains as a constant stimulus to the vascular and rage reaction, resulting in eventual pathophysiological and pathoanatomic changes. Levi suggests that emotional stress triggers sympatho-adreno-medullary and related physiological changes of relatively short duration.[136] If repeated often enough over lengthy periods and of increasing intensity, he sees these as etiological in the development of essential hypertension.

Geiger and Scotch in 1963 reviewed the biological, epidemiological, psychological, and sociocultural factors relating to the etiology of hypertension.[72,207] In concluding, these authors found ample room for further research. Essential hypertension as a pathological entity with a well-established etiological and physiochemical mechanism still required clarification. They questioned to what extent essential hypertension was related to one or more primary disease processes yet to be identified, and also whether it might not represent a variation on a norm. More research was required in establishing a hereditary basis for hypertension through the study of first-degree relatives and controls. Longitudinal studies were necessary to establish the natural history and progress of the disease. These authors saw the implication of sociocultural factors as an open question. They noted that age, sex, and other variables were more than biological, inasmuch as they served as the bases for personal interaction in a culture and family and consequently were precursors of sociocultural and personality factors, which assumed possible significance in their own right. They raised the still intriguing question whether many of the psychological variables associated with hypertension might not be more directly related to the lability of blood pressure frequently observed in the prehypertensive in-

dividual. Finally, they considered the stress factors relating to the onset of hypertension and the adaptive behavior of individuals to these and to the subsequent disease course.

Groen, following Page's[164] Mosaic theory of essential hypertension, suggests that the reactivity of the central nervous system under the influence of genetic and environmental influences is the main causal factor in a constellation of multiple factors associated with the development of hypertension.[79,164] He cites the following: (1) Hypertension is an exaggeration and intensification of normal reaction patterns of the organism; (2) It follows in the wake of repeated and prolonged conflicts; (3) It occurs in individuals predisposed to react to conflicts with key persons in certain ways, a pattern which is both genetically determined and environmentally conditioned; (4) These individuals demonstrate personality traits which include compulsivity, rigidity, sensitivity, a need for love, a fear of losing love, a tendency to dominate, a tendency toward aggression, and a tendency to inhibit the acting out of aggressive impulses; (5) Hypertension is precipitated in a conflict situation in which active aggression is inhibited; (6) Exacerbations of conflict lead to exacerbation of blood-pressure response; (7) The more severe the personality disorder and the more intense the conflict situation, the more malignant is the course of hypertension; and (8) The greater the sensitivity and the greater the reactivity associated with a greater tendency to inhibit motor discharges, the more likely will the reaction be channelled through the limbic system, the hypothalamic vasomotor center, the sympathetic nervous system, the heart, and the smooth muscles of the renal and splanchnic arterioles, leading to increased peripheral resistance. Groen sees this in terms equivalent to a displacement phenomenon in which the organism reacts to a symbolic stress via a neurovisceral route as opposed to reacting to a physical stress via a neuromuscular route. He indicates that changes in the environmental conditions, the use of central-acting tranquilizers, and peripheral-acting blocking agents together with supportive psychotherapy have ameliorating effects on hypertension.

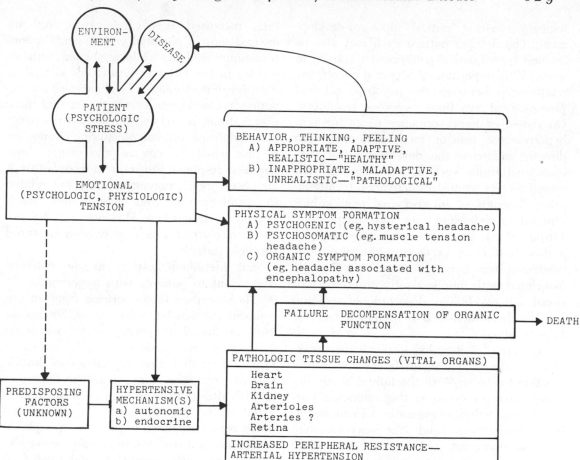

Figure 26–2. Psychophysiological relationships in patients with essential hypertension.

Reiser, in reviewing his own and others' work, identifies three phases of hypertension; Phase 1: preceding the manifestation of the clinical disease; Phase 2: the onset of the disorder; and Phase 3: the continuing course of the disease once it has become established (see Figure 26–2).[182–185] For each of the phases, he suggests that the underlying pathophysiological mechanisms may differ. For example, the importance and relative influence of variables, such as sodium metabolism, emotional influences, neurogenic and hormonal mechanisms in the mediation of the psychophysiological process may change as the disease progresses. With his associates, he has recorded the difference in the labile blood-pressure responsivity of normotensives and patients labelled prehypertensive, as contrasted to the limited responsivity of blood pressure to a structured experimental interpersonal stress in patients with well-established

essential hypertension.[186,187,228,249] In the predispositional phase, Reiser considers both genetic factors and experiential constitutional factors (deriving from the conditioning of the organism during its prenatal, perinatal, and early neonatal experience through the shaping and reinforcement of visceral functions) as contributing to the establishment of a latent but potentially pathogenic hypertensive pressor mechanism. For example, he cites the infant's crying reaction to nonspecific stress as involving a Valsalva response causing an increased intrathoracic pressure, a decreased ventricular filling, a decreased cardiac output, an increased heart rate, and an increased peripheral resistance in order to maintain the perfusion pressure of vital organs. Behavioral shaping of such a response pattern might occur through chance experiences affecting the organism in which emotions and their defenses become annealed with specific physiological patterns at "critical" phases of development. The defense pattern itself may also be learned from familial patterns of reactivity to stress. With repetition of stressful events, the relationship between the psychological and physiological reactions becomes reinforced. On the other hand, presence of an inherent hyperreactive pressor mechanism may also directly influence the development of psychological traits, such as ego defenses, that would protect against its activation by attenuating closeness of interpersonal relationships (insulating defenses) (see also Chapter 28, Introduction). This vascular hyperreactivity in and of itself, or as a reflection of total central-nervous-system hyperreactivity, may then be associated with independently observed emotional and psychological patterns of response in individuals identified as prehypertensive or hypertensive.

In Phase 2, Reiser hypothesizes the breakdown of the critical ego-defensive systems in reaction to stress. With the failure of ego defenses, changes occur in the autonomic outflow tracts, including sympatho-adreno-medullary mechanisms and the hypothalamic anteropituitary adrenal cortical axis. Affect and regressive changes occur in a large number of ego functions including attention, perception, cognition, and intellectual functions. These also influence and are in turn influenced by autonomic and/or hormonal reactions. At this point, cyclical interactions are recognized in which not only do psychological processes influence physiological ones but the changes in the latter directly affect and compromise the former.

In Phase 3, the process developed during Phase 2 becomes fixed resulting in an individual who is different both physiologically and psychologically from what he was in Phase 1. In this Phase entirely new patterns of behavior and reactions prevail.

EMOTIONS

Rennie identified that blood-pressure elevation related to anxiety and depression in patients.[188] Later Ax associated increased diastolic blood pressure with decreased heart rate, increased skin conductance, and increased muscle potential with anger.[9] In contradistinction, fear, while associated with increases in the latter two variables as well as with respiratory rate, did not produce an elevation in blood pressure. On the basis of these observations, he related anger to a discharge of epinephrine and norepinephrine as opposed to fear which he saw as producing an epinephrine response. Funkenstein recorded similar observations, suggesting anger-out related to norepinephrine while anger-in and anxiety related to epinephrine. However, specific biochemical correlates have never been measured for these states.[68]

Saul identified hostility as the essential component in patients with hypertension.[200, 201] He described this as arising from an unresolved relationship with the mother resulting in conflicts over passivity-activity, dependence-independence, and sexuality. Miller suggested that repression of hostile emotion was the core factor in hypertension.[149] Moses observed both rage and resentment as the psychic correlates of elevated blood pressure related to increased peripheral resistance, in distinction to blood-pressure elevations secondary to anxiety and related to increased stroke volume and heart rate without a change in peripheral resistance.[157] Both Schachter and Van der Valk identified fear, anger, and hostility as more intense and associated with greater elevations in hypertensives as compared with normotensive controls.[202, 242] Kaplan et al. extended these observations by demonstrating hostile content in samples of verbal productions and hypnotic dreams of patients with hypertension.[108] Using Rorschach factors, Brower correlated higher diastolic blood pressures in relationship to lower adjustment to reality.[24] Graham and coworkers related elevations in blood pressure in hypertensive subjects with the attitude of having to be on guard against bodily assault.[75] Moos and Engel, studying response specificity to stress in hypertensives vs. arthritics, demonstrated sustained elevation in blood pressure in the former and greater muscle reactivity in the latter.[155] In addition, they showed that arthritics could adapt for blood pressure but not muscle tension where the reverse prevailed for hypertensives. Weiner et al. studying cardiovascular responses in hypertensive and peptic-ulcer patients to TAT (Thematic apperception test) cards noted that these related to the interaction of the subject and experimenter.[249] Subjects with essential hypertension were remarkably unreactive as a group and this lack of physiological responsiveness was related to the nature of the interaction. McKegney and Williams showed that patients with hypertension, as opposed to those without, had greater increases in blood pressure during a personal discussion phase of the interview.[141,258] Williams et al. in further work suggested that blood-pressure elevation during an interview was related to the intensity of interviewer–subject interaction.[257] Silverstone and Kissin demonstrated that patients with essential hypertension tended to be more field dependent than patients with peptic ulcer.[216] Goldstein et al. showed that field-dependent subjects have higher GSRs (Galvanic Skin Response) at rest, and do not discriminate on a physiological level as well between conditional and other similar stimuli.[73] Sapira et al. in showing films of "good" and "bad" doctor–patient relationships to hypertensive and normotensive subjects, found that the hypertensives tended to deny seeing any difference between the two doctors.[198] These studies suggest that the hypertensive patient may be more vulnerable to external threats and therefore perceptually tend to screen out potentially noxious stimuli as a behavioral response protecting his hyperactive pressor system.

PERSONALITY

Dunbar pioneered the work in relating personality styles to specific illness constellations.[54] She identified lifelong patterns of anxiety, perfectionism, compulsivity, and difficulty with authority figures as the psychological components of the individual with hypertensive disease. Gressell et al. and Saslow et al. identified obsessive-compulsive behavior and subnormal assertiveness.[78,199] They also

noted that this correlation prevailed regardless of the type of hypertension. Ostfeld and Lebovits, using Rorschach and MMPI tests, also found no difference between patients with renal and essential hypertension.[160] Noting that blood-pressure responses during periods of life stress were also similar in the two diseases they concluded that personality and attitude factors were etiologically not related to essential hypertension. On the other hand, Koster, emphasizing differences found among patients with essential hypertension, suggested that it is basically several different diseases, each with its own peculiar physiology and psychology.[125] Davies, using the Eysenck Personality Inventory, found no correlations with neurotic traits among patients with hypertension, although he found correlations with body weight, arm circumference, body build, and a family history of cardiovascular disease.[43]

To summarize these studies, it is suggested that individuals with hypertension cope with stresses likely to precipitate emotional feelings (anger, anxiety, sadness) with repressive and protective psychological defenses leading to behavior patterns that include altered perception, especially in the area of interpersonal relationships. When stress factors break through these defenses, aggravation and exacerbation of hypertension occurs.

ENVIRONMENTAL FACTORS

Investigators have been concerned with the identification of environmental stress and its relationship to the development and/or exacerbation of hypertension. Wolf et al. studied fifty-eight patients with hypertension and reported that they met day-to-day threats and challenges with restrained aggression, simultaneously displaying a vascular reaction characterized by elevated blood pressure and vasoconstriction of both afferent and efferent renal glomerular arterioles.[265] Even after sympathectomy, they observed that hypertensives continued to respond to threatening situations with constriction of the afferent arteriole although the efferent arteriolar reaction was abolished. Reiser et al. associated emotionally charged life situations with the course of the disease and the precipitation of malignant hypertension.[185] Harris et al., studying "pre-hypertensives" (patients with labile blood-pressure responses) and matched controls, found that the former were less well-controlled, more impulsive, more egocentric, and less adaptable in stressful situations.[85] Henry et al., using an ingenious intercommunicating box system, studied the social response of two groups of mice, differently raised, to the effect of crowding and competition.[93] Mice isolated from weaning to maturity showed profound physical signs and pathology in addition to markedly elevated blood pressure. In addition, the deprived mice demonstrated an inability to respect each other's need for territory and to control aggression. Subsequently, they observed that susceptible mice subjected to psychosocial stimulation showed increases in catecholamine-forming enzymes. They suggest that the increase in these enzymes may be neuronally mediated and that unlike epinephrine and norepinephrine, enzyme changes may take a long time to develop.[94] Henry and Cassel in a review article suggested that repeated arousal of the defense alarm response may be one mechanism for elevated blood pressure.[92] In man, such arousal may occur when previous socially sanctioned patterns of behavior, to which the organism has become adapted during critical early learning periods, can no longer be used to express normal behavioral urges. Difficulties in adaptation and status ambiguity may result in years of repeated arousals of vascular, autonomic, and hormonal function due to the organism's perception of events as threatening. This may lead to progressive and irreversible disturbances.

Kasl and Cobb reported that blood-pressure levels were higher among workers during an anticipation of job loss, unemployment, and probationary reemployment than after later stabilization.[109] Men, whose blood pressure remained higher for a longer time, were subject to greater unemployment, manifested lower ego resilience, and reported longer-lasting subjective stress.[264] Harburg, Schull, et al.

in a pilot study, identified that the proportions of persons with hypertensive levels were significantly greater in a high-stress area than in a low-stress one.[84,206] The stresses identified included: ecological, personal-interpersonal (making a living, marital, early family life, neighborhood, race relations, life situations, status striving, resentment, self-esteem), and health risks (family history of cardiovascular disease, weight, smoking, infrequent use of medical aids). Sokolow et al. studied blood pressure responses automatically recorded every thirty minutes in hypertensives who concurrently kept a log of events and completed mood checklists.[220] The highest systolic and diastolic levels correlated with times of reported anxiety, time pressure, and alertness.

Although some workers have identified specific environmental stresses as directly affecting blood-pressure responses, a current interpretation is that hypertension develops as a consequence of the manner in which a genetically vulnerable individual perceives an environmental threat, and the defensive patterns that he gradually adopts determine the complex somatopsychosocial relationships.

THERAPY

Shapiro, working in the field of hypertension for the past thirty years, has been, perhaps, the most important pioneer in therapeutic developments.[209–212] Advocating supportive psychotherapy, together with the use of antihypertensive agents, he has achieved an amelioration of symptoms and a slowing of disease progression by assisting the patient in identifying and avoiding noxious stimuli and learning how to adjust to his environment and the limitations of disease. He has found therapy to be most effective when it is transmitted in a supportive, nonthreatening, and nonauthoritative doctor–patient relationship. Wolff and Lindeman, and Sokolow and Perloff have reviewed the pharmaceutical agents used in the control of hypertension.[267, 219] Relaxation methods have enjoyed limited popularity from time to time. Jacobson and Raab have been proponents of these, both noting beneficial results for patients with cardiovascular disease.[100,177,179] Gantt has advocated therapy through conditioning techniques.[69] Most recently Miller, DiCara, and their co-workers at Rockefeller University[150, 151,45] have demonstrated effective conditioning of blood pressure in laboratory animals. More limited success has been obtained with human subjects.[14,211,212] The relationships of these techniques to the control of hypertension by meditational experiences remains to be elucidated.

Conclusions

During the past thirty years, workers in the field have adopted a multi-factorial genesis for the ill-defined condition called "essential hypertension." First and foremost, a primary genetic predisposition on the basis of geographic, racial, and family studies has been suggested as necessary, but not sufficient, for the development of hypertension. Environmental studies have implicated early developmental factors, especially those relating to mother–child interaction. Of considerable interest has been the observation of the alterations in perception that seem to occur in patients with hypertension in the course of the disease, suggesting that these may represent an attempt to protect a vulnerable hyperreactive pressor mechanism. Increasing attention is presently directed at the early conditioning of autonomic responses in an attempt to explain the repeated association of emotional and psychological traits with hypertension. The emotions most often identified have been those of anxiety and hostility or anger, where expression is frequently repressed. Obsessive and compulsive personality patterns have also been identified. Depressive reactions have frequently been observed to correlate with the development and/or exacerbation of hypertension. Secondary to the development of the disease, altered physiological and behavioral patterns have been hypothesized and attributed to secondary effects of the process, especially on the heart, brain, and kidneys. Such effects may include deterioration of perceptual

and cognitive functions. Stress relative to specific environmental factors has been identified as relating to the development and/or exacerbation of hypertension in genetically and psychologically vulnerable individuals. Therapeutic approaches include the combination of peripheral antihypertensive agents and psychotherapy. Several investigators have suggested the possible benefit of antidepressants when depression coexists. There is considerable excitement about the potential use of operant conditioning in modifying autonomic activity. Whether these will prove effective for all phases of the illness remains questionable.

⟨ Special Psychological Aspects of Diagnosis and Treatment

The investigation and treatment of cardiovascular disorders frequently involves specialized procedures and approaches which, in themselves, contribute to the precipitation of emotions and the erection of defenses against them. Catheterization, implantation of a pacemaker, intensive care units, and cardiac surgery are among these.

Cardiac Catheterization

Greene et al. have observed that patients undergoing cardiac catheterization exhibit four behavioral patterns: (1) anxious-engaged; (2) anxious not-engaged; (3) depressed; and (4) calm.[76] All of these conditions showed elevated free fatty acids. Cortisol was elevated in both anxious groups, whereas growth hormone was elevated only in the anxious not-engaged group. Neither the depressed nor the calm group demonstrated elevations in cortisol or growth hormone. A follow-up study of twenty-two patients indicated significantly greater mortality among the anxious not-engaged and depressed groups.[76] These observations indicate the stress that catheterization has for patients and how reaction patterns may be characterized by both psychological and physiological measures. They also suggest the possible prognostic value of the identification of patients' reactions to catheterization in terms of subsequent survival.

Pacemakers

Several investigators have studied reactions of patients requiring the implantation of cardiac pacemakers.* Noting the initial anxieties of patients relative to the underlying cardiac disease and arrhythmias, they have delineated the concerns of these patients about relying on an artificial mechanical instrument, its unpleasant side effects, the possibility that batteries run out, and possible complications resulting from implantation. Blacher and Basch have identified three phases in the acceptance of pacemakers by patients: (1) the preoperative, characterized by concern with life and death, confrontation with the mystique of medical technology, fear of dependence on an artificial device that could fail, guilt, and pessimism; (2) the immediate posthospital phase characterized by depression; and (3) a later phase in which there has been acceptance of the pacemaker and the pursuance of normal activities, control and mastery of feelings, and preoccupation with physical sensations, fantasies, and denial.[17] Crisp and Stonehill, comparing patients with external and internal pacemakers, noted that the former exhibited greater distress, and suggested that patients with implanted pacemakers were able to make greater use of denial as a defense mechanism in coping with an incurable disease.[39,225]

The Intensive Care Unit (ICU)

As hospitals are absorbing the technological advances that applied scientific research and methodology brought to medicine, specialized units have been established to cope with acute and specific problems. These intensive care units (ICU) and coronary care units (CCU) have evolved from hospital wards or recovery rooms into highly complex and specially constructed acute emergency units, requiring

* See references 17, 39, 47, 77, and 225.

skilled nursing and medical technicians to operate the monitors, defibrillators, respiratory and suction apparatuses, and hypothermia units. In many ways, these units have become the symbol of the new frontier in medicine, its technological coming of age. As such they present a new unknown for the patient, his family, and the medical staff. Simultaneous with the development of these units, the hospital staff has noted an increasing incidence of behavioral disturbances among patients admitted to them, a phenomenon that Nahum has aptly identified as one of the "new diseases of medical progress."[158] Consequently, the ICUs and CCUs have become foci of interest for the behavioral scientist in observing and identifying possible explanations for these syndromes that are estimated to occur 40–60 percent of the time. Kornfeld has developed four categories for the behavior observed in these units:[123]

1. **Behavioral reactions** associated with the medical and surgical illness and/or arising from metabolic, circulatory, or toxic factors.

Hackett and his group, who have compiled extensive observations of patients in CCUs, emphasize the psychological reactions to illness of the patients admitted to the CCU.[33, 34,82,83] Noting that one-third of patients admitted to CCUs were referred for psychiatric consultation, Cassem and Hackett classified the reactions as anxiety, depression, and behavior disorder (see Figure 26–3).[32] Anxiety was related to impending death or death heralds of pain, breathlessness, weakness, and new complications. Anxiety was most manifest in the first two CCU days. Depression was seen as representing injuries to the self-esteem and was observed on the third to fourth CCU day, whereas behavioral disorders had a bimodal distribution during the whole CCU period, with the primitive defense of denial most present on the second day and more sophisticated defenses, appropriate to the patient's personality style, emerging after the fourth day. The defensive behavior described included denial of illness, inappropriate euphoric or sexual responses, and projection of hostile dependent conflicts. These observations raise interesting questions about the pro-

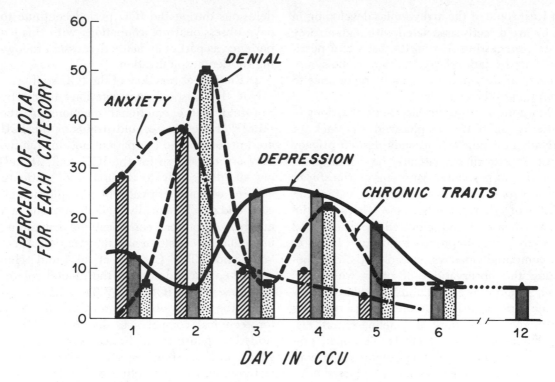

Figure 26–3.   Psychological responses in a coronary care unit.

tective role of denial. In the days following the catastrophic onset, denial of anxiety would seem to serve a protective function for the patient. Later, as his physiological course has stabilized, denial of illness may keep him from accepting and conforming to medical and rehabilitative routines. Cassem and Hackett specify psychiatric intervention in the CCU as including medication to diminish anxiety, explanatory clarification, environmental manipulations, bolstering of optimism, elaborating on the patient's anticipations, confrontation, and hypnosis. That these techniques may be of value is proved by their finding of three times less mortality in the referred group as compared with nonreferred CCU groups.

Organic brain syndromes, usually acute, may be associated with the cardiac dysfunction and present with symptoms and signs of impairment in the cognitive functions. These may also result from drugs administered to the patient. Occasionally withdrawal states from alcohol, barbiturates, or other drugs are observed three to five days following admission of a patient to the ICU.

2. **Psychiatric reactions** to the unique and unfamiliar environment of the ICU.

McKegney has studied the emotional reaction of the patient to acute and catastrophic illness in the ICU setting.[139,140] Identifying the initial anxiety and subsequent depression experienced by these patients, he stressed not only deficits in the physical environment, but also emphasized problems relating to the medical personnel, and the interactions between these and the patient and his family. Crucial for the patient's adjustment in the ICU is the relationship established with the medical and nursing attendants and the acceptance by the relatives of the ICU environment and the patient's condition.

Not least among the hazards of the ICU environment are emergency situations and their associated procedures. Arrhythmias are not uncommon and often demand dramatic intervention of cardioversion either by drugs or electrical defibrillation.[166] For the patient, this means additional medications with their potential untoward effects and/or the preparation for light anesthesia and electrical shock.

At least some of the arrhythmias developing in ICUs are directly associated with high-anxiety states, suggesting that on the basis of a possible causal relationship, attention to the symptoms of anxiety may be equal in importance to attention to the arrhythmia.[134]

Margolis, in studying psychotic reactions in patients in ICUs, emphasized the lack of privacy at a time when many desired privacy most.[145] For these patients, he noted a diminution of psychotic symptoms on transfer to private rooms. Studies of patients witnessing deaths of other patients in the ICU by Bruhn et al. demonstrated elevated systolic blood pressures and symptoms of anxiety.[28] Leigh et al. compared open vs. closed ICUs, corroborating the observations of other workers.[133] They found that closed units provided privacy at the expense of human interactions, resulting in increased feelings of loneliness and displacement of hostile feelings. The open unit was observed as providing greater social contact with associated freedom of expression of hostile feelings, while the lack of privacy resulted in higher levels of "shame" anxiety. On the basis of these and other observations, they suggested that some individuals will do better in one setting and/or that an ideal CCU could be designed to provide for both togetherness and privacy. Some units have already incorporated this plan with folding partitions that can be closed at the time of nursing procedures, and open at other times to provide for communication with other patients.

3. **Psychiatric reactions** produced by the ICU environment and experience that manifest themselves after discharge from the unit.

Klein et al., and Dominian and Dobson have found heightened anxiety, associated with cardiovascular distress, in patients at the time of and following discharge from the ICU.[121,48] Correlating these emotional changes with increased urinary catecholamines, Klein subsequently demonstrated that cardiovascular complications were reduced in patients prepared for transfer and followed by the same nurse and physician throughout hospitalization.

Kimball has observed that many patients experiencing delirium with hallucinations and delusions during the ICU period continue to have obsessional preoccupations with this experience as part of an acute depression following sudden hospitalization.

4. **Emotional reactions** of the ICU staff.

Not the least of considerations found by Kornfeld is the emotional reactions of the staff.[123] If the stresses and strains of the ICU are burdensome to the patient and his family, they are equally so for the ICU staff, attending simultaneously to a number of patients, each of whom is critically ill, and physiologically and psychologically labile to any one of a number of potential complications demanding immediate recognition and intervention. Vreeland and Ellis, Cassem et al., and Hay and Oken, have described the pivotal role of the nurse in the ICU.[246,33,87] They have compared the nurse's objective role, i.e., the need for technical competence, decisive and controlled response to a chronic state of emergency, and constant vigilance, with her subjective one, i.e., interacting with patients and relatives, handling the fatigue and brusqueness of physicians, and containing her own emotions. They have proposed that these factors be considered in the training and scheduling of nurses. Some hospitals now arrange for intermittent rotation of ICU nurses to general-nursing floors and for the opportunity to ventilate feelings in group discussion with nurses and administrators within their own hospital as well as from other centers.

Attention to these environmental and personnel factors is needed as a crucial prelude for the patient's hospitalization and eventual rehabilitation and adjustment.

Cardiovascular Surgery

Since cardiac surgery was first performed, severe behavioral postoperative states have been observed. Blachly and Starr have given the name postcardiotomy delirium to these states.[19] This condition is described as occurring suddenly three to five days following surgery after an untoward early postoperative period. The delirium is marked by increasing confusion, progressing to delusions and hallucinations. Blachly and associates attribute this condition to an abnormal metabolic state and postulate the presence of psychotoxic metabolites.[18,197]

Studies have suggested that not only the physical condition but the psychological condition of the individual faced with surgery strongly influences the success or failure of cardiac surgery in terms of morbidity and mortality. Attempts to gain a clearer understanding of these conditions have focused on various aspects of the patient's hospital and surgical course. Janis has observed that the way in which a patient handles anxiety before an operation affects his postoperative course.[102] Patients who denied or showed little or no anxiety and those who manifested overwhelming anxiety sustained greater postoperative morbidity than those patients who admitted to anxiety and demonstrated moderately intact and mature defenses in coping with it.

Abram has verified that patients with high anxiety preoperatively are more likely to experience a postcardiotomy delirium.[1] He explains the occurrence of this psychoticlike state as a defense against the anxiety over the possibility of death. Meyer et al. have suggested that this condition arises out of the patient's misperceptions in the early postoperative period, occurring while he is still under the influence of anesthesia and adjunctive agents such as the anticholinergics.[148,100] They also postulate that in his semidrugged state the individual misperceives what is going on in an unfamiliar environment, picking up fragments from this which he may subsequently attempt to fit together in what is projected as an unreal delusional sequence.

Kornfeld et al. emphasized the possible contributing effects of the recovery room (RR) or ICU.[123,124] Here was an environment of simultaneous sensory overstimulation and monotony in terms of the repetitive beeping sounds of cardiac monitors, the hissing of oxygen and suction apparatuses, the intermittent clacking of automatic blood-pressure recordings.[272] The patient was constantly aroused by nursing staff carrying out necessary medical observations and procedures. Sleep was only possible in short sequences. The patient's communication was disrupted because of oxygen masks, tracheotomies, and the suppression of cognitive processes (orientation, memory, concentration, and abstraction) associated with analgesics and sedatives. In the case of cardiac surgery, the environment becomes further distorted by the introduction of hypothermia, and, for the coronary patient in rarer instances, by the use of hyperbaric chambers.[217,238] Not only was the patient estranged from those in the immediate environment by machines and sounds, but in a large measure, the ICU was similarly isolated from the rest of the world. Windows in these units were rare. Lights were kept on at all times obliterating day-night sequences, distorting circadian rhythms, and ultimately the patient's time sense and orientation. Clocks and calendars were absent. Regular meal times were not observed. Familiar objects were nowhere to be seen. The personnel was strangely garbed and masked. Other patients were perceived as moaning heaps of white, while physically close enough at hand to compromise privacy, frequently far distant in a communicative sense. No wonder then that patients admitted to these units often experienced confusion, disorientation, misperceptions, and, less frequently, manifested delusional and hallucinatory behavior associated with agitation interfering with medical care. In rarer instances, the disruptive behavior resulted in patients' ripping off intravenous and monitor attachments and fleeing from the unit followed by a melange of attendants to the startled attention of the other patients. Kornfeld's vivid description went beyond mere observation. He suggested a number of remediable factors which have since been introduced into the ICU that presumably have led to the reduction in the incidence of these behavioral states.

Kimball et al. following patients undergoing cardiac surgery, observed that the delirium identified by Blachly and others is almost always preceded by symptoms and signs suggesting progressive cognitive dysfunction from the first postoperative day, and is most frequent in individuals who reported prior compromise of cerebral functions.[118,120] Early symptoms and signs included restlessness, agitation, mild confusion, complaints, and little or no sleep. These occurred in patients whose operative experience and postoperative course had been more severe. In other studies, Kimball found that patients who preoperatively denied anxiety and yet manifested considerable agitation, and those with marked depression were more likely to experience adjustment difficulties in the postoperative period and sustained greater morbidity and mortality.[116,117] These patients responded to cognitive deficits with heightened anxiety and depression which further compromised their ability to cope with the stresses of the postoperative environment. With increasing sleep deficits and the not infrequent complications, mild confusion became gross disorientation with increasing agitation, which, if left untreated, resulted in delusional and hallucinatory states (see Figure 26-4). Patients who had fairly successful life patterns before surgery enjoyed lower mortality, although those who had used illness as a means of adjusting to life situations showed greater morbidity postoperatively and had poorer overall results.

Kennedy and Bakst identified six groupings of patients preoperatively as having predictive significance in terms of postoperative adjustment and outcome.[114] Focusing on patients' expectations of surgery, they observed that patients with a long history of unsatisfactory life conditions approached surgery consciously expressing a death wish. On the other hand, patients with congenital cardiac defects expressed optimism, viewing the repair as something owed to them and that correction would make them rightfully healthy. Patients who had used their illness in making life adjustments feared and later experienced profound readjustment problems when they no longer had severe disability to rely upon in negotiating their demands. Knox's experience with patients he classified as neurotics or hysterics on the basis of interviews and performance on the M-R section of the Cornell Medical Index showed similar poor postoperative adjustment.[122]

Tufo et al. have correlated aberrant postoperative behavior with demonstrated neurological deficits and neuropathological lesions.[240] Furthermore, they have shown that patients who had long intervals on extracorporeal circulation and who had sustained blood pressures below 60 mm. Hg. were more vulnerable to postoperative delirium. Heller et al. demonstrated that patients with longer bypass times were more vulnerable to developing delirium, raising the interesting hypothesis of the possible role of the lung in metabolizing substances that, when accumulated, are toxic to brain function.[90]

Precise explanation for the various correlations are still in the process of evolution based upon more intensive research. Efforts are in progress to identify biological correlates of the emotional and behavioral states. Such studies suggest, but do not conclusively prove, that the manner in which individuals confront experiences influence their subsequent psychological and physiological behavior in identical ways. For instance, a possible explanation why depressed patients are more likely to die is that the depressed state prevents them from augmenting sufficient physiological defenses to sustain the stress of the operative procedure.[175] However, it is possible that depressed states and their biological correlates vary considerably from one individual to another.

Identifying in vulnerable patients preoperatively signs and symptoms of organicity, overwhelming anxiety and/or depression, and considering appropriate preoperative and/or postoperative intervention may help to diminish postoperative morbidity. Attention to the individual's expectations may be all important in whether or not he makes a satisfactory response. If expectations are unrealistic, if the patient expects rebirth and rejuvenation, and discovers in its place continued limitation and restriction, recovery and rehabilitation will be retarded. The preoperative and rehabilitative efforts of the staff need to include the family, especially the spouse. Attention to vocational, social, and domestic (including marital) expectations of the patient and his family is their responsibility. Without such attention, the social reintegration of the patient will be less than ideal and fraught with superimposed

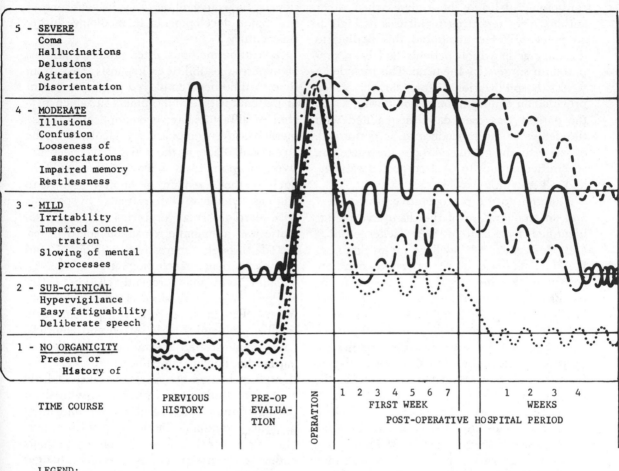

Figure 26–4. Course of mental status of patients undergoing heart surgery.

frustrations. The efforts of the staff do not cease with the event of successful surgery. The long road to recovery has only just begun, the twists, turns, and detours are many and can only be approached and overcome by the continued support, understanding, and foresight of the team.

Lazarus and Hagens have demonstrated that patients who underwent a preoperative interview with a psychiatrist had lower mortality and morbidity than matched patients who were not afforded this experience.[131] This observation has recently been substantiated by Layne and Yudofsky.[130] Kimball noted in his original series of fifty-four patients that there was no occurrence of post-cardiotomy delirium at a time when other authors were reporting incidences as high as 40 percent.[116] He attributed this finding to the manner in which patients had been prepared for surgery by the team. This included a week's hospitalization before surgery which provided an equilibration period during which the patient was seen daily, acquainted with the details of the procedure to be performed, exposed to the recovery room, instructed in several techniques to be used postoperatively, and talked with a psychiatrist.

Attention to the postoperative environment and an amelioration of the disruptive factors identified by Kornfeld,[123,124] Heller et al.,[90] and McKegney,[140,141] will go far in diminishing the incidence of postoperative delirium. Instructing the nursing staff in the ICU in the use of a scale similar to the Eleven Item Behavioral Rating Scale will lead to the early detection of cognitive deficits and will prevent gross behavioral disturbance through the appropriate intervention.[176] Judicious and cautious use of phenothiazines to diminish the anxiety underlying or associated with aberrant behavior, whatever its cause, has helped greatly in controlling behavior and bringing relief to the disturbed patient.[20] Preparation of the patient for release as well as admission to the ICU, as stressed by Klein, will help prevent the occurrence of transfer anxiety, when the patient suddenly feels abandoned and on his own.[121]

Lastly, for the physician and the team that works with these patients and wishes to sensitize himself to the subjective concerns of the patient undergoing cardiac surgery, reading of Rachel MacKenzie's *Risk*[142] is essential.

Behavior and Conditioning Techniques

During the past decade, innovative research, based on new laboratory techniques, has led to renewed interest in the potential role of conditioning in the understanding and treatment of autonomic dysfunctions. Although this research is in its infancy and still of more theoretical interest than of practical application, enough experimental work has been accomplished to suggest that an extension of these techniques may become one of the major developments in medicine during this century.

Relaxation methods, often under conditions of hypersuggestibility or hypnosis, have from time to time been employed in the treatment of patients with chronic illness in which psychological factors have been implicated. These methods, given emphasis by Jacobson in the 1930s, and Raab in the 1960s, have been derived in part from behavior therapy.[101,177] Such methods remain in limited use. Raab emphasized the use of "retreats" by patients with cardiovascular problems in which somatic and autonomic relaxation could be effected through "regressive" individual and group experiences, including mud baths.

Gantt, and more recently Rifkin (after Wolpe), have emphasized classical conditioning methods in their work with patients with cardiac problems.[69,189,270] Aiken and Henrichs have demonstrated relaxation techniques in patients following open-heart surgery.[4] Although in limited use, partly because of little contact of students and physicians with them during training, the use of specific and more general conditioning methods have an important place in the rehabilitation of patients enduring disease processes in which changes in habits are deemed essential to their continued effectiveness and survival.

Most exciting is the work performed by Miller and his colleagues, Banuazizi, Carmona, and DiCara in operant conditioning or instrumental learning.[150-152,46] In instrumental, as opposed to classical conditioning, reinforcement or reward may strengthen any immediately preceding response. In classical conditioning the reward achieves its desired effect only when the response to be learned is already elicited by an unconditional stimulus. Miller explains the relationship between these methods as different manifestations of the same basic phenomenon under different conditions. He identifies similar laws as effecting both types of learning and assumes that there is essentially only one kind of learning.

Using curarized rats in order to ablate the

affect of skeletal on visceral responses to be conditioned by instrumental learning, Miller and Trowill were able to demonstrate that increases or decreases in heart rate could be effected, using as a reward direct stimulation of the rewarding areas of the brain or as punishment a mild pain stimulus to the tail.[150,239] Subsequently Miller and DiCara were able to effect greater changes in these responses through the techniques of shaping and to demonstrate that learning can be both brought under the control of a discriminative stimulus and retained. They were then able to show that operantly learned behavior under the influence of curare could be carried over to the noncurarized state, supporting the contention that this learning is effected directly through the visceral system rather than indirectly through the effect of learned motor behavior on visceral functions as summarized by Katkin and Murray.[110] Such learning was also demonstrated to be specific for the condition rewarded and not generalized to other autonomic functions. In other words, cardiovascular functions such as blood pressure and heart rate could be independently conditioned in either direction. However, DiCara has observed greater "emotionality" occurring in animals conditioned to increase their heart rate, as compared to those conditioned to decelerate their heart rate following instrumental conditioning. To date, operant learning, while it occurs, has been poorer in the noncurarized state than the curarized one, a phenomenon explained by Miller on the basis that the later state eliminates sources of distractability and variability. Because of initial success in effecting brain wave activity and associated behavior through instrumental learning techniques, Miller and his colleagues are at present attempting to modify the activity of a specific part of the vagal nucleus directly which holds potential for the instrumental regulation of cardiac activity.

The implications of this work are several. Understanding the individual specificity with which organisms react to similar stresses through their autonomic nervous system may be tentatively explained on the basis of the at first casual juxtaposition of a chance stress with such a response at a particularly vulnerable time in the development or structuring of that autonomic function under a specific environmental situation in which the gross behavior associated with the autonomic response was wittingly or unwittingly rewarded (reinforced).

With improvement and perfection of these techniques, their theoretical potential for use in altering visceral dysfunctions is viewed as unlimited. This has especial potential for cardiovascular disorders such as cardiac arrhythmias and hypertension, where preliminary human trials have suggested their applicability. Frazier et al. have shown that discriminative avoidance conditioning leads to changes in the rate of response, the speed of the detection response, and the probability of signal detection, noting associated changes in heart rate, pulse pressure, skin resistance, and 17-hydroxycorticosteroid, epinephrine, and norepinephrine excretions.[62] Headrick et al., with augmented sensory feedback techniques, effected heart-rate increases.[88] They cited three dependent factors: (1) amount of training time required; (2) feedback; and (3) motivation. Weiss and Engel have reported success in using operant techniques in treating cardiac arrhythmias, work that has yet to be replicated by others.[251] Plumlee has described increases in blood pressure under operant learning and Benson et al., and Shapiro et al., have achieved significant decreases in systolic blood pressures with these methods used on patients with essential hypertension.[174,14,212] Whether these techniques will achieve long-term results awaits further trials and observations. In concluding this brief discussion, the authors are reminded of the long-observed changes in autonomic responses occurring in transcendental meditation or yoga.[42]

(Bibliography

1. ABRAM, H. S. and B. F. GILL. "Predictions of Postoperative Psychiatric Complications," *N. Engl. J. Med.*, 265 (1961), 1123–1128.

2. ADAMS, F. H. and A. J. MOSS. "Physical Activity of Children with Congenital Heart Disease," *Am. J. Cardiol.*, 24 (1969), 605–606.

3. ADSETT, C. A. and J. G. BRUHN. "Short-term Group Psychotherapy for Post-myocardial Infarction Patients and Their Wives," *Can. Med. Assoc. J.*, 99 (1968), 577–584.

4. AIKEN, L. H. and T. F. HENRICHS. "Systematic Relaxation as a Nursing Intervention Technique with Open Heart Surgery Patients," *Nurs. Res.*, 20 (1971), 212–217.

5. ALEXANDER, F. "Emotional Factors in Essential Hypertension," *Psychosom. Med.*, 1 (1939), 173–179.

6. ALEXANDER, H., DE M. "A Few Observations on the Blood Pressure in Mental Disease," *Lancet* (July 5, 1902), 18–20.

7. ALTSCHULE, M. D. *Bodily Physiology in Mental and Emotional Disorders*, pp. 23–24. New York: Grune & Stratton, 1953.

8. ARLOW, J. A. "Anxiety Patterns in Angina Pectoris," *Psychosom. Med.*, 14 (1952), 461–468.

9. AX, A. F. "The Physiological Differentiation between Fear and Anger in Humans," *Psychosom. Med.*, 15 (1953), 433–442.

10. BAHNSON, C. B. and W. I. WARDWELL. "Parent Constellation and Psychosexual Identification in Male Patients with Myocardial Infarction," *Psychol. Rep.*, 10, 3-V10 (Monograph Suppl.) (1962), 831–852.

11. BAKKER, C. B. and R. M. LEVENSON. "Determinants of Angina Pectoris," *Psychosom. Med.*, 29 (1967), 621–633.

12. BARNES, R. and W. SCHOTTSTAEDT. "The Relation of Emotional State to Renal Excretion of Fluids and Electrolytes in Patients with Congestive Heart Failure," *Clin. Res.*, 6 (1958), 224.

13. BENDIAN, J. and J. GROEN. "A Psychological-Statistical Study of Neuroticism and Extraversion in Patients with Myocardial Infarction," *J. Psychosom. Res.*, 7 (1963), 11–14.

14. BENSON, H., D. SHAPRIO, B. TURSKY et al. "Decreased Systolic Blood Pressure through Operant Conditioning Techniques in Patients with Essential Hypertension," *Science*, 173 (1971), 740–741.

15. BILODEAU, C. B. and T. P. HACKETT. "Issues Raised in a Group Setting by Patients Recovering from Myocardial Infarction," *Am. J. Psychiatry*, 128 (1971), 73–78.

16. BINGER, C. "On So-called Psychogenic Influences in Essential Hypertension," *Psychosom. Med.*, 13 (1951), 273–276.

17. BLACHER, R. S. and S. H. BASCH. "Psychological Aspects of Pacemaker Implantation," *Arch. Gen. Psychiatry*, 22 (1970), 319–323.

18. BLACHLY, P. H. "Open Heart Surgery: Physiological Variables of Mental Functioning," *Int. Psychiatry Clin.*, 4 (1967), 133–155.

19. BLACHLY, P. H. and A. STARR. "Post-cardiotomy Delirium," *Am. J. Psychiatry*, 121 (1964), 317–375.

20. ———. "Treatment of Delirium with Phenothiazine Drugs following Open Heart Surgery," *Dis. Nerv. Syst.*, 27 (1966), 107–110.

21. BOLT, W., M. F. BELL, and J. R. HARNES. "A Study of Mortality in Moderate and Severe Hypertension," *Trans. Assoc. Life Ins. Med. Dir. Am.*, 41 (1958), 61.

22. BOYLE, E., JR. "Biological Patterns in Hypertension by Race, Sex, Body Weight, and Skin Color," *JAMA*, 213 (1970), 1637–1643.

23. BROD, J. "Haemodynamics and Emotional Stress," *Bibl. Psychiatr.*, 144 (1970), 13–33.

24. BROWER, D. "The Relation between Certain Rorschach Factors and Cardiovascular Activity before and after Visuo-Motor Conflict," *J. Gen. Psychiatry*, 37 (1947), 93–95.

25. BROZEK, J. "Personality Differences between Potential Coronary and Noncoronary Subjects," *Ann. N.Y. Acad. Sci.*, 134 (1966), 1057–1064.

26. BRUHN, J. G., B. CHANDLER, M. C. MILLER et al. "Social Aspects of Coronary Heart Disease in Two Adjacent Ethnically Different Communities," *Am. J. Public Health*, 57 (1966), 1493–1506.

27. BRUHN, J. G., B. CHANDLER, and S. WOLF. "A Psychological Study of Survivors and Nonsurvivors of Myocardial Infarction," *Psychosom. Med.*, 31 (1969), 8–19.

28. BRUHN, J. G., A. E. THURMAN, JR., B. C. CHANDLER et al. "Patients' Reactions to Death in a Coronary Care Unit," *J. Psychosom. Res.*, 14 (1970), 65–70.

29. BRUNNER, H. R., J. H. LARAGH, L. BAER et al. "Essential Hypertension: Renin and Aldosterone, Heart Attack and Stroke," *N. Engl. J. Med.*, 286 (1972), 441–449.

30. CAFFREY, B. "A Multivariate Analysis of Sociopsychological Factors in Monks with Myocardial Infarctions," *Am. J. Public Health*, 60 (1970), 452–458.

31. CASSEL, J., S. HEYDEN, A. G. BARTEL et al. "Incidence of Coronary Heart Disease by Ethnic Groups, Social Class, and Sex," *Arch. Intern. Med.*, 128 (1971), 901–906.

32. CASSEM, N. H. and T. P. HACKETT. "Psychiatric Consultation in a Coronary Care Unit," *Ann. Intern. Med.*, 75 (1971), 9–14.

33. CASSEM, N. H., T. P. HACKETT, C. BASCOM et al. "Reactions of Coronary Patients to the Coronary Care Unit Nurse," *Am. J. Nursing*, 70 (1970), 319–324.

34. CASSEM, N. H., H. A. WISHNIE, and T. P. HACKETT. "Response of Coronary Patients to Last Rites," *Postgrad. Med.*, 45 (1969), 147–152.

35. CHAGAN, M., T. HANES, D. O'NEILL et al. "The Intellectual and Emotional Development of Children with Congenital Heart Disease," *Guys Hosp. Rep.*, 100 (1951), 331–341.

36. CHAMBERS, W. N. and M. F. REISER. "Emotional Stress in the Precipitation of Congestive Heart Failure," *Psychosom. Med.*, 15 (1953), 38–60.

37. CLEVELAND, S. E. and D. L. JOHNSON. "Personality Patterns in Young Males with Coronary Disease," *Psychosom. Med.*, 24 (1962), 600–610.

38. COHEN, S. and O. A. PARSONS. "The Perception of Time in Patients with Coronary Artery Disease," *J. Psychosom. Res.*, 8 (1964), 1–7.

39. CRISP, A. H. and E. STONEHILL. "Aspects of the Psychological Status of Patients Treated with Cardiac Pacemakers," *Postgrad. Med.*, 45 (1969), 423–427.

40. CROOG, S. H. and S. LEVINE. "Social Status and Subjective Perceptions of 250 Men after Myocardial Infarction," *Public Health Rep.*, 84 (1969), 989–997.

41. CROOG, S. H., D. SHAPIRO, and S. LEVINE. "Denial among Male Heart Patients: An Empirical Study," *Psychosom. Med.*, 33 (1971), 385–397.

42. DATEY, K. K., S. N. DESHMUKH, C. P. DALVI et al. " 'Sahvasan': A Yogic Exercise in the Management of Hypertension," *Angiology*, 20 (1969), 325–333.

43. DAVIES, M. "Blood Pressure and Personality," *J. Psychosom. Res.*, 14 (1970), 89–104.

44. DAWBER, T. R. and W. B. KANNEL. "Atherosclerosis and You: Pathogenic Implications from Epidemiologic Observations," *J. Am. Geriatr. Soc.*, 10 (1962), 805–821.

45. DiCARA, L. V. and N. E. MILLER. "Instrumental Learning of Systolic Blood Pressure Responses by Curarized Rats; Dissociation of Cardiac and Vascular Changes," *Psychosom. Med.*, 30 (1968), 489–494.

46. ————. "Long-Term Retention of Instrumentally Learned Heart-Rate Changes in the Curarized Rat," *Comment. Behav. Biol.*, 2 (1968), 19–23.

47. DLIN, B. M. and H. K. FISCHER. "Psychologic Adaptation to Pacemaker and Open Heart Surgery," *Arch. Gen. Psychiatry*, 19 (1968), 599–610.

48. DOMINIAN, J. and M. DOBSON. "Study of Patients' Psychological Attitudes to a Coronary Care Unit," *Br. Med. J.*, 4 (1969), 795–798.

49. DONALDSON, J. F. "Patterns of Disease in Rhodesia Central Africa," *J. Med.*, 17 (1971), 51–53.

50. DOYLE, J. T., T. R. DAWBER, W. B. KANNEL et al. "Cigarette Smoking and Coronary Heart Disease," *N. Engl. J. Med.*, 266 (1962), 796–801.

51. DREYFUSS, F., H. DASBERG, and M. I. ASSAEL. "The Relationship of Myocardial Infarction to Depressive Illness," *Psychother. Psychosom.*, 17 (1969), 73–81.

52. DREYFUSS, F., J. SHANAN, and M. SHARON. "Some Personality Characteristics of Middle-Aged Men with Coronary Artery Disease," *Psychother. Psychosom.*, 14 (1966), 1–16.

53. DRUSS, R. G. and D. S. KORNFELD. "The Survivors of Cardiac Arrest," *JAMA*, 201 (1967), 291–296.

54. DUNBAR, F. *Emotions and Bodily Changes*, pp. 331–361. New York: Columbia University Press, 1954.

55. ELIASSON, S., B. FOLKOW, P. LINOGREN et al. "Activation of Sympathetic Vasodilator Nerves to the Skeletal Muscle in the Cat by Hypothalamic Stimulation," *Acta Physiol. Scand.*, 27 (1953), 18–37.

56. ENGEL, G. L. "Sudden and Rapid Death during Psychological Stress," *Ann. Intern. Med.*, 74 (1971), 771–782.

57. EPSTEIN, F. H. "Epidemiologic Aspects of Atherosclerosis," *Atherosclerosis*, 14 (1971), 1–11.

58. ERIKSON, E. *Childhood and Society*, pp.

247–274. New York: Norton, 1963.

59. FISHER, S. H. "Psychological Factors and Heart Disease," *Circulation*, 27 (1963), 113–117.

60. Fox, H. M. "Physiological Response of the Adrenal to Psychological Influences as Indicated by Changes in the 17-Hydroxycorticosteroid Excretion Pattern," in G. E. W. Walstenholme, ed., *Ciba Foundation Colloquia on Endocrinology*, Vol. 8, p. 612. London: Churchill, 1955.

61. Fox, H. M., B. J. MURAWSKI, G. W. THORN et al. "Urinary 17-Hydroxycorticoid and Uropepsin Levels with Psychological Data. A Three-Year Study of One Subject," *Arch. Intern. Med.*, 101 (1958), 859–871.

62. FRAZIER, T. W., H. WEIL-MALHERBE, and H. S. LIPSCOMB. "Psychophysiology of Conditioned Emotional Disturbances in Humans," *Psychophysiology*, 5 (1969), 478–503.

63. FRIEDMAN, E. H. and H. K. HELLERSTEIN. "Occupational Stress, Law School Hierarchy, and Coronary Artery Disease in Cleveland Attorneys," *Psychosom. Med.*, 30 (1968), 72–86.

64. FRIEDMAN, M., S. O. BYERS, R. H. ROSENMAN et al. "Coronary-Prone Individuals (Type A Behavioral Pattern) Growth Hormone Response," *JAMA*, 217 (1971), 929–932.

65. FRIEDMAN, M. and R. H. ROSENMAN. "Association of Specific Overt Behavior Pattern with Blood and Cardiovascular Findings," *JAMA*, 169 (1959), 1286–1296.

66. ———. "Overt Behavior Pattern in Coronary Disease: Detection of Overt Behavior Pattern A in Patients with Coronary Disease by a New Psychophysiological Procedure," *JAMA*, 173 (1960), 1320–1325.

67. FRIEDMAN, M., R. H. ROSENMAN, R. STRAUS et al. "The Relationship of Behavior Pattern A to the State of the Coronary Vasculature," *Am. J. Med.*, 44 (1968), 525–537.

68. FUNKENSTEIN, D. H., S. H. KING et al. "The Experimental Evocation of Stress," in *Symposium on Stress*, p. 304. Washington: Army Medical Service Graduate School, 1953.

69. GANTT, W. H. "The Meaning of the Cardiac Conditioned Reflex," *Cond. Reflex*, 1 (1966), 139–143.

70. GARFINKEL, L. "The Association between Cigarette Smoking and Coronary Heart Disease and Other Vascular Diseases," *Bull. N.Y. Acad. Med.*, 44 (1968), 1495–1501.

71. GARNER, H. H. and M. A. FALK. "Recognizing the Patient with Pseudoangina," *Geriatrics*, 25 (1970), 87–92.

72. GEIGER, H. J. and N. A. SCOTCH. "The Epidemiology of Essential Hypertension. I. Biologic Mechanisms and Descriptive Epidemiology," *J. Chronic Dis.*, 16 (1963), 1151–1182.

73. GOLDSTEIN, H. S., H. PARDES, A. M. SMALL et al. "Psychological Differentiation and Specificity of Response," *J. Nerv. Ment. Dis.*, 151 (1970), 97–103.

74. GORDON, T. "Mortality Experience among Japanese in the United States, Hawaii, and Japan," *Public Health Rep.*, 72 (1957), 543–553.

75. GRAHAM, D. T., J. D. KABLER, and F. K. GRAHAM. "Physiological Response to the Suggestion of Attitudes Specific for Hives and Hypertension," *Psychosom. Med.*, 24 (1962), 159–169.

76. GREENE. W. A., G. CONRON, D. S. SCHALCH et al. "Psychological Reactions with Changes in Growth Hormone and Cortisol Levels: A Study of Patients Undergoing Cardiac Catheterization," *Psychosom. Med.*, 32 (1970), 599–614.

77. GREENE, W. A. and A. J. MOSS. "Psychosocial Factors in the Adjustment of Patients with Permanently Implanted Cardiac Pacemakers," *Ann. Intern. Med.*, 5 (1969), 897–902.

78. GRESSEL, G. C., F. O. SHOBE, G. SALLOW et al. "Personality Factors in Arterial Hypertension," *JAMA*, 140 (1949), 265–272.

79. GROEN, J. J., J. M. VAN DER VALK, A. WELNER et al. "Psychobiological Factors in the Pathogenesis of Essential Hypertension," *Psychother. Psychosom.*, 19 (1971), 1–26.

80. GROLLMAN, A. "Effect of Psychic Disturbances on the Cardiac Output, Blood Pressure, and Oxygen Consumption in Man," *Am. J. Physiol.*, 89 (1929), 584–593.

81. HACKETT, T. P. and N. H. CASSEM. "Factors Contributing to Delay in Responding to Signs and Symptoms of Acute Myocardial Infarction," *Am. J. Cardiol.*, 24 (1969), 651–658.

82. HACKETT, T. P., N. H. CASSEM, and H. A. WISHNIE. "The Coronary Care Unit: An Appraisal of Its Psychological Hazards," *N. Engl. J. Med.*, 279 (1968), 1365–1370.

83. ———. "Detection and Treatment of Anxiety in the Coronary Care Unit," *Am. Heart J.*, 78 (1969), 727–730.

84. HARBURG, E., W. J. SCHULL, J. C. ERFURT et al. "A Family Set Method for Estimating Heredity and Stress. I. A Pilot Study of Blood Pressure Among Negroes in High and Low Stress Areas. Detroit 1966–1967," *J. Chronic Dis.*, 23 (1970), 69–81.

85. HARRIS, R. E., M. SOKOLOW, L. G. CARPENTER, JR. et al. "Response to Psychologic Stress in Persons Who Are Potentially Hypertensive," *Circulation*, 7 (1953), 874–879.

86. HATCH, F. T., P. K. REISSELL, T. M. W. POON-KING et al. "A Study of Coronary Heart Disease in Young Men. Characteristics and Metabolic Studies of the Patients and Comparison with Age-Matched Healthy Men," *Circulation*, 33 (1966), 679–703.

87. HAY, D. and D. OKEN. "The Psychological Stresses of Intensive Care Unit Nursing," *Psychosom. Med.*, 34 (1972), 109–118.

88. HEADRICH, M. W., B. W. FEATHER, and D. T. WELLS. "Unidirectional and Large Magnitude Heart Rate Changes with Augmented Sensory Feedback," *Psychophysiology*, 8 (1971), 132–142.

89. HEINE, B. E., P. SAINSBURY, and R. C. CHYNOWETH. "Hypertension and Emotional Disturbance," *J. Psychiatr. Res.*, 7 (1969), 119–130.

90. HELLER, S. S., K. A. FRANK, J. R. MALM et al. "Psychiatric Complications of Open-Heart Surgery," *N. Engl. J. Med.*, 283 (1970), 1015–1020.

91. HELLERSTEIN, H. K. and E. H. FRIEDMAN. "Sexual Activity and the Post-Coronary Patient," *Arch. Intern. Med.*, 125 (1970), 987–999.

92. HENRY, J. P. and J. C. CASSEL. "Psychosocial Factors in Essential Hypertension. Recent Epidemiologic and Animal Experimental Evidence," *Am. J. Epidemiol.*, 90 (1969), 171–200.

93. HENRY, J. P., J. P. MEEHAN, and P. M. STEPHANS. "The Use of Psychosocial Stimuli to Induce Prolonged Hypertension in Mice," *Psychosom. Med.*, 29 (1967), 408–432.

94. HENRY, J. P., P. M. STEPHANS, J. AXELROD et al. "Effect of Psychosocial Stimulation on the Enzymes Involved in the Biosynthesis and Metabolism of Noradrenaline and Adrenaline," *Psychosom. Med.*, 33 (1971), 227–237.

95. HICKAM, J. B., W. H. CARGILL, and A. GOLDEN. "Cardiovascular Reactions to Emotional Stimuli: Effect on Cardiac Output, Arteriovenous Oxygen Difference, Arterial Pressure, and Peripheral Resistance," *J. Clin. Invest.*, 27 (1948), 290–323.

96. HINKLE, L. E. "Some Social and Biological Correlates of Coronary Artery Disease," *Soc. Sci. Med.*, 1 (1967), 129–139.

97. HINKLE, L. E., L. H. WHITNEY, E. W. LEHMAN et al. "Occupation, Education and Coronary Heart Disease," *Science*, 161 (1968), 238–246.

98. HOVARTH, S. M. "Cardiac Disease in the Context of the Future Environment," *Environ. Res.*, 2 (1969), 470–475.

99. IBRAHIM, M. A., C. D. JENKINS, J. C. CASSEL et al. "Personality Traits and Coronary Heart Disease," *J. Chronic Dis.*, 10 (1955), 255–271.

100. ITIL, T. and M. FINK. "Anticholinergic Drug-Induced Delirium: Experimental Modification, Quantitative EEG, and Behavioral Correlations," *J. Nerv. Ment. Dis.*, 142 (1966), 492–507.

101. JACOBSON, E. *Progressive Relaxation*. Chicago: University of Chicago Press, 1938.

102. JANIS, I. L. *Psychological Stress. Psychoanalytic and Behavioral Studies of Surgical Patients*. New York: Wiley, 1958.

103. JENKINS, C. D. "Psychologic and Social Precursors of Coronary Artery Disease (Part 1)," *N. Engl. J. Med.*, 284 (1971), 244–255.

104. ———. "Psychologic and Social Precursors of Coronary Artery Disease (Concluded)," *N. Engl. J. Med.*, 284 (1971), 307–317.

105. JENKINS, C. D., S. J. ZYZANSKI, and R. H. ROSENMAN. "Progress toward Validation of a Computer-Scored Test for the Type A Coronary-Prone Behavior Pattern," *Psychosom. Med.*, 33 (1971), 193–202.

106. JENKINS, C. D., S. J. ZYZANSKI, R. H. ROSENMAN et al. "Association of Coronary-Prone Behavior Scores with Recurrence of Coronary Heart Disease," *J. Chronic Dis.*, 24 (1971), 601–611.

107. KANNEL, W. B., J. LeBAUER, T. R. DAWBER et al. "Obesity and Coronary Heart Disease," *Circulation*, 35 (1967), 734–744.

108. KAPLAN, S. M., L. A. GOTTSCHALK, E. B.

MAGLIOCCO et al. "Hostility in Verbal Productions and Hypnotic Dreams of Hypertensive Patients," *Psychosom. Med.*, 23 (1961), 311–322.

109. KASL, S. V. and S. COBB. "Blood Pressure Changes in Men Undergoing Job Loss: A Preliminary Report," *Psychosom. Med.*, 32 (1970), 19–38.

110. KATKIN, E. S. and N. E. MURRAY. "Instrumental Conditioning of Autonomically Mediated Behavior: Theoretical and Methodological Issues," *Psychol. Bull.*, 70 (1968), 52–68.

111. KATZ, L. N. "The Mechanism of Cardiac Failure," *Circulation*, 10 (1954), 663–679.

112. KATZ, L. N., S. S. WINTON, and R. MEGIBOW. "Psychosomatic Aspects of Cardiac Arrhythmias," *Ann. Intern. Med.*, 27 (1947), 261–274.

113. KEITH, R. A. "Personality and Coronary Heart Disease: A Review," *J. Chronic Dis.*, 19 (1966), 1231–1243.

114. KENNEDY, J. A. and H. BAKST. "The Influence of Emotions on the Outcome of Cardiac Surgery: A Predictive Study," *Bull. N.Y. Acad. Med.*, 42 (1966), 811–849.

115. KEYS, A. "Diet and the Epidemiology of Coronary Heart Disease," *JAMA*, 164 (1957), 1912.

116. KIMBALL, C. P. "Psychological Responses to the Experience of Open-Heart Surgery. I," *Am. J. Psychiatry*, 125 (1969), 348–359.

117. ———. "The Experience of Open-Heart Surgery. II. Determinants of Post-operative Behavior," *Proc. 8th Europ. Conf. Psychosom. Med.*, 1970. *Psychother. Psychosom.*, 18 (1970), 259–274.

118. ———. "The Experience of Open-Heart Surgery. III. Toward a Definition and Understanding of Post-cardiotomy Delirium," *Arch. Gen. Psychiatry*, 27 (1972), 57–63.

119. KIMBALL, C. P., D. M. QUINLAN, F. OSBORNE et al. "The Experience of Cardiac Surgery. V. Psychological Patterns and Prediction of Outcome," *Proc. 9th Europ. Conf. Psychosom. Med.*, Vienna, 1972. *Psychother. Psychosom.*, 22 (1973), 310–319.

120. KIMBALL, C. P. and J. V. MAGNUSON. "Depression and Contraception," in P. Zuspan and M. D. Lindeheimer, eds., *Medical Complications of Pregnancy*. New York: Lea & Feiber, forthcoming.

121. KLEIN, R. F., V. A. KLINER, D. P. ZIPES et al. "Transfer from a Coronary Care Unit," *Arch. Intern. Med.*, 122 (1968), 104–108.

122. KNOX, S. J. "Psychiatric Aspects of Mitral Valvotomy," *Br. J. Psychiatry*, 109 (1963), 656–668.

123. KORNFELD, D. S. "Psychiatric Problems of an Intensive Care Unit," *Med. Clin. North Am.*, 55 (1971), 1353–1363.

124. KORNFELD, D. S., S. ZIMBERG, and J. R. MALM. "Psychiatric Complications of Open-Heart Surgery," *N. Engl. J. Med.*, 273 (1965), 287–292.

125. KOSTER, M. "Patterns of Hypertension," *Bibl. Psychiatr.*, 144 (1970), 1–8.

126. LACEY, J. I., D. E. BATEMAN, and R. VAN LEHN. "Autonomic Response Specificity: An Experimental Study," *Psychosom. Med.*, 15 (1953), 8–21.

127. LACEY, J. I. and R. VAN LEHN. "Differential Emphasis in Somatic Response to Stress," *Psychosom. Med.*, 14 (1952), 71–81.

128. LARAGH, J. H. "The Pill, Hypertension, and the Toxemias of Pregnancy," *Am. J. Obstet. Gynec.*, 109 (1971), 210–213.

129. ———. "Mechanisms of Edema Formation and Principles of Management," *Am. J. Med.*, 21 (1956), 423.

130. LAYNE, O. L., JR. and S. C. YUDOFSKY. "Post-operative Psychosis in Cardiotomy Patients," *N. Engl. J. Med.*, 284 (1971), 518–520.

131. LAZARUS, H. R. and J. H. HAGENS. "Prevention of Psychosis following Open-Heart Surgery," *Am. J. Psychiatry*, 124 (1968), 1190–1195.

132. LEBOVITS, B. Z., R. B. SCHKELLE, A. M. OSTFELD et al. "Prospective and Retrospective Psychological Studies of Coronary Heart Disease," *Psychosom. Med.*, 29 (1967), 265–272.

133. LEIGH, H., M. HOFER, J. COOPER et al. "A Psychological Comparison of Patients in 'Open' and 'Closed' Coronary Care Units," (Am. Psychosom. Ann. Meet., Abstract), *Psychosom. Med.*, 33 (1971), 476.

134. LEON, A. S. and W. B. ABRAMS. "The Role of Catecholamines in Producing Arrhythmias," *Am. J. Med. Sci.*, 262 (1971), 9–13.

135. LEUTSCHER, J. A. and B. B. JOHNSON. "Observations on the Sodium-Retaining Corti-

coid (Aldosterone) in the Urine of Children and Adults in Relation to Sodium Balance and Edema," *J. Clin. Invest.*, 33 (1954), 1441–1446.

136. LEVI, L. "Emotional Stress and Sympatho-Adrenomedullary and Related Physiological Reactions with Particular Reference to Cardiovascular Pathology," *Bibl. Psychiatr.*, 144 (1970), 38–51.

137. LILJEFORS, I. and R. H. RAHE. "An Identical Twin Study of Psychosocial Factors in Coronary Heart Disease in Sweden," *Psychosom. Med.*, 32 (1970), 523–542.

138. LYNN, D. B., H. H. GLASER, and G. S. HARRISON. "Comprehensive Medical Care for Handicapped Children: III. Concepts of Illness in Children with Rheumatic Fever," *Am. J. Dis. Child*, 103 (1962), 120.

139. McKEGNEY, F. P. "The Intensive Care Syndrome. The Definition, Treatment and Prevention of a New 'Disease of Medical Progress'," *Conn. Med.*, 30 (1966), 633–636.

140. ———. "After the Coronary Care Unit: Three Transitions," in M. A. F. Pranulis, ed., *After the Coronary Care Unit—Then What?*, pp. 3–13. Proceedings of a symposium sponsored by the Greater Bridgeport Heart Association, December 3, 1969. Bridgeport, Conn.: Connecticut Regional Medical Program.

141. McKEGNEY, F. P. and R. B. WILLIAMS. "Psychological Aspects of Hypertension. II. The Differential Influence of Interview Variables on Blood Pressure," *Am. J. Psychiatry*, 123 (1967), 1539–1545.

142. MacKENZIE, R. *Risk*. New York: Viking, 1971.

143. MAI, F. M. M. "Personality and Stress in Coronary Disease," *J. Psychosom. Res.*, 12 (1968), 275–287.

144. MAINZER, F. and M. KRAUSE. "Influence of Fear on Electrocardiogram," *Br. Heart J.*, 2 (1940), 221–230.

145. MARGOLIS, G. J. "Postoperative Psychosis on the Intensive Care Unit," *Compr. Psychiatry*, 8 (1967), 227–232.

146. MARRIOTT, H. J. L. and P. M. NIZET. "Physiological Stimuli Simulating Ischemic Heart Disease," *JAMA*, 200 (1967), 139.

147. MERRILL, A. J. "Edema and Decreased Renal Blood Flow in Patients with Chronic Congestive Heart Failure," *J. Clin. Invest.*, 25 (1946), 389–400.

148. MEYER, B. C., R. S. BLACHER, and F. BROWN. "A Clinical Study of Psychiatric and Psychological Aspects of Mitral Surgery," *Psychosom. Med.*, 23 (1961), 194–218.

149. MILLER, M. L. "Blood Pressure Findings in Relation to Inhibited Aggressions in Psychotics," *Psychosom. Med.*, 1 (1939), 162–172.

150. MILLER, N. E. "Learning of Visceral and Glandular Responses," *Science*, 163 (1969), 434–445.

151. MILLER, N. E. and A. BANUAZIZI. "Instrumental Learning by Curarized Rats of a Specific Visceral Response, Intestinal or Cardiac," *J. Compr. Physiol. Psychol.*, 65 (1968), 1–7.

152. MILLER, N. E. and A. CARMONA. "Modification of a Visceral Response, Salivation in Thirsty Dogs by Instrumental Training with Water Reward," *J. Compr. Physiol. Psychol.*, 63 (1967), 1–6.

153. MINC, S. "Psychological Factors in Coronary Heart Disease," *Geriatrics*, 20 (1965), 747–755.

154. MINC, S., G. SINCLAIR, and R. TAFT. "Some Psychological Factors in Coronary Heart Disease," *Psychosom. Med.*, 25 (1963), 133–139.

155. MOOS, R. H. and B. T. ENGEL. "Psychophysiological Reactions in Hypertensive and Arthritic Patients," *J. Psychosom. Res.*, 6 (1962), 227–241.

156. MORDKOFF, A. M. and O. A. PARSONS. "The Coronary Personality: A Critique," *Psychosom. Med.*, 29 (1967), 1–14.

157. MOSES, L., G. E. DANIELS, and J. L. NICKERSON. "Psychogenic Factors in Essential Hypertension: Methodology and Preliminary Report," *Psychosom. Med.*, 18 (1956), 471–485.

158. NAHUM, L. H. "Madness in the Recovery Room from Open Heart Surgery or 'They Kept Waking Me Up'," *Conn. Med.*, 29 (1966), 771–772.

159. OLIN, H. S. and T. P. HACKETT. "The Denial of Chest Pain in 32 Patients with Acute Myocardial Infarction," *JAMA*, 190 (1964), 977–981.

160. OSTFELD, A. M. and B. Z. LEBOVITS. "Personality Factors and Pressor Mechanisms in Renal and Essential Hypertension," *Arch. Intern. Med.*, 104 (1959), 59–68.

161. PAFFENBARGER, R. S., JR. "Chronic Disease

in Former College Students. VI. Implications for College Health Programs," *J. Am. Coll. Health Assoc.*, 16 (1967), 51–55.

162. PAFFENBARGER, R. S., JR., J. NOTKIN, D. E. KRUEGER et al. "Chronic Disease in Former College Students. II. Methods of Study and Observations on Mortality from Coronary Heart Disease," *Am. J. Public Health*, 56 (1966), 962.

163. PAFFENBARGER, R. S., JR., P. A. WOLF, J. NOTKIN et al. "Chronic Disease in Former College Students. I. Early Precursors of Fatal Coronary Heart Disease," *Am. J. Epidemiol.*, 83 (1966), 314–328.

164. PAGE, I. H. In Ciba Symposium, *Hypertension*. Berlin: Springer, 1966.

165. PAUL, O. "Myocardial Infarction and Sudden Death," *Hosp. Practice*, 6 (1971), 91–108.

166. PAULK, E. A., JR. "Clinical Problems of Cardioversion," *Am. Heart J.*, 70 (1965), 248–274.

167. PELSER, H. E. "Psychological Aspects of the Treatment of Patients with Coronary Infarct," *J. Psychosom. Res.*, 11 (1967), 47–49.

168. PENAZ, J. "The Blood Pressure Control System: A Critical and Methodological Introduction," *Bibl. Psychiatr.*, 144 (1970), 125–150.

169. PERLMAN, L. V., S. FERGUSON, K. BERGUM et al. "Precipitation of Congestive Heart Failure: Social and Emotional Factors," *Ann. Intern. Med.*, 75 (1971), 1–7.

170. PETERS, J. P. "The Problem of Cardiac Edema," *Am. J. Med.*, 12 (1952), 66–76.

171. PICKERING, G. *The Nature of Essential Hypertension*. London: Churchill, 1961.

172. PINDERHUGHES, C. A. and C. A. PERLMAN. "Psychiatric Aspects of Idiopathic Cardiomyopathy," *Psychosom. Med.*, 31 (1969), 57–67.

173. PITTS, R. F. "Some Reflections on Mechanisms of Action of Diuretics," *Am. J. Med.*, 24 (1958), 745–763.

174. PLUMLEE, L. A. "Operant Conditioning of Increases in Blood Pressure," *Psychophysiology*, 6 (1969), 283–290.

175. PRICE, D. B., M. THALER, and J. W. MASON. "Preoperative Emotional States and Adrenal Cortical Activity," *Arch. Neurol. Psychiatry*, 77 (1957), 646–656.

176. QUINLAN, D. M., C. P. KIMBALL, and F. OSBORNE. "The Experience of Open Heart Surgery. IV. Assessment of Disorientation and Dysphoria Following Cardiac Surgery," *Arch. Gen. Psychiatry*, 31 (1974), 241–244.

177. RAAB, W. *Organized Prevention of Degenerative Heart Disease: A Challenge to American Medicine and Economy*. Burlington, Vt.: Queens City Press, 1962.

178. ———. "Emotional and Sensory Stress Factors in Myocardial Pathology," *Am. Heart J.*, 72 (1966), 538–564.

179. ———. "The Preventable Neurogenic Causes of Hypoxic Myocardial Disease," *Med. Psicosomatica (Rome)*, 11 (1966), 1–30.

180. ———. "Correlated Cardiovascular Adrenergic and Adrenocortical Responses to Sensory and Mental Annoyances in Man: A Potential Accessory Cardiac Risk Factor," *Psychosom. Med.*, 30 (1968), 809–818.

181. REES, W. D. and S. G. LUTKINS. "Mortality of Bereavement," *Br. Med. J.*, 4 (1967), 13–16.

182. REISER, M. F. "Theoretical Considerations of the Role of Psychological Factors in Pathogenesis and Etiology of Essential Hypertension," *Bibl. Psychiatr.*, 144 (1970), 117–124.

183. REISER, M. F., A. A. BRUST, and E. FERRIS. "Life Situations, Emotions and the Course of Patients with Arterial Hypertension," *Psychosom. Med.*, 13 (1951), 133–139.

184. REISER, M. F., R. B. REEVES, and J. ARMINGTON. "The Effect of Variations in Laboratory Procedure and Experimenter upon the Ballistocardiogram, Heart Rate, and Blood Pressure of Healthy Young Men," *Psychosom. Med.*, 17 (1955), 185–199.

185. REISER, M. F., M. ROSENBAUM, and E. B. FERRIS. "Psychologic Mechanisms in Malignant Hypertension," *Psychosom. Med.*, 13 (1951), 147–159.

186. REISER, M. F., M. THALER, and H. WEINER. "The Experimental Manipulation of Projective Stimuli in the Study of Psychophysiological Responses," *Psychosom. Med.*, 17 (1955), 480.

187. REISER, M. F., H. WEINER, and M. THALER. "Patterns of Object Relationships and Cardiovascular Responsiveness in Healthy Young Adults and Patients with Peptic Ulcer and Hypertension," *Psychosom. Med.*, 19 (1957), 498.

188. RENNIE, T. A. "Personality in Hypertensive

States," *N. Engl. J. Med.*, 221 (1939), 448–456.

189. RIFKIN, B. F. "The Treatment of Cardiac Neurosis Using Systematic Desensitization," *Behav. Res. Ther.*, 6 (1968), 239–241.

190. RISEMAN, J. E. F. "Management after the Acute Coronary Attack," *Vasc. Dis.*, 3 (1966), 315–319.

191. RODDA, B. E., M. C. MILLER, 3RD, and J. G. BRUHN. "Prediction of Anxiety and Depression Patterns among Coronary Patients Using a Markov Process Analysis," *Behav. Sci.*, 16 (1971), 482–489.

192. ROSEN, J. L. and G. J. BIBRING. "Psychological Reactions of Hospitalized Male Patients to Heart Attacks," *Psychosom. Med.*, 28 (1966), 808–821.

193. ROSENBERG, S. G. "Patient Education Leads to Better Care for Heart Patients," *HSMHA Health Rep.*, 86 (1971), 793–802.

194. ROSENMAN, R. H. and M. FRIEDMAN. "The Central Nervous System and Coronary Heart Disease," *Hosp. Practice*, 5 (1971), 87–97.

195. ROSENMAN, R. H., M. FRIEDMAN, and S. O. BYERS. "Glucose Metabolism in Subjects with Behavior Pattern A and Hyperlipemia," *Circulation*, 33 (1966), 704–707.

196. ROSENMAN, R. H., M. FRIEDMAN, C. D. JENKINS et al. "The Prediction of Immunity to Coronary Heart Disease," *JAMA*, 198 (1966), 137–140.

197. SACHDEV, N. S., C. C. CARTER, R. L. SWANK et al. "Relationship between Post-Cardiotomy Delirium, Clinical Neurological Changes and EEG Abnormalities," *J. Thorac. Cardiovasc. Surg.*, 54 (1967), 557–563.

198. SAPIRA, J. D., E. T. SCHEILP, R. MORIARTY et al. "Differences in Perception between Hypertensive and Normotensive Populations," *Psychosom. Med.*, 33 (1971), 239–250.

199. SASLOW, G., G. C. GRESSEL, F. O. SHOBE et al. "Possible Etiologic Relevance of Personality Factors in Arterial Hypertension," *Psychosom. Med.*, 12 (1950), 292–302.

200. SAUL, L. J. "Hostility in Cases of Essential Hypertension," *Psychosom. Med.*, 1 (1939), 153–161.

201. SAUL, L. J., E. SHEPPARD, D. SELBY et al. "The Quantification of Hostility in Dreams with Reference to Essential Hy-

pertension," *Science*, 119 (1954), 382–383.

202. SCHACTER, J. "Pain, Fear, and Anger in Hypertensives and Normotensives," *Psychosom. Med.*, 19 (1957), 17–29.

203. SCHNEIDER, D. E. *The Image of the Heart.* New York: International Universities Press, 1956.

204. SCHNEIDER, R. A. and V. M. ZANGARI. "Variations in Clotting Time, Relative Viscosity and other Physiochemical Properties of the Blood Accompanying Physical and Emotional Stress in the Normotensive and Hypertensive Subject," *Psychosom. Med.*, 13 (1951), 289–303.

205. SCHOTTSTAEDT, W. W., W. J. GRACE, and H. G. WOLFF. "Life Situations, Behaviour, Attitudes, Emotions, and Renal Excretion of Fluid and Electrolytes, I–V," *J. Psychosom. Res.*, 1 (1956), 75–83.

206. SCHULL, W. J., E. HARBURG, J. C. ERFURT et al. "A Family Set Method for Estimating Heredity and Stress: II. Preliminary Results of the Genetic Methodology in a Pilot Survey of Negro Blood Pressure, Detroit, 1966, 1967," *J. Chronic Dis.*, 23 (1970), 83–92.

207. SCOTCH, N. A. and H. J. GEIGER. "The Epidemiology of Essential Hypertension. II. Psychological and Sociocultural Factors in Etiology," *J. Chronic Dis.*, 16 (1963), 1183–1213.

208. SELYE, H. *The Stress of Life*, pp. 128–148. New York: McGraw-Hill, 1956.

209. SHAPIRO, A. P. "Psychophysiologic Pressor Mechanisms and Their Role in Therapy," *Mod. Treat.*, 3 (1966), 108–117.

210. SHAPIRO, A. P., M. ROSENBAUM, and E. B. FERRIS. "Relationship Therapy in Essential Hypertension," *Psychosom. Med.*, 13 (1951), 140–146.

211. SHAPIRO, D., B. TURSKY, E. GERSHON et al. "Effects of Feedback and Reinforcement on the Control of Human Systolic Blood Pressure," *Science*, 163 (1969), 588–590.

212. SHAPIRO, D., B. TURSKY, and G. E. SCHWARTZ. "Control of Blood Pressure in Man by Operant Conditioning," *Circ. Res.*, 27, *Suppl.* 1 (1970), 27–41.

213. SHEKELLE, R. B., A. M. OSTFELD, B. Z. LEBOVITS et al. "Personality Traits and Coronary Heart Disease: A Re-examination of Ibrahim's Hypothesis Using Longitudinal Data," *J. Chronic Dis.*, 23 (1970), 33–38.

214. SHEKELLE, R. B., A. M. OSTFELD, and O. PAUL. "Social Status and Incidence of

Coronary Heart Disease," *J. Chronic Dis.*, 22 (1969), 381–394.

215. SILVERMAN, A. J., S. I. COHEN, and G. D. ZUIDIMAN. "Psychophysiological Investigations in Cardiovascular Stress," *Am. J. Psychiatry*, 113 (1957), 691–693.

216. SILVERSTONE, S. and B. KISSIN. "Field Dependence in Essential Hypertension and Peptic Ulcer," *J. Psychosom. Res.*, 12 (1968), 157–161.

217. SILVERSTONE, J. T., M. M. TANNAHILL, and J. A. IRELAND. "Psychiatric Aspects of Profound Hypothermia in Open-Heart Surgery," *J. Thorac. Cardiovasc. Surg.*, 59 (1970), 193–200.

218. SJOERDSMA, A. "Relationships between Alterations in Amine Metabolism and Blood Pressure," Society of Actuaries. The Build and Blood Pressure Study, 1959. *Circ. Res.*, 9 (1961), 734–745.

219. SOKOLOW, M. and D. PERLOFF. "The Choice of Drugs and the Management of Essential Hypertension," *Prog. Cardiovasc. Dis.*, 8 (1965), 253–277.

220. SOKOLOW, M., D. WERDEGAR, D. B. PERLOFF et al. "Preliminary Studies Relating Portably Recorded Blood Pressures to Daily Life Events in Patients with Essential Hypertension," *Bibl. Psychiatr.*, 144 (1970), 164–189.

221. STAMLER, J. "Cigarette Smoking and Atherosclerotic Coronary Heart Disease," *Bull. N.Y. Acad. Med.*, 44 (1968), 1476–1494.

222. ———. The Primary Prevention of Coronary Heart Disease," *Hosp. Practice*, 6 (1971), 49–61.

223. STEAD, E. A., JR., J. V. WARREN, A. J. MERRILL et al. "Cardiac Output in Male Subjects as Measured by Technique of Right Atrial Catheterization. Normal Values with Observations on the Effect of Anxiety and Tilting," *J. Clin. Invest.*, 24 (1945), 326–331.

224. STEVENSON, I. P., C. H. DUNCAN, and H. G. WOLFF. "Circulatory Dynamics before and after Exercise in Subjects With and Without Structural Heart Disease during Anxiety and Relaxation," *J. Clin. Invest.*, 28 (1949), 1534–1543.

225. STONEHILL, E. "The Role of Denial in Incurable Disease: Psychological Adaptation to Long-term Cardiac Pacemakers," *Bibl. Psychiatr.*, 144 (1970), 151–163.

226. STORMENT, C. T. "Personality and Heart Disease," *Psychosom. Med.*, 13 (1951), 304–313.

227. SYME, S. L. "Psychological Factors and Coronary Heart Disease," *Int. J. Psychiatry*, 5 (1968), 429–433.

228. THALER, M., H. WEINER, and M. F. REISER. "Exploration of the Doctor–Patient Relationship through Projective Techniques. Their Use in Psychosomatic Illness," *Psychosom. Med.*, 19 (1957), 228–239.

229. THOMAS, C. B. "Observations on Some Possible Precursors of Essential Hypertension and Coronary Artery Disease," *Bull. Johns Hopkins Hosp.*, 89 (1951), 419–441.

230. ———. "Characteristics of the Individual as Guideposts to the Prevention of Heart Disease," *Ann. Intern. Med.*, 47 (1957), 389–401.

231. ———. "Characteristics of Smokers Compared with Nonsmokers in a Population of Healthy Young Adults, Including Observations on Family History, Blood Pressure, Heart Rate, Body Weight, Cholesterol and Certain Psychologic Traits," *Ann. Intern. Med.*, 53 (1960), 697–718.

232. ———. "The Precursors of Hypertension," *Med. Clin. North Am.*, 45 (1961), 259.

233. ———. "Psychophysiologic Aspects of Blood Pressure Regulation: The Clinician's View," *Psychosom. Med.*, 26 (1964), 454–461.

234. ———. "Psychophysiological Aspects of Blood Pressure Regulation: A Clinician's View," *J. Chronic Dis.*, 17 (1964), 599–607.

235. ———. "The Precursors of Hypertension and Coronary Artery Disease: Insights from Studies of Biological Variation," *Ann. N.Y. Acad. of Sci.*, 134 (1966), 1028–1040.

236. ———. "Developmental Patterns in Hypertensive Cardiovascular Disease: Fact or Fiction?" *Bull. N.Y. Acad. of Med.*, 45 (1969), 831–850.

237. THOMAS, C. B. and B. H. COHEN. "The Familial Occurrence of Hypertension and Coronary Artery Disease with Observations Concerning Obesity and Diabetes," *Ann. Intern. Med.*, 42 (1955), 90–126.

238. THURSTON, J. G. B. "A Controlled Trial of Hyperbaric Oxygen in Acute Myocardial Infarction—Preliminary Results," *Am. Heart Assoc. (Abstract in circulation)*, 40 *Suppl.* 3 (1969), 203.

239. Trowill, J. A. "Instrumental Conditioning of the Heart Rate in the Curarized Rat," *J. Compr. Physiol. Psychol.*, 63 (1967), 7–11.

240. Tufo, H. M., A. M. Ostfeld, and R. Shekelle. "Central Nervous System Dysfunctioning following Open-Heart Surgery," *J. Am. Heart Assoc.*, 212 (1970), 1333–1340.

241. Vanderhoof, E., J. Clancy, and R. S. Engelhart. "Relationship of a Physiological Variable to Psychiatric Diagnoses and Personality Characteristics," *Dis. Nerv. Syst.*, 27 (1966), 171–177.

242. Van der Valk, J. M. "Blood-Pressure Changes under Emotional Influences in Patients with Essential Hypertension and Control Subjects," *J. Psychosom. Res.*, 2 (1957), 134–144.

243. Van der Valk, J. M., and J. J. Groen. "Personality Structure and Conflict Situation in Patients with Myocardial Infarction," *J. Psychosom. Res.*, 11 (1967), 41–46.

244. von Eiff, A. W. "The Role of the Autonomic Nervous System in the Etiology and Pathogenesis of Essential Hypertension," *Jap. Circ. J.*, 34 (1970), 147–153.

245. Voors, A. W. "Lithium in the Drinking Water and Atherosclerotic Heart Death: Epidemiologic Argument for Protective Effect," *Am. J. Epidemiol.*, 92 (1970), 164–171.

246. Vreeland, R. and G. L. Ellis. "Stresses on the Nurse in an Intensive Care Unit," *JAMA*, 208 (1969), 332–334.

247. Walter, P. F., S. D. Reid, and N. K. Wenger. "Transient Cerebral Ischemia Due to Arrhythmia," *Ann. Intern. Med.*, 72 (1970), 471–473.

248. Weinberger, M. H., R. D. Collins, A. J. Dowdy et al. "Hypertension Induced by Oral Contraceptives Containing Estrogen and Gestragen," *Ann. Intern. Med.*, 71 (1969), 891–902.

249. Weiner, H., M. T. Singer, and M. F. Reiser. "Cardiovascular Responses and Their Psychological Correlates. I. A Study in Healthy Young Adults and Patients with Peptic Ulcer and Hypertension," *Psychosom. Med.*, 24 (1962), 477–498.

250. Weiss, B. "Electrocardiographic Indices of Emotional Stress," *Am. J. Psychiatry*, 113 (1956), 348–351.

251. Weiss, T. and B. F. Engel. "Operant Conditioning of Heart Rate in Patients with Premature Ventricular Contractions," *Psychosom. Med.*, 33 (1971), 301–321.

252. Wells, R. L. "The 'Unemployable' Cardiac Patient," *JAMA*, 218 (1971), 247.

253. Wendkos, M. H. "The Influence of Autonomic Imbalance on the Human Electrocardiogram. I. Unstable T-Waves in Precordial Leads from Emotionally Unstable Persons without Organic Heart Disease," *Am. Heart J.*, 28 (1944), 549–567.

254. Wendkos, M. H. and R. Logue. "Unstable T-Waves in Leads II and III in Persons with Neurocirculatory Asthenia," *Am. Heart J.*, 31 (1946), 711–723.

255. Werko, L. "Can We Prevent Heart Disease? Multifactorial Physical, Environmental, Hereditary, Clinical Factors Are Identified," *Ann. Intern. Med.*, 74 (1971), 278–288.

256. White, K. "Angina Pectoris and Angina Innocens," *Psychosom. Med.*, 17 (1955), 128–138.

257. Williams, R. B., Jr., C. P. Kimball, and H. N. Willard. "The Influence of Interpersonal Interaction Upon Diastolic Blood Pressure," *Psychosom. Med.*, 32 (1972), 194–198.

258. Williams, R. B., Jr., and F. P. McKegney. "Psychologic Aspects of Hypertension. I. The Influence of Experimental Interview Variables on Blood Pressure," *Yale J. Biol. Med.*, 38 (1965), 265–273.

259. Williamson, J., J. Mitchell, S. Kreider et al. "Assessing End Results for Heart Failure Patients Selected from a Coronary Care Unit," *Am. Fed. Clin. Res. Natl. Meet.*, May 1968, Abstract. *Clin. Res.*, 16 (1968), 367.

260. Wincott, E. A. and F. I. Caird. "Return to Work after Myocardial Infarction," *Br. Med. J.*, 2 (1966), 1302–1304.

261. Wishnie, H. A., T. P. Hackett, and N. H. Cassem. "Psychological Hazards following Coronary Infarct," *JAMA*, 215 (1971), 1292–1296.

262. Wolf, G. A. and H. G. Wolff. "Studies on the Nature of Certain Symptoms Associated with Cardiovascular Disorders," *Psychosom. Med.*, 8 (1946), 293–319.

263. Wolf, S. "Psychosocial Forces in Myocardial Infarction and Sudden Death," *Circulation*, 39, *Suppl.* 4 (1969), 74–83.

264. WOLF, S., P. V. CARDON, JR., E. M. SHEPARD et al. *Life Stress and Essential Hypertension: A Study of Circulatory Adjustment in Men.* Baltimore: Williams & Wilkins, 1955.

265. WOLF, S., J. B. PFEIFFER, H. S. FIPLEY et al. "Hypertension as a Reaction Pattern to Stress: Summary of Experimental Data in Variations in Blood Pressure and Renal Blood Flow," *Ann. Intern. Med.*, 29 (1948), 1056–1076.

266. WOLF, S. and E. SHEPARD. "An Appraisal of Factors that Evoke and Modify the Hypertensive Reaction Pattern," *Assoc. Res. Nerv. Ment. Dis. Proc.*, 29 (1950), 976–984.

267. WOLFF, F. W. and R. D. LINDEMAN. "Effects of Treatment in Hypertension. Results of a Controlled Study," *J. Chronic Dis.*, 19 (1966), 227–240.

268. WOLFF, H. G. "Life Stress and Cardiovascular Disorders," *Circulation*, 1 (1949), 187–203.

269. WOLFF, K. "Angina Pectoris and Emotional Disturbances," *Dis. Nerv. Syst.*, 30 (1969), 401–404.

270. WOLPE, J. *Psychotherapy by Reciprocal Inhibition*, pp. 139–165. Stanford: Stanford University Press, 1958.

271. YAMORI, Y., W. LOVENBERG, and A. SJOERDSMA. "Norepinephrine Metabolism in Brainstem of Spontaneously Hypertensive Rats," *Science*, 170 (1970), 544–546.

272. ZISKIND, E. and T. AUGSBURG. "Hallucinations in Sensory Deprivation," *Dis. Nerv. Syst.*, 28 (1967), 721–726.

CHAPTER 27

PSYCHOLOGICAL ASPECTS OF GASTROINTESTINAL DISORDERS*

George L. Engel

❡ Introduction

THIS CHAPTER is intended to summarize the present status of our knowledge with respect to the interrelationships of psychic and somatic processes as they affect gastrointestinal activity. Furthermore, it offers a clinical classification of the varieties of gastrointestinal disturbances which may result directly or indirectly from psychological influences.

Historically, there have been two major approaches to psychosomatic research. The psychoanalytic approach, exemplified by the work of Franz Alexander,[8,10,7] by elucidating

the nature of unconscious mental processes, identified specific psychodynamic tendencies that are intimately related to gastrointestinal activity in a developmental as well as functional sense. While such data originated in the course of the psychoanalytic treatment of neurotics and led to the now familiar concepts of the oral and anal phases of psychosexual development, the application of the same method to patients with gastrointestinal disorders served to highlight more explicit etiological relationships between such unconscious psychodynamic influences and gastrointestinal symptoms.† Furthermore, psychoanalytic theory and method have made the development of other techniques possible, such as the various projective and other testing instruments of the clinical psychologist, whereby the uncon-

---

* This chapter is a revised version of the author's chapter "Psychological Processes and Gastrointestinal Disorders" which appeared in M. Paulson, ed., *Gastroenterologic Medicine*, Philadelphia: Lea & Febiger, 1969. It is used here by permission.

†See references 7, 20, 94, 96, and 158.

scious psychic processes can be identified and studied.

During the same period, Harold Wolff, Stewart Wolf, and others at Cornell University approached the problem through direct observation and measurement of physiological change in the exposed gut of fistulous subjects and related these changes to concomitant psychological states.[56,161,162] These correlative psychophysiological and biochemical studies have provided a basis for delineating the somatic parameters more precisely in terms which can be related to concurrent psychological and behavioral variables.[162] Some efforts have been made to combine the two approaches, that is, to make physiological or biochemical measurements in the course of psychoanalysis, but these have involved such technical and theoretical difficulties as to seriously limit the value of the results so obtained.[104, 108,138] In addition to these approaches, careful clinical—including epidemiological—studies of individuals and populations of patients correlating the course of disease with psychological and social factors, continue to be an indispensable source of new knowledge in this area. Less distinction between the approaches is made today than two decades ago, and the student of gastrointestinal disorders draws upon multiple perspectives and overlapping approaches.

(Specific Relationships Between Psychological Processes and the Gastrointestinal Tract

The most significant contribution of psychoanalysis to gastroenterology was the demonstration of the role of feeding and elimination in the psychological and social development of the child. The relevant points may be summarized as follows:

1. The newborn infant's cycle of hunger → crying → nursing → satiation → sleep → hunger → and so on, constitutes an important, biological influence regulating the first establishment of a relationship between the neonate and its mother. In the course of mounting hunger and then nursing, the infant periodi-cally achieves relief of tension in the mother's arms, laying the basis for the ultimate association in the nervous system of an intrinsic drive (hunger) and its relief through an environmental influence (mother). This is a reciprocal process, the mother being required to recognize and respond appropriately to the infant's cues indicating hunger and the infant being required to fit into the mother's particular patterns of nursing. If successful, it is a source of mutual gratification; if unsuccessful, it becomes a source of tension and frustration for both infant and mother. The consequence of this dependence on the feeding cycle for the psychobiological unit of mother and child is that for the infant many of the first learning experiences, i.e., the first awareness of the mother as part of an outer environment, and the early associations of comfort and discomfort, may be experienced in the oral intaking terms of the nursing experience. This is responsible for the fact that one prominent psychological perspective of the young infant is an oral one, namely, that which is perceived as good or desirable is taken in, while that which is felt as bad is spit out or refused. Evident in infancy in such literal behavioral terms as mouthing, sucking, and tasting everything in reach, this is also manifest in later life as a general psychodynamic tendency which is capable of influencing the content of thought and the nature of behavior, if not the actual activity of the gastrointestinal tract itself. This is revealed in the oral mannerisms of sucking, mouthing, and chewing pencils, pipes, cigarettes, knuckles, gum, and what not, in such familiar oral terms of endearment and pleasure as "How sweet!", "I could eat you up," or of displeasure (distaste!) as, "You make me sick (to my stomach)," "I can't stomach that," as well as in the language used to designate certain personality traits, as "sour," "greedy," "sweet," etc. In a broader context, the feeding experiences of infancy also provide a nidus around which may cluster a whole complex of associations related to such fundamental human needs as to be taken care of, supported, and nurtured, the so-called dependency needs, and hence the classical psychodynamic association, "oral-dependent."

2. With the eruption of teeth and the transition from sucking to chewing comes another contribution of a body activity to psychic development, namely, the expression of aggression and hostility in oral terms, namely, biting, tearing, and even consuming cannibalistically. Again, human behavior and language amply attest to the universality of such psychodynamic tendencies. "Gnashing the teeth," or "clenching the jaw with rage," or "biting sarcasm" (from the Greek, "sarkazo," to tear flesh), and many other expressions may be cited. Characteristically, the thwarting of oral needs, literally or figuratively, may elicit aggressive impulses, to take by force that which is not given, or to force the others to give, expressed literally by the child (and symbolically by the adult) through grabbing, tearing, biting, or holding firmly with the teeth. Greed, envy, possessiveness, spite, bitterness, sarcasm, vindictiveness, all are words that convey such oral aggressive meaning.

3. Since the infant cannot survive or develop without food and cannot feed in the absence of a nurturing person (mother), it is clear that these oral-dependent and oral-aggressive tendencies must be present and operative in all individuals. But what originally was essential for survival, eventually loses such imperative qualities and the associated patterns of behavior must give way to other patterns more acceptable to society. Critical for the course of such developmental achievements are the strength or the driving quality of the original feeding impulses, the degree to which the mother succeeds or fails in gratifying the primary oral needs, the range of other biological and psychological gratifications that are available to or provided for the developing infant, and the environment's standards and expectations as to manner, degree, and circumstance of oral expression and behavior (the interpersonal and social forces). The child in time internalizes these external demands, expectations, and standards and he learns, so to speak, the conditions under which he can prosper and be loved and those under which he is frustrated or rejected. In brief, through the processes of socialization he not only learns that the reality of his particular life situation requires compromises, delays, and the weighing of the consequences of his wishes, impulses, and acts, but in so doing he is repeatedly subject to intrapsychic as well as interpersonal conflict.

The presence of a legacy of past as well as of current conflict is a fact of psychic life. It is a fundamental premise of psychoanalysis that those psychodynamic tendencies which must be denied expression for any reason, may nonetheless continue as unconscious forces to exert an influence on mentation and behavior, an influence which may be reflected in various bits of derived behavior, including changes in gastrointestinal function. It is assumed that unconscious oral-dependent or oral-aggressive impulses, if not successfully gratified by psychological or social devices may be accompanied by physiological changes in the stomach appropriate to preparing to take food into the stomach. Evidence that such indeed is the case in infancy, when affection and aggression are literally expressed in oral terms, is found in the results of a study of concomitant behavior and gastric secretion in a fifteen to eighteen-month-old infant with a gastric fistula.[56] When this baby was relating to a familiar experimenter either with affection and pleasure or with rage, the rate of hydrochloric acid secretion by the stomach was high. On the other hand, when the experimenter was a stranger from whom she typically withdrew and whom she ignored completely, becoming totally inactive, sometimes to the point of falling asleep, the secretion of gastric acid virtually ceased, even remaining unresponsive to histamine. When the familiar experimenter reappeared, she characteristically exhibited signs of exuberant joyful recognition, and a copious secretion of gastric juice ensued. The maximum rates of acid secretion during a sustained joyfully affectionate relationship, or during intense rage approached those observed during sham feeding. In brief, this study[56] appeared to establish that at the level of development characteristic of this child (actually closer to ten to twelve months in development than to her chronologic age of fifteen to eighteen months) active relating patterns, whether affectionate or hostile, were

accompanied by the increments in gastric secretion comparable to what occurred when
the stomach was preparing to receive food; in
the absence of both food and meaningful
human relationship, stomach activity virtually
ceased. Similar findings have been reported in
a pair of twins a year and a half old, one with
a gastric fistula and the other normal.[28]

Comparable psychophysiological studies of
a four-year-old child demonstrated the dissociation between behavior and gastric secretion
that takes place upon the development of
more sophisticated mental means of relating
and communicating, including language. This
child showed a low basal level of secretion of
acid and pepsin when she was relating comfortably and happily with the experimenter
withdrawing gastric juice. This contrasts with
the high secretion found in the younger infant
under such circumstances. On the other hand,
when the four-year-old had to make an effort
to relate, as with a new experimenter, gastric
secretion rose, as it did also when she was
angry or anxious. Secretion was low when she
became detached or withdrawn.[55]

Studies of adults with a gastric fistula also
indicate rise in gastric secretion during rage,
both expressed and suppressed, and a fall during dejection and withdrawal.[141,164,162] Depression and "giving up" experimentally induced through hypnosis in adult volunteers
also has been found to be associated with a
decline in the rate of gastric acid secretion.[86]

4. Like feeding, elimination constitutes another physiological pattern, the development
and control of which eventually involves a reciprocal relationship between mother and
child. In earliest infancy defecation is controlled by an innate reflex which automatically
empties the bowel when it reaches a critical
degree of fullness. Presumably the infant has
no psychic engagement in this process other
than in terms of what pleasant or unpleasant
sensations may accompany such peristaltic
activity. However, toward the end of the first
year and for a variable period thereafter, most
infants not only appear to experience pleasure
in the act of defecation but may also come to
regard their feces with interest, if not decided
pleasure. Certainly they manifest no disgust.

Ultimately, however, the child must learn to
control defecation and restrict his pleasure in
feces in a manner prescribed by the child-rearing practices of his particular group, which
may range from highly exacting to excessively
lenient. Ultimately feces become objects of
loathing and disgust, though this attitude is
more pronounced toward another's bowel
movements than one's own. This constitutes
another important reciprocal relation between
mother and child that is geared closely to an
intrinsic biological rhythm in the child. To aid
her child to achieve bowel control, the mother
must learn the physiological cues that the
child emits and which indicate his readiness to
defecate, while the child must learn from the
mother's response that his physiologically derived sensations call for a specific toileting
action. As with nursing, this reciprocal situation is mutually gratifying when successful but
fraught with complications when mother or
infant fail to respond properly to each other.
The latter incompatibility may range from the
mother who misses all the cues and fails to put
the baby on the pot to the mother who interprets the wrong cues and puts the baby on the
pot at the wrong times. The tensions which
may develop between mother and child with
such stressful learning failures constitute the
basis for explicit psychophysiological relationships between behavior on the one hand and
variations in bowel activity on the other. In
addition, the failure to resolve successfully the
inevitable incompatibility between the wishes
to enjoy feces and the bowel movement, and
the necessity to conform to parental requirements may perpetuate such underlying psychodynamic pressures and exert a distinctive
influence on personality development, contributing to the development of the so-called
"anal traits" of exaggerated orderliness, perfectionism, punctuality, and pedantry. These
are seen as defenses against a persistent unconscious wish to be free to soil. Once again,
the persistence of unconscious psychodynamic
tendencies must be emphasized, exerting an
influence on mentation and behavior, and
sometimes on bowel function as well. As will
be discussed later, bowel symptoms are common in persons with these characteristics,

called "anal" in psychoanalytic terminology.

The utilization of concepts of bowel activity as a vehicle for the expression of aggression is amply attested to by familiar anal and fecal swear words and gestures. Increased physiologic activity of lower bowel has been noted during expression of anger in fistula subjects.[161]

5. By virtue of the pleasurable sensations which originate during sucking, eating, and defecation, and the intimate role of feeding and excremental activities in the development of affectual relationships, it should not be surprising that both ends of the gastrointestinal tract are capable of being endowed by the child with sexual meaning. Concepts of oral or anal intercourse and oral or anal pregnancy and birth are a common part of the fantasy life or misinterpretation of children. How such ideas, when unresolved, may serve to provoke gastrointestinal symptoms, will be discussed later.*

(Classification of Psychological Phenomena in Relation to the Gastrointestinal Tract

Psychogenic Disorders

These include two groups of disorders. One refers explicitly to symptoms ascribed by the patient to the abdomen or gastrointestinal tract which, in fact, constitute psychic phenomena involving intrapsychic representations of gastrointestinal function and process. In such disorders, the gastrointestinal tract per se either is not primarily involved, or is responding in a normal manner to a stimulus, as for example, nausea or vomiting in response to a disgusting idea. Within this category are conversion reactions, somatic delusions, and hypochondriacal phenomena.

The second group comprises bizarre and inappropriate patterns of feeding or elimination which represent either inadequate or undifferentiated behavior patterns and/or are the logical consequences of bizarre (psychotic) ideation. These include anorexia nervosa, pica, food faddism, encopresis, psychogenic megacolon, compulsive use of laxatives or enemas, and other bizarre feeding or bowel behavior. Some persons in this group are psychotic.

* For a more detailed consideration of these concepts, the reader is referred to reference 48.

Psychophysiological Disorders

These involve mainly the physiological concomitants of affects, e.g., rage, anxiety, shame, guilt, etc. The involvement of the gastrointestinal tract may be direct, through its innervations, or indirect, through other general physiological or biochemical processes. Important here is that in the presence of preexisting organic vulnerabilities or latent defects such physiological or biochemical processes may serve to precipitate manifest organic disease.

Somatopsychic-Psychosomatic Disorders

These are organic disorders, the predisposing conditions for which not only are present or acquired early in infancy but also have influenced psychological development in specific ways. Such disorders may become manifest any time in life but the individual bearing the predisposing biological factor, though always vulnerable, will only develop the manifest disorder if certain environmental—including psychological—stresses occur. Included in this category are the conditions classically considered in the past as psychosomatic, i.e., duodenal ulcer and ulcerative colitis, as well as others such as coeliac (malabsorption) syndrome, regional enteritis, and achalasia.

(Psychogenic Disorders

The psychogenic disorders contribute disproportionately to the number of patients presenting with complaints presumably originating from the gastrointestinal tract. Anorexia, bulimia, nausea, vomiting, dysphagia, abdominal pain, bloating, aerophagia, rectal incontinence, diarrhea, constipation, and pruritus ani all are symptoms which may be psychogenic in origin rather than the consequences of intrinsic disorder of the gastrointestinal system. Before discussing specific syndromes and symptoms, however, it is necessary to elucidate some underlying psychic mechanisms, including conversion and delusion, and to relate these to the syndromes of hysteria, hypochondriasis, and schizophrenia.

Conversion Reactions

Conversion reactions[48,49,53] comprise a major category of psychogenic disturbances, experienced or manifested in somatic terms. As a psychological process, conversion represents a means of dealing with stress which makes use of the fact that it is possible to express ideas symbolically through body activities or sensations. The gesture is a familiar example of how a body movement may be used to communicate an idea or a wish and to relieve tension. The typical conversion reaction, however, occurs when the wish, idea, or fantasy in question not only cannot be consciously expressed, but cannot even be consciously acknowledged. Under such circumstances the idea may achieve expression in the form of a sensation or a body activity which symbolically represents the idea in question, and yet at the same time effectively prevents it from being acted upon. As a means of dealing with psychological stress and resolving intrapsychic conflict, such symbolic use of the body replaces both acting on the wish and consciously entertaining it as a thought or fantasy, both of which are felt as threatening. By this means, psychological compensation is maintained although at the expense of some abnormal utilization of the body part selected for this purpose. The result is a somatic symptom based on psychological misuse of the body part, not on disease of the part so involved. Physical examination, therefore, demonstrates no organic defect directly related to the symptom.

The common conversion reactions involve a great variety of body parts and functions, all of which share the following: (1) they are accessible to voluntary control (motor) or awareness (sensation); (2) they had been involved in some way in human relationships in the course of development; and (3) they are capable of being imagined in the form of some concepts of the body image or a function thereof. Each conversion manifestation characteristically is overdetermined, meaning that multiple factors are involved in determining the choice of the particular bodily expression used. The expression which proves to be the most satisfactory psychologically is the one which can most economically symbolize these multiple determinants.

We may best illustrate conversion by a hypothetical example. As pointed out earlier, circumstances may encourage some children excessively to endow the act of eating or swallowing with sexual or aggressive fantasies or wishes which then become a source of conflict. When later in life some provoking circumstance serves to activate such an unconscious impulse, as, for example, the equating of the act of eating with an infantile primitive wish to bite aggressively or to use the mouth for sexual purposes, the conflict evoked may serve to block the impulse from coming to consciousness as a thought or a wish, as well as prevent the overt act. Instead, it may appear in its symbolic form as a conversion symptom, as anorexia, dysphagia, nausea, vomiting, or pain. In such a case the disturbing wish or fear, namely, to bite, to perform fellatio, to be bitten or be sucked on, has been effectively disposed of and has been "converted" to a bodily activity which symbolically means, "I can't eat (swallow)," or "I throw up what I swallow." This forms one basis for such conversion symptoms as anorexia, dysphagia, nausea, or vomiting. Such an inhibition of the processes of eating, swallowing, or retaining that swallowed is a symbolic substitute for the forbidden idea, an idea which in fact had originally related not to food in its literal sense but rather to some unacceptable sexual or aggressive wish which, in the course of development, acquired a link to the act of eating or swallowing. The person so afflicted not only keeps the forbidden idea from conscious awareness by literally not eating, swallowing, or retaining, but he also broadcasts to the world that he does not take anything into his mouth; when he does do so, he has difficulty swallowing it or he regurgitates it. In this symptomatic act the disturbing motivation is contained as "I wish to bite, to take the penis in the mouth, to swallow the loved (or hated) person," etc., implementation of which is blocked. Thus he simultaneously expresses the wish symbolically, yet makes it impossible for the wish to be acted upon.

How the conversion is experienced by the patient and communicated to others is in part determined by the characteristics of the society in which the patient lives and in part by the nature of his thought processes and capacity for reality testing. "Styles" of conversion reactions change with changing times and attitudes, so that certain patterns common in a past generation now are rare. The Victorian swoon is a good example. Modern health and medical consciousness contributer to a tendency to manifest conversion symptoms in keeping with the popular concepts of what physicians expect of physically sick patients. The more capable the patient is of retaining accurate reality orientation, the more likely will the conversion symptom be communicated in such terms. In contrast, the psychotic patient whose thought processes and reality capacities are defective is more likely to experience and communicate conversion symptoms in bizarre terms, approaching true somatic delusions, and to offer bizarre explanations for the symptoms.

The positive identification of a bodily symptom as a conversion reaction requires considerable diagnostic skill. The common practice of depending solely upon the ruling out of organic factors as the means of diagnosing conversion is hazardous. Not only may some organic defects be extremely difficult to demonstrate but also conversion symptoms and organic processes may coexist. *In the absence of positive psychological criteria, conversion cannot be invoked as the explanation of a symptom, even when all other data indicating organic defect are negative.*

The conversion symptom always has its sources in the history of the individual's past human relationships and in the types of bodily activities or experiences which had been in-

volved in the gratifications and conflicts that marked these relationships. A skillfully conducted interview is the keystone to the diagnosis of conversion.

Conversion reactions may occur under a wide variety of stressful circumstances and in persons of the most varied psychological characteristics, from the essentially healthy individual to the psychotic. They are most common in and characteristic of *hysteria,* a condition in which there is a predilection toward use of the body for expression of feelings, wishes, and ideas. But it is not correct to assume that conversion reactions occur only among hysterics.

A less common syndrome than hysteria is *hypochondriasis,* marked by the occurrence of unpleasant bodily sensations, as itch, formication, crawling, pulling, fullness, pain, and other peculiar sensations or by the persistent idea of the presence of an organic disease, as cancer, tuberculosis, syphilis, etc. The latter represent disturbed ideas but may include as well symptoms related to the disease in question, as, for example, fullness, bloating, anorexia, etc., associated with the idea of stomach cancer. Hypochondriacal symptoms characteristically have an insistent, demanding, nagging, torturing, and even persecuting quality and are the source of great distress to the patient, who pleads for relief. They involve especially the skin, abdomen, nose, rectum, and genitals. Peculiar and persistent sensations in the rectum are especially characteristic. At times hypochondriacal symptoms assume the quality of somatic delusions. Thus, the patient may experience or interpret sensations to mean that something is growing inside, that his insides are rotting away, that a body part is changing shape, that bugs are crawling under the skin, etc.

Specific gastrointestinal conversion symptoms have their origins in the psychodynamic factors discussed earlier. They include the whole range of oral and anal, aggressive and sexual fantasies of which the child is capable. Thus anorexia, bulimia, hypophagia, nausea, vomiting, and bloating may relate to conflicts over unacceptable wishes to be nursed like a baby, to bite or swallow aggressively, to use the mouth for sexual purposes, concepts of oral pregnancy or birth, and many others.

Some general clinical characteristics of individual conversion symptoms that are manifest as gastrointestinal symptoms follow.

ANOREXIA

As a conversion symptom, anorexia is likely to be described in complex terms and to be expressed as an active distaste for food, or dislike of eating rather than merely as an absence of appetite. It may be directed toward certain foods and not others, especially foods capable of symbolic meaning, such as liquid egg white, scum on milk, rare meat, etc. There may be a preference for "baby" foods. It may occur only in certain settings or with certain people and be totally absent at other times or under different circumstances. Occasionally the complaint of anorexia does not correspond with the observed nutritional status, the patient maintaining or even gaining weight by virtue of eating more than he realizes. Appetite may be present, even ravenous, only to disappear upon the sight or odor of food, or at the time when meals are served, returning when the meal is over.

BULIMIA

Certain types of sporadic overeating, often followed by self-induced vomiting, may be regarded as conversion reactions. In these cases the act of gorging, the manner of biting, chewing, and swallowing the food, and even the choice of food so consumed are determined by their symbolic defensive function in dealing with threatening aggressive or sexual wishes. The induction of vomiting sometimes represents an attempt to undo the symbolic act.

DRY MOUTH, BURNING OR PAINFUL TONGUE

Such symptoms are occasionally brought about through the conversion mechanisms. On examination mouth moisture is seen to be ample and no changes in the tongue are evident. Such a sensation of dry mouth may symbolize fear or may be a defense against an oral sexual wish. The conversion symptom, burning tongue, may reflect a conflict either about the use of the tongue in speaking, such

as to utter burning, sharp, or acid words of attack, or about its use as a sexual organ. The common expression, to be "burnt" refers to being caught and hurt or punished for committing a forbidden act. Pain in the tongue may reflect symbolically the notion "I will bite my tongue rather than say that."

NAUSEA AND VOMITING

As conversion symptoms these share many of the characteristics already described for anorexia. The symptom may be unrelated to eating, and may either precede or follow food intake. The vomiting may be relatively unproductive, yielding only mucus or a small amount of bile-stained gastric juice. Retching and gagging may be prominent, at times occurring merely on the sight of food or when food enters the mouth or posterior pharynx. Food may be taken into the mouth gingerly, in small morsels, and kept in the forepart of the mouth for a long time, the act of swallowing evoking a gag. Morning nausea, gagging, and vomiting may indicate unconscious pregnancy fantasies in men as well as women. Similar symptoms at night may reflect an unconscious wish for or fear of an oral sexual experience.

DYSPHAGIA

The idea as well as the act of swallowing is discomforting. It may include the feeling that the food cannot be taken into the mouth, cannot be passed into the pharynx, and, if it is swallowed, that it will stick in the gullet. Observed eating, the patient may pucker his face, chew very slowly and gingerly, keep the bolus in the forepart of the mouth, and act as if it is very difficult to move it into the vault. Indeed, he may spit it out. Here an inhibition of the volitional part of swallowing is quite evident. Food is experienced as sticking high in the gullet. The difficulty in swallowing may be restricted to particular items of food or may include everything swallowed, liquid as well as solid. Conversion dysphagia may involve all consistencies of food rather than showing the usual progression of difficulty, from solid to soft, and then liquid that is more characteristic of organic obstructions. Achalasia is classified as a somatopsychic-psychosomatic disorder and will be discussed later.

GLOBUS HYSTERICUS

This conversion reaction, a sensation of a lump in the throat usually at the suprasternal notch, is unrelated to eating and usually does not interfere with swallowing, though the patient may fear that it will.

ABDOMINAL BLOATING

This term covers a number of entities. Some patients complain that the abdomen is enlarged, but this is not confirmed upon examination. This false perception of abdominal distention usually is accompanied by unpleasant abdominal sensations, sometimes specified as gurgling or movement and sometimes interpreted by the patient as indicating a cancer. Complaints of belching, flatus, and indigestion are common. Such persons are usually blatantly hysterical or hypochondriacal. Evidence for an underlying pregnancy fantasy is usually not hard to come by.

The second type is called nongaseous abdominal bloating and is produced by simultaneously thrusting the lumbar spine forward and relaxing the abdominal musculature.[16] The lumbar lordosis is often so great that the hand may easily be passed beneath the spine of the reclining patient. This type of muscular bloating typically appears and disappears rapidly, often within seconds. It characteristically disappears during sleep. These patients, almost always women, also are obviously hysterical, with unconscious pregnancy fantasies, intense longing to be pregnant, or actual delusions of pregnancy.

Air swallowing (aerophagia) is a third mechanism of bloating and will be discussed under Psychophysiological Disorders.

CONSTIPATION AND DIARRHEA

As conversion symptoms these are concerned mainly with that segment of lower bowel which is under more or less voluntary control. Conversion constipation is secondary to an inhibition of the act of defecation rather than to an intrinsic disturbance in bowel motility, though the latter may develop in time as

well. The history generally will reveal considerable variability in bowel behavior, with an inability to defecate at certain times or in certain settings, as in strange and unclean bathrooms, in the presence of others, etc. Its sporadic appearance may be correlated with the threatening emergence of anal soiling or sexual impulse.

Diarrhea as a conversion symptom most often consists merely of the complaint of several stools a day, but these are usually relatively formed. It is uncertain whether true diarrheal stools ever result from a conversion mechanism.

PRURITUS ANI

As a conversion reaction, this symptom is more common among men than women (who are more likely to complain of pruritus vulvae). It rather typically reflects unconscious erotic anal fantasies, including a wish for anal masturbation. In some instances the unconscious latent homosexual implications contribute to a paranoid attitude, a fear of anal attack, or the delusion that another man threatens such an attack. The existence of such paranoid tendencies must always be carefully searched for before the male patient with pruritus ani is subjected to rectal examination or proctoscopy.

PAIN*

Probably the most common conversion symptom encountered in medical practice is pain. Conversion pain may be experienced in any part of the body and therefore must be distinguished from pain that indicates organic disorder. The topic of pain is treated fully in Chapter 34 of this volume.

In differentiating conversion pain from pain of other origin, it is necessary to explore the patient's background not only for the specific psychodynamic factors which are especially conducive for the choice of pain, rather than some other symptom, but also to determine that it is in fact conversion pain. A careful description of the pain is of high importance in differentiating the two varieties of pain. In

---

* See references 45, 47, 53, 114, and 143.

general, the conversion pain differs from the pain of a discrete organic process in respect to its quality, timing, location, radiation, and the nature of the provoking and alleviating factors. The latter reflect the characteristics of the neural input as determined by the pathophysiological processes at the periphery and confer upon the pain experience those distinctive qualities which enable one to differentiate the pain of biliary colic, for example, from that of peptic ulcer.[54] This may be referred to as "the peripheral signature" and it is the deviation from such discrete patterns which usually first alerts the physician to the possibility that the pain is not originating from a peripheral site. Occasionally, however, the patient with a conversion pain, having been subjected to pointed and directive interview experiences, may present a description indistinguishable from some classical organic syndrome. The same may hold true of the patient whose conversion pain actually was preceded by some painful illness, as biliary colic or duodenal ulcer, or of the patient who has an intimate knowledge of such syndromes through close contact with another patient, or through the familiarity that results when the patient is a physician or nurse. Ordinarily, conversion pain is described either with vivid imagery or very vaguely. Such complex pain descriptions as "burning like a fire," "like being stabbed with a knife," "like being tied in a knot," "wrung like a mop," reflect the idiosyncratic psychological meaning of the pain to the sufferer and are of value in suggesting the diagnosis.

⟨ Disorders of Eating and Elimination Secondary to Psychopathological States

There are a variety of patients who exhibit inappropriate or bizarre patterns of eating or elimination which are secondary to psychopathological states. These differ from conversion reactions as described above in that they represent more complex disturbances in the behavior associated with eating and elimination rather than involving the use of a body part or function in a symbolic and defensive manner. Such disturbances may range from inadequate or undifferentiated eating or elimination behavior to behavior which is determined by bizarre (psychotic) ideation but is logical in the framework of that ideation though inappropriate or strange by ordinary standards. For the most part, this group of patients make themselves evident by the obvious peculiarity of their ideas about or manner of eating or moving their bowels, though these may easily be overlooked if the examining physician neglects to obtain a precise description of these acts or to explore the patient's explanation for his complaint of "no appetite," "sick to the stomach," "constipation," or "diarrhea."

Anorexia Nervosa

Typically a disorder of young people, usually beginning during adolescence, and far more common among girls than boys, anorexia nervosa generally presents as profound weight loss and emaciation secondary to a failure to eat. This syndrome is described fully in Chapter 32 of this volume.

Pica, Food Faddisms, and Other Peculiar Dietary Habits; Laxative and Enema Addiction

This group ranges from children (and a rare adult) who exhibit a defect or perversion in the ability to discriminate the edible from the inedible to persons whose food habits are determined by bizarre or peculiar modes of thinking. As a whole these patients have not been very extensively studied. The first group includes the childhood syndrome of pica and those who habitually consume hair and other items, leading to bezoar formation. By and large these are grossly disturbed people.

Food faddism, vegetarianism, addiction to peculiar diets, morbid concern over contamination of food, harmful ingredients, artificial additives, etc., and excessive use of laxatives or enemas may present as thoroughly rationalized behavior, or in relationship to some gastrointestinal complaint which the patient usually explains in terms of his idiosyncratic concepts. Such patients are unlikely to consult physicians about their theories of diet or digestion. Indeed, they commonly have a low regard for the medical profession and may withhold such information. More often they offer such traditional complaints as lack of appetite, nausea, vomiting, eructation, bloating, abdominal rumbling, "indigestion," excessive gas, diarrhea, or constipation, but a less directed inquiry which permits the patient to elaborate his own ideas about his difficulty quickly reveals these to be expressions of more complex and pathological ideation. In brief, they reflect morbid psychological concepts of something "bad" or destructive within the body, which in actuality represent displacements of "bad" or disturbing thoughts or fantasies. Accordingly, the patient sees certain foods or the contents of the bowel as positively bad or dangerous, not simply as disagreeing with him—a contrast to patients with specific food intolerances. Instead, they espouse complex and bizarre theories as to the mode of action of the food on the body or mind, and sharply divide foods into beneficial and harmful categories. Some may indulge in compulsive and excessive catharsis, or use of enemas or colonic irrigation as means of getting rid of the "bad" that is inside. Secondary nutritional deficiencies and electrolyte imbalances may result from such self-imposed dietary restrictions or excessive purging.[33]

More detailed psychological inquiry usually establishes that these strange notions are not restricted to the functions of the gastrointestinal system but extend to many other spheres as well. Thus these people may also exhibit eccentricities in dress, manner, behavior, and belief systems, and belong to crank or fringe groups. Some are obviously schizophrenic, while most reveal at least an inclination toward the persecutory delusional attitude of the paranoid. In general, they feel strongly about their theories, which are not easily modified by any argument no matter how sound.

Encopresis and Psychogenic Megacolon

Encopresis,[17,126,38] or "fecal soiling," like its urinary counterpart, enuresis, with which it is occasionally associated, represents a complex psychologically determined failure or lapse in toileting. It consists of the passage of stools of normal or near-normal consistency into clothes, bed clothes, or any receptacle not intended for such purposes. It typically begins in childhood either as a failure to achieve proper toileting or as a loss of previously achieved bowel control. Less frequently it extends into adulthood, unless one includes in this category patients who become incontinent in the course of organic brain disease. Severely withdrawn, catatonic schizophrenics and other disturbed psychotics may also relinquish normal standards.

Among children encopresis may take the form either of the promiscuous and casual expulsion of feces whenever the impulse so moves or of prolonged retention of stool, with leakage of feces or periodic huge movements. The latter may be associated with enormous distention of the colon, sometimes designated as *psychogenic megacolon*. This may be distinguished from *aganglionic megacolon* (Hirschsprung's disease) by the following characteristics.[126] It begins at an age when neuromuscular control is to be expected; the child is encopretic (as defined above); there are periodic voluminous bowel movements either spontaneously or after an enema; defecation may occur in supine and standing positions; the rectum commonly is packed with feces; episodes of intestinal obstruction do not occur; the course is relatively benign; and the spastic rectal segment characteristic of Hirschsprung's disease does not occur.

Of the many variables involved in the genesis of encopresis, toilet training and possibly some intrinsic factors enhancing the meaning of the bowel movement for the child appear to be the most important.[17] The reader is referred to pp. 656–657 for a discussion of such factors in child development.

Giant megacolon or megasigmoid may

occur in chronically institutionalized psychotic, mentally deficient, or brain-damaged patients. It is thought to reflect a neglect to respond to defecation stimuli, leading to the accumulation of enormous fecal masses. Major complications include sigmoid volvulus, secondary toxemia, and perforation of a stercoraceous ulcer. Subtotal colectomy may be necessary.[38,149,93]

Feeding and Bowel Disorders with Psychosis

Reference already has been made to the role of psychotic ideation in the genesis of some of these disorders. It suffices to add here only that such occur most commonly in the syndromes of paranoid schizophrenia and endogenous depression where delusions of internal persecutors are not uncommon. The paranoid may complain of bowel symptoms, including bizarre rectal sensations, while the depressed person typically suffers with anorexia and constipation which at times may be considerable.

⟨ Psychophysiological Disorders

Psychophysiological gastrointestinal disorders include concomitants of affect, local defense reactions, or the expressions of drive patterns. Interactions between such physiological processes and other preexisting or concurrent somatic processes may result in organic pathology.

Physiological Concomitants of Affects

It has been known for centuries that intense or prolonged unpleasant emotions may be accompanied by gastrointestinal symptoms associated with changes in gastrointestinal function. Changes in secretory patterns, blood flow, and motility have been demonstrated in the esophagus, stomach, small bowel, and colon during spontaneous as well as evoked emotions, but so far there is little information as to how to relate such physiological changes to the symptoms experienced during affect experience.* Hence, at the present time little is known about the clinical significance of such physiological changes, at least as they involve otherwise normal gut. The story may be different in the presence of preexisting defect or abnormality, as will be discussed below.

Be that as it may, it is important from the practical clinical point of view to appreciate that the patient who presents with such gastrointestinal complaints as change in appetite, nausea, vomiting, cramps, diarrhea, or constipation may be undergoing psychological stress, and be experiencing anxiety, shame, guilt, depression, or anger. When consulting a physician, some patients place the major emphasis on their physical symptoms rather than on their emotional state. At times this is a way of avoiding having to face the underlying psychological issues, while at other times it reflects the patient's expectation that the physician will be more attentive to somatic than to psychological complaints. By conducting a more thorough interview, the physician will usually be able to establish that the patient is experiencing a significant psychological stress, such as a frustrating life situation, a recent or impending loss, or an interpersonal conflict, and that he is also exhibiting other psychological or physiological expressions of affect. Thus, the patient experiencing realistic or neurotic anxiety is likely, at the same time, to reveal some of the usual circulatory and respiratory concomitants of anxiety, such as palpitation, tachycardia, cold moist hands, sighing respiration, etc., as well as to be beset with anxious or phobic concerns of one sort or another. The depressed patient may appear lethargic, inactive, burdened, slowed down, and may acknowledge feeling blue, discouraged, pessimistic, helpless, or hopeless.

In general, it is not difficult to identify the patient whose gastrointestinal symptoms are reflections of the physiological concomitants of an affective response to psychological stress. However, it cannot be emphasized too

* See references 12, 15, 56, 68, 86, 104, 110, 130, 131, 138, and 162.

strongly that a direct cause-and-effect relationship is not necessarily justified when gastrointestinal symptoms follow a psychological stress, for it is also entirely possible for an organic gastrointestinal disorder to develop under quite the same circumstances. For this reason, the most meticulous care must be taken in the study and examination of the patient whose gastrointestinal symptoms appear during or after a period of obvious psychological stress, so as not to overlook these occasions when a somatic lesion develops as well. Awareness of this possibility is generally sufficient to alert the physician to be comprehensive in his inquiry. One should be especially wary of patients who are insistent on ascribing their symptoms to psychological stress, for just as some patients emphasize somatic processes in order to avoid facing their psychological problems, so, too, may patients fearful of organic disease, especially cancer, set up the smoke screen of alleged psychological causes to hide from themselves and their physician the organic state they fear more.

Another potential source of error in the differential diagnosis of gastrointestinal disturbances accompanying affects and psychological distress concerns the patient who is experiencing an affective response to an *occult organic process*. A notorious offender in this regard is *carcinoma of the body or tail of the pancreas*, though other types of intraabdominal neoplasm may also be responsible.[72,91] Prominent complaints among patients with such occult disorders are irritability, anxiety, depression, or hypochondriacal concern, as well as the gastrointestinal complaints commonly associated with such affective states. The high frequency with which abdominal or back pain eventually occurs in pancreatic cancer is the most important clue to the correct diagnosis. In all likelihood, the important factors in the prominence of psychological symptoms in pancreatic carcinoma and other occult disorders are the vagueness and intractability of the symptoms, and the difficulty in reaching a definitive diagnosis. Diagnostic or therapeutic uncertainty on the part of the physician is another potent source of psychological stress to such patients.

Local Defense Reactions

In addition to the more or less nonspecific physiological patterns of affects already referred to, there are also local defense patterns involving the surfaces and the portals of entry into the body, such as upper gastrointestinal tract, respiratory passages, lower bowel, lower urinary tract, skin, and conjunctivae.[163,164] All of these local reactions constitute well-defined riddance patterns designed to cope with noxious agents, be they irritating chemical substances, poisons, foreign bodies, or microorganisms. However, identical responses may also be provoked by a learned stimulus that indicates the threat of such a noxious agent, as well as by a stimulus that is symbolic of a past danger. It has now been suggested experimentally[106] that specific visceral and glandular responses can be learned. Such local responses to learned or symbolic stimuli include surface changes, to dilute, wash away, neutralize, or digest the noxious material, and motor activity to keep out or expel the noxious agent. Surface charges include edema, vascular engorgement, and hypersecretion and may involve the skin, the conjunctivae, and the mucous membranes of nasal and upper respiratory passage, bronchi, esophagus, stomach, and colon. Motor activity includes spasm, hyperperistalsis or reverse peristalsis of the smooth muscles of esophagus, stomach, bronchial tree, sigmoid, and rectum. Accordingly, individuals may respond to certain symbolic stimuli with such manifestations as engorgement and congestion of the nasal passages, nausea and vomiting, esophageal spasm, pylorospasm, diarrhea, etc. Presumably the stimulus is symbolically experienced as justifying such local defense reactions, either because it is capable of being so represented mentally or because it was in some way in the past associated with a situation in which such reactions had been activated by a noxious agent. For example, nausea and vomiting may ensue upon eating contaminated fish, on the sight or odor of fish, at the thought of eating fish in the same setting where the fish was first eaten, or upon the anniversary of the original experience. Such gastrointestinal reactions may occur in response to foods that fall under cultural, religious, or family taboos, unfamiliar foods, foods from filthy sources, foods with disagreeable sensory properties, and foods simply with unpleasurable associations.[85]

The psychological mechanisms involved in such reactions are closely related to the conversion reactions involving the same systems and in some instances the two cannot be distinguished (see pp. 659–661). The example of nausea and vomiting just cited does not, strictly speaking, constitute a conversion reaction as we have defined it. But were fish, be it the animal, the word, or the idea, to be equated symbolically with an unconscious conflict (e.g., a conflict over a wish to take the penis in the mouth), then the reaction pattern more properly constitutes a conversion.

Displaced or Incomplete Drive Patterns

Some somatic reactions do not constitute expressions of defense but of incomplete or substitute drive activities where the full expression of drive is blocked by conflict or by external restraints. Thus, increased secretory and motor activity of the stomach or of the bowel may reflect oral or anal drive activity which for some reason cannot adequately be expressed in psychological or behavioral terms. It is uncertain how often such processes are productive of symptoms in a person with a normal gastrointestinal tract. Presumably, prolonged tension of such origin could contribute to hyperemia, hypersecretion, or hypermotility with consequent symptoms of dyspepsia, heart burn, gas cramps, constipation, or diarrhea. It is also conceivable, but as yet unproven, that such psychophysiological influences may play a role, directly or indirectly, in the variations in symptomatology of such conditions as esophagitis, hiatus hernia, diverticulosis, and even tumors. For example, in the presence of a hiatus hernia, hypersecretion of gastric acid so induced may contribute to the symptoms of peptic esophagitis; with a bowel tumor, increased motor activity may give rise to the first symptoms of the developing bowel obstruction.

Some disturbances are due to the inhibition of a drive action after the physiological process has been initiated. This is exemplified in the gastrointestinal tract by "air swallowing" or aerophagia (with bloating and eructation). The syndrome may occur in some individuals when a stong need to discharge feelings by speaking has to be suppressed. Normally during speaking a small amount of air is taken into the esophagus at the beginning of inspiration and this is used for phonation during the balance of inspiration. If some of the motor actions of speaking are carried out at the same time that actual phonation is inhibited, then the air may be swallowed instead of expelled. Clinically one notes audible swallowing of air and frequent belching during periods when the patient remains silent while struggling to keep from exploding with a verbal torrent. Once encouraged to vocalize what is being held back, the episode may quickly subside.

Complications of Affect Concomitants

Reference has already been made to some of the complications which may develop when psychophysiological reactions involve gut which already is the site of structural abnormalities. For completeness, mention must also be made of the role of psychological stress responses acting in a nonspecific way to alter resistance of the body to physical stressors or latent intrinsic metabolic or cellular defects. Empirically, it has been noted that a wide variety of organic disorders become manifest in settings in which individuals psychologically "give up" upon encountering some life situation with which they are unable to cope. The corresponding affect states are best described as "helplessness" and "hopelessness."[132] Infections, neoplasia, metabolic disorders, and degenerative changes all have been noted to emerge under such circumstances. It is hypothesized that some biological changes occurring during the psychobiological state of "giving up" may, in as yet unidentified ways, constitute conditions permissive or precipitating for the onset of the somatic disease, so long as the necessary predisposing organic factors already exist. On the other hand, in the absence of such somatic determinants, no somatic disorder develops, though the psychological state is nonetheless manifest in terms of affects and behavior, often experienced by the patient as depressive. Sometimes more discrete psychopathological states develop instead of somatic disorder.[2]

Such relationships, while as yet unexplained, underscore again the practical necessity to deal with somatic and psychological phenomena in a unified fashion. All persons experiencing psychological decompensation in response to stress must be considered also as potentially having organic disease, rather than solely as being candidates for psychophysiological disorder. Accordingly, somatic symptoms occurring under such circumstances must be carefully evaluated. Gastric or bowel cancer, benign gastric ulcer, intestinal tuberculosis, active amoebic colitis in a chronic carrier, acute pancreatitis[146] and even appendicitis have been reported under such circumstances.[117]

(Somatopsychic-Psychosomatic Disorders

In this grouping belong certain conditions which in the past have been designated as "psychosomatic diseases," as well as some not heretofore so considered. This sequence of terms is intended to convey two basic notions as to the etiopathogenesis of these disorders. The first is that the primary factor in the genesis of the disorder is a somatic process which not only is responsible for the nature of the final organic state, e.g., duodenal ulcer, but also is capable of contributing directly or indirectly to the development of specific psychological characteristics. Some of the ways in which gastrointestinal processes may influence psychic development have already been discussed. The second is that these psychological features define, in a more or less specific way, the circumstances which prove psychologically stressful for the individual, and hence the psychodynamic conditions under which the organic process may become activated. The

sequence of the term "somatopsychic-psychosomatic," thus has developmental and chronological implications. It specifies the primacy and the necessity of the somatic factor in the genesis of the ultimate lesion as well as its influence on psychic development. At the same time it specifies the influence of psychic factors on the ultimate emergence of the somatic lesion. To fulfill these requirements, the somatic factor must be present and exerting an influence from very early in life, placing it in the category of a genic, congenital, or early acquired defect.[50,108]

This formulation gives due emphasis to the evidence that a somatic factor (the constitutional factor of Franz Alexander) is necessary before a particular psychodynamic complex can give rise to a particular disease.[9] But it goes further than the classical psychosomatic concept in that it proposes that the demonstrated psychological similarities of patients with each of these disorders reflects in addition a contribution of the somatic factor to psychological development as well. It is in these regards that these disorders differ from those designated more simply as psychogenic and psychophysiological. The following clinical features characterize the disorders which are classified as somatopsychic-psychosomatic:

1. The disease may make its first appearance at any age, from earliest infancy to old age. Its occurrence in the neonatal period, though rare, may be regarded as evidence for the overriding importance of the somatic factor in these cases. Ordinarily, the peak incidence of first attacks is during adolescence and early adulthood.

2. Once initiated, the disorder is characteristically chronic or recurring. Though some remissions may be complete, with no evidence of residual structural change, the capacity for relapse is ever present, provided the appropriate pathogenic conditions recur.

3. Psychological stress is an important contributing factor for the development of the manifest disorder. Furthermore, careful clinical psychological study reveals for each illness an impressive consistency, not only in respect to the psychological characteristics of the patients so afflicted but also in the particular

psychodynamic settings that are stressful in provoking, as well as helpful in relieving, attacks.

The following gastrointestinal disorders are here classified as somatopsychic-psychosomatic, though the data justifying such a categorization are more complete for the first three than the others: duodenal ulcer, ulcerative colitis, celiac-sprue syndrome, regional enteritis and colitis (Crohn's disease), irritable bowel syndrome (spastic colon, mucous colitis), and achalasia.

Duodenal Ulcer*

The work and ideas of Mirsky elucidating the pathogenesis of duodenal ulcer provides the paradigm for the somatopsychic-psychosomatic concept.[107,108,150]

PATHOGENESIS

Most patients with duodenal ulcer characteristically have large and chronically hypersecreting stomachs.[24,30,79,108] Some active ulcer patients show a low secretory capacity, ascribed by some to accompanying gastritis.[73,167] But while duodenal ulcer will not develop in the absence of acid and pepsin, hypersecretion alone is not sufficient for ulcer formation. Thus, while duodenal ulcer patients are relatively high acid and pepsin secretors, not all hypersecretors have ulcers. Yet, as Mirsky has shown, those persons with consistently higher gastric secretory capacities, as evidenced by plasma pepsinogen values above the median for the total population, constitute the subgroup from which the bulk of actual and potential duodenal ulcer patients are

---

* Comparable physiological and psychological data are not available concerning benign gastric ulcer and hence this discussion is limited to duodenal ulcer. While the presence of acid gastric juice apparently is necessary for gastric-ulcer formation, chronic hypersecretion is not characteristic of gastric ulcers, except for those occurring in the immediate prepyloric region. Rather there is evidence that factors decreasing the competence of gastric mucosa to contain an acid solution are implicated.[163] The same probably holds true for so-called stress ulcers, or acute gastric mucosal bleeding, associated with burns or trauma, though ulcers occurring after head trauma sometimes are accompanied by a sharp rise in acid secretion.[39,105]

drawn. In addition, the same distribution of plasma pepsinogen levels holds for children as for adults, suggesting that the tendency toward higher secretory patterns is established early and presumably maintained into adult life.[108]

These findings identify at least one of the somatic factors in the genesis of duodenal ulcer. Whether the large stomach with its big parietal cell mass and its generally increased secretory potential is a genically determined anatomical characteristic, or whether the stomach hypertrophies in response to some primary central nervous system influences operating from birth, cannot be answered. There is a significantly higher concordance of ulcer disease among monozygotic than dizygotic twins and a highly significant excess of ulcers among close relatives.[36,35,112] Relatives without ulcer show a highly significant increase in hydrochloric acid response to maximal histamine stimulation when compared with controls.[59] Individuals who are blood group O and nonsecretors of blood group antigens are much more liable to duodenal ulcer.[37] While such findings indicate a genetic factor, Pearl et al. have produced a marked and sustained increase in the parietal cell mass in cats by continuing anterior hypothalamic stimulation for four to six weeks.[120] This suggests that increased functional demand, for whatever reason, may also contribute to the development of a hypersecretory capacity. Whichever factors may be operating it is known that infants differ in their patterns of feeding activity, but whether those with the more active gastric secretory potential are also the ones with a more vigorous drive to nurse has not yet been studied. Be that as it may, such a possibility provides the basis for an attractive hypothesis relating ulcer predisposition with incompatibilities between mother and infant in the early nursing relationship. As has already been discussed (see pp. 654–655), the repetitive sequences of hunger crying → feeding by mother → satiation → sleep reflect one parameter of a rising and falling psychic tension, regulation of which is achieved in relationship with another human being, the nursing adult. The drive aspect of this has been designated as *oral*, since the tension can be relieved only by oral activities, namely nursing and related processes. The hypothesis suggests that the infant with the more active gastric secretory pattern behaves more of the time like a hungry infant than does the normo- or hyposecreting infant. Furthermore, it proposes not only that infants differ in the vigor of this oral drive but also that mothers differ in their ability and capacity to satisfy the oral drive. Thus, one may postulate a range of possible mother–infant relationships as shown in Table 27–1.

TABLE 27–1. **Relationship of Infant's Oral Drive to Mother's Ability to Gratify It**

INFANT'S ORAL DRIVE	MOTHER'S ABILITY TO GRATIFY ORAL NEEDS	INFANT'S ORAL SATISFACTION
1. High	High	May be achieved
Medium	High	Will be achieved
Low	High	Will be achieved
2. High	Medium	Will not be achieved
3. Medium	Medium	May be achieved
Low	Medium	Will be achieved
4. High	Low	Will not be achieved
Medium	Low	Will not be achieved
5. Low	Low	May be achieved

According to this schema, when the mother's ability to gratify oral needs matches or exceeds that of the infant, then the infant will have a good chance of satisfaction and hence a better opportunity to gain confidence that oral tensions will not become intolerable or remain unrelieved. On the other hand, when the ability of the mother to satisfy the oral drive is relatively lower than the need of the infant, the latter repetitively or chronically will be exposed to periods of oral tension and will have difficulty gaining confidence that the environment can be depended upon to fulfill these needs. Furthermore, this schema allows

for the possibility that even a mother with an excellent integrative capacity and without any basic hostile or rejecting attitudes toward her infant may not succeed in satisfying the physiological and psychological needs of an excessively orally demanding hypersecreting infant. Such failure on the part of the mother may also prove to be frustrating to her and hence may provoke in her a hostile or rejecting attitude toward her infant. Thus, relative incompatibilities between infant needs and maternal capacities may serve to intensify and entrench in the developing child strong oral-dependent wishes, expressed ultimately as a lack of confidence in the ability or willingness of the environment to provide and in a corresponding need in one way or another to compensate for this. Such tensions, projected over the entire developmental span of the child, may be expected to exert a significant influence on the ultimate psychic structure of the adult.

This hypothesis corresponds closely to what has long been known psychologically about the ulcer and ulcer-prone patient. So-called oral character traits and conflicts around the dependent-independent axis, though expressed in many different ways, are prominent characteristics of duodenal ulcer patients. But not all persons with such psychological characteristics develop ulcer or are ulcer prone. Whether or not a duodenal ulcer develops later in life is dependent upon still another factor, namely, the secretory capacity of the stomach, the greatest potential for ulcer formation being among those who are hypersecretors and were orally frustrated in infancy. In this way we can understand how some hypersecretors, by virtue of adequate nurturing, may develop neither noticeable psychological distortions nor duodenal ulcer; how hypersecretors and some normosecretors with adequate mothering may be highly ulcer prone; and how other normosecretors with inadequate mothering may develop psychological traits indistinguishable from those found among ulcer patients, yet never develop ulcer. It is not the gastric hypersecretion alone which is the decisive determinant in the psychological development but the success or failure of the transaction between mother and child around this need–frustration cycle. If the infant with hypersecreting stomach is adequately satisfied, his psychological development will be less influenced by the kinds of distortions which result when such oral needs are chronically or recurrently unsatisfied. Hence he will be less ready in later life to experience situations as threatening his inner sense of security or his confidence in the environment as a source of support. On the other hand, hypersecreting infants less adequately handled may suffer on both scores and hence be more vulnerable to ulcer formation. This would explain not only the occurrence of hypersecretors (as determined by plasma pepsinogen) without ulcer, but also the occurrence of ulcer among those with pepsinogen levels more near the median.

While the secretory capacity of the stomach and the psychological status together determine the individual's vulnerability to duodenal ulcer formation, these do not determine whether or when an ulcer will develop. This is dependent on current psychosocial factors and the degree to which they are psychologically stressful for the particular individual. Thus it is possible for one individual with relatively high ulcer vulnerability to go through life without ever developing an ulcer, while another, who may even have a lesser vulnerability, may experience repeated bouts of ulcer activity. The psychosocial situations specifically stressful for each individual make up the precipitating circumstances determining the point in time at which an ulcer ultimately forms in the ulcer-prone person.

Strong support for this formulation comes from a study in which it was possible to distinguish, by purely psychological means, the hypersecretors from the hyposecretors and to predict among whom peptic ulcer developed in a stressful situation.[150,168] From a group of over 2000 army inductees, sixty-three were selected with high serum-pepsinogen values and fifty-seven with low pepsinogen levels. Not only could these two populations be distinguished by psychological criteria (without prior knowledge of the pepsinogen values), but also the three soldiers who subsequently were found to have evidence of healed ulcer,

and the six who developed active ulcer during the induction period, all fell in the upper 15 percent, eight in the upper 5 percent of pepsinogen values.* Of relevance to these findings are the experiments of Ader on gastric erosions in the acid-secreting portion of the stomach provoked by subjecting rats to physical restraint for six hours.[3–6] These studies demonstrated that, while animals with high plasma pepsinogen were more likely to develop erosions than were those with low levels, high pepsinogen was neither necessary nor sufficient. Taking advantage of the known twenty-four-hour activity cycle of rats, it was hypothesized that restraint instituted during a period of activity would be more "stressful" than during a period of quiescence. When rats were restrained under these two conditions it was found that all the rats who developed erosions had high pepsinogen levels and had been restrained during a period of activity.

PSYCHOLOGICAL CHARACTERISTICS OF THE GASTRIC HYPERSECRETOR AND DUODENAL-ULCER POPULATION

The classical psychodynamic formulation of the peptic ulcer patient was developed by Alexander and has been confirmed and elaborated by others.† Mirsky has shown that comparable psychological features characterized about 85 percent of the hypersecretor group whether or not they had had active ulcer to the time he examined them. As has already been stated, similar features may be expected as well among some individuals who are neither hypersecretors nor have ulcers.[150] Among identical twins discordant for ulcer, the twin with the peptic ulcer displays these psychological features more prominently than the twin without ulcer.[36]

The basic psychodynamic trends in the hypersecretor-duodenal ulcer group cluster

---

* The fact that the hyposecretors also fall into a discrete group in terms of psychological characteristics is of theoretical interest. Furthermore, not only are these characteristics essentially the same as those that have been noted among patients with pernicious anemia but also the extreme hyposecretors (achylia gastrica) constitute the population in which pernicious anemia ultimately may develop.[150]

† See references 9, 65, 81, 82, 87, 97, 107, 108, 129, 150–152, and 157.

around strong needs to be taken care of, to lean on others, to be fed, to be nurtured, to have close body contact of a succoring type. Many developmental factors serve to determine how such a central organizing psychodynamic tendency is eventually expressed. By way of emphasis, several caricatures of hypersecretor ulcer-prone patients may be drawn to indicate how these underlying dependent wishes may be organized.[82,87]

The Pseudoindependent. His underlying dependent needs may be largely or completely denied and an opposite facade presented. These patients then appear as highly independent, self-reliant, aggressive, controlling, and overactive. Men present a caricatured "hypermasculine" facade, while the women show strong "masculine"[*] identifications. Such persons ridicule the necessity for rest, relaxation, or vacations, and are contemptuous of those they consider weak and dependent. In Western society these characteristics are peculiarly in keeping with success in the business and professional world. The interpersonal relationships of these patients are controlling rather than warm. By dominating or controlling behavior they force others to provide their wants and in this way succeed in keeping unconscious the gratification of their dependent needs. The spouse, for example, is likely to be the long-suffering, self-denying provider, while the patient sees himself as powerful and self-sufficient. The following case[47] illustrates this situation. They are vulnerable to ulcer disease early in life and vascular disease later on.

Mr. D., a forty-eight-year-old consulting engineer, had ulcer symptoms on and off since age twenty.[†] The twelfth of fourteen children born of immigrant parents, he was a completely self-made man. With a harsh, exacting father and an overburdened mother, his childhood was marked by premature assumption of work responsibilities and denial of the usual childhood gratifications. He early strove for and achieved a status of such social and occupational independence that he could claim he was beholden to no one. His greatest success was as a consultant who "cured sick industries," a situation in which he could feel that the entire organization depended upon him. Indeed, he only accepted such consulting positions under the condition that he take orders from no one. Aggressive, dominating, constantly on the go, involved in many ventures at a time, he never rested or took vacations. Indeed, when a well-intentioned physician advised that he buy a farm as a means of relaxation, he converted it into a successful business venture.

Supporting this facade of ruthless independence were a coterie of assistants, secretaries, and sycophants who were kept on the go doing his bidding, and a wife to whom he cynically assigned the task of catering to his needs at home and toward whom he felt no affection. He divorced his first wife and left his children when she became too preoccupied with their care, marrying a second woman who would devote herself to gratifying his needs.

The intense drive to be cared for and supported, a need of which he was completely oblivious, was revealed not only by the efficient machinery he set up to assure this, as described above, but also by numerous side remarks and slips of the tongue. He repeatedly spoke of what a good cook his mother was and made invidious comparisons with his two wives. Of one he said, "She just puts on a God-damn salad with a couple of leaves." He derived much pleasure from feeding and caring for the farm animals, saying, "I treated them better than myself," but quickly philosophized that "there is danger in taking care of someone so well that they never take care of themselves."

Ulcer symptoms first developed soon after being drafted into the Army in World War I when he could not control his environment. Subsequently, symptoms occurred when his wife or his staff failed him, when threatened by reverses beyond his control, and between jobs. As he grew older, he subtly shifted toward a more obviously dependent relationship with an older business executive in whose or-

---

[*] By culturally bound definitions.

[†] The role of pain from a glomus tumor was a variable in this case not discussed in this summary.

ganization he, for the first time, took a permanent position. His most severe ulcer symptoms occurred after this man died and was succeeded by his son, who deprecated our patient.

The Passive-Dependent. The underlying dependent needs are overtly expressed and to a considerable degree are conscious as well. These persons, some of whom may be fairly successful, are outwardly compliant, passive, ingratiating, eager to perform for others; yet they are also clinging, dependent, and may even be demanding in a passive-aggressive way. They tend to get into social and interpersonal relationships in which they can depend on a nurturing figure or a paternal, supportive social organization. The men may show strong feminine identifications.*

The patient was a fifty-two-year-old black laborer born and raised on a farm in the South, the middle child of thirteen children. He was much attached to his mother, but felt discriminated against by his father and brothers. He was the hardest working and most conscientious of all the children. At twenty-one years of age he married a motherly, dependable type of girl. Mild, transient epigastric distress first developed when the patient became worried over his wife's frequent pregnancies. Because of lack of economic opportunity in the South, the patient moved his family to Cincinnati and obtained work in a railroad roundhouse, where he remained twenty years. His bosses gradually entrusted him with more responsibilities without commensurate salary increase. Fellow workers soon came to know that he would finish the work that they had left undone. This caused the patient to feel resentful toward them, but he was not able to summon up enough aggressiveness to object. By hard work and careful saving he and his wife built their own home and successfully raised a family of five children. When this house burned to the ground, his wife was badly injured, and two grandchildren were

* By culturally bound definitions.

burned to death. He struggled to reaccumulate his fortune, but was discouraged by increased responsibilities at his job without a raise and by the failure of his wife to recover from her injuries. During this period, symptoms of a duodenal ulcer started. Epigastric pain was experienced at work when he felt imposed upon by his boss or fellow workers, and it was accentuated at home when his wife was forced to take to bed. A rather meek, effeminate individual, he became quite dependent on the therapist and was never able to express any aggression toward his doctors, illustrated by the fact that he was unable to interrupt his visits to his former doctor, "because I don't want to hurt his feelings."[82]

The Acting Out. In this group the dependent needs are taken care of by blatant acting out and/or by insistent demanding. These are, psychologically speaking, the most immature patients; their character is marked by the infantile trait of "I want what I want when I want it," even if this involves asocial, antisocial, or criminal behavior that disregards the needs and rights of others and of sociey. Irresponsible, with little investment in achievement, they may drift from job to job and are often unemployed. Addiction to tobacco, alcohol, and drugs is common. In their relationships they are parasitic and without consideration of others.

The patient was a thirty-eight-year-old man whose childhood was unhappy and deprived. Before he was three years old his parents separated and he was placed in an orphanage. Later, he never got a permanent job or settled down, but drifted around the country working spasmodically as a peddler or dishwasher. His first marriage was unhappy. Ulcer symptoms and chronic alcoholism developed in conjunction with economic difficulties and incompatibility with his wife. He married a second time to a motherly type of wife, but his ulcer was reactivated and later perforated while she was pregnant. Following an operation it was quiescent for a short period during which he obtained a temporary job as a cook. When his employer, in desperation over the manpower shortage, made the patient night manager of the restaurant the ulcer began to bleed.[82]

These caricatures serve to highlight the extremes of the types that are most vulnerable psychologically and hence most likely to develop active ulcer. While all share the same underlying psychodynamic tendencies, among many these are much more subtly manifest or defended against. Indeed, some hypersecretors even have evolved such effective and socially acceptable psychological and social devices to assure satisfaction of needs, and are so well buffered against stress, that they may never develop an ulcer or do so only during some extreme stress, as the death of the beloved spouse or the threatened loss of a business. On the other hand, there are extreme hypersecretors who, though psychologically fairly well adjusted, have such a low threshold for ulcer formation that ulcer symptoms occur in response to relatively minor variations in their life situations.

The Nature of the Pathogenic Psychological Stress

Effective frustration of dependent needs is the common denominator of the psychological stresses leading to activation of duodenal ulcer. This may include any of the vicissitudes of life which result in brief or prolonged periods of deprivation. It may be a feeling revived by virtue of passing through the anniversary of a previous frustration. It may also be brought on by some symbolic stimulus and the development of an intrapsychic conflict evocative of such frustration. In brief, the precipitating events are characterized by their capacity to mobilize fears of loss of love or security through intensification or frustration of persistent infantile, passive dependent wishes, usually with feelings of helplessness and anger.[132]

Awareness of the psychological and social devices characteristically utilized by these patients to assure gratification of dependency needs is useful to the physician in anticipating what will be stressful for any particular hypersecretor ulcer-prone patient. Thus, as illustrated in the preceding examples, the pseudo-independent person is likely to have ulcer activity when his own efforts no longer succeed in forcing others to provide, or when external circumstances beyond his control become frustrating. The passive-dependent person may develop ulcer symptoms when the person or organization upon whom or which he is dependent refuses or fails to satisfy his needs. The acting-out or demanding person will get symptoms when he is forcibly restrained from acting out, as when jailed, or when supplies of his needs simply are not forthcoming. Groen suggests that the rising incidence of peptic ulcer among men in the twentieth century may be related to the fact that the specific conflict situation is linked with the social structure of twentieth-century Western society. Only in this culture is work so important as a way to obtain recognition and increase self-esteem, while the emancipation of women renders them less available to some men for gratification of dependent needs.[70]

In most cases the sequence of events in response to such a psychological stress is for the patient: (1) to intensify the psychological and social devices that he characteristically utilizes to assure gratification of needs; (2) when these fail, to experience increasing anger, which, however, usually must be suppressed or denied if it threatens the sources of supply still further; (3) then, to turn on to the self or internalize the aggressive impulse, with the development of corresponding feelings of guilt; and finally (4) when he no longer feels able to cope, to give up, with feelings of helplessness in some, hopelessness in others. Once symptoms begin, this sequence may be terminated or reversed by the altered expectation from the self and the changed behavior of the environment toward the patient. The exact point in this sequence when ulcer activity begins has not yet been clearly delineated.

Relation Between Psychological Stress and Ulcer Activation

Little is known concerning this relation. While there is considerable support for the thesis of Alexander that both increased dependent needs and aggression are accompanied by increased gastric secretions (as if the need for support is to be satisfied symbolically by preparation for eating and the aggression acted out by a symbolic cannibalism of the loved and hated object), as yet there has been no definite demonstration that actual ulcer formation is indeed preceded by a significant increase in gastric secretion.* In general, basal acid secretion is alleged to be the same during periods of ulcer activity as during quiescence,† though in some subjects healing following a severe, protracted episode may be accompanied by a fall in the high hydrochloric acid output.[99] Basal hydrochloric acid secretion is said to be more variable among duodenal ulcer patients than nonulcer patients, but whether gastric secretion of ulcer patients is more responsive to stress is a matter of disagreement.[66,110,165] Clearly, the Alexander thesis requires that the specific psychodynamic situation be associated with increased gastric secretion and that both regularly precede ulcer activation. No appropriate test of this assumption has yet been accomplished.

Garma has introduced another psychological construct which may have relevant pathophysiological implications. He invokes a primitive, infantile fantasy, namely that in the face of oral frustration the archaic concept of the frustrating provider (mother) is revived as a bad object inside, to be extruded or destroyed. This view evolves purely from psychoanalytic data, but it does suggest the possibility of an underlying physiological process, namely, forceful gastric contractions periodically subjecting the duodenum to jets of highly acid gastric juice which cannot be neutralized by available enteric juice.[44,65] Wolf reports such forceful gastric contractions up to the point of tetany, along with increased secretion in an ulcer patient during a stress interview.[162] Smith et al. showed a marked increase in gastric and duodenal motor activity occurred upon administration of an acid–barium meal among ulcer patients, but not among normal

subjects.[137] Rhodes demonstrated that the duodenal mucosa of patients with high levels of gastric secretion is exposed to much longer and more profound fluctuations in acidity than is that of normals, further indicating that alternation between spasm and rapid emptying may be a significant variable.[66,77–79,125]

Some alteration in the mucous barrier or in other determinants of tissue resistance or of vascularity as nonspecific biological concomitants of the affects of giving up cannot be excluded.[50,132] The roles of newly identified hormones, such as vasoactive intestinal hormone, gastric inhibitory hormone, motilitin, and others in the pathogenesis of ulcer is a new chapter yet to be considered by psychosomatic investigators.

IMPLICATIONS FOR TREATMENT

From the discussion just presented, it should be evident that any activity on the part of the physician (or others) which assures gratification of the patient's dependent needs without, at the same time, undermining his pride and self-respect, such as it is, should have a salutary effect in reversing the conditions which led to ulcer activation. Clearly this requires an understanding by the physician of the psychological and social resources peculiar to each patient. He must know, for example, to what extent and under what circumstances the pseudoindependent patient will permit himself to be controlled by the physician. The clinician must know who in the family or among friends is acceptable to and capable of supporting the patient. He must recognize that for the pseudoindependent patient, respite may not be achieved by rest or inactivity but by permission to engage in some other activity, to escape temporarily. He must know that the passive-dependent patient may need a much longer period of babying and indulgence, but also that a few of these patients are insatiable in their needs to be taken care of. He must recognize that the excessively passive-dependent patient may respond to surgery by prolonged invalidism even though the ulcer heals, while the guilt-ridden patient may have intractable pain long after the ulcer is healed. Attention to such details will greatly widen

* See references 9, 56, 108, 110, 141, 143, 161, and 162.

† See references 66, 95, 99, 108, 110, 141, 143, and 145.

the range of effectiveness of drugs and diet beyond that achieved by neutralization of gastric acid.

The somatopsychic-psychosomatic concept also should make it evident that no form of psychotherapy can be expected to eliminate the underlying somatic determinants, that is, the life-long chronic hypersecretion and the as yet unidentified factors determining the vulnerability of the duodenal mucosa. On the other hand, psychotherapy, including psychoanalysis, may be expected to improve in some individuals significantly the capability of the individual to manage his life, to deal with unconscious conflicts, and to gratify needs in personally and socially acceptable ways. None of these, however, can be expected to protect him from the vicissitudes of life and hence it is possible that even the best adjusted hypersecretor may under sufficient provocation develop a duodenal ulcer.

Nonspecific Inflammatory Bowel Disease

ULCERATIVE COLITIS

As a chronic or remitting disorder involving primarily the mucosa and submucosa of the large bowel—and occasionally of the small bowel as well—ulcerative colitis fulfills all the criteria of a somatopsychic-psychosomatic disorder as outlined above. Clinically, there is evidence that the capacity to develop the disorder is present early in life, though as yet no biological index, corresponding to the hypersecretory state so characteristic of the duodenal ulcer-prone population, has been identified. A significant familial occurrence supports the view of a genetic relationship, probably involving a polygenic inheritance with the interaction of several genes.[88,113,135] Dick et al. demonstrated persistence of mucosal abnormality even during symptomfree periods; it would be interesting to know whether such changes antedate the onset of symptoms.[34] Burch suggests that extrinsic factors, including psychological stress, disturb an endogenous defense mechanism directed against a forbidden clone derived from a gene mutation, and thereby bring about activation of the dis-

ease.[23] Shorter et al.[133] propose that the inflammatory reaction results from the establishment early in life of a state of hypersensitivity to antigens of bacteria normally present in the individual's gastrointestinal tract and that the pathological and clinical features of inflammatory bowel disease then result from a predominantly cell-mediated hypersensitivity reaction to the bowel wall. They discuss how various factors, including psychic insult, may trigger the breakdown of defenses in such "immunologically primed" patients to produce the overt disease. Engel had suggested earlier from clinical, psychological, and pathological data that the disease may result from "unidentified changes which alter relationships in the colon so that it responds to its own flora as pathogens."[41] Spontaneous occurrence of ulcerative colitislike lesions in gibbons in response to psychological stress has recently been reported.[52,56]

The manifest disease may develop at any age, including neonatally, and once initiated may be marked by remissions and relapses, or by a chronic unremitting course. When one carefully studies the setting in which symptoms develop and remit, there is a clear-cut chronological relationship between psychological stress and onset or exacerbation on the one hand, and psychological support and remission on the other. Furthermore, there is a consistency not only in the nature of the circumstances which are likely to be psychologically stressful or helpful, but also in the psychological characteristics of ulcerative colitis patients as a group. For the most part, these characteristics antedate the development of the active disease, though they may, in certain respects, also become exaggerated in the presence of the symptomatic bowel disorder. To what extent the as yet unidentified biological preconditions for the bowel disease contribute distinctively to the psychological development of the patients can, at present, only be conjectured.

Summary of Psychological Data. In 1955 we summarized the available knowledge about the psychological features of ulcerative colitis patients beginning with the first study by Murray in 1930.[41] Since then numerous clinical reports have largely confirmed those formulations;* so too has psychological testing using projective techniques.[18,157] On the other hand, studies comparing ulcerative colitis patients with "controls" (usually other gastroenterology or general medical patients) using MMPI (Minnesota Multiphase Personality Inventory), or various ratings of psychological abnormality have failed to reveal differences; indeed, one group using such an approach pronounced colitis patients to be "supernormal"![57,154,64] For the most part such studies can be criticized on the basis of a naive conceptualization, that ulcerative colitis is a "psychogenic disease" caused by psychic disturbances, and therefore should demonstrate more rampant psychopathology than the control patients. Furthermore, the psychological procedures used have not been sufficiently specific to detect the personality features reported by clinicians to characterize ulcerative colitis patients. These characteristics, as described below, may differ in degree from patient to patient but still provide a reliable overview of what to expect upon the psychological study of such patients. Among the more important variables accounting for differences between patients are the sex and age at which the colitis began.[18]

Personality Structure. A high proportion of ulcerative colitis patients are described as manifesting so-called obsessive-compulsive character traits, including neatness, orderliness, punctuality, conscientiousness, indecision, obstinacy, and conformity. A few are conspicuously messy and dirty. Along with these are often noted a guarding of affectivity, overintellectualization, rigid attitudes toward morality and standards of behavior, meticulousness of speech, avoidance of "dirty" language, defective sense of humor, obsessive worrying, and timidity. Some are petulant, querulous, demanding, and provocative, but by and large well-directed aggressive action and clear-cut expressions of anger are uncommon. Many investigators have been impressed with the extreme sensitivity of these patients, their almost uncanny perception of hostile or

* See references 18, 19, 32, 58, 63, 71, 83, 84, 92, 111, 134, 142, and 157.

rejecting attitudes in others. They are easily hurt, constantly alert to the attitudes and behavior of others toward them, and they tend to brood and withdraw. Much activity is devoted to warding off or avoiding rebuffs, manifest in some patients by placating attitudes, submission, politeness, attempts to please and conform, in other patients by attempts to deny or ignore by remaining proud, nonchalant, haughty, and aloof.

Some patients give an outward appearance of energy, ambition, and efficiency, but this often proves to cover feelings of inferiority, an acute sense of obligation, a need to experience some sense of security. By and large they avoid chances and do not deal daringly with their environment. Such people are often admired for their virtue, morality, and high standards. They are more likely to seek achievements in the intellectual sphere and to eschew modes of life demanding vigorous physical activity. It must be emphasized that such characteristics are entirely compatible with effective accomplishment, and indeed some noted scientists, artists, writers and even a few athletes have been numbered among ulcerative colitis victims. While good statistical data are not available, it is a clinical impression that the disorder is relatively less common in the lower socioeconomic bracket and in the intellectually less well endowed.[1]

Relationship with People. The patient with ulcerative colitis reveals a rather consistent pattern of interpersonal relationship, a pattern which originates in the relationship with the mother (see below). On the one hand, he appears to have a quite "dependent" relationship with one or two key persons, usually a parent or parent figure; on the other hand, he has a limited capacity to establish warm, genuine friendships with others.

Close scrutiny reveals that the patient often lives through a key figure who at the same time lives through him. Often this is the mother or a mother substitute. The patient appears to use the key figure as though a part of his equipment for dealing with the external world. He leans on the key figure for guidance, advice, and direction; he is reluctant to take initiative or to plan independent action, and he tends to act out the wishes, conscious and unconscious, of the key figure. At the same time this is a highly ambivalent relationship, one within which overt expressions of hostility are fraught with great danger, for to be rejected may induce overwhelming feelings of helplessness. This type of relating reflects a fixation at a symbiotic level of object relationship and is a recurring feature in the majority of patients. The quality of expectation from the key figure (mother) is magical, imperious, and omnipotent. In most cases it is clear that it is not only the patient but the maternal figure who needs the mutual symbiosis.

This pattern of relating may be carried over into the relationship with the physician. Ordinarily, the patient either becomes very "dependent" upon his physician or establishes no relationship or, at best, a very superficial one. Further, the patients who do develop a "dependent" relationship in general fare better than those who do not. Once established, it is difficult for the patient to relinquish the relationship and remain in good health. A disruption of the doctor–patient contact is not infrequently followed by some relapse of symptoms.[122,20]

Mothers: Psychological Characteristics and the Symbiotic Relationship. The nature of the relationship with the mother is of decisive importance in understanding the psychology of the ulcerative colitis patient. There is also an impressive consistency in the description of the mothers of patients with ulcerative colitis, although women patients describe their mothers differently from the way men do. This consistency is confirmed by direct observation of the mothers and by projective testing of the children.[111,18]

In general, the mothers are described as controlling and dominating. Women patients are likely to see their mothers as powerful and overwhelming figures, who make them feel helpless and dependent. They often describe their mothers as cold, unaffectionate, punitive, rigid, strict, and judgmental. The men, although describing similar domination, are more likely to find this acceptable and to portray their mothers as kind, considerate women who worry constantly about their well-being.

Women more often portray themselves as in competition or combat with the mother, while the men more readily capitulate and give in. Despite these different attitudes of the men and women toward their mothers, one readily finds many similarities among the mothers. In general they are either unhappy, pleasureless, gloomy women with no great zest or enjoyment in life, or hard-driving, businesslike, perfectionistic women who are active and concerned with many outside interests but often dissatisfied with their own or others' accomplishments. They tend to be worrisome, complaining, pessimistic, and often hypochondriacal. Expression of genuine warmth, affection, and understanding comes with difficulty. A high proportion show moderate to severe obsessive-compulsive traits; a smaller proportion show pathologically disordered behavior or eccentric preoccupation with collections of odds and ends. A few are psychotic characters or frankly psychotic, usually paranoid. Many of these mothers are described as depressive.

A prominent feature is the mother's propensity to assume the role of a martyr, often mobilizing thereby guilty reactions from the patient.

The persisting symbiotic nature of the patient's relationship with the mother is reflected in the patient's exquisite sensitivity to the mother's feelings and behavior. The patient often behaves as if he cannot distinguish his own feelings from his mother's. Patients comment on their sensitivity to mother's sigh, disapproving look, or change in posture or facial expression, as well as to verbal expressions of distress. Some patients, especially the men, submit passively and obediently to the mother's domination. Others, while submitting, do so with the complaint that mother won't permit them to do otherwise or that they can't stand mother being upset. In general, the patient feels under great pressure from the mother to perform, whether it be in the sense of general social achievement or in ways peculiarly designed to meet the mother's emotional needs or alleviate her guilt, shame, or anxiety. This may lead the patient to manipulate others so that mother will be spared distress. In other words, the patient "learns" the conditions under which he will be spared rejection. Mother's love is conditional on his fulfilling her requirements. In the mutual symbiosis the patient may unconsciously act on the underlying wishes or needs of the mother, even to the extent of remaining ill.

Notable is the need of these mothers to be in control of their children even after they are grown up. Many insist on taking care of their ill adult sons or daughters even when spouses are willing and available.

Fathers. In general, the woman patient is inclined to portray her father as a gentle, kind, passive, usually ineffective man to whom she is quite attached, while the male patient is likely to describe his father either as brutal, punitive, threatening, coarse, and very masculine, or occasionally as passive and weak, and unable to stand up to the mother. The man may see his father as threatening and abusive to the mother, in which case he becomes excessively submissive to both parents. Not uncommonly the male patient feels that his father compared him unfavorably to a more masculine brother who more adequately fulfilled the father's ideal. The woman, on the other hand, often complains that the father did not adequately protect her from mother's aggression, that he let her down.

We have seen two men patients whose symbiotic object relationship was with the father and not the mother. In both cases the son was attempting to fulfill the ambition for physical accomplishment of a father who was frustrated by crippling in adolescence. Superficially these two patients presented as very active, even adventurous men. In both the disease began when they disappointed the father by failing in an important competitive sport event.

Family Dynamics. A study of families with children with ulcerative colitis has characterized these families as "restricted."[80] They reveal a marked inability to engage in or even recognize opportunities for behavior outside the pattern of their own immediate lives. They are limited in the range of interaction, careful in dealing with each other, and they handle a variety of situations in a similar fashion. This was seen as a false solidarity or pseudomutuality. More family studies are needed.

Sexual and Marital Adjustment. In general, these patients tend toward inadequate sexual development. Interest and participation in sexual activity tend to be relatively low. Most of the women are frigid, and even those who experience orgasm do so infrequently. A few patients engage in little or no heterosexual activity even when married. Many acknowledge a preference to being fondled or cuddled, more like a child, and largely reject any genital approach. They are prone to regard sexual activity in anal terms, using such terms as "dirty," "soiling," "disgusting," "unclean," etc., and are squeamish about body contact, secretions, and odors. Excessive bathing, use of deodorants, concern about being malodorous or dirty may be present even in the absence of bowel symptoms, and may be used as rationalization to avoid sexual contact. In the marital relationship the spouse commonly fulfills the role of the succoring, sustaining mother or takes a role subordinate to the mother. Sometimes it is a mother-in-law, who closely resembles the mother, who is the real object for the patient. Under such circumstances the spouse often is related to more like a sibling than a marital partner.

The Nature of the Significant Psychological Stress. In establishing exactly the time of onset of the disease, it is necessary to establish the first clear deviations from usual bowel activity. Many patients are found to have had rectal bleeding or abrupt severe constipation for days, weeks, or even months before diarrhea begins. When the onset of disease is accurately established, it is often found that the time interval between a psychologically stressful circumstance and the onset of the first symptom of the colitis is a matter of hours or a day or two. On the other hand, there are cases where the onset is rather gradual and not easily timed. Here one deals not with a well-defined stressful experience but rather with a gradually changing psychic status during which symptoms gradually and sometimes intermittently develop. The latter is typical of colitis developing during adolescence. In general, psychologically stressful events are likely to fall into the following categories: (1) real, fantasied, or threatened interruption of a key relationship; (2) demands for performance which the patient feels incapable of fulfilling, especially when support had already been withdrawn or when disapproved activities are involved; and (3) overwhelming threat from or disapproval by a parental figure. As a rule hostility and rage toward the disappointing figure is repressed. Common to all these circumstances is an acute or gradually developing feeling on the part of the patient that he has become helpless to cope with what is happening. The disease becomes active in the course of "giving up" psychologically, which is marked by the affect of helplessness. Patients verbalize giving up in such terms as "too much," "despair," "nothing left I could do," "helpless," "overwhelmed," etc.

The following vignettes illustrate patterns of onset and typical precipitating, psychological stress.

Case 1. Constipation and Bleeding. A thirty-one-year-old married woman became pregnant a few months after the birth of her first baby. The first pregnancy had been a deliberate and successful attempt to hold her husband, who had become interested in another woman. To have two babies so close together, however, seemed more than she could cope with. Shortly after she missed her first period she became constipated and noted the passage of bright red blood. For the next six months she continued to pass fresh blood, with and without feces, one to three times a day. Stools remained formed and somewhat constipated, often with fresh blood on the surface. True diarrhea developed six months after the bleeding began, as the inevitability of the second baby became undeniable and the implications overwhelming.

Case 2. Acute Constipation. A twenty-one-year-old married woman was awaiting the return from overseas of her soldier husband, whose train reached the city that day. After keeping her waiting four to five hours while he visited his mother, he appeared at the door, and without further elaboration announced that he wished a divorce. On this note he left. The same day she was seized with terrific cramplike pain in the left lower quadrant of the abdomen and an urge to defecate, but she was unable to do so. She was admitted to a hospital where she was given eight enemas in two days before any relief was achieved. Following this she had formed stools, three to four times a day, for a month, when small amounts of blood were first noted. Thereafter she passed blood and mucus four to five times a day, stools became semiformed, then grossly diarrheal and bloody.

Case 3. Bloody Diarrhea. A twenty-nine-year-old woman married when she discovered she was two months pregnant. She hoped to hide the premarital conception from her puritanical mother by saying the baby was born prematurely. Gestation actually was seven months, so the baby was born five months after the marriage. Two days after the baby was brought home and her mother arrived to help, she had abrupt onset of chills, fever, and diarrhea which became grossly bloody in a few days.

Case 4. Insidious Diarrhea. A fifteen-year-old girl noted over a period of two months a gradual increase in the frequency of her bowel movements, which remained, however, formed but soft. This coincided with the first emergence of the typical conflicts of adolescence. She was then in an automobile accident, which involved no serious injury but did bring up some problems of adolescent acting out. Immediately after the accident her bowel movements became watery and frankly bloody.

Case 5. Tenesmus and Cramps. Immediately following the death of her brother, a thirty-one-year-old unmarried woman developed postprandial distention, belching, mild lower abdominal cramps, and tenesmus associated with the passage of small amounts of blood, mucus, and flatus. Her stool remained formed and hard, and she was constipated for a month. Thereafter she had one to three semisolid fecal movements with blood.

In general, the older the patient at the time of onset of the disease the more likely is the precipitating circumstance to be a major external event. Thus, a fifty-year-old chairman of a university department experienced his first attack, which was fatal, soon after the death of both his parents in a fire. His wife, who would have been his source of support, lost her mother around the same time.

At the present time there is no information as to why this psychobiological state of giving up and helplessness is associated with activation of the ulcerative colitis process. Of interest is the fact that if the patient becomes angry and aggressive, and does not give up, but instead feels guilty, he is more prone to develop headache than activation of colitis.[42] Indeed, the appearance of headaches in a heretofore acutely ill colitis patient is a good prognostic sign.

Three incidents from Case 1 (above) illustrate this:

October 31, 1947—headache: The patient had been free of bowel symptoms for three months. Her two-and-a-half-year-old son defecated in his crib and smeared the feces. "I was awfully mad and gave him a spanking. That night I had a migraine attack. The next morning I still had a headache. Then I realized how guilty I was feeling for spanking him. Shortly thereafter my headache disappeared."

August 20, 1954—bleeding: The patient and her husband bought a building lot, but it turned out that the real estate man tricked them. The patient became very angry with him and told him how she felt. He was unmoved. "I got so mad, and there was absolutely nothing I could do about it." Now they faced the loss of their precarious financial reserves. By that evening she was bleeding.

March 28, 1951—headache terminating attack of colitis: The patient began to bleed on February 20, 1951, when she realized a business venture of her husband was going to fail. She had increasing bleeding and diarrhea and after a couple of weeks it became necessary to confine her to bed at home. At my suggestion another doctor saw her at home, but she had the feeling, "you are leaving me flat." I called her by phone daily, but she was apathetic and relatively uncommunicative. The other internist and I considered hospitalization but decided to delay it as long as possible to keep the financial burden at a minimum. On March 28, 1951, she called me for the first time and said firmly and belligerently, "You must put me in the hospital; I am too sick." On admission I was astonished to discover that she was not suffering primarily from diarrhea but from a severe, left-sided migraine headache, with nausea and vomiting. Her opening remark was an unprecedented: "I don't like you." Her headache subsided by noon and within two days she had formed stools without blood.

In general patients who are good at differentiating their feelings have little difficulty in identifying the affective state most conducive to relapse. Thus one woman claimed the anxiety associated with long-standing phobic symptoms never precipitated colitis symptoms; nor did bursts of rage expressed to her estranged husband. The dangerous period was when she ceased trying to cope actively with these stresses and gave up, sometimes taking to her bed to "sleep it off" only to awaken with cramps or bleeding.

Implications for Treatment.[43,83,84,88] The physician who understands the basic psychological processes operating in these patients is much better equipped to do what is helpful and to avoid doing what is harmful.

The first step in the treatment of an acutely ill patient is to establish a relationship. This is best achieved through the sensitive quality of the physician's first inquiry and his prompt attention to relief of discomfort. Thereafter, constant awareness of the patient's needs and of his characteristic ways of functioning is of the utmost importance in enabling the patient to utilize the relationship with his physician as a means of reestablishing his psychological equilibrium and health. In many respects, this is the keystone of the whole treatment program, and if the initial step is unsuccessful, the whole treatment program may fail.

The physician who undertakes the care of the patient with ulcerative colitis assumes a very complex responsibility, for if he succeeds in this first step of establishing a relationship with the patient, he must be aware that in so doing he is, in part at least, taking over the role of the key figure. This means that while this relationship may be a powerful factor in initiating recovery, its disruption may carry with it the equally great danger of precipitating a relapse. The patient, for some time at least, remains just as vulnerable to a disturbance in his relationship with his physician as he was to a disturbance in his original key relationship. He quickly comes to endow his physician with omniscient and omnipotent qualities. He literally expects the physician to know more of his needs and wants than he himself reveals. Therefore, the doctor must attend closely and respond appropriately to the patient's communications of needs and of sources of discomfort, even when these are not verbally conveyed. This demands patience, a willingness to devote time to the patient, and, most important, the capacity to appreciate and accept the patient's need to have tangible demonstration of the physician's reliability, even in respect to such seemingly minor details as punctuality, following through on promises, and availability for help. Simply the assurance that the physician can be reached at any time can be a powerful source of help, even if this resource is never actually used. It is difficult to overemphasize the importance of these small details, which are perceived by the patient as indices of the doctor's successful and effective participation in his care.

A patient (Case 1, above) had a serious relapse when she had called her physician to check on her medication schedule only to discover that he was out of town and unavailable for a week. When she became my patient we had a standing arrangement whereby she could call me anytime day or night, even when I was away from the city. She called infrequently and then only to report some considerable symptom or a disturbing situation. A relapse occurred following a remission of almost a year when the patient moved into a house in a new suburban tract only to discover that the phone company had not yet laid the cables and hence she would be without a phone for an uncertain period. Symp-toms promptly subsided when I was able to prevail upon the phone company to put in an emergency line and she once again knew she could reach me.

The management of the family is another important consideration. Awareness of the kind of relationship that exists with other members of the family, especially with the mother or the spouse, prepares the physician for the kinds of difficulties which may arise. Usually the important other figure is experiencing a considerable amount of guilt concerning the illness of the patient and may have a strong need to reassert her control both over herself and the patient. It is important that the physician not take a retaliative or a punitive attitude toward the other members of the family. On the other hand, to the patient he must appear stronger than any member of the family. Occasionally, for example, we find the patient making demands, such as to leave the hospital or change medication, which, in fact, reflect not the patient's needs or concerns but rather those of some other family figure. For the physician not to accede to such requests may be a great relief to the patient, for by asserting his medical authority the physician protects the patient from what actually may have been a frightening prospect.

While this approach is predicated on a psychotherapeutically oriented perspective, it is well to recognize that some patients can profit from more systematic psychotherapy in the hands of a skilled therapist.[83,84] The capacity of a patient to so benefit must be evaluated by the psychiatrist, but care must be exercised that the referral to a psychiatrist, even when initiated by the patient, is not interpreted by the patient as a rejection by the internist or gastroenterologist. The latter, by all means, should maintain an active involvement with the patient so that beginning psychotherapy is seen as an addition, not a replacement.

In one study, in which patients receiving psychotherapy in addition to medical therapy were matched with patients receiving medical therapy alone, pretreatment criteria favoring good response to psychotherapy were identified.[83] These included: (1) the presence of an obvious precipitating event, especially if recognized by the patient; (2) depression traceable to loss, as compared to depressive apathy; (3) the unconscious use of diarrhea and bleeding as substitutes for rage and as means of punishment, in contrast to regarding the illness without shame or guilt as a justification to remain helpless and make demands on others; and (4) a wish to become independent.

In recognizing the role of psychotherapy in the treatment of these patients, one should also have very clearly in mind what psychotherapy can and what it cannot be expected to accomplish. There is no evidence at the present time that psychotherapy, no matter how intensive, can eliminate the biological defect underlying colitis. Therefore, an expectation of complete cure is unjustified. While remission and complete healing are common, psychotherapy cannot ensure against recurrence in the face of sufficient stress. The major contribution that psychotherapy can make is the modification of the basic psychological structure so as to render the individual less vulnerable to the types of situations in which the disease becomes manifest. These particularly concern the capacity of the patient to develop human relationships and to tolerate their loss or the threat of their loss. Successful psychotherapy usually brings about a significant improvement in the patient's techniques of dealing with the early parental figures, as well as some resolution of early conflicts. With this one generally sees a gradual emancipation from parental figures and an increasing capacity to establish satisfying and enduring relationships with others. But, as with any person, there may still occur events with which the patient feels he has no effective means of coping and under such circumstances the disease may resume. In general, however, we find that the patient who has achieved some successful psychotherapeutic response has more chance of maintaining a remission. But it is of the utmost importance that the patient, embarking on psychotherapy, clearly understands that psychotherapy cannot eliminate the potential for colitis, otherwise even a mild relapse may be felt as a personal failure or destroy the patient's confidence in the therapist, thereby constituting a major stress capable of provoking a massive recurrence. Many of the serious relapses during or upon termination of psychotherapy or psychoanalysis have been of this nature and have led to an unjustified pessimism as to the effectiveness of this approach.

As to modalities of psychotherapy, insight therapy is more useful with the relatively more active, independent patients, while patients who are strongly symbiotic or transitional are helped more by support, catharsis and suggestions than interpretation. Best results are obtained by therapists who rate high in interest in the patient, empathic understanding, and optimism about results, and with patients who are most hopeful about being helped and who can develop a warm trusting working alliance with the therapist. The ability of the therapist to "fit" or match himself to the fluctuating dependency needs of the patient is important. Symbiotic patients improve when their therapists are able to tolerate their infantile dependent needs without rejection, impatience, or arbitrary corrective attitudes. The papers by Karush et al., and by Groen et al. are excellent sources of information about the psychotherapy of ulcerative colitis patients.[83,84,71]

In considering the usual indications for ileostomy and colectomy, namely, intractable diarrhea, recurring fistulae or abscesses, massive hemorrhage, rectal incontinence, and threat of cancer, it is important to appreciate how stressful it is for these patients not to have complete control over their bowel activity, whether it be in the form of unpredictable bleeding, diarrhea, or cramps. With his great need to maintain control over his thoughts, acts, and body, and to perform well, incapacity on this score is often felt as a true inadequacy, for which the patient often inappropriately assumes responsibility. Hence the removal of the offending colon and the construction of an artificial anus (ileostomy) over which the patient generally has much better control often has a more salutary effect psychologically than had been anticipated by the patient, his family or physician, all of whom tend to view the procedure primarily in terms of its mutilating effect. Hence the psychotherapist is well advised to keep in mind not only these indications for surgery, but also the contribution he can make in preparing the patient for operation and the postoperative adjustment. Above all must he appreciate that recourse to surgery does not constitute a failure of psychotherapy or grounds for relinquishing his therapeutic role. There is great advantage for the prospective ileostomy patient to meet a successful ileostomy patient and to learn at first hand the gains as well as the realistic problems of ileostomy. Additional help may be provided through participation in the activities of the Ileostomy Clubs, which constitute a resource not only for practical information but also for group activity which is psychologically sound for these patients. Their slogan HELP (Help, Encouragement, Learning, Participation) clearly reflects an intuitive grasp of the basic human and psychological needs of the ulcerative colitis patients.

Ulcerative Enteritis. That the same pathological process may also involve the terminal ileum has been known for a long time. Less well known is that it may develop in a previously healthy ileum after colectomy and ileostomy have been performed, and under the same types of psychologically stressful situations as had previously led to the activation of the ulcerative colitis. The entire small bowel may rarely be so involved. Swelling of the stoma with partial obstruction, profuse watery drainage, or perforation may ensue. Edema, petechial hemorrhages, and ulceration of the protruded mucous membrane may be noted.

The risk of this complication provides further reason why a continuing supportive or psychotherapeutic approach is called for, even after colectomy and ileostomy, especially with the patient who has been in psychotherapy.

REGIONAL ENTERITIS AND COLITIS (CROHN'S DISEASE)

While not the subject of as extensive psychological inquiry as ulcerative colitis, the available data indicate many similarities between patients with regional enteritis and those with ulcerative colitis.[*] This is not surprising, considering the fact that although clearly differentiated on pathological grounds, there is nonetheless a tendency for the two diseases to occur in the same family suggesting a common genetic factor.[14,90,135] Furthermore, now that it is being appreciated that a similar pathological process may affect the large bowel (granulomatous colitis, Crohn's disease of the colon), it is clear that at least some of the colitis patients studied psychologically in the past actually belonged in this category. The several patients that this writer has studied who later proved to have the granulomatous form of colitis did not appear to differ psychologically from those who had classical ulcerative colitis. The resemblance is greatest in respect to the prominence of obsessive-compulsiveness, the patterns of relating, and the vulnerability to object loss and subsequent development of giving up as the setting in which onset or relapse of active disease occurs. Compared to ulcerative colitis patients, some authors feel patients with Crohn's disease are relatively more flexible[60] and more active,[119] but the only systematic comparative study suggests no differences.[102] Hence, until more information is available, it seems warranted to use the data on ulcerative colitis as a rough guide for the management of these patients as well. More detailed study is called for.

Possible Somatopsychic-Psychosomatic Conditions

There are a number of other conditions which possibly can be classified under the heading of somatopsychic-psychosomatic disorders but which have not yet been sufficiently studied to justify the claim.

CELIAC SPRUE[†]

It is currently believed that celiac disease of childhood and many instances of so-called

---

[*] See references 31, 67, 90, 139, and 156.
[†] See references 22, 61, 69, 98, 118, 123, and 145.

idiopathic steatorrhea of adulthood represent the same disorder, hence the term "celiac sprue." In both diseases identical and to a large extent reversible damage to the small intestinal mucosa is produced by low-molecular-weight glutamine-rich polypeptides, isolated from the breakdown products of gluten, the water-insoluble protein moiety of wheat. Many adult patients give a history of celiac disorder early in childhood, while proven childhood celiacs, allegedly recovered, may as adults still show absorption defects, typical histopathological changes, and reactivity to gluten, with intermittent mild symptoms of malabsorption.[98] Evidence for a genetic determinant has been brought forth,[22,145] leading to the suggestion of an inborn deficiency in the intestinal mucosa of a peptidase that hydrolyzes the peptides of gluten.[61,101,76]

The natural history of spontaneous remissions despite the presence of dietary gluten in the childhood form of the disease, and the poor correlation between symptoms and the presence of typical histopathological changes suggests that the underlying mucosal defect and the presence of gluten in the diet may be necessary but not sufficient for the development of the malabsorption syndrome. Individuals appear to differ in sensitivity to gluten, and symptoms may also correlate more with the extent of the intestine involved than with the severity of the lesion on biopsy.[100] The effects of gluten are more marked on proximal than on distal intestine, presumably a reflection of declining concentration of the noxious polypeptides. The great majority of patients show prompt marked clinical improvement on strict glutenfree diets with reversal of epithelial changes more complete distally than proximally. But returning gluten to the diet does not necessarily reactivate symptoms even though biopsy evidence of damage may be demonstrated. Hence some have suggested that psychological stress may be a contributing factor.[118,123] Among children a disturbance in the mother–child relationship, including changes in patterns of handling and feeding, appear to be associated with exacerbations, while remissions have been brought about through improving the mother–child

relationship, even without removing gluten from the diet.[123] Among adults, with and without a childhood history, onset or recurrences are noted in settings in which real or threatened loss of support eventuates in psychological "giving up" with feelings of sadness, despair, and helplessness. These are psychological states in which Sadler and Orton have demonstrated decreased absorption of amino acids in a surgically isolated loop of ileum in a man who did not have celiac-sprue syndrome.[131]

Suggestive data on this interrelationship between the intrinsic intestinal defect, dietary gluten, and psychological factors have been provided by Grant's double-blind study of eight patients with adult celiac disease, four of whom were known to have had childhood celiac disease and three of whom had a history compatible with childhood celiac disease.[69] Placed on a gluten-free diet, all patients showed remission of symptoms and improvement in absorption. Then, in a double-blind fashion they were given capsules containing either gliadin (a derivative of gluten containing the glutamine-rich polypeptides) or an inactive material. The occurrence of symptoms was noted and the psychological state evaluated. Gliadin capsules were administered a total of thirty-one periods during five of which typical malabsorption symptoms developed. All of these occurred within days of the onset of a psychological upset, generally characterized by some loss, defeat, discouragement, or helplessness. On *no* occasion did gliadin alone induce symptoms in a patient who otherwise was emotionally composed. On the other hand, bowel symptoms also occurred during periods when the patient was similarly upset but was *not* receiving gliadin. Notable, however, was the fact that under such conditions the symptoms were those of a nonspecific, nonfoul watery diarrhea, sometimes with mucus, and did not include the typical bloating or the foul smelling, pale, copious stools typical of malabsorption. These observations suggest an interaction between at least three factors in the production of the full-blown malabsorption syndrome: (1) an intrinsic intestinal defect; (2) gliadin in the diet; and

(3) some effect mediated through psycho-physiological or neurogenic influences.

The data available are insufficient to justify any statement concerning distinctive psychological characteristics of this group of patients. Paulley emphasizes querulousness and extreme rigidity among the more disturbed patients and perhaps a higher incidence of psychotic, often delusional and paranoid features.[118] We have been impressed with the immaturity and dependency of the adults with a childhood history of celiac disorder as well as their unusual vulnerability to loss of love objects. Prugh, in his study of children, emphasizes the prominence of obsessive-compulsive traits, and the controlling and ambivalent nature of the mother's relation with her child, and points to evidence that such attitudes of the mother antedated the birth of the child.[123] He describes the children on the surface to be passive, often withdrawn, inhibited personalities, with a tendency toward obsessive-compulsive features. Overt expressions of aggression or self-assertion seem to be difficult for these children. As infants, they were fussy, irritable, and cried a great deal, even before the onset of the celiac symptoms. Somatic effects of multiple nutritional deficiencies as well as of the psychological responses to diarrhea and other debilities must not be underestimated in evaluating some of these descriptions.

IRRITABLE BOWEL SYNDROME*

This is the classical "functional" bowel disorder, characterized by alternating diarrhea and constipation, abdominal cramps, flatulence, and at times increased mucus in the stools. Some investigators differentiate two groups, i.e., spastic colon and functional diarrhea.[27] Those with spastic colon have lower abdominal pain and cramps as their main symptom, and in addition have constipation which alternates with diarrhea or with periods of normal bowel movements. Patients with functional diarrhea have little or no abdominal pain, their chief symptom being constant or intermittent diarrhea. Many are overtly

anxious and their symptoms may more properly be classified as instances of diarrhea as a physiological concomitant of affect, though it remains obscure why some anxious people have diarrhea and others do not. Both neural and hormonal mechanisms have been postulated. Accelerated transport of intestinal contents, through increased peristalsis induced by increased sensitivity to cholecystikinin, by gastro-ileal or gastro-colic reflexes or by higher neurogenic effects may induce diarrhea simply by overloading the absorptive capacity of the colon.[74,128,148] Both with spastic colon and with functional diarrhea it has been claimed that the colon reacts excessively to parasympathetic stimulation as compared to the colon of patients without bowel disorder or with ulcerative colitis, but some writers disagree.[12,15,27] They point out that the increase in intraluminal pressure is a function of the mechanics of intraabdominal pressure recording, important factors being resistance to expulsion and the consistency of the stools.[128,148] While pressures are low with diarrhea and high with constipation, the increased activity in painless diarrhea may reflect a control mechanism for handling excessive intestinal contents by segmentation rather than by inhibition.[128,147] Such findings give further reason to regard patients with painless diarrhea as belonging to a different group from the rest of those with irritable colon syndrome.

Be that as it may, there is virtually universal acceptance of the view that bowel symptoms in both types are somehow brought about by psychological influences.† This has led to the classification of irritable colon syndrome as a "psychogenic" or "psychophysiological" disorder, the inference being that the bowel disorder can be accounted for by chronic and excessive parasympathetic stimulation psychophysiologically determined. This is almost certainly an oversimplification. The virtually lifelong symptomatic history of many of these patients suggests that there may be as yet unidentified organic factors influencing the bowel response to psychological stress. Until more definitive data are available, it seems

---

* See references 9, 11, 13, 15, 27, 89, 128, 147, 148, and 155.

† See references 11, 13, 27, 89, 128, 148, and 155.

prudent not to exclude such primary organic determinants; hence its classification here as a "somatopsychic-psychosomatic" rather than psychophysiological disorder.

Because there is no clear organic criterion for the diagnosis of irritable bowel syndrome, which even gastroenterologists make largely by exclusion, existing data on the psychological characteristics of patients with this syndrome are highly dependent upon the population utilized. In general they have been patients referred to a psychiatrist after the gastroenterologist has ruled out other explanations of the symptoms, and often because he has been impressed by evidence of neurotic difficulties. Early published series may well have included patients who now would be recognized as suffering from lactase deficiency or adult celiac syndrome. Hence it is likely that patients so far reported on have been selected to begin with because of manifest emotional problems, and are neither a representative population nor even necessarily all have irritable bowel syndrome. With this caveat it is claimed that patients with spastic colon are more inclined to be rigid, obsessional, and compulsive individuals while those with functional diarrhea may show more diffuse free-floating or phobic anxiety as well. Many tend to be orderly, methodical, conscientious, precise, preoccupied with cleanliness, tidiness, regularity, punctuality, and schedules, and it is not surprising that some gravitate to work roles in which such qualities are valued as accounting, bookkeeping, filing, library work, etc. Such patients place a high premium on intellectual control and performance and are very restrained in expression of emotions, be they pleasurable or unpleasurable. By the same token, they tend, on the one hand, to maintain a cold, intellectual almost impervious air toward the emotional turmoil of others, while, on the other, to be extremely sensitive to hostile or rejecting behavior, or emotional outbursts when directed toward them. In the latter respect they appear as hypersensitive and easily hurt to the point at times of paranoid suspiciousness. Important in the underlying psychodynamics are conflicts about giving and receiving, and the control of aggression.[9] Distrustful and fearful of rejection, especially if aggressive or sexual impulses are displayed, they tend to hold on to what they possess, not to give. Some are stingy, stubborn, and parsimonious, while others overdo the guise of generosity (reaction formation) but as a result constantly feel unappreciated and disappointed that the recipient is not more grateful. Feelings of depression are common, and there is a relatively high incidence of significant clinical depression.

It has been suggested that the alternations between constipation and diarrhea characteristic of these patients reflect shifts between psychologically holding back and maintaining control, on the one hand, and letting go in an unconscious, aggressively soiling or depreciatingly giving way on the other.[9] It is of interest that headaches commonly accompany the controlled, constipated phase, which is marked not only by guilt-determined inhibition of action but also by the use of the head (intellect). In general, diarrhea is most prominent at times when emotional tension is most evident.

ACHALASIA (CARDIOSPASM)*

Though not accepted by all, the association between psychological stress and onset or exacerbation of cardiospasm has been proposed for many years. However, the disorder is relatively uncommon and hence the information available is insufficient to document more than the fact of a high incidence of psychological disturbances among the sufferers and a chronological correlation between psychological stress and episodes of the disorder. The fact that the disease may have its onset at any age, though it is rare in infancy and childhood, that it most commonly develops in early adult life, that there is a familial incidence, and that there is evidence of a disturbance in the intrinsic parasympathetic innervation of the esophagus all favor some intrinsic organic process present or acquired early in life. Patients with achalasia have an elevated level of resting lower esophageal sphincter pressure and incomplete sphincter relaxation with swal-

* See references 29, 103, 108, 130, 136, 153, and 159.

lowing. The available evidence indicates that this is caused by the loss of β-adrenergic inhibitory activity and that denervation of the sphincteric muscle is of primary importance.[109,29] The difficulty in swallowing is accentuated during emotional upset but as yet too few patients have been studied in detail to provide any general psychological characterization as a group.

❮ Bibliography

1. ACHESON, E. D. and M. D. NEFZGER. "Ulcerative Colitis in the United States Army in 1944. Epidemiology: Comparisons between Patients and Controls," *Gastroenterology*, 44 (1963), 7–19.

2. ADAMSON, J. D. and A. H. SCHMALE. "Object Loss, Giving Up and the Onset of Psychiatric Disease," *Psychosom. Med.*, 27 (1965), 557–576.

3. ADER, R. "Plasma Pepsinogen Level as a Predictor of Susceptibility to Gastric Erosions in the Rat," *Psychosom. Med.*, 25 .(1963), 221–232.

4. ———. "Gastric Erosions in the Rat. Effects of Immobilization at Different Points in the Activity Cycle," *Science*, 145 (1964), 406–407.

5. ———. "Behavioral and Physiological Rhythms and the Development of Gastric Erosions in the Rat," *Psychosom. Med.*, 29 (1967), 345–353.

6. ADER, R., C. C. BEELS, and R. TATUM. "Blood Pepsinogen and Gastric Erosions in the Rat," *Psychosom. Med.*, 22 (1960), 1–12.

7. ALEXANDER, F. "The Influence of Psychologic Factors upon Gastrointestinal Disturbances: General Principles, Objectives and Preliminary Results," *Psychoanal. Q.*, 3 (1934), 501–539.

8. ———. "Gastrointestinal Neuroses," in S. Portis, ed., *Diseases of the Digestive System*, 1st ed., pp. 206–226. Philadelphia: Lea & Febiger, 1941.

9. ———. *Psychosomatic Medicine.* New York: Norton, 1950.

10. ———. "Emotional Factors in Gastrointestinal Disturbances," in S. Portis, ed., *Diseases of the Digestive System*, 3rd ed., pp. 228–252. Philadelphia: Lea & Febiger, 1953.

11. ALMY, T. P., F. K. ABBOT, and L. E. HINKLE. "Alterations in Colonic Function in Man under Stress. IV. Hypomotility of the Sigmoid Colon and Its Relationship to the Mechanism of Functional Diarrheas," *Gastroenterology*, 15 (1950), 95–113.

12. ALMY, T. P., L. E. HINKLE, B. BERLE et al. "Alterations in Colonic Function in Man under Stress. III. Experimental Production of Sigmoid Spasm in Patients with Spastic Constipation," *Gastroenterology*, 12 (1949), 437–449.

13. ALMY, T. P., F. KERN, and M. TULIN. "Alterations in Colonic Function in Man under Stress. II. Experimental Production of Sigmoid Spasm in Healthy Persons," *Gastroenterology*, 12 (1949), 425–436.

14. ALMY, T. P. and P. SHERLOCK. "Genetic Aspects of Ulcerative Colitis and Regional Enteritis," *Gastroenterology*, 15 (1966), 757–763.

15. ALMY, T. P. and M. TULIN. "Alterations in Colonic Function in Man under Stress: I. Experimental Production of Changes Simulating the 'Irritable Colon'," *Gastroenterology*, 8 (1947), 616–626.

16. ALVAREZ, W. C. "Hysterical Type of Non-Gaseous Abdominal Bloating," *Arch. Intern. Med.*, 84 (1949), 217–245.

17. ANTHONY, E. J. "An Experimental Approach to the Psychopathology of Childhood; Encopresis," *Br. J. Med. Psychol.*, 30 (1957), 146–175.

18. ARTHUR, B. "Role Perceptions of Children with Ulcerative Colitis," *Arch. Gen. Psychiatry*, 8 (1963), 536–545.

19. ASKEVOLD, F. "Studies in Ulcerative Colitis," *J. Psychosom. Res.*, 8 (1964), 89–100.

20. BACON, C. "Typical Personality Trends and Conflicts in Cases of Gastric Disturbances," *Psychoanal. Q.*, 3 (1934), 540–557.

21. BARKER, W. F. "Family History of Patients with Ulcerative Colitis," *Am. J. Surg.*, 103 (1962), 25–26.

22. BOYER, P. H. and D. H. ANDERSON. "A Genetic Study of Celiac Disease," *Am. J. Dis. Child.*, 91 (1956), 131–136.

23. BURCH, P. R. J., F. T. deDOMBAL, and G. WATKINSON. "Aetiology of Ulcerative Colitis. II. A New Hypothesis," *Gut*, 10 (1969), 277–284.

24. CARD, W. L. and I. N. MARKS. "The Relationship between the Acid Output of the Stomach following 'Maximal' Histamine

Stimulation of the Parietal Cell Mass," *Clin. Sci.*, 19 (1960), 147–163.

25. CHAUDHARY, N. A. and S. C. TRUELOVE. "Human Colonic Motility: A Comparative Study of Normal Subjects, Patients with Ulcerative Colitis, and Patients with Irritable Bowel Syndrome," *Gastroenterology*, 40 (1961), 1–17.

27. ———. "The Irritable Colon Syndrome," *Q. J. Med.*, 31 (1962), 307–316.

28. CODDINGTON, D. "Study of an Infant with a Gastric Fistula and Her Normal Twin," *Psychosom. Med.*, 30 (1968), 172–192.

29. COHEN, S. and Z. W. LIPSHUT. "Lower Esophageal Sphincter Dysfunction in Achalasia," *Gastroenterology*, 61 (1971), 814–820.

30. COX, A. S. "Stomach Size and Its Relation to Chronic Peptic Ulcer," *Arch. Pathol.*, 54 (1952), 407–422.

31. CROCKET, R. W. "Psychiatric Findings in Crohn's Disease," *Lancet*, 1 (1952), 946–949.

32. DANIELS, G. E., J. F. O'CONNOR, A. KARUSH et al. "Three Decades in the Observation and Treatment of Ulcerative Colitis," *Psychosom. Med.*, 24 (1962), 85–93.

33. DEGRAFF, J. and M. A. M. SCHUURS. "Severe Potassium Depletion Caused by Abuse of Laxatives," *Acta Med. Scand.*, 166 (1960), 407–422.

34. DICK, A. P., L. P. HOLT, and E. R. DALTON. "Persistence of Mucosal Abnormality in Ulcerative Colitis," *Gut*, 7 (1966), 355–360.

35. DOLL, R. and J. BUCH. "Hereditary Factors in Peptic Ulcer," *Ann. Eugen.*, 15 (1950), 135–146.

36. EBERHARD, G. "Peptic Ulcer in Twins. A Study in Personality Heredity and Environment," *Acta Psychiatr. Scand.*, 44, *Suppl.* 205 (1968), 7–118.

37. EDWARDS, H. H. "The Meaning of the Associations between Blood Groups and Disease," *Ann. Hum. Genet.*, 29 (1965), 77–83.

38. EHRENTHEIL, O. F. and E. P. WELLS. "Megacolon in Psychotic Patients," *Gastroenterology*, 29 (1955), 285–294.

39. EISENMAN, B. and R. L. HEYMAN. "Stress Ulcers—A Continuing Challenge," *N. Engl. J. Med.*, 282 (1970), 372–374.

40. ENGEL, G. L. "Studies of Ulcerative Colitis. II. The Nature of the Somatic Processes and the Adequacy of Psychosomatic Hy-

potheses," *Am. J. Med.*, 16 (1954), 416–433.

41. ———. "Studies of Ulcerative Colitis. III. The Nature of the Psychologic Processes," *Am. J. Med.*, 19 (1955), 231–256.

42. ———. "Studies of Ulcerative Colitis. IV. The Significance of Headaches," *Psychosom. Med.*, 18 (1956), 334–346.

43. ———. "Studies of Ulcerative Colitis. V. Psychological Aspects and Their Implications for Treatment," *Am. J. Dig. Dis.*, 3 (1958), 315–337.

44. ———. "Review of A. Garma, 'Peptic Ulcer and Psychoanalysis'," Nerv. Ment. Dis. Monograph no. 85. *Am. J. Dig. Dis.*, 4 (1959), 829–831.

45. ———. "Psychogenic Pain and the Pain-Prone Patient," *Am. J. Med.*, 26 (1959), 899–918.

46. ———. "Biologic and Psychologic Features of the Ulcerative Colitis Patient," *Gastroenterology*, 40 (1961), 313–317.

47. ———. "Guilt, Pain and Success. Success Facilitated by the Pain of a Glomus Tumor and Peptic Ulcer," *Psychosom. Med.*, 24 (1962), 37–48.

48. ———. *Psychological Development in Health and Disease*, pp. 29–104. Philadelphia: Saunders, 1962.

49. ———. *Psychological Development in Health and Disease*, pp. 364–380. Philadelphia: Saunders, 1962.

50. ———. *Psychological Development in Health and Disease*, pp. 381–401. Philadelphia: Saunders, 1962.

51. ———. "A Reconsideration of the Role of Conversion in Somatic Disease," *Compr. Psychiatry*, 9 (1968), 316–326.

52. ———. "Psychological Factors in Ulcerative Colitis in Man and Gibbon," *Gastroenterology*, 57 (1969), 362–365.

53. ———. "Pain" in C. M. MacBryde and R. S. Blacklow, eds., *Signs and Symptoms: Applied Pathologic Physiology and Clinical Interpretation.* 5th ed., pp. 44–61. Philadelphia: Lippincott, 1970.

54. ———. "Conversion Symptoms," in C. M. MacBryde and R. S. Blacklow, eds., *Signs and Symptoms: Applied Pathologic Physiology and Clinical Interpretation.* 5th ed., pp. 650–668. Philadelphia: Lippincott, 1970.

55. ENGEL, G. L., F. REICHSMAN, and D. ANDERSON. "Behavior and Gastric Secretion. III. Cognitive Development and Gastric Secre-

tion in Children with Gastric Fistula," *Psychosom. Med.*, 33 (1971), 472–473.

56. ENGEL, G. L., F. REICHSMAN, and H. SEGAL. "A Study of an Infant with a Gastric Fistula. I. Behavior and the Rate of Total Hydrochloric Acid Secretion," *Psychosom. Med.*, 18, (1956), 374–398.

57. FELDMAN, F., D. CANTOR, S. SOLL et al. "Psychiatric Study of a Consecutive Series of 34 Patients with Ulcerative Colitis," *Br. Med. J.*, 1 (1967), 14–17.

58. FINCH, S. M. and J. N. HESS. "Ulcerative Colitis in Children," *Am. J. Psychiatry*, 118 (1962), 819–826.

59. FODOR, O., S. VESTEA, S. URCAN et al. "Hydrochloric Acid Secretion Capacity of the Stomach as an Inherited Factor in the Pathogenesis of Duodenal Ulcer," *Am. J. Dig. Dis.*, 13 (1968), 260–265.

60. FORD, C. V., G. A. GLOBER, and P. CASTELNUOVO-TEDESCO. "A Psychiatric Study of Patients with Regional Enteritis," *JAMA*, 208 (1969), 311–315.

61. FRAZER, A. C. "The Present State of Knowledge of the Celiac Syndrome," *J. Pediatr.* 57 (1960), 262–276.

62. FRENCH, J. M., C. F. HAWKINS, and W. T. COOKE. "Clinical Experience with the Gluten-Free Diet in Idiopathic Steatorrhea," *Gastroenterology*, 38 (1960), 592–595.

63. FREYBERGER, H. "The Doctor–Patient Relationship in Ulcerative Colitis," *Psychother. Psychosom.*, 18 (1970), 80–89.

64. FULLERTON, D. T., E. J. KOLLAR, and A. B. CALDWELL. "A Clinical Study of Ulcerative Colitis," *JAMA*, 181 (1962), 463–471.

65. GARMA, A. *Peptic Ulcer and Psychoanalysis.* Nerv. Ment. Dis. Monograph no. 85, 1958.

66. GOLDMAN, M. C. "Gastric Secretion during a Medical Interview," *Psychosom. Med.*, 25 (1963), 351–356.

67. GRACE, W. J. "Life Stress and Regional Enteritis," *Gastroenterology*, 23 (1953), 542–553.

68. GRACE, W. J., S. WOLF, and H. G. WOLFF. *The Human Colon.* New York: Hoeber, 1951.

69. GRANT, J. M. "Studies on Celiac Disease. I. The Interrelationship between Gliadin, Psychological Factors, and Symptom Formation," *Psychosom. Med.*, 21 (1959), 431–432.

70. GROEN, J. J. "The Psychosomatic Specificity Hypothesis for the Etiology of Peptic Ulcer," *Psychother. Psychosom.*, 19 (1971), 295–305.

71. GROEN, J. J. and D. BIRNBAUM. "Conservative (Supportive) Treatment of Severe Ulcerative Colitis. Methods and Results," *Israel J. Med. Sci.*, 4 (1968), 130–139.

72. GULLICK, H. D. "Carcinoma of the Pancreas. A Review and Critical Study of 100 Cases," *Medicine*, 38 (1959), 47–84.

73. GUNDRY, R. K., R. M. DONALDSON, C. A. PINDERHUGHES et al. "Patterns of Gastric Acid Secretion in Patients with Duodenal Ulcer: Correlations with Clinical and Personality Features," *Gastroenterology*, 52 (1967), 176–184.

74. HARVEY, R. F. and A. E. READ. "Effects of Cholecystokinin on Colonic Motility and Symptoms in Patients with the Irritable Bowel Syndrome," *Gut*, 13 (1972), 837–838.

75. HISLOP, I. G. and A. K. GRANT. "Genetic Tendency in Crohn's Disease," *Gut*, 10 (1969), 994–995.

76. HOFFMAN, H. N., E. E. WOLLEAGER, and E. GREENBERG. "Discordance for Non-Tropical Sprue (Adult Celiac Disease) in a Monozygotic Twin Pair," *Gastroenterology*, 51 (1966), 36–42.

77. HUNT, J. N. "Inhibition of Gastric Emptying and Secretion in Patients with Duodenal Ulcer," *Lancet*, 1 (1957), 132–134.

78. ———. "The Influence of Hydrochloric Acid on Gastric Secretion and Emptying in Patients with Duodenal Ulcer," *Br. Med. J.*, 1 (1957), 681–684.

79. ———. "Some Notes on the Pathogenesis of Duodenal Ulcer," *Am. J. Dig. Dis.*, 2 (1957), 445–453.

80. JACKSON, D. and I. YALOM. "Family Research in the Problem of Ulcerative Colitis," *Arch. Gen. Psychiatry*, 15 (1966), 410–418.

81. KAPLAN, H. "The Psychosomatic Concept of Peptic Ulcer," *J. Nerv. Ment. Dis.*, 123 (1956), 93–111.

82. KAPP, F., M. ROSENBAUM, and J. ROMANO. "Psychological Factors in Men with Peptic Ulcers," *Am. J. Psychiatry*, 103 (1947), 700–704.

83. KARUSH, A., G. E. DANIELS, G. F. O'CONNOR et al. "The Response to Psychotherapy in Chronic Ulcerative Colitis. I. Pretreatment Factors," *Psychosom. Med.*, 30 (1968), 255–276.

84. ———. "The Response to Psychotherapy in Chronic Ulcerative Colitis. II. Factors Arising from the Therapeutic Situation," *Psychosom. Med.*, 31 (1969), 201–226.

85. KAUFMAN, W. "Some Emotional Uses of Food," *Conn. Med.*, 23 (1959), 158–161.

86. KEHOE, M. and W. IRONSIDE. "Studies on the Experimental Evocation of Depressive Responses Using Hypnosis. II. The Influence of Depressive Responses upon the Secretion of Gastric Acid," *Psychosom. Med.*, 25 (1963), 403–419.

87. KEZUR, E., F. KAPP, and M. ROSENBAUM. "Psychological Factors in Women with Peptic Ulcers," *Am. J. Psychiatry*, 108 (1951), 368–373.

88. KIRSNER, J. B. "Ulcerative Colitis, Mysterious, Multiplex and Menacing," *J. Chronic Dis.*, 23 (1971), 681–684.

89. KIRSNER, J. B. and W. L. PALMER. "The Irritable Colon," *Gastroenterology*, 34 (1958), 491–501.

90. KIRSNER, J. B. and J. A. SPENCER. "Family Occurrence of Ulcerative Colitis. Regional Enteritis and Ileocolitis," *Ann. Intern. Med.*, 59 (1963), 133–144.

91. KOHN, L. "The Behavior of Patients with Cancer of the Pancreas," *Cancer*, 5 (1952), 328–330.

92. KOLLAR, E. J., D. T. FULLERTON, R. DICENSO et al. "Stress Specificity in Ulcerative Colitis," *Compr. Psychiatry*, 5 (1964), 101–112.

93. KRAFT, E., N. FINBY, P. T. EGIDIO et al. "The Megasigmoid Syndrome in Psychotic Patients," *JAMA*, 195 (1966), 1099–1101.

94. LEVEY, H. B. "Oral Trends and Oral Conflicts in a Case of Duodenal Ulcer," *Psychoanal. Q.*, 3 (1934), 574–582.

95. LEVIN, E., J. B. KIRSNER, and W. L. PALMER. "Twelve-Hour Nocturnal Gastric Secretion in Uncomplicated Duodenal Ulcer Patients: before and after Healing," *Proc. Soc. Exp. Biol. Med.*, 69 (1948), 153–157.

96. LEVINE, M. "Pregenital Trends in a Case of Chronic Diarrhea and Vomiting," *Psychoanal. Q.*, 3 (1934), 583–588.

97. LIEBERMAN, M. A., D. STOCK, and R. WHITMAN. "Self-Perceptual Patterns among Ulcer Patients," *Arch. Gen. Psychiatry*, 1 (1959), 167–176.

98. LINDSAY, M. K. M., B. E. C. NORDIN, and A. P. NORMAN. "Late Prognosis in Celiac Disease," *Br. Med. J.*, 2 (1956), 14–18.

99. LITTMAN, A. "Basal Gastric Secretion in Patients with Duodenal Ulcer: A Long-Term Study of Variations in Relation to Ulcer Activity," *Gastroenterology*, 43 (1962), 166.

100. MACDONALD, W. C., L. L. BRANDBORG, A. L. FLICK et al. "Studies of Celiac Sprue. IV. The Response of the Whole Length of the Small Bowel to Gluten-Free Diet," *Gastroenterology*, 47 (1964), 573–589.

101. MACDONALD, W. C., W. O. DOBBINS, and C. E. RUBIN. "Studies of the Familial Nature of Celiac Sprue Using Biopsy of the Small Intestine," *N. Engl. J. Med.*, 272 (1965), 448–456.

102. MCKEGNEY, F. P., R. O. GORDON, and S. M. LEVINE. "A Psychosomatic Comparison of Patients with Ulcerative Colitis and Crohn's Disease," *Psychosom. Med.*, 32 (1970), 153–166.

103. MCMAHON, J. M., F. I. BRACELAND, and H. J. MOERSCH. "The Psychosomatic Aspects of Cardiospasm," *Ann. Intern. Med.*, 34 (1951), 608–631.

104. MARGOLIN, S. G. "The Behavior of the Stomach during Psychoanalysis," *Psychoanal. Q.*, 20 (1951), 349–369.

105. MENGUY, R. "Acute Gastric Mucosal Bleeding," *Ann. Rev. Med.*, 23 (1972), 297–312.

106. MILLER, N. "Learning of Visceral and Glandular Responses," *Science*, 163 (1969), 434–445.

107. MIRSKY, I. A. "Psychoanalysis in the Biological Sciences," in F. Alexander and H. Ross, eds., *Twenty Years of Psychoanalysis*, pp. 155–176. New York: Norton, 1953.

108. ———. "Physiologic, Psychologic and Social Determinants in the Etiology of Duodenal Ulcer," *Am. J. Dig. Dis.*, 3 (1958), 285–314.

109. MISIEWICZ, J. J., S. L. WALLER, P. P. ANTHONY et al. "Achalasia of the Cardia: Pharmacology and Histopathology of Isolated Careiac Sphincteric Muscle from Patients with and without Achalasia," *Q. J. Med.*, 38 (1969), 17–30.

110. MITTLEMAN, B. and H. G. WOLFF. "Emotions and Gastrointestinal Function," *Psychosom. Med.*, 4 (1942), 5–61.

111. MOHR, G. J., I. M. JOSSELYN, J. SPURLOCK et al. "Studies in Ulcerative Colitis," *Am. J. Psychiatry*, 114 (1958), 1067–1076.

112. MONSON, R. R. "Familial Factors in Peptic

Ulcer. I. The Occurrence of Ulcer in Relatives," *Am. J. Epidemiol.*, 91 (1970), 453–459.

113. MORRIS, P. J. "Familial Ulcerative Colitis," *Gut*, 6 (1965), 176–178.

114. NOORDENBOS, W. *Pain.* Amsterdam: Elsevier, 1959.

115. PAULLEY, J. W. "Regional Ileitis," *Lancet*, 1 (1948), 923.

116. ———. "Chronic Diarrhoea," *Proc. R. Soc. Med.*, 42 (1949), 241–244.

117. ———. "Psychosomatic Factors in the Aetiology of Acute Appendicitis," *Arch. Middlesex Hosp.*, 5 (1955), 35–41.

118. ———. "Emotion and Personality in the Etiology of Steatorrhea," *Am. J. Dig. Dis.*, 4 (1959), 352–360.

119. ———. "Crohn's Disease," *Psychother. Psychosom.*, 19 (1971), 111–117.

120. PEARL, J. M., W. P. RITCHIE, R. B. GILSDORF et al. "Hypothalamic Stimulation. Feline Gastric Mucosa Cellular Populations," *JAMA*, 195 (1966), 281–284.

121. PILOT, M. L., A. MUGGIA, and H. M. SPIRO. "Duodenal Ulcer in Women," *Psychosom. Med.*, 29 (1967), 586–597.

122. POSER, E. G. and S. G. LEE. "Thematic Content Associated with Two Gastrointestinal Disorders," *Psychosom. Med.*, 25 (1963), 162–173.

123. PRUGH, D. G. "A Preliminary Report on the Role of Emotional Factors in Idiopathic Celiac Disease," *Psychosom. Med.*, 13 (1951), 220–241.

124. REINHART, J. B. and R. A. SUCCOP. "Regional Enteritis in Pediatric Practice," *J. Am. Acad. Child Psychiatry*, 7 (1968), 252–281.

125. RHODES, J., H. T. APSIMON, and J. H. LAWRIE. "pH of the Contents of the Duodenal Bulb in Relation to Duodenal Ulcer," *Gut*, 7 (1966), 502–508.

126. RICHMOND, J. B., E. J. EDDY, and S. D. GARRARD. "The Syndrome of Fecal Soiling and Megacolon," *Am. J. Orthopsychiatry*, 24 (1954), 391–401.

127. RIEMER, M. D. "Ileitis—Underlying Aggressive Conflicts," *N.Y. State J. Med.*, 60 (1960), 552–557.

128. RITCHIE, J. A. and M. S. TUCKEY. "Intraluminal Pressure Studies at Different Distances from the Anus in Normal Subjects and in Patients with Irritable Colon Syndrome," *Am. J. Dig. Dis.*, 14 (1969), 96–106.

129. ROSENBAUM, M. "Psychosomatic Aspects of Patients with Peptic Ulcer," in E. Wittkower and R. A. Cleghorn, eds., *Recent Developments in Psychosomatic Medicine*, pp. 326–344. Philadelphia: Lippincott, 1954.

130. RUBIN, J., R. NAGLER, H. N. SPIRO et al. "Measuring the Effect of Emotions on Esophageal Motility," *Psychosom. Med.*, 24 (1962), 170–176.

131. SADLER, H. H. and A. V. ORTEN. "The Complementary Relationship between the Emotional State and the Function of the Ileum in a Human Subject," *Am. J. Psychiatry*, 124 (1968), 1375–1384.

132. SCHMALE, A. H. "Giving Up as a Final Common Pathway to Changes in Health," *Adv. Psychosom. Med.*, 8 (1972), 20–41.

133. SHORTER, R. G., K. H. HINZENGA, and R. J. SPENCER. "A Working Hypothesis for the Etiology and Pathogenesis of Nonspecific Inflammatory Bowel Disease," *Am. J. Dig. Dis.*, 17 (1972), 1024–1032.

134. SIFNEOS, P. E. *Ascent from Chaos. A Psychosomatic Case Study.* Cambridge: Harvard University Press, 1964.

135. SINGER, H. C., J. G. D. ANDERSON, H. FRISCHER et al. "Familial Aspects of Inflammatory Bowel Disease," *Gastroenterology*, 61 (1971), 423–430.

136. SLESINGER, M. H., M. DAVIDSON, J. H. PERT et al. "Recent Advances in the Physiology of the Esophagus," *N.Y. State J. Med.*, 55 (1955), 2747–2754.

137. SMITH, H. W., E. C. TEXTER, J. H. STICKLEY et al. "Intraluminal Pressures from the Upper Gastrointestinal Tract. II. Correlations with Gastroduodenal Motor Activity in Normal Subjects and Patients with Ulcer Distress," *Gastroenterology*, 32 (1957), 1025–1047.

138. STEIN, A., M. R. KAUFMAN, H. D. JANOWITZ et al. "Changes in Hydrochloric Acid Secretion in a Patient with a Gastric Fistula during Intensive Psychotherapy," *Psychosom. Med.*, 24 (1962), 427–458.

139. STEWART, W. A. "Psychosomatic Aspects of Regional Ileitis," *N.Y. State J. Med.*, 49 (1949), 2820–2824.

140. STOUT, G. and R. L. SYNDER. "Ulcerative Colitis-like Lesion in Siamang Gibbons," *Gastroenterology*, 57 (1969), 256–261.

141. SUN, O. C. H., H. SHAY, B. DLIN et al. "Conditioned Secretory Response of the Stomach Following Repeated Emotional

Stress in a Case of Duodenal Ulcer," *Gastroenterology*, 35 (1958), 155–165.

142. SUNDBY, H. S. and A. M. AUESTAD. "Ulcerative Colitis in Children. A Follow-Up Study with Special Reference to Psychosomatic Aspects," *Acta Psychiatr. Scand.*, 43 (1967), 410–423.

143. SZASZ, T. S. *Pain and Pleasure*. New York: Basic Books, 1957.

144. SZASZ, T. S., E. LEVIN, J. B. KIRSNER et al. "The Role of Hostility in the Pathogenesis of Peptic Ulcer," *Psychosom. Med.*, 9 (1947), 331–336.

145. THOMPSON, M. W. "Heredity, Maternal Age and Birth Order in Aetiology of Celiac Disease," *Am. J. Hum. Genet.*, 3 (1951), 159–166.

146. TRIPP, L. E. and D. P. AGLE. "Acute Pancreatitis as a Psychophysiologic Response: A Case Study," *Am. J. Psychiatry*, 124 (1968), 1253–1260.

147. TRUELOVE, S. C. "Movements of the Large Intestines," *Physiol. Rev.*, 46 (1966), 457–512.

148. WANGEL, A. G. and D. J. DELLER. "Intestinal Motility in Man. III. Mechanisms of Constipation and Diarrhea with Particular Reference to the Irritable Colon Syndrome," *Gastroenterology*, 48 (1965), 69–84.

149. WATKINS, G. L. and G. A. OLIVER. "Giant Megacolon in the Insane," *Gastroenterology*, 48 (1965), 718–727.

150. WEINER, H., M. THALER, M. F. REISER et al. "Etiology of Duodenal Ulcer. I. Relation of Specific Psychological Characteristics to Rate of Gastric Secretion (Serum Pepsinogen)," *Psychosom. Med.*, 19 (1957), 1–10.

151. WEISMAN, A. D. "A Study of the Psychodynamics of Duodenal Ulcer Exacerbations," *Psychosom. Med.*, 18 (1956), 2–42.

152. ———. "The Psychiatric Management of Duodenal Ulcer," *Int. Record Med.*, 170 (1957), 568–575.

153. WEISS, E. "Cardiospasm," *Am. J. Dig. Dis.*, 3 (1958), 275–284.

154. WEST, K. L. "MMPI Correlates of Ulcerative Colitis," *J. Clin. Psychol.*, 26 (1970), 214–219.

155. WHITE, B. V., S. COBB, and C. JONES. *Mucous Colitis. A Psychological Medical Study of 50 Cases*, Psychosom. Med. Monograph, NRC, 1939.

156. WHYBROW, P. C., F. J. KANE, and M. A. LIPTON. "Regional Ileitis and Psychiatric Disorder," *Psychosom. Med.*, 30 (1968), 209–221.

157. WIJSENBEEK, H., B. MAOZ, I. NITZAN et al. "Ulcerative Colitis, Psychiatric and Psychologic Study of 22 Patients," *Psychiatr. Neurol. Neurochir.*, 71 (1968), 409–420.

158. WILSON, G. "Typical Personality Trends and Conflicts in Cases of Spastic Colitis," *Psychoanal. Q.*, 3 (1934), 558–573.

159. WINKELSTEIN, A. "Psychogenic Factors in Cardiospasm," *Am. J. Surg.*, 12 (1931), 135–138.

160. WLODEK, G. K. "Gastric Mucosal Competence and Its Role in the Etiology of Peptic Ulcers," *Can. Med. Assoc. J.*, 99 (1968), 483–488.

161. WOLF, S. "Physiology of the Mucous Membranes and Direct Observations on Gastric and Colonic Function in Man," in S. Portis, ed., *Diseases of the Digestive System*, 3rd ed., pp. 183–208. Philadelphia: Lea & Fe'iger, 1953.

162. WOLF, S. and H. G. WOLFF. *Human Gastric Function*. London: Oxford University Press, 1947.

163. WOLFF, H. G. "Stress and Adaptive Patterns Resulting in Tissue Damage in Man," *Med. Clin. North Am.*, 39 (1955), 783–797.

164. ———. "The Mind-Body Relationship," in L. Bryson, ed., *An Outline of Man's Knowledge*, pp. 41–72. New York: Doubleday, 1960.

165. WOLFF, P. and J. LEVINE. "Nocturnal Gastric Secretion of Ulcer and Non-Ulcer Patients under Stress," *Psychosom. Med.*, 17 (1955), 218–226.

166. WOLOWITZ, H. M. and S. WAGONFELD. "Oral Derivatives in the Food Preferences of Peptic Ulcer Patients. An Experimental Study of Alexander's Psychoanalytic Hypothesis," *J. Nerv. Ment. Dis.*, 146 (1968), 18–23.

167. WORMSLEY, K. G. and M. I. GROSSMAN. "Maximal Histalog Test in Control Subjects and Patients with Peptic Ulcer," *Gut*, 6 (1965), 427–432.

168. YESSLER, P. G., M. F. REISER, and D. M. RIOCH. "Etiology of Duodenal Ulcer. II. Serum Pepsinogen and Peptic Ulcer in Inductees," *JAMA*, 169 (1959), 451–456.

CHAPTER 28

PSYCHOSOMATIC ASPECTS
OF BRONCHIAL ASTHMA[*]

Peter H. Knapp

⟨ Introduction

OBSERVATIONS bearing on the role of psychological factors in bronchial asthma have a long history. Hippocrates allegedly said "The asthmatic must guard against anger." Distinguished clinicians in the 18th century contributed anecdotal evidence about the role of emotions in precipitating or aggravating the disorder. As recently as 1971 a critical review of respiratory function in asthma remarked that "many asthmatic persons are somewhat unstable and it is admitted that the course of the disease may be affected by emotional or environmental factors."[10]

In the late 1930s, a group of psychiatric clinicians, most of them psychoanalytically inspired, along with physiologists and other basic scientists, turned their attention to a group of chronic diseases of unknown etiol-

ogy. Bronchial asthma was an early object of this psychosomatic scrutiny. The monograph on asthma by French and Alexander[23] reported a series of twenty-six cases treated by psychoanalysis, and surveyed the psychosomatic evidence then extant. Since that time the continuously expanding number of reports has been reviewed by Leigh,[47] Freeman et al.,[21] and Kelly.[38]

Various psychosomatic theories have been proposed, the best known of which is the thesis that asthma represents a "suppressed cry for the mother," originally stated by E. Weiss[89] and elaborated by French and Alexander.[23] Such views have seldom been rigorously tested, and still less solidly confirmed, although a thorough experiment in blind diagnosis from edited protocols, designed by Alexander and his colleagues to put his theories to test, did yield support for his original hypothesis about asthma.[6] Most of the reported studies have involved clinical and predominantly psychotherapeutic approaches,

[*] Supported in part by Grant MH 11299–05. Grateful acknowledgment is made of the criticism and assistance of A. A. Mathé, and L. Vachon.

the ultimate effects of which could only be ascertained by painstaking investigation over a long time. They have also frequently failed to explain their conceptual basis, and to specify by just what means and to what extent events in the psychological-social sphere are conceived as interacting with pulmonary processes. Finally they have often neglected to encompass knowledge about the complex pathophysiological aspects of asthma itself, which has undergone remarkable growth in the past decade.

This chapter will survey relatively recent work in four areas: (1) *Biological observations* which have thrown light on the pathogenesis of bronchial asthma and on pathways leading from brain to peripheral pulmonary tissues, in other words on potential psychosomatic mechanisms; (2) *psychophysiological studies*, offering evidence that short-term psychological influences, possibly utilizing such pathways, may contribute to acute exacerbations and remissions in asthmatic subjects; (3) *psychosocial studies*, suggesting that certain personality constellations, possibly extending short-range influences into chronic states of readiness, may correlate with the disorder; and (4) studies of *therapy*, examining various psychotherapeutic approaches to asthma, their limitations, and potential future directions.

❨ Biological Observations

The basic pathophysiological defect in bronchial asthma is reversible obstruction of the small airways. Presumably it results from smooth muscle spasm, edema of bronchiolar mucosa, hypersecretion, or possibly all three. A consequence of such obstruction is heightened resistance to the flow of air. Increase in airway resistance—or decrease in its reciprocal, airway conductance—is an essential index of asthmatic dysfunction. Without evidence about air flow, which many clinical reports lack, it is difficult to make meaningful statements about physical changes in an asthmatic patient.

Methods of assessing respiratory function have advanced rapidly in the past two decades. Relatively simple and easily applied techniques for estimating air flow, i.e. the timed vital capacity tracing and the peak-flow meter, suffer from some inaccuracy and are to a large extent dependent on voluntary effort. Since 1956 they have gradually been replaced by the whole-body plethysmograph which yields a rapid accurate sampling of airway conductance, corrected for lung volume, largely independent of effort. This was first applied to the study of psychiatric patients by Ottenberg and Stein,[71] later by Heim et al.,[30] Luparello,[50] and others. The instrument is cumbersome, expensive and requires some skilled cooperation. Additional techniques provide greater flexibility, i.e., flow-volume measurement, and the recently introduced respiratory resistance unit, which allows breath-by-breath assessment of total respiratory resistance.[25]

Studies of gas exchange and of total, as well as regional ventilation have also thrown light on asthma. Dudley and Martin and their colleagues, working with normal subjects, have demonstrated marked sensitivity of numerous respiratory indices to hypnotically induced emotion and pain.[18]

Their techniques and the previously mentioned measures of airway resistance all interfere with free bodily movement and occlude the mouth. As yet there is no satisfactory noninvasive way of monitoring the respiratory functions crucial to asthma. Useful approximations can be obtained by pneumograph tracings of external chest movement, calibrated against other respiratory indices. Heim et al.[31] have applied this approach to speaking subjects, and a number of groups are working with still greater refinements, integrating thoracic and abdominal tracings and using a sensitive magnetic pneumograph.[61]

Taken as a whole, these physiological methods have clarified the enormous range in severity of pulmonary dysfunction in asthma, which may or may not correlate with a patient's subjective impressions. They have shown complex impairments of elasticity and regional ventilation, the clinical significance of which is not entirely clear. Exercise also has a puzzling relationship to asthma, at times alleviating and at times aggravating the disorder.[10] Of great importance is the remarkably protracted and persistent impairment of pulmonary function following a severe attack.[53] Equally important is the well-established phenomenon of impaired gas exchange in asthma of more than mild degree. Decrease in arterial oxygen concentration appears early in severe attacks and requires careful monitoring; the concentration of CO_2 rises as a late manifestation when attacks continue and worsen. It can increase alarmingly, adding a marked respiratory acidosis to the effects of hypoxia, dehydration, and exhaustion, with which the patient is struggling; it may require correction by administration of bicarbonate.[65] Despite recent advances in pharmacotherapy, such severe episodes of *status asthmaticus* remain a frequent, life-threatening complication of the disease, calling for competent and vigilant therapeutic management.

The factors initiating all of these pulmonary changes are still obscure. Two pathogenetic views exist, each supported by a body of evidence and often zealous, if not myopic, proponents: the allergic-immunologic and the neurogenic.

The view of asthma as basically an allergic disorder has been paramount during most of this century. Clinically it is well known that asthmatics tend to have a family history of allergic sensitivity. Careful epidemiological studies support the concept of an hereditary predisposition,[78] although a recent study of 7000 twin pairs in Sweden by Edfors,[19] indicated that concordance for asthma in identical twins is only 18 percent, a surprisingly low figure which suggests a far greater role for environmental factors than had been thought previously.

In so-called "extrinsic" asthma, comprising possibly 40–60 percent of cases, a specific antibody, reagin, is demonstrable in the blood serum and is also present in the bronchial tissue of the predisposed individual. Binding of antigen to this specific antibody (immediate hypersensitivity, type I) results in the release of several substances, or mediators. These are still not fully understood. Histamine, serotonin, and bradykinin have been implicated,

as has a less clearly identified, slow reacting substance probably released from polymorphonuclear leucocytes.[70] So, more recently, have prostaglandins. Mathé and his colleagues, measuring airway conductance, found that ten asthmatic subjects were almost 8000 times more sensitive to prostaglandin F_2a than were ten matched control subjects.[58]

Factors governing the release and activity of such substances have also not been completely elucidated, particularly in the substantial proportion of cases where no extrinsic allergens can be demonstrated. Pulmonary infections are frequently associated with asthma, but it is not always known whether these constitute specific or nonspecific precipitants, or complications developing after the asthmatic process is already underway.

A crucial question for our purposes is whether the immunologic-allergic responses of the body are independent of influences from the brain. There is evidence to indicate a connection. Hypothalamic lesions or electrical stimulation of hypothalamic areas can induce changes not only in the autonomic nervous system but in immunologic reactivity. Tuberal lesions have proved capable of protecting the rat against fatal anaphylactic shock.[51] Anterior, but not posterior, hypothalamic lesions have had similar protective effects in the guinea pig.[85] In that species they have led to a significant decrease in circulating antibodies.[82] It may thus, in Szentivanyi's words, "be possible to profoundly alter the anaphylactic reactivity" of various animal species.[83]

Immunological and allergic factors may thus interact with neurophysiological and neurochemical influences on the pulmonary tree. The latter are complex in their own right. The role of the parasympathetic nervous system is a case in point. Vagal stimulation and parasympathomimetic agents produce an asthmalike response of the bronchial tree. Vachon et al.[87] have elicited a short-lived and mild but definite decrease in airway conductance in normal subjects by sudden immersion of their heads in water, apparently eliciting a vagal response via a central link, the so-called "diving reflex."[77]

These more or less pure parasympathetic

nervous effects tend to be transient and relatively mild. Airway-conductance deficits of from 15 to 20 percent are the rule. (We shall see that this holds also for effects of simple suggestion, which may also be vagally mediated.) Moreover, pharmacological blockade of the parasympathetic nervous system, or even vagotomy, have not proved effective in treating asthma. The theory that asthma represents a "vagotonic" disorder, prevalent at the turn of the century, was largely eclipsed in succeeding years by immunological advance.

However, careful experiments by Gold and his colleagues[24] have forced a reconsideration of the role of the vagus. Using dogs allergic to known antigens, they demonstrated that vagal blockade, both afferent and efferent, could eliminate the experimentally induced sharp rise in airway resistance. They showed furthermore, that unilateral challenge of one lung with antigen resulted in bilateral bronchoconstriction, also inhibited by vagal blockade on the challenged side. They concluded that "vagally mediated reflex broncho constriction, possibly arising from epithelial irritant receptors, is a major component of acute, antigen-induced canine asthma."[24] Only further investigation can tell whether these striking findings will be applicable in human asthmatic disease.

Advancing knowledge about the sympathetic nervous system adds to this picture of intricately balanced adaptive regulation of airway caliber. Ahlquist's formulation of alpha- and beta-adrenergic receptors, as two systems which have both overlapping and antagonistic functions, has drawn attention to the role of these receptors in asthma.[4] Some evidence has been offered[7] that the human lung has alpha adrenergic receptors, stimulation of which, contrary to usual thinking about adrenergic activity, can induce mild broncho constriction, although other evidence is contradictory on this point.[26] What is unequivocal is the fact that beta-adrenergic agents have maximal bronchodilating action, tending to override parasympathetic activity.[91] The most widely used, potent, short-range agent, having predominantly beta-adrenergic activity, is isoproterenol.

These facts have led to another line of investigation. Szentivanyi, working with mice, which usually show little allergic reactivity, exposed them to *Bordetella pertussis* and found that they then developed marked sensitivity to histamine and to various antigens.[83,84] He suggested that this altered state was an animal model of "beta-adrenergic blockade" and proposed a sweeping hypothesis: namely, that the key feature in human asthma was such a "blockade" of beta receptors, leaving the lungs prey to bronchoconstrictive reaction upon exposure to allergens, as well as to other noxious stimuli, including cold, infection, and emotional arousal.

Human studies yield some support for the clinical importance of this concept. It is well known that asthmatics are dangerously sensitive to the beta-adrenergic blocking agent, propranolol. Although earlier investigations using relatively insensitive methods failed to show a pulmonary effect in normal subjects,[93] McNeil and Ingram, using the body plethysmograph to measure five normal subjects, produced beta blockade by propranolol and found marked increase in airway resistance, varying from 40 to over 100 percent.[56] These findings in normal subjects of responses which approached the asthmatic range are unusual. They support the possibility, which is though by no means a certainty, that deficient beta-adrenergic responsivity could play a part in asthma. If so, we should note, it would not necessarily represent a fixed receptor lesion, but might equally well result from a reversible deficiency of circulating catecholamines (as suggested by Mathé.)[57,59,60] Conceivably this could play a role in the nocturnal incidence of many asthmatic attacks, although evidence is unclear on this point.[1,67]

Understanding is still incomplete of the additional steps mediating cellular responses following the action of catecholamines at receptor sites. The second messenger system, adenosine monophosphate (cyclic AMP), is probably involved;[84] and other messenger systems may play various roles (as indicated in the earlier reference to prostaglandins). For present purposes it is important to indicate the existing pathways that link brain processes with those occurring at the peripheral cellular level.

Obviously all these facts have important pharmacological implications. As noted, atropine and antihistamine drugs have only limited influence on the asthmatic process, in contrast to the powerful short-term effects of beta-adrenergic agents, notably isoproterenol. In severe asthma, one encounters limits posed by excitatory adrenergic side effects, particularly cardiovascular ones, as well as by the still puzzling phenomenon of "fastness" to adrenergic agents. Other drugs, such as aminophylline and especially corticoid substances, have important bronchodilatory action. The latter, as we shall see later, have their own complications, although so far no satisfactory substitute has been found for them.

An intriguing speculation is that tricyclic antidepressant drugs, thought to mobilize catecholamine stores in the brain, might have some beneficial central and also peripheral effect in asthma; preliminary evidence supports such a possibility,[8,62] though the putative mode of action is obscure.

To summarize: Physiological regulation of lung function represents a complex adaptive balance; its accurate study is necessary to provide precise knowledge about the wide range of pathophysiological respiratory function encountered in asthma.

Immunologic-allergic reactions can lead to a broncho obstructive asthmatic response. However, it seems unlikely that they are the sole cause of asthma, particularly in the substantial number of chronic asthmatics without clear evidence of extrinsic allergy. There is reason to believe that immunological systems may be integrated with the parasympathetic nervous system centrally or peripherally or both. Nervous influences may augment or decrease the final broncho obstructive process.

The sympathetic nervous system may also be important in the etiology of asthma. Relative deficiency of beta-adrenergic function may aggravate the disorder because of failure to counteract persistence of basic immunologic and/or parasympathetic nervous activity. A second, radical hypothesis is that some sort of "beta-adrenergic deficit" is fundamental in

asthma, allowing allergic as well as other noxious influences to produce the disorder. A third, more general possibility is that there is a reciprocal balance between bronchodilating (beta-adrenergic) and bronchoconstrictive (immunologic and parasympathetic) influences, both having links to the brain; and that asthma may represent an acute or chronic imbalance between the two.

Clearly mechanisms are available permitting psychological factors to play a role in asthma, either in conjunction with allergy or possibly at times by themselves. We next must ask what is the psychophysiological and psychosocial evidence for their activity.

⟮ Psychophysiological Observations

Acute Exacerbation and Remission

The physiological considerations just mentioned may throw light on a paradox that has puzzled students of asthma. Acute attacks often occur in a setting of turmoil and anxiety, both in adults[43] and children.[28] Hahn found elevations in both heart rate and skin temperature in asthmatic, as compared with normal, children and concluded that there was sustained activation of some parts of the sympathetic nervous system.[28] One is faced with the troublesome question of why the asthmatic patient, in a state of turmoil and arousal, does not "cure himself."

Experimental stress should throw some light on this matter. Mathé and Knapp[59,60] used as stressful stimuli a film and a mathematical task carried out under negative criticism. No effort was made to differentiate the "first-day" stress from these experimental stimuli. Their subjects were eight mild asthmatics free of symptoms and not requiring medicine, and eight comparison subjects matched for age and socioeconomic status. All dietary and activity factors relevant to catecholamine excretion were controlled. Asthmatics and normals alike responded with increase in heart rate, blood pressure, and circulating corticoids under stress as compared to the control day. As expected, asthmatics differed significantly in their respiratory responses, showing a decrease in airway conductance, as well as slowing of respiration. In addition they showed a highly significant difference in free fatty acid response and epinephrine excretion. Both of these measures were elevated in the control subjects under stress but remained strikingly constant in the asthmatic subjects. Subjectively the asthmatics also reported increases in anxiety and in overall affect but differed on one emotional dimension: they reported significantly less anger in the provoking experimental circumstances. A partial repetition of this work, confirming the faulty mobilization of epinephrine excretion, has been recorded by Bernstein and Greenland.[11] These findings are consistent with the view that some kind of adrenergic defect does play a role in acute asthma.

Physiological considerations are also important in evaluating studies of *learning* in bronchial asthma. Classical conditioning of asthma was reported by Noelpp-Eschenhagen and Noelpp[68] who exposed guinea pigs to an allergic stimulus, provoking a dyspneic asthmalike response; later this was obtained merely by introducing the animals to the experimental chamber. More recently Justesen, Braun, et al.[37] described similar conditioned "asthma" in guinea pigs and used a variety of pharmacological influences to affect this response. Both of these studies must be questioned, however, in the light of the careful work of Ottenberg and Stein[72] and of Stein and Schiavi.[75,82] These authors showed that the preponderant effect observed in attempts at conditioning is hyperventilation, presumably as part of a diffuse stress reaction. By careful measurement of airway resistance they were able to identify an apparently true asthmatic response and to obtain this in a small number of animals as a true learned response. However, it readily extinguished, and extrapolation to the human disorder is difficult.

In humans, Dekker, Pelser, and Groen[16] attempted to show conditioning. However, their results were inconstant and their measurement technique, the timed vital capacity, was relatively crude. Effects of suggestion or pseudo-

conditioning could not be excluded in those cases who did show some increase in timed vital capacity. Sloanaker and Luminet[79] used a classical paradigm, exposing subjects in a closed-breathing circuit to a parasympathomimetic stimulus (mecholyl) preceded by a tone. In a small number of instances they obtained a possible conditional asthmalike response, but, again, chance or suggestive effect could not be excluded. We must conclude that there is no convincing evidence for classical conditioning in the strict sense as a cause of bronchial asthma in the human. The possibility remains that classical sequences, such as strong emotions associated with prior asthma, may serve as conditional triggering stimuli for subsequent attacks.

An alternative approach is found in the operant paradigm. Vachon[86] used the respiratory resistance unit, which gives a breath-by-breath feedback of information; this was computer processed and fed back to subjects. He worked with two groups of mild asymptomatic asthmatics, fifteen in one and thirteen in another. They were instructed to keep a red light on, programmed to flash when their resistance fell below a critical level. They were also given a monetary reward. The result was a "learned" drop in airway resistance in both groups of experimental subjects. They differed significantly from control subjects exposed to the same situation but given purely random reinforcement. The decrease in resistance was modest, about 15 percent. How reproducible and lasting, in short, how clinically significant the change was, remains to be determined, as does the question of whether its extent can be increased.

Suggestion (which perhaps should be regarded as a variant of learning, capitalizing on either acquired associations, or implied reinforcement, or both) has also intrigued students of asthma ever since Sir James McKenzie's vivid description in 1886 of "rose asthma" (that is, acute coryza and respiratory congestion accompanied by wheezing) induced in a young woman by the sight of a paper rose.[55] Dekker and Groen[15] reported a number of attacks in subjects, which followed exposure to pictorial or verbal suggestions of objects or substances to which they were sensitive. Their results were not uniform; the extent and mechanism of the asthmalike response remain unclear. Luparello et al.[50] and McFadden, Luparello, and Lyons[54] carried out body plethysmographic studies of forty subjects exposed to saline aerosol, suggesting that it was either an allergenic precipitant to which they had been found sensitive, or a bronchodilator. In approximately half of their subjects they found clear-cut changes in airway conductance in the suggested direction. The effect was blocked by atropine, pointing to an acute vagal influence. Weiss[90] was unable to confirm this suggestive effect in children, possibly because he used less sensitive measures. White[92] also, using the less sensitive timed vital capacity, attempted by hypnosis to influence asthmatics suffering from clinical disease. As a group they reported subjective relief, but gave no objective evidence of improved pulmonary function.

Environmental change has played a time-honored role with asthmatics, particularly children. Many clinical observations have indicated that when a child is sent away from his family, whether to a hospital, school, or camp, his asthma improves, at least initially. The suspicion followed that one might be removing the child from noxious interaction with family members, especially his mother. Abramson and Peshkin have even talked of the beneficial effects of "parentectomy."[3]

An obvious question is whether social or allergenic factors were changed. Lamont[46] and his collaborators hospitalized children allegedly sensitive to house dust in their homes. The investigators then secured house dust from each home and distributed it copiously in each child's hospital room. In nineteen of twenty cases no asthma ensued. Purcell et al.[73] carried out an even more rigorous experiment with thirty-five children. They paid their parents to take a vacation away from home, and brought in an experienced nurse to make daily measurements of medication, respiratory symptoms, and peak air flow. Though some children seemed to have mild anticipatory anxiety, at times accompanied by symptoms, the main effect was, as predicted, im-

provement in their asthmatic status in the absence of their parents. Again this was modest in scope and occurred in about half of their subjects. It was of further interest that, on the basis of a brief specially designed diagnostic interview, the authors were able to predict with a high degree of success which children would show improvement and which would not.

Such observations on separation from the home environment fit with earlier reports of Purcell, Bernstein, and Bukantz,[73] indicating that two types of children appeared to be admitted to the Children's Asthma Research Hospital in Denver. They labelled these rapid remitters and steroid dependent, respectively. The former cleared up rapidly; the latter had persistent intractable symptoms and required continued steroid medication. The authors found more obvious neurotic difficulties, both in the children and in their families, in the rapid remitters. They postulated two distinct types of asthma, one more psychosocial in origin, the other more biological. However, one cannot be sure that they ruled out more subtle emotional conflicts, perhaps deep-seated and masked by denial, nor that they excluded a possible physiological chain of events which kept children bound to maintenance steroids, partly on an iatrogenic basis. We will see a similar debate about long-term personality trends in asthmatics. It is worth noting that Kinsman, Luparello, and their colleagues,[39] studying acute symptom patterns in adults, rather than finding simple dichotomous distribution, noted a complex patterning of subjective symptomatology, based around five clusters of symptoms: panic-fear, irritability, hyperventilation–hypercapnia, bronchoconstriction, and fatigue.

To *summarize*: Acute changes in airway conductance can occur in response to psychosocial stimuli in certain subjects. Presumably these are mediated by the parasympathetic nervous system, that is, vagal influences on the upper airways.

Somewhat more sustained changes in airway conductance, probably involving altered neuroendocrine balance, may be related to specific impairment of epinephrine mobilization. Conceivably this may be a function of altered patterns of arousal, in particular partial mobilization of aggressive impulses along with inhibition of their full expression.

These findings point to avenues whereby learning may influence moment-to-moment airway patency. Classical conditioning has yet to be demonstrated to play a significant role in human asthma, although its participation in triggering attacks cannot be excluded. Possibly more important is the role of operant learning, in which subjects achieve change to gain reinforcement. Preliminary evidence suggests that this can influence airway resistance, though the extent and lasting nature of the effect remains to be shown.

Regardless of the exact nature of mediating pathways, there is strong evidence that remission of asthma may be brought about in certain subjects by interruption of on-going pathogenic interaction, especially with parental figures. The assertion remains open, but not proved, that these subjects represent a distinct subgroup, comprising about 50 percent of severe perennial asthmatics; they may have prominent "neurotic" elements in their exacerbations, in contrast to other patients with a more permanent "organic" basis.

❡ Psychosocial Observations

Long-term Factors in Bronchial Asthma

It seems wise to return to the assumption stated earlier that asthma as a long-term disorder almost invariably requires some biological vulnerability, hereditary or (conceivably in some instances) acquired in early years. The classical life history is that of a child with a positive family history who develops allergic manifestations, usually eczema, in his first year of life, followed by respiratory difficulty, coming on gradually in the second or third year, often associated with infection, which then develops into typical periodic obstructive disease running its complex fluctuating course.

Although the predisposition is probably always lifelong, many major variations occur in its course. Approximately half of the children with infantile eczema do not develop asthma. A crucial study of family differences among those who do and those who do not has been undertaken, but not yet completed, by Meijer.[63] Asthmatics change with chronological age. There is allegedly a preponderance of males among asthmatic children, and of females among adults, though recent accurate studies bearing on this distribution are not available. We do know that some children "grow out" of asthma in adolescence. While they are growing out, others are "growing in." Asthma in midlife seems to have special features. It may run an acute, even fatal course; often it seems to resemble a midlife depression, as illustrated in cases described by Knapp and Nemetz.[43–45] Recovery, when it takes place, may seem relatively complete. Often in such cases a strong family history is absent. As with many chronic diseases, a sudden onset relatively late in life may carry an improved prognosis, providing the patient weathers the acute phase successfully.

Other specific features have been sought in populations of asthmatic patients. Studies purporting to show EEG abnormality have been reviewed by Leigh and Pond,[48] who conclude that asthmatics are not different from other "psychiatric" patients; the authors explicitly leave open the rather tenuous possibility that all such patients may differ from "normals."

The incidence among different cultural groups is unclear. Anecdotal reports have suggested a higher frequency of asthma among Puerto Rican immigrants to large inner cities, such as New York and Boston. However, valid epidemiologic evidence has not been forthcoming; and the relative role of sociocultural stress, as against air pollution, inadequate heating, infection, dietary deficiency, and other factors, cannot be ascertained.

The family structure of asthmatics has been a focus of much attention. A number of studies have dealt with mother and child. The early notion of a "rejecting" mother[64] yielded to that of an "engulfing" one.[2] An investigation by Block et al.[12] suggests that clinicians working with asthma are not in complete agreement about maternal characteristics, raising the possibility of more than one subgroup of mothers and children. Freeman and her colleagues[21] bring evidence that there may be a reciprocal relationship between the allergic potential of a child and psychopathology in the mother. The authors suggest two types of disease, one primarily biogenic, the other sociogenic. This and other efforts to dichotomize the population of asthmatic mothers and children—as in the work of Purcell, Bernstein and Buchantz[73] already mentioned—risk overlooking the role of denial. Some mothers may have a powerful need to overemphasize putative biological contributions to the children's illness and to minimize psychosocial conflict. Jacobs and his colleagues in two studies[33,34] tested young adult males with hay fever and mild asthma, using selected indices of biological reactivity, along with a battery of projective tests administered on a "blind basis." The subjects perceived their mothers retrospectively as controlling or rejecting or both; their feelings in this respect differentiated them from the healthy comparison group. It was possible, on a basis of both "allergic potential" alone and "psychologic potential" alone, for blind judges successfully to select individuals who showed actual manifestations of allergic disease. Jacobs' hypothesis was additive: that both psychological and biological factors are widely distributed in the allergic population and that their combined strength determines the severity of the disorder.

We are entering an area which requires complex estimates of family constellations and inner psychological processes. Surface factors may directly contradict and mask hidden elements. Objective methods to measure such balanced forces are not available, and we must rely on more subjective clinical judgments. These have come chiefly from psychoanalytically oriented investigations of a small number of cases. Some of these are summarized below, recognizing their limitations but feeling that their insight cannot be ignored. It remains to be seen whether future large-scale, methodologically more refined, studies will verify them.

Examining a small number of children in psychoanalytically oriented psychotherapy and in psychoanalysis, Jessner and her associates[35,36] found evidence of continuing oscillation between attempts on the part of the asthmatic patient to separate from the mother and to achieve intense erotized closeness. Sperling[80] elaborated this pattern, underlining the existence of faulty differentiation between mother and child. She felt that mothers of asthmatic children, like those of young patients with other psychosomatic diseases, could tolerate their child only when ill. This viewpoint, phrased in other terms, suggests that the mother may inadvertently provide powerful sustained reinforcement of the asthmatic process.

Fathers may play an important auxiliary role. Jacobs' retrospective studies with allergic subjects suggest that fathers of asthmatics tend to be absent in one or another way, either physically out of the home, aloof, or ineffective, so that they fail to correct the imbalance between mother and child.[33,34]

These findings might lead one to expect consistent *characterological* features in patients suffering from asthma, and there is clinical evidence that these do exist. Some of them center around conflictual concerns which are relatively specific and perhaps have a somatopsychic basis: sensitivity to odors, concern about water, sleep, crying, and use of the voice. Stein and Ottenberg[81] and Herbert[32] offer evidence that asthmatics as a group have a heightened sensitivity to odors, which at times antedates the onset of asthmatic symptoms. McDermott and Cobb[52] reported that fears of water or of drowning were more common and intense in asthmatics than in comparison subjects, thus partially confirming what a number of clinicians, for example Deutsch[17] reported. Excessive secretion in the respiratory tract can lead to a state in which the individual feels close to drowning in his own fluids, and such experiences could well mold the anxieties of the asthmatic.

Asthmatic attacks tend to develop at night, often waking the sufferer from sleep, frequently being interwoven with bizarre sleep patterns. It has not been possible to identify asthma clearly with the REM phase of sleep,[29] nor with variations of the diurnal cycle of catecholamine or cortisol secretion, although all of these features may play some role.

Early studies of asthmatics suggested that weeping, crying, and related vocalization were often stirred up, yet were conflictual and not easily expressed. Such "suppressed crying," as French and Alexander put it in their familiar formulation,[23] might be part of the acute process of asthma, though obviously not specific for that disorder alone. Concern with the voice and the process of speech itself seems at times to be closely related to asthmatic symptoms, possibly connected with inhibition of powerful primitive aggressive impulses, as Bacon[9] speculates. Knapp[41] and Nemetz[44] reported a number of cases in which episodes of aphonia were strikingly interwoven with asthmatic symptomatology. They discussed the possibility, raised by earlier clinicians,[69] that sensitizing life experiences, including close interpersonal experiences with an individual suffering from respiratory disease, might contribute to the later development of asthma as a form of primitive or "pregenital" conversion symptom. Occasional reports keep this possibility alive; for example, a striking case mentioned by Lofgren,[49] in which a patient had been nearly strangled in childhood, and an example of Coolidge's of asthma in three successive mother-daughter generations.[14]

These reported conflicts influence other habitual character traits. Alternation of asthmatic symptoms with overt psychotic manifestations may occur, although this appears to be the exception, not the rule.[43] Chessick et al. reported that the most frequent chronic disease among narcotic addicts at the U. S. Public Health Hospital, Lexington, Kentucky was asthma.[13]

Other clinical observations have suggested that asthmatics as a group have unusually strong passive and dependent personality traits, reflecting needs to maintain gratification and support from key persons in their environment. This form of personality organization is obviously not unique to asthmatics. At times, furthermore, it appears to be subjected to a kind of personality "counterrevolution" in which a surface picture of marked assertiveness becomes dominant, perhaps assisting the individual in some way to overcome his illness. Frequent anecdotal reports describe children hospitalized for asthma, recovering symptomatically from their disorder and becoming aggressive behavior problems. The more frequent finding is that hints of hidden aggressive impulses, appearing only briefly, are followed by intensification of asthma, often with evidence of guilty depressive feeling. In a study of psychoanalytic material from one patient, two psychoanalysts using a model of primitive impulse-arousal plus failure of psychological defenses, studied notes of sessions immediately before twenty-five exacerbations of asthma and twenty-five comparison sessions from the same period of the treatment. Notes were edited to remove medical cues; as a further control they were given to two allergist-internists who attempted the same task. The psychoanalysts were able to select "asthmatic" contexts from neutral comparison contexts with significant success, whereas the allergists' results were only at a chance level.[42]

A clinical hypothesis to account for these observations is that many asthmatics have a deep and early developmental personality defect, which leaves them both attached to a parental figure and subject to powerful aggressive impulses of an early infantile type. Some of these may have a particularly sadistic flavor. The hidden sadistic components have been striking in a series of our patients[41] studied psychoanalytically. Full emergence of such impulses would threaten their "partial symbiotic" attachment, so that when aggression is aroused it is in some way "switched off" and results in asthma. (One is tempted to speculate about connections with a possible parallel defect in adrenergic catecholamine mobilization mentioned earlier.) It is interesting that detailed biographical material of a famous asthmatic, Marcel Proust, supports this picture of a passive loving son attached to and deeply identified with his mother. He showed unmistakable evidence of hidden sadistic perverse impulses.[41]

To *summarize*: Long-term psychological or social patterns associated with asthma can be defined only tentatively. There appears to be an interaction between hereditary vulnerability and the early environment. The exact nature of their respective roles is uncertain; so is the question of whether we are dealing with a simple dichotomy of allergic versus sociopsychologic cases, as advocated by some, or with a more variable spectrum.

Concerns with odors and water, and conflicts over crying and over use of the voice may be partly related to heightened somatic responsivity in a somatic subject. Other characterological features, although colored by somatic illness, often antedate it and appear related to early experience with the human environment. These pertain to fears of separation from the mother, and to primitive impulses often of a sadistic destructive nature, deeply hidden and defended against by passive, dependent, and masochistic personality organization. Such traits are not unique for asthmatics but may interact with other factors localizing a somatic process in the pulmonary system, and thus contribute to the overall picture of the disease.

❰ Therapeutic Considerations

If, indeed, we are dealing with a lifelong, often life-threatening disorder, having multiple etiologic factors and running a fluctuating course, the problem of evaluating therapy is inevitably difficult.

These considerations apply to all therapy in bronchial asthma, including reports of medical measures. As Bates, Macklem, and Christie remark:[10] "In no other common disorder have so many different therapeutic approaches been adopted and it is suspicious that many of these are credited with improving the condition." They add that "spontaneous improvement and remission are common, often occurring independently of any change in treatment," though one must add that a careful search for any change in life situation must be conducted before one can be sure change is entirely "spontaneous." If there is any truth to the assertion that asthmatics are sensitive to personal relationships, the influence of these

must be considered in reports of success with allergic or other measures. In all assessments of therapeutic results the severity of cases treated must be carefully specified, as well as the amount and kind of all modalities of treatment. Therapy which produces amelioration must be distinguished from therapy which approaches long-range cure. As a rule, ethical considerations demand, at least in patients with asthma of any severity, that some medical allergic management go along with psychotherapy.

A particular problem is posed by steroid medications. In the short run these have changed the picture of the management. Terrifying episodes of *status asthmaticus* can be brought under control and immediate dangers to life greatly diminished. However, the long-term effects are far from clear. Schneer[76] cites evidence that mortality in children with asthma is as great a decade after the introduction of steroids as it was before their advent. Certainly the persistent complications and side effects, i.e., electrolyte imbalance, hypertension, or tendency to peptic ulcer, present hazards. They are compounded by the states of dependence which patients develop. These appear to have a clearly physiological basis. Removal of steroids leads to a characteristic state of lassitude and weakness, and in asthmatics, a proneness to explosive and drastic exacerbation, sometimes itself fatal. Yet occasionally in our experience, possibly aided by a variety of therapeutic modalities, including careful medical weaning, also with psychotherapeutic support, patients who have been receiving large amounts of steroid medication do recover and function without the need for medication.

Antidepressive Measures

These have been tried in a sporadic fashion with asthmatics. In sudden late-life asthma, electric shock has been occasionally used, although there are no systematic evaluations of its effect. Experimental evidence of possible bronchodilatory effects of antidepressant medication has led to clinical reports of their use, though these are scattered and inconclusive.[62]

Suggestive Measures, Hypnosis

Although hypnosis may be unable to affect the fully established pathophysiological process, it is possible that hypnotherapy may have long-term benefits. Falliers[20] studied 120 asthmatic patients, using 115 control subjects, also suffering from asthma. The experimental group was treated with brief rapid-induction hypnosis at weekly intervals. Control subjects were treated with body relaxation. Both groups showed improvement, the females significantly more with hypnosis. By the end of a year in the hypnotized group 59 percent were better and 8 percent worse; the control-group figures were 43 percent better and 17 percent worse; the difference between the groups was significant at the 5-percent level. One patient in each group was dead. One cannot exclude a general "physician-interest" effect, and it would be interesting to know more about the exact characteristics of the patients involved. Nevertheless, a beginning in the study of an important treatment modality is represented here.

Relaxation

This form of quasisuggestive therapy has also been tried, mostly with children. A study by Alexander et al.[5] shows some effects, mostly in mild cases, of relaxation instructions, relayed to the subjects in different ways. The approach has a certain logic. Clinically many asthmatics state that if they can only "relax," their tightness, wheezing, and congestion seem to improve. It will be necessary to await further results before we can fully assess the clinical importance of this approach.

Behavior Modification

There are only a few systematic studies of this form of treatment. Walton[88] used Wolpe's method of "reciprocal inhibition" successfully with one case. Moore[66] extended his observations in a controlled study, comparing systematic "desensitization" with two other treatment modalities, simple suggestion and a relaxation therapy. She studied twelve subjects, half of them children, in a balanced incomplete block design so that two forms of treatment were given to every patient, and each of the three treatments could be compared in eight subjects. All three forms of treatment led to some subjectively reported improvement. Significantly more improvement in peak air flow, the physiological measure used, was found in the group which had reciprocal inhibition. The strength of this study lies in the fact that the patients were their own controls. However, the numbers were small. A major share of the variance was contributed by two subjects who received reciprocal inhibition as their first treatment, and had a rather marked effect from it. It is possible that individual differences in such a small group of subjects still played a major role. Few details were given about the initial status of the patients and the severity of their illness. The study needs replication, but is nevertheless a model for systematically controlled investigation of therapeutic approaches in this area.

Operant Conditioning

This method, using the biofeedback model, is technically available after the initial studies of Vachon,[86] but it has not yet been systematically applied as a therapy.

Group Therapy

Groen[27] reports an intensive group-therapy experience in the Netherlands. It involved weekly meetings with patients and an extensive supportive medical and milieu regime. Results were positive, but the large number of variables involved makes definitive assessment difficult.

Long-term Psychoanalytically Oriented Psychotherapy

This method was applied to the original series of twenty-six adults and children reported by French and Alexander.[23] They described substantial improvement in their series but did not give detailed physiological or other follow-up data. The approach has also been applied to severely incapacitated patients by Knapp,[40,41] Sperling,[80] and others. One can argue logically that such a long-term approach is indicated if one accepts the evidence of early disturbance in mother-child relationships and deep, primitive personality disorganization in many asthmatic patients. The classical analytic approach must be modified, most observers state, as many individuals suffer from severe personality disturbances. It is necessary to think of severe asthmatics as suffering from "borderline" or "narcissistic" disturbance, though this may be masked by many effective areas of functioning. Different strategies are possible within this general psychoanalytic framework, such as the more egonurturant empathic approach advocated by some, or a more confrontative and active attack on the defensive and gratifying "use" of symptoms by a subject, as advocated by Sperling.[80] No real evidence can decide between these, considering the lack of definitive long-term assessment of all therapeutic results with asthma.

In *conclusion*: Given the tentative nature of therapeutic evidence, what should a psychiatrist advise for an asthmatic? He is probably wisest if he approaches patients with this "psychosomatic" disorder on the basis of their obvious psychopathology. As with all forms of psychiatric treatment at this time, he must be guided by his own beliefs and experience, and must try to carry out therapy systematically with the hope that time and the accumulation of clinical knowledge will make it possible to sort the wheat of results from the chaff of claims.

Two contrasting cautions are important: the psychiatrist should respect the potential seriousness of the biological process and utilize sophisticated medical knowledge, which in most cases means a sophisticated medical colleague, as part of the total treatment plan. Yet he should respect the remarkable capacity of psychological conflict to lurk behind a screen of "real" physiological symptoms; he must be prepared to stick to his insight when he senses such conflict, though the patient, the family, and even the attending physician may rationalize it away as an unfortunate by-product of physical suffering. Time-limited and controlled approaches are valuable for purposes of comparative study, particularly of mild cases; but in severe asthma one faces a complicated problem of long-term management, and a long-term relationship with an individual whose somatic and psychic difficulties are extraordinarily intertwined.

(Bibliography

1. ABBASY, A. S., M. S. FAHMY, and M. M. KANTOUSH. "The Adrenal Glucocorticoid Function in Asthmatic Children," *Acta Paediatr. Scand.*, 56 (1967), 593–600.
2. ABRAMSON, H. A. "Evaluation of Maternal Rejection Theory in Allergy," *Ann. Allergy*, 12 (1954), 129.
3. ABRAMSON, H. A. and M. M. PESHKIN. "Group Psychotherapy of the Parents of Intractably Asthmatic Children," *J. Childr. Asthma Res. Inst. Hosp.*, 1 (1961), 77.
4. AHLQUIST, R. P. "The Adrenergic Receptors," *J. Pharm. Sci.*, 55 (1966), 359–67.
5. ALEXANDER, B. "Systematic Relaxation in Asthmatic Children," *Psychosom. Med.*, 34 (1972), 389.
6. ALEXANDER, F., T. M. FRENCH and G. POLLOCK. *Psychosomatic Specificity*, Vol. 1, *Experimental Study and Results*. Chicago: University of Chicago Press, 1968.
7. ANTHRACITE, R. F., L. VACHON, and P. H. KNAPP. "Alpha-adrenergic Receptors in the Human Lung," *Psychosom. Med.*, 33 (1971), 481–489.
8. AVNI, J. and I. BRUDERMAN. "The Effect of Amitryptymine on Pulmonary Ventilation and the Mechanics of Breathing," *Pharmacologia*, 14 (1969), 184–192.
9. BACON, C. "The Role of Aggression in the Asthmatic Attack," *Psychoanal. Q.*, 25 (1956), 309–324.
10. BATES, D. V., P. T. MACKLEM, and R. V. CHRISTIE. *Respiratory Function in Disease*, Philadelphia: Saunders, 1971.
11. BERNSTEIN, I. L. and R. GREENLAND. "Catechol Excretion in Asthma," (Abstract), *Fed. Proc.*, 32 (1973), 813.
12. BLOCK, J., E. HARVEY, P. H. JENNING et al. "Clinicians' Conceptions of the Asthmato-

genic Mother," *Arch. Gen. Psychiatry*, 15 (1966), 610.

13. CHESSICK, R. D., M. D. KURLAND, R. M. HUSTED et al. "The Asthmatic Narcotic Addict," *Psychosomatics*, 1 (1960), 346.

14. COOLIDGE, J. C. "Asthma in Mother and Child as a Special Type of Intercommunication," *Am. J. Orthopsychiatry*, 26 (1956), 165.

15. DEKKER, F. and J. GROEN. "Reproducible Psychogenic Attacks of Asthma," *J. Psychosom. Res.*, 1 (1956), 58–67.

16. DEKKER, F., H. E. PELSER, and J. GROEN. "Conditioning as a Cause of Asthmatic Attacks," *J. Psychosom. Res.*, 2 (1957), 96.

17. DEUTSCH, F. "Basic Psychoanalytic Principles in Psychosomatic Disorders," *Acta Ther.*, 1 (1953), 102–111.

18. DUDLEY, D. L., T. H. HOLMES, C. J. MARTIN et al. "Changes in Respiration Associated with Hypnotically Induced Emotion Pain and Exercise," *Psychosom. Med.*, 26 (1964), 46–57.

19. EDFORS-LUBS, M. L. "Allergy in 7000 Twin Pairs," *Acta Allergol.* 26 (1971), 249–285.

20. FALLIERS, C. J. "Hypnosis for Asthma—A Controlled Study," *Br. Med. J.*, 31 (1968), 476–479.

21. FREEMAN, E. H., B. F. FEINGOLD, K. SCHLESINGER et al. "Psychological Factors in Allergy: A Review," *Psychosom. Med.*, 26 (1964), 543–575.

22. FREEMAN, E. H., F. J. GORMAN, M. T. SINGER et al. "Personality Variables and Allergic Skin Reactions: A Cross Validation Study," *Psychosom. Med.*, 29 (1967), 312–332.

23. FRENCH, T. M. and F. ALEXANDER. "Psychogenic Factors in Bronchial Asthma," *Psychosom. Med. Monogr.*, 4 (1941), 2–94.

24. GOLD, W. M., G. R. KESSLER, and D. Y. C. YU. "Role of Vagus Nerves in Experimental Asthma in Allergic Dogs," *J. Appl. Physiol.*, 33 (1972), 719–725.

25. GOLDMAN, M., R. J. KNUDSON, J. MEAD et al. "A Simplified Measurement of Respiratory Resistance by Forced Oscillation," *J. Appl. Physiol.*, 28 (1970), 113.

26. GRIECO, M. H., R. N. PIERSON, and F. X. PI SUNYER. "Comparison of the Circulatory and Metabolic Effects of Isoproterenol, Epinephrine and Methoxamine in Normal and Asthmatic Subjects," *Am. J. Med.*, 44 (1968), 863.

27. GROEN, J. "Experience with and Results of Group Therapy with Bronchial Asthma," *J. Psychosom. Res.*, 4 (1960), 191.

28. HAHN, W. "Automatic Responses of Asthmatic Children," *Psychosom. Med.*, 28 (1966), 323.

29. HARTMAN, E. *The Biology of Dreaming.* Springfield, Ill.: Charles C. Thomas, 1967.

30. HEIM, E., H. CONSTANTINE, P. H. KNAPP et al. "Airway Resistance and Emotional States in Bronchial Asthma," *Psychosom. Med.*, 29 (1967), 450–467.

31. HEIM, E., P. H. KNAPP, L. VACHON et al. "Emotion, Breathing and Speech," *J. Psychosom. Res.*, 12 (1968), 261–274.

32. HERBERT, M., R. GLICK, and H. BLACK. "Olfactory Precipitants of Bronchial Asthma," *J. Psychosom. Res.*, 11 (1967), 195–202.

33. JACOBS, M. A. et al. "Incidence of Psychosomatic Predisposing Factors in Allergic Disorders," *Psychosom. Med.*, 28 (1966), 679–695.

34. JACOBS, M. A., L. S. ANDERSON, H. D. EISMAN et al. "Interaction of Psychologic and Biologic Predisposing Factors in Allergic Disorders," *Psychosom. Med.*, 29 (1967), 572–585.

35. JESSNER, L. "The Psychoanalysis of an Eight-Year-Old Boy with Asthma," in H. I. Schneer, ed., *The Asthmatic Child*, pp. 118–137. New York: Harper & Row, 1963.

36. JESSNER, L., J. LAMONT et al. "Emotional Impact of Nearness and Separation for the Asthmatic Child and His Mother," in *The Psychoanalytic Study of the Child*, Vol. 10, p. 353–375. New York: International Universities Press, 1955.

37. JUSTESEN, D. R., E. W. BRAUN, R. G. GARRISON et al. "Pharmacologic Differentiation of Allergic and Classically Conditioned Asthma in the Guinea Pig," *Science*, 170 (1970), 864–866.

38. KELLY, E. "Asthma and Psychiatry," *J. Psychosom. Res.*, 13 (1969), 377.

39. KINSMAN, R. A., T. J. LUPARELLO, K. O'BANION et al. "Multidimensional Analysis of the Subjective Symptomatology of Asthma," *Psychosom. Med.*, 35 (1973), 250–266.

40. KNAPP, P. H. "The Asthmatic Child and the Psychosomatic Problem of Asthma," in H. I. Schneer, ed., *The Asthmatic Child*, pp. 234–255. New York: Harper & Row, 1963.

41. ———. "The Asthmatic and His Environ-

ment," *J. Nerv. Ment. Dis.*, 149 (1969), 133.

42. KNAPP, P. H., C. MUSHATT, and S. J. NEMETZ. "The Context of Reported Asthma during Psychoanalysis," *Psychosom. Med.*, 32 (1970), 167–188.

43. KNAPP, P. H. and S. J. NEMETZ. "Personality Variations in Bronchial Asthma: A Study of 40 Patients: Notes on the Relationship to Psychosis and the Problem of Measuring Maturity," *Psychosom. Med.*, 19 (1957), 443–465.

44. ———. "Sources of Tension in Bronchia Asthma," *Psychosom. Med.*, 19 (1957), 443.

45. ———. "Acute Bronchial Asthma: 1. Concomitant Depression and Excitement and Varied Antecedent Patterns in 406 Attacks," *Psychosom. Med.*, 22 (1960), 42–56.

46. LAMONT, J. "Psychosomatic Study of Asthma," *Am. J. Psychiatry*, 114 (1958), 890.

47. LEIGH, D. "Asthma and the Psychiatrist. A Critical Review," *Int. Arch. Allergy*, 4 (1953), 227.

48. LEIGH, D. and D. A. POND. "The Electroencephalogram in Cases of Bronchia Asthma," *J. Psychosom. Res.*, 1 (1956), 120.

49. LOFGREN, J. B. "A Case of Bronchial Asthma with Unusual Dynamic Factors Treated by Psychotherapy and Psychoanalysis," *Int. J. Psycho-anal.*, 42 (1961), 414–423.

50. LUPARELLO, T. J., H. A. LYONS, E. R. BLEECKER et al. "Influences of Suggestion on Airway Reactivity in Asthmatic Subjects," *Psychosom. Med.*, 30 (1968), 819–825.

51. LUPARELLO, T. J., M. STEIN, and C. D. PARK. "Effect of Hypothalamic Lesions on Rat Anaphylaxis," *Am. J. Physiol.*, 207 (1964), 911–914.

52. McDERMOTT, N. T. and S. COBB. "A Psychiatric Survey of 50 Cases of Bronchial Asthma," *Psychosom. Med.*, 1 (1939), 203–244.

53. McFADDEN, E. R., JR., R. KISER, and W. J. DeGROOT. "Acute Bronchial Asthma," *N. Engl. J. Med.*, 288 (1973), 221–225.

54. McFADDEN, E. R. JR., T. LUPARELLO, H. A. LYONS et al. "The Mechanisms of Action of Suggestion in the Induction of Acute Asthma Attacks," *Psychosom. Med.*, 31 (1969), 134–43.

55. MacKENZIE, J. N. "The Production of 'Rose Asthma' by an Artificial Rose," *Am. J. Med. Sci.*, 91 (1886), 45.

56. McNEIL, R. S. and C. G. INGRAM. "Effect of Propanolol on Ventilatory Function," *Am. J. Cardiol.*, 18 (1966), 473–475.

57. MATHÉ, A. A. "Decreased Circulating Epinephrine Possibly Secondary to Decreased Hypothalamic Adrenomedullary Discharge; A Supplementary Hypothesis of Bronchial Asthma Pathogenesis," *J. Psychosom. Res.*, 15 (1971), 349–359.

58. MATHÉ, A. A., P. HEDQVIST, A. HOLMGKEN et al. "Bronchial Hyperactivity to Prostoglandin F$_2$ and Histamine in Patients with Asthma," *Br. Med. J.*, 36 (1973), 193–196.

59. MATHÉ, A. A. and P. H. KNAPP. "Decreased Plasma Free Fatty Acids and Urinary Epinephrine in Bronchial Asthma," *N. Engl. J. Med.*, 281 (1969), 234–238.

60. ———. "Emotional and Adrenal Reactions to Stress in Bronchial Asthma," *Psychosom. Med.*, 33 (1971), 323.

61. MEAD, J., N. PETERSON, and G. BRIMBY. "Pulmonary Ventilation Measured from Body Surface Movements," *Science*, 156 (1967), 1383.

62. MEARES, R. A., J. E. MILLS, T. B. HORVATH et al. "Amitryptillene and Asthma," *Med. J. Aust.*, 2 (1971), 25–28.

63. MEIJER, A., and P. H. KNAPP. "Asthma Predictors in Infantile Atopic Dermatitis," *J. Psychosom. Res.*, in press.

64. MILLER, H. and D. W. BARUCH. "Psychiatric Studies of Children with Allergic Manifestations. I. Maternal Rejection: A Study of 63 Cases," *Psychosom. Med.*, 10 (1948), 275–278.

65. MITHOEFER, J. C., R. H. RUNSER, and M. S. KARETZKY. "Use of Sodium Bicarbonate in the Treatment of Acute Bronchial Asthma," *N. Engl. J. Med.*, 272 (1965), 1200–1203.

66. MOORE, N. "Behavior Therapy in Bronchial Asthma—A Controlled Study," *J. Psychosom. Res.*, 9 (1967), 257–77.

67. MORRIS, H. G., G. ROCHE, and M. R. EARLE. "Urinary Excretion of Epinephrine and Norepinephrine in Asthmatic Children," *J. Allergy Clin. Immunol.*, 50 (1972), 138–145.

68. NOELPP-ESCHENHAGEN, I. and B. NOELPP. "New Contributions to Experimental Asthma," *Progr. Allergy*, 4 (1954), 361.

69. OBERNDORF, C. P. "The Psychogenic Factors

in Asthma," *N.Y. J. Med.*, 35 (1935), 41–48.

70. ORANGE, R. P., M. D. VALENTINE, and K. F. AUSTEN. "Release of Slow-Reacting Substance of Anaphylaxis in the Rat: Polymorphonuclear Leukocyte," *Science*, 157 (1967), 318–319.

71. OTTENBERG, P. and M. STEIN. "Psychological Determinants in Asthma," *Trans. Acad. Psychosom. Med.*, (5th Annual Meeting) (1958), 122.

72. ———. "Learned Asthma in the Guinea Pig," *Psychosom. Med.*, 20 (1958), 395.

73. PURCELL, K., L. BERNSTEIN, and S. BUKANTZ. "A Preliminary Comparison of Rapidly Remitting and Persistently Steroid Dependent Asthmatic Children," *Psychosom. Med.*, 23 (1961), 305.

74. PURCELL, K., K. BRADY et al. "Effect on Asthma in Children of Experimental Separation from the Family," *Psychosom. Med.*, 31 (1969), 144–164.

75. SCHIAVI, R. C., M. STEIN, and B. B. SETHI. "Respiratory Variables in Response to a Pain-Fear Stimulus and in Experimental Asthma," *Psychosom. Med.*, 23 (1961), 485.

76. SCHNEER, H. I., ed. *The Asthmatic Child.* New York: Harper & Row, 1963.

77. SCHOLANDER, P. F. "The Master Switch of Life," *Sci. Am.*, 209 (1963), 92–107.

78. SCHWARTZ, M. "Heredity in Bronchial Asthma: A Clinical and Genetic Study of 191 Asthma Probands and 50 Probands with Baker's Asthma," *Acta Allergol.* 5, Suppl. 2 (1952), 1.

79. SLOANAKER, J. and D. LUMINET. "Classical Conditioning in Bronchial Asthma." Unpublished Ph.D. dissertation, Boston University, 1961.

80. SPERLING, M. "A Psychoanalytic Study of Bronchial Asthma in Children," in H. I. Schneer, ed., *The Asthmatic Child.* New York: Harper & Row, 1963.

81. STEIN, M. and P. OTTENBERG. "The Role of Odors in Asthma," *Psychosom. Med.*, 20 (1958), 60.

82. STEIN, M. and R. SCHIAVI. "Respiratory Disorders," in A. M. Freedman, and H. I. Kaplan, eds., *Comprehensive Textbook of Psychiatry*, pp. 1068–1071. Baltimore: Williams & Wilkins, 1967.

83. SZENTIVANYI, A. "The Beta Adrenergic Theory of the Atopic Abnormality in Bronchial Asthma," *J. Allergy*, 42 (1968), 203–232.

84. ———. "Effect of Bacterial Products and Adrenergic Blocking Agents on Allergic Reactions," in M. Samter, ed., *Immunologic Disease*, pp. 356–374. Boston: Little Brown, 1971.

85. SZENTIVANYI, A. and G. FILLIP. "Anaphylaxis and the Nervous System: 2," *Ann. Allergy*, 16 (1958), 143–151.

86. VACHON, L. "Visceral Learning of Respiratory Resistance," (Abstract), *Psychosom. Med.*, 34 (1972), 471–472.

87. VACHON, L., C. J. BROTMAN, and P. H. KNAPP. "Bronchial Tree Response to the Diving Reflex," (Abstract), *Psychosom. Med.*, 31 (1969), 447.

88. WALTON, D. "Application of Learning Theory to a Case of Bronchial Asthma," in H. Eyesenck, ed., *Behavior Therapy and the Neuroses.*, pp. 188–189. Oxford: Pergamon, 1960.

89. WEISS, E. "Psychoanalyse eines Falles von Nervösen Asthma," *Int. Z. Psychoanal.*, 8 (1922), 440–445.

90. WEISS, J. H. "Effects of Suggestion on Respiration in Asthmatic Children," *Psychosom. Med.*, 32 (1970), 409–415.

91. WIDDICOMBE, J. G. "Regulation of Tracheobronchial Smooth Muscle," *Physiol. Rev.*, 43 (1963), 1.

92. WHITE, H. "Hypnosis in Bronchial Asthma," *Psychosom. Res.*, 5 (1961), 272.

93. ZAID, G. and G. N. BEALL. "Bronchial Response to Beta Adrenergic Blockade," *N. Engl. J. Med.*, 275 (1966), 580–584.

CHAPTER 29

DISORDERS OF
IMMUNE MECHANISMS

Raul C. Schiavi and Marvin Stein

IN RECENT YEARS immunology has progressed from description of the immune reaction to cellular and molecular analysis of the underlying mechanisms. The fields of microbiology, biochemistry, and biophysics as well as other biological disciplines have developed and applied specialized quantitative techniques which have led to the understanding of immune processes at the organ, tissue, cellular, and subcellular levels. Immune phenomena were initially considered in relation to infectious diseases, and as having a protective and adaptive function. As more knowledge was gathered, it appeared that immune mechanisms may also be involved in the development of various pathological states. Allergic disorders were among the first to be considered as pathological manifestations of immune processes. Since 1950, with the explosive expansion of information and techniques in the field of immunology, considerable data has been acquired, indicating that immune processes are involved in a wide range of path-

ological and clinical disorders, including autoimmune diseases, neoplasia, and organ transplants. Although clinicians now have an increased understanding of the immunological basis of a variety of illnesses, little attention has been paid to the psychophysiological aspects of immune processes. The immune system, similar to the nervous and endocrine systems, plays an important role in biological adaptation, contributing to the maintenance of homeostasis and to the establishment of body integrity. The similarity between the function of the immune and central nervous systems maintaining the integrity of the organism in relation to the external environment has recently been pointed out by Salk.[106]

The observation that emotions modify host resistance to infection and that they may influence the development and course of some hypersensitive reactions and autoimmune and neoplastic diseases have led some investigators to propose that immune processes play a significant role in the mediation of psychological influences in some physical illnesses. This chapter will review clinical and experimental findings concerned with the influence of psychosocial processes on immunological reactions. There is an extensive literature in the area of serum proteins and immunological responsivity in psychiatric disorders which has been recently reviewed;[10,125,131] these data will not be presented here.

⟨ Immune Response

Before considering specific immune disorders, it is important to have an understanding of the concepts of immune response.[1,39,122] The immune response may be thought of as a complex specialized reaction developed against foreign proteins or polysaccharide substances known as antigens. The response is specific for each antigen and usually becomes more intense and highly specific with each repeated exposure to the specific antigen.

Immune responses consist of an afferent phase, a central phase, and an effector phase. The borders between these various phases are not clearly delineated. During the afferent phase antigen is processed and identified as foreign; during the central phase various processes occur primarily in the lymphoid tissues which amplify the recognition signal; and in the effector phase appropriate cells are mobilized to react against the antigen. The response may be recognized at the effector level either as specific humoral antibodies elaborated by lymphoid cells, or by an action of specific cells (e.g., lymphocytes or macrophages) on the relevant antigen. Circulating antibodies are usually produced in response to a soluble antigen, whereas cell-mediated immunity develops in response to an antigen fixed in the tissue. The humoral antibody response and the cell-mediated response will be briefly reviewed.

Humoral Antibody Response

Soluble antigen passes to the medulla of lymph nodes or the red pulp of the spleen where it is taken up by macrophages. These cells then appear to send a message to plasma-cell precursors, which lie in close proximity to the macrophages at the cortico-medullary junction of lymph nodes and in the red pulp of the spleen. The plasma-cell precursor, probably lymphocytes, proliferate into antibody-producing cells (plasma cells). Plasma cells contain all of the systems required for the synthesis and secretion of proteins. This class of proteins produced by plasma cells is known as antibodies since they react directly with antigens. They are primarily γ globulins and, because of their immunological function, are referred to as immunoglobulins. There are at least five classes and several subclasses of immunoglobulins in man. The three major classes are designated IgM, IgG, and IgA.

The IgM antibodies are extremely efficient in binding to particulate antigens such as bacteria and erythrocytes, but not as efficient in binding to particulate antigens, such as toxins. The IgG system can bind to soluble antigens, and antibodies are produced for long periods of time. The cells of the IgA, and perhaps of the IgE system, produce molecules capable of binding to skin and mucous membranes. Reagins which have been classified as IgE antibodies are associated with anaphylactic phenomena such as hay fever and asthma. After the interaction of antigen and IgA or IgE antibodies, histamine and other pharmacological agents are locally released.

Cell-Mediated Immune Response

If antigen is fixed in tissues, such as a tissue homograft, or in a modified part of the body's own tissues, such as skin treated with a simple chemical sensitizing agent, the response is of a different type than that of the humoral antibody response. It appears that small lymphocytes passing through the tissues are sensitized peripherally and then pass down to a local lymph node where they enter the free area of the cortex follicles. The small lymphocytes proliferate at this point and become differentiated into large cells with easily identifiable characteristics. After a few days some of the lymphocytes become immunologically active leaving the local lymphoid tissue to go to other lymph nodes where other immunologically active lymphocytes are propagated. At this point, the immunologically active cells can be found in the peripheral blood and pass to the graft where they can initiate the process of graft rejection or react with an antigen deposit in peripheral tissue to produce an inflammatory response such as that which occurs in chemical contact sensitivity or the tuberculin reaction. Immunological responses carried out by sensitized cells in the absence of circulating antibody include delayed sensitivity, transplantation immune reactions, and various autoimmune phenomena. The cellular systems capable of carrying out these processes may form part of a surveillance system the function of which may be to eliminate cells arising as a result of mutation, e.g., neoplastic cells.

◖ Infectious Diseases

The concept of multiple causation of disease is well illustrated by the observation that colonization of an organism by bacteria does not necessarily result in illness. Clinically, it has been noted for many years that infectious diseases are the result of host–microorganism interaction. In order to understand the disease process, it is necessary to investigate the aspects which determine the capability of the microorganism to initiate infection and those which influence the host response to the infection. A great deal of attention has been devoted clinically and in the laboratory to the identification of microorganisms involved in infectious diseases and there has been growing interest in the factors which modify host resistance. Among these, psychosocial influences have been shown to play a role in infectious diseases.[32] For example, several studies have shown that psychological variables influence the rate of recovery from infectious mononucleosis[40] and influenza,[50] and the development of lesions due to herpes simplex virus.[38] Psychological factors have also been demonstrated to modify the onset and course of pulmonary tuberculosis[43] and experimentally it has been shown that the tuberculin reaction can be inhibited by means of hypnosis.[8]

There are, however, few data regarding the physiological mechanisms involved in the mediation of psychological factors on host resistance in man. The study of Meyer and Haggerty[79] represents one of the few attempts to consider immune variables in relation to psychological influences on infectious diseases. They studied prospectively members of sixteen families for a one-year period with systematic throat cultures for β hemolytic streptococci, periodic measurement of antistreptolysin-O-antibody titers, and clinical evaluation of illness. It was found that acute or chronic family stresses not only were important factors determining whether the individual became a host for the streptococcus, or became ill following colonization, but also that psychological stress influenced the proportion of persons in whom there was a rise of antistreptolysin O following infection.

In addition to clinical observations, there is a growing body of experimental data supporting the hypothesis that psychosocial factors play a role in infectious diseases. Rasmussen and collaborators,[53,54,98,99] in an extensive series of studies, have primarily employed avoidance-learning procedures as the experimental model for investigating the effects of psychological stress. This procedure requires mice to jump a barrier once every five minutes at the presentation of a signal to avoid an electric shock delivered to their paws, a response the animals quickly learn to perform. Daily exposure for six-hour periods to these conditions resulted in an increased susceptibility to herpes simplex virus,[99] poliomyelitis virus,[54] coxsackie B,[53] and polyoma virus infection.[98] Physical restraint also was found to increase the susceptibility of mice to herpes simplex virus,[99] while high-intensity sound stress resulted in a transient diphasic susceptibility pattern in mice inoculated intranasally with vesicular stomatitis virus.[52] In monkeys acute avoidance stress was found to decrease their susceptibility to poliomyelitis.[75] Social factors such as the effect of differential housing have been studied, and it has been shown that mice housed alone were significantly more susceptible to encephalomyocarditis virus and less susceptible to Plasmodium berghei than animals housed in groups.[33]

In summary, both clinical and experimental observations demonstrate that psychosocial factors influence infectious diseases. The experimental procedures which have demonstrated psychosocial influences on host response to infection have also been shown to modify a variety of immune processes. These studies will be reviewed in a later section.

⟨ Allergic Disorders

Hypersensitivity refers to a state of enhanced reactivity to a foreign substance acquired by previous exposure to the same or a related substance.[88] Allergy is frequently used synonymously with hypersensitivity and has come to be considered a clinical state in which individuals react in an intense and frequently injurious manner to a substance that usually has no effect on most people. A wide range of antigens are capable of inducing the hypersensitive response and the term allergen is used generically. Hypersensitive reactions are of two major types. Immediate hypersensitivity in which the response takes place within seconds or moments after exposure to the allergen and is always associated with humoral antibodies. This type of reaction occurs in anaphylaxis and in various allergic clinical states such as asthma, hay fever, eczema, and urticaria.

The other type of hypersensitive reaction occurs two to three days after exposure to the antigen and is referred to as delayed hypersensitivity. In this reaction there are no humoral antibodies, and it is a cell-mediated immune response. As mentioned earlier, the tuberculin reaction typifies delayed hypersensitivity. Clinically, contact allergy occurring in response to poison ivy, poison oak, or contact with certain drugs is a manifestation of a delayed hypersensitive reaction.

Considerable clinical evidence suggests that psychological factors are related to the precipitation of many allergic disorders including bronchial asthma. The literature on the role of psychological influences on bronchial asthma is reviewed in Chapter 28 of this volume and the present discussion will focus only on the relationship of emotional factors to allergic processes in general.

It has been repeatedly demonstrated that periods of life change and stress antedate the onset of many allergic episodes and that a variety of emotional states may trigger the onset of symptoms.[30,62] Sensitivity to allergens has not been demonstrated to be quantitatively stable with time and in a number of instances it has been demonstrated to increase in association with emotional distress.[101] More than twenty years ago, Holmes et al.[47] demonstrated that naturally occurring and experimentally induced emotional distress enhanced the intensity of allergic rhinitis and the magnitude of the response of the nasal mucosa of patients with hay fever exposed to a standard amount of pollen. The evidence suggested that parasympathetic activity mediated the psychological influences in the nasal mucous membranes. Since that time, a body of information has been gathered from the fields of pharmacology, immunology, and pulmonary physiology, substantiating the influence of the autonomic nervous system on vascular, mucosal, and muscular changes occurring in target organs during the hypersensitive reaction. Mediating mechanisms involved in the precipitation of at least some allergic and asthmatic episodes probably include the autonomic and endocrine systems interacting with allergic inflammatory processes. It has been postulated that increased parasympathetic activity leading to bronchoconstriction and to an increase in bronchial mucous secretion mediates behavioral influences in the precipitation of asthmatic attacks.[71,102,124]

Several investigators studied[9,31,51] the relationship between psychological factors and biological susceptibility as two sets of independent variables predisposing to allergic illnesses. The results have shown that both emotions and immune mechanisms contribute to the development of susceptibility to allergy although the mode of interaction is still unclear. The findings have also suggested that failure to take into account the immunological heterogeneity of allergic patients may have been one important source of inconsistency in earlier psychosomatic investigations.

Implicit in a number of psychological studies of hypersensitive patients is the possibility that emotional factors not only interact with an already established allergic substrate, but that they may also directly influence the development of an allergic diathesis. There is, at present, no solid clinical evidence; limited experimental data will be reviewed later.

(Autoimmune Diseases

It is well known that antibodies are not usually developed against an individual's own tissues. Burnet and Fenner[13] emphasized this phenomenon when they discussed the concept of self-recognition, i.e., the ability of the mechanisms responsible for antibody production to distinguish "self" from "not self." In view of the previous discussion of the immune response, the formation of antibodies which would react with the body's own tissues would be extremely destructive. Usually a substance is only antigenic when foreign to a specific organism. In rare instances cells are antigenic in the organism from which they arise. The antibodies which develop are known as autoantibodies and the immunizing process is referred to as autoimmunization. Autoimmune disease is defined as an illness in which autoantibodies or a sensitized lymphocyte reacts with host tissue. It is important to note that there is no conclusive evidence indicating that the autoantibody or lymphocyte is the causative agent. Autoantibodies could be causative, a result of autoimmune disease, or only a concomitant part of the illness.[35]

It has been suggested that autoimmunity is a result of immunologic hyperactivity in response to the release of a sequestered antigen or due to proliferation of "forbidden clones" of antibody-producing cells. Both of these theories have been thoroughly discussed.[12,35,122] Another hypothesis is that autoimmune disease is a result of a state of immunological deficiency, and several theories have been proposed to explain the pathogenic mecha-

nism of the deficient state.[35] Among these is the suggestion that a latent virus, mycoplasma, or bacterium may become pathogenic and alter the immunological mechanism resulting in the production of autoantibodies. The autoantibody may be an attempt of the organism to protect itself and may not represent the primary pathogen.

A number of clinical entities in man are now considered to be autoimmune diseases and include systemic lupus erythematosus, rheumatoid arthritis, chronic glomerulonephritis, thyroiditis, and hemolytic anemia.[80] In addition, autoimmunity has been implicated in the pathogenesis of scleroderma, myasthenia gravis, and ulcerative colitis. There is evidence strongly suggesting that the tissue in rheumatoid arthritis is involved in a chronic immune response. The profuse lymphocytic infiltration of synovial tissue in rheumatoid arthritis and the immune complexes found in the synovial fluid support this hypothesis. The specific aspects of the altered cellular antigen have not as yet been demonstrated, but a chronic viral infection is one of the major possibilities. It is likely that one of the many viruses capable of slow atypical infection may modify the antigenicity of the synovial cells and result in an immune reaction. It has been speculated that a similar immune process is involved in other collagen vascular diseases such as scleroderma, dermatomyositis, and systemic lupus erythematosus.

Solomon has reviewed the extensive literature concerned with the psychophysiological aspects of autoimmune diseases.[113,114] Among autoimmune diseases, rheumatoid arthritis has been the disorder most frequently considered in psychosomatic investigations. Several investigators[82,84,85] have studied the influences of psychosocial factors in relation to rheumatoid arthritis and have assessed personality traits in arthritic patients. Although no consistent personality pattern in rheumatoid patients emerges from these studies, the findings convincingly document the importance of emotional factors in the course of the disease. Patients have been described as predominantly perfectionistic, self-conscious, introverted, and inhibited in relation to various comparison groups. Moos and Solomon[84,85] in a controlled study found that patients with rheumatoid arthritis were significantly more masochistic and self-sacrificing and showed difficulties in recognizing and expressing hostility. They also studied the relation between psychological factors and rapidity of progression of the disease,[83] and functional incapacity[86] and response to medical treatment.[117] Patients with poor prognosis and less satisfactory response were significantly more anxious and depressed, and demonstrated more social alienation and less adequate coping and adaptive mechanisms.

Several authors[113,114] have drawn attention to similarities in the role of psychological factors in patients with rheumatoid arthritis and patients with other autoimmune disorders. Stressful life events, such as the loss or threatened loss of a significant relationship, were reported to precede not only the onset of rheumatoid arthritis, but also of systemic lupus erythematosus.[69,93] Furthermore, similarities were found in the personality characteristics of patients with these two disorders. Patients with ulcerative colitis, a disease in which anticolon antibodies have been demonstrated, have also been described as showing certain obsessive-compulsive traits[113,114] which resemble to some degree the personality factors described in arthritic patients. The meaning of personality factors in the various autoimmune disorders is, however, not certain and requires further study.

Solomon has[113,114] advanced the theory that the central-nervous-system control of immune mechanisms plays an important role in the mediation of the effect of psychological factors in autoimmune disease. This theory rests on evidence that autoimmune diseases are the result of a state of immunological incompetence, and it has been proposed that the immune deficient state may be the consequence of the activation of the adrenocortical system due to emotional influences. A deficient immunological state may prevent elimination of self-reacting immunologic competent cells, or it may permit the formation of soluble antigen–antibody complexes resulting in the production of tissue injury and inflammation.

◖ Organ Transplants

In the 1960s, considerable progress has been made in the area of organ transplantation and there are a number of excellent reviews which consider the immunological aspects.[42,48,108] The greatest success has been with the kidney, while transplantation of other organs e.g., liver, heart, or lungs, has been far less successful. A great deal of attention has been paid to the mechanisms responsible for failures in the acceptance of grafted organs. Peter B. Medawar and his co-workers were the first to demonstrate that the homograft reaction is mediated by immune mechanisms. It has been demonstrated that skin homografts are rejected by the cell-mediated immune response as described earlier. The rejection of other grafts such as the kidney involves both humoral and cellular immune mechanisms. Hume[49] has described the mechanism of primary acute rejection of the kidney. Antigens migrate from the donor kidney to local lymph nodes where they encounter immunocompetent plasma cells. In the lymph node humoral antibodies and sensitized lymphocytes are produced and migrate back to the donor kidney. The sensitized lymphocytes and humoral antibodies react to the kidney cells resulting in the characteristic pathological features of the rejection crisis. Progress has been made in the use of immunosuppressive agents which inhibit the immune mechanisms involved in organ rejection while leaving all other immune responses intact.[111]

Attention has also been drawn to the role of psychosocial factors in relation to organ transplantation. It has been shown experimentally that in mice subjected to chronic avoidance learning, there is a prolongation of skin homograft survival time.[128] This effect is probably mediated by a modification of immune mechanisms as a result of the psychological stress produced by the avoidance learning.

Clinically, some investigators have reported that stressful life events, intense anxiety and depression precede some rejection crisis following renal homo-transplantation.[6,14,23,58] Patients who died following kidney transplantation were observed to experience feelings of abandonment, emotional tensions, and grief to a degree not evidenced among patients who survived. Various pathophysiological processes may be directly responsible for the patient's death, including disturbances in electrolyte balance, hemorrhage, cardiovascular complications, and infection. The possibility that immune processes may participate in some rejection crises associated with psychological trauma deserves consideration. At present, however, there are no data reported in this regard.

(Cancer

The natural history of neoplastic diseases is in many ways similar to the interaction between host and microorganisms in infectious diseases. The genetic characteristics of both participants, as well as a variety of internal and external factors, determine the outcome of the relation between the host and living pathogenic cells. There is a growing body of knowledge that immune mechanisms may be involved in both the development and outcome of neoplasia. It has been shown that many experimental cancers in animals contain new antigens. In addition, it has also been demonstrated that the majority of carcinogenic agents decrease the overall immunological capacity before the onset of cancer.[7,118] There are many reports suggesting immunological deficiency in man as a prerequisite for progressive neoplasia.[27,34] It is of interest that the relation of immunological mechanisms to cancer has been further supported by some observations on immunosuppressive techniques utilized in organ transplants.[49] It has been found that there is a marked increase in the incidence of tumors in approximately 6–8 percent of transplant patients maintained on immunosuppressive drugs. Furthermore, it appears that in some instances when the immunosuppressive treatment is stopped, the tumors that developed while on immunosuppression rapidly regress.

As pointed out above, a variety of internal and external host factors appear to play a role in the development, course, and outcome of neoplastic disorders. Among these factors psychosocial influences have been shown, both experimentally and clinically, to be determinants in neoplasia.[17]

Experimentally, considerable evidence demonstrates that early experiential factors not only have a profound influence on behavior and on the endocrine and immunological responsiveness of small mammals, but that they also influence the development and course of experimentally induced cancer. Furthermore, the findings show that the outcome of the relation between the host and the neoplastic process depends upon the species and the nature of the experimental intervention. Brief daily handling and mild electric shock administered early in life, for instance, modify the rate of tumor development and the survival of rats injected with Walker-256 sarcoma.[2] Infantile stimulation also shortens the survival time of mice after transplantation of lymphoid leukemia,[66] but does not modify the mortality rate of murine leukemia virus.[32] Similarly, differential housing and sex-segregated groupings modify the incidence of mammary carcinomas in mice,[74] decrease the survival time to injections of subcellular leukemia material,[22] but do not influence the development of Walker sarcoma tumors.[32]

Clinically, a number of investigators have reported a relationship between certain premorbid factors and personality types, and the development of cancer.[4,17,41,65] Kissen and collaborators,[59–61] for example, have conducted an extensive series of studies on the role of personality factors in lung cancer. They have repeatedly observed that lung cancer patients have less ability for emotional discharge than noncancer patients, as assessed clinically and measured by the Maudsley Personality Inventory. In addition, they have found significant differences between the same lung-cancer patients and controls in the reported incidence of certain environmental factors such as adverse episodes in childhood and adulthood. Bahnson and Bahnson[5] also have claimed that certain features such as depression, denial, and repression exist to a pathological extent as premorbid characteristics in patients with cancer.

By and large, the studies concerned with premorbid factors in cancer are retrospective in nature and, therefore, are limited by the inability to control for distortions due to the effect of immediate precipitating factors and the psychological impact of the disease. Some investigators have focused on the role of emotional factors during the immediate premorbid phase. Their findings have demonstrated that depression, hopelessness, inability to express hostile feelings, and object loss may play an important role in influencing the onset of the neoplasia or the course and outcome of the disease. An illustrative example is given by an interesting predictive study conducted by Schmale and Iker[110] on fifty-one females with cervical cellular cytology, indicating suspicion of cervical cancer identified during routine screening procedures. The investigators were able to make a significantly high number of correct predictions regarding the diagnostic outcome of cone biopsy of the cervix, based on the clinical assessment of feelings of hopelessness during the previous six months. Assuming that a causal relationship exists between emotional factors and the onset and development of neoplasia, a question that has attracted considerable interest is concerned with the nature of the physiological processes involved. The growing information on the immunological aspects of cancer raises the possibility that immunological mechanisms play an important role in the mediation of emotional influences on susceptibility to neoplastic disease. The extensive literature on the psychophysiological aspects of cancer has been thoroughly reviewed.[4,17]

(Psychosocial Factors and Immune Processes

It is of considerable interest that some of the psychosocial situations, which have been demonstrated to modify the susceptibility to infection and the development of neoplasia, have also been found to have a profound influence on immune processes. Avoidance learning, for example, decreases the susceptibility of mice to passive anaphylaxis.[100] Overcrowding, but not the stress of electric shock, initiated prior to immunization of rats with flagellin, a bacterial antigen, reduced both the primary and secondary antibody response.[112] Vessey[123] found that grouped mice have significantly lower titers of circulating antibodies than isolated mice and, by identifying social rank, he demonstrated that dominant mice had higher titers than the other mice in their groups. In primates, exposure to a complex pattern of visual, auditory, and somasthetic stimulation was observed to increase plasma cortisol levels markedly and to decrease the circulating antibody response to immunization with bovine serum albumin.[46] A number of reports in the Russian literature have considered the effect of psychological mechanisms on antibody titers.[21,67,87,107] Petrovskii,[95] for example, studied changes in agglutinin titers associated with behavioral disturbances induced in immunized dogs and baboons by stressful stimuli or by conflict-conditioning techniques. He observed a parallelism between the intensity and duration of the behavioral disturbances and the fall in circulating antibody titers. It is to be noted that under certain conditions psychological stimulation can enhance the immune response. Brief handling of rats, for instance, during the preweaning period was found to increase both the primary and secondary antibody response to flagellin immunization.[115]

The physiological mechanisms which mediate the psychosocial influences on host resistance are complex and in need of further clarification. It seems reasonable to speculate that the demonstrated effect of psychosocial stress on the modified susceptibility to some viral infections and neoplastic processes may be due to the suppression of immediate and delayed hypersensitive mechanisms.

There is evidence that the hormonal and reticulo-endothelial systems are involved in the mediation of psychological influences. Avoidance learning or confinement is accompanied by adrenal hypertrophy, lymphocytopenia and a slowly developing involution of the thymus and spleen occurring in temporal relation with the increase in susceptibility to viral infection.[76] The pituitary-adrenocortical system which is known to be altered by psychosocial stimulation, has been the focus of considerable attention because of evidence primarily derived from pharmacological studies that adrenal steroids may modify susceptibility to infectious disease, alter immune reactions, or depress inflammatory responses.[20,45,57] In addition, both psychological stress and adrenocortical steroids have been reported by some investigators,[15,105] although not by others,[116] to suppress interferon production, a nonspecific protein directly involved in host resistance to viral infection.

Whether changes in endogenous adrenal hormones, occurring in response to environmental stimulation, are responsible for some of the effects of host resistance and immune processes requires further analysis in the context of the different experimental models investigated. Based on studies conducted with stressed, adrenalectomized animals, it appears that adrenal steroids are responsible for the increased resistance to passive anaphylaxis,[121] while the retarded rate of disappearance of vesicular stomatitis virus from the site of inoculation and the increased susceptibility to this viral agent seems independent of adrenal activity.[132] These findings clearly demonstrate the complexity of the field.

Little information is available on the role played by other hormonal systems and physiological processes in the mediation of psychological and environmental stimulation. Probably only after careful elucidation of the physiological correlates of psychosocial intervention and their interaction with the pathophysiological processes underlying a given pathogenic stimulus, will it be possible to predict the response of an organism to specific experimental conditions.

❴ The Central Nervous System and Immune Processes

Recently the neurophysiological mechanisms that might mediate the psychosocial influences on immunological reactions have been experimentally studied. At the turn of the century the central nervous system (CNS) was considered to be involved in the development of immune phenomena. The brain was thought to be the target organ initiating the anaphylactic reaction. A series of studies conducted between 1910 and 1920 demonstrated, however, that the characteristic signs of anaphylaxis could occur in decerebrated guinea pigs and dogs. With the development of immunological and biochemical techniques, an impressive amount of knowledge on the cellular and chemical aspects of immune processes was acquired, and the participation of the CNS was largely overlooked. The consideration of the integrative capacity of the CNS on a variety of physiological processes has stimulated a renewed interest in the role of the CNS in immune processes.

Studies of the effect of sectioning the spinal cord on immunogenesis have shown changes such as decreased antibody formation following sensitization[11] and lowered histamine sensitivity.[16] These findings may be the secondary result, however, of peripheral disturbances in temperature control and blood circulation.

The effect of midbrain lesions on the course of anaphylaxis in the guinea pig has been investigated by Freedman and Fenichel.[29] Bilateral electrolytic lesions at the level of the superior colliculus involving the reticulothalamic tracts and deep tegmental nuclei inhibited anaphylactic death. Szentivanyi and Filipp[120] were among the first to study the role of the hypothalamus on anaphylaxis. They demonstrated that lethal anaphylactic shock in the guinea pig and the rabbit can be prevented by bilateral focal lesions in the tuberal region of the hypothalamus. Luparello, Stein, and Park[68] investigated the effect of hypothalamic lesions on rat anaphylaxis and found that anterior, but not posterior, hypothalamic lesions inhibited development of lethal anaphylaxis in the rat. In a recent study reported by Macris, Schiavi, et al.,[72] it has been shown that lesions in the anterior hypothalamus of actively immunized guinea pigs afforded significant protection against lethal anaphylaxis. Lesions in the median and posterior basal hypothalamus did not modify anaphylactic reactions.

Little is known about the mechanisms involved in the antianaphylactic effect of hypothalamic lesions. Filipp and Szentivanyi[26] have reported that circulating as well as tissue-fixed antibodies were markedly reduced in guinea pigs injured in the tuberal region. Low precipitin levels were observed in sensitized animals following hypothalamic lesions as evidenced by the Ring test. Korneva and Khai[63] also found that lesions in the posterior ventral hypothalamus of rabbits completely suppressed the production of complement-fixing antibodies and induced a prolonged retention of the antigen in the blood. In cases where the areas of destruction were localized in other parts of the hypothalamus, the thalamic structure, the caudate nucleus, and the posterior commissure, the course of immune processes was similar to that in control animals. It has been found that anterior hypothalamic lesions in the guinea pig were associated with significantly lower circulating antibody titers.[72]

The significance of the low-circulating antibodies in the decreased anaphylactic response remains to be determined. If the antianaphylactic effect was due solely to diminished antibody production, then no protection would be expected in animals passively immunized with antibody levels that are sufficient to produce lethal anaphylaxis. Szentivanyi and Filipp[120] have reported that guinea pigs passively sensitized with homologous as well as with heterologous (rabbit) serum are protected by hypothalamic lesions. These investigators did not identify the hypothalamic structures damaged by the lesions nor did they quantify the amount of antibodies injected to the animals. Macris, Schiavi, et al.[73] investigated the effect of hypothalamic lesions in guinea pigs passively immunized with heterologous (rabbit) antiovalbumin. Significant protection against passive lethal anaphylaxis was found in the animals with anterior but not with posterior hypothalamic lesions.

There are several mechanisms that may be involved in the protective action of anterior hypothalamic lesions in addition to their effect on circulating antibodies. The lesions may interfere with antibody binding to host tissues; they may alter the content and release of histamine and other mediator substances by the tissues; or they may diminish the responsiveness of the target tissue to the pharmacological agents liberated by the antigen–antibody reaction. Several studies have reported that the CNS modified the susceptibility of animals to histamine which, in the guinea pig, is the main agent responsible for the acute anaphylactic reaction. Whittier and Orr[126] found that bilateral lesions of the caudate nuclei of rats were associated with a significant increase in survival time following the intraperitoneal administration of histamine phosphate; sham operations and lesions in the cerebral cortex did not modify the time of survival. Przbylski[97] investigated the effect of the removal of the region of quadrigeminal bodies and of the cerebral cortex on histamine toxicity in guinea pigs. The animals in which the quadrigeminal bodies were removed showed a decreased susceptibility to histamine when administered either intravenously or by the inhalation of an aerosol. Removal of the cerebral cortex did not modify the reactivity of the animals.

Schiavi, Adams, and Stein[109] studied the effect of bilateral electrolytic lesions in the anterior and posterior medial hypothalamus of guinea pigs on histamine toxicity as measured by dose–mortality curves and the LD_{50}. The animals with anterior lesions were afforded significant protection against histamine toxicity. The mechanism by which anterior hypothalamic lesions modifies the susceptibility of the animals to exogenous histamine is not apparent from this study. Máslinski and Karczewski[77,78] extensively investigated the effect of electrical stimulation of the brain of guinea pigs with current intensities above and below the seizure threshold on the susceptibility of the animals to histamine. They found that electrical stimulation of guinea pigs through temporal electrodes with a 50-100 Hz. current at levels between 8 and 10 milli amp. has a marked protective effect against lethal histamine shock. These investigators demonstrated that the decrease in histamine susceptibility was transitory and was associated with a marked decrease in the bronchospastic effect of histamine. Karczewski[55] found that the parameters of electrical stimulation effective against lethal histamine shock also induced a marked depression of the electrical activity of the afferent and efferent fibers of the vagus. This and other observations led him to postulate that the modified histamine susceptibility following brain stimulation could be due to a reduced physiological tone of the airways leading to a reduced response to the constricting stimuli. A study by Mills and Widdicombe[81] conducted on vagotomized guinea pigs provided evidence that a vagal reflex is partially responsible for the bronchoconstriction occurring in anaphylaxis and following intravenous administration of histamine. A decreased response to bronchoconstricting agents due to an autonomic imbalance induced by the anterior hypothalamic lesions deserves further consideration.

Extensive work has demonstrated that the hypothalamus is intimately involved with autonomic nervous activity. Several lines of evidence[127,129,130] indicate that bronchomotor tone is the result of a balance between parasympathetic and sympathetic influences. Damage to the region of the anterior hypothalamus, which is thought to mediate primarily parasympathetic responses[36,37] may decrease vagal bronchoconstrictor tone resulting in the predominance of bronchial adrenergic β-receptor activity. In keeping with this hypothesis, inhibition of vagal activity[44,56] or β-adrenergic stimulation[3] decrease histamine induced bronchoconstriction while blockage of β receptors potentiate histamine bronchospasm.[70]

Szentivanyi[119] has postulated that the hyperreactivity observed in bronchial asthma may be due to the reduced functioning of the β-adrenergic system leading to α-adrenergic dominance and the consequent increase in bronchial responsiveness to the various pharmacological mediators. Orange and Austen have reported[92] that increased intracellular levels of cyclic adenosine-3'5'-mono-phosphate (cyclic AMP) following activation of β-adrenergic receptors inhibit the IgE mediated immunological release of histamine and "slow reactive substance" (SRS-A) from lung tissues. Hypothalamic lesions may produce a functional imbalance in the two adrenergic effector systems or increase the levels of cyclic AMP resulting in an inhibition of release of histamine and SRS-A; at present, however, there are no data to support these possibilities.

The influence of the CNS on immune mechanisms may be due, at least in part, to changes in neuroendocrine function induced by the destruction of specific hypothalamic structures. It has been shown in the rat[18,28] that the anterior medial hypothalamus is involved in the regulation of the secretion of thyroid stimulating hormone (TSH) by the hypophysis. Electrolytic lesions in this area induce low plasma levels of TSH and decreased thyroid function. A number of investigators have demonstrated in the rat and guinea pig a relationship between thyroid physiology and immune processes. It has been noted[64] that the resistance to the anaphylactic reaction is increased in thyroidectomized rats. Similar findings were observed by Nilzen in the guinea pig following thyroidectomy or administration of I.[131] Suppression of thyroid activity inhibits local and systemic anaphylaxis, abolishes circulating precipitins, and decreases the susceptibility of the animals to exogenous histamine.[89–91] Little is known about the effect of anterior hypothalamic lesions on thyroid function in the guinea pig.

Hypothalamic lesions can also modify ACTH secretion and blood corticoid levels. Adrenal steroids have been found to have a protective effect against anaphylactic shock in the rat and an inhibitory effect on antibody formation in rats and guinea pigs.[19,103] Adrenocortical hormones (ACTH) also have a profound action on the metabolism and effects of histamine. They have inhibitory effects on histamine decarboxylase activity,[94] tissue binding of newly formed histamine[108] and on the amount of histamine released by the tissues.[133] Although adrenal steroids have a protective effect against histamine toxicity in mice and rats, they do not appear to modify significantly the susceptibility of guinea pigs to anaphylaxis and to exogenous histamine.

It has been suggested that the protective effect of anterior lesions may also be due to simultaneous changes in thyroid and adrenocortical function. Filipp and Mess[24] reported that exogenous administration of thyroxin partially restored the sensitivity to anaphylaxis of actively immunized guinea pigs with lesions in the tuberal area of the hypothalamus. In another study[25] the same authors investigated the combined effect of thyroxin and metopirone, an inhibitor of adrenocorticol hormone synthesis, on the anaphylactic response of sensitized guinea pigs with lesions in the tuberal region. The observation that the administration of both substances completely abolished the protective effect of the lesions led the investigators to postulate that the antianaphylactic effect of hypothalamic damage is due to the combined effect of decreased thyroid function and increased adrenocortical activity. There have been very few studies concerned with the neuroendocrine effects of localized hypothalamic damage in guinea pigs. Additional information is necessary on plasma levels of thyroid, adrenocortical, and adrenomedullary hormones in guinea pigs with well defined hypothalamic lesions effective in decreasing anaphylactic reactivity.

Concluding Remarks

This chapter has reviewed the effect of psychosocial influences on infectious diseases, allergic disorders, autoimmune diseases, organ transplantation, and cancer. Clinical and experimental data have been presented which suggest that the effect of psychosocial factors on these disorders is due at least in part to an alteration in immunological mechanisms. The role of the CNS in relation to immune processes has also been discussed. The complexity of the psychophysiological processes involved in the role of psychosocial factors on immune disorders has been emphasized.

Bibliography

1. ABRAMOFF, P. and M. LAVIA. *Biology of the Immune Response.* New York: McGraw-Hill, 1970.
2. ADER, R. and S. B. FRIEDMAN. "Differential Early Experiences and Susceptibility to Transplanted Tumor in the Rat," *J. Comp. Physiol. Psychol.,* 59 (1965), 361–364.
3. AVIADO, D. M. "Antiasthmatic Action of Sympathomimetics: A Review of the Literature on Their Bronchopulmonary Effects," *J. Clin. Pharmacol.,* 10 (1970), 217–221.
4. BAHNSON, C. B. "Second Conference on Psychophysiological Aspects of Cancer," *Ann. N.Y. Acad. Sci.,* 164 (1969), 307–634.
5. BAHNSON, C. B. and M. B. BAHNSON. "Role of the Ego Defenses: Denial and Repression in the Etiology of Malignant Neoplasia," *Ann. N.Y. Acad. Sci.,* 125 (1966), 827–845.
6. BASCH, S. H. "The Intrapsychic Integration of a New Organ: A Clinical Study of Kidney Transplantation," *Psychoanal. Q.,* 42 (1973), 364–384.
7. BERENBAUM, M. C. "Effects of Carcinogens on Immune Processes," *Br. Med. Bull.,* 20 (1964), 159–164.
8. BLACK, S., J. H. HUMPHREY, and J. S. F. NIVEN. "Inhibition of Mantoux Reaction by Direct Suggestion under Hypnosis," *Br. Med. J.,* 1 (1963), 1649–1652.
9. BLOCK, J. "Further Consideration of Psychosomatic Predisposing Factors in Allergy," *Psychosom. Med.,* 30 (1968), 202–208.
10. BOCK, E., B. WEEKE, and O. J. RAFAELSEN. "Serum Proteins in Acutely Psychotic Patients," *J. Psychiatr. Res.,* 9 (1971), 1–9.
11. BOGENDÖRFER, L. "Über den Einfluss des Zentralnervensystems auf Immunitätsvorgänge: Beziehungen des Sympathicus zum Zustandekommen der Agglutination," *Arch. Exp. Pathol. Pharmakol.,* 133 (1928), 107–110.
12. BURNET, F. M. *The Clonal Selection Theory of Acquired Immunity.* Nashville, Tenn.: Vanderbilt University Press, 1959.
13. BURNET, F. M. and F. FENNER. *The Production of Antibodies.* Melbourne: McMillan, 1941.
14. CASTELNUOVO-TEDESCO, P., ed. *Psychiatric Aspects of Organ Transplantation.* New York: Grune & Stratton, 1971.

15. CHANG, S. S. and A. F. RASMUSSEN. "Stress-Induced Suppression of Interferon Production in Virus Infected Mice," *Nature*, 205 (1965), 623–624.

16. COOPER, I. S. "Neurological Evaluation of Cutaneous Histamine Reaction," *J. Clin. Invest.*, 29 (1950), 465–469.

17. CRISP, A. H. "Some Psychosomatic Aspects of Neoplasia," *Br. J. Med. Psychol.*, 13 (1970), 313–331.

18. DEJONG, W. and J. MOLL. "Differential Effects of Hypothalamic Lesions on Pituitary-Thyroid Activity in the Rat," *Acta Endocrinol. (Kbh.)*, 48 (1965), 522–535.

19. DEWS, P. B. and C. F. CODE. "Effect of Cortisone on Anaphylactic Shock in Adrenalectomized Rats," *J. Pharmacol. Exp. Therap.*, 101 (1951), 9.

20. ———. "Anaphylactic Reactions and Concentrations of Antibodies in Rats and Rabbits. Effect of Adrenalectomy and of Administration of Cortisone," *J. Immunol.*, 70 (1953), 199–206.

21. DZHUMKHADE, A. P. "Role of Conditioned Reflexes in Production of Antibodies," *Zh. Vyssh. Nerv. Deiat.*, 10 (1960), 599–601.

22. EBBESEN, P. and R. RASK-NIELSEN. "Influence of Sex-Segregated Grouping and of Inoculation with Subcellular Leukemic Material on Development of Non-Leukemic Lesions in DBA/2, BALB/C and CBA Mice," *J. Natl. Cancer Inst.*, 39 (1967), 917–925.

23. EISENDRATH, R. M. "The Role of Grief and Fear in the Death of Kidney Transplant Patients," *Am. J. Psychiatry*, 126 (1969), 129–135.

24. FILIPP, G. and B. MESS. "Role of the Thyroid Hormone System in Suppression of Anaphylaxis Due to Electrolytic Lesion of the Tuberal Region of the Hypothalamus," *Ann. Allergy*, 27 (1969), 500–505.

25. ———. "Role of the Adrenocortical System in Suppressing Anaphylaxis after Hypothalamic Lesion," *Ann. Allergy*, 27 (1969), 607–610.

26. FILIPP, G. and A. SZENTIVANYI. "Anaphylaxis and the Nervous System, Part III," *Ann. Allergy*, 16 (1958), 306–311.

27. FISHERMAN, E. "Does the Allergic Diathesis Influence Malignancy?" *J. Allergy*, 31 (1960), 74–78.

28. FLORSHEIM, W. H. "The Effect of Anterior Hypothalamic Lesions on Thyroid Function and Goiter Development in the Rat," *Endocrinol.*, 62 (1958), 783–789.

29. FREEDMAN, D. X. and G. FENICHEL. "Effect of Midbrain Lesions on Experimental Allergy," *Arch. Neurol. Psychiatry*, 79 (1958), 164–169.

30. FREEMAN, E. H., B. F. FEINGOLD, K. SCHLESINGER et al. "Psychological Variables in Allergic Disorders: A Review," *Psychosom. Med.*, 26 (1964), 543–575.

31. FREEMAN, E. H., F. J. GORMAN, M. T. SINGER et al. "Personality Variables and Allergic Skin Reactivity," *Psychosom. Med.*, 29 (1967), 312–322.

32. FRIEDMAN, S. B. and L. A. GLASGOW. "Psychologic Factors and Resistance to Infectious Disease," *Pediatr. Clin. North Am.*, 13 (1966), 315–335.

33. FRIEDMAN, S. B., L. A. GLASGOW, and R. ADER. "Psychosocial Factors Modifying Host Resistance to Experimental Infections," in C. B. Balmson, ed., *Second Conference on Psychophysiological Aspects of Cancer. Ann. N.Y. Acad. Sci.*, 164 (1969), 381–393.

34. FUDENBERG, H. H. "Immunologic Deficiency, Lymphoma and Autoimmune Diseases: Observations, Implications, Speculations," *Arthritis Rheum.*, 9 (1966), 464–472.

35. ———. "Are Autoimmune Diseases Immunologic Deficiency States?" in R. A. Good and D. W. Fisher, eds., *Immunobiology*, pp. 175–183. Stamford, Conn.: Sinauer Associates, 1971.

36. GELLHORN, E. *Autonomic Imbalance and the Hypothalamus*. Minneapolis: University of Minnesota Press, 1957.

37. GELLHORN, E., H. NAKAO, and E. S. REGATE. "The Influence of Lesions in the Anterior and Posterior Hypothalamus on Tonic and Phasic Autonomic Reactions," *J. Physiol.*, 131 (1956), 402–423.

38. GEOCARIS, K. "Circumoral Herpes Simplex and Separation Experiences in Psychotherapy," *Psychosom. Med.*, 23 (1961), 41–47.

39. GOLD, E. R. and D. B. PEACOCK. *Basic Immunology*. Bristol, England: John Wright, 1970.

40. GREENFIELD, N. S., R. ROESSLER, and A. P. CROSLEY. "Ego Strength and Length of Recovery from Infectious Mononucleosis," *J. Nerv. Ment. Dis.*, 128 (1959), 125–128.

41. HAGNELL, O. "The Premorbid Personality of

Persons Who Develop Cancer in a Total Population Investigated in 1947 and 1957," *Ann. N.Y. Acad. Sci.*, 125 (1966), 846–855.

42. HASEK, M., A. LENGEROVÁ, and T. HRABA. "Transplantation Immunity and Tolerance," *Adv. Immunol.*, 1 (1961), 1–56.

43. HAWKINS, N. G., R. DAVIES, and T. H. HOLMES. "Evidence of Psychosocial Factors in the Development of Pulmonary Tuberculosis," *Am. Rev. Tuberc. Pulmon. Dis.*, 75 (1957), 5–10.

44. HERXHEIMER, H. "Bronchoconstrictor Agents and Their Antagonists in the Intact Guinea Pig," *Arch. Int. Pharmacodyn. Ther.*, 106 (1956), 371–380.

45. HICKS, R. "The Effects of Drug-Induced Adrenocortical Deficiency and of Mineralocorticoid Drugs on Anaphylaxis in the Guinea Pig," *J. Pharm. Pharmacol.*, 20 (1968), 497–504.

46. HILL, C. W., W. E. GREER, and O. FELSENFELD. "Psychological Stress, Early Response to Foreign Protein and Blood Cortisol in Vervets," *Psychosom. Med.*, 29 (1967), 279–283.

47. HOLMES, T. H., T. TREUTING, and H. G. WOLFF. "Life Situations, Emotions and Nasal Disease," *Psychosom. Med.*, 13 (1951), 71–82.

48. HUME, D. M. "Immunological Consequences of Organ Homotransplantation in Man," *Harvey Lect.*, 64 (1968–1969), 261–388.

49. ———. "Organ Transplants and Immunity," in R. A. Good and D. W. Fisher, eds., *Immunobiology*, pp. 185–194. Stamford, Conn.: Sinauer Associates, 1971.

50. IMBODEN, J. B., A. CARTER, and E. C. LEIGHTON. "Convalescence from Influenza: A Study of the Psychological and Clinical Determinants," *Arch. Intern. Med.*, 108 (1961), 115–123.

51. JACOBS, M. A., L. S. ANDERSON, H. D. EISMAN et al. "Interaction of Psychologic and Biologic Predisposing Factors in Allergic Disorders," *Psychosom. Med.*, 29 (1967), 572–585.

52. JENSEN, M. M., and A. F. RASMUSSEN, JR. "Stress and Susceptibility to Viral Infections: II. Sound Stress and Susceptibility to Vesicular Stomatitis Virus," *J. Immunol.*, 90 (1963), 21–23.

53. JOHNSON, T., J. F. LAVENDER, E. HULLIN et al. "The Influence of Avoidance-Learning Stress on Resistance to Coxsackie B. Virus in Mice," *J. Immunol.*, 91 (1963), 569–575.

54. JOHNSON, T. and A. F. RASMUSSEN, JR. "Emotional Stress and Susceptibility to Poliomyelitis Virus Infection in Mice," *Arch. Gesamte Virusforsch.*, 18 (1965), 392–398.

55. KARCZEWSKI, W. "The Electrical Activity of the Vagus Nerve After an 'Antianaphylactic' Stimulation of the Brain," *Acta. Allergol. (Kbh)*, 19 (1964), 229–235.

56. KARCZEWSKI, W., P. S. RICHARDSON, and J. G. WIDDICOMBE. "The Role of the Vagus Nerves in Determining Total Lung Resistance and Histamine-Induced Bronchoconstriction in Rabbits," *J. Physiol.*, 181 (1965), 20P.

57. KASS, E. H. "Hormones and Host Resistance to Infection," *Bacteriol. Rev.*, 24 (1960), 177–185.

58. KEMPH, J. P. "Renal Failure, Artificial Kidney and Kidney Transplant," *Am. J. Psychiatry*, 122 (1966), 1270–1274.

59. KISSEN, D. M. "Relationship between Lung Cancer, Cigarette Smoking, Inhalation, and Personality," *Br. J. Med. Psychol.*, 37 (1964), 203–216.

60. ———. "Psychosocial Factors, Personality and Lung Cancer in Men Aged 55–64," *Br. J. Med. Psychol.*, 40 (1967), 29–43.

61. KISSEN, D. M. and L. L. LESHAN, eds. *Psychosomatic Aspects of Neoplastic Disease*. London: Pitman, 1964.

62. KNAPP, P. H. and S. J. NEMETZ. "Acute Bronchial Asthma: I. Concomitant Depression and Excitement and Varied Antecedent Patterns in 406 Attacks," *Psychosom. Med.*, 22 (1960), 42–56.

63. KORNEVA, E. A. and L. M. KHAI. "Effect of Destruction of Hypothalamic Areas on Immunogenesis," *Fed. Proc. (Transl. Suppl.)*, 23 (1964), T88–92.

64. LEGER, J. and G. MASSON. "Factors Influencing an Anaphylactoid Reaction in the Rat," *Fed. Proc.*, 6 (1947), 150–151.

65. LESHAN, L. L. "An Emotional Life-History Pattern Associated with Neoplastic Disease," *Ann. N.Y. Acad. Sci.*, 125 (1966), 780–793.

66. LEVINE, S. and C. COHEN. "Differential Survival to Leukemia as a Function of Infantile Stimulation in DB A/Z Mice," *Proc. Soc. Exp. Biol. Med.*, 102 (1959), 53–54.

67. LUKÝANENKO, V. L. "The Conditioned Reflex Regulation of Immunological Reactions," *Zh. Mikrobiol. Epidemiol. Immunobiol.*, 30 (1959), 53–59.

68. LUPARELLO, T. J., M. STEIN, and D. C. PARK. "Effect of Hypothalamic Lesions on Rat Anaphylaxis," *Am. J. Physiol.*, 207 (1964), 911–914.

69. McCLARY, A. R., E. MEYER, and D. J. WEITZMAN. "Observations on the Rôle of Mechanism of Depression in Some Patients with Disseminated Lupus Erythermatosus," *Psychosom. Med.*, 17 (1955), 311–321.

70. McCULLOCH, M. W., C. PROCTOR, and M. J. RAND. "Evidence for an Adrenergic Homeostatic Bronchodilator Reflex Mechanism," *Europ. J. Pharmacol.*, 2 (1967), 214–223.

71. McFADDEN, E. R., JR., T. LUPARELLO, H. A. LYONS et al. "The Mechanism of Action of Suggestion in the Induction of Acute Asthma Attacks," *Psychosom. Med.*, 31 (1969), 134–143.

72. MACRIS, N. T., R. C. SCHIAVI, M. D. CAMERINO et al. "Effect of Hypothalamic Lesions on Immune Processes in the Guinea Pig," *Am. J. Physiol.*, 219 (1970), 1205–1209.

73. ———. "Effect of Hypothalamic Lesions on Passive Anaphylaxis in the Guinea Pig," *Am. J. Physiol.*, 222 (1972), 1054–1057.

74. MARCHANT, J. "The Effects of Different Social Conditions on Breast Cancer Induction in Three Genetic Types of Mice by Dibenz (A,H) Anthracene and a Comparison with Breast Carcinogenesis by 3-Methylcholanthrene," *Br. J. Cancer*, 21 (1967), 576–585.

75. MARSH, J. T., J. F. LAVENDER, S. S. CHANG et al. "Poliomyelitis in Monkeys: Decreased Susceptibility after Avoidance Stress," *Science*, 140 (1963), 1414–1415.

76. MARSH, J. T. and A. F. RASMUSSEN, JR. "Response of Adrenal, Thymus, Spleen and Leucocytes to Shuttle Box and Confinement Stress," *Proc. Soc. Exp. Biol. Med.*, 104 (1960), 180–183.

77. MÁSLIŃSKI, C. and W. KARCZEWSKI. "Prevention of So-Called Histamine Shock by Stimulation of the Brain with Electric Current: Preliminary Communication," *Acta. Physiol. Pol.*, 6 (1955), 372–376.

78. ———. "The Protective Influences of Brain Stimulation by Electric Current on Histamine Shock in Guinea Pigs," *Bull. Acad. Pol. Sci.*, 5 (1957), 57–62.

79. MEYER, R. J. and R. J. HAGGERTY. "Streptococcal Infections in Families: Factors Altering Individual Susceptibility," *Pediatrics*, 29 (1962), 539–549.

80. MIESCHER, P. A. and H. J. MÜLLER-EBERHARD, eds. *Textbook of Immunolopathology*. New York: Grune & Stratton, 1968.

81. MILLS, J. E. and J. G. WIDDICOMBE. "Role of the Vagus Nerves in Anaphylaxis and Histamine-Induced Bronchoconstrictions in Guinea Pigs," *Br. J. Pharmacol.*, 39 (1970), 724–731.

82. MOOS, R. H. "Personality Factors Associated with Rheumatoid Arthritis: A Review," *J. Chronic Dis.*, 17 (1963), 41.

83. MOOS, R. H. and G. F. SOLOMON. "Personality Correlates of the Rapidity of Progression of Rheumatoid Arthritis," *Am. Rheum. Dis.*, 23 (1964), 145–151.

84. ———. "Psychologic Comparisons between Women with Rheumatoid Arthritis and Their Non-Arthritic Sisters: I. Personality Test and Interview Rating Data," *Psychosom. Med.*, 27 (1965), 135–149.

85. ———. "Psychologic Comparisons between Women with Rheumatoid Arthritis and Their Non-Arthritic Sisters: II. Content Analysis of Interviews," *Psychosom. Med.*, 27 (1965), 150–164.

86. ———. "Personality Correlates of the Degree of Functional Incapacity of Patients with Physical Disease," *J. Chronic Dis.*, 18 (1965), 1019–1038.

87. MONAENKOV, A. M. "The Influence of Changes in the Activity of the Cerebral Hemispheres in Immunological Reactions," *Zh. Mikrobiol. Epidemiol. Immunobiol.*, 12 (1956), 88–89.

88. MOVAT, H. Z. *Inflammation, Immunity and Hypersensitivity*. New York: Harper & Row, 1971.

89. NILZEN, A. "The Influence of the Thyroid Gland on Hypersensitivity Reactions in Animals: I," *Acta Allergol. (Kbh)*, 7 (1955), 231–234.

90. ———. "The Influence of the Thyroid Gland on Hypersensitivity Reactions in Animals: II," *Acta Allergol. (Kbh)*, 8 (1955), 57–60.

91. ———. "The Influence of the Thyroid Gland on Hypersensitivity Reactions in

Animals: III," *Acta Allergol. (Kbh)*, 8 (1955), 103–111.

92. ORANGE, R. P. and F. AUSTEN. "Chemical Mediators of Immediate Hypersensitivity," in R. A. Good and D. W. Fisher, eds., *Immunobiology*, pp. 115–121. Stamford, Conn.: Sinauer Associates, 1971.

93. OTTO, R. and I. P. MACKAY. "Psychosocial and Emotional Disturbance in Systemic Lupus Erythematosus," *Med. J. Aust.*, 2 (1967), 488–491.

94. PARROT, J. L. and C. LABORDE. "Inhibition d'histidine-décarboxylase par la cortisone et par le salicylate de sodium," *J. Physiol.*, 53 (1955), 441–442.

95. PETROVSKII, I. N. "Problems of Nervous Control in Immunity Reactions: II. The Influence of Experimental Neurosis on Immunity Reactions," *Zh. Mikrobiol. Epidemiol. Immunobiol.*, 32 (1961), 1451–1458.

96. PORTER, J. C. "Secretion of Corticosterone in Rats with Anterior Hypothalamic Lesions," *Am. J. Physiol.*, 204 (1963), 715–718.

97. PRZBYLSKI, A. "Effect of the Removal of Cortex Cerebri and the Quadrigeminal Bodies Region on Histamine Susceptibility of Guinea Pigs," *Acta. Physiol. Pol.*, 13 (1962), 535–541.

98. RASMUSSEN, A. F. JR. "Emotions and Immunity," in C. B. Bahnson, ed., *Second Conference on Psychophysiological Aspects of Cancer. Ann. N.Y. Acad. Sci.*, 164 (1969), 458–462.

99. RASMUSSEN, A. F. JR., J. T. MARSH, and N. Q. BRILL. "Increased Susceptibility to Herpes Simplex in Mice Subjected to Avoidance-Learning Stress or Restraint," *Proc. Soc. Exp. Biol. Med.*, 96 (1957), 183–189.

100. RASMUSSEN, A. F., JR., E. T. SPENCER, and J. T. MARSH. "Decrease in Susceptibility of Mice to Passive Anaphylaxis Following Avoidance-Learning Stress," *Proc. Soc. Exp. Biol. Med.*, 100 (1959), 878–879.

101. REES, W. L. "Physical and Emotional Factors in Bronchial Asthma," *J. Psychosom. Res.*, 1 (1956), 98–114.

102. ———. "The Role of the Autonomic Nervous System in Asthma and Allied Disorders," *J. Psychosom. Res.*, 9 (1965), 159–163.

103. ROSE, B. "Hormones and Allergic Responses," in J. H. Shaffer, G. A. LoGrippo, and M. W. Chase, eds., *International Symposium on Mechanisms of Hypersensitivity*, pp. 599–634. London: Churchill, 1959.

104. RUSSELL, P. S. and A. P. MONACO. "The Biology of Tissue Transplantation," *N. Engl. J. Med.*, 271 (1964), 502, 553, 610, 664, 718, 776.

105. RYTEL, M. W. and E. D. KILBOURNE. "The Influence of Cortisone on Experimental Viral Infection," *J. Exp. Med.*, 123 (1966), 767–775.

106. SALK, J. "Theoretical Psychophysiological Considerations," in Bahnson, C. B., ed., *Second Conference on Psychophysiological Aspects of Cancer. Ann. N.Y. Acad. Sci.*, 164 (1969), 590–610.

107. SAVCHUK, O. Y. "The Reflex Mechanism of the Formation of Antibodies," *Zh. Mikrobiol. Epidemiol. Immunobiol.*, 29 (1958), 123–131.

108. SCHAYER, R. W., J. K. DAVIS, and R. L. SMILEY. "Binding of Histamine in Vitro and Its Inhibition by Cortisone," *Am. J. Physiol.*, 182 (1955), 54–56.

109. SCHIAVI, R. C., J. ADAMS, and M. STEIN. "Effect of Hypothalamic Lesions on Histamine Toxicity in the Guinea Pig," *Am. J. Physiol.*, 211 (1966), 1269–1273.

110. SCHMALE, A. H. and H. P. IKER. "The Affect of Hopelessness in the Development of Cancer: I. The Prediction of Uterine Cervical Cancer in Women with Atypical Cytology," *Psychosom. Med.*, 26 (1964), 634–635.

111. SCHWARTZ, R. S. and Y. BOREL. "Principles of Immunosuppressive Drug Action," in P. A. Miescher and H. J. Müller-Eberhard, eds., *Textbook of Immunopathology*, Vol. 1, pp. 227–235. New York: Grune & Stratton, 1968.

112. SOLOMON, G. F. "Stress and Antibody Response in Rats," *Arch. Allergy*, 35 (1969), 97–104.

113. ———. "Emotion, Stress, the Central Nervous System and Immunity," in C. B. Bahnson, ed., *Second Conference on Psychophysiological Aspects of Cancer. Ann. N.Y. Acad. Sci.*, 164 (1969), 335–343.

114. ———. "Psychophysiological Aspects of Rheumatoid Arthritis and Autoimmune Disease," in O. W. Hill, ed., *Modern Trends in Psychosomatic Medicine*, pp. 189–216. New York: Appleton-Century-Crofts, 1970.

115. SOLOMON, G. F., S. LEVINE, and J. K.

KRAFT. "Early Experience and Immunity," *Nature*, 220 (1968), 821–822.

116. SOLOMON, G. F., T. MERIGAN, and S. LEVINE. "Variation in Adrenal Cortical Hormones within Physiological Ranges, Stress and Interferon Production in Mice," *Proc. Soc. Exp. Biol. Med.*, 126 (1967), 74–79.

117. SOLOMON, G. F. and R. H. MOOS. "Psychologic Aspects of Response to Treatment in Rheumatoid Arthritis," *Gen. Pract.*, 32 (1965), 113–115.

118. STJERNSWARD, J. "Age-Dependent Tumor Host Barrier and Effect of Carcinogen-Induced Immunodepression on Rejection of Isografted Methylcholanthrene-Induced Sarcoma Cells," *J. Natl. Cancer Inst.*, 37 (1966), 505–512.

119. SZENTIVANYI, A. "The Beta Adrenergic Theory of the Atopic Abnormality in Bronchial Asthma," *J. Allergy*, 42 (1968), 203–232.

120. SZENTIVANYI, A. and G. FILIPP. "Anaphylaxis and the Nervous System, Part II," *Ann. Allergy*, 16 (1958), 143–151.

121. TREADWELL, P. E. and A. F. RASMUSSEN, JR. "Role of the Adrenals in Stress-Induced Resistance to Anaphylactic Shock," *J. Immunol.*, 87 (1961), 492–497.

122. TURK, J. L. *Immunology in Clinical Medicine.* New York: Appleton-Century-Crofts, 1969.

123. VESSEY, S. H. "Effects of Grouping on Levels of Circulating Antibodies in Mice," *Proc. Soc. Exp. Biol.*, 115 (1964), 252–255.

124. WAN, W. C. and M. STEIN. "Effect of Vagal Stimulation on the Mechanical Properties of the Lungs in Guinea Pigs," *Psychosom. Med.*, 30 (1968), 846–852.

125. WEIL-MALHERBE, H. and S. I. SZARA. *The Biochemistry of Functional and Experimental Psychoses.* Springfield, Ill.: Charles C. Thomas, 1971.

126. WHITTIER, J. R. and A. ORR. "Hyperkinesia and Other Physiologic Effects of Caudate Deficit in the Adult Albino Rat," *Neurology*, 12 (1962), 529–539.

127. WIDDICOMBE, J. G. "Regulation of Tracheobronchial Smooth Muscle," *Physiol. Rev.*, 43 (1963), 1–37.

128. WISTAR, R. T. and W. H. HILDERMANN. "Effect of Stress on Skin Transplantation Immunity in Mice," *Science*, 131 (1960), 159–160.

129. WOLLCOCK, A. J., P. T. MACKLEM, J. C. HOGG et al. "Influence of Autonomic Nervous System on Airway Resistance and Elastic Recoil," *J. Appl. Physiol.*, 26 (1969), 814–818.

130. WOLLCOCK, A. J., P. T. MACKLEM, J. C. HOGG et al. "Effect of Vagal Stimulation on Central and Peripheral Airways in Dogs," *J. Appl. Physiol.*, 26 (1969), 806–813.

131. WYATT, R. J., B. A. TERMINI, and J. DAVIS. *Biochemical and Sleep Studies of Schizophrenia: A Review of the Literature— 1960–1970.* Schizophrenia Bulletin, Issue no. 4. Washington, D.C.: Natl. Clearinghouse for Mental Health Information, Fall 1971.

132. YAMADA, A., M. JENSEN, and A. F. RASMUSSEN, JR. "Stress and Susceptibility to Viral Infections: III. Antibody Response and Viral Retention during Avoidance Learning Stress," *Proc. Soc. Exp. Biol. Med.*, 116 (1964), 677–680.

133. YAMASAKI, H. and T. YAMAMOTO. "Inhibitory Effect of Adrenal Glucocorticoids on Histamine Release," *Jap. J. Pharmacol.*, 13 (1963), 223–224.

CHAPTER 30

MUSCULOSKELETAL DISORDERS

Donald Oken

❲ Introduction

THIS CHAPTER will discuss five clinical disorders: psychogenic rheumatism, occupational cramp, rheumatoid arthritis, parkinsonism, and gout. It is immediately apparent, therefore, that its title is a misnomer in one important sense. The basic pathophysiological processes involved in at least three of these disorders almost certainly lie outside the musculoskeletal system. A more accurate title might have referred to disorders with predominant musculoskeletal manifestations. The logic of their selection based on common symptomatic features is reinforced by a significant resemblance among the psychological factors that have been found associated with each.

The fact that the psychological findings reported for these disorders overlap poses questions about their precision, if not their validity. The similarities, however, may be quite real. If so, this raises a suspicion that the findings are similar for the same reason that the disorders are, i.e., their shared manifestations. The presence of any disease that causes severe limitation of motility, as well as pain and related symptoms in the muscles and joints, will produce psychological reactions to these symptoms. Perhaps the greatest problem in obtaining and interpreting data on patients with musculoskeletal disorders lies in separating these consequences of disease from factors which are antecedent. Some of the data does bear on factors antedating onset and these are of particular interest. But the entire subject area contains a wealth of findings that merit interest, and illustrate both the successes and difficulties of the psychosomatic approach.

Prior to the consideration of the disorders themselves is a section which reviews the available data in the area of basic psychophysiology most relevant to the musculoskeletal system, i.e., muscle tension. The rationale for this choice can be questioned for the very reason and to the same degree that the chapter may be mislabeled. Nevertheless, muscle tension does seem to have direct relevance to two of the disorders, and indirect relevance to at least two others. It also represents an important area of psychophysiology in its own right. Other relevant areas of psychophysiology will not be neglected, but will be considered in direct relation to the disorders in which they may be implicated.

❰ Basic Psychophysiology

It hardly needs to be pointed out that posture, gait, facial expression, and gestures represent basic characteristics of the personality. Individuals have their own relatively unique styles of motor expression which are readily recognizable both to themselves and those who know them. The style of a person's motor activity also provides revealing manifestations of his psychological attributes. Many studies (reviewed by Plutchik[208]) are unanimous in showing that motor expression reliably communicates characteristic attitudes.

Freud pioneered our understanding of the significance of "meaningless" motor acts as manifestations of specific unconscious motivational forces.[79,80] Psychoanalysts who followed have provided further insights about the meanings behind various movements and postures. The individualized nature of these activities makes an ideographic clinical approach such as psychoanalysis the most appropriate method for their psychological study. No comparable method existed on the motor side for a long time. Now an ingenious beginning toward a science of "Kinesics" has been launched by Birdwhistell.[17,18]

Expressive behavior has obvious relevance to both normal personality and psychopathology, the domain of psychiatry. The psychosomatic approach requires a focus on psychophysiological mechanisms, rather than motor behavior. Within this framework, our interest is in muscle tension.

Muscle Tension

The term "tension," with its inherent dual meaning of a psychological as well as muscular phenomenon, implies the existence of a psychosomatic relationship. While this may be revealing in a very general sense, a scientific understanding of that relationship requires specific, precise definition of both its psychological and somatic components. The vagueness of the term tension to represent a psychological phenomenon is obvious. It may be less evident that there has been considerable variation in its use on the somatic side as well.[13,86] The common feature which appears to underlie these various usages is skeletal muscle contraction; and it seems most sensible to define muscle tension simply in that way.[86] In so doing we bypass issues of central neurophysiological states, and ignore the highly unlikely possibility that differing types of contraction exist.

This still leaves the problem of operational definition. The methods used to measure muscle tension have varied widely. As early as 1942, R. C. Davis catalogued six different modes of measurement, each including multiple differing techniques.[55] Davis' careful analysis led him to conclude that the best method is the electronically integrated electromyogram (EMG) recorded from electrodes on the skin. There is now general agreement with his viewpoint that the surface EMG represents the most definite, sensitive, reliable, and practically useful method of measuring muscle tension.[13] A manual providing a detailed description of the technique is available.[53] Care must be exerted to choose electronic components with appropriate characteristics.[99] With such equipment, the EMG is a direct, linear correlate of isometric skeletal muscle contraction over most of its range.[53,115,144] It appears also to correlate with subjective feelings of muscle tension.[226]

Nevertheless other methods continue to be used. Among these are a resonance technique which records combined motion and tension;[263] eye-blink rate;[176] the speed and accuracy of fine psychomotor activity;[237] the aftercontraction phenomenon;[233] several techniques for quantifying movement,[228,229] including a "motility bed";[249] and many others. All may have value. But they are measuring different phenomena than the muscle action potentials which the EMG detects. They *cannot* be considered equivalent either to the EMG or to one another.[55,86]

Another problem lies in the choice of the muscle groups to be measured. Factor analyses applied to data from several independent studies show convincingly that a *general factor* of muscle tension does exist.[13,108,198,258] This indicates that there is a tendency for tension to occur to a similar degree in muscles throughout the body. However, this tendency is limited. The general factor neither includes all muscles nor does it represent close to all the variance of those it does include. Additional factor clusters also emerge from the analyses that represent more localized patterning of tension. Moreover, it has been demonstrated that *response specificity* occurs for the muscles as well as autonomic variables.[90,240] This phenomenon, originally identified by Lacey, represents the tendency for individuals to react physiologically to differing stimuli in a preferential fashion, with maximum response in a particular, differing response system.[136–138] The determinants, or even correlates, of the "choice" of a specific site of muscular responsivity remain unknown. *Stimulus specificity*, the patterning of responses due to the specific effects of a given stimulus, also seems to occur.[136,137] The study by Voas also indicated that muscle tension measured in seven separate sites varied not only for different individuals but within the same individual during different conditions.[255] In any single research, therefore, confidence can be placed on the findings *only* as they apply to those muscles specifically measured. Very few studies have included EMG's from multiple sites. Yet the results from one or two sites are frequently interpreted as if they represented a valid index of generalized tension. One of the favored sites is the frontalis. Here the dangers of erroneous extrapolation are especially great, for this muscle seems to be one of those least related to the general tension factor.[13] In a few instances there are several studies focused on a given research question which together include sufficient sites to permit a reasonable capacity to infer that generalized tension has been demonstrated. There are also, of course, questions for which measurement of tension in only a single site is relevant. If, for example, one wishes to know if a symptom arises from muscle tension, then the tension at its locus represents the only relevant measure.

Additional methodological problems arise about the selection of variables for analysis. Is the variable of choice the resting EMG level, or that reached after stimulation? Is it the mean response or the peak? Is duration of response more important than its magnitude, or, returning to the matter of the locus of response, is it better to know when tension involves a greater number of muscle areas or the body as a whole? There are no a priori answers. All these indices have been used. Any of them may be valid (i.e., relevant) to a *given* problem. At times, the use of several adds up to a broader understanding. But the lesson is clear; each study must be examined carefully to learn precisely what was measured and how, and the results interpreted in those terms.

Muscle Tension and Personality

Systematic attempts to understand the relation of specific personality traits to muscle tension began to develop around the turn of the century. One of the first was provided by William James, who divided people into hyper- and hypoactive types;[120] the former being excitable, hypermotile, and tense, and the latter phlegmatic, calm and relaxed. Many other observers have suggested a similar dichotomy, often emphasizing that hyperactivity occurred at times of emotional stimulation. These and related studies have been the subject of an extensive review by Iris Balshan Goldstein.[86]

It seems likely that emotional "excitability" corresponds closely to what we would now term "trait anxiety." To be distinguished from the state of anxiety, this term refers to the characterological tendency to respond with anxiety to many situations, including those of low threat, i.e., a chronic proneness to anxiety.[247] The threshold may be so low that anxiety is experienced even at seeming rest. Using this better defined concept, Balshan Goldstein found that normal women, scoring high on trait anxiety scales, had higher levels of tension (in sixteen muscles) during noise stimulation than did those with low scores.[13] This greater responsiveness was negatively related to scores for *restraint*, and positively to scores for *general activity* in the Guilford-Zimmerman Temperament Survey, but not to any of its other trait variables. In a later very similar study, this time using a patient group, Balshan Goldstein found the same relationship between EMG-measured tension and trait anxiety.[87] Rossi also demonstrated a relation between these two variables.[225] Trait anxiety has also been related to eye-blink rate, a measure that has been proposed as an index of overall tension.[145,177]

In both of Balshan Goldstein's studies, tension levels at rest were very low for all groups. Malmo also believes that stressful stimulation usually is required to bring out the higher tension levels of more anxious people.[156] Others have suggested that anxious individuals will have significantly greater tension even at rest.[168] The explanation for the discrepancy may lie in the degree of success in creating sufficiently non-stimulating conditions. The anxiety-inducing effects of exposure to the psychosomatic laboratory itself makes it difficult to achieve truly basal conditions.[227]

Trait anxiety would be expected to be associated with evidences of maladjustment. This too has been shown to relate to muscle tension. Duffy found that children with lower ratings of adjustment in nursery school manifested higher pressure in squeezing a hand dynamometer.[58] Adults with increased EMG tension (in the arm, shoulder and back) have been noted to react to minor environmental changes with anger and irritation.[151] Similarly, Wenger found that boys judged to be most tense physically tended to be emotional, irritable, aggressive, and unstable,[257] and that ratings of tension in children correlated with emotionality, carelessness, distractibility, and impulsiveness.[258] There is evidence of the same relationship in laboratory settings as well.[152,159]

Lacey has reported data suggesting that impulsivity and hyperkinetic traits are associated with tendencies to exhibit bursts of sympathetic-like activity, or continuous oscillatory changes, in *autonomic* variables.[139] Although he did not measure muscle tension, its correlation with these behaviors has just been indicated. Lacey's interesting idea remains conjectural, however, since the only attempt at replication has proved negative.[265]

The interrelationships among autonomic variables, muscle tension, and personality represents a barely touched-upon subject that may have considerable significance. One interesting possibility is opened by the study of Kempe.[130] This revealed contrasting traits between individuals whose stress response was primarily autonomic and those who tended to develop generalized muscle tension. Those with tension responses tended to be aloof, to deny emotion, and to intellectualize easily. The autonomic responders were emotional, insecure, and prone to worry. Although stress does have some tendency to result in a generalized "activation" of all physiological responses (as will be considered shortly), there is also evidence that the autonomic and muscle systems may have a reciprocal relationship under some circumstances. Malmo and Shagass noted this reciprocity between heart rate, and both motor responses and EMG levels in the arm in a group of psychiatric patients exposed to a painful stimulus.[161]

In this latter study, some of the motor responses were "defensive," i.e., they served to terminate the painful stimulus. This raises the issue of the role of psychological defense in producing muscle tension. The traits reported by Kempe to characterize those who respond to stress with generalized muscle tension suggest a personality in which defenses against affects are predominant. This is an issue of great importance. The control of affect, particularly anger, has been postulated as a major pathogenic mechanism in several of the musculoskeletal disorders to be discussed in subsequent sections.

This relationship has been suggested by many psychoanalytic observations. Abraham reported in 1913 that "during analysis patients show inhibitions of those bodily movements which derive from a *repressed* [my emphasis] erotic pleasure in movement."[1] Ferenczi noted the frequent reciprocity between thought and action, and observed that many patients exhibit stiffness of the limbs during a state of resistance, which disappears following its resolution.[70] The tendency for the affect-controlled compulsive character to manifest generalized muscular rigidity was explored in detail by Reich, who clarified its ties to the rigidity of defense in the important term "character armor."[215] He pointed out how physical relaxation can result in a loosening of defenses and freeing of affective expression. Similarly, Barlow reported that following relaxation "one may see uncontrollable reactions, such as laughter and weeping."[14] Fenichel comments that "pathogenic defense always means the blocking of certain movements." He reported that a patient "who can no longer avoid seeing an interpretation is correct, but nevertheless tries to, frequently shows cramping of his entire muscular system or of certain parts of it."[69] The most detailed psychoanalytic studies were carried out by Felix Deutsch who reported on the presence of individually characteristic infantile postures and movements associated with the regressive nature of the psychoanalytic situation.[57] A portion of what he observed were defensive movements, e.g., rigidity related to the *suppression* of thoughts, a point also emphasized by Ascher.[8] In sum, these observations focus on the role of muscle tension in relation to defense, and often specifically in relation to control of affective expression. Plutchik summarizes the implication of these and other studies in much the same way.[208] He comments also on the ubiquity of reference to this connection in everyday language (being rigid, keeping one's chin up, etc.). There is, in addition, the familiar observation that being self-protectively "on guard" in the face of danger is associated with muscular tenseness. Also consistent with the reciprocity noted by Kempe[130] are Kepecs' psychoanalytic observations of a reciprocity between muscle and secretory activity, including weeping and exudation into the skin.[131] He suggests that when the muscles are about to be activated during rage but this undergoes inhibition, the result may be actual weeping or weeping lesions of the skin.

An attempt was made by the Michael Reese group to obtain experimental verification of the relationship between muscle tension and "control." In the initial study a series of hospitalized depressed patients were selected for study because of the motoric disturbances found in this type of disorder. These patients were exposed to a stressful situation, and one designed to stimulate efforts at self-control, while EMG recordings were obtained from seven muscles.[241] The temporary activation of efforts at self-control did not elevate muscle tension. However, there were a number of significant correlations between tension in four muscles (frontalis, trapezius, quadriceps, and particularly the biceps) and several personality trait measures that seem consistent with the postulated relationship. Tension in these muscles was greater in the patients who were characterologically less emotional, less anxious, more prone to use fantasy than action, and who had a more rigid definition of their body boundaries. An attempt to replicate these findings on a different study population, a mixed group of psychiatric outpatients, failed.[107] A careful analysis of the discrepancies suggests that their major source lay in the differences between the psychological characteristics of the patients in the two studies.[107,108] Whatever the explanation, one can only conclude that the clinical observation that defensive character armoring is reflected in elevated levels of muscle tension remains unverified in the laboratory.

The basis for selection of a measure of body boundary definiteness stemmed from the work of Fisher and Cleveland. These researchers have conducted a number of studies of body image focused on the degree to which an individual conceives of his body boundary as representing a distinct barrier between internal and external interchanges. They developed the hypothesis that a high "barrier" measure is associated with exterior psychosomatic disorders, including *arthritis*, and with greater reactivity of the physiological systems nearer the surface of the body. In several studies, it was found that subjects with a high barrier score developed greater levels of muscle tension in response to stressful stimulation than did those with a low barrier score. Details of their work and that of others on this subject are available in two books.[73,75]

Stress, Arousal, Emotion, and Defense

There is solid evidence that the psychological stress response is accompanied by an increase in muscle tension in most people. In Duffy's studies, the greatest rises in tension occurred with emotional stress.[59] It has been repeatedly demonstrated that when elevations of muscle tension occur during interviews, specifically stressful material is being discussed.* In one interesting study, jaw muscle tension was high following criticism by the therapist, but fell after praise, in *both* the patient and therapist.[158]

Not only does tension increase under stress, it spreads to involve larger areas of the body. There is a tendency for an individual to lose his ability to discretely utilize specific muscles required for appropriate action, and for tension to spread progressively from that site. Luria's classical studies demonstrated that affectively meaningful stimuli produced a disorganization of purposeful responses in the hand, which became impulsive and tremulous; there was "overflow" of tension to the muscles of the nonactive hand.[152] Factor analyses of the data collected in the Michael Reese studies mentioned above also revealed that muscle responses became more diffuse as stress intensified.[108]

There is a school of thought which asserts that there are no real physiological differences among the various states of affect associated with stress, nor indeed among these and other states of heightened motivation and mental effort. All such states are seen as representing points of elevation along a single continuum. Their qualitative differences are ascribed to added cognitive elements and components of "directionality" (approach avoidance). The central underlying phenomenon has been termed "arousal" or "activation," the former

emphasizing its behavioral properties, the latter its neurophysiological ones. A detailed consideration of this theory and the evidence upon which it is based is available,[61,157] and does not concern us here.

What we do need to note is that the theory postulates that the level of muscle tension (along with manifestations of sympathetic nervous system activity) parallels the level of activation. Consistent with this are the findings of increased tension associated with learning, motivation, difficulty of mental work, reaction time, attention, thinking, etc. (References to this work can be found in Balshan Goldstein's review.[86]) Certainly emotional stresses of essentially every kind have been demonstrated to be associated with increased muscle tension. One interesting exception is the occurrence of a precipitous drop in tension, to the point of physical collapse, associated with sudden surges of intense emotion, the phenomenon known as *tonusverlust*.[254]

Levels of activation may be applied not only to classify stimuli (stronger stimuli being more activating) but to characterize individuals as well. There is a tendency for people to retain their respective ranks in their levels of muscle tension across a variety of stimulus situations.[58,60] Individuals at the poles of such a ranking would presumably be the same ones identified by the hyper- vs. hypoactive personality typology already described.

While activation theory may have value in understanding states of affective arousal in general, there are sound reasons for looking beyond it to more specific issues. As Lacey has so well clarified for autonomic responses, specific "fractionation" of the general response occurs, with variations ascribable to the stimulus, to the individual, and probably to the quality of the internal response state evoked.[136,137] It has been indicated already that the tendency for muscles to react in a generalized fashion is not a strong one, and that there is distinct evidence that more discrete response patterns occur. It is now a commonplace laboratory observation that rises in muscle tension during arousal often can be demonstrated *if* the "correct" muscle is found, but this site will vary among individuals.

* See references 52, 114, 159, 162, and 238.

Whatever activation theory does explain, it necessarily begs questions relevant to the occurrence of specific sites of tension in specific people under specific circumstances, compelling us to look further.

Anxiety plays a special role in the psychological stress response, being both an indicator of its presence and a precursor of further response.[96] Hence it is not surprising that anxiety is the affect most clearly implicated in stress-associated rises in muscle tension. Motor hyperactivity and "nervous" mannerisms are widely accepted as evidence of everyday anxiety. Tremor, purposeless movements, restlessness, and other motor symptoms are regular features of clinical states of anxiety. Cameron's systematic analysis of symptoms occurring in patients with anxiety revealed that the "skeletal muscle pattern" represented the largest subgroup.[32] Balshan Goldstein concluded from her extensive review that muscle tension tends to be high, "particularly in disorders in which anxiety is the major concomitant."[86] In studies of the stress responses of psychiatric patients belonging to several diagnostic categories, Malmo and Shagass found that the degree of anxiety paralleled the extent of the rise in muscle tension, regardless of the diagnosis (with some exceptions among chronic schizophrenics).[156,159,163,164] Two separate studies of hypnotically induced emotions demonstrated that rises in muscle tension were greater following an anxiety or fear suggestion than one for depression.[50,169] A detailed laboratory study of muscle tension in psychiatric outpatients by the Michael Reese group, involving multiple psychological variables, revealed that the increases in muscle tension occurring with stress were related most closely to ratings of anxiety.[242] Both Jacobson and Wolpe consider muscle tension as an inherent component of the state of anxiety, so that their anxiety treatment techniques are based on tension reduction.[117,269]

Anxiety also causes a prolongation of the muscle-tension response to stressful stimulation.[14,51,163] The exaggerated startle reaction so typical of anxiety seems to be due to this rather than an increased magnitude of response. Anxious patients manifested a continu-ing rise in tension following a sudden noise stimulus at a time when the responses in normals were falling and had almost disappeared.[54]

Anger also is relevant. The subjective sense of increased tension associated with rising anger is a familiar experience. A specific attempt to differentiate the physiological patterns specifically characteristic of fear vs. anger revealed that both were associated with elevated frontalis tension, with the levels during anger exceeding those for fear.[11]

The state of frustration may not be identical to that of anger, but it is certainly one closely akin. In his thoughtful review, Plutchik marshalled a substantial body of evidence linking frustration and conflict to muscle tension.[208] He cites a variety of studies which confirm the observable link between frustration, anger, and hypermotility, and of tension arising in situations where internal conflicts block action. From these and other data he concludes that chronic muscular tensions represent "a continuous state of readiness, indicating present day conflict or frustrations" that "reflect attitudes which are usually verbally unexpressed." Freeman also felt frustration and conflict were central to the development of muscle tension.[76]

If we take a second look at the studies of stress, maladjustment and trait anxiety, it becomes apparent that irritation, irritability, impatience, and similar states are frequently part of the reported affective reactions. Given the complexity of human beings, states in which a single "pure" affect develop are rare. Experience in the psychosomatic laboratory confirms this; even with the specific attempt to stimulate a given affect, mixed states occur.[202] Certainly the physiological features of anxiety, anger, and other affects overlap, requiring great sophistication in research methodology to delineate their minor, quantitative differences.[11] It may be that each affect is associated with a somewhat specific *patterning* of tension, i.e., with prediliction for certain muscle groups. Bull has suggested that feeling states arise secondarily as the perception of the patterned muscular responses which, she feels, represent the primary emotional state, a derivative of the James-Lange theory.[31] The term she uses for emotional states is "attitude," one that has both affective and positional connotations.

But in every situation of stress and affect arousal it is equally certain that the reaction also will include elements of ego defense. It is impossible to conceive of a state of stress in human beings unaccompanied by the mobilization of *defenses and coping mechanisms.* The states of frustration and conflict, discussed above, also include a component of defense. Even simpler demands for performance, problem solving, attention, etc., necessarily call forth adaptive efforts. Thus we are brought back again to the possible role of *control* and defense mechanisms in the production of muscle tension, especially when it is sustained. It is possible that it is these processes, rather than the affect, that is the crucial factor in stress-induced tension.

The two studies[107,241] which attempted specifically to identify the role of *control* were, as indicated, negative. The focus of these was on relatively conscious and immediate exertions of control efforts, i.e., self-control. Perhaps a better definition of control related to more automatic processes, or a focus on other defense and coping mechanisms, especially those linked to character, might have better payoff. One report, which touches on this subject, linked the responsiveness of frontalis muscle tension to ego strength, as measured by the MMPI (Minnesota Multiphasic Personality Inventory).[224] Given the known inverse relationship of ego strength to such factors as trait anxiety, which correlate with muscle tension, this seems puzzling. The explanation may lie in the greater defensive response of the high ego-strength subjects. Unfortunately the design of the study included no observations of this dimension.

Any stressful situation will inevitably tend to cause rises in all these factors concomitantly, i.e., a mixture of various affects, defenses, and coping maneuvers. A researcher will therefore find the *explanatory* variables he happens to look for.[203] The present state of our knowledge suggests that all these factors may bear a relationship to muscle tension.

It seems sensible to view tension as representing a final common pathway of peripheral response which is related to a variety of central psychological states. Within this very general situation, it may be that differential patterning of muscle response occurs in relation to specific states. To determine if this is so requires more sophisticated research which can examine a variety of psychological factors simultaneously, each in relation to tension measures taken from many muscles. Until then, we are left with many interesting conjectures but only a few dependable conclusions.

Psychiatric Disorders

There is one direction in which many findings do converge. Every one of the aforementioned factors suggests that elevated muscle tension should be found in psychiatric patients. Who, if not psychiatric patients, are prone to manifest anxiety, conflict, stress sensitivity, etc.? The verification of this is ample. The overall picture shows that patients with essentially every disorder exhibit a heightened muscle tension under many conditions. In fact, several of the studies already discussed have used patient groups precisely for this reason. Therein lies the problem. In such instances it is difficult to discern if the findings bear a relationship to the disorder per se. The burden of proof must rest in the other direction, given the widespread presence of elevated tension across diagnostic groups.

Several of Malmo's studies have specifically suggested that anxiety is the primary significant factor.[156,159,164] Also consistent is Martin's finding that "dysthymic" (anxious, depressed, and/or obsessional) neurotics displayed significantly more forearm and frontalis tension at rest than did hysterics.[168] A similar comparison by Balshan Goldstein revealed like differences which, however, were small and not statistically significant.[88] There seems little point, therefore, in discussing the many studies in which mixed, nonspecified or anxious patient groups have been studied.

Several studies focusing on *schizophrenia* have pointed to elevated levels of tension in these patients, at least under "resting" conditions. Whatmore and Ellis found resting EMG tension recorded from four areas (forehead, jaw, forearm, and leg) to be higher in a group of twenty-one schizophrenics than in ten normal controls.[259] The nature of the patient group was not specified beyond statements that they had "clear-cut" diagnoses, and were "without signs of deterioration." Malmo and his coworkers compared neck and forearm EMG levels in seventeen *chronic* schizophrenics, with groups of "acute psychotics," neurotics, and normal controls.[165] All patient groups had high levels of tension at rest, whereas the normals did not. Stressful stimulation produced an increase in tension for all groups, but the rise was significantly lower for the chronic schizophrenics than the other patient groups, with the normals falling between. The schizophrenics were especially less responsive if the stimulus was brief. Very similar results to those of Malmo were obtained by Williams using a resonance (non-EMG) technique.[263]

In a previous study from the same laboratory, "early" schizophrenics were found to be similar to *very* anxious neurotics. Both showed high levels of neck tension in response to painful stimulation. The schizophrenics, however, manifested poor discrimination among the various levels of stimulus intensity. Martin also reported that early schizophrenics were significantly more tense (frontalis and forearm EMG) than normals.[168] But the difference was present at rest and disappeared following stimulation.

In a complex and methodologically sophisticated study, Balshan Goldstein compared muscle tension in psychotics, neurotics, patients with character disorders, and normal controls.[88] All groups included contained fifteen subjects, and both sexes. The psychotics were *not chronic* and included ten schizophrenics. The EMG records were obtained from seven muscles at rest and in response to a noise stimulus. The psychotics had generally higher tension levels at rest, and distinctly greater responses to the noise. The differences were significant for the sternocleidomastoid, frontalis, biceps, and forearm extensor muscles, especially the forearm. Both the normals

and patients with character disorders had low levels and responses, while the neurotics fell between. This study incorporated a unique feature in that the neurotic and psychotic groups were equated for their levels of anxiety on the Taylor MAS scale (manifest anxiety scale). Thus their differences in tension seem reliably related to the diagnostic difference itself. This is the only study about which such a statement can be made with confidence.

Whatmore and Ellis also conducted studies of *depression*. In their initial project, six severely retarded patients, as well as thirteen patients with agitated or mixed pictures, were compared with matched controls.[260] All were female. Resting EMG recordings (forehead, jaw, forearm, and leg) revealed high tension in all areas, with the greatest differences in the jaw muscles, and the least in the frontalis. The highest levels occurred in the *retarded* depressives. On the basis of these data Whatmore and Ellis formulated a theory that persistent muscular hypertension at rest, which they termed "hyperponesis," reflected a central neurophysiological state that was an inherent aspect of the depressive disorder. This formulation, however, is not only vague but loses some credibility from their own previous similar findings in schizophrenics, of which they make no mention. Nevertheless their data, particularly those in retarded patients, are of great interest.

In their second project, five previously studied severely retarded depressed patients were followed with the same measures longitudinally through remissions and relapses.[261] Increased tension was again demonstrated during periods of depression. Although the levels decreased temporarily during successful treatment, they soon returned to the previous high levels which persisted "indefinitely." In one patient, a relapse was just preceded by an increase above the already elevated level. Whatmore and Ellis interpret these data as further support for their concept of "hyperponesis."

Martin and Rees found increased forearm tension in female depressives during a reaction-time test, compared to controls.[170] While patients' mean reaction times were slower, some of their responses were as fast as the normals, suggesting that the difference may have been due to reduced motivation.

The degree of elevation in forearm tension was found to correlate with the severity of depression in a group of patients (of both sexes) studied by Noble and Lader.[201] Tension correlated also with the level of anxiety. In contrast to Whatmore and Ellis' findings, the elevated resting level dropped significantly following electroconvulsive therapy (ECT). Mental arithmetic produced an increase in tension to about the same levels both before and after ECT, the extent of the change being greater afterwards because of the lower resting level. A positive relationship between the intensity of depression and the level of resting tension in the forearm, and to some extent the frontalis, was found also in another study of depressed patients, by Rimón et al.[219] This was more certain for males than females. Jaw tension however, which Whatmore and Ellis reported as showing the highest levels,[260] had a negative relationship with the severity of depression in both sexes. The posttreatment data are confusing. Patients who made a good recovery showed an increase in tension, while those who had a poor recovery had a decrease.

Data on depressives was obtained also in the aforementioned study by Balshan Goldstein.[88] Tension levels were recorded from seven muscles in *nonpsychotic* depressed patients and matched groups of nondepressed neurotics and controls. Each contained thirteen women and eight men. Following a stimulus, the depressed patients had significantly higher levels of tension in the trapezius and frontalis; in the forearm the difference fell just short of significance. Similar, but insignificant, differences were present at rest. No differences in jaw tension were found, a result in accord with the findings of Rimón[219] but directly contrary to those of Whatmore and Ellis.[260] It seems likely that Goldstein's subjects were less severely depressed than those in either of these two studies, which had included psychotic patients. Whatmore and Ellis' patients also were older, a factor which Rimón found to be associated with higher levels of tension.[219]

The problem of relating specific *sites* of ten-

sion to specific disorders is illustrated by the data on the forearm extensors. Elevated tension in these muscles is the most reliable finding in depressives, having been reported in all the studies discussed above. However, it has also been reported to occur in schizophrenics in three separate studies.[88,165,259]

A recent study has demonstrated a decrease in the postural reflex activity of the shoulder (supraspinatus) in depressed patients. This correlated, in general, with the level of depression.[10] These findings fit with the commonly observable slumped posture of depressives. An essential point is that this interesting technique is entirely different from that used in the other studies considered above.

It might be mentioned also that psychotics of all types are said to differ from neurotics in having significant disturbances of *fine* psychomotor activity.[132] Finally, it should be noted that characteristic microscopic muscle lesions and an elevation in circulating levels of certain muscle enzymes have been reported to occur in patients with a variety of *acute* psychoses.[72,173,174]

Conclusions

It seems possible to come to a few general conclusions despite the differing and somewhat confusing nature of this array of data:

1. There is a tendency for individuals to be characterized by different levels of muscle tension and to maintain this relative level in various situations. Perhaps the best personality correlate of higher levels of tension is the tendency to experience anxiety and to manifest other forms of emotional hyperreactivity.

2. Individuals have a proclivity to develop tension, when stimulated, primarily in specific sites characteristic for themselves. Under conditions of increased arousal, tension tends to become progressively more generalized, and the differences among individuals thus tend to disappear.

3. Under stressful conditions, particularly those which induce anxiety, muscle tension rises. At high anxiety levels this increase in

response is likely to be accompanied by its prolongation in time, and by its spread, leading to disruption of motor coordination. The relationship of stress-induced tension with heightened anxiety is clearest, but it may be related also to anger and other affects, to the mobilization of certain defenses, to the state of conflict or frustration, or to all of these.

4. Patients with psychiatric disorders of every type are likely to exhibit high levels of muscle tension, especially after stressful stimulation. It is uncertain if this relates to the disorders themselves or is merely a reflection of anxiety and the other factors just mentioned. Increased tension may be especially characteristic of two disorders, schizophrenia and the depressions, above and beyond the presence of anxiety. For the depressions, where the evidence seems particularly strong, the level of tension seems to parallel the severity of the disorder, even in the presence of overt psychomotor retardation.

5. No convincing evidence yet exists to relate specific patterns or sites of muscle tension to specific affect states or to specific psychiatric diagnostic entities, despite several interesting suggestions. This state of knowledge may be partly a product of the fact that few studies have obtained tension measures from more than a limited number of sites.

6. Clarification of many of these problems seems amenable to research embodying now existing technical and methodological knowledge.

These conclusions reflect the substantial body of research on the basic psychophysiology of muscle tension. None of them bears directly on the role of muscle tension in the musculoskeletal disorders. They do, however, have some relevance to the psychological characteristics which have been suggested as playing a significant role in these disorders, as will be seen. There are also a few studies in which tension measures have been made directly in patients with given disorders. These will be considered, as appropriate, within the following sections which deal with each disorder.

❴ Psychogenic Rheumatism

While the term "rheumatism" lacks precise meaning, that very quality may have a particular aptness in grouping together a grab bag of disabilities which have common underlying features. The complaints may include a variety of aches, pains, weakness, stiffness, and other uncomfortable sensations in the muscles or joints, as well as subjective swelling, tenderness, and limitation of motion. These may involve a single area, several, or occur "all over" the body, and they may be migratory. The diagnosis of psychogenic rheumatism is applied to such disorders in which the symptoms and disability occur in the absence of established "organic" disease or are significantly out of proportion to its extent. Clinically, the complaints often have a vague or odd quality, may not conform to expected anatomic distributions, and may be unrelieved by analgesics or physical therapies. Abnormal, sometimes bizarre, posture and movements may develop. However, the symptoms can closely mimic known *organic* diseases.

The overall incidence of minor isolated rheumatic symptoms must be 100 percent. (Who has not had unexplainable aches and pains?) But there are no clear figures for the prevalence of disability significant enough to require diagnostic labeling. It is established that this disorder occurs frequently enough to comprise a major portion of the patients with diagnosed rheumatic disease. In several large series, reviewed by Boland, it consistently ranked among the top three causes of rheumatic disease, along with rheumatoid and osteoarthritis.[22] The incidence seems to be particularly high in military personnel, where figures as high as 34 and 42 percent of the admissions to special rheumatic centers have been reported.[21,22] In this setting, its onset is especially common just prior to overseas or combat duty.[110]

Some further idea of the vast extent of rheumatic disease and its disability, particularly in the military, is provided by data on veterans' pensions. In 1931 (an era when the number of veterans was far fewer than it is today and their care was far less complete) the Federal government was providing pensions to more than 35,000 disabled veterans in this category, at an annual cost exceeding 10 million dollars![110]

Classification and Mechanisms

Boland, who provides one of the best general reviews of the subject, refers to the disorder also as "psychoneurotic musculoskeletal complaints."[22] He does so to emphasize the very high incidence of coexisting neurotic symptoms and predisposing "neurotic traits" he finds to be characteristic. Ehrlich also describes it as a form of psychoneurosis.[64] The studies on which this impression is based, however, lacked adequate controls, and the ubiquity of psychiatric symptoms when these are skillfully sought after makes one cautious about this viewpoint. It seems likely that many cases of lesser severity which do not require referral to a rheumatologist or psychiatrist will fail to demonstrate overt psychopathology.

Boland classifies psychogenic rheumatism into three subtypes: (1) pure; (2) superimposed (functional overlay); and (3) residual (functional prolongation).[22] The last most often follows trauma, while the superimposed type is usually associated with more minor rheumatic diseases, rather than with a serious articular disease such as rheumatoid arthritis. *Fibrositis* is traditionally included as one minor condition particularly prone to psychogenic overlay. But there is good reason to question whether this entity exists at all. Its diagnosis is based on subjective complaints. Though nodules are sometimes palpable, Halliday has pointed out that these can be found (as?) often, if sought for, in *a*symptomatic individuals.[103] In one study cited by Boland, 70 percent of cases labeled as fibrositis showed "significant psychiatric disorders."[22] Although acknowledging the difficulties in diagnosis, Hench and Boland suggest that, with care, the two can be differentiated clinically.[110] They characterize fibrositis as having more localized and definite symptoms which are highly responsive to external temperature and humidity (rather than to mood, distraction, or emotional stress), as having a better response to the usual therapies, as associated with less disability, and as occurring in less neurotic patients who are more calm and cooperative during examination, and who may evidence a more "objective" attitude about their illness.

Halliday, the earliest serious student of the problem, classified fibrositis as one of three types of psychogenic rheumatism. The others were hysterical pains, seen most often in people in hazardous occupations, and symptoms arising as manifestations of a psychoneurotic anxiety state or psychotic depression.[103] Paul, who studied back pain, divided that condition into four categories.[205] These included: (1) pain due to muscle tension "of conversion origin;" (2) pain of conversion origin without increased muscle tension; (3) pain due to muscle tension of "anxiety-tension origin;" and (4) any of these with associated back disease or injury.

Each of these classifications has some heuristic value, but a fully satisfactory taxonomy remains to be developed. One problem centers around symptoms arising from conversion (hysterical) mechanisms. Because they represent psychogenic rather than psychophysiological disturbances, conventionally these are excluded from the "psychosomatic" category. This may be entirely appropriate for such curious and blatant examples of hysteria as camptocormia,[231] or the "stiff-man" syndrome.[85] But it is likely that more minor conversion mechanisms are involved in some of the ordinary disorders diagnosed as psychogenic rheumatism. This may occur as a secondary elaboration of symptoms which initially developed on a psychophysiological basis. Faulty postural compensations also can add a significant element to symptoms which arose originally on a psychological basis.[211]

Nevertheless in most instances the major pathogenic mechanism seems to be a psychophysiological one, i.e., elevated muscle tension. Of the several major clinical disorders considered in this chapter in which increased muscle tension has been hypothesized to be the significant mechanism, the evidence seems by far most dependable for psychogenic rheumatism. Clear signs of localized muscle tension are often readily apparent in the physical examination of patients with the symptoms of psychogenic rheumatism. This clinical finding has been confirmed by EMG measures.* Particularly relevant is the phenomenon termed "symptom specificity," elucidated by the excellent research of Malmo and Shagass.[160] Symptom specificity refers to the fact that the stress response of some individuals is characterized by a distinct predilection for hyperactivity in a given muscle (or autonomic variable) leading to symptoms directly referable to that increased activity. Thus, patients with a history of head and neck pains responded to psychological stress with greater rises in neck-muscle tension than did controls or patients with cardiovascular symptoms, while the latter patients had the greatest cardiovascular changes. In longitudinal studies, several headache patients manifested periods of increased head and neck tension occurring during stress, and it was at such times that episodes of their typical pain occurred.[52,160, 162,238]

Rinehart, disciple of Jacobson's "progressive relaxation," also identifies elevated muscle tension as the primary issue in psychogenic rheumatism.[220] His entirely anecdotal report loses all credibility, however, by lumping together *all* rheumatic disease (including rheumatoid and osteoarthritis) as having the identical pathophysiology and pathogenesis, as does the entire school of "progressive relaxation" by its indiscriminate implication of muscular hypertension as being the central defect in a large array of disease processes.[118]

Psychogenesis

There are few disorders in which patients' use of symbolic *organ language* is as conspicuous as in psychogenic rheumatism. One is struck, as were Halliday, Weiss, and Paul, by these patients' references to themselves, their reactions, and their world in terms replete with musculoskeletal connotations.[102,205,256]

* See references 52, 140, 160, 162, 211, and 238.

They are people who "wouldn't stoop" to certain behavior, even when they meet "stiff" situations, as might a "spineless" person; they manage somehow to "limp along" and "not buckle," even when things are a "pain in the neck," etc.

Two themes are especially prominent in their expressions: *anger* and *its control*. These same issues were identified by Weiss as the characteristic feature of forty patients with varied rheumatic symptoms.[256] His interviews revealed "chronic resentment" and "smoldering discontent" to be their "special emotional problem." They were "burned up" and "aching to" express their hostility, but were unable to do so because of repressing forces. Weiss went on to comment that muscles "serve as the means for defense and attack in the struggle for existence," and that chronic muscle tension arises when the expression of aggression is inhibited.

The very careful study of seventy-five diverse backache patients led Holmes and Wolff to quite similar conclusions, despite their different (nonpsychoanalytic) frame of reference.[114] They were able to discern a common "basic personality" characterized by an "action orientation" going back to childhood, and by a "basic insecurity" which had led to a wary, tentative, "on-guard" approach to people and life situations. These patients had many obsessive-compulsive character traits and a strong need to "keep the peace." Episodes of back pain occurred in life situations in which they felt disapproved, unreceiving of deserved praise, or criticized despite their efforts, and thus felt "anger and resentment" over being taken advantage of, but could not take action without increasing their insecurity. They dealt with this conflict by being even more "on guard." Support for this formulation came from EMG measures taken during interviews. Striking increases in muscle tension occurred during the discussion of stressful events of the specific type noted, which were especially prone to occur when the current life situation was of the same nature.

Something very like the "on-guard" attitude seems to characterize the response of these patients during medical examinations. Hench and Boland describe the attitude of "touch me not" as being sufficiently typical to constitute a clue to diagnosis.[110] The obsessive-compulsive traits also were noted by both Halliday and by Rinehart.[102,220] This makes sense, given the psychodynamic relationships of such defenses to the control of anger, and their common "anal" genetic origin—a shorthand designation for a developmental period in which the main issue is the mastery and control of *muscular* activity.

However, the clinical descriptions provided in these and several other reports include some patients who have manifest anxiety. This was the major quality communicated in Boland's descriptions, as already noted. The question therefore exists whether it is the anger, its control, or anxiety over that or other conflicts, which is the relevant factor. Basic research, as I have noted in an earlier section, leaves this matter open. Perhaps the wisest present position that can be taken is that one must determine individually for each patient the psychological factors that are involved in *his* increased muscle tension.

Chapman makes the interesting observation that these disorders occur mainly in muscles that have important uses in animals, but are of lesser importance in man.[34] Just why a given site is involved in a given person is not always clear. What psychological factors contribute to the "symptom specificity"? Sometimes the specific symbolic meanings of the part seem to be involved. These may become apparent in the organ language used to describe the symptoms. One interesting lead is provided by experimental findings which suggest that hostility is related to tension in the arm, and that, in women, sexual problems are related to leg tension.[166,238] Further work of this type is needed.

Treatment

As always, good treatment rests on accurate diagnosis. Little can be added to Halliday's advice that this requires establishing *what kind* of a person this is, why did he take ill *when* he did, and in the *manner* that he did.[102] In many mild cases, the kind of doctor-patient relationship inherent in this approach itself leads to a reduction in the intensity of conflicts, allowing for recovery. At an early stage the usual simpler techniques of symptomatic relief, reassurance, support, ventilation, and environmental manipulation usually suffice. Muscle relaxants may be very useful for the anxious patient, especially if these also have "tranquilizer" effects.[206] These agents require more cautious use in rigidly controlled patients, who suffer from generalized muscle tension. "Relaxation" may have a paradoxical effect by threatening such patients with an inability to maintain their defenses.[234]

Major and prolonged illnesses represent a far more difficult problem. There is great value in early intervention before symptoms have become fixed and elements of secondary gain are superimposed. As Hench and Boland understate it: "Our pleasure at being able to reassure soldiers . . . that they do not have arthritis . . . and need not fear the presence of a crippling disease is tempered by the difficulty in helping them develop insight and to accept the diagnosis."[110] Physical and pharmacological therapies specifically associated with "organic" forms of arthritis should be avoided, since the patient uses these to reinforce his denial of the psychogenic nature of his illness. The physician's firmness in this regard does not require being argumentative and must be combined with an accepting open attitude to the patient. The treatment of persistent symptoms in its further details merges into the entire body of techniques of psychotherapy.

Special therapeutic techniques designed specifically to reduce muscle tension promise usefulness in those many instances where muscular hypertension can be implicated. These include "autogenic training," "progressive relaxation," hypnosis, and the "reciprocal inhibition," associated with behavior therapies.[117,154,269] All of these techniques have been reported to produce significant immediate relaxation in selected individual instances during training sessions. This has been confirmed by EMG measures. But it is yet far from clear how much generalization occurs to situations outside sessions, whether reports of outside subjective improvement are also associated with demonstrable reductions in EMG levels, or how widely applicable such methods are to different patients.[140] The body of literature on these techniques is very large, but almost none of the "research" reports can be said to embody even the most minimal principles of scientific methodology, though beginnings are being made.

❲ Occupational Cramp

The occupational cramps include a large number of functional disorders characterized by the impairment of a specific learned occupational motor skill. The dysfunction typically is associated with muscle spasm, and pain or severe discomfort of the involved part, although the specific clinical features vary. An excellent brief review of the subject is available.[183]

The varieties of cramp are apparently as numerous as there are occupational motor acts. Some thirty-four varieties affecting the upper extremity alone have been delineated, ranging from telegraphist's, to cigar maker's, to violinist's cramp![183] The various forms seem to have much in common. The incidence of each seems merely to reflect the prevalence of the skill. For this reason writing is by far most often affected.

Writer's cramp is well known and certainly the best studied of these disorders. Crisp and Moldofsky have reviewed the subject extensively.[48] It exists essentially in all cultures. Its incidence is reported as being 0.1 percent of "neuropsychiatric cases," though the meaning of this figure is obscure, given the impossibility of defining the base. Mild cases are probably quite numerous. As with the other occupational cramps, its psychogenic nature is evident from the fact that a specific skill is involved, while unrelated activities involving the same muscles and movements are spared or minimally affected. The disability tends to increase with stress, and concomitant neurotic symptoms are usually found.

Many psychologists would formulate the origins of the disorder as a "faulty learning experience." This viewpoint has become more attractive because of the resurgent interest in the application of learning models to behavioral disorders. But the idea is not new, and corresponds closely to that held by Pierre Janet. Techniques of "reeducation" have, indeed, proved somewhat efficacious. This is more likely to be the case when they are combined with other techniques of effective psychotherapy. Partly, such reeducation may be required because of the superimposition of secondary maladaptive compensatory positions and movements, which do represent a form of erroneous learning. Frustration and anxiety over anticipated failure play a role in this development. In any event, the faulty-learning-habit explanation begs the questions of *why* the learning was deviant, and why the disorder developed *when* it did.

Psychiatrists have tended generally to classify writer's cramp as a psychoneurotic symptom, though most formulations have been vague. Most writers have tended to view it as an hysterical symptom, though noting that it might occur in conjunction with an obsessional state.[48] Cameron viewed it as an hysterical symptom related to ambivalence over the writing activity,[33] and Glover felt it represented an hysterical conversion mechanism.[84]

Crisp and Moldofsky present compelling arguments for placing it instead in the psychosomatic (psychophysiological) category.[48,183] Careful study revealed that their patients lacked the classical hysterical features, i.e., they were neither bland nor manipulative. In fact, obsessive-compulsive traits were usual. Secondary gain played a minimal role; the actual inability to write was rare. Instead, there was a "continuing unresolved ambivalence" over writing, with expressed resentment over having to do so. Symptomatic exacerbations corresponded closely with periods of intensified resentment. Thus, the disorder seems to represent a concomitant of affective disturbance, rather than a neurotic defense against it. Finally, a physiological disturbance of the motor system does seem to be present and to extend beyond the symptom. Von Reis has provided EMG evidence of widespread muscle tension throughout the arm of the involved hand, occurring even at rest.[216]

Crisp and Moldofsky's experience also underlines the value of an overall treatment program which combines psychotherapy with both relaxation exercises and reeducation. They emphasize that the *transference relationship* plays a key role in the effectiveness of treatment, sufficiently so that it can be used as a predictor of therapeutic success.[48]

❲ Rheumatoid Arthritis

Rheumatoid arthritis (RA) is an inflammatory disorder of connective tissue, with polyarthritis as its most characteristic feature. The arthritis has a predilection for the more peripheral and smaller joints, and is typically symmetrical. The pathological process in the joints is one of acute proliferative inflammation which attacks the synovial membrane. This results in the formation of a granulomatous pannus, with damage and destruction of the underlying cartilage. Adhesions and scar formation tend to occur, eventuating in disability and deformity which may be crippling. Any of the connective tissues throughout the body may be involved in a similar inflammatory process. Constitutional symptoms are common. The typical course of the disease is dominated by unexplained exacerbations and remissions, which may be total. Attacks may vary greatly in the severity of the arthritis and other symptoms, and there are marked differences in the long-term course of those afflicted.

The disease is worldwide, though it may be less common in the tropics. It occurs at all ages, the most common onset being the mid-30s. Females are affected about two and one half times more frequently than men, with onset in middle age not uncommon. It is generally said to occur in approximately 3 percent of the population. Precise figures, however, are uncertain because of its episodic and varying course, even with the arduous development of standard diagnostic criteria.[16,19,120,236] It has been suggested that RA may be a much more common and benign disorder overall than is generally believed.[43]

Rheumatoid arthritis is classified as one of the *collagen* or connective tissue diseases, grouped together because of their common histopathological features, symptoms, therapeutic response to steroids, and other similarities. The etiology of all these disorders is unknown. There are strong indications that alterations in the immune response are involved. Even if this is confirmed, the causative factors that initiate and underlie this immunological disturbance require clarification.

Genetic factors also have been implicated, since RA has a high familial incidence; but such a finding can arise from environmental as well as genetic factors, and definitive data are lacking.[42,43] Genetic explanations are inadequate to explain certain peculiarities of its familial incidence, for example its increased frequency in spouses.[16,42,180]

Psychosomatic Correlations; the "RA Personality"

The notion that RA might be a psychosomatic disorder is an ancient one. Paulus Aegineta, who lived in the sixth or seventh century, ascribed attacks to "sorrow, care, watchfulness and other passions of the mind."[253] In modern times, well over 100 papers and books have appeared which have linked psychological and social factors to the disease. The bulk of this work has been examined in several thoughtful and comprehensive reviews.* The book by Prick and Van de Loo, published in 1964, contains summaries of most of the then available studies, including many by European workers not included in other sources.[212] Further information is provided by the *Annual Rheumatism Review*, published since 1935.

The vast preponderance of reports which deal directly with the role of psychological factors in RA are in agreement that stress is associated with attacks, if not the origin of the disease. Much of this material, unfortunately, is anecdotal and impressionistic. It is little different from what has been reported for innumerable other disease states. Seemingly

---

* See references 133, 179, 187, 236, and 267.

every type of stressful situation has been implicated. On the other hand, the most extensive clinical epidemiological study of arthritis thus far carried out, reported a failure to find evidence of stressful situations associated with the onset of RA.[142] It is difficult to place much reliance on this report either, however, because of the grossly superficial methods used to collect the psychological data.

Some studies have attempted to go beyond this level of generality to identify personality features that might characterize the RA patient. This work has provided descriptions of these patients as shy, leading quiet lives, and feeling inadequate and inferior;[36,103,148] as self-sacrificing and needing to serve others;[105,125,222] as conscientious, dutiful and compulsive;[47,103,125] as having a strict, rigid, moralistic conscience;[27,103] and as manifesting a tendency to depression.[20,39,150,253] This offers too much diversity to indicate that there is any one simple overt "RA personality type."

Still other studies have probed deeper to attempt to identify underlying conflicts and defenses. These suggest that there may well be specific psychological attributes which characterize RA patients at this deeper level. A preponderance of this work suggests in a variety of ways that the central issue for these patients relates to the *control or containment of anger.** Thus, RA patients are felt to have a great deal of unconscious or unexpressed anger;† but they sharply restrict their overt expressions of hostility (and other emotions);‡ and avoid situations likely to result in disagreement;[15,25,27,172] because anger, they report, "is likely to make their joints worse."[39] Swaim links the recovery from RA to the patient's capacity to develop a satisfactory overall philosophy of life leading to a state of spiritual harmony. It would be easy to dismiss this as unscientific and irrelevant, were it not for the fact that this author is a renowned rheumatologist, and that his approach involves persuading his patients to "give their *resentments* to God."[250] (My emphasis.)

RA patients also have been reported to en-

gage in a great deal of physical activity in the form of sports and hard work.[15,37,58] The preference for these activities is reported to go back to childhood, and has been interpreted as representing a preferred method for safely discharging aggression.§ Thus it has been suggested that RA may be precipitated when this channel for discharge becomes blocked.[47,125,150]

Arthritics of both sexes have been reported also to suffer from disturbances in sexual identification.¶ In the females, this has been described as having the features of a classical masculine protest reaction, which seems linked to their involvement in active physical sports as girls.[125]

Perhaps fears of disagreements and the need to maintain tight emotional control explain their reported difficulty in establishing close relationships,[15,25,150,172] and also their shy, quiet attributes already mentioned. Most of the other overt personality traits noted (being compulsive, self-sacrificing and depressed, having a strict conscience, etc.) are equally consistent with conflicts over hostility and aggression, as these can be understood within a psychoanalytic framework. The seemingly diverse overt personality traits, therefore, exhibit psychodynamic coherence.

Another reported finding is a frequent history of separation or loss of a parent figure during childhood.# It has been suggested that grief and separation are important antecedent stresses in relation to the development of an attack.[81,147,243] In two studies, however, the control groups showed an equal or higher incidence of early parental loss.[135,221]

All these trends were noted by King in his 1955 review.[133] Justifiably, he was critical of methodological deficiencies in all the studies then available. Most were impressionistic and lacked control for bias; almost none used comparison groups; diagnosis was loose; and all were retrospective and thus potentially interpretable in terms of the consequences of RA, etc. Yet, as King indicated, there is an

---

* See references 20, 39, 47, 123, 125, 150, and 222.
† See references 20, 125, 149, 150, and 172.
‡ See references 20, 39, 47, 104, 125, 150, and 172.

§ See references 15, 25, 38, 47, 125, 150, and 172.
¶ See references 15, 25, 125, 147, 172, and 253.
\# See references 15, 20, 25, 36, 146, 150, 222, and 243.

impressive consistency to this work, especially in the prominence of problems related to aggression.

The attempt to develop a comprehensive, coherent schema, that utilized psychoanalytic insights, in order to explain the genesis of RA and other psychosomatic diseases reached its acme in the work of Franz Alexander and his co-workers.[3] For over thirty years this group carried out a series of intensive studies of patients with several psychosomatic disorders to elicit a "specific dynamic configuration" characterizing each. It was their view that such a configuration, in combination with certain equally specific but unknown somatic factors, led to susceptibility to the disease. The disorder would then appear in situations whose nature was specifically such as to severely aggravate the conflict nuclear to the configuration.

The formulation developed for RA indicated that these patients: (1) had overprotective, restrictive parents who stimulated rebellious feelings together with heightened anxiety over the expression of these; (2) the rebellion was discharged in childhood via sports and physical activity, associated in women with a masculine protest reaction; (3) progressively in later life hostility was expressed through masochistic self-sacrifice which served to control the environment while denying hostility (benevolent tyranny); (4) an interruption in the availability or success of this pattern led to rising anger and increased conflict over its expression; (5) this led to simultaneous increased tension in both sets of opposing (because of the conflict) muscles; and (6) this led somehow to arthritis.[3,125]

Methodological considerations momentarily aside, the formulation has an elegant quality in its internal consistency and its integration of diverse observational data. Its correctness, moreover, need not be limited by its etiological implications. There is no reason why this formulation cannot be correct at the *descriptive* level, even if it proves inadequate at the *explanatory* level. The two are separable. The former requires merely establishing that the postulated psychodynamic features are characteristic of RA patients. Validation of the latter requires additional data demonstrating that these characteristics existed prior to the onset of the disease, and represented necessary and/or sufficient factors for its occurrence.[179] Whether this formulation will be acceptable even in this limited descriptive sense depends ultimately on one's willingness to accept conceptualizations of human behavior in psychoanalytic terms. One can only note that for clinicians with this orientation who have actual experience working with arthritics, the formulation does seem remarkably applicable to many RA patients.

The study on which it is based does, of course, exhibit grave methodological faults. The patients were interviewed with full knowledge of their diagnosis and of the personality traits reported by previous investigators, and no control groups were used. Some reassurance is provided by a later systematic validation study conducted by the Alexander group.[4] Using eighty-three patients representing seven major psychosomatic disorders for which formulations had been developed, "blind" diagnoses were made on case records from which medical diagnostic clues were deleted. Psychoanalytic judges were able to make the correct diagnosis significantly more often than at chance expectancy, and also significantly better than could a group of internists judging the same data. The degree of success in identifying the RA patients was particularly high.

Additional confirmation comes from studies carried out by Cleveland and Fisher utilizing psychological test data. They compared RA patients with a matched control group of patients suffering from back pain, utilizing a battery of projective tests, such as Rorschach, TAT (thematic apperception test), and DAP (draw-a-person), to elicit unconscious fantasies.[36] The fantasies of the RA patient "were so unique that three psychologists were able to differentiate with only one error" the RA patients from the controls. During interviews the RA patient was noted to be an "overtly calm" person who "rarely expresses or feels anger." But the test data revealed that "covertly he seems to be containing a large amount of hostile feelings." The RA patients displayed evidence of a relatively unique body image, characterized "as a kind of hollow container filled with uncontrolled fluid material and surrounded by a hard, unpenetrable surface." This external "barrier" quality was conceptualized as playing a major role in the defense against hostile expression.

Cleveland and Fisher also compared RA with ulcer patients.[37] Both groups evidenced strong hostility. But the RA patients were distinctive in their use of physical activity as a technique for handling this, and they more frequently gave a history of greater participation in rugged physical activity during early life. Subsequent studies utilizing similar test data have confirmed the findings with regard both to body image and contained hostility.[194,195,264] The general nature of these findings is also remarkably consistent with the early, less systematic Rorschach studies of Booth.[26,27]

Further information has been provided by the series of careful psychosocial studies carried out by Cobb, King, and their associates, using sophisticated survey research methods.[42,44,134] These data confirmed previous observations that RA is more prevalent in the lower classes.[134] (As one observer has put it, "RA seems to be a disease of losers . . . all evidences of the disease were commoner in those with low incomes or little education."[35]) Discrepancy between income and education, which King and Cobb point to as an indicator of social-status stress, was especially associated with RA. Other indices of social stress also were more common.[134]

Certain factors appeared prevalent specifically in *women* with RA.[42] They had come from parental homes with high social-status stress; they reported mother's authority and discipline as more arbitrary and controlling; their recalled reaction to this was high covert hostility but very low overt resistance and aggressiveness; and they evidenced strong identification with mother despite her negative image. As adults, the conflicts over the control of anger remained in evidence, and they manifested evidence of poorer mental health functioning. Their own marriages too were likely to be with husbands of incongru-ent social status, and to be characterized by much hostility. Men married to these women are more likely to have peptic ulcers.[42] Taken all together, these data on women are in remarkable agreement with the psychoanalytically derived formulation of the Alexander group. The information regarding the families of origin is of special interest in that it represents reasonably objective evidence of stress *antecedent* to the disease onset.

Cobb and his associates also report that RA patients had a higher incidence of divorce but put up with an unsatisfactory marriage longer than those free of the disease. They interpret this as evidence of the suppression of hostility.[44] A Swedish study failed to confirm the higher divorce rate for RA patients.[109] The implication that this represents refutation, however, is incorrect, pointing up an important methodological clarification about this type of research. Divorce and similar social indices represent culture-bound phenomena with multiple determinants. Within any one society, divorce can be interpreted as an evidence of interpersonal disturbance. The fact that it does not occur differentially in another society may merely mean that other cultural determinants there make it sufficiently accessible or inaccessible to its members, so that psychological factors become irrelevant. In such a culture interpersonal difficulties, when present, will be evidenced in alternative aspects of social behavior. The data of Cobb et al.[44] deserve the test of replication within the United States; but this would represent their only valid test.

It seems appropriate at this point to mention the reported relationship of RA to schizophrenia. Two studies have suggested that the disorders rarely occur simultaneously. In one study, not a single case of arthritis was found among 2200 patients at a mental hospital.[200] In another, only twenty arthritics were found among more than 15,000 hospitalized psychotics.[95] Both studies exhibit serious methodological deficiencies.[133,236] Yet, the magnitude of these findings is impressive. If they are correct, it is difficult to interpret their meaning. Some observers have suggested that RA patients are, underneath, seriously disturbed psychologically,[149,199] and that RA may thus constitute an organismic defense against psychosis.[199]

Objective Tests

The aforementioned studies by Cobb, King, et al.[42,44,134] and by Cleveland and Fisher represented a major advance in methodological sophistication. Nevertheless, these too had shortcomings that have been pointed out by Scotch and Geiger.[236] In an effort to introduce greater precision, a number of investigators have carried out a series of studies using better defined samples and better control groups, and relying on objective psychological tests, usually the MMPI.

The choice of such tests deserves comment. They can be easily and directly scored, have well-established baseline data on large normal and other samples, and provide concrete quantifiable data. They can provide measures of static traits or trait clusters, including nomothetic expressions of underlying motivational forces (e.g., hostility, dependency) one at a time. These data are important, valid and reliable. But they are simply not relevant to every problem. These tests do not provide information about dynamic relationships among motivational forces and defenses, nor their ideographic expressions. They cannot provide any direct information about the presence of a complex psychodynamic configuration of the type proposed by Alexander. Some reviewers have reacted to "projective" psychological tests as if that adjective represented the converse of objective, i.e., as if data derived from such instruments lacks validity.[236,267] Projective tests are, of course, less precise and quantifiable. But, in fact, the concern of such critics with the validity of projective methods seems to reflect their skepticism about the acceptability of psychodynamic conceptualizations per se. Both types of tests are valid. Each has its disadvantages as well as advantages, and the appropriateness of each varies with the purposes for which they are used.

A number of studies have utilized the MMPI. An almost universal finding is elevation of the "neurotic triad" of the hypochondriasis, hysteria, and depression scales.* It seems clear that the RA patient describes himself as characterized by neurotic trends. On the other hand, the scale elevations are less than those found in neurotic patients, and the picture is inconsistent with the view that RA patients are seriously disturbed and near psychotic.[150,199] The fact that these findings are indistinguishable from those in neurotic patients has been interpreted as running counter to the expectation that a specific RA personality pattern exists.[267] A question also can be raised as to whether these abnormal MMPI findings merely reflect the presence of the symptoms and disability which RA produces. To get more information on this, several investigators have carried out item analyses to determine if the scale elevations result entirely from responses which reflect these manifestations of the disease. The results have been conflicting.[197,209,268]

Bourestom and Howard described similarities in the MMPI-scale elevations among patients with RA, multiple sclerosis, and spinal-cord injuries.[29] They also found overall differences which "support the hypothesis of some specific personality correlates associated with the three disabilities."[29] In addition, sex-linked differences were found within each group, and the male arthritics seemed somewhat different from all other groups. Nalven analyzed MMPI responses in terms of hostility, and also obtained scores on three special hostility scales. The data failed to provide evidence of increased hostility in RA patients but did suggest that they had the problem of overcontrol of hostility.[197] Geist used projective tests and a questionnaire battery as well as the MMPI.[81] His MMPI data indicated neurotic trends similar to the earlier studies. The other instruments revealed signs of inhibited chronic aggression in the RA patients. They also indicated the presence of obsessive compulsive defenses, participation and interest in sports prior to disease onset, and a suggestion that the families of origin were characterized by matriarchal discipline. Unfortunately his sam-

* See references 29, 81, 189, 197, 209, 262, and 268.

ple was relatively small (twenty-two), and his questionnaire lacked external validation.

Robinson and his co-workers used Catells' *16 Personality Factor Inventory* (16PF) to study patients with recent ("new") as well as long-standing ("old") RA, and similar matched groups of tuberculosis, diabetes, and hypertension patients.[223] The new RA patients differed little from the other new disease groups, but did show deviations from the test norms indicating neurotic trends similar to that revealed by the MMPI. In contrast to the other illness groups, the new and old RA patients were significantly similar to one another, which these authors interpreted as evidence supporting the existence of an RA personality type. As a whole, the RA patients manifested emotional instability, introversion, guilt, and depression proneness, exaggerated dependency needs, and trends toward compulsivity and tension. This combination, they concluded, reflects "a person who restricts his emotional expression, including expression of aggression."[223]

The 16PF was used also by Moldofsky and Rothman in a complex study of symptoms, treatment and personality in a group of RA patients.[185] The patients as a group had test scores which, compared to norms, revealed low ego strength, emotional instability, dependency, and conformity, i.e., again, similar findings to the MMPI studies. The investigators concluded from this that there was no specific RA personality. The personality traits did not show any relationship to disease activity, but patients on steroids manifested more severe emotional symptoms. Wolff comments that "the results obtained in these two 16PF studies differed considerably, strongly suggesting that large variations in personality patterns exist in RA."[267] Here again, the nature of the data does not seem to be considered sufficiently.

The most creatively designed studies utilizing the MMPI were carried out by Moos and Solomon.[189-192] They scored the MMPI on a variety of derived scales developed to reveal underlying personality traits, as well as on the conventional scales, and also utilized ratings and content analyses of interviews. Women with RA were compared with their healthy sisters, and with other female relatives. The patients displayed more compliance-subservience, depression, conservatism-security, and sensitivity to anger than did their sisters.[190] They also manifested clear and striking differences from their sisters in their self-descriptions, in the extent of their masochism, self-sacrifice, and denial of hostility, in their perceptions of the amount of rejection they perceived from their mothers and of the strictness of their fathers.[191] Compared with female relatives in general, the patients scored higher on scales reflecting physical symptoms, depression and apathy, psychological rigidity, and neurotic symptoms indicative of anxiety, masochism, self-alienation and over-compliance. No clear differences in physical interests or activity could be elicited. The RA patients also displayed some similarities to patients with other psychosomatic conditions. As the authors note, this finding cannot be interpreted merely as lack of specificity, for it was not general. There were similarities to both ulcer and hypertension patients, but in entirely *different* ways. The point is that the dynamic formulations for different disorders do overlap, not merely because they lack precision but also because each is a constellation of transacting traits which include some common elements.

This work provides meaningful information about personality in RA that goes well beyond the earlier, less sophisticated MMPI studies. At the same time, it is entirely consistent with that work in revealing the general pattern of nonspecific neurotic symptoms characteristic of the RA patient. As did some earlier workers, Moos and Solomon carried out a careful item analysis to see if this was explainable on the basis of RA symptoms alone, which substantiated the impression that it was not.[189] (They also cite an unpublished study by D. Cohen that provided a similar result.) Moos and Solomon take pains to point out, however, that this tendency of the RA patient to display neurotic symptoms could be a nonspecific consequence of the presence of a painful, disabling disease. They reaffirm the point, made by every serious student of the problem, that the interpretation of reported distinctive personality findings requires longitudinal studies to determine if these existed antecedent to the onset, and there are absolutely no such data as of 1972.

A later study carried out by Meyerowitz, Jacox, and Hess is of special interest because of its methodological approach.[180] Detailed psychological test and clinical studies were carried out on eight sets of female monozygotic twins, discordant for RA. No consistent differences in personality could be found. There was nothing distinctive about the patients' conflicts or handling of hostility. *Both* groups showed a conspicuous preference for physical activity, and a need to serve and take responsibility for others. The single consistent difference pertained to the involvement of the ultimately affected twin, prior to disease onset, in events experienced as "demanding and restricting." To these, the patients responded "with their characteristic heightened activity, but increasing stress was experienced to the point of being unable to cope."[179]

In a subsequent review, Meyerowitz points to the importance of distinguishing such contributions to disease onset from those purporting to explain etiology, as well as from those which merely delineate the effects of psychological factors upon the course of the disease.[179] Nevertheless, this finding is strongly reminiscent of the etiological specificity hypothesis proposed for RA by Graham and Grace.[93,94] These latter investigators proposed that psychosomatic disorders are characterized by the presence of a distinctive "attitude" prior to the disease onset. The latter was defined as a feeling state combined with a disposition towards some action. A concomitant specific physiological state is proposed, which is implicated in the pathogenesis of the given disorder. For RA, the attitude is defined as follows: "Felt tied down and wanted to get free (felt restrained, restricted, confined, and wanted to be able to move around)."[94] The problems of evaluating the retrospective report of this particular attitude provided by a patient currently affected by the characteristic effects of RA are too obvious to detail.

Subgroups

An apposite criticism of many of the reported studies is their failure to provide a detailed description of the particular patients studied.[187,236] The specific characteristics of a given sample can affect the data in significant ways. Findings may derive from characteristics of the sample entirely extraneous to the presence of RA. As well as being misleading, these may obscure the manifestations of factors that are specific to the disorder. There is also the possibility that seeming discrepancies among studies may reflect the existence of variants of the disorder (subgroups), each of which has differing psychological characteristics. The most obvious example of this relates to the sex of the patients studied. Most studies have been restricted to a single sex, or have failed to consider the male and female patients separately.[187] Yet in two instances already mentioned, where both sexes were included and their data were compared, differences were found.[29,42] One would hardly expect otherwise. If psychological factors are involved in RA, their role is complex and related to deeper layers of the personality where sex-linked motivations and characteristics exist. At the least, similar dynamic forces will manifest themselves differently within the total psychological economies of men and women. It is possible also that the relevant factors themselves differ for the two sexes.

The importance of elucidating characteristics to identify still other possible subgroups is well illustrated by the careful study of Rimón.[218] This Finnish researcher conducted detailed physical and psychiatric examinations of 100 female clinic patients with RA, and compared them to the same number with other "somatic diseases." He identified fifty-five of the RA patients in whom there was a correlation between emotional conflict situations and the disease onset, and thirty-three in whom there was no such correlation. (The balance represented an inbetween situation.) There were significant differences between the two. In the group where the disease onset followed a significant conflict, recurrences also tended to follow similar conflict situations, and the course of the disease was one of sudden onset with distinct and often acute symptoms and a much more rapid progression. The patients had few affected relatives. In the group without conflict correlation, the onset was slow and the progression of symptoms delayed, and these patients had a relatively high family incidence of RA. This latter group had an evident incapability of expressing hostile feelings. (For the whole group, "problems in aggression dynamics were of minor incidence" at the "rational" level, again suggesting the irrelevance of data at this level.) A detailed look at ten patients, whose disease had a malignant progression, revealed that half had an exceptionally heavy genetic predisposition, while the other half manifested a great "psychic vulnerability." The latter was indicated by evidence of ego disorganization with overt depression. This research, therefore, suggests that two separate groups of people have a predilection to develop RA. In one, heredity plays the major role, whereas for the other psychological stress is the significant factor; the disease progresses differently for each.

Additional confirmation will be required before we can accept Rimón's findings as generally valid. There are data available from an earlier study by King and Cobb which furnish indirect support for some of Rimón's findings.[135] They compared thirty-two severe RA patients, 25 percent of them hospitalized, with a group of normal controls, and also with data obtained previously on a group of normals and twenty-one patients diagnosed as having mild RA. The severe cases showed poorer maternal identification and felt a lack of a positive relationship with their mothers, perceiving her as giving insufficient attention and affection. They viewed both parents as having been strict and uncompromising. In contrast, the mild cases were like the controls. If we assume that these psychosocial variables parallel psychological stress proneness, then their more severe disease seems to match the more acute and rapid disease progression in Rimón's comparable group.

Also somewhat confirmatory is a study by Moos and Solomon which found that patients with greater functional incapacity from their disease had poorer ego strength and evidences of a variety of abnormal personality traits, as measured by the MMPI.[192] These researchers took pains to match the two groups on many variables, but their efforts failed on one. The more incapacitated group had a shorter duration of illness, and since the groups were matched for the stage of disease, this means the rate of progression had been more rapid in that group. The greater psychopathology which they manifested is thus consistent with Rimón's data. Another study by the same investigators indirectly points in a different direction.[245] In asymptomatic relatives of RA patients, those who lacked the serum rheumatic factor had greater evidence of emotional disturbance on the MMPI. This led the investigators to conclude that only those individuals who have the hereditary predisposition *and* experience emotional distress are likely to develop RA.

Regardless of the plausibility of that suggestion, the important issue is the need for further studies like that of Rimón which attempt to delineate subgroups. A further illustration of this approach, as well as the use of an anteriospective design, is provided by the work of Moldofsky and Chester who observed two contrasting pain patterns in a group of sixteen RA patients.[184] In patients manifesting the "synchronous" pattern, changes in arthritic symptoms occurred concomitantly with, or just after, mood changes, primarily those of anxiety or hostility. Patients with the "paradoxical" pattern were characterized by an inverse relationship between joint symptoms and feelings of hopelessness. No clinical or socioeconomic variables differentiated the two groups. However, the paradoxical group demonstrated a less favorable outcome when followed longitudinally.

Studies which focus on treatment outcome can contribute to the same end. Factors which are discovered to predict differential responsiveness to differing therapies may serve as clues to subgroups basic to the disorder itself. McGlaughlin et al. found personality differences between patients who responded well to

ACTH (adrenocorticotropic hormone) and those who do not.[172] Those who had good dream recall, indicating a higher level of ego function, responded better. Apropos of the point made earlier, there also were differences between the findings for the male and female patients. The characteristic conflict in both was between hostility and dependency; but the males dealt with this by compulsive defenses and withdrawal, whereas the females relied more on physical activity and on the control of others through self-sacrifice.

A study carried out by Wolff is also of interest in its predictive design, as well as its use of a measure of "pain sensitivity range" he developed.[266] Lower preoperative pain sensitivity served to predict a more favorable outcome to surgical rehabilitative procedures. It seems likely, however, that this variable is more relevant to rehabilitation potential in general than to RA or any subtypes which it may include.

Mechanisms

Any theory which postulates that psychological factors play an etiological role in RA must account for a psychophysiological mechanism through which these factors produce its characteristic joint lesions. The psychoanalytically oriented investigators of RA typically have suggested that conflict over the expression of hostility causes increased muscle tension, and that this leads somehow to the joint pathology. Studies were conducted by two of these research groups dealing with the first part of this proposed chain of events, i.e., the psychophysiology of muscle tension in RA patients. Morrison, Short, Ludwig, et al. studied thirty-four RA patients, using both surface and needle EMG.[193] Half of the RA patients evidenced inconstant spontaneous spiking in some muscles adjacent to the affected joints, when they were apparently relaxed. The normals showed no such activity.

Gottschalk and his co-workers, associates of Alexander, carried out two studies.[91,92] In the first, multiple handwriting variables were measured in RA patients, in a mixed group of fifteen psychiatric patients that contained nine

hypertensives, and in fifteen normal subjects.[91] *Both* patient groups exhibited greater variability on several measures than did the normal subjects. These data were interpreted as evidence of a disturbance in the synergistic use of muscles related to neurotic conflict or pent-up aggression. In their second study, EMG records were obtained on groups of equal size (six) of RA patients, RA patients in psychoanalysis, hypertensives, and normal subjects.[92] Initially, measures were taken from the forearm muscles at rest, and during actual and imagined movements. The RA patients in analysis and the controls showed generally lower tension than the medically treated RA patients and the hypertensives. It was concluded that both RA and hypertension are associated with increased muscle tension and that this may be reduced by psychoanalysis. The second part of this study recorded arm and leg tension in the patients in analysis before and after emotional stress. There were marked reactions "partly predictable" from knowledge of the analysis. "In general," when defenses allowed expression of hostile impulses the tension decreased, and when there was inadequate means of coping with these impulses, the tension rose.

Surprisingly, there seem to be but two subsequent studies on this issue. Southworth obtained surface EMG recordings from the trapezius and frontalis in patients with RA and those with peptic ulcer before and after a stressful word association test.[246] The only difference was in a more prolonged elevation subsequent to the stress in the RA group, confined to the trapezius. (Moos and Engel interpreted this as a "lack of adaptation," i.e., perseveration, in the muscle responses of arthritics, and suggest that findings might have been enhanced had "symptomatic" muscles been selected for study.[188]) The word association data failed to indicate conflicts over aggression in either group; conflicts over dependency were equally present in both. However, a computed overall "emotional disturbance score" correlated negatively with trapezius tension, which Southworth interprets as evidence that discharge via emotional and muscular tension are inversely related.

Moos and Engel carried out a study of their own.[188] They attempted to determine if hypertensives and RA patients would demonstrate "response specificity" (see p. 728). A complex conditioning technique was used to study twelve female patients in each group. No conditioning occurred. The RA patients showed generally higher tension in their symptomatic muscles, and greater reactivity in both symptomatic and asymptomatic muscles, as measured by EMG. They also demonstrated a failure to "adapt" (i.e., a persisting response) in their muscle responses, although their blood pressure responses did adapt; hypertensives displayed the reverse.

Even if we accept these findings, major problems arise with regard to their interpretation. First, the presence of acute arthritis or any painful process is associated with splinting of the involved part by increased muscle tension. Hence increased tension, specifically around a symptomatic joint, may be a consequence rather than a cause of arthritis. The only finding that even partly confronts this issue is a mention by Morrison et al. of a single instance in which occasional spikes recorded from a resting muscle preceded by one week the appearance of arthritis in the adjacent joint.[193] Second, and more important, among the various extraarthritic manifestations of RA is a *myositis* associated with round-cell infiltration, indistinguishable from that found in the other collagen diseases.[113] There is at least as much reason to implicate this as the basis for increased muscle tension as a psychophysiological mechanism.

To clarify the relationship of conflicts over the expression of anger to muscle tension in RA will require studies made during periods of total remission or, better still, prior to the initial onset of the disease. (Data from normal subjects who do not develop RA may not be adequate, since RA patients could differ in the presence of just such a relationship.) A longitudinal approach allowing for observations antecedent to onset will also answer the question as to whether the psychological findings arise as the result of the disorder or precede it. Every thoughtful student of the field has emphasized the need for such longitudinal studies, while recognizing the immense practical problems which have precluded their accomplishment thus far.

The hypothesis that muscle tension represented the pathogenic link between psychological factors and arthritis seemed plausible at the time it was proposed. Since then, our knowledge of RA has vastly increased. If RA is a systemic disease of collagen tissue, as we now believe, that hypothesis no longer seems adequate. An acceptable psychosomatic theory must account for the specific pathogenic process central to a disease, as Engel has pointed out so beautifully.[66–68] This viewpoint in no way affects the validity of any of the above mentioned psychological findings per se, which either may play no etiological role, or may do so via another pathogenic mechanism.

One such alternative mechanism has, in fact, been proposed. There is accumulating evidence strongly suggesting that all of the collagen disorders, RA among them, represent "autoimmune" diseases.[115] Although the initiating mechanism remains obscure, a hypersensitivity mechanism seems to be involved in their pathogenesis. Consistent with this, the serum of RA patients typically (though not invariably) contains a macroglobulin "rheumatoid factor." This has been identified as a complex of an unknown 19S macroglobulin with normal gamma globulin, suggesting that it represents an immune reaction to the patient's own serum protein. Solomon and Moos have suggested that RA may arise via stress-induced alterations of immunological mechanisms.[244] They have marshalled data from a large variety of studies which suggest that emotional factors can alter immune mechanisms.[244] Among these was Fessel's work demonstrating elevated 19S protein in stressed prisoners,[71] and their own demonstration of elevated immunoglobulins in psychiatric patients. Hendrie et al. also found elevated gamma globulin levels in female psychiatric patients, but not in males, and confirmed Solomon's finding that this bore no specific relation to schizophrenia.[112] The relevance of this body of research to RA is entirely indirect. Thus Solomon and Moos label their hypothesis a "speculative theoretical interpretation."[244] However it clearly merits further pursuit, using both RA patients and experimental animals.[6,111]

This new approach, as well as the whole thread of the discussion in this section, tells us a good deal about the present state of the field. The evolution of psychosomatic research on RA has reached the stage of progress which provides a clear guideline for its future direction. The major focus of future research must be on the painstaking clarification of mechanisms through which psychological and somatic processes interface. These must be chosen in terms of their relevance to the best available knowledge of the pathogenic processes centrally involved in the disorder.

(Parkinsonism

The parkinsonian syndrome is a progressive neurological disorder manifested by muscular tremor, weakness, and rigidity, often associated with autonomic symptoms, that arises from abnormalities of the basal ganglia. In some instances, lesions result from an attack of encephalitis, and, less commonly, trauma, toxins, neurosyphilis, and possibly arteriosclerosis have been implicated. But there remain a large group of patients, most likely a majority, in whom no such specific cause is found, and where the disorder is ascribed to *ideopathic* degeneration of the basal ganglia. Under these circumstances it has been suggested that the disorder may belong to the *psychosomatic* category. The basis for this viewpoint came from a number of observations that: (1) the onset followed emotional stress; (2) that those afflicted had a characteristic personality configuration; and (3) that psychiatric symptomatology is frequently exhibited.

An early impetus for this viewpoint came from Jeliffe, who described the "obvious resemblances" between parkinsonians and catatonics.[121] He indicated that, in both, the motility disturbances served to bind unconscious hostility;[121] and likened the parkinsonian posture to that of a boxer.[123]

Jackson and his co-workers, although taking a more traditional *organic* stance regarding etiology, observed that "the direct exciting causes are as a rule psychogenic."[116] They called attention to the great frequency and variety of psychiatric symptoms found in the disorder, noting that often these *preceded* the neurological signs. Depression was by far the commonest finding in their large series of patients, but many other symptoms were noted, including delusions, hallucinations, and agitation. It seems likely that some of the striking nature of these findings resulted from sampling bias, i.e., the authors were located at a state hospital. A more recent and conservative study carried out by Schwab, Fabing, and Prichard also emphasized the number and variety of psychiatric symptoms to be found in parkinsonians.[235] These neurologists grouped the psychiatric disturbances into four categories: (1) unrelated, e.g., antedating the disorder; (2) reactive; (3) secondary to medication; and (4) paroxysmal, often associated with oculogyric crises and attributed to the CNS (central nervous system) pathology. The latter included episodes of anxiety, depression, compulsive acts, agitation, paranoia, and other symptom clusters.

The Parkinsonian Personality

The first major systematic studies of psychogenesis were carried out by Booth.[26-28] Several series of patients, both here and in Germany, were studied by clinical interviews as well as the Rorschach. For the first time, control groups were utilized. From these data Booth concluded definitely that a "specific personality type" was to be found. He described this as characterized by an "urge to action" through motor activity and industriousness, and by a "striving for independence, authority and success within a rigid, usually moralistic, behavior pattern." He adds that "the balance between success, aggression, and morals appears to be unusually delicate."[28] Of special interest to us, Booth's controls included a group of patients with rheumatoid arthritis. He was struck by their many similarities to parkinsonians. Both disorders, he concluded, are dominated by an urge for independent action in which "obstacles are likely to provoke aggressiveness," and both are subject to conflicts between these feelings and a strict rigid conscience.[27] The difference lay in their emotional relationships. Whereas the arthritics had a "*defensive* attitude against emotional involvement and outside influences," the parkinsonians were "*activated* by emotional experience coming from the environment"[26] (my emphases). Booth's work represents one of the rare instances in which subtle psychological differences among given "psychosomatic" diseases have been dissected from their similarities. (These studies also included hypertensives, and delineated a different personality constellation for that disorder which will not be considered here).[27] Unfortunately, methodological flaws open all of Booth's work to question, i.e., the patients were interviewed and tested by him alone, and his interpretations were made with full foreknowledge of the nature of the diagnoses.

Three clinical studies provided additional data that coincide with Booth's findings. Unfortunately, all are mere anecdotal reports devoid of controls. Mitscherlich reported on the presence of chronic emotional tension in relation to aggression, leading to "readiness to motor activity without the possibility to realize it," resulting in a personality presenting as "coolness."[182] Shaskan et al. regarded the needs for conformity and "virtuousness" to be so great as to produce an "unusually satisfactory" adjustment to the disease (a finding that seems at considerable variance from that of most observers).[239] Sands considered these needs as sufficiently striking to characterize parkinsonians as having a "masked personality."[232] The last two investigators emphasized that intense anxiety, anger, and conflict lay beneath the superficial calm and conformity.

Machover, who like Booth utilized Rorschach data, failed to confirm these observations.[154] He found *no* evidence of any consistent personality picture. What little homogeneity he did elicit was limited to signs of cognitive interference, dependence, affective instability, inertia, and passivity—data at

considerable variance with the industriousness and striving for independence reported by Booth. These were related to the duration of the disease and were explained as the consequences of *living with* a disabling disease that severely constrained activity. Unfortunately, he failed to use controls.

Stronger support for these negative findings have come from the program of well-designed studies of Riklan, Diller, and their associates. Their findings, together with a comprehensive review of the background of the problem, have been collected in an excellent monograph.[217] Extensive data were derived from systematic interviews with both patients and family members; from detailed clinical observations and examinations; and from a battery of psychological tests, both objective and projective, which tapped cognitive as well as personality attributes; and from controls. These data led to the conclusion that parkinsonians do *not* reveal distinctive behavioral features. Neither a "parkinsonian personality," nor even a typical reaction to the disease (such as reported by Machover) was found. Impairment in perceptual-cognitive functions was sometimes present but this covaried with the *severity* of the neurological impairment, not its duration. The investigators tend to view it as due to the disease process itself, not its symptoms.

Support for the findings in the cognitive area comes from a study by Talland.[252] On the basis of a specially selected group of cognitive tests "No definite signs of impairment could be established." Patients off medication generally did better on all tests, suggesting that some of the defects observed clinically might be due to drug effects. Talland was by no means unaware of the existence of patients with severe intellectual impairment. But he differentiates these few from parkinsonians generally, and suggests that they may represent an etiologically distinct subgroup in which the pathological process directly disrupts brain functions. Riklan and his co-workers extended this line of thinking even further. The diversity of their findings led them to conclude that "parkinsonism refers to a number of complex and composite neurological syndromes," and, "it would be theoretically inconsistent and practically useless to propose that parkinsonian patients define an entity generalizing its own behavioral characteristics."[217] Here precisely lies the nub of a problem in accepting their negative findings as the final word on the question of a parkinsonian personality. Each subtype of the disorder has special features which act to obscure any held in common. If a specific personality configuration should exist, its presence can only be determined by eliminating these extraneous sources of variance. This requires the selection of uniform subgroups for study. The first task is to exclude patients whose disease arises from known exogenous factors, as well as all those in whom there is any evidence of intellectual or other diffuse neurological impairment. Demographic variables should then be used to create still more homogeneous subgroups. Even then, problems remain. One is left with patients whose impairment varies in extent and locus, and whose psychological reactions to these differ. Perhaps the question will only be answered when longitudinal prospective studies can be done. In any event, the present weight of the evidence favors caution about the existence of a parkinson-specific personality.

In contrast, the influence of psychological factors on parkinsonian symptoms, is an established fact. Symptoms frequently are increased in the presence of strong emotion, stress, and fatigue.[24,235] This tells us nothing about etiology, since all diseases necessarily are responsive to psychological influence. A disorder of the CNS itself would seem especially likely to exhibit a sensitivity to emotional arousal. The CNS is characterized by rich interconnections among its parts, and the hypothalamic and limbic structures which subserve emotion have known effects upon the musculature.[83,155] Clinically this is apparent in the familiar extrapyramidal side effects of the phenothiazines. Nor can we make any etiological inferences from the symptomatic improvement that can result from psychotherapy.[167]

However it is difficult indeed to explain away the careful report by Grinker and Spie-gel of the development of the full-blown parkinsonian syndrome in cases of *combat exhaustion*.[97] These patients were indistinguishable from typical "organic" parkinsonians, except that the entire picture rapidly disappeared with psychiatric treatment. A report also has appeared in which parkinsonian symptoms developed during the course of a schizophrenic illness, and disappeared following a lobotomy concomitant with symptomatic recovery from the psychosis.[100] Psychodynamic study of this patient suggested that "the parkinson syndrome may have developed as a defense against the patient's violent hostility" (reminiscent of the aforementioned formulations of Jeliffe[121] and Booth[26-28]) as well as serving regressive needs.

Somatopsychic Correlations

Cooper's development of a stereotactic neurosurgical approach to parkinsonism which involves the production of lesions in the thalamus and corpus pallidum, provides a new avenue for increasing our understanding of the functions of these parts of the brain.[46] This work has been the subject of an excellent review by Crown, (which also considers some of the material covered above).[49] In the *cognitive* sphere the findings are reasonably definite. There are transient losses postoperatively, which seem more related to verbal skills with left-sided lesions, and to performance and visual-motor skills with those on the right side.[171,217] More important, no permanent cognitive defects can be ascertained.[9,217]

A detailed clinico-pathological correlational study is available which clarifies some of the subtle language and speech effects of thalamic surgery.[230]

Some interesting findings emerge with regard to *personality* effects following surgery, though these are far from clear. Riklan and Levita mention only two changes which seemed to be persistent. These were a defect in body image and a reduction in perceptual integration and nonspecific drive or energy.[217] The latter, according to these workers, may reflect reduced kinesthetic feedback to the reticular activating system, a kind of relative sensory deprivation. This intriguing hypothesis receives some support from another of their studies. In a group of parkinsonians, a negative correlation was demonstrated between "activation level" (as measured by skin resistance) and the degree of voluntary motor impairment.[207]

The reports of *mood* changes after surgery are somewhat conflicting. McFie comments on the "improved emotional reactions *following the alleviation of symptoms*" (my emphasis), and on the frequency of overt euphoria which he linked to right-sided surgery.[171] He likens the reaction to that found with leukotomy. Hays also found euphoria to be the commonest affective reaction.[106] However he attributed this to the specific CNS effects of the surgery, and found that it was *not* related to the degree of improvement. In contrast, Asso found that most affective changes were those of anxiety or depression, and that euphoria was rare.[9] Unfortunately, there is no direct way to compare these studies. Uniform rating scales were not used, nor is it clear if there were equivalent preoperative levels of depression or expectancies of benefit from the surgery in the three groups.

Obviously, we have still much to learn about the role of these brain structures in personality and mood.

⟪ Gout

Gout is a disorder of uric acid metabolism in which symptoms arise from the formation of urate deposits in various body areas. The usual site for deposition is one or more of the joints, producing an acute, often exquisitely painful arthritis. Chronic joint deformities occasionally eventuate. The other major sites are the subcutaneous tissues, giving rise to the development of nodular *tophi*, and the kidneys, resulting in nephritis and stone formation. The metabolic dyscrasia is ordinarily manifested by an elevated concentration of uric acid in the blood and other body fluids, but may only be evident in other subtler but measurable abnormalities (e.g., an increased

size of the uric acid pool). Most research has identified the major metabolic defect as being an overproduction of uric acid, though its decreased conversion or excretion, or both, may also play a role.[251]

Dietary overindulgence (increased purine intake), alcohol, exercise, and certain drugs can increase uric acid levels transiently to precipitate an acute attack. (The classically ascribed causative role of venery, however, seems dubious!) Trauma, infection, surgery, and other physical stressors also may act as precipitants. So can acute emotional stress. Sydenham, himself a victim, as quoted by Talbott, advised gout sufferers to "keep the mind quiet."[251] However, it is now well substantiated that these factors have relevance only to the precipitation of acute attacks, and only to a small minority of these, whereas the pertinent issue for the disorder is a metabolic fault, in which such factors play no important role.

The disease was known as early as the fifth century B.C., when it was described by Heiron, a resident of ancient Syracuse. Its hereditary nature has been recognized nearly as long. Modern studies, while confirming the genetic factor, have amplified our understanding of it in important ways. It is likely that multiple genes are involved, and that their effects are simply additive rather than interactive.[77] The heritability factor has been quantified as ranging from approximately one fifth to one third, and being distinctly less important for males than females.[77,196] Twin studies together with those of family incidence suggest strongly that, for males, environmental influences may outweigh the genetic as determinants of uric acid levels.[77,196]

The relevance of this sex difference becomes apparent in the fact that more than 95 percent of gout occurs in men. Mean uric acid levels in males are approximately 5 mg. percent, a value about 1 mg. percent higher than that for women beginning from puberty. The difference converges somewhat in late life because of a rise in the level for women at menopause.[181] The precipitation of uric acid in the tissues is, of course, a function of its concentration. As levels progressively exceed its solubility (ca. 6.4 mg. percent) there is a parallel increase in the probability that crystallization and deposition will occur.

The observation that the disease is more common among the affluent, eminent, and successful also goes back to antiquity. With the clarification of the role of uric acid, it has become possible to examine this relationship more closely. A substantial number of modern studies have provided both confirmation of its general validity, and a clarification that the crucial issue is not socioeconomic status per se, but the psychological characteristics of drive achievement and leadership. The latter, of course, build the path to success and prominence. Mueller and his associates have provided an extensive review of this work.[196]

The relationship with social status has been demonstrated in a variety of groups. Uric acid levels were found to be higher in executives than both craftsmen and normal controls, and higher in medical than high school students.[7,63] Within a single plant, Oak Ridge, the highest mean values were found in the Ph.D. scientists and the lowest in craftsmen, with the supervisors and inspectors falling in between.[40] Dodge and Mikkelson, as cited by Mueller,[196] found the age corrected urate levels of professionals and executives to be higher than those of workers in unskilled jobs and farmers. State white-collar employees had a higher mean level than the general population.[141]

By comparing subsamples within some of these and similar groups, it has become possible to delineate the role of *achievement-related behavior* from overall socioeconomic characteristics, since each group is more-or-less homogeneous with regard to the latter. Thus, in a Scottish study, the top executives had urate levels exceeding those found in those of lower rank.[7] Executives enrolled in a summer Executive Development Program, and thus presumably of greater ambition, had uric acid levels exceeding those of an unselected group of executives.[186] Among the state employees, those with the greatest number of job changes (considered to be an index of upward mobility) had the higher levels. In a study of a group of men anticipating job

termination, those with high uric acid levels were more likely to resign early to find another job.[129]

Even closer to the point, within a sample of university professors, interview ratings of achievement motivation were found to correlate at a level of $r = 66$ with serum uric acid values.[30] Similarly, Jenkins et al. found significant correlations, within a large group of supermarket employees, between serum urate levels and test items related to drive, competitiveness and challenging life circumstances, as cited by Mueller from a personal communication.[196] Further confirmation is provided by a pilot study that utilized a measure of the motivational trait free from overt achievement behavior. Patients with gout and hyperuricemia had measurably higher levels of *need achievement* than did a control group of social work students.[196]

The relationship holds also in regard to educational variables. The uric acid levels of high school and college students were positively related to the extent of their extra curricular activities, including those of a social and nonathletic type, and with test measures of achievement motivation.[63,190,127,128] There does not appear to be any simple relationship of uric acid to grades.[128] However, high school students with poor grades turned out to be more likely to go to college if they had high uric acid levels than if they did not, and within this group, uric acid levels correlated with the length of time they remained in college.[126] Approached from the other side, students attending or planning to attend college had higher uric acid values than those without such plans, above and beyond any association with grades.[128]

A few reports have appeared that fail to demonstrate relationships between uric acid and social class.[2,175,210] But, as of 1971, the weight of the evidence is so preponderant, both in numbers of studies and their meaningful consistencies, that it is difficult to be skeptical. It should be emphasized, however, that, with a single exception, all the findings involve studies done exclusively on *men*. Given the sex incidence of hyperuricemia and gout, this is not surprising. Moreover, the apparently greater role of genetic factors in women may dilute the effect of other variables, including those related to achievement. The one study done on women did show a suggestive relationship. In nursing students, a positive association was found between uric acid and extracurricular activities.[90] It will be important to learn if this relationship does indeed hold true also for women.

In one of the aforementioned studies, uric acid measures were taken also on a group of women, the subjects' spouses. Because achievement indices were recorded only for their husbands, this study provides no contribution to the question of the relationship of this variable in women. These data are helpful in another way. The uric acid levels of the executives' and professionals' wives did *not* exceed that of the wives of the less skilled workers. Thus, there is further support for believing that it is not their living styles (dietary and drinking habits etc.), nor other aspects of social class per se which are involved in the elevated uric acid levels found in their husbands. It might be added that various details of design in several of the other studies mentioned above lead to further confidence that such exogenous factors are not responsible for the findings.

There is one additional facet of this whole body of research that is of unique significance. Because the subjects had hyperuricemia but not gout, the psychological findings cannot be ascribed to any secondary effects of suffering from that disease. In this sense, this is prospective research, free from the potential error inherent in the retrospective method.

Assuming that the relationship between uric acid and achievement behavior and/or motivation does exist, how are we to understand it? The possibility arises that uric acid overproduction is a concomitant of chronic stress arising from the drive to success and the effort attendant upon its achievement. There are two studies which provide direct evidence that short-term psychological stress is associated with a rise in uric acid. In a group of Navy frogmen during training, Rahe and his co-workers[213,214] found uric acid elevations just prior to the start of training (the familiar pre-experimental anticipation effect that occurs in many stress variables.[227]) Rises in uric acid also occurred during periods when the trainees approached demanding tasks with an "optimistic" attitude, while drops were noted during a period when they felt "overburdened" and less assured of success.[213,214] Similar findings occurred in a study of stably employed men experiencing job loss because of a plant closing.[129] Anticipation of job loss was associated with elevations of uric acid which dropped following new employment. The duration of the rise tended to parallel the length of time it had taken to find the new job. Of special interest, those men who resigned prior to termination to obtain a new job had *stable* higher uric acid levels. This latter behavior not only implies greater achievement drive, it also suggests a greater degree of optimism. Furthermore, for a small subgroup in which psychological measures could be made reliably, a combined rating of sadness, low self- steem, and anxiety correlated negatively with uric acid levels.

Thus, these studies contribute to the understanding of the relationship of uric acid to transient emotional states, as well as to the larger body of work on its relationship to enduring personality traits. They also provide an intriguing lead for better delineating *achievement* drive in terms of the attitude associated with it. Additional confirmation of this lead can be found in closer scrutiny of some of the previously mentioned studies of the achievement trait. More frequent job change seems interpretable in terms of optimism and a sense of active mastery, as well as of upward mobility. So does the willingness to attempt college. Moreover the uric acid levels in college professors, which were positively correlated with ratings of achievement motivation, were concomitantly negatively correlated with reported feelings of being overburdened and worried about their jobs. Also consistent with this point is the finding that high school students with lower uric acid levels had more unrealistic vocational expectations and aspirations than those with high levels (the degree to which such goals are unrealistic being a concomitant of achievement avoidance).[128]

It would be difficult to overestimate the importance of this type of clarification. Such traits as *drive, achievement,* and *leadership* represent global qualities which may subsume or even obscure more narrowly and precisely defined personality attributes. It is essential to separate the latter from the grosser traits within which they are imbedded. (An excellent example of such an endeavor is to be found in Jenkin's delineation of the separate traits included within the *coronary-prone personality.*[124]) The justification for this viewpoint comes not only from considerations of logic but from its demonstrated payoff. Thus, in several of the studies reported, cholesterol levels were measured also and showed a very different relationship with the psychological variables than did uric acid.[129,196,214,216] In general the relation of cholesterol to the personality continuum of the optimism sense of mastery vs. less assured overburdened was just opposite to that for uric acid. Since coronary disease is accompanied by elevation in the mean levels both of cholesterol and uric acid,[83] the clarification of the differential personality correlates of the two substances is of considerable interest.

The correlation between personality traits and biochemical or physiological variables does not, of course, indicate a causal relationship. Either or both may be mere derivative products of other, more central factors. Even if the relationship were causal, the psychological variable need not be the primary factor. As a matter of fact, Orowan has offered the interesting converse hypothesis that uric acid acts as an endogenous cortical stimulant.[204] Consistent with this is the positive relationship between uric acid and IQ levels.[175,248] However, this correlation, albeit statistically significant, is very low ($r \cong 0.1$),[248] and, in any event, this hardly constitutes validation of the hypothesis.

Clearly there remains much work to be done. In this instance such a statement is no mere cliché. Rather it reflects an existing stage of accomplishment, important not merely in itself but in the clear directions it provides for further research. The elucidation of the relationship of uric acid and personality represents one of the brighter areas of psychosomatic research.

❨ Bibliography

1. ABRAHAM, K. (1913) "A Constitutional Basis of Locomotor Anxiety," in *Selected Papers on Psychoanalysis,* pp. 235–243. London: Hogarth, 1949.

2. ACHESON, R. M. and W. O'BRIEN. "Some Factors Associated with Serum Uric Acid in the New Haven Survey of Joint Disease," in P. H. Bennett and P. Wood, eds., *Population Studies of the Rheumatic Diseases,* pp. 365–370. Amsterdam: Excerpta Medica Foundation, 1968.

3. ALEXANDER, F. *Psychosomatic Medicine.* New York: Norton, 1950.

4. ALEXANDER, F., T. FRENCH, and G. H. POLLOCK. *Psychosomatic Specificity.* Chicago: University of Chicago Press, 1968.

5. ALLPORT, G. W. and P. VERNON. *Studies in Expressive Movement.* New York: Macmillan, 1933.

6. AMKRAUT, A. A., F. SOLOMON, and C. KRAEMER. "Stress, Early Experience and Adjuvant-Induced Arthritis in the Rat," *Psychosom. Med.,* 33 (1971), 203–214.

7. ANUMONYE, A., J. DOBSON, S. OPPENHEIM et al. "Plasma Uric Acid Concentrations among Edinburgh Business Executives," *JAMA,* 208 (1969), 1141–1148.

8. ASCHER, E. "Motor Attitudes and Psychotherapy," *Psychosom. Med.,* 11 (1949), 228–234.

9. ASSO, D., S. CROWN, J. A. RUSSELL et al. "Psychological Aspects of the Stereotactic Treatment of Parkinsonism," *Br. J. Psychiatry,* 115 (1969), 541–553.

10. AVNI, J. and J. CHACO. "Objective Measurements of Postural Changes in Depression." Paper presented at the Annual Meeting of the American Psychosomatic Society, Boston, April 1972. Unpublished.

11. AX, A. F. "The Physiological Differentiation between Fear and Anger in Humans," *Psychosom. Med.,* 15 (1953), 433–442.

12. AX, A. F., J. BAMFORD et al. "Autonomic Response Patterning of Chronic Schizophrenics," *Psychosom. Med.,* 31 (1969), 353–364.

13. BALSHAN, I. D. "Muscle Tension and Personality in Women," *Arch. Gen. Psychiatry*, 7 (1962), 436–448.

14. BARLOW, W. "Anxiety and Muscle Tension," in D. O'Neill, ed., *Modern Trends in Psychosomatic Medicine*. New York: Hoeber, 1955.

15. BENNETT, L. A. "The Personality of the Rheumatoid Arthritis Patient." Master's thesis, McGill University, Montreal, 1952. Unpublished.

16. BENNETT, P. and P. H. N. WOOD, eds., *Population Studies of the Rheumatic Diseases*, International Congress Series no. 148. Amsterdam: Excerpta Medica Foundation, 1968.

17. BIRDWHISTELL, R. L. *Introduction to Kinesics*. Louisville: University of Louisville Press, 1952.

18. ———. *Kinesics and Context*. Philadelphia: University of Pennsylvania Press, 1970.

19. BLAND, J. H., ed. "Symposium on Rheumatoid Arthritis," *Med. Clin. North Am.*, 52 (1968), 477–769.

20. BLOM, G. E. and G. NICHOLLS. "Emotional Factors in Children with Rheumatoid Arthritis," *Am. J. Orthopsychiatry*, 24 (1954), 588–600.

21. BOLAND, E. W. "Psychogenic Rheumatism: The Musculoskeletal Expression of Psychoneurosis," *Calif. Med.*, 68 (1948), 273–279.

22. ———. "Psychogenic Factors in Rheumatic Disease," in J. L. Hollander, ed., *Arthritis and Allied Conditions*, 6th ed. Philadelphia: Lea & Febiger, 1960.

23. BOLAND, E. W. and W. P. CORR. "Psychogenic Rheumatism," *JAMA*, 123 (1943), 805–809.

24. BOMAN, K. "Effect of Emotional Stress on Spasticity and Rigidity," *J. Psychosom. Res.*, 15 (1971), 107–112.

25. BOOTH, G. "Personality and Chronic Arthritis," *J. Nerv. Ment. Dis.*, 85 (1937), 637–662.

26. ———. "Objective Techniques in Personality Testing," *Arch. Neurol. Psychiatry*, 42 (1939), 514–530.

27. ———. "Organ Function and Form Perception," *Psychosom. Med.*, 8 (1946), 367–385.

28. ———. "Psychodynamics in Parkinsonism," *Psychosom. Med.*, 10 (1948), 1–14.

29. BOURESTOM, N. C. and M. T. HOWARD. "Personality Characteristics of Three Disability Groups," *Arch. Phys. Med. Rehabil.*, 46 (1965), 626–632.

30. BROOKS, G. W. and E. MUELLER. "Serum Urate Concentrations among University Professors," *JAMA*, 195 (1966), 415–418.

31. BULL, N. *The Attitude Theory of Emotion*. New York: Coolidge Foundation, 1951.

32. CAMERON, D. E. "Observations on the Patterns of Anxiety," *Am. J. Psychiatry*, 101 (1944), 36–41.

33. CAMERON, N. *The Psychology of Behavior Disorders*. Boston: Houghton Mifflin, 1947.

34. CHAPMAN, A. H. *Management of Emotional Disorders: A Manual for Physicians*. Philadelphia: Lippincott, 1962.

35. CHRISTIAN, C., ed. "Nineteenth Rheumatism Review," *Arthritis Rheum.*, 13 (1970), 474–711.

36. CLEVELAND, S. and S. FISHER. "Behavior and Unconscious Fantasies of Patients with Rheumatoid Arthritis," *Psychosom. Med.*, 16 (1954), 327–333.

37. ———. "A Comparison of Psychological Characteristics and Physiological Reactivity in Ulcer and Rheumatoid Arthritis Groups: I. Psychological Measures," *Psychosom. Med.*, 22 (1960), 283–289.

38. CLEVELAND, S., E. E. REITMAN, and E. J. BREWER, JR. "Psychological Factors in Juvenile Rheumatoid Arthritis," *Arthritis Rheum.*, 8 (1965), 1152–1158.

39. COBB, SIDNEY. "Contained Hostility in Rheumatoid Arithritis," *Arthritis Rheum.*, 2 (1959), 419–425.

40. ———. "Hyperuricemia in Executives," in J. H. Kellgren, ed., *The Epidemiology of Chronic Rheumatism*, pp. 182–196. Philadelphia: Davis, 1963.

41. ———. *The Frequency of Rheumatic Diseases*. Cambridge, Mass.: Harvard University Press, 1969.

42. COBB, SIDNEY and T. LINCOLN. "On the Frequency of Individuals Who Suffer Occasional Attacks of Rheumatoid Arthritis," *Arthritis Rheum.*, 3 (1960), 48.

43. COBB, SIDNEY, M. MILLER, and M. WIELAND. "On the Relationship between Divorce and Rheumatoid Arthritis," *Arthritis Rheum.*, 2 (1959), 414–418.

44. COBB, SIDNEY, W. J. SCHULL, E. HARBURG et al. "The Intrafamilial Transmission of Rheumatoid Arthritis," *J. Chronic Dis.*, 22 (1969), 195–296.

45. COBB, STANLEY, W. BAUER, and I. WHITING. "Environmental Factors in Rheumatoid

Arthritis," *JAMA*, 113 (1939), 668–670.

46. COOPER, I. S. *The Neurosurgical Alleviation of Parkinsonism.* Springfield, Ill.: Charles C. Thomas, 1956.

47. CORMIER, B. M. and E. WITTKOWER. "Psychological Aspects of Rheumatoid Arthritis," *Can. Med. Assoc. J.*, 77 (1957), 533–541.

48. CRISP, A. H. and H. MOLDOFSKY. "A Psychosomatic Study of Writer's Cramp," *Br. J. Psychiatry*, 111 (1965), 841–858.

49. CROWN, S. "Psychosomatic Aspects of Parkinsonism," *J. Psychosom. Res.*, 15 (1971), 451–459.

50. DAMASER, E. C., R. SHOR, and M. ORNE. "Physiological Effects during Hypnotically Requested Emotions," *Psychosom. Med.*, 25 (1963), 334–343.

51. DAVIDOWITZ, J., A. N. BROWN-MAYERS, R. KOHL et al. "An Electromyographic Study of Muscular Tension," *J. Psychol.*, 40 (1955), 85–94.

52. DAVIS, F. H. and R. B. MALMO. "Electromyographic Recording during Interview," *Am. J. Psychiatry*, 107 (1951), 908–915.

53. DAVIS, J. F. *Manual of Surface Electromyography.* Montreal: Allan Memorial Institute of Psychiatry, 1952.

54. DAVIS, J. F., R. B. MALMO, and C. SHAGASS. "Electromyographic Reaction to Strong Auditory Stimulation in Psychiatric Patients," *Can. J. Psychol.*, 8 (1954), 177–186.

55. DAVIS, R. C. "Methods of Measuring Muscular Tension," *Psychol. Bull.*, 39 (1942), 329–346.

56. DECKER, J. L. "The Epidemiology of Hyperuricemia: A Summary," in G. Katona and J. R. Gill, eds., *Panamerican Rheumatology*, pp. 74–75. Amsterdam: Excerpta Medica Foundation, 1969.

57. DEUTSCH, F. "Analysis of Postural Behavior," *Psychoanal. Q.*, 16 (1947), 195–213.

58. DUFFY, E. "The Measurement of Muscular Tension as a Technique for the Study of Emotional Tendencies," *Am. J. Psychol.*, 44 (1932), 146–162.

59. ———. "The Relation between Muscular Tension and Quality of Performance," *Am. J. Psychol.*, 44 (1932), 535–546.

60. ———. "Level of Muscular Tension as an Aspect of Personality," *J. Gen. Psychol.*, 35 (1946), 161–171.

61. ———. *Activation and Behavior.* New York: Wiley, 1962.

62. DUNBAR, H. F. *Emotions and Bodily Changes.* New York: Columbia University Press, 1954.

63. DUNN, J., W. G. BROOKS, J. MAUSNER et al. "Social Class Gradient of Serum Uric Acid Levels in Males," *JAMA*, 185 (1963), 431–436.

64. EHRLICH, G. E. "Psychosomatic Aspects of Musculoskeletal Disorders," *Postgrad. Med.*, 38 (1965), 614–619.

65. ELEFTHERIOU, B. and J. P. SCOTT. *The Physiology of Aggression and Defeat.* New York: Plenum, 1971.

66. ENGEL, G. L. "Studies of Ulcerative Colitis: I. Clinical Data Bearing on the Nature of the Somatic Process," *Psychosom. Med.*, 16 (1954), 496–501.

67. ———. "Studies of Ulcerative Colitis: II. The Nature of the Somatic Processes and the Adequacy of Psychosomatic Hypotheses," *Am. J. Med.*, 16 (1954), 416–433.

68. ———. "Studies of Ulcerative Colitis: III. The Nature of the Psychologic Processes," *Am. J. Med.*, 19 (1955), 231–256.

69. FENICHEL, O. *The Psychoanalytic Theory of Neurosis.* New York: Norton, 1945.

70. FERENCZI, S. (1919) "Thinking and Muscle Innervation," in J. Rickman, ed. *Further Contributions to the Theory and Technique of Psychoanalysis*, pp. 230–232. New York: Basic Books, 1952.

71. FESSEL, W. J. "Mental Stress, Blood Proteins and the Hypothalamus," *Arch. Gen. Psychiatry*, 7 (1962), 427–435.

72. FISCHMAN, D. A., H. MELTZER, and R. POPPEI. "Disruption of Myofibrils in the Skeletal Muscle of Psychotic Patients," *Arch. Gen. Psychiatry*, 23 (1970), 503–513.

73. FISHER, S. *Body Experience in Fantasy and Behavior.* New York: Appleton-Century-Crofts, 1970.

74. FISHER, S. and S. E. CLEVELAND. "A Comparison of Psychological Characteristics and Physiological Reactivity in Ulcer and Rheumatoid Arthritis Groups: II. Differences in Physiological Reactivity," *Psychosom. Med.*, 22 (1960), 290–293.

75. ———. *Body Image and Personality*, 2nd ed. New York: Dover, 1968.

76. FREEMAN, G. L. "Postural Tensions and the Conflict Situation," *Psychol. Rev.*, 46 (1939), 226–240.

77. FRENCH, J. G., H. J. DODGE, M. O. KJELS-
BERG et al. "A Study of Familial Aggregation of Serum Uric Acid Levels in the
Population of Tecumseh, Michigan, 1959–
60," *Am. J. Epidemiol.*, 86 (1967), 214–
224.

78. FRENCH, T. and L. SHAPIRO. "The Use of
Dream Analysis in Psychosomatic Research," *Psychosom. Med.*, 11 (1949),
110–112.

79. FREUD, S. *The Problem of Anxiety*. New
York: Norton, 1936.

80. ———. (1901) *The Psychopathology of
Everyday Life*, in J. Strachey, ed., *Standard Edition*, Vol. 6. London: Hogarth,
1953.

81. GEIST, H. *The Psychological Aspects of
Rheumatoid Arthritis*. Springfield, Ill.:
Charles C. Thomas, 1966.

82. GELLHORN, E. *Physiological Foundations of
Neurology and Psychiatry*. Minneapolis:
University of Minnesota Press, 1953.

83. GERTLER, M. M., S. M. GARN, and S. A.
LEVINE. "Serum Uric Acid in Relation to
Age and Physique in Health and in Coronary Heart Disease," *Ann. Intern. Med.*, 34
(1951), 1421–1431.

84. GLOVER, E. *Psycho-analysis*. London: Staples Press, 1949.

85. GOLD, S. "Psycho-Genesis in the 'Stiff-Man
Syndrome'," *Guys Hosp. Rep.*, 114 (1965),
279–285.

86. GOLDSTEIN BALSHAN, I. "Role of Muscle
Tension in Personality Theory," *Psychol.
Bull.*, 61 (1964), 413–425.

87. ———. "Physiological Responses in Anxious
Women Patients," *Arch. Gen. Psychiatry*,
10 (1964), 382–388.

88. ———. "The Relationship of Muscle Tension and Autonomic Activity to Psychiatric
Disorders," *Psychosom. Med.*, 27 (1965),
39–52.

89. GOLDSTEIN BALSHAN, I., R. R. GRINKER, SR.,
H. A. HEATH et al. "Study in Psychophysiology of Muscle Tension: I. Response
Specificity," *Arch. Gen. Psychiatry*, 11
(1964), 322–330.

90. GORDON, R. E., R. LINDEMAN, and K. GOR-
DON. "Some Psychological and Biochemical
Correlates of College Achievement," *J.
Am. College Health Assoc.*, 15 (1967),
326–331.

91. GOTTSCHALK, L., M. SEROTA, and K. ROMAN.
"Handwriting in Rheumatoid Arthritics,"

Psychosom. Med., 11 (1949), 354–360.

92. GOTTSCHALK, L., H. SEROTA, and L. SHAP-
IRO. "Psychologic Conflict and Neuromuscular Tension," *Psychosom. Med.*, 12
(1950), 315–319.

93. GRACE, W. J. and D. GRAHAM. "Relationship
of Specific Attitudes and Emotions to Certain Bodily Diseases," *Psychosom. Med.*,
14 (1952), 243–251.

94. GRAHAM, D. T., R. M. LUNDY, L. S. BEN-
JAMIN et al. "Specific Attitudes in Initial
Interviews with Patients Having Different
'Psychosomatic' Diseases," *Psychosom.
Med.*, 24 (1962), 257–266.

95. GREGG, D. "The Paucity of Arthritis among
Psychotic Cases," *Am. J. Psychiatry*, 95
(1939), 853–856.

96. GRINKER, R. R., SR., S. J. KORCHIN,
H. BASOWITZ et al. "A Theoretical and
Experimental Approach to Problems of
Anxiety," *Arch Neurol. Psychiatry*, 76
(1956), 420–431.

97. GRINKER, R. R., SR. and J. SPIEGEL. *War
Neurosis in North Africa: The Tunisian
Campaign*. New York: Josiah Macy Foun-
dation, 1943.

98. GROKOEST, A. W., I. SNYDER, and R.
SCHLAEGER. *Juvenile Rheumatoid Arthritis*. Boston: Little, Brown, 1962.

99. GROSSMAN, W. I. and H. WEINER. "Some
Factors Affecting the Reliability of Surface
Electromyography," *Psychosom. Med.*, 28
(1966), 78–83.

100. GUGGENHEIM, P. and L. COHEN. "A Case
of Schizophrenia in which Manifestations
of Parkinsonism Appeared during the
Course of the Psychosis and Disappeared
after Lobotomy," *Psychosom. Med.*, 20
(1958), 151–160.

101. GUTMAN, A. B., ed. "Proceedings of Conference on Gout and Purine Metabolism,"
Arthritis Rheum., 8 (1965), 589–910.

102. HALLIDAY, J. L. "Psychological Factors in
Rheumatism," *Br. Med. J.*, 1 (1937), 213–
217; 264–269.

103. ———. "The Concept of Psychogenic
Rheumatism," *Ann. Intern. Med.*, 15
(1941), 666–677.

104. ———. "The Psychological Approach to
Rheumatism," *Proc. R. Soc. Med.*, 35
(1942), 455–457.

105. ———. "Concept of a Psychosomatic
Affection," *Lancet*, 2 (1943), 692–696.

106. HAYS, P., et al. "Psychological Changes

following Surgical Treatment of Parkinsonism," *Am. J. Psychiatry*, 123 (1966), 657–663.

107. HEATH, H. A., D. OKEN, and W. G. SHIPMAN. "Muscle Tension and Personality," *Arch. Gen. Psychiatry*, 16 (1967), 720–726.

108. HEATH, H. A., D. OKEN, and W. G. SHIPMAN et al. "Three Factor Analyses of Electromyographic Data Under Varying Conditions," *Multivariate Behav. Res.*, 2 (1967), 263–280.

109. HELLGREN, L. "Marital Status in Rheumatoid Arthritis," *Acta Rheumatol. Scand.*, 15 (1969), 271–276.

110. HENCH, P. S. and E. W. BOLAND. "The Management of Chronic Arthritis and Other Rheumatic Diseases among Soldiers of the United States Army," *Ann. Intern. Med.*, 24 (1946), 808–825.

111. HENDRIE, H. C., F. PARASKEVAS, and J. D. ADAMSON. "Stress, Immunoglobulin Levels and Early Polyarthritis," *J. Psychosom. Res.*, 15 (1971), 337–342.

112. ———. "Gamma Globulin Levels in Psychiatric Patients," *Can. Psychiatr. Assoc. J.*, 17 (1972), 93–97.

113. HOLLANDER, J. L., ed. *Arthritis and Allied Conditions: A Textbook of Rheumatology*, 6th ed. Philadelphia: Lea & Febiger, 1960.

114. HOLMES, T. H. and H. WOLFF. "Life Situations, Emotions, and Backache," *Psychosom. Med.*, 14 (1952), 18–33.

115. INMAN, V. T., H. J. RALSTON, J. B. DE C. M. SAUNDERS et al. "Relation of Human Electromyogram to Muscular Tension," *Electroencephalogr. Clin. Neurophysiol.*, 4 (1952), 187–194.

116. JACKSON, J. A., G. B. M. FREE, and H. V. PIKE. "The Psychic Manifestations in Paralysis Agitans," *Arch. Neurol. Psychiatry*, 10 (1923), 680–684.

117. JACOBSON, E. *Progressive Relaxation*. Chicago: University of Chicago Press, 1938.

118. JACOBSON, E., ed. *Tension in Medicine*. Springfield, Ill.: Charles C. Thomas, 1967.

119. JAMES, W. *The Principles of Psychology*. New York: Holt, 1890.

120. JEFFREY, M. R. and J. BALL. *The Epidemiology of Chronic Rheumatism*. Philadelphia: Davis, 1963.

121. JELLIFFE, S. E. "The Mental Pictures in Schizophrenia and in Epidemic Encephalitis," *Am. J. Psychiatry*, 6 (1926), 413–465.

122. ———. "The Parkinsonian Body Posture," *Psychoanal. Rev.*, 27 (1940), 467.

123. JELLIFFE, S. E. and W. A. WHITE. *Diseases of the Nervous System*. Philadelphia: Lea & Febiger, 1935.

124. JENKINS, C. D., S. J. ZYZANSKI, and R. H. ROSENMAN. "Progress toward Validation of a Computer-Scored Test for the Type A Coronary-Prone Behavior Pattern," *Psychosom. Med.*, 33 (1971), 193–202.

125. JOHNSON, A. M., L. SHAPIRO, and F. ALEXANDER. "Preliminary Report on a Psychosomatic Study of Rheumatoid Arthritis," *Psychosom. Med.*, 9 (1947), 295–300.

126. KASL, S. V., G. W. BROOKS, and SIDNEY COBB. "Serum Urate Concentrations in Male High School Students, a Predictor of College Attendance," *JAMA*, 198 (1966), 713–716.

127. KASL, S. V., G. W. BROOKS, and W. RODGERS. "Serum Uric Acid and Cholesterol in Achievement Behavior and Motivation: I. The Relationship to Ability, Grades, Test Performance, and Motivation," *JAMA*, 213 (1970), 1158–1164.

128. ———. "Serum Uric Acid and Cholesterol in Achievement Behavior and Motivation: II. The Relationship to College Attendance, Extracurricular and Social Activities, and Vocational Aspirations," *JAMA*, 213 (1970), 1291–1299.

129. KASL, S. V., SIDNEY COBB, and G. W. BROOKS. "Changes in Serum Uric Acid and Serum Cholesterol in Men Undergoing Job Loss," *JAMA*, 206 (1968), 1500–1507.

130. KEMPE, J. E. "An Experimental Investigation of the Relationship Between Certain Personality Characteristics and Physiological Responses to Stress in a Normal Population." Ph.D. dissertation, Michigan State University, 1956. Unpublished.

131. KEPECS, J. G. "Some Patterns of Somatic Displacement," *Psychosom. Med.*, 15 (1953), 425–432.

132. KING, H. E. "Psychomotility: A Dimension of Behavior Disorder," *Proc. Am. Psychopathol. Assoc.*, 58 (1969), 99–128.

133. KING, S. H. "Psychosocial Factors Associated With Rheumatoid Arthritis," *J. Chronic Dis.*, 2 (1955), 287–302.

134. KING, S. H. and SIDNEY COBB. "Psychosocial Factors in the Epidemiology of Rheumatoid Arthritis," *J. Chronic Dis.*, 7 (1958), 466–475.

135. ———. "Psychosocial Studies of Rheumatoid Arthritis: Parental Factors Compared in Cases and Controls," *Arthritis Rheum.*, 2 (1959), 322–331.

136. LACEY, J. I. "Psychophysiological Approaches to the Evaluation of Psychotherapeutic Process and Outcome," in E. A. Rubinstein and M. B. Parloff, eds., *Research in Psychotherapy*, pp. 160–208. Washington, D.C.: American Psychological Association, 1959.

137. ———. "Somatic Response Patterning and Stress: Some Revisions of Activation Theory," in M. H. Appley and R. Trumbull, eds., *Psychological Stress*, pp. 14–37. New York: Appleton-Century-Crofts, 1967.

138. LACEY, J. I., D. E. BATEMAN, and R. VANLEHN. "Autonomic Response Specificity," *Psychosom. Med.*, 15 (1953), 8–21.

139. LACEY, J. I. and B. LACEY. "The Relationship of Resting Autonomic Activity to Motor Impulsivity," *Res. Publ. Assoc. Res. Nerv. Ment. Dis.*, 36 (1956), 144–209.

140. LADER, M. H. and A. M. MATTHEWS. "Electromyographic Studies of Tension," *J. Psychosom. Res.*, 15 (1971), 479–486.

141. LANESE, R. R., G. GRESHAM, and M. D. KELLER. "Behavioral and Physiological Characteristics in Hyperuricemia," *JAMA*, 207 (1969), 1878–1882.

142. LEWIS-FANNING, E. "Report on an Enquiry into the Aetiological Factors Associated with Rheumatoid Arthritis," *Ann. Rheum. Dis.*, 9 (1950), Suppl.

143. LINDSLEY, D. B. "Emotion," in S. S. Stevens, ed., *Handbook of Experimental Psychology*, pp. 473–516. New York: Wiley, 1951.

144. LIPPOLD, O. C. J. "The Relation between Integrated Action Potentials in a Human Muscle and Its Isometric Tension," *J. Physiol.*, 117 (1952), 492–499.

145. LOVAAS, O. I. "The Relationship of Induced Muscular Tension, Tension Level, and Manifest Anxiety in Learning," *J. Exp. Psychol.*, 59 (1960), 145–152.

146. LOWMAN, E. W., ed. *Arthritis: General Principles, Physical Medicine, Rehabilitation*. Boston: Little, Brown, 1959.

147. LOWMAN, E. W., S. MILLER, P. LEE et al. "Psycho-Social Factors in Rehabilitation of the Chronic Rheumatoid Arthritic," *Ann. Rheum. Dis.*, 13 (1954), 312–316.

148. LUDWIG, A. O. "Emotional Factors in Rheumatoid Arthritis," *Physiother. Rev.*, 29 (1949), 339–342.

149. ———. "Psychogenic Factors in Rheumatoid Arthritis," *Bull. Rheum. Dis.*, 2 (1952), 33–34.

150. ———. "Rheumatoid Arthritis," in E. D. Wittkower and R. A. Cleghorn, eds., *Recent Developments in Psychosomatic Medicine*, pp. 232–244. Philadelphia: Lippincott, 1954.

151. LUNDERVOLD, A. "An Electromyographic Investigation of Tense and Relaxed Subjects," *J. Nerv. Ment. Dis.*, 115 (1952), 512–525.

152. LURIA, A. *The Nature of Human Conflicts*. New York: Liveright, 1932.

153. LUTHE, W., ed. *Autogenic Training: Psychosomatic Correlations*. New York: Grune & Stratton, 1964.

154. MACHOVER, S. "Rorschach Study on the Nature and Origin of Common Factors in the Personalities of Parkinsonians," *Psychosom. Med.*, 19 (1957), 332–338.

155. MACLEAN, P. D. "The Limbic ('Visceral Brain') in Relation to Central Gray and Reticulum of the Brain Stem," *Psychosom. Med.*, 17 (1955), 355–366.

156. MALMO, R. B. "Symptom Mechanisms in Psychiatric Patients," *Trans. N.Y. Acad. Sci.*, 18 (1956), 545–549.

157. ———. "Activation: A Neuropsychological Dimension," *Psychol. Rev.*, 66 (1959), 367–386.

158. MALMO, R. B., T. J. BOAG, and A. A. SMITH. "Physiological Study of Personal Interaction," *Psychosom. Med.*, 19 (1957), 105–119.

159. MALMO, R. B. and C. SHAGASS. "Physiologic Studies of Reaction to Stress in Anxiety and Early Schizophrenia," *Psychosom. Med.*, 11 (1949), 9–24.

160. ———. "Physiologic Study of Symptom Mechanisms in Psychiatric Patients under Stress," *Psychosom. Med.*, 11 (1949), 25–29.

161. ———. "Studies of Blood Pressure in Psychiatric Patients under Stress," *Psychosom. Med.*, 14 (1952), 82–93.

162. MALMO, R. B., C. SHAGASS, and F. H. DAVIS. "Symptom Specificity and Bodily Reactions during Psychiatric Interview," *Psychosom. Med.*, 12 (1950), 363–376.

163. MALMO, R. B., C. SHAGASS, and J. F. DAVIS. "A Method for the Investigation of Somatic Response Mechanisms in Psychoneurosis," *Science*, 112 (1950), 325–328.

164. ———. "Electromyographic Studies of

Muscular Tension in Psychiatric Patients under Stress," *J. Clin. Exp. Psychopathol.*, 12 (1951), 45–66.

165. MALMO, R. B., C. SHAGASS, and A. SMITH. "Responsiveness in Chronic Schizophrenia," *J. Pers.*, 19 (1951), 359–375.

166. MALMO, R. B., A. A. SMITH, and W. A. KOHLMEYER. "Motor Manifestation of Conflict in Interview: A Case Study," *J. Abnorm. Soc. Psychol.*, 52 (1956), 268–271.

167. MARSCHALL, W. "The Psychopathology and Treatment of the Parkinsonian Syndrome and Other Post-Encephalitic Sequelae," *J. Nerv. Ment. Dis.*, 84 (1936), 27–45.

168. MARTIN, I. "Levels of Muscle Activity in Psychiatric Patients," *Acta Psychol. (Amst.)*, 12 (1956), 326–341.

169. MARTIN, I. and H. J. GROSZ. "Hypnotically Induced Emotions," *Arch. Gen. Psychiatry*, 11 (1964), 203–213.

170. MARTIN, I. and L. REES. "Reaction Times and Somatic Reactivity in Depressed Patients," *J. Psychosom. Res.*, 9 (1966), 375–382.

171. McFIE, J. "Psychological Effects of Stereotaxic Operations for the Relief of Parkinsonian Symptoms," *J. Ment. Sci.*, 106 (1960), 1512–1517.

172. McLAUGHLIN, J. T., R. N. ZABARENKO, P. B. DIANA et al. "Emotional Reactions of Rheumatoid Arthritics to ACTH," *Psychosom. Med.*, 15 (1953), 187–199.

173. MELTZER, H. Y. and W. ENGEL. "Histochemical Abnormalities of Skeletal Muscle in Acutely Psychotic Patients," *Arch. Gen. Psychiatry*, 23 (1970), 492–502.

174. MELTZER, H. Y. and R. MOLINE. "Muscle Abnormalities in Acute Psychoses," *Arch. Gen. Psychiatry*, 23 (1970), 481–491.

175. MERSY, D. J., T. AUYONG, and R. EELKEMA. "Relationship of Serum Urate Levels to Occupation and Mental Retardation," *Psychosomatics*, 9 (1968), 199–201.

176. MEYER, D. R. "On the Interaction of Simultaneous Responses," *Psychol. Bull.*, 50 (1953), 204–220.

177. MEYER, D. R., H. P. BAHRICK, and P. M. FITTS. "Incentive, Anxiety, and the Human Blink Rate," *J. Exp. Psychol.*, 45 (1953), 183–187.

178. MEYEROWITZ, S. "Editorial: Psychosocial Factors in the Etiology of Somatic Disease," *Ann. Intern. Med.*, 72 (1970), 753–754.

179. ———. "The Continuing Investigation of Psychosocial Variables in Rheumatoid Arthritis," in A. Hill, ed., *Modern Trends in Rheumatology*, pp. 92–105. New York: Appleton-Century-Crofts, 1971.

180. MEYEROWITZ, S., R. JACOX, and D. W. HESS. "Monozygotic Twins Discordant for Rheumatoid Arthritis: A Genetic, Clinical and Psychological Study of 8 Sets," *Arthritis Rheum.*, 11 (1968), 1–21.

181. MIKKELSEN, W. M., H. DODGE, and H. VALKENBURG. "The Distribution of Serum Uric Acid Values in a Population Unselected as to Gout or Hyperuricemia," *Am. J. Med.*, 39 (1965), 242–251.

182. MITSCHERLICH, M. "The Psychic State of Patients Suffering from Parkinsonism," in A. Jores and H. Freyberger, eds., *Advances in Psychosomatic Medicine*, pp. 317–324. New York: Brunner, 1961.

183. MOLDOFSKY, H. "Occupational Cramp," *J. Psychosom. Res.*, 15 (1971), 439–444.

184. MOLDOFSKY, H. and W. J. CHESTER. "Pain and Mood Patterns in Patients with Rheumatoid Arthritis," *Psychosom. Med.*, 32 (1970), 309–318.

185. MOLDOFSKY, H. and A. I. ROTHMAN. "Personality, Disease Parameters and Medication in Rheumatoid Arthritis," *Arthritis Rheum.*, 13 (1970), 338–339.

186. MONTOYE, H. J., J. A. FAULKNER, H. J. DODGE et al. "Serum Uric Acid Concentration among Business Executives," *Ann. Intern. Med.*, 66 (1967), 838–850.

187. MOOS, R. H. "Personality Factors Associated With Rheumatoid Arthritis: A Review," *J. Chronic Dis.*, 17 (1964), 41–55.

188. MOOS, R. H. and B. T. ENGEL. "Psychophysiological Reactions in Hypertensive and Arthritic Patients," *J. Psychosom. Res.*, 6 (1962), 227–241.

189. MOOS, R. H., and G. SOLOMON. "Minnesota Multiphasic Personality Inventory Response Patterns in Patients with Rheumatoid Arthritis," *J. Psychosom. Res.*, 8 (1964), 17 28.

190. ———. "Psychologic Comparisons between Women with Rheumatoid Arthritis and Their Non-arthritic Sisters: I. Personality Test and Interview Rating Data," *Psychosom. Med.*, 27 (1965), 135–149.

191. ———. "Psychologic Comparisons Between Women with Rheumatoid Arthritis and Their Non-arthritic Sisters: II. Content Analysis of Interviews," *Psychosom. Med.*, 27 (1965), 150–164.

192. ———. "Personality Correlates of the Degree of Functional Incapacity of Patients with Physical Disease," *J. Chronic Dis.*, 18 (1965), 1019–1038.

193. Morrison, L. R., C. L. Short, A. O. Ludwig et al. "The Neuromuscular System in Rheumatoid Arthritis," *Am. J. Med. Sci.*, 214 (1947), 2–49.

194. Mueller, A. D. and A. M. Lefkovits. "Personality Structure and Dynamics of Patients with Rheumatoid Arthritis," *J. Clin. Psychol.*, 12 (1956), 143–147.

195. Mueller, A. D., A. M. Lefkovits, J. E. Bryant et al. "Some Psycho-social Factors in Patients with Rheumatoid Arthritis," *Arthritis Rheum.*, 4 (1961), 275–282.

196. Mueller, E. F., S. V. Kasl, G. W. Brooks et al. "Psychosocial Correlates of Serum Urate Levels," *Psychol. Bull.*, 73 (1970), 238–257.

197. Nalven, F. B. and J. O'Brien. "Personality Patterns of Rheumatoid Arthritic Patients," *Arthritis Rheum.*, 7 (1964), 18–28.

198. Nidevar, J. E. *A Factor Analytic Study of General Muscle Tension.* Ph.D. dissertation, University of California at Los Angeles, 1959. Unpublished.

199. Nissen, H. A. "Chronic Arthritis and Its Treatment," *N. Engl. J. Med.*, 210 (1934), 1109–1115.

200. Nissen, H. A. and K. A. Spencer. "The Psychogenic Problem (Endocrinal and Metabolic) in Chronic Arthritis," *N. Engl. J. Med.*, 214 (1936), 576–581.

201. Noble, P. J. and M. H. Lader. "An Electromyographic Study of Depressed Patients," *J. Psychosom. Res.*, 15 (1971), 233–239.

202. Oken, D. "An Experimental Study of Suppressed Anger and Blood Pressure," *Arch. Gen. Psychiatry*, 2 (1960), 441–456.

203. ———. "The Role of Defense in Psychological Stress," in R. Roessler and N. S. Greenfield, eds., *Physiological Correlates of Psychological Disorder*, pp. 193–210. Madison: The University of Wisconsin Press, 1962.

204. Orowan, E. "Origins of Man," *Nature*, 175 (1955), 683–684.

205. Paul, L. "Psychosomatic Aspects of Low Back Pain," *Psychosom. Med.*, 12 (1950), 116–124.

206. ———. "Mephenesin in Anxiety-tension States," *Psychosom. Med.*, 14 (1952), 378–382.

207. Ploski, H., E. Levita, and M. Riklan.
"Impairment of Voluntary Movement in Parkinson's Disease in Relation to Activation Level, Autonomic Malfunction, and Personality Rigidity," *Psychosom. Med.*, 28 (1966), 70–77.

208. Plutchik, R. "The Role of Muscular Tension in Maladjustment," *J. Gen. Psychol.*, 50 (1954), 45–62.

209. Polley, H., W. M. Swenson, and R. M. Steinhilber. "Personality Characteristics of Patients with Rheumatoid Arthritis," *Psychosomatics*, 11 (1970), 45–49.

210. Popert, A. J. and J. Hewitt. "Gout and Hyperuricaemia in Rural and Urban Populations," *Ann. Rheum. Dis.*, 21 (1962), 154–163.

211. Price, J. P., M. H. Clare, and F. H. Ewerhardt. "Studies in Low Backache with Persistent Muscle Spasm," *Arch. Phys. Med.*, 29 (1948), 703–709.

212. Prick, J. J. G., and K. Van de Loo. *The Psychosomatic Approach to Primary Chronic Rheumatoid Arthritis.* Philadelphia: Davis, 1964.

213. Rahe, R. H. and R. Arthur. "Stressful Underwater Demolition Training. Serum Urate and Cholesterol Variability," *JAMA*, 202 (1967), 1052–1054.

214. Rahe, R. H. et al. "Serum Uric Acid and Cholesterol Variability," *JAMA*, 206 (1968), 2875–2880.

215. Reich, W. *Character-Analysis*, 2nd ed. New York: Orgone Institute Press, 1949.

216. Reis, G. von. "Electromyographical Studies in Writer's Cramp," *Acta. Med. Scand.*, 149 (1954), 253–260.

217. Riklan, M. and E. Levita. *Subcortical Correlates of Human Behavior.* Baltimore: Williams & Wilkins, 1969.

218. Rimón, R. "A Psychosomatic Approach to Rheumatoid Arthritis: A Clinical Study of 100 Female Patients," *Acta Rheumatol. Scand.*, (Suppl). 13 (1969), 1–154.

219. Rimón, R., A. Stenback, and E. Huhmar. "Electromyographic Findings in Depressive Patients," *J. Psychosom. Res.*, 10 (1966), 159–170.

220. Rinehart, R. E. "Physiologic Approach to Rheumatic Disease," in E. Jacobson, ed., *Tension in Medicine*, pp. 55–70. Springfield, Ill.: Charles C. Thomas, 1967.

221. Robb, J. H. and B. S. Rose. "Rheumatoid Arthritis and Maternal Deprivation: A Case Study in the Use of a Social Survey," *Br. J. Med. Psychol.*, 38 (1965), 147–159.

222. ROBINSON, C. E. G. "Emotional Factors and Rheumatoid Arthritis," *Can. Med. Assoc. J.*, 77 (1957), 344–345.

223. ROBINSON, H., R. KIRK, and R. GRYE. "A Psychological Study of Rheumatoid Arthritis and Selected Controls," *J. Chronic Dis.*, 23 (1971), 791–801.

224. ROESSLER, R., A. ALEXANDER, and N. GREENFIELD. "Ego Strength and Physiological Responsivity: I," *Arch. Gen. Psychiatry*, 8 (1963), 142–154.

225. ROSSI, A. M. "An Evaluation of the Manifest Anxiety Scale by the Use of Electromyography," *J. Exp. Psychol.*, 58 (1959), 64–69.

226. RUESCH, J. and J. FINESINGER. "The Relation between Electromyographic Measurements and Subjective Reports of Muscular Relaxation," *Psychosom. Med.*, 5 (1943), 132–138.

227. SABSHIN, M., et al. "Significance of Pre-experimental Studies in the Psychosomatic Laboratory," *Arch. Neurol. Psychiatry*, 78 (1957), 207–219.

228. SAINSBURY, P. "Muscle Responses: Muscle Tension and Expressive Movement," *J. Psychosom. Res.*, 8 (1964), 179–185.

229. SAINSBURY, P. and W. R. COSTAIN. "The Measurement of Psychomotor Activity: Some Clinical Applications," *J. Psychosom. Res.*, 15 (1971), 487–494.

230. SAMRA, K., M. RIKLAN, E. LEVITA et al. "Language and Speech Correlates of Anatomically Verified Lesions in Thalamic Surgery for Parkinsonism," *J. Speech Hear. Res.*, 12 (1969), 510–540.

231. SANDLER, S. A. "Camptocormia, or the Functional Bent Back," *Psychosom. Med.*, 9 (1947), 197–204.

232. SANDS, I. "The Type of Personality Susceptible to Parkinson Disease," *J. Mt. Sinai Hosp.* (N.Y.), 9 (1942), 792–794.

233. SAPIRSTEIN, M. R. "The Effect of Anxiety on Human After-Discharges," *Psychosom. Med.*, 10 (1948), 145–155.

234. SARWER-FONER, G. J. "Psychoanalytic Theories of Activity-Passivity Conflicts and the Continuum of Ego Defenses," *Arch. Neurol. Psychiatry*, 78 (1957), 413–418.

235. SCHWAB, R. S., H. FABING, and J. PRICHARD. "Psychiatric Symptoms and Syndromes in Parkinson's Disease," *Am. J. Psychiatry*, 107 (1950), 901–907.

236. SCOTCH, N. A. and H. GEIGER. "The Epidemiology of Rheumatoid Arthritis," *J. Chronic Dis.*, 15 (1962), 1037–1067.

237. SEASHORE, R. H. "Work and Motor Performance," in S. Stevens, ed., *Handbook of Experimental Psychology*, pp. 1341–1362. New York: Wiley, 1951.

238. SHAGASS, C. and R. B. MALMO. "Psychodynamic Themes and Localized Muscular Tension during Psychotherapy," *Psychosom. Med.*, 16 (1954), 295–314.

239. SHASKAN, D., H. YARNELL, and K. ALPER. "Physical, Psychiatric and Psychometric Studies of Post-Encephalitic Parkinsonism," *J. Nerv. Ment. Dis.*, 96 (1942), 652–662.

240. SHIPMAN, W. G., H. HEATH, and D. OKEN. "Response Specificity Among Muscular and Autonomic Variables," *Arch. Gen. Psychiatry*, 23 (1970), 369–377.

241. SHIPMAN, W. G., D. OKEN, I. BALSHAN GOLDSTEIN et al. "Study in Psychophysiology of Muscle Tension: II. Personality Factors," *Arch. Gen. Psychiatry*, 11 (1964), 330–345.

242. SHIPMAN, W. G., D. OKEN, and H. HEATH. "Muscle Tension and Effort at Self-Control during Anxiety," *Arch. Gen. Psychiatry*, 23 (1970), 359–368.

243. SHOCHET, B. R., E. T. LISANSKY, A. F. SCHUBERT et al. "A Medical-Psychiatric Study of Patients with Rheumatoid Arthritis," *Psychosomatics*, 10 (1969), 271–279.

244. SOLOMON, G. F. and R. MOOS. "Emotions, Immunity and Disease," *Arch. Gen. Psychiatry*, 11 (1964), 657–674.

245. ———. "The Relationship of Personality to the Presence of Rheumatoid Factor in Asymptomatic Relatives of Patients with Rheumatoid Arthritis," *Psychosom. Med.*, 27 (1965), 350–360.

246. SOUTHWORTH, J. A. "Muscular Tension as a Response to Psychological Stress in Rheumatoid Arthritis and Peptic Ulcer," *Genet. Psychol. Monogr.*, 57 (1958), 337–392.

247. SPIELBERGER, C. D. "Theory and Research on Anxiety," in C. D. Spielberger, ed., *Anxiety and Behavior*, pp. 3–20. New York: Academic, 1966.

248. STETTEN, D. and J. HEARON. "Intellectual Level Measured by Army Classification Battery and Serum Uric Acid Concentration," *Science*, 129 (1959), 1737.

249. STONEHILL, E. and A. H. CRISP. "Problems in the Measurement of Sleep with Particular Reference to the Development of a Motility Bed," *J. Psychosom. Res.*, 15 (1971), 495–499.

250. SWAIM, L. J. *Arthritis Medicine and the Spiritual Laws.* Philadelphia: Chilton, 1962.

251. TALBOTT, J. H. *Gout,* 2nd ed. New York: Grune & Stratton, 1964.

252. TALLAND, G. A. "Cognitive Function in Parkinson's Disease," *J. Nerv. Ment. Dis.,* 135 (1962), 196–205.

253. THOMAS, G. W. "Psychic Factors in Rheumatoid Arthritis," *Am. J. Psychiatry,* 93 (1936), 693–710.

254. TYNDEL, M. "The Other Side of A One-Sided Approach," *Am. J. Psychiatry,* 127 (1971), 1101.

255. VOAS, R. B. "Generalization and Consistency of Muscle Tension Levels." Ph.D. dissertation, University of California at Los Angeles, 1952. Unpublished.

256. WEISS, E. "Psychogenic Rheumatism," *Ann. Intern. Med.,* 26 (1947), 890–900.

257. WENGER, M. A. "Some Relationships between Muscular Processes and Personality and Their Factorial Analysis," *Child Dev.,* 9 (1938), 261–276.

258. ———. "An Attempt to Appraise Individual Differences in Level of Muscular Tension," *J. Exp. Psychol.,* 32 (1943), 213–225.

259. WHATMORE, G. B. and R. M. ELLIS, JR. "Some Motor Aspects of Schizophrenia: An EMG Study," *Am. J. Psychiatry,* 114 (1958), 882–889.

260. ———. "Some Neurophysiologic Aspects of Depressed States: An Electromyographic Study," *Arch. Gen. Psychiatry,* 1 (1959), 70–80.

261. ———. "Further Neurophysiologic Aspects of Depressed States," *Arch. Gen. Psychiatry,* 6 (1962), 243–253.

262. WIENER, D. N. "Personality Characteristics of Selected Disability Groups," *Genet. Psychol. Monogr.,* 45 (1952), 175–255.

263. WILLIAMS, J. G. L. "Use of a Resonance Technique to Measure Muscle Activity in Neurotic and Schizophrenic Patients," *Psychosom. Med.,* 26 (1964), 20–28.

264. WILLIAMS, R. and A. KRASNOFF. "Body Image and Physiological Patterns in Patients with Peptic Ulcer and Rheumatoid Arthritis," *Psychosom. Med.,* 26 (1964), 701–709.

265. WILLIAMS, T. A., J. SCHACHTER, and R. ROWE. "Spontaneous Autonomic Activity, Anxiety, and 'Hyperkinetic Impulsivity'," *Psychosom. Med.,* 27 (1965), 9–18.

266. WOLFF, B. B. "Experimental Pain Responses as Predictors of Outcome of Surgical Rehabilitation in Rheumatoid Arthritis," (Abstract), *Arthritis Rheum.,* 11 (1968), 519–520.

267. ———. "Current Psychosocial Concepts in Rheumatoid Arthritis," *Bull. Rheum. Dis.,* 22 (1972), 656–660.

268. WOLFF, B. B. and R. FARR. "Personality Characteristics in Rheumatoid Arthritis," (Abstract), *Arthritis Rheum.,* 7 (1964), 354.

269. WOLPE, J. *Psychotherapy by Reciprocal Inhibition.* Stanford: Stanford University Press, 1958.

CHAPTER 31

OBESITY

Albert J. Stunkard

Obesity is a condition characterized by excessive accumulations of fat in the body. By convention, obesity is said to be present when body weight exceeds by 20 percent the standard weight listed in the usual height-weight tables.[38] This index of obesity, however, is only an approximate one at lesser degrees of overweight, since bone and muscle can make a substantial contribution to overweight. In the future, diagnosis will probably be based upon newer and more accurate methods of estimating body fat.[6] Skin-fold calipers are already gaining acceptance because of their convenience and because much of the excess fat is localized in subcutaneous tissue.[48,49] But for most clinical purposes the eyeball test is still the most reasonable: "If a person looks fat he is fat."

(Epidemiology

Strikingly little information is available about the prevalence of obesity. Since most good diagnostic methods are too cumbersome for use in large-scale studies, much of our information is derived from height-and-weight data of poor quality, averaged over populations, and subjected to the criterion of 20 percent over standard weight. The data we have suggest that prevalence of obesity reaches a peak at age forty when 35 percent of men and 40 percent of women can be so designated. Prevalence has been increasing slightly for men, and decreasing slightly for women, during the past thirty years.[38,41]

There have been studies of more limited populations utilizing more reliable data and permitting more valid inferences. Unfortunately these studies have differed in their criteria of obesity, making their data difficult or impossible to use for comparisons among studies. These studies show a striking effect of age, with a monotonic increase in the prevalence of obesity between childhood and age fifty, and a twofold increase between ages twenty and fifty.[40] At age fifty, prevalence falls sharply, presumably because of the very high mortality of the obese from cardiovascular disease in the older age groups. Since these studies use the height-weight criterion, and since the fat content of the body increases per unit weight with age, these studies almost certainly underestimate the prevalence of obesity in older persons. The increasing use of skin-fold calipers should soon be providing far more satisfactory data.

All studies that have compared the sexes report a higher prevalence of obesity among women; this discrepancy is particularly pronounced after age fifty because of the higher mortality rate among obese men in that age group.

Social factors exert a powerful influence on the prevalence of obesity. In many countries undernutrition limits the development of obesity. Freed of this constraint in the affluence of American society, many ethnic groups show a marked increase in the prevalence of obesity during their first generation in this country. Thereafter, a variety of social influences combine to radically reduce the prevalence of obesity. One study reported a fall from 24 to 5 percent between the first and fourth generations in this country.[19]

The most striking antiobesity influence is that of socioeconomic status. Figure 31–1 shows that obesity is six times as common among women of low status as among those of high status in New York City.[19] A similar,

though weaker, relationship was found among men. Two findings suggest that a causal relationship underlies these correlations. First, as Figure 31–1 shows, social class of origin is almost as closely linked to obesity as is the subject's own social class. Although obesity could conceivably influence a person's own social class, his obesity can hardly have influenced the social class of his parents. Furthermore, obesity is far more prevalent among lower-class children than it is among upper-class children; highly significant differences are already apparent by age six.[58] Similar analyses have shown that social mobility, ethnic factors, and generational status in the United States also influence the prevalence of obesity.[19]

⟮ Genetics

The existence of numerous forms of inherited obesity in animals, and the ease with which adiposity can be produced by selective breeding, make it clear that genetic factors can play a determining role in obesity.[33,35] These fac-

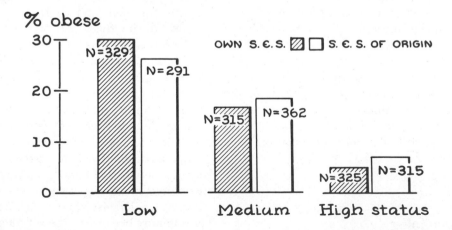

Figure 31–1. Decreasing prevalence of obesity with increasing socioeconomic status (S.E.S.) among women in New York City. Socioeconomic status of origin is almost as strongly linked to obesity as is the person's own socioeconomic status.[19] (Reprinted from P. B. Goldblatt, M. E. Moore, and A. J. Stunkard, "Social Factors in Obesity," *Journal of the American Medical Association*, 192 (1965), 1039–1044. Copyright © 1965 by the American Medical Association.)

tors must also be presumed to be important in human obesity, although clear-cut evidence of genetic transmission has been obtained only in such rare conditions as the Laurence-Moon-Biedl syndrome.

A number of studies have confirmed the layman's impression that obesity "runs in families." In one study obesity was reported in the offspring of approximately 80 percent of obese-x-obese matings, in 40 percent of obese-x-nonobese matings, and in no more than 10 percent of nonobese-x-nonobese matings.[33] In another series, Davenport reported that among fifty-one children of slender parents none was of more than average weight and most were slender; among thirty-seven children of obese parents, on the other hand, none was slender, all were of at least average weight, and a third were obese.[13] But such figures inevitably confuse genetic and environmental influences. Although there have been efforts to separate these influences—by studies of twins and of adopted children—none has elucidated the mechanism of transmission nor provided more than rough estimates of the relative contribution of inheritance.[63] Because so many nongenetic factors can influence body weight, it is generally agreed that overweight per se is an unsatisfactory phenotype for the study of the genetics of human obesity.

Interest is now shifting to the transmission of somatotypes. Their relevance is clear from Seltzer and Mayer's demonstration that obesity occurs with much greater frequency in some physical types than others.[48] Obese adolescent girls, for example, show extremely low ratings for ectomorphy; the presence of even a moderate degree of ectomorphy appeared to protect against obesity. It has been estimated that two-thirds of women in the general population may be sufficiently ectomorphic to receive significant protection against obesity. Preliminary studies by Withers suggest that somatotypes are heritable, particularly father–daughter transmission of mesomorphy and mother–son transmission of endomorphy.[64] Further investigations of the inheritance of body types, and of their relation to obesity are sorely needed.

❲ Obesity in Childhood

The obesity of persons who were obese in childhood—the so-called "juvenile-onset obese"—differs from that of persons who became obese as adults. Juvenile-onset obesity tends to be more severe, more resistant to treatment, and more likely to be associated with emotional disturbances.

Obesity that begins in childhood shows a very strong tendency to persist. Long-term prospective studies in Hagerstown, Maryland, have revealed the remarkable degree to which obese children become obese adults. In the first such study, 86 percent of a group of overweight boys became overweight men, as compared to only 42 percent of boys of average weight.[2] Even more striking differences in adult weight status were found among girls: 80 percent of overweight girls became overweight women, as compared to only 18 percent of average weight girls. A later study showed that the few overweight children who reduced successfully had done so by the end of adolescence. The odds against an overweight child becoming a normal weight adult, which were 4:1 at age twelve, rose to 28:1 for those who did not reduce during adolescence.[57] An even more recent study, which used a longer interval (thirty-five years) and, unfortunately, different (more rigid) criteria for obesity, found the difference in adult weight status continuing to grow: 63 percent of obese boys became obese men, as compared to only 10 percent of average weight boys.[1]

A brilliant series of studies of adipose tissue has recently helped to explain the remarkable persistence of juvenile-onset obesity. Many obese persons, particularly those with juvenile-onset obesity, show a marked increase in total number of adipocytes in subcutaneous tissue and in other depots.[20] Whereas the average nonobese person has a total of $25–30 \times 10^9$ adipocytes, obese persons may have five times this number. The average lipid content of the adipocytes of normal-weight and obese persons varies to a far smaller degree: 0.7 μg. for the nonobese and 1.0 μg for the obese.

With weight reduction, individual cells shrink greatly, but the total adipocyte number remains constant. A number of animal studies suggest that early in life adipose tissue grows both by increasing cell size and increasing cell number. If feeding patterns are changed during the first three weeks of a rat's life, there will be marked changes in cell number.[27] But when the animal is made obese in adult life, he grows no new adipocytes, the ones he has simply enlarge.

These studies of cellularity in obesity focus attention on the influence early feeding patterns have on the later development of obesity. Adipocyte size and number may be another factor that influences hypothalamic activity and feeding behavior. Obese persons who have lost weight but whose increased number of adipocytes persists tend to overeat and thus refill these extra cells. We have no biochemical data as yet to indicate the nature of the signal from adipose tissue to the hypothalamus.

⟮ Etiology

What causes obesity? In one sense the answer is quite simple—eating more calories than are expended as energy. In another sense, the answer still eludes us. For we do not know why some people eat more calories than they expend. But we are making progress. We no longer, for example, expect to find *the* cause of obesity, and we are far more aware than were our predecessors of the many factors involved in the regulation of body weight.

Our increased awareness of the problem's complexity has resulted in the development of an appealing framework for considering the etiology of obesity. Obesity may profitably be viewed as the end product of a disturbance in energy balance, or in the regulation of body weight. This view has helped us organize current information about obesity and has encouraged and informed the search for new information. I will consider at some length what is now known about the regulation of body weight, to understand better how six

disparate factors may influence this regulation. I have already discussed three of these, the genetic, social, and developmental. I will take up the other three later i.e., physical activity, brain damage, and emotional problems.

The Regulation of Body Weight

An average nonobese man stores fat to the extent of about 15 percent of his body weight, enough to provide for all of his caloric needs for nearly a month. This same man consumes approximately one million calories a year. His body fat stores remain unchanged during this time, because he expends an equal number of calories. An error of no more than 10 percent in either intake or output would lead to a thirty-pound change in body weight within this year.

Rats who are force-fed or deprived of food rapidly return to their normal body weights when permitted to return to ad libitum feeding.[12] Similar studies of man are extraordinarily difficult to carry out. Yet in the rare instances when the body weight of human volunteers has been experimentally altered, it, too, rapidly returned to normal values. Sims found that normal-weight volunteers who were fattened by overfeeding and underactivity returned to their normal body weight soon after returning to their usual patterns of eating and activity.[51] Keys' classic study of experimental semistarvation showed a similar rapid return to normal body weight when the subjects were permitted free access to food.[26] Clearly body weight is regulated with the greatest precision in all nonobese animals, including man. This regulation has been described in detail in two recent scholarly reviews,[21,28] as has the powerful glucostatic theory of the regulation of food intake.[34]

As befits such a vital function, the neural control of food intake is widely distributed throughout the brain. Within the limbic system alone six thousand different sites have been found to influence eating behavior.[43] Nevertheless, certain structures seem to play a more important part than others.

The discovery that two different hypothalamic areas control hunger and satiety—one in the lateral hypothalamus mediating the former, the other in the ventromedial nucleus mediating the latter—initiated our current understanding of these clearly separable functions. More recent anatomic studies have identified extrahypothalamic structures which play a part as important as that of the hypothalamus in the regulation of food intake. Feeding, for example, is controlled by a diffuse circuit that links the forebrain limbic system (and particularly areas in the amygdala) and the globus pallidus to the midbrain tegumentum via the lateral hypothalamus. The satiety area in the ventromedial hypothalamus similarly links forebrain limbic structures and the head of the caudate nucleus to the midbrain. There are also more direct connections between the feeding and satiety systems, for example, the inhibitory fibres that run from the ventromedial to the lateral hypothalamic areas.

Noradrenalin serves as a major neurotransmitter in both the feeding and satiety systems. Alpha- and beta-adrenergic subsystems have recently been identified, although their precise functions and locations are still unclear.[21]

Most of our information about the role of the central nervous system in food intake regulation has been obtained experimentally, by destroying or stimulating certain areas electrically or chemically. But what signals normally activate this complex neural apparatus?

A common-sense view holds that we stop eating at the end of a meal because we have replenished some nutrient that had been depleted. And we become hungry again when the nutrient, which had been restored by the meal, is once again depleted. Specifically it has been proposed that some metabolic signal, derived from food that has been absorbed, is carried by the blood to the brain. There this signal activates receptor cells, probably in the hypothalamus, to produce satiety. Hunger is the consequence of the decreasing strength of this same metabolic signal, secondary to the depletion of the critical nutrient.

Four classical theories of hunger and satiety have been based upon this argument, differing from each other only in the nature of the signal to which they ascribe primary significance.

The thermostatic theory, for example, proposes that postprandial increases in hypothalamic temperature mediate satiety; hunger results from a decrease in temperature at this site.[4] Lipostatic,[24] aminostatic,[37] and glucostatic[34] theories each assign the critical regulatory role to blood-borne metabolites of fat, protein, and carbohydrate.

Although each of these theories explains some of the many phenomena involved in the control of food intake, the glucostatic theory has had by far the greatest predictive power. It starts, as do the others, with the assumption that the signal to the central nervous system comes from one of the three major foodstuffs, i.e., fat, carbohydrate, or protein, or from a metabolic product of one of them. When we consider that the body stores of the key nutrient must be significantly depleted in the hours between meals, we must rule out the role of fat and protein. For such a tiny fraction of the total body stores of both these is used up in those few hours that it is very unlikely that any brain center could detect the change.

With carbohydrates the situation is quite different. The body as a whole can store only very small amounts and the liver, which is the principal storage site of readily available carbohydrate, can actually store no more than half the body's daily requirement of calories. In the few hours between meals, therefore, an enormous percentage of the body's carbohydrate stores is used up. Any center sensitive to the depletion of carbohydrate stores should have no trouble in detecting a depletion of this size, and in letting the brain know that more carbohydrate is needed.

According to the glucostatic theory, depletion of carbohydrate stores is signalled by the amount of "available glucose" in the circulating blood; a fall in the level of available glucose, signaled to hypothalamic glucoreceptors, becomes the signal for hunger. An increase in available glucose, with carbohydrate repletion, activates the hypothalamic satiety areas, and terminates eating. The heuristic value of this theory was demonstrated when hypothalamic "glucoreceptors" first postulated by Mayer[34] but unknown at the time that he proposed the theory, were discovered.

The vigor of the glucostatic theory, twenty years after it was first proposed, is manifested by the many studies it continues to stimulate. Direct measurements of the electrical activity of the hypothalamus have confirmed the findings of earlier, indirect studies of the influence of intravenous glucose. Glucose infusion increases electrical activity in the ventromedial area, and decreases such activity in the lateral area in accordance with the prediction that glucose should increase satiety and decrease hunger.[6] Another line of evidence in support of the glucostatic theory has been derived from studies using the nonmetabolizable glucose analogue 2-deoxy-D-glucose (2-DG). Administration of 2-DG to animals produces decreased intracellular utilization of glucose, particularly in the brain. Such a decrease in available glucose, a classic example of the signal postulated by the glucostatic theory, pro-duces a prompt and significant increase in food intake.[52] Recently Russek has proposed an imaginative variation of the glucostatic theory.[45] He has amassed considerable evidence in support of the idea that the primary site of glucoreception is not in the hypothalamus, but in the liver.

Despite the attractiveness of the glucostatic theory, it shares with all single-factor theories the difficulty of encompassing the many events involved in the regulation of food intake. Figure 31–2 shows, in schematic outline, the many variables that must be considered in this regulation.[53]

In addition to this general problem, single-factor theories of the control of food intake encounter also two specific problems. First, how can a mechanism of short-term, meal-to-meal, control of food intake account for the remarkable stability of body weight over long

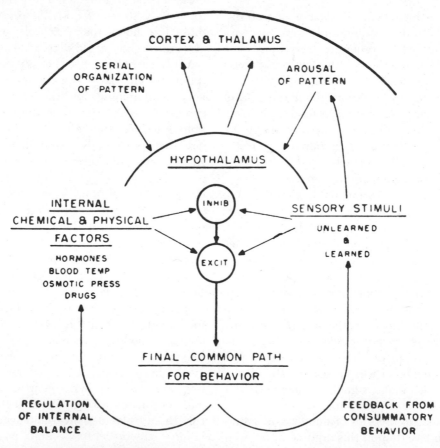

Figure 31–2. Scheme of the factors contributing to the regulation of body weight.[53] (Copyright 1954 by the Amer. Psychol. Assoc. Reprinted by permission.)

periods of time, and in the face of often marked short-term fluctuations? Second, how can a single-factor theory, or indeed any physiological theory, account for the function of satiety? For satiety occurs very soon after the beginning of a meal, when only a small proportion of the total caloric intake of the meal can have been absorbed. If satiety were based solely on the limited information about food intake available at that point, it could contribute little or nothing to the regulation of food intake.

Recent work by LeMagnen has further documented just how imprecise the mechanism of satiety really is.[28] He has shown that when animals feed ad libitum, meal size bears little relation to the length of the preceding period of food deprivation. But meal size does determine, quite precisely, the length of time until the next meal. The energy needs of the body determine when a meal is initiated, but not the size of the meal. In other words, what is regulated is meal-interval, not meal-size. Or, in the regulation of food intake, hunger is controlled precisely, satiety only approximately.

Man's ability to alter the interval between meals is sharply limited by the routines of daily life. As a consequence, he is forced to rely primarily on changes in meal size to regulate his food intake. Thus the imprecise mechanism of satiety is burdened even more heavily in man than in animals. If satiety depended solely on humoral factors such as ingested glucose or other nutrients, it would be hopelessly inadequate to the task of regulating food intake.

If humoral factors do not terminate eating, what does? "A full stomach" may be a better answer than we would have thought even a few years ago. Certainly common sense and personal experience suggest that the smell and taste of food, and the feeling of a full stomach, play a part in satiety. Recent systematic clinical investigations support this view. In man as in animals, gastric filling, quite irrespective of the nutritive value of the meal, is the major determinant of satiety in single-meal experiments.[22] The neural mechanism that mediates this response has also recently been demonstrated: gastric distention and direct stimula-

tion of the mechanoreceptors of the stomach wall increase the firing rate of single units within the ventromedial nucleus.[3]

Although the nutritional value of the meal, as we have noted, plays little or no part in satiety in single-meal experiments, man seems to learn (as do other animals) to change his food intake and even his meal size, in response to changes in energy expenditure and in the character of his food. Is this learning? If so, how does he learn?

Alimentary Learning

An understanding of the mechanism for adjusting food intake, and particularly changes in meal size and frequency, has long eluded us. Our areas of ignorance are still vast. But some recent discoveries have made it possible to entertain a theory which would have been untenable until now. I propose that the adjustment of meal size and meal frequency is a learned process involving Pavlovian, or respondent, conditioning. In this theory oral and gastric factors serve as conditioned stimuli, while humoral factors absorbed from the gastrointestinal tract serve later as the unconditioned stimuli. This sequence can account both for the termination of eating early in the process of food absorption from the intestine and for the long-term adjustment of meal size to changing caloric needs.

Until recently this theory had an apparently fatal flaw. The interval between presentation of the postulated conditioned stimuli and presentation of the unconditioned stimuli may well be an hour long. Pavlov showed early in this century that classical conditioning cannot occur if the interval exceeds a few seconds.

The idea that the interval between conditioned and unconditioned stimuli (the CS-US interval) could not exceed a few seconds went unchallenged through fifty years of research on conditioning. Then two lines of investigation produced evidence demolishing this constraint. In a little-noticed paper in *Science*, Garcia reported a striking exception to the belief that the CS-US interval cannot exceed a few seconds in duration.[15] Using saccharine as the conditioned stimulus, and x-radiation (and the consequent radiation sickness) as the unconditioned stimulus, he was able to produce in rats a conditioned aversion to saccharine with CS-US intervals of *hours* in length. Further studies showed that, in contrast to the frequent CS-US pairings necessary to produce most conditioned responses, such aversion can occur with only one pairing of CS and US. Finally, and again in contrast to the usual conditioned response, the aversion is remarkably resistant to extinction.[16]

More recently, Rozin has shown that positive reinforcers can produce food *preferences*, "specific hungers," under conditions similar to those in which aversive reinforcement produces aversions.[44] It has been known for years that animals deficient in thiamine select diets that contain thiamine (even if only a trace) out of a wide variety of possible foods. Rozin showed that this preference results from two factors: (1) a learned aversion, of the type demonstrated by Garcia, to diets that do not contain thiamine, and (2) the positively reinforcing effect of the vitamin on the vitamin-deficient animal. Learning about beneficial consequences over long CS-US intervals is clearly weaker than learning about the aversive consequences. We do not know the upper limit of the interval between the conditioned stimulus of thiamine ingestion and the unconditioned stimulus of well-being, but it can hardly be shorter than many minutes, and it may be as long as hours.

The food preferences and aversions demonstrated by Rozin and Garcia seem to represent a special form of Pavlovian conditioning which, for convenience, we may call "alimentary learning." The distinctive features of "alimentary learning" are: (1) the conditioned stimulus must be either taste or smell; (2) the unconditioned stimulus must be a general body state, either a dysphoric one such as radiation sickness, fever, nausea or, on the other hand, a euphoric one such as is presumably produced by thiamine repletion; (3) the learning can occur with unusual rapidity, after as few as one CS-US pairing, (4) the CS-US intervals can be as long as ten hours; and (5) these conditioned responses are unusually resistant to extinction.

The food preferences and aversions which have taught us about "alimentary learning" are of great importance in their own right. Furthermore, they have freed us from those constraints of Pavlovian conditioning which have limited our understanding of control of food intake. But I believe that they are best understood as special cases of a more general phenomenon. The primary purpose of "alimentary learning" may be the mediation of satiety. I see "alimentary learning" as a bridge between the long-term, physiological regulation of food intake based upon humoral factors, and the short-term cessation of eating based on gastric filling. If this view is even approximately correct, then impaired "alimentary learning" may underlie the eating disorders found in obesity. An impairment of satiety surely plays a major role in these disorders.

Physical Activity

The only component on the energy-expenditure side of the caloric ledger that both fluctuates and is under voluntary control is physical activity. As such, it is a vital factor in the regulation of body weight. Indeed, the marked decrease in physical activity in affluent societies seems to be the major factor in the recent rise of obesity as a public health problem. Obesity is a rarity in most underdeveloped nations, and not solely because of malnutrition. In some rural areas, a high level of physical activity is at least as important in preventing obesity. Such levels of physical activity are the exception in this country. If the trend exemplified by automatic can openers and mechanized swizzle sticks continues, we may succeed in reducing our energy expenditure to near basal levels. Among many obese women, the trend is already far advanced.

Figure 31–3 shows marked reduction of physical activity of a group of Philadelphia housewives; this reduction is so great as to account almost entirely for their excess weight.[11] But such low levels of physical activity are not present among all obese persons. Figure 31–3 shows that the differences in physical activity among the men were so small

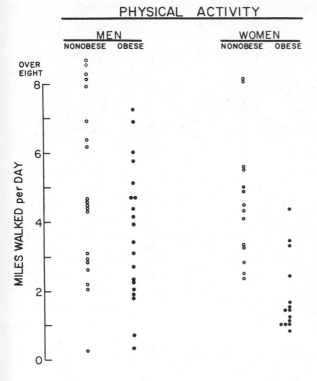

PHYSICAL ACTIVITY

MEN
NONOBESE · OBESE

WOMEN
NONOBESE · OBESE

MILES WALKED per DAY

Figure 31–3. Comparison of the physical activity of obese and nonobese men and women. Each point represents the average distance walked each day by each subject, as measured by a mechanical pedometer. Most obese women walked shorter distances than nonobese women. Among men, there is less difference in the distances walked.[11] (Reprinted by permission from *N. Engl. J. Med.*, 263 (1960), 935–946.)

that the additional energy expended by obese subjects in moving their heavier bodies produced a caloric expenditure equal to that of nonobese men.

Until quite recently, physical inactivity was considered to cause obesity primarily via its restriction of energy expenditure. There is now good evidence that inactivity may contribute also to an increased food intake. Although food intake increases with increasing energy expenditure over a wide range of energy demands, intake does not decrease proportionately when physical activity falls below a certain minimum level,[36] as shown in Figure 31–4. In fact, restricting physical activity may actually *increase* food intake! Conversely,

when sedentary persons increase physical activity, their food intake may decrease. The mechanism involved in this intriguing control are still unclear, but its great therapeutic potential makes it worthy of careful study.

Disorders in the Regulation of Body Weight

Our general understanding of the regulation of body weight was greatly advanced during the late 1940s when it was discovered that destruction of the satiety areas of the hypothalamus could produce obesity. Many of the features of the disordered food intake produced by these lesions were described by Neal Miller in 1950 in a paper with the trenchant title, "Decreased Hunger and Increased Food Intake in Hypothalamic Obese Rats."[39] This remarkably prescient report described for the first time the peculiar feeding behavior of rats made obese by hypothalamic lesions.

The cardinal feature of the rats' behavior was that they overate when food was freely available, but when an impediment was placed in the way of their eating, they not only decreased their food intake, but actually decreased it to a far lower level than that of control rats without hypothalamic lesions. Furthermore, it seemed to make little difference what kind of impediment was used; motivation to work for food was impaired in every manner of task that could be devised. These rats seemed to be relatively unresponsive to all physiological cues about their nutritional state, and they responded imperfectly to signals both of satiety and of deprivation.

On the other hand, the obese rats seemed hyperresponsive to the taste of food and to its availability. They increased their overeating when fat and sweet substances were added to their diet, and radically restricted intake when the palatability of their food was decreased by the addition of quinine. Similar eating patterns have been reported in a wide variety of animals when they became obese for natural reasons, such as in the genetically determined yellow obese mouse, in the rat when it becomes obese with aging, and even in the dor-

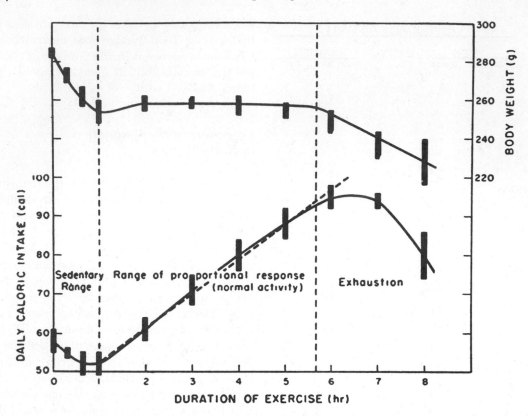

Figure 31–4. Caloric intake and body weight as functions of duration of exercise in adult rats. Within the range of normal physical activity, food intake increases with increasing physical activity and body weight remains stable. In the sedentary range of activity, however, decreasing physical activity is associated with *increased* food intake and an increase in body weight.[36] (Copyright © 1967 by the Amer. Assoc. Advance. Science. Reprinted by permission.)

mouse during the hyperphagia which precedes its hibernation.

The impaired satiety found in different forms of experimental obesity also characterizes the eating patterns of many obese persons. In the exceptional instance this disorder results from unequivocal hypothalamic damage as a result of a strategically placed tumor or vascular lesion;[55] usually we do not know the cause of this impaired satiety. Such persons characteristically complain of being unable to stop eating; it is the unusual obese person who reports being driven by hunger or who eats in ravenous manner. Instead, obese persons seem inordinately susceptible to food cues in their environment, to the palatability of foods, and to the inability to stop eating if food is available.

Bruch has documented these problems of the obese without brain damage in her vivid descriptions of their misperception of important visceral events.[7] Some obese persons, who are also neurotic, have difficulty in identifying hunger and satiety. They frequently seem unable to distinguish between hunger and other kinds of dysphoria. Bruch has linked this "conceptual confusion" to severe deficits in identity and to feelings of personal ineffectiveness.[7] She has convincingly described the need on the part of these patients for external signals to tell them when to eat and when to stop eating. Strong support for Bruch's position has come from a recent study which shows that neurotic obese persons have a strong response bias that impairs their perception of gastric motility.[59] Unfortunately, correction of the bias did not result in weight loss.

Schachter has reported a long series of experiments documenting that obese persons are unusually susceptible to all kinds of "external" stimuli to eating, while they remain relatively unresponsive to the usual "internal," i.e., physiological, signals of hunger.[47] In one comparison with normal-weight controls, obese subjects overate a palatable ice cream and underate an unpalatable one. Similarly, they overate in an experimental setting when food was in front of them, while they underate when getting additional food required no more than opening a refrigerator door. Their eating was even influenced inordinately by what time of day they thought it was.

These findings suggest the ways in which social factors may influence the prevalence of obesity. For the ways in which a culture makes food available (and relatively less available) to its obesity-prone, "externally controlled" members may well determine the degree to which such individuals overeat.

Disorders in the Regulation of Body Weight, Emotional Determinants

Many obese persons report that they often overeat and gain weight when they are emotionally upset. But it has proved singularly difficult to proceed from this provocative observation to an understanding of the precise relationship between emotional factors and obesity.

The most clear-cut evidence of how emotional factors influence obesity has come from two small subgroups of obese persons, each characterized by an abnormal and stereotyped pattern of food intake.[55] About 10 percent of obese persons, most commonly women, manifest a "night-eating syndrome" characterized by morning anorexia, and evening hyperphagia with insomnia. This syndrome seems to be precipitated by stressful life circumstances and, once present, tends to recur daily until the stress is alleviated. Attempts at weight reduction when the syndrome is present have an unusually poor outcome and may even precipitate a more severe psychological disturbance.

The "binge-eating syndrome," found in fewer than 5 percent of obese persons, is one of the rare exceptions to the pattern of impaired satiety.[55] It is characterized by the sudden, compulsive ingestion of very large amounts of food in a very short time, usually with great subsequent agitation and self-condemnation. It too appears to represent a reaction to stress. But in contrast to the night-eating syndrome, these bouts of overeating are not periodic and they are far more often linked to specific precipitating circumstances. Binge eaters can sometimes lose large amounts of weight by adhering to rigid and unrealistic diets, but such efforts are almost always interrupted by a resumption of eating binges.

(Complications

Troublesome as obesity may be from a cosmetic standpoint, it is the serious health hazards associated with it that have warranted its description as the nation's greatest preventable cause of death. This effect is largely the result of obesity's impact on the cardiovascular diseases which now cause half the deaths in this country.

Effects on Mortality

The evidence is strong that obesity adversely affects morbidity and mortality rates. The death rate from a variety of diseases is significantly higher among obese persons, and the rate increases in proportion to the severity of the obesity and to its duration during adult life.[23,31] Sudden death is particularly closely linked to obesity.[10] Furthermore, obese persons who lose weight and maintain the loss show radically reduced mortality rates. For women, the rate after weight reduction was as low as if they had never been obese.[31]

This evidence of the direct effect of obesity on mortality is matched by evidence of its indirect effect. Two of the most potent risk factors for coronary artery disease, i.e., adult-onset diabetes and hypertension, are also highly correlated with obesity. Here again, weight reduction has a powerful effect: 75 percent of adult-onset diabetics may discontinue medication, and the blood pressure of 60 percent of hypertensives returns to normal levels after significant weight loss.[23]

In recent years, arguments against the importance of obesity in coronary disease have been raised on the basis of data from prospective population studies. These studies report that, if such associated conditions as hypertension and elevated cholesterol and triglyceride levels are factored out, obesity is a poor, and often a very poor, predictor of coronary disease.[10,50] But since obesity contributes to both hypertension and to disorders of lipid metabolism, such an analysis may not be justified. Furthermore, many laboratory studies have demonstrated how obesity may contribute to coronary disease. Adult-onset obesity predisposes to a response to a carbohydrate load characterized by hyperglycemia, hyperinsulinism, and hypertriglyceridemia, all implicated in the pathogenesis of atherosclerosis.

Keys' seven-country study is worthy of note.[25] Although coronary heart disease was only weakly correlated with obesity, it was closely correlated with the saturated fatty acid content of the diet. The very high percentage of calories from this source in the American diet suggests that treatment of obesity should include restriction of saturated fatty acids as well as of calories.

Physical and Laboratory Abnormalities

The most serious physical manifestation of obesity, and the only one which is (very rarely) life-threatening, is the encircling of the thorax with fatty tissue together with pressure on the diaphragm from below due to intraabdominal accumulations of fat. The result is reduced respiratory excursion, with dyspnea on even minimal exertion. In very obese persons, this condition may progress to the so-called "Pickwickian syndrome," characterized by hypoventilation with consequent hypercapnia, hypoxia, and, finally, somnolence.[9]

Severe obesity leads to a variety of orthopedic disturbances, including low-back pain, aggravation of osteoarthritis, particularly of the knees and ankles, and often enormous calluses over the feet and heels. Even mild degrees of obesity are associated with amenorrhoea and other menstrual disturbances. Subcutaneous fat is an excellent heat insulator, and the skin of obese persons is often warm and sweaty, particularly after meals. Hyperhidrosis leads to intertrigo in the pendulous folds of tissue, making itching and skin disorders common. Mild to moderate edema of the feet and ankles often occurs, probably due to venous obstruction; diuretics are not indicated. What is most notable about all of these complications is the ease with which they can be controlled and eliminated by weight reduction, often of only a moderate degree.

Blood pressure elevations are frequently found in obese persons, often due to an artifact, i.e., the presence of masses of subcutaneous tissue between the blood pressure cuff and the brachial artery. This problem can sometimes be overcome by using a wider blood-pressure cuff. But any serious doubt as to the existence of hypertension should be resolved by direct intraarterial measurement, particularly before starting specific antihypertensive therapy.

Hyperuricemia is sometimes found in obesity, and it may reach a significant degree in persons who fast intermittently. When obesity has produced respiratory distress, hypercapnia may develop along with a respiratory acidosis.

A particular problem in the laboratory evaluation of obesity is the impaired glucose tolerance, and even fasting hyperglycemia, that occurs in many obese persons without a family history of diabetes. The high insulin levels in the fasting state and after a glucose load, usually associated with obesity,[46] are related to the presence of muscle and adipose tissue resistance to carbohydrate metabolism. The precise relationship between tissue resistance and insulin levels is not clear. It may be that tissue resistance signals the pancreas to produce more insulin, or that a high-calorie diet may increase insulin production, with tissue resistance a secondary phenomenon. However these questions are finally resolved, the response to weight reduction is highly gratifying. Most such abnormalities disappear completely unless the patient is truly diabetic.

Plasma-lipid levels are often moderately

elevated in the obese; again both cholesterol and triglyceride levels decline with weight reduction.

Emotional Disturbances

Numerous reports on psychological disturbances among the obese have flooded the literature, making it difficult even for the expert to reconcile the varied and conflicting observations. Many of the problems are the result of difficulties in establishing suitable control groups. It has generally turned out that the better the control group the less the evidence for distinctive psychological features and disabilities. The view that obese persons have a specific personality pattern is no longer held.

Carefully controlled studies do show that the obese have a higher degree of psychopathology than do the nonobese. The differences, however, are relatively small for the obese population as a whole.[40] For certain subgroups, on the other hand, the differences may be quite significant. Prominent among these are young women of upper- and middle-socioeconomic status. The reasons for the special vulnerability of these groups are of interest.

Since both obesity and emotional disturbance are common among persons of lower socioeconomic status, any association between the two in this stratum is quite likely to be coincidental. Higher up on the socioeconomic ladder, however, obesity is far less prevalent and the sanctions against it far stronger. There is also far less emotional disturbance at this level. As a result, when obesity and emotional disturbance coexist in this group, the likelihood that they are associated is far higher. Among young, upper-class women any obesity is very often closely linked to neurosis. What is the nature of this linkage?

Of the various emotional disturbances to which obese persons are subject, only two are specifically related to their obesity. The first is overeating, the second, disturbance in body image.[57,62]

The obese person whose body image is disturbed characteristically feels that his body is grotesque and loathesome, and that others view it with hostility and contempt. This feeling is closely associated with self-consciousness and impaired social functioning. It would seem reasonable to suppose that all obese persons have derogatory feelings about their bodies. Such is not the case. Emotionally healthy obese persons have no body-image disturbances, and, in fact, only a minority of neurotic obese persons have such disturbances. The disorder is confined to those who have been obese since childhood; less than half, even among these juvenile-onset obese, suffer from it. But it is in the group with body image disturbances that neurosis is closely related to obesity and this group contains a majority of obese persons with specific eating disorders.

The extent and severity of complications following weight reduction programs have been the subject of controversy in recent years. It now appears that as many as half of patients routinely treated for obesity by family physicians may develop mild anxiety and depression.[63] In addition, a high incidence of emotional disturbance has been reported among obese persons undergoing long-term, in-hospital treatment by fasting or severe caloric restriction.[17,18] These complications should be balanced against the likelihood of a decrease in anxiety and depression among those who diet successfully. Such newer treatments as behavior modification and intestinal by-pass surgery appear to carry less risk of emotional disturbance.

Obese persons with extensive psychopathology, those with a history of emotional disturbance during dieting, or those in the midst of a life crisis should attempt weight reduction, if at all, cautiously and under careful supervision. For others, the possibility of complications need not preclude treatment when it is indicated.

❰ Treatment

General Considerations

Weight reduction confers such great benefits upon obese persons, and it is apparently so simple, that we might expect to find large numbers of formerly fat people. How can obese people fail to reduce?

The best evidence is that they not only can, but do, fail. Perhaps the large number of women who try to reduce without medical assistance, on diets and advice from the women's magazines, have success. But most obese persons will not enter outpatient treatment for obesity; of those who do, most will not lose a significant amount of weight; and of those who do lose weight, most will regain it.[56] Furthermore, these poor results are due not to failure to implement any simple therapy of known effectiveness but to the fact that no simple or generally effective treatment exists. Obesity is a chronic condition, resistant to treatment, and prone to relapse.

The basis of weight reduction is utterly simple, i.e., establish a caloric deficit by bringing intake below output. All of the many treatment regimens have as their goal this simple task. Perhaps its very simplicity helps to account for an unfortunate aspect of treatment. Unable to understand why his patients cannot carry out this task, the physician often reacts punitively towards them. We have recently become aware that intense discrimination is practiced against obese persons, that it begins in childhood, and that it is continued throughout life to a degree that approaches that practiced against other minority groups.[14] Before undertaking treatment of an obese person, the physician should assure himself that he will not add to this burden. For given the low probability that sustained weight reduction can be achieved, it may be wisest to try to dissuade the patient from a treatment that may come to nothing more than still another experience of failure for him and a source of frustration for his physician.

The simplest way to reduce caloric intake is by means of a low-calorie diet. The best long-term effects are achieved with a balanced diet that contains readily available foods. For most people, the most satisfactory reducing diet consists of their usual foods, in amounts determined with the aid of tables of food values available in standard works.[35,54] Such a diet gives the best chance of long-term mainte-

nance of the weight lost during dieting. But it is precisely the most difficult kind of diet to follow during the period of weight reduction.

Many obese persons find it easier to use a novel or even bizarre diet of which there have been a profusion in recent years. Whatever effectiveness these diets may have is due in large part to their monotony—almost anyone will get tired of almost any food if that is all that he gets to eat. As a consequence, when he stops the diet and returns to his usual fare, the incentives to overeat are multiplied.

Fasting, which results in rapid weight loss, has had a considerable vogue as a treatment for obesity in recent years. Many obese persons find it relatively easy to tolerate. After two or three days without food, hunger decreases radically and the patient is able to get along well, as long as he remains in an undemanding environment. For some massively obese persons, or for the occasional patient in whom rapid weight loss is indicated, it has some small rationale. However follow-up studies of persons who have undergone long-term fasts, show that almost all regain at least all of the weight they lost.[30] Short-term (ten-day) intermittent fasts, by moderately obese persons, appear to have had somewhat better results, but adequate follow-up studies are not available. Because of the occasionally serious complications of fasting, this treatment should be carried out in a hospital.

Effective pharmacological treatment of obesity is largely confined to the amphetamines. These agents suppress appetite and, when used in conjunction with diet in a carefully planned treatment program, they may have limited usefulness. This usefulness is seriously limited, however, by the fact that the initial dose loses its effectiveness within a few weeks. Effectiveness can be restored by an increase in dose—a course that has been so frequently pursued by unscrupulous "diet doctors" and unsupervised dieters as to cast serious doubt on whether these drugs have any place in the treatment of obesity. In the face of today's widespread drug abuse, the mild and transient value of amphetamines in the treatment of obesity is probably outweighed by the danger posed by their abuse. This seems to be the view of the Bureau of Narcotics and Dangerous Drugs which is now taking away from physicians the option of prescribing amphetamines for obesity.

Thyroid or thyroid analogues are indicated for the occasional obese person with hypothyroidism, and probably not otherwise. Bulk producers may have limited value in eliminating the constipation that follows a marked decrease in food intake, but their effectiveness in weight reduction is doubtful. Four controlled studies of chorionic gonadotropin have found it to be ineffective in the recommended dosage.

Increased physical activity is frequently recommended as a part of weight-reduction regimens, but its usefulness has probably been underestimated even by many of its proponents. Since caloric expenditure in most forms of physical activity is directly proportional to body weight, obese persons expend more calories with the same amount of activity than do those of normal weight. Furthermore, as mentioned earlier, increased physical activity may actually cause a *decrease* in the food intake of sedentary persons.[35,36] This combination of increased caloric expenditure and (probably) decreased food intake makes an increase in physical activity a highly desirable feature of any weight-reduction program.

Treatment of obesity has generally followed a traditional medical model in which an authoritarian physician prescribes a diet and appetite-suppressing medication. The patient loses weight, if at all, largely to please the doctor and to meet his expectations. When the relationship is terminated or attenuated, the patient discontinues the diet and regains weight.

Until recently a surgical treatment for obesity would have seemed highly improbable. Within the past decade, however, a number of surgeons have attempted to treat obesity by decreasing food absorption via an intestinal bypass that short-circuits most of the absorptive surface of the intestine. Early results were discouraging. Although the first jejunocolic shunts produced large amounts of weight loss, there was a high incidence of sometimes lethal complications; the reestablishment of intestinal continuity was followed by rapid weight gain. More recently, experience with a jejunoileal shunt has been more promising.[42] Complications have been fewer and less severe. Furthermore, the discovery of a critical length of absorptive surface that will maintain body weight at approximately normal levels has made a second operation, to restore intestinal continuity, unnecessary. Despite these advances, a jejunoileal shunt is fraught with many dangers and should still be considered an investigative procedure. Until further information is available, it seems wisest to limit it to carefully selected patients with massive obesity that has proved uncontrollable by other methods.

Group therapy extends the number of obese patients the physician can treat and probably also increases the effectiveness of treatment. One convincing study showed that patients treated in groups lost more weight than those treated individually on each of three regimens: anorexigenic agents, placebo capsules, and no medication.[29] Evidence for the greater effectiveness of group over individual therapy for obesity is sufficient to encourage the family physician to attempt this modality, and the psychiatrist can provide valuable consultative help in encouraging such an undertaking.

Group methods are being applied by two different kinds of nonmedical groups with promising results. Each may provide useful adjuncts to medical treatment. TOPS (Take Off Pounds Sensibly), a self-help group with a membership of over 350,000, has over 15,000 chapters in all parts of the country and welcomes collaboration with physicians.[60] The TOPS program suffers from a high rate of drop-outs but those who remain may lose encouraging amounts of weight. Membership is almost exclusively female, and predominantly middle-aged and middle-class; such persons would seem to be good candidates for the program. Weight Watchers, a commercial organization, has been less carefully studied than TOPS. But the size of its membership—over two million—must provide a measure of satisfaction with its results. Both organizations provide powerful vehicles for introducing safe new measures for the control of obesity.

Specialized Psychotherapeutic Techniques

Information about reducing diets is so widely available that only those who have already failed to lose weight on their own come to the doctor's office. And only the medical-treatment failures reach the psychiatrist. This process of selection makes it easy to understand why there is no evidence that psychodynamic psychotherapy is any more effective than other, less expensive, aids to weight reduction. Less understandable is the widespread belief in the efficacy of such psychotherapy.

Another unsupported belief is that there is value in uncovering the unconscious causes of overeating so that the patient no longer resorts to this form of response to conflict (according to the psychodynamic model proposed for the resolution of neurotic symptoms). Obese patients may produce interesting fantasies and memories in response to the therapist's interests, but, with one exception discussed below, such production is rarely useful in producing favorable changes in behavior. Many obese persons seem particularly vulnerable to the overdependency upon the therapist and inordinate regression which can occur during the uncovering psychotherapies. Psychodynamic psychotherapy probably cannot modify the symptom choice of persons who overeat in response to stress. Years after successful psychotherapy *and* successful weight reduction, persons who overeat under stress continue to do so.

Despite these limitations, psychodynamic psychotherapy has a place in the management of obesity, and an important place in the treatment of some carefully selected obese persons. Furthermore, obese persons may seek psychotherapy for other reasons than their obesity; helping them to cope with their obesity may help them resolve their other problems. We have noted that many obese persons overeat under stress. When psychotherapy can help them to live less stressful and more gratifying lives, they are less apt to overeat. They may reduce and sometimes stay reduced.

These benefits are not less significant for being nonspecific results of treatment.

Two conditions may constitute specific indications for psychodynamic psychotherapy: disturbances in body image and the binge-eating syndrome. Both have been successfully treated, with enduring weight losses. Neither condition has been influenced by other forms of treatment including, significantly, weight reduction. Psychotherapy of patients with these conditions frequently requires years to ensure lasting results. The process may be facilitated by modifications in traditional technique designed to minimize intellectualization and regression, to cope with the "conceptual confusion" described earlier, and to increase the patient's often seriously inadequate sense of personal effectiveness. Bruch has provided excellent descriptions of such measures in her extensive writings.[8]

Behavior modification has recently been applied to the control of obesity, and it has already proven a major advance in treatment. Within four years of its introduction in 1967, every one of seven controlled studies demonstrated that behavior modification was more effective than a wide variety of alternative treatments.[56] It is particularly important for psychiatrists to know of these developments, for they have lagged in their appreciation of the potential of behavior modification. The discipline has been developed largely by psychologists, educators, and social workers. The extent to which the medical profession has defaulted is nowhere better illustrated than in behavioral therapy of the "medical" problem of obesity. Physicians participated in only one of the first nine applications of behavior modification to obesity.[56]

Stuart has recently published an extensive description of the application of behavior modification to the control of obesity.[54] A brief outline of a typical program[56] consists of the following four elements:

1. Description of the behavior to be controlled. Patients are asked to keep daily records of the amount, time, and circumstances of their eating. The immediate results of this time-consuming and inconvenient procedure

frequently are grumbling and complaints. But most patients acknowledge, often reluctantly, that keeping these records proves very helpful, particularly in increasing their awareness of how much they eat, the speed with which they eat, and the large variety of environmental and psychological situations associated with eating.

2. Modification and control of the discriminative stimuli governing eating. Most patients report that their eating takes place in a wide variety of places and at many different times during the day. It has been postulated that these times and places become so-called discriminative stimuli for eating. In an effort to decrease the potency of the discriminative stimuli, patients are encouraged to confine eating, including snacking, to one place. In order not to disrupt domestic routines of the housewives, who form such a large part of the patients so far treated in these programs, the kitchen is usually selected as the site for eating. Further efforts to control discriminative stimuli include using distinctive table settings, perhaps an unusually colored place mat and napkin. In addition, patients are encouraged to make eating a pure experience, unaccompanied by other activities such as reading, watching television, or arguing with their families.

3. Development of techniques to control the act of eating. Specific techniques are utilized to help patients decrease the speed of their eating, to become aware of all the components of the eating process, and to gain control over these components. Exercises include counting each mouthful of food eaten during a meal, placing utensils on the plate after every third mouthful until that mouthful is chewed and swallowed, and introducing a two-minute interruption of the meal.

4. Prompt reinforcement of behaviors that delay or control eating. A reinforcement schedule, using a point system, is particularly helpful in the control of eating behavior. Exercise of the suggested control procedures during a meal earns the patient a certain number of points. By this means, rapid reinforcement of the behavior is achieved. The points can then be converted into various other reinforcers, such as money or gifts from the spouse.

ℂ Conclusion

Obesity, a condition characterized by excessive accumulations of fat, is profitably viewed as a result of a disturbance in the regulation of body weight. This disturbed regulation can result from several different kinds of causes: genetic and developmental, social and emotional, physical (inactivity) and neural (impaired brain function). The relative contributions of these different influences probably varies among different obese persons.

We have strong evidence that obesity adversely affects morbidity and mortality, particularly in this country and probably because of the high saturated fatty acid content of the diet by means of which most Americans become obese. Obesity is also closely associated with many physical disabilities. The increased morbidity, mortality, and physical disability are all reversed by successful weight reduction. Because of these evident health benefits, and for cosmetic reasons, and because weight reduction should be easy, large numbers of obese persons are always trying to diet. For the most part they are unsuccessful. The poor results of weight-reduction efforts are due not to failure to implement any therapy of known effectiveness but to the fact that no simple or generally effective treatment exists. Obesity is a chronic condition, resistant to treatment, and prone to relapse.

New therapies, developed within the past decade, have achieved somewhat better results than the older ones. Most promising among these is behavior modification, which has proved more effective than a number of alternative measures. Intestinal by-pass surgery may, for the first time, offer some hope to massively obese persons who are willing to accept its risks. Lay groups may provide a useful vehicle for the introduction of new treatments as they are developed. But the main hope for control of obesity lies in a better understanding of the factors that regulate body weight. Fortunately research into this problem is proving increasingly fruitful.

❰ Bibliography

1. ABRAHAM, S., G. COLLINS, and M. NORD-SIECK. "Relationship of Childhood Weight Status to Morbidity in Adults," *HSMA Health Reports*, 86 (1971), 273–284.

2. ABRAHAM, S. and M. NORDSIECK. "Relationship of Excess Weight in Children and Adults," *Publ. Health Rep.*, 75 (1960), 263–273.

3. ANAND, B. K. and R. V. PILLAI. "Activity of Single Neurons in the Hypothalamic Feeding Centers: Effect of Gastric Distention," *J. Physiol. (Lond.)* 192 (1967), 63–77.

4. BROBECK, J. "Neural Control of Hunger, Appetite and Satiety," *Yale J. Biol. Med.*, 29 (1957), 565–574.

5. BROWN, K. A. and R. MELZACK. "Effects of Glucose on Multiunit Activity in the Hypothalamus," *Exp. Neurol.*, 24 (1969), 363–373.

6. BROZEK, J., ed. "Body Composition" in *Annals of the New York Academy of Sciences*, Vol. 110, entire issue. New York: The Academy, 1963.

7. BRUCH, H. "Conceptual Confusion in Eating Disorders," *J. Nerv. Ment. Dis.*, 133 (1961), 46–54.

8. ———. "The Practical and Psychological Aspects of Weight Change" and "Evaluation of a Psychotherapeutic Concept," in H. Bruch, *Eating Disorders: Obesity and Anorexia Nervosa, and the Person Within*, pp. 309–333 and 334–376. New York: Basic Books, 1973.

9. BURWELL, S. "Extreme Obesity Associated with Alveolar Hypoventilation—a Pickwickian Syndrome," *Am. J. Med.*, 21 (1956), 811–818.

10. CHIANG, B. N., L. V. PERLMAN, M. FULTON et al. "Predisposing Factors in Sudden Cardiac Death in Tecumseh, Michigan: A Prospective Study," *Circulation*, 41 (1970), 31–37.

11. CHIRICO, A. M. and A. J. STUNKARD. "Physical Activity and Human Obesity," *N. Engl. J. Med.*, 263 (1960), 935–946.

12. COHN, C. and D. JOSEPH. "Influence of Body Weight and Body Fat on Appetite of 'Normal' Lean and Obese Rats," *Yale J. Biol. Med.*, 34 (1962), 598–607.

13. DAVENPORT, C. B. *Body Build and Its Inheritance*, Publication no. 329. Washington, D.C.: Carnegie Institute, 1923.

14. DWYER, J. T., J. J. FELDMAN, and J. MAYER. "The Social Psychology of Dieting," *J. Health Soc. Behav.*, 11 (1970), 269–287.

15. GARCIA, J., D. J. KIMELDORF, and E. L. HUNT. "Conditioned Aversion to Saccharine Resulting from Exposure to Gamma Radiation," *Science*, 122 (1955), 157–158.

16. ———. "The Use of Ionizing Radiation as a Motivating Stimulus," *Psychol. Rev.*, 68 (1961), 383–395.

17. GLUCKSMAN, M. L. and J. HIRSCH. "The Response of Obese Patients to Weight Reduction: I. A Clinical Evaluation of Behavior," *Psychosom. Med.*, 30 (1968), 1–11.

18. GLUCKSMAN, M. L., J. HIRSCH, R. S. McCULLY et al. "The Response of Obese Patients to Weight Reduction: II. A Quantitative Evaluation of Behavior," *Psychosom. Med.*, 30 (1968), 359–374.

19. GOLDBLATT, P. B., M. E. MOORE, and A. J. STUNKARD. "Social Factors in Obesity," *JAMA*, 192 (1965), 1039–1044.

20. HIRSCH, J. and J. L. KNITTLE. "Cellularity of Obese and Nonobese Human Adipose Tissue," *Fed. Proc.*, 29 (1971), 1516–1521.

21. HOEBEL, B. "Neural Control of Food Intake," *Annu. Rev. Physiol.*, 33 (1971), 533–568.

22. JORDAN, H. A. "Voluntary Intragastric Feeding: Oral and Gastric Contributions to Food Intake and Hunger in Man," *J. Comp. Physiol. Psychol.*, 68 (1969), 498–506.

23. KANNEL, W. B., G. PEARSON, and P. M. McNAMARA. "Obesity as a Force of Morbidity and Mortality in Adolescence," in F. P. Heald, ed., *Nutrition and Growth*, pp. 51–71. New York: Appleton-Century-Crofts, 1970.

24. KENNEDY, G. C. "The Role of Depot Fat in the Hypothalamic Control of Food Intake in the Rat," *Proc. R. Soc. Lond. (Biol.)*, 140 (1953), 578–592.

25. KEYS, A. "Coronary Heart Disease in Seven Countries," *Circulation*, Vol. 41, no. 4 and Vol. 42 Supplements, April (1970).

26. KEYS, A., J. BROZEK, A. HENSCHEL et al. *The Biology of Human Starvation*, 2 vols. Minneapolis: University of Minnesota Press, 1950.

27. KNITTLE, J. L. and J. HIRSCH. "Effect of

Early Nutrition on the Development of the Rat Epididymal Fat Pads: Cellularity and Metabolism," *J. Clin. Invest.*, 47 (1968), 2091–2098.

28. LeMagnen, J. "Advances in Studies on the Physiological Control and Regulation of Food Intake," *Prog. Physiol. Psychol.*, 4 (1971), 203–261.

29. London, A. M. and E. D. Schreiber. "A Controlled Study of the Effects of Group Discussions and an Anorexiant in Outpatient Treatment of Obesity with Attention to the Psychological Aspects of Dieting," *Ann. Intern. Med.*, 65 (1966), 80–92.

30. MacCuish, A. C., J. F. Munro, and L. J. P. Duncan. "Follow-up Study of Refractory Obesity Treated by Fasting," *Br. Med. J.*, 1 (1968), 91–92.

31. Marks, H. H. "Influence of Obesity on Morbidity and Mortality," *Bull. N.Y. Acad. Med.*, 36 (1960), 296–312.

32. Mayer, J. "Correlation between Metabolism and Feeding Behavior and Multiple Etiology of Obesity," *Bull. N.Y. Acad. Med.*, 22 (1957), 744–761.

33. ———. "Genetic Factors in Obesity," *Ann. N.Y. Acad. Sci.*, 131 (1965), 412–421.

34. ———. "Some Aspects of the Problem of Regulation of Food Intake and Obesity," *N. Engl. J. Med.*, 274 (1966), 610–616, 662–673, 722–731.

35. ———. *Overweight: Causes, Cost, and Control*, pp. 1–218. Englewood Cliffs, N.J.: Prentice-Hall, 1968.

36. Mayer, J. and D. W. Thomas. "Regulation of Food Intake and Obesity," *Science*, 156 (1967), 328–337.

37. Mellinkoff, S. M., M. Frankland, D. Boyle et al. "Relationship between Serum Amino Acid Concentration and Fluctuations in Appetite," *J. Appl. Physiol.*, 8 (1956), 535–538.

38. Metropolitan Life Insurance Company. "New Weight Standards for Men and Women," *Statis. Bull.*, 40 (1959), 1–4.

39. Miller, N. E., C. J. Bailey, and J. A. F. Stevenson. "Decreased Hunger and Increased Food Intake in Hypothalamic Obese Rats," *Science*, 112 (1950), 256–259.

40. Moore, M. E., A. Stunkard, and L. Srole. "Obesity, Social Class and Mental Illness," *JAMA*, 181 (1962), 962–966.

41. National Center for Health Statistics. *Weight by Height and Age of Adults—United States 1960–63*. Series 11, no. 14. Washington: Department of Health, Education, and Welfare, 1966.

42. Payne, J. H. and L. T. DeWind. "Surgical Treatment of Obesity," *Am. J. Surg.*, 118 (1969), 141–147.

43. Robinson, B. W. and M. Mishkin. "Alimentary Responses Evoked from Forebrain Structures in Macaca Mulatta," *Science*, 136 (1962), 260–263.

44. Rozin, P. "Thiamine Specific Hunger," in W. Heidel, ed., *Handbook of Physiology*, sect. 6. Physiology of the Alimentary Canal, pp. 411–431. Washington: American Physiological Society, 1967.

45. Russek, M. "Hepatic Receptors and the Neurophysiological Mechanisms Controlling Feeding Behavior," *Neurosci. Res.*, 4 (1971), 213–282.

46. Salans, L. B., J. L. Knittle, and J. Hirsch. "The Role of Adipose Cell Size and Adipose Tissue Insulin Sensitivity in the Carbohydrate Intolerance of Human Obesity," *J. Clin. Invest.*, 47 (1968), 153–165.

47. Schachter, S. "Some Extraordinary Facts about Obese Humans," *Am. Psychol.*, 26 (1971), 129–144.

48. Seltzer, C. C. and J. Mayer. "Body Build and Obesity—Who Are the Obese?" *JAMA*, 189 (1964), 677–684.

49. ———. "A Simple Criterion of Obesity," *Postgrad. Med.*, 38 (1965), 101–107.

50. Simborg, E. W. "The Status of Risk Factors and Coronary Heart Disease," *J. Chron. Dis.*, 22 (1970), 515–552.

51. Sims, E. A. H. and E. S. Horton. "Endocrine and Metabolic Adaptation to Obesity and Starvation," *Am. J. Clin. Nutr.*, 21 (1968), 1455–1470.

52. Smith, G. P. and A. N. Epstein. "Increased Feeding in Response to Decreased Glucose Utilization in the Rat and Monkey," *Am. J. Physiol.*, 217 (1969), 1083–1087.

53. Stellar, E. "The Physiology of Motivation," *Psychol. Rev.*, 61 (1954), 5–22.

54. Stuart, R. B. and B. Davis. *Slim Chance in a Fat World: Behavioral Control of Obesity*, pp. 1–240. Champaign, Ill.: Research Press, 1971.

55. Stunkard, A. J. "Eating Patterns and Obesity," *Psychiatr. Q.*, 33 (1959), 284–295.

56. ———. "New Therapies for the Eating Disorders: Behavior Modification of Obesity and Anorexia Nervosa," *Arch. Gen. Psychiatry*, 26 (1972), 391–398.

57. STUNKARD, A. J. and V. BURT. "Obesity and the Body Image: II. Age at Onset of Disturbances in the Body Image," *Am. J. Psychiatry*, 123 (1967), 1443–1447.

58. STUNKARD, A. J., E. D'ACQUILI, S. FOX et al. "The Influence of Social Class on Obesity and Thinness in Children," *JAMA*, 221 (1972), 579–584.

59. STUNKARD, A. J. and S. FOX. "The Relationship of Gastric Motility and Hunger," *Psychosom. Med.*, 33 (1971), 123–134.

60. STUNKARD, A. J., H. LEVINE, and S. FOX. "The Management of Obesity: Patient Self-help and Medical Treatment," *Arch. Intern. Med.*, 125 (1970), 1067–1072.

61. STUNKARD, A. J. and M. McLAREN-HUME. "The Results of Treatment for Obesity: A Review of the Literature and Report of a Series," *Arch. Intern. Med.*, 103 (1959), 79–85.

62. STUNKARD, A. J. and M. MENDELSON. "Obesity and the Body Image: I. Characteristics of Disturbance in the Body Image of Some Obese Persons," *Am. J. Psychiatry*, 123 (1967), 1296–1300.

63. STUNKARD, A. J. and A. J. RUSH. "Dieting and Depression Re-examined: A Critical Review of Reports of Untoward Responses to Weight Reduction for Obesity," *Ann. Int. Med.*, 81 (1974) 526–533.

64. WITHERS, R. F. L. "Problems in the Genetics of Human Obesity," *Eugen. Rev.*, 56 (1964), 81–90.

CHAPTER 32

ANOREXIA NERVOSA

Hilde Bruch

ANOREXIA NERVOSA" is a misleading name for the condition to which it is applied. The severe weight loss and emaciation in a typical case are not due to a true loss of appetite; on the contrary, these patients are frantically preoccupied with food and eating. Their refusal to eat stands in the service of a relentless pursuit of thinness which appears to be the driving motive. Actually, this preoccupation with the body and its size is a late step in an individual's struggle to establish a sense of control and identity. Concern with control and size are the key issues in the classical anorexia nervosa syndrome, to which I shall refer here as "genuine," or "primary anorexia nervosa."[6,7]

There are other cases of psychological emaciation where the symbolic meaning of the eating function itself is interpreted in a distorted way, at times associated with a true loss of appetite. The weight loss of such patients may reach the same order of magnitude as in the genuine syndrome, but they are distinctly different in their behavior and psychological concerns. After the condition has existed for any length of time, they look deceptively like true anorexia nervosa, and the different clinical pictures have been continuously confused.

Such patients exhibit an atypical picture of anorexia nervosa. It is important to make the distinction because the therapeutic needs differ, according to the underlying problems.

⟮ History of Concept

Anorexia nervosa became a modern clinical entity with the reports by Gull[25] in England, and Lasègue[30] in France, just 100 years ago, and the picture has remained alive in medical thinking. Occasional references to a condition of self-inflicted starvation have been discovered in the older literature. Richard Morton[33] is commonly credited with the earliest medical report, in 1689, of what he called a "Nervous Consumption." His crisp description, "a skeleton only clad with skin," immediately evokes the most dramatic aspect of the condition. The medical literature of the eighteenth and nineteenth centuries contains occasional references to self-inflicted emaciation which have been mentioned in several recent monographs.[4,38,43]

In spite of the rarity of anorexia nervosa and its short history, there exists an amazingly large literature. I shall refer only to a few authors who have contributed to the understanding of this enigmatic condition. Since its discovery a certain atmosphere of controversy attached itself to the discussion. Lasègue considered some hysterical disturbance in the digestive tract to be the starting symptom, and named the condition accordingly, anorexie hystérique. Gull attributed the want of appetite to "a morbid mental state—I believe, therefore, that its origin is central and not peripheral." He described as the outstanding symptom emaciation associated with amenorrhea, constipation, loss of appetite, slow pulse and respiration, and absence of somatic pathology. He commented on the restless activity: "It is curious to note the persistent wish to be on the move, though the emaciation was so great."[26]

Considerable contradiction and confusion has been expressed in the literature during these past 100 years. Some of this may well be related to the tendency to explain all cases through the same mechanism, and the unwillingness to concede that the same surface picture, namely emaciation due to restricted food intake, may be a manifestation of different underlying factors. The whole issue became even more confused when Simmonds,[41] a pathologist, reported destructive lesions in the pituitary gland of an emaciated woman who had died following pregnancy and delivery. Until then, the assumption that anorexia nervosa was caused by psychological factors had been unchallenged. Following Simmonds' publication, in 1914, the whole approach changed and every case of malnutrition was explained as caused by some endocrine deficiency, resulting in increasing vagueness in what was considered to deserve the diagnosis, anorexia nervosa.

It was only during the 1930s that persistent efforts were made to distinguish a psychological anorexia nervosa syndrome from the so-called Simmonds disease. Once it had been reestablished that anorexia nervosa was a disease of psychological origin, publications with this orientation appeared in a steady stream, without diminishing the confusion. It was assumed that patients with such a weight loss were "fundamentally alike clinically" and that

they suffered from "concealed conflicts." The ambition was to explain the whole complex picture through one specific psychodynamic formulation; this resulted in imposing stereotyped explanations on a condition that defies such a simplistic approach.

Some of the "key" publications, illustrating the evolution of the concept, were collected in a monograph by Kaufman and Heiman;[27] though published in 1964, the most recent paper reviewed was originally published in 1943. I shall focus here mainly on publications of the 1960s and 1970s. Two main trends can be recognized: (1) the older approach of dealing with the chief symptom, i.e., the symbolic significance of the "oral" component; and (2) the approach concerned with the personality of the patient, disturbances in ego functions, and interpersonal relations.

Symptomatic Approach

Psychoanalytic studies with focus on the disturbed eating often included psychogenic vomiting and other forms of neurotic eating disturbances. Basically, they all rest on Freud's assumption that impairment in the nutritional instinct was related to the organism's failure to master the sexual excitation. This one-sided emphasis on the "oral" component, with neglect of other important aspects, has contributed to the confusion with which we are confronted today. Classical psychoanalysis viewed the whole problem as symbolically expressing an internalized sexual conflict. The high point of this approach is a paper published in 1940, by Waller, Kaufman, and Deutsch,[46] that "psychological factors have a certain specific constellation centering around the symbolization of pregnancy fantasies involving the gastrointestinal tract." The concept that anorexia nervosa was an expression of repudiation of sexuality, specifically of "oral impregnation" fantasies, has since dominated clinical thinking. Even today "oral impregnation" is the one psychodynamic issue most persistently looked for.

Modern psychoanalytic thinking has turned away from this merely symbolic, and often rather analogistic etiological approach, and

focusses more on the nature of the parent–
child relationship from its beginning. Nemiah[34]
considered the excessive dependency, un-
questioning obedience, and wilted kind of
passivity in anorexia nervosa to be the expected outcome of a mother's overprotective
attitude. Meyer and Weinroth[32] pointed to
factors that served to precondition the eating
experience in the future anorexic, and felt that
the onset at the time of puberty had given rise
to an erroneous evaluation of the oedipal conflicts in the genesis of anorexia nervosa, and
that the problem needed to be connected with
the effects of earlier preoedipal experiences.

With this increasing emphasis on early development, and on behavior and attitudes not
directly related to food, recent psychoanalytic
studies are approaching the views that have
been expressed by authors quoted in the next
section since the early 1930s. There are, of
course, still reports in the old orientation.
Thomae's monograph,[43] published in 1961, is
written in the classical psychoanalytic tradition and gives the impression of belonging to
a bygone era of medical and psychoanalytic
thinking, claiming that "obviously it is a drive
disturbance—and that oral ambivalence underlies the whole symptomatology."

Personality Problems

A few analysts recognized quite early that
the focus on the eating function failed to deal
with the underlying disturbances in the total
personality. Meng[31] compared the regression
in anorexia nervosa to what is observed in
psychosis. He focused on the deformation in
the ego structure, that in neurosis the ego is
essentially normal though the symptoms are
an expression of inner conflicts. In psychosis,
however, the ego is defective in its primary
structure, even though external factors play
also a role. Eissler[20] referred to Meng's concept of "deformation of the ego" as applicable
to his own observations on a patient who
complained that "her mind was in the mind of
other people." Eissler felt that this weak and
stunted ego had evolved out of the past interactional patterns between mother and child,
and that this attitude was different from the

dependency on the mother so frequently encountered in neurotics. Nicolle[35] differentiated between true anorexia nervosa and noneating related to hysteria or other neurotic
disorders. She drew attention to the potentially schizophrenic aspects of true anorexia
nervosa, with shallowness of feelings and cooling off in emotional awareness, as has also
been described in the early diagnosis of
schizophrenia.

Probably the most detailed account of the
inner experiences of an anorexic patient was
given by Binswanger in his report "Der Fall
Ellen West."[2] This woman had great artistic
abilities, wrote poetry, and kept a diary, before and after she became sick, and Binswanger reconstructed from this her psychological
development. After graduation from high
school she took up horseback riding and attained great skill, doing it in the same over-
intense way with which she approached every
task. In her nineteenth year, she noticed the
beginning of a *new anxiety*, namely the *fear of
becoming fat*. She had developed an enormous appetite and grew so heavy that her
friends would tease her. Immediately thereafter she began to castigate herself, denying
herself sweets and other fattening foods, drop-
ping supper altogether, and went on long exhausting walks. Though she looked miserable,
she was only *worried about getting too fat* and
continued her endless walks. Parallel to this
fear of becoming fat, her desire for food increased. The persisting conflict between the
dread of fatness and the craving for food overshadowed her whole life. After many years of
illness she wrote: "It is this external tension
between wanting to be thin and not to give up
eating that is so exhausting. In all other aspects I am reasonable, but I know on this
point I am crazy. I am really ruining myself in
this endless struggle against my nature. Fate
wanted me to be heavy and strong, but I want
to be thin and delicate."

Recent Contributions

There has been a definite change in the
whole approach since about 1960, with convergence of opinion that a true anorexia ner-

vosa syndrome needs to be differentiated from unspecific types. Reports in the past were usually based on a few patients only and authors would draw generalized conclusions from this limited experience. King[29] reported in 1963 from Australia on twenty-one patients, twelve of whom exhibited great similarities, a specific syndrome of primary anorexia nervosa which needed to be differentiated from abstinence from food as a secondary symptom. In 1969 Dally[19] reviewed the course of illness since 1940 of 140 female patients in whom the diagnosis of anorexia nervosa had been made at a teaching hospital in England. He reevaluated these patients and subdivided them into "obsessional" and "hysterical" groups, with seventy-four and thirty patients, respectively. The refusal to eat, because of fear of possible weight gain or loss of self-control, was the outstanding feature in the obsessional group. In addition, there was a group with mixed etiology, thirty-six patients representing a secondary form of the illness, with loss of appetite, complaint of abdominal fullness, decreased activity because of lack of energy. Ushakov[45] reporting on sixty-five patients from Moscow, considers anorexia nervosa a separate nosological entity, different from unspecific cases of food refusal in various psychiatric conditions. Leading in the psychopathology is the desire to be thin which he conceives of as an expression of a supervalent thought. The manifest picture is usually preceded by behavior changes over a year or two; after that the need to be thin, the fear of gaining weight, overshadows all other symptoms. Selvini[38] considers the "combination of conscious and stubborn determination to emaciate herself, despite the presence of an intense interest in food" as characteristic for anorexic girls, and that this constellation distinguishes true anorexia from other forms of psychological malnutrition. Reports by Russell[37] and Crisp[16] in England, and Theander[42] in Sweden, give similar definitions of anorexia nervosa, as "a morbid fear of being fat," or "a state of weight phobia," combined with "anorexic behavior."

I have quoted only a few of the authors who in recent years reexamined the concept of anorexia nervosa. Independently they arrived at comparable formulations, with agreement that there is a genuine syndrome, characterized by "fear of fatness," which is related to preexisting underlying disturbances. They are also in good agreement with my own formulation of the essential aspects of anorexia nervosa.

(Primary Anorexia Nervosa

Anorexia nervosa has always been considered a rare disease; there is a general impression that it is on the increase. In my own experience, based on seventy-five cases (sixty-five females, ten males) seen between 1942 and 1972, the increase is due mainly to more cases of primary anorexia nervosa. Among the sixty-five female patients, fifteen were rated as showing the atypical picture, and fifty the primary syndrome. More than half of the atypical patients were seen before 1960, whereas the great majority (86 percent) of the primary group developed the syndrome after 1960. Somatically, there is little difference between the two groups; in both there is a significant weight loss without organic explanation. The average weight loss in the primary group was 45 lbs (36.5 percent), and 48 lbs (38 percent) in the atypical group. The age of onset in the primary group was on the average 15.9 (10–26) years, and 20.3 (13–28) years in the atypical group. There is some overlap, with the youngest in the atypical group only thirteen years old, and a few in the primary group over twenty years. In the primary group six girls were still in prepuberty. The age of menarche was approximately the same in both groups, 12.6 and 12.4 respectively, with a range from 10 to 16 years. Amenorrhea was a consistent symptom in the primary group, but occurred less regularly in the atypical group. The decisive differences are in the psychological constellation.

The leading dynamic issue in the genuine syndrome is fear of fatness; the angry refusal to eat stands in the service of maintaining an extreme degree of thinness. For a dynamic understanding, which is necessary for pertinent treatment, it is essential to isolate in each individual case the focal point of the functional disturbances, to recognize the crucial problems with which a patient struggles, and to identify his tools for dealing with them. Such an evaluation implies a clear-cut distinction between the dynamic issues of the developmental impasse which has resulted in anorexia nervosa, and the secondary, even tertiary problems, symptoms and complications that develop in its wake. Most patients come to psychiatric attention only after they have been sick for a considerable period of time, and after various futile treatment efforts. It is necessary to reconstruct the behavior and problems of a patient, and the patterns of family interaction and concern, *before* the illness became manifest. In genuine or primary anorexia nervosa the main issue is a struggle for control, for a sense of personal identity, competence, and effectiveness. Many of these youngsters had tried for years to make themselves over, to be "perfect" in the eyes of others. Concern with thinness and food refusal are late steps in this maldevelopment. The underlying personality difficulties had been camouflaged during childhood by their over-compliant behavior.

The true syndrome is amazingly uniform.[12] Three areas of disordered psychological functioning can be recognized: (1) a disturbance in body image and body concept of delusional proportions; (2) inaccurate and confused perception and cognitive interpretation of stimuli arising in the body, with failure of recognition of signs of nutritional needs as the most pronounced deficiency; and (3) a paralyzing sense of ineffectiveness which pervades all thinking and activities.

Body-Image Disturbances

Of pathognomic significance for true anorexia nervosa is the vigor and stubborness with which the often gruesome emanciation is defended as normal and right, as not too thin, and as the only possible security against the dreaded fear of being fat. Cachexia may occur to the same pitiful degree in patients with the atypical syndrome, but they will complain about the weight loss. The true anorexic is identified with her skeletonlike appearance, actively maintains it, and does not "see" the abnormality.[11]

A woman twenty years old, progressing well in therapy, admitted, "I really cannot see how thin I am. I look into the mirror and still cannot see it; I know I am thin because when I feel myself I notice that there is nothing but bones." Another girl, age nineteen, also doing well in therapy, showed her physician two photographs taken on the beach, one when she was fifteen and of normal weight, and the other when seventeen and quite cachectic, admitting that she had trouble seeing a difference though she knew there was one. When she looks at herself in a mirror she sometimes can see that she is too thin, "but I can't hold onto it." She may remember it for an hour and then begins to feel again that she is much larger; there was an inner mechanism that kept on "inflating" her self-image. Only through looking in the mirror could she "let the air out again."

The misperception of their size is preceded by an exaggerated intepretation of any curve and increasing weight as excessive and too fat. One later anorexic girl described this process. She had experienced any bodily changes during puberty with intense discomfort, and began to deny that she had breasts or a rounded buttocks, and maintained this denial over the years, long before her anorexic symptoms began. Like many others she developed a negative phantom, *not seeing* and accepting her figure as it matured.

A realistic body image is a precondition for recovery in anorexia nervosa. Many patients will gain weight for a variety of reasons but no real or lasting cure is achieved without correction of the body image misperception. The resolution of this denial was studied through self-image confrontation in one case by Gottheil and co-workers.[24] After repeated self-confrontation this patient began to see how thin she was, more strikingly on video tape than by looking into the mirror. Gradually a change in her body image occurred so that thinness became ugly rather than comforting to her. The same change occurs in patients during psychotherapy, without such direct confrontation.

Another disturbance is the failure of experiencing the body as being their own. Not uncommonly, anorexics conceive of the whole illness as something that "happened to me," not as themselves having stopped eating. As they come to recognize this they will make comments like, "I realize now I was hurting my parents by not eating; the more they worried about me the more I was hurting them," without awareness that they themselves underwent this ordeal of starvation.

A male anorexic who had been sick since age twelve and who had successfully resisted all treatment efforts, weighing less than 50 lbs at age eighteen, expressed this even more clearly. Throughout this time he had struggled and fought against any effort to *make* him eat. Gradually he developed a real fear of the scale. "I feel I get evaluated by it and then I am panicky. If I gain, *they* are so proud; if I lose, my mother blows her head off. It is always somebody else's business." Talking about his parents he used the expression, "After all, I am their property." It was only after considerable therapeutic progress that he began to conceive of his body and its functions as his own; only then could he let go of his long-standing symptoms. When he was transferred to an open ward he expressed his satisfaction as, "I am free, *I own my body*—I am not supervised any more by nurses or by mother." His attitude towards his weight and what he ate underwent a complete change. "Now if I lose weight it makes me feel sick, that I am losing something that is *mine*."

Misperception of Bodily Functions

The symptom that arouses most concern, compassion, frustration, and rage is the anorexic's refusal to eat. It is this abstinence from food which is reflected in the name, "anorexia." However, the underlying disturbance is more akin to the inability to recognize hunger than to a loss of appetite. Awareness of hunger and appetite in the ordinary sense seems to be absent, and a patient's sullen statement: "I do not need to eat" is

probably an accurate expression of what he feels and experiences most of the time. This deficit in recognizing signs of nutritional need, and the confusion in hunger awareness, are part of the essential underlying personality disturbances, which are closely related to other developmental deficits.

In a study of gastric motility Silverstone and Russell[40] found that anorexic patients, though their gastric activity was similar to that found in normal subjects, usually denied sensations of hunger, or feeling anything, though they could sense the contractions. Coddington and Bruch[14] observed that anorexic individuals, when measured amounts of food were introduced into the stomach, were significantly more inaccurate in identifying the amounts than normal, and also obese subjects. This suggests some abnormality in the perception and interpretation of enteroceptive stimuli.

Since curtailment of the caloric intake is the outstanding clinical symptom, there have been unending discussions whether these patients suffer from a true loss of appetite, stubbornly refuse to eat, repress the sensation of hunger, or fail to act on its urges. Much more than dietary restriction is involved. The whole eating pattern, food preferences and tastes, eating habits and manners, become disorganized, with bizarre and rather outlandish practices developing as the illness persists.

Characteristic is the paradox of food refusal while frantically preoccupied with eating. Most develop unusual, even bizarre, highly individualistic food habits, usually restricting themselves to proteins only. Invariably they will eat more and more slowly, taking hours to finish a meal, however small. This dawdling and the continuous preoccupation with food is commonly observed during starvation. In an experimental study of semistarvation, carried out during World War II on a group of healthy young men, they would "toy" with their food and dawdle for almost two hours over a meal as the starvation progressed, though there was no diminution in the desire for food which was also the dominant topic of all conversation and thinking.[22] Much of what has been called "anorexic behavior," the obsessive ruminative preoccupation with food, narcissistic self-absorption, infantile regression, etc., appear identical with what is observed in starvation due to food shortages, though, of course, the victims will eat whatever they can find, in contrast to the starving anorexic who lives in the midst of plenty but whose fear of losing control and other internal inhibitions make him reject food that is constantly offered, even forced on him. Though without true hunger awareness the anorexic behaves like a starving organism.

Anorexics will complain of feeling "full" after a few bites of food, or even a few drops of fluid. One gains the impression that this sense of fullness is a phantom phenomenon, projection of memories of formerly experienced sensations. An eighteen-year-old girl, intelligent and articulate, but obsessed with her size and eating, felt so little differentiated from others that she would assume the identity of whomever she was with and feel "full" by watching others eat, "having people eat for me," without having eaten herself. She spoke of "keeping my mind eternally occupied with what size I am, always hoping I will become smaller. If I must eat—that takes so much mental energy to decide what, how much, and why must I."

The nutritional disorganization has two phases, absence or denial of desire for food, and uncontrollable impulses to gorge oneself, usually without awareness of hunger, and often followed by self-induced vomiting. Patients identify with the noneating phase, defending it as the realistic expression of their physiological need. In contrast, they experience the overeating as a submission to some compulsion to do something they do *not* want to do, and they are terrified by the loss of control during such eating binges. They express it as "I do not dare to eat. If I take just one bite I am afraid that I will not be able to stop." In about a quarter of the cases of primary anorexia nervosa uncontrolled eating binges and vomiting occur as leading symptoms, but fear of not being able to control their eating seems to be present in all.

In advanced stages of emaciation true loss of appetite may result from the severe nutritional deficiency, similar to the complete lack of interest in food in the late stages of starvation during a famine. This indifference to food must be differentiated from the spirited way with which the anorexic defends his noneating before the stage of extreme marasmus has been reached.

In their fight against fatness, in an effort to remove unwanted food from their bodies, many resort to self-induced vomiting and enemas, or the excessive use of laxatives, and, increasingly often, of diuretics, which may result in serious disturbances in the electrolyte balance. Although the urgent need to keep the body weight low is given as the motive, other aspects must be considered, namely that here too disturbances in the cognitive awareness of bodily sensations play a role.

Another characteristic manifestation of falsified bodily awareness is *hyperactivity*, the denial of fatigue, which impressed the earlier writers[26] but which has scarcely been mentioned in the recent psychoanalytic literature. It has often been claimed that the actual amount of exercise may not be large but only seems remarkable in view of the severe undernutrition. Through pedometric measurements Stunkard and his co-workers[3] could demonstrate that anorexia patients were indeed hyperactive, walking an average of 6.8 miles per day, despite their emanciation, while women of normal weight walked on the average 4.0 miles per day. Patients who continue in school will spend long hours on their homework, intent on having perfect grades.

Drive for activity continues until the emaciation is far advanced. The subjective feeling is one of not being tired, of wanting to do things, and this stands in marked contrast to the lassitude, fatigue, and avoidance of any effort that is symptomatic for undernutrition in chronic food deprivation, and is regularly complained of by patients in the atypical group. This paradoxical sense of alertness must also be considered an expression of conceptual and perceptual disturbances in body awareness.

One might also consider the failure of sexual functioning and the absence of sexual feelings as falling within the area of perceptual and conceptual deficits, though Russell[37] discusses the possibility of primary gonadal failure contributing to the loss of sexual interest. He observed that though most of the actions of the anterior pituitary gland are preserved during the state of starvation, there is a growing body of evidence that the release of gonadotropin is impaired and does not correct itself spontaneously after the malnutrition has been corrected.

Other bodily sensations are also not correctly recognized or responded to, and they appear also deficient in identifying emotional states. One may consider the limited range with which they describe feelings of anxiety or other emotional reactions as belonging to this failure in perception or cognitive interpretation of feeling states. Even severe depressive reactions may remain masked.

Others will misinterpret their abilities and total functioning. A seventeen-year-old girl, who had gone on a diet when she learned that her boyfriend at college was dating other girls, felt for the first time "she was getting results" when her declining weight aroused concern. She became convinced that her body had magical qualities. She had started compulsive walking rituals and would walk whether it was hot or raining, or a thunderstorm threatened. She would walk for many miles even though she was increasingly cachectic. "My body could do anything—it could walk forever and not get tired. I have the will power to walk as far as I want any time—no matter what the weather is. I felt very powerful on account of my body. My only weakness was my mind." She felt the same about her weight: "This is something I can control. I still don't know what I look like or what size I am—but I know my body can take anything." She was rather contemptuous of people who expressed concern about her health.

A sixteen-year-old anorexic girl, when at her lowest weight, was afraid of being "strong." Her ideal was to be weak and ethereal so that she could accept everybody's help without feeling guilty. Her deepest desire was to be blind; then she would show how noble she was in the face of suffering, and would be respected by everybody for this nobility. There was no realistic awareness of what it would be like to be blind, of not being able to see. In spite of this desire for "weakness" she was extremely active and perfectionistic, and would not permit herself to go to sleep until she had done calesthenics to the point of her muscles hurting.

Changes in this distorted self-awareness are necessary milestones on the road to recovery. To quote from one patient who was doing well, "I took a walk—not to wear myself out or to prove 'I could make it' but just to enjoy the bright blue sky and the pretty yellow flowers. I seemed to do it without this 'double track' thinking."

Ineffectiveness

The third outstanding feature is a *paralyzing sense of ineffectiveness*, which pervades all thinking and activity of anorexic patients. They experience themselves as acting only *in response* to demands coming from others, and *not* doing anything *because they want to*. While the two other characteristics are readily recognized, this deficiency is camouflaged by the enormous negativism and stubborn defiance of these patients. Its paramount importance was recognized in the course of extended psychotherapy. Once defined, this sense of helplessness can be identified readily early in treatment and be communicated to the patient.

This deep sense of ineffectiveness seems to stand in contrast to the vigorous behavior and the reports of normal early development which supposedly had been free of difficulties and problems to an unusual degree. These girls were described as having been outstandingly good children, obedient, clean, eager to please, helpful at home, precociously dependable, and excelling in school work. They were the pride and joy of their parents, and great things were expected of them. After a childhood of robotlike obedience, the tasks of adolescence appear insurmountable and reveal them as deficient in initiative and autonomy. Once this lack has been defined, a detailed history will reveal many subtle indications earlier in life, though parents find it difficult to accept that their well-balanced daughter should have been so troubled and under such strain.

It had always been a puzzle that this serious illness is usually precipitated by some commonplace event or trivial remark. Most give a fairly definite time of onset and usually recall the event that had made them feel "too fat" and not respected. Frequently this occurred when confronted with new experiences, such as going to camp in the younger group, or entering a new school or going to college later. In this new situation they feel embarrassed about being "chubby" and afraid of not being able to make new friends. An early signal of something wrong with their drastic dieting is that weight loss does not lead to better social relationships, but to increasing social withdrawal, often extreme isolation.

Whenever there is a detailed examination of the factors surrounding the "sudden onset" one will find that the urgent need to lose weight is a cover-up symptom, expressing an underlying fear of being incompetent, "a nothing," of not getting or even deserving respect. In this desperate worry they gain a sense of accomplishment from manipulating their eating and weight.

Family Transactions

Patterns of disturbed interaction were recognized only through intensive therapeutic contact with these families. Crisp[17] reviewed the older literature and found little consistency in the studies which dealt mainly with the disturbed patterns after onset of the anorexia. There was little agreement between investigators concerning the nature of the premorbid phenomena and influences, and the social background. Some authors, Crisp among them, have been impressed by the high proportion of patients coming from prosperous and professional homes. Ushakov[45] reports the same from Russia and speaks of the prosperous and good living conditions and the highly cultural backgrounds of these adolescents. In my own observation, more than half of the primary group were of upper-class background, with more than 10 percent belonging to the "super rich." In the atypical group middle- and lower-class status was more frequent.

The families are of small size which was more pronounced in the primary than in the atypical group, but without describable "hardfact" characteristics, except that the age of the parents at birth of the anorexic-to-be was rather high, about thirty years, a fact also commented on by others. About half of the patients were first-born children, and the position most frequently observed was that of being the older of two daughters, with a conspicuous paucity of sons. This too has been observed by others who speak of the anorexic family as being woman-dominated. The marriages appeared to be stable, at least in formalistic terms, with only two or three instances of divorce before or at the time of onset of the illness. Most parents emphasized the stability, even happiness, of their homes.

Reconstruction of the early development revealed that they had been well cared-for children to whom many advantages and privileges had been offered. Yet, on closer contact, it could be recognized that encouragement or reinforcement of self-expression had been deficient, and thus reliance on their own inner resources, ideas or autonomous decisions had remained undeveloped. Pleasing compliance had become their way of life, and they had functioned with the facade of normalcy, which, however, turned into indiscriminate negativism when progressive development demanded more than conforming obedience. No general picture can be given for the premorbid personalities in the atypical group.

Evidence of disregard of the patient's needs and emotions could be readily recognized in joint family sessions. With all the apparent benevolence, these parents appeared to be impervious to the emotional needs and reactions of their children. At times there was a shocking discrepancy between the bland and unobservant attitude of the parents, and the evidence of the serious physical and emotional illness in the patient.

With widely varying individual features, several common aspects could be recognized. The parents emphasized the normality of their family life, sometimes with frantic stress on "happiness," and they emphasized the superiority of the now sick child over her siblings. The fathers, despite social and financial success, which was often considerable, felt in some sense "second best," and were enormously preoccupied with outer appearances, expecting proper behavior and measurable achievement from their children. The mothers had often been women of achievement, or career women frustrated in their aspirations, but who had been conscientious in their concept of motherhood. This description applies probably to many "success-oriented" upper-middle-class families; these traits are probably more pronounced in anorexia nervosa, with greater imperviousness to a child's authentic need.

In order to visualize how a family, without dramatic signs of discord, fails to transmit to a child, an adequate sense of self-effectiveness, a simplified model of personality development was constructed.[10] Behavior, from birth on, needs to be differentiated into two forms, namely that *initiated* in the individual, and that *in response* to external stimuli. For a normal development it appears to be essential that there are sufficient *appropriate* responses to clues originating in the child, in addition to stimulation from the environment. If responses to child-initiated clues are continuously inappropriate or contradictory, a sense of ownership of his own body fails to develop; instead, such an individual will experience himself as not in control of his body and its functions, lacking awareness of living his own life. This is the basic psychic orientation in anorexia nervosa. The gross deficit in initiative and active self-awareness may not become manifest until puberty makes new demands, and the impact of new bodily urges provokes a feeling of helplessness, *of not owning his own sensations and his own body*.

The early feeding histories which have been reconstructed in great detail are conspicuous by their blandness. The child never gave any trouble and ate exactly what was put before him, without fussing about food. Some mothers would report how they always "anticipated" their child's needs, never permitting him to "feel hungry," that means without opportunity of developing guideposts for control from within.

Distorting feeding experiences may occur together with distortions in verbal communication, with direct mislabeling of a child's feeling states, such as that he *must* be hungry (or cold, or tired) regardless of his own sensations. This mislabeling may also apply to a child's role in the family, and his feelings and moods. Thus he comes to mistrust the legitimacy of his own feelings and experiences; in order to maintain even an unstable equilibrium with the people on whom he is most dependent, he is obliged to accept these distorted conceptions about his body, and is thus prevented from developing a clearly differentiated body scheme and sense of competence.

Sexual Adjustment and Problems

Since puberty is the characteristic time of onset it has been generally assumed that anorexia nervosa is in some way related to sexual problems. Crisp[18] observed that the later anorexic girl is heavier at birth than her sisters, and tends to have an early menarche, and that this premature demand for sexual adjustment precipitates the illness. In my group, menarche occurred at a normal age; in two instances of monozygotic twins the later anorexic twin had been smaller at birth, with menarche at a later age than the healthy twin.[8]

In psychoanalytic teaching the rejection of food has been equated with the rejection of and disgust with sex, and unconscious fear of impregnation has been considered the specific conflict situation. This type of sexual anxiety may play a role in atypical cases of anorexia, but it is rarely encountered in the primary form. Selvini,[38] too, found impregnation fantasies only rarely; when they were uncovered they were not related to true sexual fears but rather a sexual symbol of more primitive experiences.

It is difficult, if not impossible, to evaluate reports about such unconscious fantasies. When not rigidly negativistic, these patients are chameleonlike in picking up cues from their therapist. If a therapist is convinced that feeling "full" after eating is the symbolic expression of an imagined pregnancy then a patient will reply, sooner or later, that this feels like having a baby in her stomach. There seems to be a tendency to confront a patient too early in treatment with specific sexual topics, before they have developed some sense of identity and self-directed independence. Such efforts lead to sterile and threatening discussions and account, in my opinion, for the fact that treatment so often bogs down in a stalemate. One of my patients married during a remission and, though still amenorrheic, became pregnant. She experienced the enlargement of her abdomen as something desirable, as entirely different from the hateful fear of her body being too big and fat.

My cautionary remarks about "explaining" anorexia nervosa as "caused" by certain unconscious fantasies do not imply, of course, that the attitude of the patients toward sex and adulthood is not seriously disturbed. Under the fragile facade of normality, their whole development has been so distorted that it would be inconceivable if they functioned normally in this area. The changes of pubescence, the increase in size, shape, and weight, menstruation with its bleeding, and new and disturbing sexual sensations, represent a danger, the threat of losing control. The frantic preoccupation with weight is an attempt to counteract this fear; rigid dieting is the dimension through which they try to accomplish control.

(Atypical Anorexia Nervosa

Much of the confusion about anorexia nervosa is due to the failure to differentiate between the genuine syndrome, i.e., the pursuit of thinness, and other conditions where the eating function is disturbed due to various symbolic misinterpretations. No general picture can be drawn for this group except that the loss of weight is incidental to other problems, is often complained of or valued only secondarily for its coercive effect. Often there is a desire to stay sick in order to remain in the dependent role, in contrast to the struggle for an independent identity in the primary group. The characteristic features of the primary syndrome are absent, namely the pursuit of thinness, delusional denial of the emaciation, hyperactivity and striving for perfection, and constant preoccupation with food. In no case of atypical anorexia nervosa were there episodes of bulimia.

The illness is as serious and treatment problems as difficult as in primary anorexia nervosa, with poor cooperation, frequent changes of physician, and impulsive breaking off of treatment. The duration of the illness appears to be approximately the same, with two patients in each group having been unsuccessfully in treatment for over ten years, with sixteen years in a woman with the atypical syndrome as the longest.

Certain subgroups of the atypical cases can be recognized. In eight patients, neurotic and hysterical symptoms were predominant, and schizoid features in six; an adolescent depression was observed in a girl of fifteen, with roots in recurrent traumatic separations during childhood. A few brief sketches follow to indicate the different flavor of the atypical disorder.

A fourteen-year-old girl felt that her symptoms, i.e., her loss of appetite and disgust with eating, had some relationship to the birth of a child to a favorite aunt, an event to which she had reacted with disgust and horror. More severe symptoms developed when a girl friend was discovered to be illegitimately pregnant. The thought that her friend had had sexual relations disgusted her, and she became preoccupied with the idea of sexual intercourse. She said she hated her parents because they had performed this act in conceiving her, and she wished she had not been born.

She had many other symptoms, became aphonic, and spoke in a whisper for over three years. At another time she began to limp and was admitted to an orthopedic hospital, where there were no organic findings, but she was discharged on crutches. At another time she complained of severe abdominal pain and a kidney stone was suspected. What was found was that she had inserted a pencil into her bladder which was removed through a superpubic incision.

Her violent temper and behavior had kept her home in a continuous state of turmoil and excitement; she refused to eat, had vomiting spells, remained up all night, and though she had been an excellent student, she had dropped out of school. After four years of invalidism, she was finally admitted to a psychiatric service for long-term treatment.

She appeared quite depressed, tense and self-absorbed, with staying sick her main preoccupation. In her damaged self-image she was an ill, crippled, and helpless child extorting irritated attention from her parents. The intrinsic therapeutic difficulty was that throughout her life she had used illness to maintain her position in the family and thus she "needed to be sick."

A thirty-two-year-old highly intelligent professional woman had been nearly continuously in treatment since age sixteen, when she had lost a considerable amount of weight. Evaluation of her long history revealed as a major theme of her life the effort to control through weakness. The noneating was a nearly accidental symptom in a woman with the pervasive hysterical character structure. She valued her low weight for its coercive effect and had gradually learned every trick to arouse attention and concern, and to keep her weight at a dangerously low level.

A nineteen-year-old girl lost 30 lbs. during her first term in college. When she was fourteen years old her mother had undergone major surgery. From then on the daughter could not eat, "Unless I could observe the exact amount mother ate." As long as she lived at home nobody had noticed this. At college she lost weight rapidly because "I did not know what mother ate." Subsequently many other phobic symptoms became manifest.

Another college student became infatuated with her physician who had suggested reducing for her when she consulted him about some other symptom. She received much praise from him for being so cooperative as her weight dropped from 160 to 110 lbs. When she consulted him again he reassured her about her weight. She felt he had rejected her, lost her appetite, and became afraid to eat, and her weight dropped to 85 lbs. Later, in psychiatric treatment, she repeated the pattern of immediate infatuation, going to great length to force her attention on her therapist and his family. She was preoccupied with being "in control," but not as a step towards independence; it was an effort to coerce her physician into permitting her clinging dependent behavior.

A twenty-nine-year-old teacher suffered a severe weight loss after having witnessed a miscarriage. She was frightened by the amount of blood, then became obsessed with the smell of blood, first could not eat meat because it smelled of blood, then all food smelled of it. After losing 20 lbs. she felt so weak that she took to a wheelchair, and with further loss she demanded bed care.

In the schizoid group the sense of reality and the misinterpretation of the whole eating function is more dramatically disturbed, often with delusional fears of eating, whereas others refuse food for being unworthy. Characteristically, these patients are often apathetic and indolent, usually indifferent towards the emaciation; they certainly will not express pride in it.

An eighteen-year-old girl was hospitalized with a severe weight loss and scruples about sin; she felt paralyzed in doing anything. She had been quite popular in high school, even had been class president, but she was continuously preoccupied with the fear of losing her friends. She began to have peculiar thoughts about food and her digestion; she felt that what she ate would affect others. Increasingly she became preoccupied with her sins and fear of punishment. She was quite depressed and suspicious, but when hospitalized she accepted nourishment, and her weight went up and she maintained it at around 100 lbs. She suffered another episode of weight loss, down to 82 lbs., when twenty-five years old, obsessed with delusions about her digestion and the influence of thoughts on her digestion.

A twenty-one-year-old college student was advised by her professor to see a psychiatrist, after he had noted changes in her behavior and peculiarities in her style of writing. Instead she just stayed home, ate less and less, and finally did not leave her bed. Her mother had died when she was quite young, and she felt uncomfortable about living with her father. She complained that he had "not welcomed her properly," when she came back from a summer vacation. She looked emaciated and was weak, after having lost 45 lbs. There was nothing conspicuous in her attitude towards eating and she gained weight steadily in the hospital, back to the previous level of 125 lbs. She also responded well to psychotherapy and was able to free herself of her hateful dependence on her father.

These few brief sketches serve to illustrate the great differences in the precipitating events and in the personality of these patients, who have little in common except a severe sense of inadequacy and discontent.

(Anorexia Nervosa in the Male

Anorexia nervosa in the male requires a separate discussion. It is much rarer than in females, and the literature on it is even more ambiguous and contradictory. One finds side-by-side statements that typical anorexia nervosa does not occur in the male, and that it is not different from that observed in the female. It has even been doubted whether it was even justified to make the diagnosis in the male. If amenorrhea is considered a cardinal symptom then males are ipso facto excluded. Defined in psychiatric terms the condition does occur in males, and the failure in pubertal development appears to be the parallel to amenorrhea in females. Both the genuine syndrome and the atypical form are observed. As in females, relentless pursuit of thinness is the outstanding

motive in primary anorexia nervosa, representing a frantic effort to establish a sense of control and identity. In the atypical picture the eating itself is disturbed with various distortions of its symbolic meaning.

Little attention has been paid to male anorexics in the modern literature; usually they are briefly mentioned in the form of an appendix or footnote. Dally[19] surveyed 140 females with anorexia nervosa for whom he established distinctly different groups. During the same period six male anorexics were observed, who were described by Dally as more heterogeneous. He noted that it was difficult to compare the course and outcome in the two sexes. Selvini[39] stated, in a recent discussion of anorexia nervosa, that the cases of undereating in males, in her observations, were all cases of pseudoanorexia, with paranoid delusions and hypochronical ideas about the digestive system.

In my group of seventy-five patients, observed between 1942 and 1972, there were ten males (13 percent) who were diagnosed as suffering from anorexia nervosa at the time of their illness. By focusing on the core dynamic issues, and by clarifying the whole life pattern, interpersonal experiences, emotional conflicts, and psychological deficits, it was possible to define the primary picture in six cases, and to differentiate them from patients with atypical food refusal (four cases) with various psychiatric disturbances and the cachexia only an incidental finding.

Atypical Picture

As in the females, the atypical cases were the first to be observed; at the time of their illness they were considered examples of the classical anorexia nervosa picture. Two of these atypical anorexics were adults, twenty-four and twenty-seven years old, respectively, when they became nervous and fearful, and began to suffer a true loss of appetite, in response to life situations which they experienced as overdemanding; the birth of the first child in one instance, and facing independent professional responsibilities in the other. Both were of good intelligence but had been "underachievers," performing below the level of their capacities, throughout their lives. One was frantic about the weight loss, the other was pathologically indifferent, not having noticed any changes in his feelings about food, and without awareness of the weight loss, except for an increasing looseness of his clothes. The older of the two men, after a seeming recovery, had a relapse six years later and died rather suddenly, without a definite cause of death being established.

The third patient, a fourteen-year-old adolescent, became preoccupied with anxieties about the body and its functions, coinciding with pubertal development. He had been an only child and somewhat obese, always clinging and extremely dependent on his mother. He complained of headaches, became depressed and moody, was irritable and became even more withdrawn than before. He developed fear of swallowing, that the food might get into his lungs and he would suffocate, and became so phobic about swallowing that he refused to eat at all. When he became a psychiatric patient he was frantic with fear about his weight loss (over 40 lbs.), and that he did not want to be skinny. He was diagnosed as suffering from a psychoneurosis, conversion type; an effort was made to contact him five years later and it was learned that he was in a state hospital with the diagnosis of schizophrenia.

In the fourth patient whose illness had begun when he was thirteen years old, immediately following his bar mitzvah, fasting was one ritual amongst many others for "atonement of his sins." This boy was completely indifferent about his body and his appearance. Like the other boy, he had stopped going to school when the symptoms developed.

None of these patients had been in psychiatric treatment before the illness, but there had been many recognized difficulties, complaints about their poor achievement, disturbances in their eating behavior, and overt sexual anxieties. The families appeared overtly disturbed.

Many case reports on individual male patients that have been published are examples of the atypical picture, though they are referred to as representing the "classical" syndrome. They are usually young adults or even middle aged, who have nothing in common except the weight loss and certain degree of "give-up-itis."

Primary Anorexia Nervosa

In contrast to the divergent atypical picture, the primary group has many features in common. The psychological issues are similar to those observed in females. Here, too, relentless pursuit of thinness is the leading motive. The youngsters are described as having done exceptionally well as children. Closer studies revealed that these accomplishments were a facade performance, an expression of compliance, and not of self-initiated and self-directed goals. In their desperate struggle to become "somebody" and to establish a sense of differentiated identity, they become overambitious, hyperactive, and perfectionistic. As in females, manipulation of their own body through noneating is a late step in this development, but the weight loss results in a desperate picture that draws attention to their plight and finally brings them into treatment.

All six boys in this group were still in prepuberty when the illness began with what looked like a deliberate decision to reduce because they felt "too fat." If the planned lower weight had been reached, it proved "not enough," because much more than weight loss had been expected. Being and staying thin became a goal in itself. Their real fear was that of not being truly respected, of not being in control but of being a helpless product of "them." Since no manipulation of the body can possibly provide the experience of self-confidence, self-respect, and self-directed identity, the pursuit of thinness becomes more frantic, the amount of food smaller and smaller, and aimless activity, to "burn off calories," more hectic.

This acute sense of dissatisfaction had occurred, in all six cases, when there was a change of the social setting, moving to a new neighborhood, change of school or going to camp or boarding school. Throughout their lives these boys had received a great deal of praise for being outstanding from their families, and also from teachers and peers. The illness became manifest when the assured status of superior achievement was threatened, when they feared they could not obtain the same prestige in the new environment. They had been success and achievement-oriented before they became sick and four had been outstanding in athletics, greatly encouraged by their fathers. As the illness progressed, with increasing social isolation, the activities tended to become aimless, no longer integrated into athletics and group activities.

In none was there a true loss of appetite, in spite of the rigid self-starvation, which is endured without definite hunger awareness. Periods of vigorous refusal to eat alternated with eating binges of unbelievable proportions, which were followed by self-induced vomiting. Bulemia with vomiting was present to various degrees in five of the six cases. Hyperactivity and drive for achievement were remarkable, with persisting superior intellectual achievement. The boys continued to go to school in spite of the severe emaciation, with some excelling even more than before though one, observed in 1970, dropped out of school for a while under the influence of alcohol and drugs.

During psychotherapy it was learned that, in spite of their excellent performance, they had suffered from severe doubts about their adequacy and competence. In spite of the stubborn, aggressive and violent negativistic behavior, they, too, suffered from a conviction of their ineffectiveness, the dread of not being in touch with or control of their own sensations and functions. The rigid control over their weight is like a magical touchstone, the tangible evidence of control over their body. The families appeared to be stable and well-functioning, but with a transactional pattern of a controlling mother superimposing her own concepts of his needs and desires upon a developing child, disregarding the clues originating within him. Since these mothers were well informed, what they superimposed was quite reasonable, not contrary to the child's physiological and developmental needs, and when young they were healthy children and offered the facade of adequate functioning. The serious deficits were in the area of autonomy and active self-awareness which came into the open when life situations arose where independence, decision making, and self-initiated behavior were expected.

The underlying dynamic picture in male and female anorexics with the primary syndrome shows great similarity. There is one point of difference, namely, in the male all cases of primary anorexia nervosa occur in prepuberty; these boys did not develop sexually until after they had recovered. This is consistent with the reports by others on young male patients. Falstein and his co-workers[21] reported on four prepubescent boys who, they felt, showed the classical picture of anorexia nervosa as the end result of diverse and multiple contributing factors. All four boys had been preoccupied with their size. Tolstrup[44] observed four males among fourteen anorexics with onset before age fourteen; the youngest was only eight years old. He felt that they showed the typical syndrome. Ushakov[45] found that admission rates for anorexia nervosa were five times higher for girls than boys in whom the illness had an early onset between ten to thirteen years of age.

The fact that anorexia nervosa in males is conspicuously less frequent than in females may well be related to the fact that it does not occur after pubescence. In addition, the characteristic slavelike attachment of a child to the mother is probably more frequent in girls, and efforts to solve psychological probems through manipulation of the body are also more common in females. It is probably unusual for a boy to be caught in this developmental impasse. But even when this type of attachment had developed, the psychobiological experience of male puberty will flood a boy with such powerful new sensations, inducing a more aggressive self-awareness which makes a type of self-assertion possible that he was not capable of achieving in prepuberty. Once boys are caught in this vicious cycle of self-starvation and distorted body experience, endocrine treatment appears ineffective, even disturbing. It becomes of value only after the underlying psychological problems have been clarified.

⟮ Psychiatric Differential Diagnosis

There has been considerable controversy about the proper psychiatric classification of anorexia nervosa. As long as the focus was on unconscious conflicts about sexuality or pregnancy, the condition was conceived of as a neurosis; this was the majority opinion until fairly recently. In a survey of thirty patients, observed between 1935 and 1959, Rowland[36] noted that the final diagnosis was a mixture of conversion hysteria, obsessive-compulsive neurosis, anxiety reactions, schizophrenia, and depressive reaction, with schizophrenia being diagnosed more often during the 1950s than during the 1930s.

Much of the old confusion was related to the fact that all cases of psychological malnutrition were lumped together, and that psychiatric diagnostic categories were conceived of as rather fixed clinical entities. Modern psychiatric thinking has undergone many changes, and questions asked today are under what conditions will a patient react in a schizophrenic, hysterical, depressive, or obsessional *fashion*, and not whether he *has* hysteria or schizophrenia, etc. Following anorexic patients over many years brings the interrelatedness of various psychiatric syndromes into the open. Not uncommonly, an early diagnosis of neurosis, in the primary as well as the atypical group, was changed to schizophrenia as the illness persisted.

Though the concept of schizophrenia has undergone many changes, no new diagnostic concept has been formulated for clinical conditions characterized by disturbances in the symbolic processes, with *deficits* in personality integration and self-awareness, reality testing and psychosocial competence. Failure in discriminating awareness of essential bodily sensations, particularly of hunger, is an outstanding deficiency in anorexia nervosa, associated with distorted concepts of one's own body

identity. It may be associated, to various degrees, with disturbances and deficiencies in the integration of other symbolic processes. Viewed from this angle, primary anorexia nervosa is more akin to potentially schizophrenic development, or borderline states, than to a neurosis, though only a few patients with primary anorexia nervosa were overtly schizophrenic at the onset of their illness, or progressed to that state of disorganization. In the beginning neurotic mechanisms, most often obsessive compulsive defenses, stand in the foreground, efforts to ward off the frightening confrontation with their complete helplessness, the falsified awareness of their own needs, and their lack of control over their bodily functions.

Depressive features deserve special evaluation; they may indicate a true depression as a primary illness, though this is a rare occurrence; more often they express the underlying despair of a schizophrenic reaction. The earliest manifestations of something wrong, preceding the actual anorexia nervosa by months or years, may be moodiness and irritability. After the condition has existed over a long period a depressive affective state is difficult to distinguish from apathy, and the corroding effects of isolation.

Recently Selvini[39] suggested subdividing patients suffering from primary anorexia nervosa according to the differences in their eating behavior and attitude. By evaluating Rorschach records for communication defects and deviances, according to the method described by Wynne and Singer,[48] she observed differences in the style of thinking in patients with different eating behavior. She found more signs of disorganized thinking in those with eating binges and vomiting, or frantically preoccupied with fear of losing control; patients with this fragmented type of thinking had a poorer prognosis than those who maintained stable control. Using the same scoring technique, I was unable to establish such differences, either on Rorschach evaluation or clinically. Two of the three girls who died had been rigid in their food restriction but never vomited, the type Selvini calls "stable anorexic." One died directly of starvation and the other of starvation and circulatory failure. In the third in whom vomiting had been a conspicuous feature, the fatal outcome was attributed to irreversible damage due to disturbances in the electrolyte balance.

Recognition of the underlying potentially schizophrenic core is essential for effective treatment. I have seen many anorexic patients where increasing isolation had progressed to apathy and withdrawal into an autistic way of life. Unfortunately, this may even happen in patients who are in treatment, with focus on their so-called conflicts, but neglecting to deal with the underlying essential problems, the ego deficiencies and incompetence in self-awareness and human relatedness. In a misguided effort, a therapist may "support" an anorexic's increasingly bizarre living arrangements, and thus become a collaborator towards an insidious schizophrenic development.

❨ Prognosis

Anorexia nervosa has always been regarded as a serious condition, with, at best, a protracted course. Little, if any, relevant information is available on how to predict the outcome in an individual case. Evaluation of the prognosis on the basis of the literature is more confusing than enlightening. Often an inaccurate picture is presented, records at a large medical center are culled from patients seen over many years and treated by many different physicians with many different approaches. One such report,[49] supposedly based on the follow-up histories of 115 patients observed at a university medical center, actually refers to only twenty-six (21 percent) of the patients who had replied to a letter of inquiry; even for them evaluation of the long-range outcome is not based on personal contact. Nothing is known about the fate of the remaining eighty-nine (79 percent) patients. Nevertheless, the authors speak of "a significant shift back to health and maintenance of weight." In a study in which contact with patients was maintained, even though they had refused psychiatric treatment, Cremerius[15] found that the

later development of fifteen patients after fifteen to eighteen years, was highly unsatisfactory. Five showed a chronic anorexic picture, though somewhat ameliorated; five had achieved a normal, even excessive weight, and some were even menstruating, but serious maladjustment and personality disturbances persisted. One patient had died from an intercurrent illness and another was hospitalized as a chronic schizophrenic. Cremerius concluded that there is no spontaneous recovery, though five patients would have given this impression on superficial contact.

Commonly weight gain is interpreted as a sign of improvement, whereas in reality it may only be a temporary remission. This is most tragically illustrated by the histories of the five patients in my group with fatal outcome.[9] Sufficient weight was regained by four, that for a while they were thought of as recovered; one, a fourteen-year-old boy, died after a few months, not from inanition but from a severe infection. Death occurred in one atypical case, a man of twenty-seven, who had become sick and lost his appetite following the birth of his first child. After several years of seeming recovery he suffered a relapse and died suddenly at age thirty-three with vague symptoms of gastric distension. A young woman, anorexic since age sixteen, had gotten married during what looked like a spontaneous recovery. Though still amenorrheic, she became pregnant and developed tetany. The child was stillborn and a relapse of the anorexic picture followed. She came for psychiatric treatment only after marked physiological changes had taken place which proved to have caused irreversible damages. She died at age twenty-two from the effects of general calcinosis (vitamin D poisoning), with cardiac and renal failure.

The two other girls had become anorexic at age eleven and fourteen, respectively, and gained satisfactorily while in some form of supportive psychiatric treatment, which had not dealt with the patient's inner sense of incompetence. When a relapse occurred two or three years later, the parents postponed asking for help. When finally hospitalized, medical intervention was not active enough, and both girls died of inanition, with weights as low as 45 and 55 lbs. There had been nothing in the early picture of these patients suggesting that they suffered from a more malignant form of the illness.

In my opinion the long-range outcome runs directly parallel to the adequacy of the therapeutic intervention. Specifically, there is little relationship between the diagnostic classification, whether psychoneurosis or schizophrenia, and the final outcome. Some, in whom the diagnosis of schizophrenia had been made quite early, did well in the long run, whereas others, with a consistent psychoneurotic picture, did poorly or even died. This applies to both the typical and atypical group.

It has been assumed that the prognosis in young prepubertal children is better than in older patients. These young patients come for treatment earlier and the therapeutic approach is more comprehensive, with active involvement of the parents. If the therapeutic intervention with the whole family is not effective, young patients may be as seriously ill as the older ones. The onset in three of the patients who died had been below age fourteen. Probably the case in my group most resistant to treatment was a young man who had become anorexic at age twelve and whose weight at age eighteen was below 50 lbs. His case is also an example of the direct relationship of the prognosis to the pertinence of the therapeutic approach. With therapy designed to meet his underlying problems, he made a good recovery and was doing well, actively involved in living, when last heard of ten years after discharge. There were several others with even longer histories of unsuccessful treatment, up to eleven years, who responded well to a change in therapeutic approach. Several reports of effective therapeutic intervention are to be found in the schizophrenia literature,[23,47] namely of patients who had been grossly neglected at the time of their anorexic illness. Without effective intervention at the crucial point of conflict and maldevelopment, the outlook is poor, in particular after secondary symptoms have developed and an anorectic way of life has been adopted.

Selvini[39] has made the same observation, that the statistical evaluation of long range results, in particular when based on weight information alone, is not only noninformative but misleading. Recovery is entirely dependent on the capacity to understand the true conflicts of the anorexic and to help him find better ways of dealing with them.

⟪ Treatment

Treatment involves two distinct tasks, the restitution of normal nutrition and the resolution of the inner psychological problems so that a patient no longer needs to abuse the eating function in futile efforts to solve his problems. For effective long-range results the two aspects should be integrated; in reality this ideal is rarely fulfilled. All too many patients are made to gain weight on a medical service, and are then discharged back to the same environment where the illness had developed. They come for psychiatric treatment only after years of such futile efforts. In others not sufficient consideration has been given to the self-perpetuating destructive effect of the nutritional deficit itself. Psychiatrists may have the unrealistic expectation that the weight will correct itself after the psychological problems have been solved; such a wait-and-see attitude where nothing is done to correct the severe malnutrition, may unnecessarily prolong the illness. A certain degree of nutritional restitution is a prerequisite for effective psychotherapy.

Since the first description of anorexia nervosa there has been continuous debate on how to accomplish the seemingly impossible task of getting food into patients who are stubbornly determined to starve themselves. This discussion has extended to what food to offer, how to feed it, where to do it, and what medication to use. The physiological principles are very simple: increase the food intake and keep these hyperactive cachectic youngsters from exhausting themselves. The question is how to persuade, trick, bribe, cajole, or force a negativistic patient into doing something he or she is determined not to do.

It is virtually impossible to draw conclusions about the effectiveness of various regimens from the literature. The case material is extremely heterogeneous, and the reports refer to patients at various stages of their illness. One reason for the confusing reports, which is rarely openly stated, is the fact that frequently the authors themselves have little experience with such patients. Rowland's survey[36] is based on the study of the case records of thirty patients who were observed in different departments of the Columbia Presbyterian Medical Center in New York, between 1936 and 1959; the figures suggest that about one patient was observed per year. A variety of methods were used, such as frequent small feeding of special preparations with high protein content, or, in contrast, tempting choices from special trays, or coercion to eat the regular hospital food, or feeding by gastric tube or threat of it, all with unpredictable results. Similarly discouraging is the survey by Browning and Miller,[5] who concluded on basis of the records of thirty-six female anorexics treated at the University Hospital of Cleveland, between 1942 and 1966, that hospitalization did little to improve the course of the disease. The deaths of three (8 percent) patients while hospitalized is reported with the implication that vigorous treatment might have hastened the fatal outcome. This might be interpreted differently, namely, that hospitalization had been postponed until the patients were in such a debilitated state that they were beyond help.

In my experience too, a brief admission to a medical service which does not have special experience in the management of anorexia, creates as many problems as it attempts to solve. The staff is as helpless and inconsistent in dealing with the deceitfulness and cunning of these patients as the family, and is apt to react with anxiety, frustration, and angry coercion. But whether hospitalization is helpful or not, in reality most patients, long before they are seen by a psychiatrist, will have been hospitalized at least once. Early in the disease the focus is on diagnostic procedures, to recognize or exclude possible organic factors. Later on, hospitalization may be necessary as a life-saving measure, when there is progressive emaciation, or acute danger to life due to electrolyte imbalance. This is particularly apt to happen in patients who use vomiting, laxatives, and diuretics, and which many will continue to use even after they have become painfully aware of the dire consequences. Under such conditions rather heroic methods may become necessary for correction of the electrolyte imbalance. In one of my patients such help came too late; extreme calcinosis had led to wide-spread irreversible changes, with cardiac and renal failure as the cause of death.

As to the medical regimen, individualization is essential. A firm attitude that eating is necessary, combined with the reassurance "We won't let you die," may produce some gain in weight. Some find it useful to prescribe certain definite amounts of high-protein high-caloric liquid nourishment which is offered as "medication," and to leave eating ordinary food to the patient's choice. Usually such a program is reinforced by the patient's knowledge that the alternative to his eating the prescribed amounts will be tube feeding. Occasionally a patient will prefer tube feeding. The boy who fasted "as atonement for his sins" required tube feeding for several years because it was "harder" and made him feel that he performed one more ritual of atonement. Other patients, though disliking the procedure, gain a sense of reassurance that someone cares for them.

The use of various medications reflects changing concepts of the etiology of anorexia nervosa. As long as it was considered of pituitary origin it was a matter of course to attempt "replacement" therapy. Prescription of thyroid was based on the assumption that a "low" basal metabolic rate indicated deficiency. Insulin was frequently given to stimulate the appetite. Endocrine products have a legitimate use in the treatment of amenorrhea, where it is possible now to produce regular bleeding. In males, with delayed puberty, testosterone may be useful, but only after the underlying condition is sufficiently corrected that its administration will not stunt the patient's growth, or precipitate an untoward psychological reaction.

In recent years the anabolic steroids have

been used as adjuncts in the rehabilitation of long-standing cases, with the achievement of impressive weight gain and greater sense of well being. However, as far as I know, no controlled studies have been reported.

The psychiatric problems have also been treated by somatic methods. Both insulin and electroshock therapy have been used, and also psychotropic drugs, in my observations with only very temporary results.

Recently a method of behavior therapy has been described, namely, permitting freely chosen activities as prompt reward for gain in weight.[3] The immediate results appear to be good and the method is recommended with much optimism. Yet one patient in the original report, with satisfactory weight gain, committed suicide after discharge, before the planned psychotherapy had been instituted.[3] Though this or similar methods have been in use for a short time only, I have had consultations on patients who had gained satisfactorily while hospitalized, even maintained the weight for a brief period after discharge, but then relapsed. Nothing had been changed in the essential family relationships, or in the patient's underlying personality structure.*

Equally enthusiastic are recent reports on crisis-induced family therapy in which the family is stimulated to change their habitual patterns of interaction.[1] These reports deal with young patients, in the beginning of their illness, before the secondary problems have become entrenched. Thus far there have been no follow-up reports, whether these dramatic rearrangements have lasting value. In young patients equally good results can be achieved by individualized psychotherapy and more conventional work with the family. The intensity of treatment for each member, the focus and its length, vary considerably. Some of these young patients can be treated effectively while living at home; in others hospitalization may be helpful to effect a gain in weight while the underlying problems are being clarified.

In many instances, when ambulatory methods have failed, when the family problems were not resolved but have disintegrated, psychiatric admission for long-term therapy becomes necessary; it is of use only if the service has a constructive therapeutic philosophy. It has been objected that psychiatric admission is superfluous, that weight gain could be accomplished in a medical service and be followed by psychotherapy on an ambulatory basis. This reflects an outdated concept of the function of a psychiatric hospital. Great benefits can be derived from the experience of living in the hospital "milieu" provided this is integrated into the therapeutic experience.

Psychotherapy also needs to be approached in an individualized way. Since patients with the atypical syndrome vary widely in their personalities, psychological problems, and the situational and precipitating factors, no generalized statement can be made about therapy except that it needs to fit the individual circumstances. The following statements apply to the more uniform picture of primary anorexia nervosa where many similarities of the problems have been recognized.

The literature on the value of psychotherapy and psychoanalysis is hopelessly inconclusive. Psychotherapy has been referred to as useless,[28] or, conversely, psychoanalysis has been praised as the best method.[43] Authors who feel that a psychotic core underlies the overt clinical picture[20,32] have expressed doubts about verbal forms of treatment resulting in meaningful changes in a condition that assumedly develops during the preverbal phase. Selvini[38] found traditional psychoanalysis ineffective and achieved increasingly better results with a more pertinent understanding of the condition, namely as a concrete use of the body in the struggle for identity. My own experiences are similar. I have found traditional psychoanalysis and "insight" giving therapies ineffective, but that good results could be achieved, even in cases who had been considered untreatable, with an appropriate change in focus by modifying psychotherapy to meet the individual need and problems of these patients.[13]

The intrinsic therapeutic task must aim at effecting a meaningful change in their self-

---

* A series of such therapeutic failures has been reported by H. Bruch, "Perils of Behavior Modification in Treatment of Anorexia Nervosa," *JAMA*, 230 (1974), 1409–1422.

concept and sense of incompetence in areas of functioning where they had been deprived of adequate early learning. There is need to evoke awareness of impulses, feelings, and needs as originating within themselves. A patient can become an active participant in the treatment approach, and thus capable of living his life with competence, even enjoyment, and self-directed, when the therapist responds with alertness and consistency, to any self-initiated behavior and expression.

This formulation is the outgrowth of continuous evaluation, over a period of thirty years, of the therapeutic process, in particular of the difficulties and failures encountered with the traditional psychoanalytic approach. Psychoanalysis has undergone many modifications during that time, and my emphasis on evoking a better functioning self-concept is in agreement with now widely accepted modifications, particularly those developed for treatment of schizophrenia, borderline states, and narcissistic characters.

The more a therapist conceives of the psychological disorder as expressing oral dependency, incorporative cannibalism, rejection of pregnancy, etc., the more likely he will follow a classical psychoanalytic model. That had been the case in patients who had been unsuccessfully in treatment for many years, who came for therapy, or whom I saw in consultation. The concept that the abnormal eating is a late and secondary step in the whole development, a frantic effort to camouflage underlying problems, or a defense against complete disintegration, has only recently been formulated for anorexia nervosa, and is not widely known.

This orientation leads to a therapeutic approach with focus on a patient's failure in self-experience and on his defective tools and concepts for organizing and expressing his own needs, and his bewilderment in dealing with others. Instead of interpreting intrapsychic conflicts and the disturbed eating function, therapy will attempt to help him deal with the underlying sense of incompetence, encourage correction of the conceptual deficits and distortions, and thus enable a patient to emerge from his isolation and dissatisfaction. The pa-

tients need help with their lacking sense of autonomy, their disturbed self-concept and self-awareness. I have been impressed how often such angry "resisting" patients, if this is communicated to them without insult to their fragile self-esteem, will become actively interested in therapy, and even will accept the need for food, instead of fighting against it.

Inability in identifying hunger and other bodily sensations is a specific deficiency. Other sensations and feeling tones too, are inaccurately perceived or conceptualized, and this is often associated with a failure in recognizing the implications of interaction with others. These patients suffer from an abiding sense of loneliness, and feel that they are not respected by others, or are insulted and abused, though the real situation may not contain these elements. The process of exploring and examining such situations and of alternatives of interpreting and reacting to them, eventually leads to a patient experiencing himself not as utterly helpless, or the victim of compulsions that overpower him. Examining their own development in this way becomes an important stimulus for their acquiring thus far deficient mental tools. The core problems, their profound sense of ineffectiveness, their lacking self-awareness of their sensations, not feeling in control, not even owning their body and its functions, were recognized as related to deficiencies in the mother–child interaction, which had been without consistent and appropriate responses to child-initiated clues. The therapeutic situation offers the chance for new experiences, where what he has to contribute is acknowledged and reinforced.

This approach involves a reformulation of the therapeutic task, that the therapist suspend his knowledge and expertise, and permit and encourage a patient to express what he experiences, without immediately explaining and labeling it. Some of the current models of psychiatric training emphasize early formulations of the underlying psychodynamic issues. Such formulations may tempt a therapist to impose premature interpretations on a patient, and thus stand in the way of learning the truly relevant facts. The therapeutic goal is to make it possible for a patient to uncover *his own* abilities, *his* resources and inner capacities for thinking, judging and feeling. Once he has experienced this capacity of self-recognition, the whole atmosphere surrounding therapy will undergo a complete change.

❰ Bibliography

1. BARCAI, A. "Family Therapy in the Treatment of Anorexia Nervosa," *Am. J. Psychiatry*, 128 (1971), 286–290.

2. BINSWANGER, L. "Der Fall Ellen West," *Schweiz. Arch. Neurol. Psychiatr.*, 53 (1944), 255–277; 54 (1944), 69–117; 55 (1945), 16–40.

3. BLINDER, B. J., D. M. A. FREEMAN, and A. J. STUNKARD. "Behavior Therapy of Anorexia Nervosa: Effectiveness of Activity as a Reinforcer of Weight Gain," *Am. J. Psychiatry*, 126 (1970), 77–82.

4. BLISS, E. L. and C. H. H. BRANCH. *Anorexia Nervosa—Its History, Psychology and Biology.* New York: Hoeber, 1960.

5. BROWNING, C. H. and S. I. MILLER. "Anorexia Nervosa—a Study in Prognosis and Management," *Am. J. Psychiatry*, 124 (1968), 1128–1132.

6. BRUCH, H. "Perceptual and Conceptual Disturbances in Anorexa Nervosa," *Psychosom. Med.*, 24 (1962), 187–194.

7. ——. "Anorexia Nervosa and Its Differential Diagnosis," *J. Nerv. Ment. Dis.*, 141 (1966), 555–566.

8. ——. "The Insignificant Difference: Discordant Incidence of Anorexia Nervosa in Monozygotic Twins," *Am. J. Psychiatry*, 126 (1969), 123–128.

9. ——. "Death in Anorexia Nervosa," *Psychosom. Med.*, 33 (1971), 135–144.

10. ——. "Hunger Awareness and Individuation," in *Eating Disorders: Obesity, Anorexia Nervosa and the Person Within*, pp. 44–65. New York: Basic Books, 1973.

11. ——. "Body Image and Self-awareness," in *Eating Disorders: Obesity, Anorexia Nervosa and the Person Within*, pp. 87–105. New York: Basic Books, 1973.

12. ——. "Primary Anorexia Nervosa," in *Eating Disorders: Obesity, Anorexia Nervosa and the Person Within*, pp. 250–284. New York: Basic Books, 1973.

13. ——. "Evolution of a Psychotherapeutic Approach," in *Eating Disorders: Obesity, Anorexia Nervosa and the Person Within*, pp. 334–377. New York: Basic Books, 1973.

14. CODDINGTON, R. D. and H. BRUCH. "Gastric Perceptivity in Normal, Obese and Schizophrenia Subjects," *Psychosomatics*, 11 (1970), 571–579.

15. CREMERIUS, J. "Zur Prognose der Anorexia Nervosa (13 fünfzehn-bis achtzehnjährige Katamnesen psychotherapeutisch unbehandelter Fälle)," *Arch. Psychiatr. Nervenkr.*, 207 (1965), 378–393.

16. CRISP, A. H. "Some Aspects of the Evolution, Presentation and Follow-up of Anorexia Nervosa," *Proc. R. Soc. Med.*, 58 (1965), 814–820.

17. ——. "Premorbid Factors in Adult Disorders of Weight, with Particular Reference to Primary Anorexia Nervosa (Weight Phobia)" (A literature review), *J. Psychosom. Res.*, 14 (1970), 1–22.

18. ——. "Reported Birth Weights and Growth Rates in a Group of Patients with Primary Anorexia Nervosa (Weight Phobia)," *J. Psychosom. Res.*, 14 (1970), 23–50.

19. DALLY, P. *Anorexia Nervosa*, New York: Grune & Stratton, 1969.

20. EISSLER, K. R. "Some Psychiatric Aspects of Anorexia Nervosa, Demonstrated by a Case Report," *Psychoanal. Rev.*, 30 (1943), 121–145.

21. FALSTEIN, E. I., S. C. FEINSTEIN, and I. JUDAS. "Anorexia Nervosa in the Male Child," *Am. J. Orthopsychiatry*, 26 (1956), 751–772.

22. FRANKLIN, J. S., B. C. SCHIELE, J. BROZEK et al. "Observations on Human Behavior in Experimental Semi-Starvation and Rehabilitation," *J. Clin. Psychol.*, 4 (1948), 28–45.

23. GIBSON, R. W. "The Ego Defect in Schizophrenia," in G. L. Usdin, ed., *Psychoneurosis and Schizophrenia*, pp. 88–97. Philadelphia: Lippincott, 1966.

24. GOTTHEIL, E., C. E. BACKUP, and F. S. CORNELISON. "Denial and Self-image Confrontation in a Case of Anorexia Nervosa," *J. Nerv. Ment. Dis.*, 148 (1969), 238–250.

25. GULL, W. W. "Anorexia Nervosa (Apepsia Hysterica, Anorexia Hysterica)," *Trans. Clin. Soc. Lond.*, 7 (1874), 22.

26. ——. "Anorexia Nervosa," *Lancet*, 1 (1888), 516.

27. KAUFMAN, R. M. and M. HEIMAN, eds. *Evolution of Psychosomatic Concepts. Anorexia Nervosa: A Paradigm.* New York: International Universities Press, 1964.

28. KAY, D. W. K. and D. LEIGH. "The Natural History, Treatment and Prognosis of Anorexia Nervosa, Based on a Study of 38 Patients," *J. Ment. Sci.*, 100 (1952), 411–431.

29. KING, A. "Primary and Secondary Anorexia Nervosa Syndromes," *Br. J. Psychiatry*, 109 (1963), 470–479.

30. LASÈGUE, C. "On Hysterical Anorexia," *Med. Times Gaz.*, 2 (1873), 265–266, 367–369.

31. MENG, H. *Psyche und Hormon.* Bern: Huber, 1944.

32. MEYER, B. C. and L. A. WEINROTH. "Observations on Psychological Aspects of Anorexia Nervosa," *Psychosom. Med.*, 19 (1957), 389–398.

33. MORTON, R. *Phthisiologica—or a Treatise of Consumptions.* London: 1694.

34. NEMIAH, J. C. "Anorexia Nervosa—a Clinical Psychiatric Study," *Medicine* (Baltimore), 29 (1950), 225–268.

35. NICOLLE, G. "Prepsychotic Anorexia," *Proc. R. Soc. Med.*, 3 (1938), 1–15.

36. ROWLAND, C. V., JR. "Anorexia Nervosa, A Survey of the Literature and Review of 30 Cases," *Int. Psychiatry Clin.*, 7 (1970), 37–137.

37. RUSSELL, G. F. M. "Anorexia Nervosa: Its Identity as an Illness and Its Treatment," in J. H. Price, ed., *Modern Trends in Psychological Medicine*, pp. 131–164. London: Butterworth, 1970.

38. SELVINI, M. P. *L'Anoressia Mentale.* Milan: Feltrinelli, 1963; London: Chaucer Publishing, 1974.

39. ————. "Anorexia Nervosa," in S. Arieti, ed., *The World Biennial of Psychiatry and Psy-* chotherapy, Vol. 1, pp. 197–218. New York: Basic Books, 1971.

40. SILVERSTONE, J. T. and G. F. M. RUSSELL. "Gastric 'Hunger' Contractions in Anorexia Nervosa," *Br. J. Psychiatry*, 113 (1967), 257–263.

41. SIMMONDS, M. "Über embolische Prozesse in der Hypophysis," *Arch. Pathol. Anat.*, 217 (1914), 226.

42. THEANDER, S. "Anorexia Nervosa. A Psychiatric Investigation of 94 Female Patients," *Acta. Psychiatr. Scand. Suppl.*, 214 (1970), 1–194.

43. THOMAE, H. *Anorexia Nervosa.* Bern-Stuttgart: Huber-Klett, 1961; New York: International Universities Press, 1967.

44. TOLSTRUP, K. "Die Charakteristika der jüngeren Fälle von Anorexia Nervosa," in J.-E. Meyer and H. Feldman, eds., *Anorexia Nervosa*, pp. 51–59. Stuttgart: Georg Thieme, 1965.

45. USHAKOV, G. K. "Anorexia Nervosa," in J. G. Howells, ed., *Modern Perspective in Adolescent Psychiatry*, pp. 274–289. Edinburgh: Oliver & Boyd, 1971.

46. WALLER, J. V., R. KAUFMAN, and F. DEUTSCH. "Anorexia Nervosa: A Psychosomatic Entity," *Psychosom. Med.*, 2 (1940), 3–16.

47. WILL, O. A., JR. "Human Relatedness and the Schizophrenic Reaction," *Psychiatry*, 22 (1959), 205–223.

48. WYNNE, L. C. and M. T. SINGER. "Thought Disorder and the Family Relations of Schizophrenics: II. Classification of Forms of Thinking," *Arch. Gen. Psychiatry*, 9 (1963), 199–206.

49. ZIEGLER, R. and J. A. SOURS. "A Naturalistic Study of Patients with Anorexia Nervosa Admitted to a University Medical Center," *Compr. Psychiatry*, 9 (1968), 644–651.

CHAPTER 33

DISTURBANCES
OF THE BODY-IMAGE

Lawrence C. Kolb

SINCE the earlier work of this writer on
this subject and publication of the chapter on "Disturbances of the Body-Image"
in the first edition of this *Handbook* in 1959,
an extraordinary interest has developed in the
body-image as concept, its relation to personality functioning and psychopathology, the use
of psychological tests to ascertain quantitatively its expressions—particularly in boundary and penetration—the confirmation and
expansion of earlier observations as related to
developmental experiences in its evolution,
and finally, the application and elaboration of
the preventive and therapeutic procedures
suggested previously as of value in clinical
practice.

Body-image disturbances now receive wide
recognition, particularly in psychiatric and
neurological practice, and in the consultive
services to medicine and surgery in general
hospitals and clinics. The psychiatrist is frequently called upon to assess the unusual
problem of the patient with such a distur-

bance and to provide an opinion as to the
nature of the clinical phenomena and the
treatment. In the general field of psychiatry,
knowledge of the body-image concept has
been applied in furthering understanding of
the bodily preoccupations in the schizophrenias, involutional psychoses, hypochondriasis, neurasthenias, and the multitude of
phenomena that occur with acute and chronic
brain disease, or result from various toxic,
metabolic, and degenerative states. Sound
data on the specific developmental factors
which predispose or determine disturbances of
the body-image in the major psychoses and
psychoneuroses are sparse.

Body-image phenomena, as observed in the
general clinic, may represent either a healthy
psychophysiological reaction, or be evidence
of psychological and emotional maladaptation. The differences between expected and
healthy presentations of body-image phenomena and their pathological variants are not
widely recognized and hence not generally

diagnosed. The distinctions between health, disease, and the rationale of much of the clinical phenomenology may only be understood in the context of the developmental process of the personality and by consideration of the detailed accounts of phantom phenomena.

The material presented in this chapter deals mainly with the general principles and phenomenology underlying body-image disturbances, discussion of disturbances which follow dismemberment or disfigurement of the body or body surface, and considerations for prognosis and treatment. The concept of the body-image is discussed in the following section.

(Historical Perspective

The first written account of body-image disturbance was that of Ambroise Paré,[102] a sixteenth-century surgeon. Noting the frequent occurrence of the phantom limb following amputation, Paré advised surgeons that this disturbance should not prevent their proceeding with additional amputation if such were indicated. It is most unlikely, however, that Paré's report was man's first awareness of this overt expression of his body-image. Recognition probably dates back to the earliest days of man, with the phenomenon providing him with an experience as impressive and of as great psychological import as his dreams and other reactions to death. Price and Twombly[111] have translated a Latin dissertation, with commentary, written on the subject by Lemos in 1798.

Following Paré, Weir Mitchell[98] provided one of the better descriptions of the phantom, observations which were noted a few years later by Jean-Martin Charcot. Head[60] was responsible for the description and development of the first basic concepts of the body schema or body-image, as well as for the interpretation of its significance for the perception of body functioning in relation to motility, localization of tactile stimuli, and the phantom phenomenon. The broader concept of body-image presently utilized in psychiatry was developed largely by Schilder.[118]

The concept of disturbances in body-image derives from observations of the affected individual's failure to perceive his body and its parts, and adapt to them as they actually exist. The outstanding examples of acute disturbances occur as a result of traumatic or surgical dismemberment, where the basic body-image persists, despite the visible or apparent loss of a body part. The phantom limb is one of the most dramatic and convincing expressions of the phenomenology. Similar disturbances are seen following radical excision of tumors or masses of the face, head, and neck; thoracoplasty; paralysis of extremities following poliomyelitis; sudden paraplegias or hemiplegias; and distortions of the body resulting from hyperadrenalism or other endocrine dysfunctioning.

At the present time, body-image disturbances may be classified as consequent to the following categories of illness: (1) disorders following neurological diseases and affecting any part of the sensory or motor system connected with movement and posture, whether involving the peripheral or the central nervous system; (2) disorders occurring with changes in the body structure as an expression of acquired or induced toxic or metabolic disorder; (3) disorders consequent to progressive deformities, occurring either late or early in life and caused by other somatic diseases; (4) disorders after acute dismemberment; and (5) disorders of personality development, including the psychoses, psychoneuroses, and psychopathic states.

Head,[60] the neurologist, visualized the body schema not simply as the integrated resultant of past sensory experiences, but more as a unity deriving from past experiences and current sensations organized in the sensory cortex. These postural schemata, often functioning outside central consciousness, were considered to be modifying impressions of incoming sensory impulses for their localization on the body surface. Also, they made possible the intricate and delicate motor activities through the constant relationship of the body to other objects. Thus Head conceptualized an area of sensorimotor functioning, a postural model of the body, which brings about the possibility of projecting the recognition of posture, movement, and locality beyond the limits of the body to the ends of instruments held in the hand, or operated by the body. Anything which participates in movement of the body was seen as added to the postural model and as becoming a part of the body schema. The postural model of the body, as described by Head, is of major importance in understanding many phenomena which occur in the area of practice shared by the fields of neurology and psychiatry, or the levels of functioning of the central nervous system.

Schilder,[118] in contrast to Head, extended the body-image concept to include not only an individual's personal or psychological investment in his body and its parts, but also a sociological meaning for both the individual and society. To Schilder, the image of the human body is that picture or scheme of our own body which we form in our minds as a tridimensional unity involving interpersonal, environmental, and temporal factors. He also related the body-image concept to curiosity, expression of emotions, social relations, duty, and even ethics. In his considerations, the borderline between body-image and the psychoanalytic concept of the ego is obscure. He specifically suggests that one go beyond the purely perceptive side of the body-image development to that of the expressive. Schilder conceived of the ego as constant and underlying throughout life, something which takes or views the body as an object toward which it has percepts, thoughts, and feelings.

Federn,[44] in discussing the individual's consciousness of himself, differentiated the ego from the body-image. He writes of the mental and bodily ego as felt separately; the mental ego is identified alone in the sleeping state, but it is experienced as inside the bodily ego when awake. According to Federn, ego is not body-image except when the body-image is invested completely with ego-feeling. Similarly, the ego, in contrast to the body-image, is considered to be capable of complete dissolution yet to have a capacity for preservation of the somatic organization which allows for proper use of the body and its perceptions. Federn equates ego-feeling with unity, in con-

tinuity, of contiguity and causality of the experiences of the individual: "The body scheme represents the constant mental knowledge of one's body; the body image is the changing presentation of the body in one's mind. Throughout the changes, the bodily ego is the continuous awareness of one's body. Image, scheme, ego, all three are themselves not somatic but mental phenomena."

Szasz[138] reviewed the thinking of Schilder and other psychoanalysts relative to the relation of the body-image and ego. He proposes that the ego relates not only to other people as objects but also to the body (of the self) as an object, with mutual interaction between the ego and the body as an object. His discussion of his position versus that of Schilder is in terms of modern theories regarding the ego, and his effort to synthesize disparate viewpoints poses an interrelation between the ego and the developing bodily functions. This interrelation could be considered theoretically as "a process of progressive mastery of the ego over the body (as an object), or, to put it more generally, as the evolution of a progressively more complex ego-body integration."

As indicated in this brief historical account, the phantom phenomenon, as representative of the body-image phenomena, was studied by surgeons and neurologists. The first theoretical explanations for the changes in modifications in the limb phantoms were derived from neurology, namely in the context of Hughlings Jackson's laws of dissolution and restitution of function consequent to lesions within the nervous system.[70] These data have never been contradicted, and the theoretical explanations advanced suffice to describe the modifications of the body's postural image organized in the sensorimotor cerebral center under ordinary conditions.

The second primary source of information on body-image has come from psychoanalysis. The observations of psychiatrists and psychoanalysts are based on studies of percepts, thoughts, and feelings toward the body, as well as personality reactions to disruptions of the body-image. Since these data represent an organization of information which occurs in the central nervous system at the highest integrative level, they may be best understood in terms of the theoretical constructs of modern psychology. Within the later framework it is possible to predicate current unusual modifications, perceptions, attitudes, or reactions to the body as consequent to the individual's previous life experiences, which determine conflict between the body-image as perceived and that maintained by the ego as ideal.

A third, and most intriguing new line of study relating to body-image, is followed extensively by Fisher and Cleveland and their colleagues[45-49] working in the field of psychology. Moving away from earlier theoretical concepts of W. Reich's armor concept, and Jung's Mandala formulation,[74] they conceived the "body boundary" as a protective psychological construct which might be related to various more or less effective modes of personality functioning, predictive of different types of personality as correlated to externally or internally manifested psychosomatic disease. These workers devised methods of scoring the Rorschach-test responses, so as to give quantitative "body boundary" and "body penetration" scores which appear to correlate well with their predictions as to aspects of personality functioning and type of psychosomatic disease. Their methods and findings are described more fully below in the section on Special Examinations.

For the purposes of this chapter, the term "body-image" includes both the postural model of the body as defined by Head, and also the perceptions, attitudes, emotions, and personality reactions of the individual in relation to his own body.

The term body-image is too broad. The phenomena largely studied by the neurologists are best designated as representative of the *body-percept*, the accumulated sensory experiencing of the body which establishes the preconscious body schema and postural model and from which emerge the body phantoms after loss of parts. The *body-concept*, on the other hand, includes those thoughts, feelings, attitudes, and memories which evolve as the individual (ego) views and experiences his body with others. The *body-ego* is the perceiving or viewing aspect of personality as it concerns the body-image. Each individual projects an idealized image of the body, the *body-ideal*, against which he measures the percepts and concepts held of his body. His ego functions to integrate the disparities within these evaluations which lead to arousal of either painful or pleasurable affect. The ego defences alleviate the painful affect.

The descriptions of the consequences of dismemberment are now sufficiently extensive to allow discrimination between healthy and pathological adaptations to modification of the body-image resulting from trauma, surgical procedures, or disturbances of the central integrating mechanism. Where the consequence of disturbance of the body-image does not follow the general expectations of the recognized healthy adaptation, the influence of neurotic or psychotic personality development or social factors will be found operative.

The discussions appearing in the succeeding portions of this chapter are arranged to help the reader gain a clear picture of the factors influencing the development of the body-image and some of the known consequences of the expression of the body-image in healthy persons in the face of the acute stress procedures. From this information, the variations which constitute pathology and pathological psychodynamics in an individual case may be inferred.

⟨ Development of the Body-Image

Over the years, the individual organizes his body-image through the integration of multiple perceptions, a process beginning with the earliest stages of development. The embryonic and infantile nervous system is exposed to proprioceptive sensory impressions from the vestibular apparatus and the receptors in muscles and joints. (The hand-to-mouth movements appearing initially *in utero* are the precursors of the complex and significant face–hand relationship.)

With the progressive acquistion of motility, the newborn acquires knowledge of his body from tactile impressions. In the sucking and feeding process, the mouth is the first area to be stimulated, regardless of whether hand, breast, or both are presented. Tactile impressions arising from the regions of the cheeks and oral cavity become closely linked with the increasingly prominent role of the hand sucking. From approximately the twelfth week following birth, the structuring of the hand-to-mouth relationship is accelerated.[53,64,90] The child begins to use both hands and arms to grasp and knead the mother's breast. From this movement, he then proceeds to use his hands to explore his own body surface and to contact others. Concomitantly, he finds that the hand can also substitute for the nipple as a pleasure part and can thereby relieve tension.

The infant's exploratory movements of the hands over his own body, the hands in contact with the mother, and their use in projecting into and grasping objects in space provide the primary kinesthetic and tactile sensations underlying the definition of the perceptual/postural model. These are the processes upon which the beginnings of self-awareness, of individuality, and the sense of the ego are founded. Important perceptions also develop in the early period from exposure to sensations which arouse varying degrees of pleasure and displeasure; stimulation by self and others, thermal stimuli, and, occasionally, direct painful contact.

In every instance, however, those sensations subserving optic, olfactory, auditory, thermal, and pain stimuli are of secondary importance to the kinesthetic and tactile exploration and perception of the body to form this model. This is in keeping with our knowledge of the embryological development of the nervous system in humans. As Langworthy[85] found many years ago, those sensory paths subserving kinesthetic and tactile activities are the first to complete myelinization.

Even the influence of visual percepts of the body must be considered as subsidiary to the kinesthetic and tactile. The fact that the congenitally blind develop the capacity for adult patterns of response to Bender's[14] test of double simultaneous cutaneous stimuli demonstrates the fundamental importance of the processes of kinesthetic and tactile sensation

in structuring the postural model to subserve location of touch on the body surface. The significance of early sensory experience for the development of the body-image is further strengthened by the observations of Pick[107] and Riese and Bruck[116] that infants and young children who sustain an amputation before the age of five do not develop a phantom extremity. Similarly, Souques and Poisot[133] and Simmel[125] have reported that children born without limbs (congenital aplasias) do not experience a phantom limb. While finding that phantoms were rarely reported if amputation was performed before the age of four, Simmel[128] did discover three subjects with phantoms, out of 135 examined, who experienced the phantom after amputation before the age of two; one was six months at the time of operation. Weinstein and Sersen,[144] on the other hand, found phantom representation in five out of thirty children with congenital limb aplasias. The descriptions of the phantom representation in these cases were obtained by a play technique with the child where he was required to determine the length of the limb, while the examiner extended the length by moving his finger down the existing limb and then beyond the stump. The reports are not those of a fully developed limb and the children generally indicated only transitory perceptions. Whether the Weinstein-Sersen account may be accepted as equivocal to those experiences of phantoms found after amputations remains for definition and verification by others.

With growth of the individual in size and shape, and with evolving capacities for intricate motor activities, the body-image is continuously modified. The progressively developed images of the body and the body parts remain as memory traces within the nervous system and reappear in states of neurological dissolution or psychological regression, as clinical observations have demonstrated. Thus in his therapeutics with hypnosis, Halpern[57] has focused on the repressed developmental aspect of the body-image. His clinical reports disclose the reemergence of transactional sequences between parents and child under hypnosis that establish and modify the body concept, and which carry the conflict situations between the growing child and parental figures. Peto,[105] too, has noted the fantasies of bodily fusion of patient and analyst into an amorphous mass during deeply regressive transference states in the second or third year of psychoanalytic psychotherapy of patients with previous acute psychosis. He interprets these experiences as regressions to the earliest stages of archaic thinking when the individual often experiences his body as fused with the body of the parent.

In addition to the modifications resulting from developmental and sensory influences, the character or quality of the body-image is also a function of the socialization experiences of the individual. The socially determined qualities commence to appear with the earliest experiences of the individual in relation to the significant person in his family or home environment. The child acquires social percepts, attitudes, and affects toward his body and its various parts, culminating from his interaction with his parents and members of his family as they represent the molding forces of the culture. The attitudes of parents impart an indelible impression on the child's concept of himself, his body, and its function. Depending on the experience with the parents, the body and body parts may be conceived as good or bad, pleasing or repulsive, clean or dirty, loved or disliked.

Among some families as well as some cultures, certain aspects of body development tend to be prized, while others are derogated. In general, these attitudes are related to the sex of the individual. Strength and prowess may be emphasized in boys and men, with a major investment in the development of strong limbs and muscles. In a similar manner, the parents and the culture may emphasize the aspects of the body-image which are regarded as qualities of beauty for girls. Apart from these sexually defined values, there are also specific body parts which may be deemphasized for both sexes. This deemphasis can manifest itself in concealment by clothing; denial through prohibitions of exposure, touch, or examination; absence of verbal communication (except in jokes); and outspoken derogation of certain body features.

Attitudes toward the body also derive from the individual's perceptions, comparisons, and identifications with the bodies of other persons. Usually, children who are accepted by and conform to their family and cultural expectations, neither over- nor under-evaluate their body. Derogatory attitudes with overcompensatory mechanisms frequently develop to obscure either actual or fantasied body defects when the child feels, or is made to feel, that his body fails to meet the expectations of those about him. Where families tend to exploit the significance of body functioning and appearance, overevaluation and reliance upon security through bodily beauty or activity inevitably follow. Should there be a disruption of the body-image, persons with such security reliance are less able to adapt and are thus more susceptible to emotional disturbances.

Insofar as knowledge of the surface of the body and its parts is concerned, the individual has many sources upon which to draw. Early, and relatively easily and quickly, he gains a concept of the orifices, including the mouth, the nose, the ears, anus, and urethra. In contrast, knowledge of the internal organs is gained from sensations of discomfort. These sensations may be displaced to the contiguous body surface, referred over related surface segmental impressions, or transferred to the surface through the mechanism of segmental pain. The incorporation of internal organs into the body-image is customarily vague, except when a sense of pain or discomfort is referred to the surface. Exploration of the body serves as the focus for establishing language and thought, spatial orientation in differentiation of laterality (left–right), and enumeration. As has been noted many times, confusion may ensue in development and reemerge in periods of personality disturbance in terms of word usage and their symbolic meaning as referrants to the body. Hirsch[63] has reported on a series of psychotic patients who equated in their illness those parts of their personality identified as "bad" with the left side of the body—the "unconscious side" as against the "accepted" or "good" parts, as reflected in the right. This kind of valued differentiation of left–right in the body-image has a long cultural heritage. Its reemergence in psychosis indicates the fluidity of ego organization—a failure to conceive the body as a whole. The influence of body knowledge and awareness on language and usage of words referring to the body is shown in such studies as that of Wright,[148] who analyzed the names of parts of the body that occur most in literature, and found a correspondence between the ratio of frequency of body parts as compared with the ratio of distribution of sensorimotor cortical representation of the same parts. He came to the conclusion that the linguistic importance of the name of the body part was related to the extent of sensorimotor experiencing of the part. In Bennett's[15] study, groups of sighted, blind, and schizophrenic subjects were requested to list spontaneously names of parts of the body, as well as other categories of names as a means of examining their body concept. Both sighted and blind subjects list the same parts preferentially in the following order: The sighted list *arm, leg, head, fist, hand, finger, eye, neck, ear, nose, toe,* and *chest.* The blind give the same listing except *neck* which is replaced in order by *mouth* and they add *heart* and *stomach.* The schizophrenic responses were very similar to those of normals excepting that *ankle* occurred less frequently. Bennett concludes from his direct approach to body naming by men, in contrast to Wright's study of word usage—as derived from a study of word frequencies as listed in books—that his findings would not substantiate the Wright correlation with sensorimotor representation. Thus he emphasized that one might not explain the differences in responding between sighted and blind regarding the occurrence of *nose* and *eye* as the parts first listed by the blind, while they are less frequently mentioned by the sighted. One may argue instead that the frequency of linguistic preference represents rather the result of the social transactional process as it concerns the body in the interface between the developing child and parents or their substitutes.

Szasz suggested an extension of the concept of the body-image or, as he calls it, the ego-body integration, to include not only the percepts, affects, and attitudes experienced historically in the life of the individual but also body parts which occur in fantasy as wish-fulfillment in defensive operations of the ego. Thus, Szasz, in broadening the concept of the perceptive ego to the expressive, would include penis-envy in females, castration in men, fetishism, and transvestism. In the case of the transvestite, he is seen as creating, with the aid of garments, a materialization of female phantom parts and an image of the body to which the ego clings.[138]

In evaluating Szasz's concept from the standpoint of human experience, the writer holds that the expression of a phantom part is of a different quality and order than that expressed in a wished-for and envied missing body part that has never been experienced in reality. Persons who have not experienced the existence of a limb do not seem to have the capacity for consciously experiencing the existence of a phantom, even though they may wish for a limb. There is a basic physiological substratum imposed upon the cerebral cortex as the result of perceptual experience which allows development of quality of experience over and beyond that observed in the case of ego-adaptive wish-fulfillments. In line with this rationale, the writer is discussing only those disturbances of the body-image which are derived from actually perceived body parts in this chapter. Disturbances representative of partial ego-adaptive mechanisms are discussed by other contributors.

❨ Physiology of the Body-Image

From a neurophysiological standpoint, the postural model of the body is maintained through integrations of spinal neural activity and those of higher cerebral levels. That modification of peripheral sensory activity may influence the subjective appreciation of the body-image is shown by the following observations. Souques and Poisot[133] found that cocainization of the peripheral nerves leads to temporary disappearance of a phantom extremity. Schilder[118] states that Gallinek and

Forster had success in removing a phantom by peripheral changes, and also that Adler and Hoff noted diminished perception of the phantom with application of ethlyl chloride to the stump. Head[60] has described the disappearance of the phantom limb following a cerebral operation. De Gutierrez-Mahoney[32] and Echols[39] reported abolition of a painful phantom by surgical excision of the posterior central gyrus. De Gutierrez-Mahoney found, on follow-up studies, that the original impression of abolition of the pain or phantom did not hold. In their study, Appenzeller and Bicknell[4] indicate that spinal-cord lesions may alter phantom sensations and at least temporarily abolish some. Centralateral parietal-lobe lesions with accompanying sensory defects may lead to permanent disappearance of the phantom experience. Yet, their study is incomplete in that neither the extent of the cerebral impairment is known, nor the length of follow-up of patients claiming complete disappearance of the phantom. Kolb[78] observed three patients after removal of the somatosensory cerebral cortex done in an attempt to eradicate a painful phantom extremity. The phantom was not lost, but it became less vivid. He also observed[78] that there are no significant modifications in phantom percepts following explorations of the stump with removal of terminal neuromata, or with rhizotomies, sympathectomies, cordotomies, injections of alcohol into neuromata, paravertebral anesthetic blocks of the sympathetic ganglia, spinal anesthesias, and prefrontal lobotomy.

The body-image is, as Schilder so properly inferred, integrated in the parietotemporal areas of the cerebral cortex. Pool and Bridges[110] have reported that unilateral surgical ablation or cortical undercutting of the parietal lobe does not destroy phantom percepts. From his study of patients with hemiplegic anosognosia, allachesthesia, and various aphasias, Anastasopoulos[3] concludes that the right parietal lobe is the major cortical area for corporeal representation. However, it would seem that imperception of the body occurs only in those with bilateral cerebral vascular lesions that have led to extensive cortical damage. Cook and Druckemiller[29] have

suggested that the body-image is represented in the cortex as the function of a widespread neural network in the postrolandic area. This network, they postulate, may be activated by stimuli from the periphery or centrally from other areas of the brain when the individual turns attention on problems of body functioning or is actively motile.

Fisher and Cleveland[46] suggested from their studies that, when the individual ascribes definitive boundaries to his body, this correlates with the relative reactivity of his body exterior to his body interior. Using the galvanic skin resistance (GSR) as a measure of reactivity, it was found that when the individual ascribed greater strength to his right versus his left side—or vice versa—there exists a variability in the relative GSR. So, too, when the head area is perceived by the individual as of large magnitude, it is characterized by a relatively lower skin resistance than the non-head area. When adjudged to be small it has a higher skin resistance relatively to other parts of the body. This work remains unconfirmed. Its explanation in terms of integration at cortical levels of brain functioning remains unknown.

(Family and Cultural Attitudes Affecting the Body-Image

Genetic and intrauterine processes and those later accidents of life in the form of traumatic or surgical experiences determine the bodily structure adapted to and perceived by the ego. From this ongoing interaction between perceived body and perceiving ego, consciously and unconsciously, there arise percepts, attitudes, and affects leading to adaptations of the body-image.

Social psychologists have advanced the hypothesis, supported by investigations, that when one's evaluation of a personal trait is unclearly defined he will depend to a large extent on the opinion given him as to that trait by "significant others." In the studies of Kipnis,[76] her subjects perceived smaller differences between themselves and their friends than between themselves and a least-liked roommate. When her subjects perceived their best friends as relatively unlike themselves, they were more inclined to change their self-evaluations than those who perceive their best friends to be like themselves. When the subjects perceived their best friends as having positive personality traits they tended to modify their self-evaluations in a positive direction. The opposite was true when the best friend was perceived as possessing negative traits. But when her subjects perceived more negative traits in their best friend than in themselves they broke off their relationships more frequently than when the friend was perceived as having more positive traits.

These findings probably bear upon the attitudinal set which confront those with obvious body deformity. The deformities bear upon the attitudes of those who relate to the deformed which, in turn, influence the development of body concept by the deformed and mutilated. Recent experimental studies support these contentions. Centers and Centers[27] analyzed the responses to questionnaire studies of groups of children and report that the presence of amputation represents a threat to the bodily integrity of the nonamputee. This reflects in his greater tendency to reject amputee children rather than nonamputees.

Gilder et al.,[54] examined the responses of a group of amputees and nonamputees when viewing the normal and amputated human figure through the distortions produced by wearing aniseikonic lenses. Generally, the change reported was that of less distortion as if the viewer unconsciously wished to deny the mutilation.

Gross deformities, such as aplasias, lend themselves to the development of body-image concepts at both the physiological and psychological levels of integration, which differ from that where there have been less serious disturbances of the body structure. The body-image of the blind, the deaf, and persons with other dysplasias has been less well studied than that of individuals who have acquired deformities as a consequence of illness, trauma, and surgical procedures.

For the most part, the influence of family attitudes on the development of disturbed body-images has been neglected in study and practice. In point of fact, however, the capacity for a satisfactory social adaptation among those with bodily defects depends more upon the family and cultural attitudes toward body structures than upon the presence of defect. When the family or social attitude toward serious body defect is constructive and supportive, there is greater possibility for successful compensatory development without personality disorder. In the family with healthy attitudes the defect is accepted, and personality development is directed by the parents along lines where other assets can be developed and strengthened. By these means the afflicted can obtain a kind of satisfaction which, to a degree, compensates for the effects of the inadequacy of the body-image. MacGregor et al.,[92] have summarized much of the existing knowledge concerning family patterns that contribute to a healthy and satisfying body-image concept.

The attitude of society toward physical disfigurement is generally that of disapproval, repulsion, and rejection. The deformed child is rejected on grounds that his deformities are due to "sins of the fathers," "punishment for wrongdoing," "incestuous parentage," etc. These myths and conceptions exist not only among the ignorant or uneducated but also among the well-educated and highly intelligent. Adoption agencies report that it is difficult to place children with deformities. For this reason, it is not an uncommon practice for agencies to offer disfigured children to people who would otherwise not be considered suitable as adoptive parents. But even under these circumstances, the agencies report that they have difficulty in finding adoptive parents for children with physical disfigurement.

The use and misuse of superstitious rationalizations regarding deformity have a psychological value in that they provide a means for expressing and projecting an individual's own conflict and fear about deformity in his body. In the case of the parents, the acceptance of these unsound and unrealistic values provides a means or an excuse to project the blame for the deformity onto another source, to strengthen their existing guilt feelings, or to support hostile or rejecting attitudes toward those whose appearance is different.

Despite evidence of social, vocational, and intellectual competency, the deformed are exposed to a kind of stereotyping which is socially disadvantageous. Pervasive as these attitudes are, there is a reality basis for the high concern manifested by patients with physical deformities. As a rule, the type rather than the severity of the deviation evokes the stereotyped responses. A receding chin is often associated with weakness or effeminacy. A large nose may assign its possessor to a minority group. Persons with protuberant ears, knock-knees, or pigeon toes are frequently ridiculed or become the butt of jokes and hostile humor. Some facial configurations precipitate immediate typing as a moron, gangster, drug addict, or sufferer of some serious disease. On the other hand, certain physical deformities carry a degree of social prestige, as the broken nose of a prize fighter or the scar resulting from a war injury.

With the birth of a deformed child, the mother usually responds with mixed feelings of humiliation, sadness, guilt, or depression. A small group of mothers consciously fail to see the defect as being as serious as other family members and the physician do. While this minority of mothers will have feelings of protectiveness toward their deformed children, they will also feel jealous toward other mothers with healthy babies. Comments about her baby's defect tend to increase the mother's sensitivity.

MacGregor et al.,[92] in their study of persons with facial deformities, point out that the attitude of the mother varies according to the sex of the child with the defect. These investigators noted that overemphasis on physical beauty by mothers led to maladjustment in daughters. The facial defect of the female child was seen as producing feelings of rejection, hostility, or guilt in the mothers. As pointed out in this study, boys born with facial deformities were less likely to suffer from such maternal attitudes. It appears that the mothers and the culture as a whole did not make a strong connection between the idea of beauty and the equally desirable idea of "masculinity."

The attitude of the mother toward the defective body of the child is strongly influenced by her perception of the attitude of the husband-father. As a rule, if his response is sympathetic and positive, she finds it easier to accept the disfigurement. However, in some cases, mothers are less anxious about the child if the husbands show more distress than they do. In other cases, the guilt feelings of the mother may become magnified when the father blames her for the defect and when she has reason to believe that there is a basis for the accusation.

If the mother has a realistic awareness of the importance of physical appearance but does not exaggerate this value to the exclusion of all other assets, it is possible for her to accept the disfigured child. In such instances, and with the help of teachers and friends, the mother can be instrumental in helping the child to compensate through good manners, gracefulness, careful grooming, and attractive clothing. The usefulness of encouraging compensating personality traits depends, however, on the genuine acceptance of the child by both parents. Otherwise, parental urgings of compensatory behavior can aggravate or increase feelings of inadequacy in the deformed.

In a study of children with excessive body sensitivity but without particular deformity, Levy[88] found that the specially conducive factors were parental oversolicitude, histories of significant illnesses and injuries in the past, exposure to sick persons or frequent discussions of illness, bodily variations differing significantly from that of peers, and special bodily values of the group subculture. Parental solicitude leading to excessive bodily concern in the child was secondary to a variety of conditions in the life of the parents. For the mother particularly, marital conflict, death of the father, difficulty with the spouse's parents or family, absence of neighbors, and narrow emotional outlets tended to cause her to focus her interest on the child. To compound this difficulty, the interest carried with it displaced hostility, and also destructive drives and the reaction-formation of protection. In sum, parental exploitation of the child to resolve emotional conflicts or satisfy ambitions, parental ignorance or immaturity linked with vacillatory overprotection, the death or deformity of siblings, miscarriage and stillbirths, and other special concerns resulting from personal experience served to sensitize the protective parent.

Observations of family life indicate that the deformed child does not receive the same treatment as the other children of the family. The afflicted child is usually treated either with greater consideration or with less approval and warmth, and sometimes even with outright hostility. The responses of the siblings are not necessarily the same as those of the mother to the child. In families where mothers reject the deformed child, the siblings may compensate by providing friendship and help to the child with a defective body. In some other families, the siblings will treat the defective child with outspoken impatience and resentment. Observations suggest that mothers and siblings have less pathogenic attitudes toward children who are accidentally deformed than to children born with a congenital defect; there also appears to be less likelihood of guilt reaction, resentment, and hostility on the part of the mothers.

Emulating the rejecting attitudes of their families and society, most patients with body defects manifest unhealthy attitudes and behavior in relation to their bodies. The majority of children are unwilling to look into mirrors, dread making trips away from home, and try to slip into corners and hide their faces from public view. Contacts at school with other children, who may jeer or ridicule them, often result in the deformed child's returning home in tears or sulking. In small children the ridicule may not at first be understood, but, once it is within the child's comprehension, it can lead to his avoidance of other children. Frequently, a deformed child will persist in questioning the parents as to why he is different and why he is the only one in the family who is different. Some children attempt to diminish the importance of the deformity by joking about it, while still others studiously avoid mentioning the subject. In every instance,

however, these types of behavior are related to the parents' behavior and attitudes concerning the deformity.

The parental attitude is a composite of the parental health and acceptance, and particularly that of the mothers. Some mothers attempt to protect their deformed children from hardship by insistence on their avoiding any activity where they might be questioned. The consequence of this isolation is that both relatives and strangers are kept from contact with the child. Another type of mother attempts to hide the defect by requiring the child to wear certain concealing clothing or to assume certain postures. In the reports of these instances, the mothers failed to recognize that this hiding was also their effort at *withdrawal*, although they did mention feelings of anxiety in the presence of strangers. In studying the children who *deny* the existence of the body defect, it has been found that their mothers attempt to deny anxiety by insistence on exposure of the child to strangers, relatives, and others. The mothers themselves are reluctant to make personal contacts or to discuss the disfigurement. When the subject of disfigurement arises in conversations, parents holding these attitudes tend to minimize their concern. Still another group of mothers compensate for their belief that the children are stigmatized by using the mechanism of "undoing." Here the deformity is spoken of as "cute," and a lack of personal concern is stressed. It is noted in these circumstances that the presence of strangers does not produce feelings of discomfort, but discussion of the defects does.

Differences between healthy and unhealthy attitudes of mothers have been comprehensively discussed by MacGregor et al.[92] Healthy mothers do not consider disfigurement as a stigma or punishment for their own behavior. They do not hide concern, and they are able to seek advice from professional persons and their acquaintances. In contrast, mothers whose behavior fits the child's pattern of "avoidance" are likely to become angry when the child fails to follow instructions to conceal the deformity. Such mothers regularly react by blaming the child when the child complains of discrimination. While the denying mother may allow the child with a defect a greater degree of freedom, his complaints of the attitudes of others usually meet with her rejection. She is inclined to "brush him off" with statements that he should learn "not to concentrate on the defect." Those mothers who "undo" the defect attempt to have the child develop a sense of distinction, which leads to impairment of reality sense.

The foregoing description of specific interaction between mother and child in relation to body structure provides the matrix from which the body-image and consequent ego attitudes and adaptation to the body-image arise. This knowledge, derived from studies of family instruction with deformed children, may well apply to children who later show body-image disturbances in the context of schizophrenic and psychosomatic conditions. Unfortunately, detailed studies are not available on the family patterning that leads to body-image disturbance under these conditions, information which is very likely crucial to understanding the personality character of the schizophrenic, whose conviction of bodily ugliness is a well-known clinical phenomenon. This knowledge is essential to formulating rational methods of prevention and treatment of the body-image disturbance.

⟦ Special Examinations for Body-Image Disturbance

Attitudes toward the body and its parts may be elicited, and ego adaptations to such attitudes may be inferred from the data provided in the course of the psychiatric anamnesis and examination. While the usual examinations and techniques underemphasize this aspect of personality, procedures are now available which may be used to assess the body-ego integration. These techniques include modifications of the regular diagnostic examination, new rating scales for measuring and appraising body cathexis, projective techniques, and specific perceptual tests.

Years ago, Levy[87] suggested a method of integrating physical and psychiatric examina-

tions for children. The child, at the termination of an ordinary physical examination and while still undressed, is asked to play the role of physician and examine his own body. The physician asks him to comment on what he has noticed about the various parts of his body, observable differences between himself and others, and preferences as to how he would like to see his body parts when he is grown. In addition to these questions, inquiry is made regarding ideas and feelings about the importance or lack of importance of height, weight, strength, and appearance. Reporting on his study, Levy noted marked discrepancies between children's attitudes toward the various body parts and their actual physical structure. The visible mouth area produced the most frequent number of responses. Eyes and hair produced frequent responses from both boys and girls. On the other hand, mammary and genital responses were more evident in boys than in girls, a finding related by Levy to the fact that there is no censor of boys in exposing these parts to nakedness. Children showing a sensitivity to secondary sexual traits appeared to have many doubts as to their sexual identity. Individual points of body sensitivity were displaced to other parts of the body by some children. Jacobson[71] also suggested a method of evaluation.

Secord and Jourard[123] developed a rating scale as a means of appraising body cathexis. Secord[122] also devised a word-association test utilizing homonyms as a means of investigating bodily concern. Secord's test discriminates three groups of individuals relative to body concern: (1) the narcissistics who overvalue and overprotect the body because of its intrinsic personal value; (2) anxious persons who register bodily concern owing to physical pain, injury, or shame; and (3) overcontrolled individuals who apparently rid themselves of body concern through denial. The first two groups in the Secord test gave numerous responses on the word-association test, in contrast with the few responses by the third group. Using two tests, the body-cathexis scale and the word association, Secord found that the narcissistic group scored high for body acceptance and high on the word association.

The scores of those with high anxiety were low on body acceptance and high on word association. Overcontrolled persons scored low on both tests. Hunt and Feldman[68] used both the body cathexis scale of Secord and Jourard, and the Draw-a-Person test to study the responses of a group of male and female psychology students. In general, they confirmed earlier findings that women cathected their bodies more highly than men as they showed greater variability in both reporting satisfaction and dissatisfaction. The group as a whole reported more favorable responses to their bodies as perceived in the present as against earlier in adolescence.

Machover[94] described the Draw-a-Person test, a projective technique which elicits unconscious attitudes and percepts of the body-image. Using this test or its modification (the Man-Woman-and-Child test), Noble et al.,[99] Kolb,[81] and Wille[146] found that some limb amputees include amputated extremities in their drawings. It has not been determined whether the amputated percept might have existed prior to amputation, nor is it known whether all amputees provide such mutilated percepts and, if this is not the case, the factors that differentiate this group from those who fail to do so.

Using the Draw-a-Person test with crippled children, Wysocki and Whitney[149] found that they express more aggression in their drawings than do noncrippled children. In expressing their aggression through the medium of this test the crippled showed a variable intensity of aggression according to the area of insult.

Centers and Centers,[26] using the same test to study the responses of amputee children, found that the majority represented themselves realistically, omitting the missing limb or including a prosthetic device. The majority then, as might be predicted, do not present in their responses to this test evidence of greater anxiety or conflict. Yet in this study, the Self-Portrait Draw-a-Person distinguishes the amputee child from the nonamputee. The amputee children more often drew self-portraits with absence of one or both hands. Also, they showed a tendency to incorporate more detail in their self-portraits than nonamputee children. While the hypothesis of the investigators is not supported by their studies, it seems evident that the projection of the body percept in drawing differs in amputee from nonamputee children.

Studies of figure drawings of patients with paralytic poliomyelitis by Johnson[73] show that this group draws significantly smaller figures than control groups of nondisabled recovered poliomyelitics. Neither group represented their defects isomorphically, although both groups drew less distortions in upper than lower extremities. As in poliomyelitis, there occurs a loss of muscle function in the absence of loss of sensation in a part of the body; changes in the body image should offer a contrast to those following cord transections or amputations. In a study by Wachs and Zaks,[142] paraplegics tended to draw figures larger than a matched control.

Figure drawings similar to Machover's[94] have been used by Abel[1] in studying patients with such facial disfigurements as congenital absence of ears, harelips, absence of the nose, scarring from burns, oversized nose, or the sequelae of facial cancers and surgical interventions. Abel has found same-sex drawings to be especially productive of information supplied by the patient. Severely disfigured persons seeking corrective (plastic) surgery portrayed their problem fully in the same-sex drawing. The mildly disfigured were less likely to do so. The projections of the face in the drawings have been categorized by Abel into the following four groups: (1) specific portrayal of the individual's disfigurement; (2) distortion of the disfigurement (a large nose for a small nose); (3) omission of all features of the face; and (4) a face with features but without disfigurement.

While Corah and Corah[30] did not discover overt portrayal of the cleft lip or palate deformity in their studies of figure drawings of a small group of children with these deformities, they do report a significant difference in the scores of these children on an index-discrepancy score, that is the Binet mental-age. Their study did not support the hypothesis that physical handicaps will be represented often in figure drawings. The question requires re-statement and restudy.

Fisher and Cleveland[48] have utilized the Rorschach test in relating a single dimension of body-image concern with the manner in which the individual sees his body damage.

Thus they correlated personal concept of boundary definiteness with the responses to the individual's percepts to the Rorschach ink-blot stimuli. Typical responses considered to equate with expression of definite body-image boundary were: "cave with rocky walls, man in armor, animal with striped skin, turtle with shell, mummy wrapped up, woman in fancy costume." Such responses, they labeled "bar-rier responses." They also defined a second boundary index termed the "penetration re-sponse" and scored by reported verbal re-sponse to the ink blots which were interpreted as emphasizing weakness, lack of substance, or penetrability of persons and objects. Here typical verbal responses were "mashed bug, person bleeding, broken body, torn coat, body seen through a flouroscope." The method of interpreting verbally reported percepts and quantitation scoring are given in detail in their book, *Body-Image and Personality*.[49] The *barrier-response* score seems not to change with time in individuals; the *penetration-response* score correlates more with change.

Patients with rheumatoid arthritis, neuro-dermatitis, and conversion symptoms involv-ing muscular functions were found to have barrier scores higher than those with gastric ulcers or spastic colitis. So, too, those with high barrier scores seem predictable to adapt more effectively to body disablement, to maintain ego integration and to communicate well in small group settings. Roughly, the scores ap-pear to distinguish between several groups with psychopathology. Schizophrenics have higher barrier and lower penetration scores while neurotics have lower barrier and in-creased penetration scores.

As Fisher[49] mentions, others have ques-tioned his assumptions that these scores repre-sent measures of body-image and suggest instead that they are indicative of cognitive or perceptual operations. However, as suggested earlier, such operations have their beginnings in the developmental processes connected with exploration of one's body. To achieve clinical validity and usefulness, more work must be done to verify and amplify the hy-potheses and findings of Fisher and co-work-ers. Others have failed to replicate these correlations.[17,41,95] Bard[11] has utilized psy-chological tests to predict psychogenic invalid-ism following radical mastectomy.

Hunt and Weber[69] have devised a Body-Image Projective Test in which varying an-terior and lateral silhouettes of the female body are presented in booklet form to women who are requested to respond to questions as they view each silhouette in turn: "What looks most like me? What I would least like to look like? What would I most like to look like?"

Perception, as related to the postural image of the body, has been studied intensively by Asch and Witkin.[6] In this work, subjects were placed in a small, tilted room and were in-structed to adjust a rod, presented on the back wall, to the true upright. Judgments were ob-tained with the body of the subject upright and with the body tilted. Striking individual differences were found in the extent to which the perceived upright is affected by the sur-rounding tilted field. Individual consistency was considerable. Witkin is continuing these studies.

Bender's[14] studies of double simultaneous stimulation of nonsymmetrical areas of the body provide a special technique of examining perception of the body-image.

During double simultaneous stimulation of the face and another part of the body, the facial stimulation is not only invariably re-ported but is consistently dominant to all other body parts. The genital region is only slightly less dominant, with the hand the least, and other body areas falling in between. Normal persons who make frequent errors in initial trials of reporting double stimulations tend to correct errors. Persons with brain dis-ease and schizophrenics appear to modify their responses less readily. Linn,[90] utilizing Bender's test in studying patients with organic brain disease, suggests that the face-hand re-sponse is fused and the hand-touch response is not discriminated verbally. Linn's patients reported through nonverbal gestures for the hand-touch test but gave oral responses in the face-touch experiment. He concludes from these observations that the hand response is not the result of extinction by more dominant face perceptions of body-image but rather a nondiscriminated manifestation of fusion of the face-hand response. Linn's hypothesis is in keeping with what is known of the early experiencing of the body by the developing perceptual ego. Pollack and Goldfarb[109] tested both institutionalized schizophrenic and nonschizophrenic children with the Bender technique. They found that, by the age of seven, all normal children perceive both face and hand stimuli within ten trials, while the pattern of response of the schizophrenic children was significantly different and more similar to that of younger children and those with mental changes due to severe brain disease.

Orbach and co-workers[101] devised a new instrument, an adjustable body distorting mirror, as a means of determining objectively the individual's internalized picture of his physical appearance. The observer is requested to adjust his reflection until it appears undistorted to himself. In their early experiments using this device they discovered that a wide range of reflections was acceptable to the various subjects as representing his body. Yet, when subjects are shown a series of distorted and undistorted photographs of themselves they accurately select that most approaching the true identity. Each subject appears to need an external reference point for body identification. Modifying the test to allow a series of judgments, they discovered that judgments of one's head and shoulders are most accurate and consistent. Next in accuracy are judgments of the vertical halves of the body. Least accurate are those of the legs and feet. It must be recognized that such judgments are based on visual stimulation alone whereas the perceptual image of the body—as mentioned earlier—is derived from kinesthetic and tactile impairment.

A later study by Cardone and Olson,[23] utilizing this device in examining the responses of a schizophrenic population, disclosed that such patients performed less accurately than healthy controls, but the patients seemed to have, in addition to the defect in body perception, also a more general perceptual impairment. Hemiplegics, too, have the latter defect but did not disclose a body perceptual impairment.

◖ Phantom Phenomena

The phantoms of amputated limbs, the first to be recognized, are also the most frequently encountered, best understood, and best described. To a lesser degree, phantoms also occur following removal of other body protuberances such as the nose, eyes, teeth, nipples, penis, and the breasts of women. Since the phantom is the expected healthy response following sudden loss of a limb, a detailed account of this phenomenon is presented as a means of describing the pathological reactions to limb mutilations.

The phantom limb or digit is almost a universal phenomenon following amputation, having been reported in as many as 98 percent of cases. Ewalt and his associates,[43] studying 2284 amputees in an American Army hospital during World War II, developed some significant data on the occurrence of the painless phantom as compared with the painful phantom. Their report shows that only eight patients of the total group complained of painful phantom limb, whereas the remainder had a painless phantom. From 22 to 64 percent of women report breast phantoms following mastectomy,[72,130] and Jarvis[72] discusses the variability in the frequency. Figures are not yet available as to the frequency of observation of the phantom of other lost body appendages.

Riddoch,[115] Henderson and Smyth,[61] and Lhermitte,[89] have provided excellent descriptions of the characteristics of the phantom delusion. They point out that the amputee is most aware of the distal portions of the phantom such as the hand and foot. They also note that following amputation, the individual initially perceives the phantom as consisting of the whole extremity. Henderson and Smyth have characterized the sensory phenomena of the phantom as consisting of three general types. The first is a mild, tingling sensation, the basic phantom phenomenon, which is dependent upon the function of the sensori-motor cerebral cortex. The second experience is a stronger, momentary pins-and-needles sensation such as that felt in the phantom when the neuromata in the stump are touched. This sensation is apparently dependent on the functional activity of the lower spinal center. The third type consists of certain superadded disagreeable or painful sensations which are described as "twisting," "burning," "pulling," "itching," or various other complaints couched in bizarre terms. These epiphenomena are discussed in the excellent clinical reports of Bailey and Moersch.[9] Fredericks[50] distinguishes usefully between the perception of the phantom limb per se and phantom-limb sensations such as tingling, pain, or other sensory phenomena occurring with the phantom. He emphasizes that phantom sensations do not exist without the percept of the phantom part.

Most phantoms, regardless of type, are intermittent and more annoying than agonizing. The introspective and observant amputee may notice aggravation of the basic tingling sensation by stimulation of the stump. The aggravation, when a leg has been lost, may also be occasioned by urination, by changes in the weather, or by emotionally disturbing incidents.

Related to these general types of sensory phenomena, especially the pins and needles, sensations referred to the phantom are most often elicited by deep pressure on the amputation stump, less often with algesic skin stimulation, and least by tactile stimulation. Erickson and his associates,[42] have demonstrated that similar sensations may be referred to the phantom by stimulating the appropriate portion of the postcentral gyrus of the cerebral cortex. Cohen and Jones[28] have described pain of cardiac origin referred to the phantom left arm. Cronholm[31] has extensively studied the sensations referred to the phantom by various stimuli applied to the amputation stump and skin areas contiguous to the stump.

The phantom is experienced as a reality, the absent extremity occasionally described as feeling swollen, numb, or tight. Following an acute traumatic dismemberment, the amputee may forget his loss and fall as he attempts to step on the foot which has been removed. It is not unusual to obtain accounts of reflex movements in the missing extremity. The amputee often describes volitional wiggling or movement of his fingers or toes and flexion of the extremity—wrist or ankle. Weir Mitchell[98] observed that the conscious awareness of the phantom may be greater than that of the contralateral intact limb. The patient, preserving an alignment of the phantom with the stump, is likely to comment upon its capacity to penetrate solid objects unaccompanied by any sensation of touching. Thus, a patient lying in bed with a mid-thigh amputation may feel as though his phantom leg is flexed at the knees and the lower part is penetrating the mattress without experiencing contact with the mattress.

The phantom extremities existing after denervations of limbs, or severance of the spinal cord, are similar in many respects to the phantoms following limb dismemberment. Patients report that they perceive the phantom extremity in positions other than those actually maintained by the intact extremity. Occasionally, they speak of a reduplication of the phantom in which one phantom coincides with the paralyzed limb and another coincides with the limb in its healthy state. Reduplication is encountered most often in patients with high cervical transverse lesions of the spinal cord or among those with lesions in the cerebral hemispheres.

Differing from the phantom produced in the amputee, the phantom of the paraplegic does not shrink away or telescope, provided the cord transaction is complete. Also, in the paraplegic, the length and position of the phantom usually remain unaltered by postural changes of the body or by vasomotor stimulation. However, paraplegic patients do report volitional movements of the phantom and occasional homolateral associated movements. As Bors[18] reports, the most frequently willed movement in the paraplegic is in the anal sphincter.

The initial perception of the phantom becomes modified through continuing experiences. With time, the patient comes to feel certain parts less vividly than others. The faintly perceived parts tend to fade away, while others persist with undiminished intensity. In the case of the extremities, the parts which recede first are the upper arm and thighs. Next to disappear are the lower arm and calf, and these are followed in turn by the joints and parts of the hands and feet. Among the last to disappear are the toes, instep, and heel, the lateral margin of the sole of the foot or the fingers, and the palm and ulnar part of the hand. The great toe, the thumb, and the index and little fingers are retained longest.

The phantom modification and dissolution take place over varying periods of time and in some amputees are fully completed. The sequence of the disappearing parts follows the well-known neurological homunculus as represented in the sensorimotor cortex. It appears that those body areas having the most cerebral representation are richly endowed with sensory fibers that make for high sensory acuity and fine discrimination. On the motor side, the areas have high innervation ratios and the capacity for discreet and skilled movements. These highly innervated parts, dominantly perceived through usage, have not only the longest phantom life but are also subject to earliest exploration and stimulation.

Telescoping is another characteristic of the reorganization of the phantom. As the distal portions of the phantom become conspicuous in relation to the proximal segments, the position of the phantom hand or foot is at first unchanged. The patient is unaware of empty spaces or gaps between the stump and the well-perceived distal portions of the extremity. Then the amputee experiences the emptiness of the inner space, and the persisting phantom seems to become disconnected. Although it remains in its customary place and position, it has no sensation of intervening segments. Subsequently, the distal phantom hand or foot approaches the stump. In some patients the distal segment of the phantom, once connected to the stump, fades away, leaving only the toes or fingers, which may also disappear in time. In other patients the phantom hand or foot may remain intact, but in these cases it is gradually displaced into the stump, with the toes or fingers protruding. Occasionally, the stump comes to enclose both the foot or the hand. It is important to note again that the phantom extremity or portions of the extremity may diminish in size. This disconnection of the phantom size, which is frequently overlooked, is only observed if the patient is requested to compare the size of the phantom to the healthy foot.

The telescoping phenomenon is never complete. The phantom may be restored to its former extent when the peripheral stump is stimulated by pressure, as with the fitting of a prosthesis and during disturbances of consciousness in the course of severe intercurrent illness. Jackson's[70] theories of dissolution and restitution of function within the nervous system, following either temporary or complete cessation of function of cortical or higher segmental areas of the brain stem, provide insight into the basis of the process. According to Jackson, a loss of the most recently acquired and most highly organized function ensues, with a reemergence of more primitive functions with later acquisition of new or reappearance of some of the lost functions. Thus earlier infantile and childhood perceptions or the lost limb are seen in the telescoping phenomena. As a whole, neurological theories lend themselves to appropriate and satisfactory explanations of the reorganization of the phantom parts representative of the postural model of the body. Neither the psychoanalytic theory of wish-fulfillment nor gestalt psychology succeeds in explaining the failure to experience the phantom extremities by those who have an aplasia of the limb from birth or an early amputation.

In the case of an acute illness effecting loss of consciousness, there is a reduction in the recently acquired modification of the body-image among those patients in whom the phantom had disappeared. The more primitive, intact body percept, which includes the phantom, reemerges. It is of interest that a paraplegic patient with phantom does not experience telescoping under these circumstances. With these patients the continuing optical image of the intact extremities prevents reorganization of the body-image.

The life of the phantom has been variously reported to persist from a period of a few months to as many as twenty or thirty years. While it is common to hear that the usual phantom disappears within two years after amputation, no firm evidence is available on the period of survival. It seems probable that the failure to reorganize the body-image with disappearance of the phantom extends over a much longer period than is usually thought.

Facial phantoms, following loss of the nose, eyes, teeth, and other portions of the face, are less frequently reported. It is uncertain whether this infrequency results from the attending physician's failure to examine completely because of psychological denial by the patient, or from psychophysiological lack of organization of this area of the body. Hoffman[65,66] pointed out that the examination for the phantom of the facial organs should be made in terms of the subjective perception of the function of the organ. This is in accord with the description of the phantom eye of patients who have lost an eye. They report scratching or itching sensations in the eyebrow, expectancy of movements of the eyeball as though the eye were present, and sometimes blinking of the phantom eye. Among patients having resections on the nose, there may be a compulsion to touch or palpate the end of the nose. Some data exist concerning facial phenomena relative to the eye, nose, and eyebrows following radical maxillectomy with enucleation of the eyeball for carcinoma of the maxillary sinus. Similar disturbances have been reported after resection of the mandible for carcinoma.

In the last decade a number of studies have been conducted to ascertain the frequency and mode of presentation of phantoms of the breast. Jarvis[72] and Simmel[130] review the literature in this area and report extensively on their own observations. Often perceived as a percept of the whole breast, or of the nipple, many patients indicate the presence of the phantom principally in sensations of itching and scratching, as heaviness, or as "full of milk." Simmel discovered that almost all women report a faint breast phantom when requested to perform a sway test by leaning forward with closed eyes and slowly swaying backward and forward. Their perception is episodic and less realistic than that of the limb and is accentuated by menstruation and changes in the weather. Anal-genital phantoms include those of the testicles, penis, and rectum. There appears to be no direct correlation between the occurrence of actual erection and the presence or absence of the flaccid or erect penis phantom. In the paraplegic patient, Bors[18] has reported that phantom sensations of the bladder and rectum are more rare than the flaccid and erect penis.

The infrequency of breast, penis, and testicle phantoms has been ascribed by Gallinek[52] to the lack of proprioceptive sensibility in immovable organs. However, the fact that they occur occasionally makes this explanation inadequate. Bressler's comment[19] that the breast is not integrated into the primitive body-image of the female child in the early years of growth and that full development occurs later seems especially pertinent. Moreover, it is not unlikely that psychosocial and cultural attitudes toward the genital and procreative organs contribute to the tendency to consciously deny the phantom phenomena that follow their loss.

Internal organs, per se, are not represented in the body-image, presumably as there is no sensing and exploration through the kinesthetic and tactile systems and other sensory during development. When, however, the individual endures pain in such organs over a prolonged period, as with a gastric ulcer, or when through surgical or traumatic means a portion of the organ is brought to the bodily surface, both perceptual and conceptual experiences take place and come to represent that aspect of the organ in the body-image. Dorpat[34] reviewed the reports of phantom sensations of internal organs at length. Druss, O'Connor, and Stern[35] report the interesting series of body-image changes noted in four women after iliostomy. These women all wished to be men. Following surgery, the iliostomy was connected with fantasies of acquiring a phallus in part fulfilling their wish and related to behavioral changes of exhibitionism, increased aggressivity, and erotisation of the stoma.

The effects of psychotomimetics, such as mescaline and D-lysergic acid diethylamide (LSD), as they induce perceptual disturbance and modify the phantom have not been elucidated. Zador[150] has described changes in the size, shape, and position of the limb phantoms of two amputees and of a patient who was paralyzed by poliomyelitis. The latter developed a phantom of a limb after an Esmarch bandage was applied. The writer and his associates have conducted a series of experiments on an amputee who continued to have pain in a phantom arm following resection of the contralateral posterior central gyrus. In this study, 18 μg of LSD administered intravenously produced no change; 86 γ of LSD led to perception of more definite form; with a larger dose (95 γ), the size of the phantom enlarged. Phantom pain was unaffected in both trials with LSD.

(Adaptation to Disturbance of the Body-Image

A series of emotional, perceptual, and psychosocial reactions are a natural consequence of disturbance of the body-image. The nature of these reactions determines whether the individual's adaptation is healthy or pathological. The existence of a phantom is the expected healthy response to amputation of a limb or body part occurring after early childhood. Similarly, patients who have undergone changes in body configuration as the consequence of metabolic disorder frequently report bodily perceptions at variance with those observed by the patient's medical attendant and his family. The reports of sudden changes in the body configuration which result in personality disturbance are in part reactions to disturbance of the body-image.

Whether a sudden change in the body-image results from a surgical procedure or from a metabolic disorder, it always arouses anxiety in the patient. The distortion of the customary body-image is experienced as a distortion of the self. In instances of dismemberment, mourning for the loss of the part, similar to that of separation from significant persons, is expected. Further complications are introduced, with resulting anxiety, as the disfigured person is threatened by fears of separation from and rejection by the significant persons upon whom he is dependent. Feelings of hostility may emerge toward these persons as part of the separation anxiety. The perceptual life of the patient is disturbed as regards his unreal appreciation of his own body and also his perceptions of other persons. Some amputees report unusual sensitivity and discomfort upon seeing other amputees. The extent of perceptual distortion among patients with body-image disturbance is not known. The unconscious mental life of the patient is also modified by the distortion of his body-image. The dream-life may become a wish-fulfilling type in which the disfigured person sees himself performing activities in which the lost part plays an active role. Repetitive dreams recapitulating the incident that led to disfigurement are associated with the affect of anxiety.

A healthy adaptation may be measured by the patient's willingness to discuss his disfigurement, dismemberment, functional loss, and the phantom and by his ability to accept offers of aid. With plastic surgery, eyeglasses, hearing aids, dentures, and other aids to social and vocational rehabilitation now widely available, the healthy person reacts by accepting his defect and cooperating with those who can assist in readaptation. Usually, the limb amputee is willing to accept the prosthesis. Similar attitudes normally obtain among those who have lost an eye and require ocular prosthesis.

Psychopathological responses to the disturbance of the body-image are manifested variously. Denial of disfigurement as a wish-fulfilling mechanism to maintain the preexisting body-image is occasionally seen, as in the failure to report the phantom after a limb amputation.

Simmel[127] suggested that denial here represents more the conscious suppression of the existence of the phantom experience. I would suggest, however, that unconscious denial does exist as well and is evident in the behavioral expressions suggesting the continuing wish-fulfillment for the absent limb. Thus, one of the unconscious manifestations of denial is the unwillingness to accept devices that aid rehabilitation. Scott[121] has reported the phenomenon of psychological denial in a manic patient (amputee) after a suicidal attempt. The question of the frequency of the phantom phenomenon and its significance as an indication of psychopathology will remain undetermined until a more systematic study has been made of other than limb amputees. The failure to report a phantom with absence of a body part must be distinguished from conditions in which the body-image never included the absent part, or where slow modification of the image took place with progressive dismemberment, as in leprosy.[125] The known causes for failure to report a phantom with absence of a body part are: (1) aplasias of the part (congenital defect); (2) amputations in infancy and early childhood; (3) loss of internal organs; (4) slow dismemberments (nonsurgical) as in leprosy; and (5) psychological denial.

The failure to reorganize the body-image over a period of time subsequent to its distortion represents a psychopathological adaptation. This maladaptation is frequent among those individuals in which the integrity of the body-image, as it existed prior to illness or trauma, is overevaluated for maintaining self-esteem. Limb amputees, in whom the presence of a limb symbolized either masculinity or femininity, generally adapt poorly to limb loss. Renneker and Cutler[113] found that successfully married women with children adapt easier and faster to the loss of the breast from mastectomy for cancer than do those who have been unmarried or whose marriages have not been successful.

Depressive reactions occur frequently as a result of the body disfigurement. Psychodynamically, these reactions represent not only a mourning for the loss of the part but have a relation to feelings of overexpectation of rejection and fear of separation from those upon whom the patient is dependent. Repression and introjection of hostile impulses toward the significant persons are part of the reaction complex. Frank paranoidal reactions are particularly apt to express themselves following surgical procedures on patients with a self-derogatory body-image. As the expectation of a satisfying social acceptance cannot possibly be met without modification of the total personality of the neurotic patient, the hostile expectation becomes focused upon the surgeon and any others involved in the corrective procedure and toward whom the patient had built up feelings of dependent hopefulness.

Complaint of pain in the phantom or in the area of the physical disturbance may serve as a symbolic expression of the anxiety over the loss and the threat to the individual's dependency needs, as well as an expression of a sadomasochistic identification, a depressive equivalent, and as a substitute obsessional symptom. The writer has found in his study of individuals with painful phantom limbs that 70 percent had lived in close association with an amputee prior to their own loss (see Table 33–1). This appears to demonstrate the high frequency of identification as a determinant for this complaint.

As Kolb[79] pointed out, the characterization of the limb amputee as a terrifying and threatening individual is well expressed in English literature by Melville's Ahab, Stevenson's Long John Silver, Barrie's Captain Hook, and Poe's General A. B. C. Smith.

Fantasies of personal mutilation, usually repressed, may become remobilized by the threat or actuality of trauma of surgical procedure. Many patients with limb phantoms disclose terrifying and superstitious rationalizations which they utilize to explain the existence of the phantom limb. Magical thinking and fantasies concerning the mishandling of the separated limb or about the nature of the phantom commonly serve a guilt-allaying function. Patients with limb amputations frequently express a desire to have the separated part disposed of tenderly and respectfully, as if it were their whole body or that of a close family member. On some occasions they may even fantasy arrangement for disposal of the

Table 33–1.   Comparison of Affirmative Answers to Certain Questions as Given to Amputees with Painful Phantom Limb* and Other Groups

GROUP	PERSONS QUESTIONED	PERCENT RESPONDING "YES" TO QUESTIONS		
		1	2	3
Amputees	22	73	25	13
Healthy	100	20	8	8
Psychoneurotic	100	33	14	9
Psychotic	100	29	9	9

Legend: Each person interviewed was requested to answer "yes" or "no" to the following questions numbered 1, 2, and 3, as indicated in the table:
  Question 1. Have you known intimately a person with an amputated limb (friend or member of family)?
  Question 2. Was the person with the amputation a member of your own family?
  Question 3. Have you lived with a person with an amputated limb?
  * Without other physical lesions.

limb. This behavior is less likely where the illness causing the loss of the limb has been prolonged and the mourning period has been worked through prior to separation.

Psychotic reactions involving distortions in body-image follow either acute trauma or prolonged somatic disease. Bender,[12] in particular, described psychotic reactions in patients suffering Paget's disease, osteogenesis imperfecta, and dwarfism. The acromegalic presents a similar symptom picture. In the slowly developing disease processes which distort the body structure either directly or through interruption of the growth process, discrepancy develops between the body-image of the sufferer and the physical personality. As Bender indicates, the sufferer is made anxious by the obscurity and mystery of the poorly understood disease process. Moreover, the patient is thwarted in all his strivings, whether social, sexual, or vocational, which were predetermined before the illness. In adolescents the conflict over the idealized image and the fixed image ensues when the developing body structure fails to conform to the wished-for or ideal image. For adults suffering any of the somatic disorders described above, the body-image

distortion by illness requires the difficult adaptation from a level of established satisfaction to one of ill-understood acceptance and accomplishment. Bychowski[22] and Eickhoff[40] reported specifically upon the body-image disturbances in adult schizophrenics; Pollack and Goldfarb[109] have studied the image in the institutionalized schizophrenic child. Kolb[79] contrasts the body-image of the schizophrenic and of the narcissistic in his discussion of responses to amputation and emphasizes, too, the often-overlooked delusions of ugliness represented in the body concept of the schizophrenic. Harris[58] initiated work on the perceptual responsivity of the same nosological group to body drawings and word representation of self.

Simmel studied extensively the body-image of the elderly,[125] those with leprosy[125] and the mental defective.[126] With regard to the leprous, Simmel's report is of particular importance as she found that those who lost fingers or toes through absorption—that is, gradually—never developed phantoms. However, if that same limb were then amputated for some cosmetic or prosthetic reason, a full phantom emerged.

Bender[13] examined the body-image disturbance in the brain-damaged, Schontz[120] in those with hemiplegia.

Pazat[103] describes the tinnitus after amputation of the auditory field by sonic traumatism as an expression of phantom in sensory area. Blank[16] has written at length on the adaptive problems of those blinded, and a number of articles have appeared discussing the problems of children and adolescents with congenital abnormalities and/or amputations.*

While not specifically concerned with body-image, the general responses to disfigurement are considered by Dembo et al.;[33] to plastic surgery by Updergraff and Menninger;[141] to hare lip and cleft palate by Brophy;[21] to the face by Baker and Smith,[10] MacGregor et al.,[92] and Meerloo;[96] to radical maxillectomy by Hoffman;[65] to rhinoplasty by Linn and Goldman;[91] to mastectomy by Renneker and Cutler;[113] and to genitalia by Heusner.[62]

¶ Prognosis

Since body-image disturbances may occur within the context of any personality structure, only general statements may be made in regard to prognosis. The outcome of this form of personality disorder is basically dependent on the meaning of the bodily defect to the individual. The extent and disabling nature of the defect and the availability of rehabilitative services have a meaning to the patient which exists, as Kubie[82] emphasizes, on several levels of psychological functioning, i.e., the reality level, the level of conscious fantasy, and that of unconscious symbolic fantasy. Depending upon the individual, the loss may have any meaning, such as a heroic sacrifice or a deserved punishment, a realization of helplessness and vulnerability, a conviction of loathsomeness, a despicable mutilation to be hidden or accepted, or a rejection of the part with defiance toward society and social customs. The meaning may be determined only

* See references 2, 38, 114, 131, and 134.

through the psychiatric study of the individual.

A productive and satisfying social existence depends on acceptance of the changed body structure and the eventual establishment of a new body-image. The need for psychiatric treatment is evident in order to modify pathological and unconscious meanings of the change in the body structure which tend to perpetuate motivations that impede maximum recovery. But this treatment alone may be ineffective if it is not coupled with the skilled help of prosthetic experts and evaluation of vocational counselors. For some patients the attitude of responsible relatives and the local society may finally decide their success or failure in readapting to productive living. In these circumstances, educational programs designed to avoid cultural stereotyping and rejection relative to one or another disability are necessary. Attempts to predict psychogenic invalidism as a consequence of the disturbance of the body-image have been made by Bard[11] in relation to mastectomy, MacGregor and Schaffner[93] in relation to nasal plastic operations, and Fisher and Cleveland[48] in relation to amputation.

¶ Treatment

Prevention of body-image disturbance includes all those measures designed to avoid genetic and constitutional defects in bodily development. Consideration extends also to the role of industry and society generally in protecting the individual against accidental trauma. The individual's own psychological capacity for protecting himself against accidental injuries is certainly a preventive to the development of the body-image disorders. However, not only is the current state of knowledge in this area inadequate, but what is known is ineffectively applied or implemented by our present social structure.

Various means exist of strengthening the body-image and thereby enhancing ego functioning and self-esteem. They reside in the use of all those therapeutic procedures which allow for increased facility in use of the body musculature as in athletic games, dance, and posture as well as the correction of bodily defects through surgery, and cosmetic and rehabilitative efforts. It is important to conceptualize their treatment as ego enhancing—thus placing their prescriptions to the forefront in the therapeutic management of all patients suffering personality disorders associated with body-image disturbance. Goertzel et al.[55] have written specifically on dance therapy in this context.

In the instance of the individual confronted with an elective surgical procedure known to produce deformity, the psychiatrist and his medical and nursing colleagues may aid in the prevention of serious disturbance through proper use of the knowledge at hand. For those undergoing amputations or exposure to medications which produce body-image disruption, the preventive effects of proper preparation include advice as to the variety of body changes that may occur. In the case of amputation, the patient should be made aware of the occurrence of the phantom. Considerate inquiry into the patient's fears and anxieties is desirable. If a limb is to be amputated, the patient's desires as to its disposal and possible burial should be ascertained. Some initial discussions of the disability, its meaning to the patient, and compensation for it are advisable.

The family and other persons who are significant to the patient should be advised as to the expected posttreatment psychological and emotional phenomena. This is important, so that their aid may be immediately enlisted in the rehabilitation process and especially in ascertaining the possibility of the operation's emotional destructiveness to the patient. Watson and Johnson[143] have emphasized the significance of the attitude of parents in determining the management of amputation in children. Despite excellent preoperative preparation of both the child and parents for amputations for a bone tumor, the postoperative syndrome was complicated and aggravated by the denying and rejecting attitudes of the parents. Treatment should be instituted as quickly as possible when disruption of the

body structure leads to personality disorder. Failure to do so can result in fixation of chronic psychopathic reactions. In panic reactions with pain after limb amputations, the writer has utilized a brief psychotherapeutic technique in which the following topics have been penetrated in successive order from the initial interview: (1) the concept of the phantom-limb phenomenon and any attendant rationalizations regarding this; (2) wishes and fears relative to the disposal of the amputated part; and (3) the significance of present and past attitudes toward the body in relation to real or fantasied experiences with significant persons. This procedure has proved effective in alleviating panic and painful complaints in a number of limb amputees, among those with facial disfigurement following surgery, and in women with breast deformity consequent to thoracoplasty. It has also been utilized in initiating psychotherapy on amputees who have remained chronically disturbed for years following their loss.

In disturbances of the body-image that have led to chronic personality disorders, whether psychoneurotic or psychotic, the choice of therapy is dependent on the particular variety of reactions suffered by the individual. Various forms of psychotherapy[5,79,81,136] including psychoanalysis, hypnosis,[25] narcosynthesis,[56,79] electroshock therapy,[108,112] frontal lobe injection,[28] and treatment with the phenothiazines and antidepressants[97] have been reported effective. Indications for and techniques of application of these treatments are presented elsewhere in this *Handbook*.

(Bibliography

1. ABEL, T. M. "Figure Drawings in Facial Disfigurement," *Am. J. Orthopsychiatry*, 23 (1953), 253–264.
2. AITKEN, G. T. "Amputation as a Treatment for Certain Lower Extremity Abnormalities," *J. Bone Joint Surg.*, 41–A (1959), 1267–1287.
3. ANASTASOPOULOS, G. "Le Lobe pariétal et l'image de notre corps," *Med. Contemp.*, 73 (1955), 143–146.

4. APPENZELLER, O. and J. M. BICKNELL. "Effects of Nervous System Lesions on Phantom Experience," *Neurology*, 19 (1969), 141–146.

5. ARENSTEN, K. "Fantomoplevelsenhos en Amputeret Behandlet med Psykoterapi," *Nord. Med.*, 39 (1948), 1613.

6. ASCH, S. E. and H. A. WITKIN. "Studies in Space Orientation: I. Perception of the Upright with Displaced Visual Fields," *J. Exp. Psychol.*, 38 (1948), 325–337.

7. ———. "Studies in Space Orientation: II. Perception of the Upright with Displaced Visual Fields and with Body Tilted," *J. Exp. Psychol.*, 38 (1948), 455–477.

8. BACHET, M. and G. PADOVANI. "Refléxions sur le traitement psychothérapique des douleurs des amputés," *Ann. Med. Psychol. (Paris)*, 1 (1951), 206–211.

9. BAILEY, A. A. and F. P. MOERSCH. "Phantom Limb," *Can. Med. Assoc. J.*, 45 (1941), 37–42.

10. BAKER, W. Y. and L. H. SMITH. "Facial Disfigurement and Personality," *JAMA*, 112 (1939), 301–304.

11. BARD, M. "The Use of Dependence for Predicting Psychogenic Invalidism following Radical Mastectomy," *J. Nerv. Ment. Dis.*, 122 (1955), 152–160.

12. BENDER, L. "Psychoses Associated with Somatic Diseases that Distort the Body Structure," *Arch. Neurol. Psychiatry*, 32 (1934), 1000–1029.

13. ———. "Body Image Problems of the Brain Damaged," *J. Soc. Issues*, 4 (1948), 84–89.

14. BENDER, M. B. *Disorders in Perception.* Springfield, Ill.: Charles C. Thomas, 1952.

15. BENNETT, D. H. "The Body Concept," *J. Ment. Sci.*, 106 (1960), 56–75.

16. BLANK, R. H. "The Challenge of Rehabilitation," *Israel Med. J.*, 20 (1961), 127–142.

17. BLATT, E. F. "Body Image and Psychosomatic Illness," *Am. Psychol. Abstr.*, 18 (1963), 401–402.

18. BORS, E. "Phantom Limbs of Patients with Spinal Cord Injury," *Arch. Neurol. Psychiatry*, 66 (1951), 610–631.

19. BRESSLER, B., S. I. COHEN, and F. MAGNUSSEN. "Bilateral Breast Phantom and Breast Phantom Pain," *J. Nerv. Ment. Dis.*, 122 (1955), 315–320.

20. ———. "The Problem of Phantom Breast and Phantom Pain," *J. Nerv. Ment. Dis.*, 123 (1956), 181–187.

21. BROPHY, T. W. "The Deformity of Hare Lip and Cleft Palate," *Dent. Summ. (Toledo)*, 29 (1909), 465–471.

22. BYCHOWSKI, G. "Disorders of the Body Image in the Clinical Pictures of the Psychoses," *J. Nerv. Ment. Dis.*, 97 (1943), 310–335.

23. CARDONE, S. S. and R. OLSON. "Psychophysical Studies of Body-image," *Arch. Gen. Psychiatry*, 21 (1969), 464–469.

24. CATH, S. H., E. GLUD, and H. T. BLANE. "The Role of the Body Image in Psychotherapy with the Physically Handicapped," *Psychoanal. Rev.*, 44 (1957), 34–40.

25. CEDERCREUTZ, C. "Hypnotic Treatment of Phantom Sensations in 100 Amputees," *Acta. Chir. Scand.*, 107 (1954), 158–162.

26. CENTERS, L. and R. CENTERS. "A Comparison of the Body-images of Amputee and Non Amputee Children as Revealed in Figure Drawing," *J. Proj. Tech.*, 27 (1963), 158–165.

27. ———. "Peer Group Attitudes toward the Amputee Child," *J. Soc. Psychol.*, 61 (1963), 127–132.

28. COHEN, H. and H. W. JONES. "Reference of Cardiac Pain to a Phantom Left Arm," *Br. Heart J.*, 5 (1943), 67–71.

29. COOK, A. W. and W. H. DRUCKEMILLER. "Phantom Limb in Paraplegic Patients. Report of Two Cases and Analysis of Its Mechanism," *J. Neurosurg.*, 9 (1952), 508–516.

30. CORAH, N. L. and P. L. CORAH. "A Study of Body-image in Children with Cleft Palate and Cleft Lip," *J. Genet. Psychol.*, 103 (1963), 133–137.

31. CRONHOLM, B. "Phantom Limbs in Amputees; A Study of Changes in the Integration of Centripetal Impulses with Special Reference to Referred Sensations," *Acta. Psychiatr. Neurol. Scand., Suppl.*, 72 (1951), 310.

32. DE GUTIERREZ-MAHONEY, C. G. "Symposium on Neuro-Surgery: Treatment of Painful Phantom Limb: Follow-up Study," *Surg. Clin. North Am.*, 28 (1948), 481–483.

33. DEMBO, T., G. LADIEU-LEVITON, and B. A. WRIGHT. "Acceptance of Loss—Amputations," in I. F. Garrett, ed., *Psychological Aspects of Physical Disability*, ser. no. 210. Washington: Federal Security Agency, Office of Vocational Rehabilitation, 1952.

34. DORPAT, F. L. "Phantom Sensations of In-

ternal Organs," *Comp. Psychiatry*, 12 (1971), 27–35.

35. DRUSS, R. G., J. F. O'CONNOR, and L. O. STERN. "Changes in Body-image following Ileostomy," *Psychoanal. Q.*, 41 (1972), 195.

36. DUKE-ELDER, P. M. and E. WITTKOWER. "Psychological Reactions in Soldiers to the Loss of Vision of One Eye, and Their Treatment," *Br. Med. J.*, 1 (1946), 155–158.

37. DUPLAY, J. and P. COSSA. "Frontal Lobe Novocaine Injections as a Therapeutic Measure," *Ann. Med. Psychol. (Paris)*, 111 (1953), 33–40.

38. EASSON, W. M. "Body-image and Self-image in Children," *Arch. Gen. Psychiatry*, 4 (1961), 619–621.

29. ECHOLS, D. H. and J. A. COLCLOUGH. "Abolition of Painful Phantom Foot by Resection of the Sensory Cortex," *JAMA*, 134 (1947), 1476–1477.

40. EICKHOFF, L. F. W. "The Aetiology of Schizophrenia in Children," *J. Ment. Sci.*, 98 (1952), 229–234.

41. EIGENBRODE, C. R. and W. G. SHIPMAN. "The Body Image Barrier Concept," *J. Abnorm. Soc. Psychol.*, 60 (1960), 450–452.

42. ERICKSON, T. C., W. J. BLECKWENN, and C. N. WOOLSEY. "Observations on the Postcentral Gyrus in Relation to Pain," *Trans. Am. Neurol. Assoc.*, 77 (1952), 57–59.

43. EWALT, J. R., G. C. RANDALL, and H. MORRIS. "The Phantom Limb," *Psychosom. Med.*, 9 (1947), 118–123.

44. FEDERN, P. *Ego Psychology and the Psychoses*. New York: Basic Books, 1953.

45. FISHER, S. "Head-Body Differentiations in Body-Image and Skin Resistance Level," *J. Abnorm. Soc. Psychol.*, 60 (1960), 283–285.

46. ———. "A Further Appraisal of the Body Boundary Concept," *J. Consult. Psychol.*, 27 (1963), 62–74.

47. ———. "The Body-Image as a Source of Selective Cognitive Sets," *J. Pers.*, 33 (1965), 536–552.

48. FISHER, S. and S. E. CLEVELAND. "An Approach to Psychological Reactivity in Terms of a Body-Image Schema," *Psychol. Rev.*, 64 (1957), 26–37.

49. ———. *Body Image and Personality*. Princeton, N.J.: Van Norstrand, 1958.

50. FREDERIKS, J. A. M. "Occurrence and Nature of Phantom Limb Phenomena following Amputation of Body Parts and following Lesions of the Central and Peripheral Nervous Systems," *Psychiatr. Neurol. Neurochir.*, 66 (1963), 73–97.

51. FREUD, A. "The Role of Bodily Illness in the Mental Life of Children," in *The Psychoanalytic Study of the Child*, Vol. 7, pp. 69–81. New York: International Universities Press, 1952.

52. GALLINEK, A. "The Phantom Limb: Its Origin and Its Relationship to the Hallucinations of Psychotic States," *Am. J. Psychiatry*, 96 (1939), 413–422.

53. GESELL, A. and F. L. ILG. *Infant and Child in the Culture of Today*. New York: Harper, 1942.

54. GILDER, R., S. V. THOMPSON, C. W. SLACK et al. "Amputation, Body-Image and Perceptual Distortion: a Preliminary Study," *Res. Rep., Nav. Med. Res. Inst.*, 12 (1954), 587.

55. GOERTZEL, V., P. R. A. MAY, J. SALKEN et al. "Body-Ego Technique: An Approach to the Schizophrenic Patient," *J. Nerv. Ment. Dis.*, 141 (1965), 53–60.

56. GUILLAUME, J. F. and G. MAZARS. "Traitement des membres fantômes douloureux par psychothérapie sous narcose ou hypnose," *Rev. Neurol.*, 79 (1947), 213–215.

57. HALPERN, S. "Body-Image Symbols of Repression," *Int. J. Clin. Exp. Hypn.*, 13 (1965), 83–91.

58. HARRIS, J. E. "Elucidation of Body-Imagery in Chronic Schizophrenia," *Arch. Gen. Psychiatry*, 16 (1967), 679–684.

59. HARVEY, F. "Some Social Aspects in the Case of Patients Undergoing Breast Surgery," *Med. Soc. Work*, 4 (1955), 99–110.

60. HEAD, H. *Studies in Neurology*. London: Oxford, 1920.

61. HENDERSON, W. R. and G. E. SMYTH. "Phantom Limbs," *J. Neurol. Neurosurg. Psychiatry*, 11 (1948), 88–112.

62. HEUSNER, A. P. "Phantom Genitalia," *Trans. Am. Neurol. Assoc.*, 75 (1950), 128–131.

63. HIRSCH, S. J. "Left, Right and Identity," *Arch. Gen. Psychiatry*, 14 (1966), 84–88.

64. HOFFER, W. "Mouth, Hand and Ego-Integration," in *The Psychoanalytic Study of the Child*, Vol. 3/4, pp. 49–56. New York: International Universities Press, 1949.

65. HOFFMAN, J. "Facial Phantom Phenomenon," *J. Nerv. Ment. Dis.*, 122 (1955), 143–151.

66. ———. "Phantom Limb Syndrome. A Critical Review of the Literature," *J. Nerv. Ment. Dis.*, 119 (1954), 261–270.

67. HUGHES, J. and W. L. WHITE. "Amputee Rehabilitation: Emotional Reactions and Adjustment of Amputees to Their Injury," *U.S. Nav. Med. Bull. Suppl.* (March 1946), 157–163.

68. HUNT, R. G. and M. J. FELDMAN. "Body-Image and Ratings of Adjustment on Human Figure Drawings," *J. Clin. Psychol.*, 16 (1960), 35–38.

69. HUNT, V. V. and M. E. WEBER. "Body-Image Projective Test," *J. Proj. Tech.*, 24 (1960), 3–10.

70. JACKSON, J. H. *Neurological Fragments: With Biographical Memoir by James Taylor, and Including the "Recollections" of the Late Sir Jonathan Hutchinson and the Late Dr. Charles Mercier.* London: Oxford University Press, 1925.

71. JACOBSON, J. R. "A Method of Psychobiologic Evaluation," *Am. J. Psychiatry*, 101 (1944), 343–348.

72. JARVIS, J. H. "Post Mastectomy Breast Phantoms," *J. Nerv. Ment. Dis.*, 144 (1967), 266–272.

73. JOHNSON, F. A. "Figure Drawings in Subjects Recovering from Poliomyelitis," *Psychosom. Med.*, 34 (1972), 19–29.

74. JUNG, C. G. *Psychology of the Unconscious.* New York: Dodd-Mead, 1931.

75. KINZEL, A. F. "Body-Buffer Zone in Violent Prisoners," *Am. J. Psychiatry*, 127 (1970), 99–104.

76. KIPNIS, D. M. "Changes in Self Concept in Relation to Perception of Others," *J. Pers.*, 29 (1961), 449–465.

77. KIRK, N. T. "The Development of Amputation," *Bull. Med. Libr. Assoc.*, 32 (1944), 132–163.

78. KOLB, L. C. "Somatic Sensory Extinction Phenomenon and Body Schema after Unilateral Resection of the Posterior Central Gyrus," *Trans. Am. Neurol. Assoc.*, 75 (1950), 138–141.

79. ———. *The Painful Phantom. Psychology, Physiology and Treatment.* Springfield, Ill.: Charles C. Thomas, 1954.

80. ———. "The Body-Image in the Schizophrenic Reaction," in A. Auerbach, ed., *Schizophrenia: An Integrated Approach*, pp. 87–97. New York: Ronald, 1959.

81. KOLB, L. C., L. M. FRANK, and E. J. WATSON. "Treatment of the Acute Painful Phantom Limb," *Proc. Staff Meet. Mayo Clin.*, 27 (1952), 110–118.

82. KUBIE, L. "Motivation and Rehabilitation," *Psychiatry*, 8 (1945), 69–78.

83. LADIEU, G., E. HANFMANN, and T. DEMBO. "Studies in Adjustment to Visible Injuries, Evaluation of Help by the Injured," *J. Abnorm. Soc. Psychol.*, 42 (1947), 169–192.

84. LAMBERT, C. N. and J. SCIARRA. "A Questionnaire Survey of Juvenile to Young Adult Amputees who had had Prosthesis Supplied Them through the University of Illinois Division of Services for Crippled Children," *J. Bone Joint. Surg.*, 41A (1959), 1437–1454.

85. LANGWORTHY, O. R. "Development of Behavior Patterns and Myelinization of the Nervous System in the Human Fetus and Infant," *Contrib. Embryol.*, 443 (1933), 1–57.

86. LEVIN, M. "The Concept of Denial and Its Limitations, with Remarks on Phantom Limb Disorientation and Perseveration," *J. Neuropsychiatry*, 2 (1961), 167–174.

87. LEVY, D. M. "Method of Integrating Physical and Psychiatric Examination with Special Studies of Body Interest, Overt Protection Response to Growth and Sex Difference," *Am. J. Psychiatry*, 9 (1929), 121–194.

88. ———. "Body Interest in Children and Hypochondriasis," *Am. J. Psychiatry*, 12 (1932), 295–315.

89. LHERMITTE, J. "L'Image de notre corps," *Nouv. Rev. Crit.*, (1939), 256 pp.

90. LINN, L. "Some Developmental Aspects of the Body Image," *Int. J. Psycho-Anal.*, 36 (1955), 36–42.

91. LINN, L. and I. B. GOLDMAN. "Psychiatric Observations Concerning Rhinoplasty," *Psychosom. Med.*, 11 (1949), 307–314.

92. MACGREGOR, F. C., T. M. ABEL, A. BRYT et al. *Facial Deformities, and Plastic Surgery.* Springfield, Ill.: Charles C. Thomas, 1953.

93. MACGREGOR, F. C. and B. SCHAFFNER. "Screening Patients for Nasal Plastic Operations," *Psychosom. Med.*, 12 (1950), 277–291.

94. MACHOVER, K. *Personality Projection in the Drawing of the Human Figure.* Springfield, Ill.: Charles C. Thomas, 1957.

95. MEDNICK, S. A. "The Body Barriers Go Rorschach: Review of Body-Image and

Personality by Fisher, S. and Seymour, S. E., 1958," *Contemp. Psychol.*, 4 (1959), 276–277.

96. Meerloo, J. A. M. "The Fate of One's Face," *Psychiatric Q.*, 30 (1956), 31–43.

97. Miles, J. E. "Psychoses with Phantom Limb Treated by Chlorpromazine," *Am. J. Psychiatry*, 112 (1956), 1027–1028.

98. Mitchell, S. W. "Phantom Limbs," *Lippincott's Mag. Pop. Lit. Sci.*, 8 (1871), 563–569.

99. Noble, D., M. E. Roudebush, and D. Price. "Studies of Korean War Casualties, Part I: Psychiatric Manifestations in Wounded Men," *Am. J. Psychiatry*, 108 (1952), 495–499.

100. Noble, D., D. B. Price, and R. Gilder. "Psychiatric Disturbances following Amputation," *Am. J. Psychiatry*, 110 (1954), 609–613.

101. Orbach, J. "Psychophysical Studies of Body-Image," *Arch. Gen. Psychiatry*, 14 (1966), 41–47.

102. Paré, A. *The Workes of That Famous Chirurgion, Ambrose Parey.* Translated out of the Latin and compared with the French by T. Johnson. London: Cotes, 1649.

103. Pazat, P. and P. Grateau. "Phantom Hearing (Tinnitus) after Amputation of the Auditory Field by Sonic Traumatism," *Rev. Otoneuroophtalmol.*, 42 (1970), 81–90.

104. Perrin, F. A. C. "Physical Attractiveness and Repulsiveness," *J. Exp. Psychol.*, 4 (1921), 203–217.

105. Peto, A. "Body-Image and Archaic Thinking," *Int. J. Psychoanal.*, 40 (1959), 223–231.

106. Pick, A. "Zur Pathologic des Bewusstseins vom eigenen Körper. Ein Beitrag an Kriegsmedizin," *Neurol. Zentralbl.*, 34 (1915), 257–265.

107. Pick, J. F. "Ten Years of Plastic Surgery in a Penal Institution," *J. Int. Coll. Surgeons*, 11 (1948), 315–319.

108. Pisetsky, J. E. "Disappearance of Painful Phantom Limbs after Electric Shock Treatment," *Am. J. Psychiatry*, 102 (1946), 599–601.

109. Pollack, M. and W. Goldfarb. "The Face-Hand Test in Schizophrenic Children," *Arch. Neurol. Psychiatry*, 77 (1957), 635–642.

110. Pool, J. L. and T. J. Bridges. "Subcortical Parietal Lobotomy for Relief of Phantom Limb Syndrome in the Upper Extremity," *Bull. N.Y. Acad. Med.*, 30 (1954), 302–309.

111. Price, D. B., N. J. Twombly. "A. Lemos: Dedolore Membri Amputati Remanente Explicatio (1798). The Phantom Limb: An Eighteenth Century Latin Dissertation Text and Translation with a Medical Historical and Linguistic Commentary," in *Languages and Linguistics*, Working Papers. Washington: Georgetown University Press, 1972.

112. Radovici, A. and N. Wertheim. "L'Electrochoc comme traitement des douleurs irreductibles. (Causalgie, Neuralgie Rebelle, Douleurs des morphinomanes. Crises subintrantes tabetiques)," *Presse Med.*, 54 (1949), 754–755.

113. Renneker, R. and M. Cutler. "Psychological Problems of Adjustment to Cancer of the Breast," *JAMA*, 148 (1952), 833–838.

114. Resnik, H. L. P. "Suicide Attempt by a Child after Amputation," *JAMA* 212 (1970), 1211–1212.

115. Riddoch, G. "Phantom Limbs and Body Shape," *Brain*, 64 (1941), 197–222.

116. Riese, W. and G. Bruck. "Le Membre fantomes chez l'enfant," *Rev. Neurol.*, 83 (1950), 221–222.

117. Ross, N. "The Postural Model of the Head and Face in Various Positions (Experiments on Normals)," *J. Gen. Psychol.*, 7 (1932), 144–162.

118. Schilder, P. *The Image and Appearance of the Human Body. Studies in the Constructive Energies of the Psyche.* London: Kegan Paul, 1935.

119. Schonfeld, W. A. "Gynecomastia in Adolescence," *Arch. Gen. Psychiatry*, 5 (1961), 68–76.

120. Schontz, F. C. "Body Concept Disturbances of Patients with Hemiplegia," *J. Clin. Psychol.*, 12 (1956), 293–295.

121. Scott, W. C. M. "Some Embryological, Neurological, Psychiatric and Psychoanalytic Implications of the Body Scheme," *Int. J. Psychoanal.*, 29 (1948), 141–155.

122. Secord, P. "Objectification of Word-Association Procedures by the Use of Homonyms: A Measure of Body Cathexis," *J. Pers.*, 21 (1952–1953), 479–495.

123. Secord, P. and S. M. Jourard. "The Appraisal of Body Cathexis: Body Cathexis and the Self," *J. Consult. Psychol*, 17 (1953), 343–347.

124. SELECKI, R. B. and J. T. HERRON. "Disturbances of the Verbal Body-Image; A Particular Syndrome of Sensory Aphasia," *J. Nerv. Ment. Dis.*, 141 (1965), 42–52.

125. SIMMEL, M. L. "Phantoms in Patients with Leprosy and in Elderly Digital Amputees," *Am. J. Psychol,* 69 (1956), 529–545.

126. ———. "Phantom Experiences in Mental Defective Amputees," *J. Abnorm. Soc. Psychol.*, 59 (1959), 128–129.

127. ———. "Phantom, Phantom Pain and 'Denial'," *Am. J. Psychother.*, 13 (1959), 603–613.

128. ———. "The Absence of Phantoms for Congenitally Missing Limbs," *Am. J. Psychol.*, 74 (1961), 467–470.

129. ———. "Phantom Experiences following Amputation in Childhood," *J. Neurol. Neurosurg. Psychiatry*, 25 (1962), 69–78.

130. ———. "A Study of Phantoms after Amputation of the Breast," *Neuropsychol.*, 4 (1966), 337–350.

131. SIMPSON, E. B. and H. F. ALBRONDA. "Psychologic Aspects of Amputation of a Lower Limb," *Lancet*, 87 (1967), 429–431.

132. SMYTHIES, J. R. "The Experience and Description of the Human Body," *Brain*, 76 (1953), 132–145.

133. SOUQUES, A. and POISOT. "Origine périphérique des hallucinations des membres amputés," *Rev. Neurol.*, 13 (1905), 1112–1116.

134. SPRING, J. M. and C. H. EPPS, JR. "The Juvenile Amputee. Some Observations and Considerations," *Clin. Pediatr.*, (Phila.), 7 (968), 76–79.

135. STERN, K., A. LARIVIERE, and G. FOUNIER. "Psychiatric Aspects of Cosmetic Surgery of the Nose," *Can. Med. Assoc. J.*, 76 (1957), 469–472.

136. STROTZKA, H. "Psychotherapie des Phantom Schmerzes," *Klin. Med.*, 3 (1948), 172.

137. SZASZ, T. S. "Psychiatric Aspects of Vagotomy: IV. Phantom Ulcer Pain," *Arch. Neurol. Psychiatry*, 62 (1949), 728–733.

138. ———. *Pain and Pleasure*, New York: Basic Books, 1957.

139. TAYLOR, J., G. HOLMES, and F. M. R. WALSHE. *Selected Writings of John Hughlings Jackson*, Vol. 1, On Epilepsy and Epileptiform Convulsions. New York: Basic Books, 1958.

140. THORNTON, G. R. "The Effect upon Judgements of Personality Traits of Varying a Single Factor in a Photograph," *J. Soc. Psychol.*, 18 (1943), 127–148.

141. UPDEGRAFF, H. L. and K. A. MENNINGER. "Some Psychoanalytic Aspects of Plastic Surgery," *Am. J. Surg.*, 25 (1934), 554–558.

142. WACHS, H. and M. ZAKS. "Studies of Body-Image in Men with Spinal Cord Injury," *J. Nerv. Ment. Dis.*, 131 (1960), 121.

143. WATSON, E. J. and A. M. JOHNSON. "The Emotional Significance of Acquired Physical Disfigurement in Children," *Am. J. Orthopsychiatry*, 28 (1958), 85–97.

144. WEINSTEIN, S. and E. A. SERSEN. "Phantoms in Case of Congenital Absence of Limbs," *Neurol.*, 11 (1961), 905–911.

145. WHITE, J. C. and W. H. SWEET. "Effectiveness of Chordotomy in Phantom Pain after Amputation," *Arch. Neurol. Psychiatry*, 67 (1952), 315–322.

146. WILLE, W. S. "Figure Drawings in Amputees," *Psychiatr. Q.*, (Suppl.), 28 (1954), 192–198.

147. WITKEN, H. *Personality Through Perception*. New York: Harper, 1954.

148. WRIGHT, G. H. "The Names of the Parts of the Body. A Linguistic Approach to the Study of the Body Image," *Brain*, 79 (1956), 188–210.

149. WYSOCKI, B. A. and E. WHITNEY. "Body-Image of Crippled Children as Seen in Draw-a-Person Test Behavior," *Percept. Mot. Skills*, 21 (1965), 499–504.

150. ZADOR, J. "Meskalinwirkung auf das Phantomglied," *Monatsschr. Psychiatr. Neurol.*, 77 (1930), 71–99.

CHAPTER 34

COMPLEX PROBLEMS OF PAIN AS SEEN IN HEADACHE, PAINFUL PHANTOM, AND OTHER STATES

Shervert H. Frazier

To the sociologist, pain and the threat of pain are powerful instruments of learning and social preservation. To the biologist, pain is a sensory signal that warns the individual when a harmful stimulus threatens injury. To the physiologist, pain is a sensation like seeing or hearing, but he tends to ignore its conscious perceptual aspects, because consciousness has as yet no physiological equivalents; one might say that he is studying the pain "signal." To the psychologist, on the other hand, the important thing about pain is the brain's translation of the signal into a sensory experience. He finds pain, like all perceptions, to be subjective, individual, and modified by degrees of attention, emotional states, and the conditioning influence of past experience. To a man with an incurable cancer, pain is a destructive force. His suffering began too late to serve as an effective warning and it did not stop after the warning had been given.

To the layman, the sensation of pain, which he has known all his life, seems a perfectly straightforward, noncontroversial matter. "Hot" and "sharp" were among the first words he learned; his earliest memories are associated with the pain of accidental injury and of parental discipline; when he was hurt, he struggled and cried out. Man has accepted these reactions as the natural manifestations of physical suffering. Experience has taught him that pain can be caused by many different kinds of stimuli, even those such as heat or pressure which are distinctly pleasant in moderate intensities. Almost all parts of his body are sensitive to pain, and he assumes that other people are equally sensitive. He knows that pain is caused by physical injury, and believes that its intensity is proportional to the force of a blow, the heat of an iron, or the depth of a wound.

While this concept of pain as a physical quantum, measurable in terms of stimulus intensity or the body's response to injury, seems a reasonable everyday interpretation, there are many situations in which it does not apply. Superficial wounds usually are more painful than deep ones, because the skin is much more richly supplied with sensory nerve endings than are the deeper tissues. Bullet wounds are usually painless, partly because the impact of the missile can temporarily paralyze nerve conduction. Most internal organs can be cut, crushed, or burned without causing distress. There also are enormous individual variations in sensitivity to pain. At one extreme are patients with such conditions as causalgia, facial neuralgia, or postherpetic pain, their skin so sensitive that the lightest touch or even a breath of air precipitates an acute exacerbation of pain. At the other extreme are those unfortunate children who can lean against a hot stove without being distressed, who constantly injure themselves because they were born without normal susceptibility to pain, i.e., congenital indifference to pain.

The obvious biological significance of pain leads one to expect that it must always occur after injury, and to conclude that the intensity of pain felt is proportional to the amount and extent of the tissue damage. Actually, in higher species at least, there is much evidence that pain is not simply a function of the amount of bodily damage alone, but rather that the amount and quality of pain felt are also determined by previous experiences and how well memory substantiates them, by an individual's ability to understand the cause of the pain and to grasp its consequences, and even by the significance of pain in one's own family or group culture.

Considerable evidence shows that persons also attach variable meanings to pain-producing situations, and that these meanings greatly influence the degree and quality of pain felt. During World War II, Beecher[2] observed the behavior of soldiers severely wounded in battle. He found that when the badly wounded were carried into combat hospitals, only one of three complained of enough pain to require morphine. Most of the soldiers either denied having any pain or had so little discomfort as to require no medication for relief. These patients were not in a state of shock, nor unusually stoic, nor totally unable to feel pain; for example, vigorous complaints about inept vein puncture were made. When Beecher returned to civilian practice as an anesthesiologist, he tested a group of patients, who had just undergone major surgery with incisions similar to the wounds received by the soldiers, to determine whether relief of pain was required. In contrast to the wounded soldiers, four of five were in such severe distress as to require relief.

Beecher concluded that "... the common belief that wounds are inevitably associated with pain, that the more extensive the wound the worse the pain, was not supported by observations made as carefully as possible in the combat zone. ... There is no simple direct relationship between the wound per se and the pain experienced. The pain is in very large part determined by other factors, and of great importance here is the significance of the wound. ... In the wounded soldier (the response to injury) was relief, thankfulness at his escape alive from the battlefield, even euphoria; to the civilian, major surgery was a depressing, calamitous event."

The importance of the meaning associated with a pain-producing situation is made particularly clear in conditioning experiments carried out by the Russian physiologist, Ivan Pavlov.[36] Dogs normally react violently when given strong electric shocks to the paw. Pavlov found, however, that if dogs were consistently presented food after each shock, the animal developed a new response. Immediately after a shock, the dog would salivate, wag its tail, and turn toward the food dish. The electric shock now failed to evoke any responses indicative of pain and became instead a signal indicating that food was on the way. The dog's conditioned behavior persisted when Pavlov increased the intensity of the electric shocks and even when they were supplemented by burning and wounding the dog's skin. Masserman carried the experiment further.[34] After cats had been taught to respond to an electric shock as a signal for feeding, they were trained to administer the shock themselves by walking up to a switch and closing it.

(The Transmission and Perception of Pain

An excellent survey of medical concepts of pain has been written by Prococci;[38] Clark and Hunt have updated these theories comprehensively.[5] In the specific sensory-transmission system, epicritic or bright pain is thought to pass readily from the dorsal root into the spinothalamic tracts to the thalamus, and thence into the sensory cortex. Pain thresholds are known to be altered by the state of excitation of the reticular system of the internuncial pool and by the state of discharge from cortical centers.

The nonspecific sensory system—the reticular activating system—is known to receive collaterals from the specific fiber pathways to convey sensations of pain, as well as other sensations. The discovery of this system and its functions provides one of the links explaining certain clinical paradoxes. This system has the capacity for the modulation of sensory attentiveness. Thus, the severely wounded soldier can be nonattentive to pain when some other state of awareness such as strong feelings, fear of death, or great joy at being alive, is overriding. It may be speculated that reactions to pain, or the seeming lack of response observed in the wounded of various nations, may be modulated by cortical influences directed to the reticular activating system and then variously fed back to both the cortex and the periphery. It is known now that, when stimu-

lated in the bulbar and reticular areas, this system is capable of blocking afferent volleys in the spinal cord. There is evidence that a physiological system exists that may either intensify or lessen an incoming sensation and, in fact, may defend the organism against too intense a stimulation or heighten its capacity to attend threats to the system.

Of particular interest to the clinician is the fact that transmission of impulses within the nonspecific activating system may be modified by pharmacological means. It appears that anesthetics exert their primary effect in blocking conscious response to noxious stimuli by dampening conduction through this system. Very likely the phenothiazine derivatives, important in clinical psychiatry, act upon this system as well. The modern psychological and pharmacological modes of sensory alarm functioning allow more comprehensive explanation of many of the variable expressions of pain found in the clinic.

No longer can complex pain problems be explained solely by relying upon the older concept of a specific sensation from the periphery to the cortex. Instead, the concept of a prolonged or intractable painful or anesthetic state is a perceptual action system designed to signal either distress or, paradoxically, gratification of pleasure.

Perceptual processes are established by repetitive experience encoded in the large cortical areas of the brain, where, in turn, the adaptive patterns of behavior are coded. To the physiological model of the systems subserving pain must be added the great modifying influences of man's cerebral cortex wherein are implanted the long and continuing experiences of suffering, and the adaptive behavioral patterns for relief that are initiated at birth and expanded, from experience, throughout life. These learning experiences occur primarily in the human environment, the surrounding persons, most notably the family, who inflict and assuage pain.

The experience of pain signifies to the patient that he is suffering structural or functional damage. When this percept is conveyed to the clinician as a complaint, the latter commonly interprets it as a consequence of a "physical" or "organic" lesion. Although the pain percept is an innate response to injury to the organism, its associated complaint in language may be modified by learning processes established by the family and the cultural environment. Through the learning experiences, a patient's complaint of pain may communicate not only a signal of bodily damage but also a message of social importance, that of a need for help or for pleasurable gratification through a supportive relationship with another person. One may intensify this conditioning through the secondary gratification obtained by the avoidance of the painful stimuli. Here is the source of the difficulty in establishing the meaning of the symptom in chronic pain conditions.

The symbolic meaning of the symptom of pain is established in the manner in which an individual has learned to complain, or not complain, and to use the symptom of pain as a means of relating himself to others. The clinician's ability to understand this meaning for each individual determines the ultimate ability to assay the proper meaning, initiate the indicated intervention, and provide the person with a rational management devoid of untherapeutic emotionality. Confronted with the complex problem of a patient complaining of a long-standing painful condition, the clinician must ascertain not only whether there exists a physical disability causing a painful percept but also: (1) Will a physical procedure relieve the symptom? (2) Is the symptom expressive of a psychiatric disability? (3) Will removal of the symptom unmask a serious personality disorder? (4) Will this, in turn, result in serious interpersonal issues and even, perhaps, in eventual medico-legal problems?

What is the investigative evidence to support the contention that the pain complaint often has meaning determined by other than the activation of a specific sensory system? Hardy, Wolff, and Goodell[28] attempted to study the response of various individuals to the measured amount of energy required to induce a threshold pain. This they did by exposing a small area of the skin to radiant heat and asking the subject to indicate the feeling of pain. Only by using trained subjects was it possible to obtain a relatively fixed pain threshold.

Various other investigators have failed to substantiate any consistency in the pain threshold, and have discovered that it might be increased as much as 40 percent by hypnosis and could be altered by analgesics as well as by suggestion. Furthermore, such studies make it apparent that in addition to the pain threshold there also is a highly variable threshold for reaction to pain that is highly individualistic. What has been learned from these careful studies is that the responses to painful stimuli vary greatly in relation to the personality makeup and emotional state of the particular individual, and also that the responses to painful stimuli vary among different individuals.

This point is illustrated by observations on various unsatisfactory therapeutic efforts. Penman[37] studied 275 patients successfully treated by alcohol injection of the Gasserian ganglion for trigeminal neuralgia. Only 20–25 percent were relieved of the pain by this procedure; 22 percent reported that they were worse off than before treatment. In the latter group there was either an obsessive preoccupation with the resulting paresthesia or an eruption of neurotic or psychotic symptoms. In the dissatisfied group were found dependent, inactive, and elderly persons, all of whom had suffered pain at least six months before treatment was given. This emphasized once again the influence of personality organization and the significance of the pain to the adaptability of the person.

That cultural influences determine the individual's reaction to pain has been demonstrated in the report by the sociologist, Zborowski,[56] who examined the attitudes of Italian, Jewish, and old American patients (those who had lived three generations in the United States) when confronted by a painful illness. Some were described by the doctors as being "emotional" in responses to pain. The underlying attitudes toward pain were different, however, in the several groups. Some patients seemed concerned mainly with the immediate fear of the pain experience and were disturbed by the actual pain sensations experienced in a given situation, while some patients reported concern about the symptomatic meaning of the pain, the significance of the pain to their health and to the welfare of their families. It was noticed that once the pain was relieved, some patients dismissed their suffering and reported contentment. Other patients were reluctant to accept drug therapy, worried over the effect of the drug upon health, were concerned that the drug would not be curative, and sometimes hid the pain-relieving medication. Finally, even if the pain were relieved, some patients were often depressed and worried, fearful that the disease was not cured.

These observations are of importance in the management of pain problems. With pain of immediate importance to the patient, the physician has to provide early and adequate relief; whereas with pain-threatened patients, one must relieve the anxiety in regard to the source of the pain, as well as the pain itself. The members of some groups are not fearful of expressing their emotions. They complain a great deal, call for help, and expect sympathy and assistance from their families. Although this behavior is approved and accepted in their culture, it is not accepted by certain other patients. The physician, too, may easily be provoked to distrust and dislike patients because they do not conform to the doctor's ideas and patterns of acceptable behavior in facing painful illness. Some more stoic patients tend to minimize responses to pain and to avoid complaining and provoking pity. They are anxious to cooperate with those who are expected to take care of them.

Whenever a patient describes a painful illness, the physician who knows that some emotional disturbance is associated in time with the onset or recurrence of his complaint should suspect that psychic processes are operative in its maintenance. Most frequently such events are the death of or separation from a parent, spouse, or lover; difficulties in relations with an employer or some parental figure; or threat of illness. Some patients with an emotionally motivated, painful complaint have intermittent attacks of pain that may be induced through discussion of the appropriate anxiety-laden topics. Others, notably those in whom the pain represents one of the symptoms of an obsessive neurosis, a hypochondriacal state, or a depression, complain of a more or less persistent symptom. In such instances, the psychic conflict is less easily identified.

Patients complaining of suffering from intractable headache, backache, atypical facial pains, pain in phantom extremities or other parts, who seem entirely undisturbed by their symptoms but suddenly grasp at the affected part when the interview is finally focused on their important personal conflict, make the difficulty apparent to the skillful examiner who should push on with further inquiries and not be distracted by the symptom. Also, in psychotherapy, patients often actively hallucinate pain in localized bodily areas before revealing the distressing interpersonal events underlying the painful experience.

❴ Headache

One of the most common pain syndromes which every psychiatrist sees in patients is headache. The terms "headache" and "head pain" refer to a variety of symptoms and syndromes of diverse origins, produced by many mechanisms. An excellent classification has been made by the Ad Hoc Committee on Classification of Headache.[1]

1. Vascular headache of migraine type
   a. classic migraine
   b. common migraine
   c. cluster headache
   d. hemiplegic and ophthalmoplegic migraine
   e. lower-half headache
2. Muscle-contraction headache
3. Combined headache, vascular and muscle contraction
4. Headache of nasal vasomotor reaction
5. Headache of delusional, conversion, or hypochondriacal states
6. Nonmigrainous vascular headaches
7. Traction headaches

8. Headache due to overt cranial inflammation
9.–13. Headache due to disease of ocular, aural, nasal, sinusal, dental, or other cranial or neck structures
14. Cranial neuritides
15. Cranial neuralgias

Psychiatric or psychogenic aspects of headache are specifically involved in the vascular, muscle contraction, combined, delusional, conversional, and hypochondriacal states, and also—to a lesser secondary extent—in the other types. An excellent review of the literature on psychogenic headache has been written by Boag.[3] Headache is a symptom, not a disease. Psychological factors may be precipitating, conversional, or a factor in the selection of the head as the body part in delusional and hypochondriacal states. In every headache problem, thorough medical and neurological evaluation should precede or be conducted concomitantly with the psychological and psychiatric evaluation. The clinical features, including major and minor criteria, physiological factors, psychological factors, and treatment will be noted only for the types of headache most likely to be seen by the psychiatrist.

Vascular Headaches of Migraine or Its Variants

CLINICAL FEATURES

Sharply defined neurological or visual prodromata usually precede the onset of a one-sided headache of two to four hours' duration. The pain is usually in the anterior part of the head, quite intense, commonly associated with nausea and vomiting. Early in the headache phase, the pain is throbbing or pulsatile. Mood disturbances may accompany the prodromal or headache phase, or both. In some patients the involved cranial artery may be visible, palpable, and tender. Neurological complications such as ophthalmoplegia, hemiplegia, and speech disorders may accompany the attack. A family history of such headaches is found in two-thirds of the patients.

Vascular headache variants are facial cephalgia, weekend headache, and menstrual headache. These types usually do not have sharply defined prodromata, may last from two to twenty-four hours, are of variable severity, and may change from throbbing to a steady ache. Cluster headaches occur in clusters of short duration, usually without prodromata, are strictly unilateral, and almost always on the same side in the anterior or orbital distribution. The pain is severe, accompanied by nasal and ocular congestion, occasionally with miosis and ptosis, and precipitated by vasodilators such as alcohol.

PHYSIOLOGICAL FACTORS

Arterial dilation and surrounding tissue reaction occur concomitantly. Often one major artery in the carotid system becomes dilated, but constriction may precede dilation. The cause of the arterial changes is not known, but evidence suggests a neurogenic factor with subsequent accumulation of tissue substances which produce small-vessel dilation, edema, and tenderness. Vasomotor centers and the cerebral cortex play a major factor in the central origin.

PSYCHOLOGICAL FACTORS

Recent studies of a series of vascular-headache patients reveal that while no single personality type predisposes to the vascular headache, many patients of the obsessional personality type may be liable because they suppress or repress anger or rage by supercontrol mechanisms. Substitutionary or compensatory perfectionism, ambition, success-striving, and excessive environmental demands may produce vulnerability to autonomic nervous system stress, as well as situational and intrapsychic conflicts. As a group, the patients are intelligent and demonstrate unusual adaptational patterns to cope with life stresses.

Difficulties in adapting to major phases of the life cycle, such as adolescence, menstruation, separation from home and family, starting work, changing jobs, marriage and parenthood, or in dealing with critical life crises, such as the death of a spouse or being passed over for promotion, may precipitate bouts of vascular headache. In many vascular-headache patients, an underlying core of depression may be demonstrated when the usual defense mechanisms are no longer successful in maintaining repression. The majority of migraine sufferers who come to psychiatrists (and certainly we see only a few of them) are from families who take great pride in attainment, follow rigid forms of behavior, and deny the expression of direct or verbal aggression. Because such families punish members who defy these standards by excluding them from the family group, any feelings of resentment or hostility toward a parent or another close person tend, therefore, to be deeply rejected or repressed, producing conflict with associated anxiety. The struggle between inevitable emerging hostility and the need to maintain the family standards in order to continue the desired relationships shapes the interpersonal matrix that triggers the headache.

Not infrequently, the anticipation of the headaches becomes a crippling life pattern, and the patient may show increasing withdrawal from personal responsibility and socialization. When psychopharmacological treatment accompanied by psychotherapy is successful, many patients find attacks of vascular headache less frequent, less severe, and life more bearable.

TREATMENT

Migraine is most successfully treated with ergotamine tartrate with caffeine. Associated symptoms may be treated with antispasmodics, antiemetics, or sedatives. Best control is attained when the medication is taken early in the prodroma stage of the headache. The variants do not respond so dramatically to ergotamine and caffeine. Cluster headaches are notorious in their difficulty of treatment; some respond to ergotamine tartrate, but many do not. Although pain relief is a major goal, narcotics are dangerous because of the recurrent nature of the illness. Psychotherapy of a joint-venture type is especially helpful in teaching the patient alternative adaptational patterns to life stresses. Psychoanalyses have been reported in detail by Brenner and associates,[4] Fromm-Reichmann,[22] Selinsky,[44] Sperling,[47,48] and Robinson.[40] Psychopharmaco-

logical treatment of depression with tricyclic antidepressants is indicated. Because the depressions are unipolar, one must try the various substances such as imipramine hydrochloride or amitriptyline hydrochloride in order to find which type of tricyclic drug is effective for a particular patient. Sufficient dosage must be utilized. Alcohol must be specifically prohibited to those persons who are sensitive to it. While the prevention of headaches is not very successful, methysergide maleate has been useful, but must be carefully monitored because of side effects and complications in therapy.[19]

Muscle-Contraction Headache

CLINICAL FEATURES

Autogenic feedback mechanisms have been reported as successful in the treatment of migraine and muscle-contraction headaches. Recurrent, of variable severity, and persisting from several hours to days, muscle-contraction headaches are described as dull, pressing, or aching. The pain is suboccipital, usually bilateral, and extends to other areas of the head, including frontal, temporal, and band-around-the-head, and may also involve the facial musculature. The scalp and neck may be tender on pressure with the hand. Prodromata are not present, and nausea and vomiting are rare. The headache may be temporally related in onset to a specific stress. Family history is usually unimpressive.

PHYSIOLOGICAL FACTORS

Ischemia is a possible factor in producing muscle contraction and pain. It is presumed that tension and emotional stress can cause muscle tightening with prolonged muscle contraction.

PSYCHOLOGICAL FACTORS

Persons of every personality type have been demonstrated to be subject to muscle-contraction headaches. States of prolonged chronic anxiety are most common. Irritability, depression, insomnia, fits of weeping, and overconcern about the opinions of others are usual accompaniments in patients with this type of headache. In the worst cases, there is severe regression with constant headache and the patient is bedridden day and night, requiring total nursing care. Invariably the family is involved, and the frequency of interpersonal conflict is high. Uncovering psychotherapy leads to denied and repressed hostile, aggressive feelings, and unacceptable sexual impulses and ideas. In the early stages, attempts to hide the weakness associated with headaches are accompanied by holding the head high or craning the neck in defiance of the urge to give up and give in. This type of psychological body language most commonly demonstrates anxiety neurosis. Characterological disorders, neuroses, body-image disorders, posttraumatic neuroses, depressions, and psychoses have frequently been identified initially as muscle-contraction headaches.

TREATMENT

Although psychiatric treatment is necessary, the first consideration is providing some respite from the pain. Antianxiety psychopharmacological substances, such as chlordiazepoxide hydrochloride, diazepam, and meprobamate in adequate dosage give much relief. Muscle relaxants such as carisoprodol may also be helpful. Heat and massage are usually beneficial if used concomitantly. These pharmacological substances and physical therapies are sustaining while the psychiatric problem is in process of definition.

The taking of a detailed history, exploring the patient's complaints with great care and precision, requires much time. The psychiatrist should evaluate the pain and explore the social, family, work, and pleasure attitudes and environment, as well as the patient's responses to stress, personality traits, long-range life goals, and habitual patterns of coping with tension in order to build, in his own mind, a model of the patient's life. Once this has been attained, the problem areas can be specifically defined. Such an evaluation may reveal a characterological disorder, a neurosis, a body-image disorder, a posttraumatic neurosis, a depression, or even a psychosis. Depending on the psychodynamic formulation of the meaning of the symptoms to a particular pa-

tient, a psychiatric treatment program can be planned and a treatment goal established. Whether the route lies with supportive psychotherapy, uncovering psychotherapy, guidance and educative approaches, or psychoanalytic investigation must be decided. One would usually strive for resolution of the patient's conflict and some modification of personality structure.

Combined Headache

Combined headache is a combination of the vascular and muscle-contraction types. A clear definition of the factors which fall into each category assists the psychiatrist to understand the physiological and psychological components, and plan a treatment program to encompass the various identifiable parts of the combination. Experience teaches that, in many instances, successful treatment of the combined-headache patient requires close collaboration between internist, neurologist, and psychiatrist, with each physician understanding the nature of the expertise and treatment plans of the others, and willing to interact in this way. When cooperation is not present, the patient collects conflicting statements, involves the physicians in devisive maneuvers, and can easily sabotage the therapeutic efforts of everyone involved.

Delusional States and Conversion

Friedman and Frazier[18] showed in 1971 in a selected series of 250 headache patients—all of whom had had previous treatments, multiple physicians, and were treatment failures by their own declarations—that 25 percent had organic brain disorders not previously diagnosed, and 28 percent had psychoses not previously diagnosed. This highly selective sample of long-term headache sufferers clearly indicated that headache can mask very severe illnesses, and that such masks are utilized defensively, for long periods of time, to avoid knowing the true cause and treatment of the symptoms. Monosymptomatic delusions of headache and body delusions occur frequently in schizophrenia, as well as in manic-depressive psychosis (bipolar), involutional melancholia, and unipolar illness.

Conversion reaction may present symptomatically as headache. The symbolic meaning of the head and its special importance have been recognized throughout history. From earliest childhood, developmental experiences involve the head-placed organs of special sense, i.e., eating and learning. Considering the head as locus of the intelligence and so many critical senses imprints the necessity of protecting it, and also defines it as the source of many conflicts.

Every psychiatrist has seen a delusional patient who concretely defines a perception in terms of the organ of perception. Similarly, our society, regarding the head as symbolic of organizer, controller, or director of the entire organism, uses the terms "headman," "headmaster," "headquarters," and "headwaiter;" or, very simply, calls the person in charge "the head." This metaphor, with some variations, is constant in everyday speech, even in regard to inanimate things and natural phenomena. The "head" is the upper end of beds, valleys, stairs, and pages; the useful section of hammers, golf clubs, and many other objects; the culminating point of cabbages, flowers, and pimples; the source of a stream; and the leading end of a ship, train, or parade. The head of the table, even when the ends are identical, is, of course, the place of prestige.

Some authors have considered headache in broad adaptational and psychogenic context. It has, for instance, been suggested that the vascular mechanisms in many headaches are related to normal circulatory changes that accompany intense and prolonged mental activity, especially in a setting of relative frustration, with the circulatory process extending beyond normal range when the activity is not brought to a resolution or conclusion. Grinker and Robbins[26] related it to the evolutionary migration of complex and integrated functions toward the head end of the organism and the complex sensory, postural, and symbolic activities integrated there. Interest in the expression of psychological and emotional tension in this part of the body has led, in turn, to consideration of postural reflexes and muscle tension. This points up a general tendency, identified in headache sufferers, both to locate the ego and psychic functions generally in the head,[23] and to elaborate further symbolic transformations of such beliefs. Wolff[54] wrote: "Since the human animal prides himself on 'using his head' it is perhaps not without meaning that his head should be the source of so much discomfort . . . or that the vast majority of discomforts and pains of the head . . . are accompaniments of resentments and dissatisfactions." Kolb,[30] observing that personal attitudes toward the head are derived from early learning and appreciation of body functioning and image, sees the expression of concerns related to intellect, brain function, or emotional capacities in terms of head-referred complaints, particularly headache. Rangell[39] and Rosenbaum[41] discuss the more complex symbolism of the headache symptom as a compromise formation representing the impulse and the defense against it. Both authors describe cases illustrating different complex patterns of interrelated defense mechanisms. Rangell notes that conversion symptoms of this type are not confined to hysterical patients but may also occur with either obsessive-compulsive neuroses or depressions.

Posttraumatic Headaches

This type of headache is reminiscent of the war neurosis and so-called "combat fatigue." Patients so afflicted often have vivid and terrifying nightmares as well as "startle" reactions, that symbolize the threat to survival experienced at the time of trauma.

Often, very careful intravenous administration of sodium pentothal or sodium amytal provides the patient with just enough sedation to release his mental controls, allowing him to talk freely of the events surrounding the traumatic accident and to abreact the terror he experienced. When this is done, several persons should be present because these patients often abreact with considerable physical and motor excitement.

One of my posttraumatic headache patients, a twenty-one-year-old Canadian farm boy, had suffered a leg fracture and toe amputation from catching his foot in a hay baler. Because of the loud noise of the machinery, his father did not hear the son's cries until the baler turned at the end of a fence row. When he saw the boy writhing in pain and in a state of shock, he shouted, "Oh, my God, he's dead!" Under amytal sedation the young man fought furiously, as if trying to free himself from the machine. Reliving the situation with great clarity, he then fainted. In the weeks after this session, the material he abreacted during the amytal interview was slowly brought to his awareness and he was relieved of his headache. The syndrome such patients suffer has a quality resembling a psychoneurotic conversion type of symptom, with the symptom as the symbolic mental representation of an unacceptable conflictual impulse.

In some cases of posttraumatic headache, the most significant component in perpetuating the symptoms is the compensation received by the patient. The most usual compensation is, quite simply, relief from disliked duties, responsibilities, or employment. The patient utilizes the accident as a means of flight from an unpleasant job or some other situation about which he has had long-harbored fantasies of escape. A second factor, desire for financial remuneration and security, is demonstrated by the fact that these patients often are employees of big corporations, the government, or other institutions which provide benefits for injured workers.

Still a third component sometimes interwoven into the continuation of symptoms is the attention, support, and solicitude these patients may long have desired, and now gain from family members or an "understanding" physician. They are, therefore, understandably reluctant to surrender a symptom that provides such remarkable profits. Such individuals tend to project, assigning their feelings and attitudes to those around them. They sense and react to the wariness and suspicion that they arouse in the physician, and in other ways also demonstrate great insecurity.

One of my posttraumatic headache patients was a forty-one-year-old chemical-industry worker who injured his knee on a cracking tower, became faint, and fell against an outside steel ladder. His faintness was associated with fear of a fatal fall off the ladder onto the ground seven or eight stories below, or into a mass of pipes, boilers, and other equipment. Immediately following his feeling of faintness, the patient developed a headache. Results of a neurological examination were negative, but after recovering from the minor knee injury, he still complained of severe head pain associated with dizziness. He found the condition so disabling that he could not leave the ground to climb into the towers as his work required.

During an amytal interview, the patient associated his fear of death from a fall with the memory of a friend's fatal plunge at the same plant six years before. He then voluntarily described a childhood experience in which he fell from a bicycle, striking his head on the pavement. He recalled his parents' oversolicitous attitude toward the minor head pains he suffered.

After the interview, the patient connected the multiple accident history with his expectation that his company would continue the compensation which he had been receiving for nine months. After short-term psychotherapy, with direct interpretation of his desire to be cared for, the patient came to understand the nature of the psychological connections he had made about the accident and returned to work with a gradually abating headache pattern.

(Hypochondriasis

Hypochondriasis, i.e., persistent pathological concern about the health of the body, is expressed in marked diffuse preoccupation about malfunctioning organs or parts. This concern tends to usurp all other interests. Although at one time the term "hypochondriacal" was used only for those patients who had no organic pathology, it is now used sometimes for those with excessive preoccupation about actual organic illness. Symptoms of the hypochondriacal state include complaints of pressure in the head, inadequate memory, inability to concentrate, irritability, poor sleep patterns, with any of these accompanied by multiple aches and pains, and all of them dwelt on and described compulsively and repeatedly.

Many of the patients have basic character defects, or a serious internal or visceral body-image problem. Although typically classified as a neurotic disorder, hypochondriasis may actually incorporate beliefs about the body which are delusional, hence psychotic.

Hypochondriasis is a compensation for serious defects in self-esteem or for unaccomplished ideals in life. Many of the patients are bored, self-centered, and lead dull, uninteresting lives. Many are victims of a series of embittering misfortunes. Their symptomatology is the somatic expression of the resentment and concern they are otherwise unable to express, and serves to maintain their balance between rationality and irrationality.

The patients usually present the physician with a list of bodily complaints in addition to headaches. Although the psychiatric approach should aim toward reeducation, it is unrealistic to expect total relief of the symptoms. In general, the prognosis is poor. It is difficult to discuss their symptomatology with them or to treat the headaches directly. After the therapist gives a long explanation of the nature of body symptoms and of how the condition might have come about, the hypochondriacal patient will say, "Well, of course, that doesn't apply to me. Now what about my headaches?"

The lesson that body symptoms can be expressions of psychological problems must be subtly taught. For the patient to acquire a new view of frustration, tension, and anxiety, the physician must maintain an objective, unemotional approach and be careful not to promise, even by implication or attitude, that the patient's physical symptoms will disappear; nor must he permit the patient to think that just visiting the physician will make the symptoms magically go away.

The physician should assume a joint-venture approach: "Yes, you have symptoms, and yes, I have some knowledge. Perhaps, working together, we may be able to understand the nature of your headaches and other symp-toms." This attitude eventually reassures the patient and enlists his cooperation. He gradually understands that the doctor will make no pronouncements, and that it is the verbal explorations between the doctor and himself which, by leading to a more lucid comprehension of his life situation and bodily complaints, may in some measure ameliorate his condition.

⟨ Causalgia and Painful Phantom

Causalgia is a posttraumatic syndrome characterized by persistent, diffuse, burning pain, which is aggravated by stimuli that may be trivial or purely emotional. The frequency of causalgic pain following nerve injury is approximately 2–5 percent in case reports, being much more common in the upper than in the lower extremities. The patient is usually debilitated by it and sometimes completely dominated by its timelessness.

Phantom pain can occur after the healing phase of an amputation or an extensive avulsion. It is described as a burning, twisting, cramping, sharp, shooting, cyclic pain perceived in the vicinity of the absent body part, usually an extremity. While the nonpainful phantom is considered to be a normal condition following amputation, the painful phantom is a pathological circumstance reported in as few as 8 (0.36 percent) of 2200 patients by Ewalt, Randall, and Morris.[6]

There are three main theories attempting to explain the phantom phenomenon and the painful phantom:

The Peripheral Theory

The peripheral theory states that persisting sensations from the nerve endings in the stump are assigned to those parts originally innervated by the severed nerves and result in these phenomena. According to this theory, a neuroma develops, scar tissue is formed, and the circulation is decreased. These factors, plus other mechanical defects and irritants, result in a constant bombardment of impulses to the conscious mind giving rise to the phantom and the pain.

The Central Theory

The central theory proposes that phantoms are due to conscious processes that are more or less independent of sensory impulses from the periphery. A question in this theory is whether awareness of the body is learned or innate. In the structural or nativistic version, the phantoms reflect the constant features of central representation of the sensory and motor systems.

The body image is built up in the early years of life from multiple postural, tactile, and visual-sensory impressions. The body image usually has the same extension as the body surface, so that with loss of a body part there is a reactivation of former perceptive patterns. The organization of these sensory impressions probably takes place in the parietotemporal cortex. With the passage of time, the phantom part shrinks as the body image is reorganized through new sensory impressions. The evidence given for this theory is the following:

1. No phantoms are found with congenital absence of limbs or early childhood amputations, evidently because the body image is not fully developed before the age of six. Also, no phantoms are seen in adults if there is long anesthesia of the limb prior to amputation.
2. The phantom is kept natural and more vivid if the patient exercises it.
3. There is increased sensitivity in the stump with a telescoped phantom than in the contralateral homologous limb. This is interpreted as reflecting central reorganization, since there are no changes in the stump to account for this heightened sensitivity.
4. Incorporation into the phantom of extra factors such as rings is observed.
5. Phantoms fade and telescope according to cortical representation. The fingers and toes are more in contact with the environment and have more nerves and cortical representation than many other body parts. Therefore, they are of greater importance in the body image, and their phantoms will persist longer.
6. Fading is considered to be due to the gradual increase of central suppression of afferent impulses as the body image is reorganized.
7. Involuntary movements of the phantom are likened to Jacksonian seizures, a central process.
8. The patient has the ability to call up the phantom at will and to move it voluntarily.
9. Phantoms may be temporarily lost after certain brain injuries or surgery only to reappear later because of central reorganization.

The Mixed Theory

The mixed theory combines the peripheral and central theories and proposes that the state of the internuncial pool is responsible for the phantom sensations. According to this theory, peripheral irritation stimulates internuncial neurons so that reverberatory, self-perpetuating circuits are set up. Impulses go peripherally and centrally from these neurons, resulting in perception of the phantom and pain. As impulses are overcome by conscious inhibition, the phantom approaches the stump. If sensations are too painful and enduring, the conscious inhibition is ineffective, and the phantom and pain persist. This accounts for the success of peripheral methods of treatment in the early stages of development of the painful phantom, and for failure later when cord and brain surgery may not work. However, the phantom pain is often unrelieved by surgical procedures. Thus, there has been more inquiry into the dynamics and motivation in phantom limbs.

One psychiatric theory proposes that the phantom is a wish-fulfilling hallucination resulting from the denial of a lost part, and that pain results from denial of the affect associated with the loss. Some psychoanalysts stress the decreased positive aspects of self-concepts, i.e., that the amputee feels castrated and deprived, and that he lacks an intact personality.

The rule of denial is also stressed, although

it is held by many that denial has a limited place in the phenomenon. Kolb[30] feels that denial does not cause the phantom, which is a healthy psychological response. Rather, those patients who do not experience a phantom are in fact denying their loss. He attributes the lower incidence of phantom breast, penis, and so forth, to the mechanism of denial. The phantoms are repressed because the patients cannot accept the loss.

Weiss and English[51] maintain that the phantom results from the amputee's narcissistic demand to retain the limb, and that the pain has the functional value of convincing him on an unconscious level that the limb is present. He manages this denial through activity.

Simmel[45] believes that the phantom is genuinely experienced and may become a focus for denial instead of being motivated by denial. Also, the emotions and anxiety associated with the body loss are not denied but rather the patient is overwhelmed by the effect.

It has been proposed that the phantom is a product of the unconscious and subject to its law. Phantoms, like dreams and hallucinations, undergo condensation, displacement, and secondary elaboration, and can pass through solid objects. Simmel explains that phantoms are lacking in early childhood amputations because there are not enough wishes about body organs at that time. Pain results from provocation of the unconscious by peripheral stimulation or by psychic conflicts between the opposed desires, regaining the loss versus adjusting to reality.

The importance of the patient's personality in his reaction to amputation or afferent denervation should not be underemphasized. In a study of combat casualties, psychiatric disturbances were related to the patient's personality and not to the nature of the injury. It is felt that the patient's emotions give force to the perceptive patterns activated by body loss, and that the variety of responses to mutilation results from the varying personalities.

The patient's attitude about his body and the emotional significance of his body parts are determined by family and cultural attitudes toward the body and its parts. His body image is reinforced by these emotions and attitudes. Therefore, on loss of certain body parts, varying emotions and reactions to the event will come into play depending on the personality makeup. The obsessional patient, for example, has considerable difficulty in adapting to any bodily change, whether it's a small dental bridge or an extremity prosthesis.

It is only natural that a patient shows some anxiety concerning an amputation. It is normal that an amputee mourns for the lost body part and is anxious about its disposal. It was found in a study of war casualties that 64 percent of the patients showed anxiety or other psychiatric symptoms, which were unobserved by ward personnel. It is abnormal, however, when an amputee has persistent pain unrelieved by narcotics and not characteristic of physical disease. Of those with a painful phantom, less than 20 percent had signs of physical disease in the stump.

Kolb[30] claims that states of fear, perception, and associated ideas influence the internuncial pool in such a way that pain results, i.e., psychic pain is projected via the internuncial pathways into the phantom, resulting in the painful phantom. In the war studies, patients with this kind of pain showed a marked psychopathology that was thought to reflect a premorbid personality disorder. They gave evidence, for instance, of reckless behavior and exhibitionism. Such patients are often hostile, demanding, and uncooperative, and complain about neglect within and outside the hospital. There seems to be a parallel between these patients and paranoids.

Kolb finds no consistent personality structure or defect, but feels that these patients are generally maladjusted to their environment and to a prosthesis. A chronic painful phantom represents an emotional response to the loss of an important body part that is significant in the patient's relationship with others. Hostile feelings with resultant guilt feelings develop toward those with whom the patient identifies as mutilating or multilated, and also toward those on whom he is dependent and whose rejection he fears. It was noted that hostility was the forbidden impulse in these amputees. The pain may symbolize punishment for these hostile and guilty emotions. Of twenty-one patients with painful phantoms, fourteen had previously had a close emotional attachment to another amputee.

Kolb[30] thinks that amputations arouse fantasies of personal mutilation which are overcome by repression. These fantasies may come to the fore after amputation, resulting in such hostility and guilt feelings that even reference to an amputee can elicit phantom pain. Pain can also be caused by mentioning a person on whom the patient depends. Besides the hostility factor, pain has the functional role of binding this person to the patient. An interesting finding is that there seems to be a correlation between loss of function and phantom pain. Patients with functioning prostheses tend to have normal phantoms, whereas those with no prostheses or only cosmetic ones show an increased incidence of pain.

An interesting psychological phenomenon found in amputees is the projection of their own defects into the environment. For example, an amputee often thinks normal people have amputations, while on closer inspection he finds this is not so. On figure drawing tests, a patient may fail to draw in the part that he lacks, or he may distort the figure in other ways. In Rorschach tests, figures are cut off. Amputees may have wish-fulfilling dreams in which the limb is present and functioning normally, or anxiety laden, repetitive dreams reexperiencing the injury leading to amputation. All these illustrations may be considered manifestations of a disturbance of body image. Haber,[27] in a study of postoperative reactions following amputation, found that some amputees try to overcompensate to make up for their loss, but others may become depressed and mournful.

Treatment

What then are some of the treatments for causalgia and the painful phantom? Initially, rapid interruption of sensory impulses could be assured by the use of local block in the area of injury, or by such modalities as rhizotomy, cordotomy, tractotomy, thalamotomy, or leucotomy. The use of ultrasound physiotherapy with the stump, psychopharmacologic agents, and psychotherapy when indicated may be helpful. Relief by the use of chlorpromazine, reserpine, and electroshock alone has been reported. Imipramine and amitriptyline have been helpful as analgesics.

The psychotherapist should investigate the overall circumstances of the patient, exploring his attitudes about the injury or amputation, preferably before an elective amputation, with a view toward understanding the patient's feelings about his body image, his associations to his body parts, and the relative value placed on body parts by himself and by his family. In addition, the patient should be given the opportunity to discuss his fantasies about the appearance of his injured extremity or about the disposal of the amputated part. Considerable time should be spent exploring the patient's attitudes towards amputees and mutilated people, and previous associations with individuals who have undergone amputation or mutilating injuries. His attitudes, as gleaned from literature, about Captain Ahab in *Moby Dick*,[35] Captain Hook, or others, should also be investigated in an effort to assess his overall feeling about bodily parts in terms of his own relative overevaluation of them.

The patient should be reassured by the surgeon or physician as to the mode of disposal of the amputated part. The damaged remaining body parts, that is, the stump or the causalgic area, should be shown to be accepted by the physician by his viewing and examining the area frequently, and thus communicating to the patient its acceptability. More important, prior to an elective amputation, the patient should be counselled that he can expect to have phantom sensations and that this is a normal phenomenon. If this is done, he may be spared much of the considerable anxiety that will occur when he awakes from the anesthetic still feeling the absent extremity.

After a satisfactory sympathectomy, causalgia patients often make a much more satisfactory social adjustment when placed on a schedule of regular supportive contact with their physicians. This medical dependent relationship offers opportunity for discussions of personal problems under the symbolic presentation of mild sedative-analgesic combinations.

⟐ Conclusion

In summary, when evaluating and treating patients with a complicated pain problem, one cannot understand the meaning of persistent, painful complaining unless one considers the meaning of the symptom and its origin in prolonged learned experiences in the patients' family, culture, and daily life. One should investigate their personality structures and those emotional stresses to which they are abnormally reactive.

⟐ Bibliography

1. AMERICAN MEDICAL ASSOCIATION. Ad Hoc Committee on Classification of Headache. "Special Report," *JAMA*, 179 (1962), 717–718.

2. BEECHER, H. K. "Pain in Man Wounded in Battle," *Ann. Surg.*, 123 (1946), 96–105.

3. BOAG, T. J. "Psychogenic Headaches," in P. J. Vinken and G. W. Bruyn, eds., *Handbook of Clinical Neurology*, Vol. 5, pp. 247–257. New York: American Elsevier, 1969.

4. BRENNER, C., A. P. FRIEDMAN, and S. CARTER. "Psychological Factors in the Etiology and Treatment of Chronic Headache," *Psychosom. Med.*, 11 (1949), 53–56.

5. CLARK, W. C. and H. F. HUNT. "Pain," in J. A. Downey and R. C. Darling, eds., *Physiological Basis of Rehabilitation Medicine*, pp. 373–401. Philadelphia: Saunders, 1971.

6. EWALT, J. R., G. C. RANDALL, and H. MORRIS. "The Phantom Limb," *Psychosom. Med.*, 9 (1947), 118–123.

7. FORRER, G. R. "Hallucinated Headache," *Psychosomatics*, 3 (1962), 120–128.

8. FRAZIER, S. H. "The Psychotherapeutic Approach to Patients with Headache," *Mod. Treat.*, 1 (1964), 1412–1424.

9. ———. "Psychotherapy of Headache," *Res. Clin. Stud. Headache*, 2 (1969), 195–220.

10. FRAZIER, S. H. and A. C. CARR. *Introduction to Psychopathology*. New York: Macmillan, 1964.

11. FRAZIER, S. H. and L. C. KOLB. "Psychiatric Aspects of Pain and the Phantom Limb," *Orthop. Clin. North Am.*, 1 (1970), 481–495.

12. FRIEDMAN, A. P. "Migraine and Tension Headaches," *Conn. State Med. J.*, 20 (1956), 440–444.

13. ———. "The Mechanism and Treatment of Migraine and Tension Headaches," *Miss. Valley Med.*, 80 (1958), 141–146.

14. ———. "Headache," in A. M. Freedman, H. I. Kaplan, and H. S. Kaplan, eds., *Comprehensive Textbook of Psychiatry*, pp. 1110–1113. Baltimore: Williams & Wilkins, 1967.

15. ———. "The Headache in History, Literature, and Legend," *Bull. N.Y. Acad. Med. 2nd Ser.*, 48 (1972), 661–681.

16. ———. "Current Concepts in the Diagnosis and Treatment of Chronic Recurring Headache," *Med. Clin. North Am.*, 56 (1972), 1257–1271.

17. FRIEDMAN, A. P. and C. BRENNER. "Psychological Mechanism in Chronic Headache," *Assoc. Res. Nerv. Dis. Proc.*, 29 (1950), 605–608.

18. FRIEDMAN, A. P. and S. H. FRAZIER. "Critique of the Psychiatric Treatment of Chronic Headache Patients," *Proc. 5th World Congr. Psychiatry, Mexico City, 1971*. New York: American Elsevier, 1973.

19. ———. Personal communications, 1973.

20. FRIEDMAN, A. P., S. H. FRAZIER, and D. SCHULTZ. *The Headache Book*. New York: Dodd-Mead, 1973.

21. FRIEDMAN, A. P. and H. H. MERRITT. *Headache: Diagnosis and Treatment*. Philadelphia: Davis, 1959.

22. FROMM-REICHMAN, F. "Contribution to the Psychogenesis of Migraine," *Psychoanal. Rev.*, 24 (1937), 26–33.

23. GITTLESON, N. L. "Psychogenic Headache and the Localization of the Ego," *J. Ment. Sci.*, 108 (1962), 47–52.

24. GRAHAM, J. R. *Treatment of Muscle Contraction Headache*. New York: Harper & Row, 1964.

25. GRINKER, R. R. and L. GOTTSCHALK. "Headaches and Muscular Pain," *Psychosom. Med.*, 11 (1949), 45–52.

26. GRINKER, R. R. and F. P. ROBBINS. *Psychosomatic Case Book*. New York: Blakiston, 1954.

27. HABER, W. B. "Reactions to the Loss of Limb: Physiological and Psychological As-

pects," *Ann. N.Y. Acad. Sci.*, 74 (1958), 14–24.

28. HARDY, J. D., H. G. WOLFF, and H. GOODELL. "Studies on Pain Sensation. I. Measurement of Pain Threshold with Thermal Radiation" (Abstract), *Am. J. Physiol.*, 125 (1939), 523–524.

29. KOLB, L. C. "Pain as a Psychiatric Problem," *Lancet*, 72 (1952), 50–54.

30. ———. *The Painful Phantom, Psychology, Physiology and Treatment.* Springfield, Ill.: Charles C. Thomas, 1954.

31. ———. "Psychiatric Aspects of the Treatment of Headache," *Neurology*, 13 (1963), 34–37.

32. ———. *Modern Clinical Psychiatry*, 8th ed. Philadelphia: Saunders, 1973.

33. MARTIN, M. J., H. P. ROME, and W. M. SWENSON. "Muscle-Contraction Headache, A Psychiatric Review," *Res. Clin. Stud. Headache*, 1 (1967), 184–204.

34. MASSERMAN, J. H. "The Neurotic Cat," *Psychol. Today*, 1 (1967), 36–39.

35. MELVILLE, H. *Moby Dick.* New York: Franklin Watts, 1967.

36. PAVLOV, I. *Experimental Psychology and Other Essays.* New York: Philosophical Library, 1957.

37. PENMAN, J. "Trigeminal Sensoz Root Injection," *Opert. Surg.*, 16 (1958), 45–51.

38. PROCACCI, P. "A Survey of Modern Concepts of Pain," in P. J. Vinken and G. W. Bruyn, eds., *Handbook of Clinical Neurology*, Vol. 1, pp. 114–146. New York: American Elsevier, 1969.

39. RANGELL, L. "Psychiatric Aspects of Pain," *Psychosom. Med.*, 15 (1953), 22–37.

40. ROBINSON, D. B. "Psychological Aspects of Migraine," *Clin. Res. Rev.*, in press.

41. ROSENBAUM, M. "Symposium; Psychogenic Headache," *Cincinn. J. Med.*, 28 (1947), 7–16.

42. SACKS, O. W. "Migraine: Intelligence, Social Class, and Family Prevalence," *Br. Med. J.*, 2 (1971), 77–81.

43. SARGENT, J. D., E. E. GREEN, and E. D. WALTERS. "Preliminary Report on the Use of Autogenic Feedback Techniques in the Treatment of Migraine and Tension Headaches," *Psychosom. Med.* (in press).

44. SELINSKY, H. "Psychologic Study of the Migrainous Syndrome," *Bull. N.Y. Acad. Med.*, 15 (1939), 757–763.

45. SIMMEL, M. L. "A Study of Phantoms after Amputation of the Breast," *Neuropsychologia*, 4 (1966), 331–350.

46. SLOANE, R. B. "Psychological Aspects of Headache," *Can. Med. Assoc. J.*, 91 (1964), 908–911.

47. SPERLING, M. "A Psychoanalytical Study of Migraine and Psychogenic Headache," *Psychoanal. Rev.*, 39 (1952), 152–163.

48. ———. "A Further Contribution to the Psycho-Analytical Study of Migraine and Psychogenic Headaches," *Int. J. Psychoanal.*, 45 (1964), 549–557.

49. STERNBACH, R. A. *Pain: A Psychophysiological Analysis.* New York: Academic, 1968.

50. TOURAINE, G. A. and G. DRAPER. "The Migrainous Patient; A Constitutional Study," *J. Nerv. Ment. Dis.*, 80 (1934), 1–23, 182–204.

51. WEISS, F. and O. S. ENGLISH. *Psychosomatic Medicine.* Philadelphia: Saunders, 1957.

52. WOLBERG, L. R. "Psychosomatic Correlations in Migraine," *Psychiatr. Q.*, 19 (1945), 60–70.

53. WOLFF, H. G. "Personality Features and Reactions of Subjects with Migraine," *Arch. Neurol. Psychiatry*, 37 (1937), 895–921.

54. WOLFF, H. G., ed. *Headache and Other Head Pain*, 2nd ed. London: Oxford University Press, 1963.

55. WOOD, E. H., A. P. FRIEDMAN, A. J. ROWAN et al. "Observations on Vascular Headache of the Migraine Type." Paper presented before the 5th Symposium of the Migraine Trust, London, September 1972.

56. ZBOROWSKI, M. *People in Pain.* San Francisco: Jossey-Bass, 1969.

CHAPTER 35

SLEEP DISORDERS AND DISORDERED SLEEP

Robert L. Williams and Ismet Karacan

❴ Introduction

Observers who enjoy speculating about such statistics have offered various estimates as to how many times the stream of EEG paper generated in sleep research would reach around the world. The fact that a recording for a single night for one subject is often a quarter-mile in length stimulates a variety of metaphors to describe this almost endless flow made possible by the technological "break-throughs" of the old dams which limited the size and scope of sleep studies. Hopefully, the thousands of miles of EEG wiggles and squiggles have produced information which can be useful to the clinician for the solution of problems he encounters in the everyday practice of medicine.

In this chapter, we will concentrate on the findings which are pertinent to sleep disorders. Under this category we will consider the so-called primary sleep disorders. These are conditions in which various abnormalities of sleep represent the cardinal and often only sign or symptom from which the patient suffers. We will discuss secondary sleep disorders in which chronic clinical problems are accompanied by specific or nonspecific sleep disturbances. Parasomnias, in which an activity normally associated with waking behavior appears during sleep, will be discussed. Sleep-modified disorders, in which the basic disorder worsens or occurs primarily in sleep, will be mentioned briefly, and additional references will be suggested for the interested reader.

The clinical information and research data about sleep disorders and disordered sleep have been organized under the categories mentioned above for convenience. In most instances, the etiology and the pathophysiological mechanisms of these conditions are unknown or only suspected. This fact makes it impossible at this time to classify them by etiology or mechanisms as is typically done for diseases which are better understood. A group of investigators in the Association for the Psychophysiological Study of Sleep has been meeting periodically during the period of preparation of this chapter in an effort to develop a standardized classification of sleep disorders and disordered sleep which would provide a common point of reference for clinicians and researchers in the field. Hopefully, a standard will be developed with which the classification used in this chapter will be compatible.

The reader unfamiliar with the terminology employed by EEG sleep researchers should consult Chapter 8 in Volume 6 of this *Handbook*. Briefly, the classification of EEG sleep stages proposed by Dement and Kleitman,[87] and used by most workers, consists of four sleep stages and the waking state: (1) wakefulness, or stage 0, which is predominantly alpha activity; (2) stage 1, a mixed-voltage fast pattern without sleep spindles; (3) stage 2, K-complex or 12–16 cycles per second (cps) spindle activity against a low-voltage background; (4) stage 3, high-voltage, 1–2 cps activity (delta waves) during no more than half of each scoring epoch; and (5) stage 4, delta activity during at least half of the scoring epoch. Conjugate, rapid eye movements (REMs), as monitored by the electrooculogram (EOG), and depressed electromyogram (EMG) activity, periodically accompany stage-1 sleep. This special form of stage-1 sleep is designated stage 1-REM. Stage 1-REM, which has also been called paradoxical sleep, typically occurs four to six times per night in healthy adults, and subjects awakened from REM sleep usually report dreams much more frequently than when awakened from non-REM (NREM) sleep.[18,87] Stages-3 and -4 sleep (slow-wave sleep) are commonly considered to be the deepest stages of sleep.

◖ Primary Sleep Disorders

Under this category, as defined above, we have included insomnia, narcolepsy, chronic hypersomnia, the Kleine-Levin and Pickwickian syndromes, sleep paralysis, and frightening dreams.

Insomnia

This is probably one of the most common problems encountered by the physician in his day-to-day practice. Until recently, the term "insomnia" was often used loosely to describe any or all of the disorders discussed in this chapter. As research has progressed, it has become possible to distinguish a number of specific entities which were once lumped together under this general term. Many authors in the past have listed physical or organic factors as primary causes of some types of insomnia. We have been able to refine our classification so that many conditions can now be considered as sleep-modified disorders, or, as in the case of insomnia accompanying depression or schizophrenia, they can be listed as secondary sleep disturbances.

We view the disorders which we shall include under this heading as a very specific type of primary sleep disorder. Primary insomniacs suffer from a persistent inability to obtain adequate sleep but they exhibit no gross physical or psychological pathology. This restricted definition of insomnia is relatively new, and as a consequence there are limited data from polygraphic studies of this condition where the more circumscribed definition has been utilized.

The incidence of insomnia has been assessed by both indirect and direct methods. There are many reports which provide indirect evidence about the prevalence of the disorder. The United States Department of Health, Education, and Welfare[90] reported a 535 percent increase in retail sales of sedatives and tranquilizers between 1952 and 1963. In 1971, the consumer newsletter *Moneysworth* stated that $170 million is spent annually in the United States on sleeping pills.[286]

More direct evidence is provided by Weiss et al.,[425] who obtained reports of sleep disturbances in 72 percent of 108 male veterans who were psychiatric outpatients, in 22 percent of 101 veterans being treated for medical complaints, and in 15 percent of 110 active Air Force personnel with no known medical or mental disturbance. They also found that sleep disturbances increased with increasing age. One should pay special attention to their finding of complaints in 15 percent of a supposedly healthy population.

In the past, the most commonly accepted etiology for most cases of insomnia was emotional disturbance. Such a conclusion was reached by a study of the case history and an examination of the psychodynamics. The hypotheses developed by these approaches had implicated almost every type of psychopathological mechanism and led to a wide range of diagnostic formulations. Insomnia has been described as a habit and a psychoneurosis,[156] a typical psychosomatic syndrome,[429] or a type of reaction formation.[361] Anxiety and fear, including fear of unconscious repressed desires, fear of homicidal or suicidal wishes, and fear of death, have all been implicated as primary causes.

Systematic studies of groups of insomniacs support the hypothesis that some are more disturbed psychologically than are noninsomniacs. Monroe[287] examined the psychological, physiological, and sleep EEG characteristics of a number of poor and good sleepers. In a questionnaire, his subjects were asked about the length of time required to fall asleep, the number of nightly awakenings, and the degree of subjective difficulty in falling asleep. Although the poor sleepers self-categorized by the questionnaire were not suffering from severe sleep disturbances and did not consider themselves insomniacs, they were found to differ significantly from good sleepers because of greater pathology on nine of the thirteen clinical scales of the MMPI (Minnesota Multiphasic Personality Inventory). They also reported significantly more somatic and emotional symptoms on the Cornell Medical Index. In a similar study, Rechtschaffen[332] was unable to detect any *significant* differences between good and poor sleepers on MMPI scores, although the poor sleepers had scores indicative of greater pathology on each of the scales. He suggested that a smaller sample size and smaller initial sleep differences between his good and poor sleepers may have prevented the detection of statistically significant differences in the MMPI scores.

Other workers[104,214] have reported results similar to those of Monroe.

Monroe[287] found that poor sleepers showed greater amounts of physiological activation than good sleepers. They exhibited greater numbers of body movements and peripheral vascular constrictions, and higher basal temperatures during sleep than the good sleepers. The poor sleepers also tended to have higher heart rates and pulse volumes. The poor sleepers appeared to be more activated—as reflected by levels of heart rate, peripheral vasoconstriction, and rectal temperature—than good sleepers, even before they retired. Rechtschaffen and Monroe[338] concluded that the persistence of physiological activation during the sleep of poor sleepers may represent a failure of the rest-inducing mechanisms of sleep rather than a continuation of the pre-sleep level.

Insomniacs have usually been classified according to the time during the sleep period when wakefulness is more troublesome. Some patients complain mainly of difficulty in falling asleep. Some complain of frequent and/or long awakenings after falling asleep. And others complain of early morning awakenings. Many clinicians are aware of patients who have of a combination of these complaints. However, if polygraphic data reported from the sleep EEG's of insomniacs can be considered more objective descriptors of the qualitative and quantitative disturbances in the sleep of insomniacs, then it becomes clear that the classification mentioned above is too simplistic. Data from the limited number of polygraphic studies which have been performed indicate that there are many different types of insomnia and various combinations of disturbances. These studies have been reviewed elsewhere.[227] As an example, we will briefly describe two studies performed in our laboratories. The first[229] was a study of "hardcore" insomniacs. We found on the second and third laboratory recording nights that eight male and two female insomniacs between the ages of thirty and fifty-five exhibited significantly longer sleep latencies and longer latencies of arising (time from morning awakening to arising) than did the age- and sex-matched controls. Insomniacs also obtained less total sleep than controls, but the large variability in the insomniacs' total sleep times prevented this difference from attaining statistical significance. There was no difference between groups in the number of awakenings, primarily because some of the controls awoke quite frequently during the night. However, the ratio of total sleep time to time in bed, which summarized the relative sleep efficiency, was significantly smaller in the insomniacs. Many insomniacs and controls failed to obtain stage-4 sleep. Most of the subjects did obtain some stage 3, and the latency to the first appearance of this stage from sleep onset was significantly longer in the insomniacs. In the insomniacs, once stage 1-REM sleep appeared it occurred at a faster pace than in the controls, with the average time between stage 1-REM intervals being consistently shorter. During the first four hours of sleep the cumulative minutes of stage 1-REM was higher for the insomniacs. After the first four hours, however, the insomniacs began to wake up and no comparison was possible for the later hours of sleep. It is nevertheless clear that insomniacs establish and maintain a higher absolute amount of stage 1-REM than controls as the night progresses.

In the second study,[221] we examined the EEG sleep patterns of eleven male insomniacs, ages thirty-four to fifty-six, and their age- and sex-matched controls. Each subject's sleep was recorded for eight consecutive nights. We found that differences among subjects in the insomniac group were significantly greater than the differences among control subjects in the percentage of stage 0 and of stage 4. This suggested that our insomniac group may have contained several different subtypes of insomniacs. Furthermore, the insomniacs varied more from night-to-night than controls in total time in bed; total sleep time; ratio of total sleep time to time in bed; sleep latency; number of stage shifts; number of awakenings; percentages of stages 1-REM, 2, and 4; latency to stage 4 from sleep onset; and the ratio of minutes of REM sleep to minutes of stage 4 sleep. These results led us to speculate that part of the insomniac's problem may be that

he can never predict whether or not he will obtain a satisfactory night of sleep.

From our studies of insomniacs, we have noted several additional factors which may contribute to the difficulties of adequately describing them. Some patients who complain of not sleeping at all have apparently normal sleep patterns in terms of the percentages of each sleep stage, but exhibit alpha activity superimposed on the delta waves. These patients are often quite resistant to pharmacological treatment. Other patients seem to exhibit greater amounts of theta and beta activity. Since these qualitative characteristics are not usually measured in the present sleep-stage scoring system they may have been overlooked in other studies.

In conclusion, insomnia has been redefined to refer to a persistent inability to obtain adequate sleep in individuals exhibiting no gross physical or psychological pathology. Judging from sales of hypnotic medications, insomnia is quite prevalent in the general population. Many early explanations of insomnia attributed it primarily to emotional disturbance, and more recent systematic studies support the conclusion that psychological factors may play a role. However, there is also evidence of a physiological basis for these patients' complaints. Their sleep is considerably disturbed, according to EEG criteria, both in terms of the kinds and amounts of sleep they obtain, the night-to-night variability of their sleep patterns, and the qualitative aspects of their EEG activity. From such studies it appears that there may be several subtypes of insomniacs. Although the study of insomnia, as we have defined it, has only just begun, it is obvious that these and future findings may have major implications for the identification of more rational therapeutic procedures for this sleep disturbance.

Narcolepsy

Although the symptom complex had been described earlier,[428] Gélineau[148] was the originator of the term "narcolepsy" to refer to a condition consisting of recurring, uncontrollable episodes of brief sleep. This syndrome has been described with increasing refinement,[2,77] and the criteria presented by Yoss and Daly[436] form the basis for present diagnoses.

In narcolepsy the primary symptom of sleep attacks is often accompanied by one or more of three associated symptoms, i.e., cataplexy, sleep paralysis, and hypnogogic hallucinations. Yoss and Daly[436] referred to this symptom complex as the "narcoleptic tetrad" and reported that 11 percent of approximately 300 narcoleptics examined at the Mayo Clinic presented the full set of symptoms.

Cataplexy, which occurred in 68 percent of Yoss and Daly's[436] patients, was first described by Loewenfeld in 1902.[253] It is characterized by brief episodes of isolated or generalized muscular weakness, and the degree of disability may range from a subjective feeling of weakness, through loss of use of one or more extremities, to almost total paralysis. Emotion-provoking events and other strong stimulations are common precipitators of these attacks, and many patients develop peculiar stratagems for avoiding or alleviating the effects of these situations.

Sleep paralysis is similar to cataplexy in that it involves loss of muscle tone. However, it is usually experienced as a full-blown paralysis of the entire body, and occurs solely during the transition between sleep and wakefulness, or vice versa. Yoss and Daly[436] reported that 24 percent of their patients experienced this symptom. As will be discussed in a later section of this chapter, this symptom has been increasingly described as an isolated symptom in otherwise normal individuals. In either case, the individual usually remains quite conscious during the attack, which may last from several seconds to several minutes. A touch will usually terminate the attack, if it has not ended spontaneously.

Visual and auditory hypnogogic hallucinations often occur during sleep paralysis attacks in these patients. Yoss and Daly[436] reported that 30 percent of the Mayo Clinic narcoleptics exhibited this symptom, while Roth and Bruhova[353] observed an incidence of 19 percent in their sample of narcoleptics. The experience is often a frightening one, but many patients appear to be aware of the hallucinatory nature of it, which has prompted Roth and Bruhova[353] to describe it as a pseudohallucination. In any case, these hallucinations are characteristically quite bizarre and kaleidoscopic in nature. Oswald[304,306] has fully discussed the psychological and neurophysiological aspects of these events.

It has become common practice to differentiate between idiopathic narcolepsy and symptomatic narcolepsy. In the former the etiology of the disorder remains unknown, while in the latter there is a history of, or an association with, some organic disorder such as trauma, encephalitis, epilepsy, etc. As will be discussed below, data from polygraphic studies of narcoleptics suggest that there may be two forms of idiopathic narcolepsy—independent narcolepsy, in which sleep attacks are the only symptom, and narcolepsy accompanied by one or more of the other symptoms in the narcoleptic tetrad.

Although no systematic studies have been made of the incidence of narcolepsy, Roth[352] has estimated the incidence to be between 0.2 and 0.3 percent. At the Mayo Clinic, 241 cases were seen from 1950 through 1954,[436] and in 1960 Yoss and Daly[439] reported that approximately 100 new cases are seen there each year. The disorder appears to be equally distributed between the two sexes, and the typical age of onset is during the second or third decade.[436] There is some evidence of a genetic basis for narcolepsy in the high incidence in certain families.[194,239,437]

Diplopia is a common and early symptom of narcolepsy in many cases,[65,232] and McCrary and Smith[268] have described two narcoleptics with altered color vision. Gunne and Lidvall[166] found narcoleptics to excrete greater amounts of noradrenaline in the urine than controls. These patients also exhibited smaller daily fluctuations of noradrenaline levels. There were no abnormalities in urine levels of dopamine, adrenaline, or vanillylmandelic acid or in cerebrospinal fluid content of 5-hydroxyindolacetic acid. Administration of 100 mg. of L-dopa or 200 mg. of DL-dopa had no alerting effects on either patients or controls. These results should be somewhat cautiously interpreted, however, for the patients had been withdrawn from various medications, including amphetamine, just twenty-four hours prior to the beginning of the study. Sjaastad et al.[383] reported increased estriol secretion in male narcoleptics, although some complicating factors did not allow them definitely to attribute this increase to the narcolepsy per se. And finally, Goodwin et al.[155] have described a narcoleptic with an extremely high sensitivity to alcohol.

The nature of the narcoleptic's symptoms may often lead to the misdiagnoses of hypothyroidism, hypoglycemia, and epilepsy,[438] and each of these disorders has at one time or another been assigned an etiological role in narcolepsy. However several lines of evidence suggest that these factors are not characteristic or critical in the etiology of the disorder. Yoss and Daly[438] have commented that lower basal metabolism rates in these patients may seem to confirm the patient's complaint of being always tired. However, if care is taken to determine basal metabolism rates during times of relaxed alertness, normal values are usually obtained. Furthermore, administration of thyroid extract has not proved effective in increasing these patients' alertness. Hypoglycemia may be diagnosed on the basis of the persistent drowsiness and periods of impaired consciousness. However, sleep attacks are often most common after meals, which would rule out hypoglycemia as a precipitator. Furthermore, some narcoleptics are actually hyperglycemic,[347] while others exhibit no differences from controls in blood glucose values during various phases of nocturnal sleep.[323]

The evidence concerning the relationship of narcolepsy to epilepsy is contradictory. Some investigators* have detected abnormal or epileptiform waveforms in the waking EEG's of narcoleptics. Others[36,76,99,145] have found most patients to have essentially normal EEG's. In Dynes and Finley's[99] study all but one of the seventeen patients with normal EEG's also suffered from cataplexy, while none of the five patients exhibiting EEG abnormalities suffered from this symptom. As a

result, the authors proposed that patients with normal EEG's be considered idiopathic narcoleptics, and those showing EEG abnormalities as symptomatic. Daly and Yoss[76] found only two grossly abnormal EEG's in a study of 100 patients during a true alert state. On the other hand, they noted that although true sleep was rare during the recordings, a majority of the patients exhibited patterns of drowsiness at some time during the recording, often from the very onset of the recording and for long periods. Daly and Yoss suggested that this persistent drowsiness may lead to the impression that the EEG shows generalized slowing. Furthermore, the EEG artifact produced by head nodding during drowsiness may be misinterpreted as evidence of an akinetic seizure. Dement and Rechtschaffen and their associates[88,89,334] have suggested that the periods of drowsiness (stage-1 sleep) observed by Yoss and Daly may in fact have been REM sleep which was undetected because eye movements were not monitored during the clinical EEG. However, Berti Ceroni et al.[31] have confirmed that prolonged periods of stage-1 sleep without eye movements may characterize the daytime EEG's of these patients.

Psychological factors have quite naturally been assigned a role in the etiology of narcolepsy because of the apparent escapism involved in the symptoms and because of the apparent psychotic nature of the hypnogogic hallucinations. Sours[390] has reviewed these propositions and particularly that concerning the relationship between narcolepsy and schizophrenia. More recently Mitchell et al.[284] reported that all of twenty-two patients had undergone prolonged periods of sleep deprivation and disturbance, in association with major life transitions, prior to the recognition of their narcolepsy. Nevertheless, both Roth[352] and Yoss and Daly,[438] who have studied large numbers of these patients, have failed to detect any consistent evidence of psychopathology. As Yoss and Daly noted,[438] the social and economic disruption in the narcoleptic's life due to his symptoms may well lead to emotional disturbance, but it remains to be shown that this disturbance is the basis of the disorder.

* See references 35, 72, 360, 395, and 414.

Although modern sleep-research techniques have been extensively applied to the study of narcolepsy since the early 1960s, their use has not yet supplied any clear-cut evidence concerning the etiology of this disorder. Use of them has, however, considerably refined the description of the various narcoleptic phenomena, and in this way will undoubtedly contribute to the ultimate explication of the etiology.

It is now rather commonly agreed that narcoleptics who experience sleep attacks and one or more of the auxiliary symptoms of the narcoleptic tetrad can be recognized on the basis of the sleep EEG.[184,334,355] Whereas the normal individual, even when napping during the day,[224] proceeds through various phases of NREM sleep before the first REM period occurs, narcoleptics with cataplexy and/or the other symptoms exhibit a very strong tendency to enter REM sleep directly from wakefulness during both daytime sleep attacks and nocturnal sleep.[*] Although this sleep-onset REM period has not characterized every recording taken from every patient, it has occurred with sufficient frequency to suggest strongly that in this type of narcolepsy there is some neurophysiological or biochemical disturbance of the REM sleep system.

Furthermore, both direct and indirect evidence indicates that cataplexy, sleep paralysis, and hypnogogic hallucinations represent dissociated forms of REM sleep. It is well known that one of the unique and reliable characteristics of normal REM sleep is the inhibition of muscle tone in some muscle groups,[199] and of tibial nerve-calf muscle and tibial-plantar electrically induced reflexes.[191] The relevance of this inhibition to cataplexy and sleep paralysis is obvious, as is the dreaming of REM sleep to hypnogogic hallucinations. In fact, it has been shown that, as in normal REM sleep, tonic EMG activity and H-reflexes are depressed during the narcoleptic's sleep-onset REM period,[189] and that motor inhibition is more pronounced during the sleep-onset REM period than during these patients' later REM periods or during the REM sleep of nor-

mals.[292] Polygraphic recordings[†] during sleep-paralysis attacks and accompanying hypnogogic hallucinations have consistently revealed patterns of REM sleep. Although the early part of a cataplectic attack may be accompanied by waking EEG patterns, REM sleep may develop if the attack lasts long enough. Most patients who exhibit sleep attacks and other symptoms of the narcoleptic tetrad have nocturnal sleep which is characterized by numerous and long awakenings, decreased sleep time, and frequent body movements, and even though these patients typically exhibit sleep-onset REM periods, they obtain essentially normal amounts of REM sleep and normal numbers of REM periods. However, there have been occasional reports of increased REM time and numbers of REM periods. On the other hand, with only one exception,[31] deep slow-wave sleep has been found to be rare or nonexistent in these patients.

Recordings of twenty-four-hour periods of patients with sleep attacks and auxiliary symptoms have revealed increased REM time, as compared to normals sleeping approximately eight hours, in many, but not all, patients.[31, 88,313] Passouant[312] and his colleagues[313, 315,316] reported that the REM sleep attacks occur approximately every two hours during the day, suggesting a continuation during the daytime of the REM cycle of normal nocturnal sleep. These investigators also noted that the frequent daytime sleep attacks and interrupted night sleep of these patients produce a polyphasic twenty-four-hour sleep pattern, which contrasts with the monophasic pattern of normal adults but resembles the typical sleep pattern of infants.

In contrast to narcoleptics with auxiliary symptoms, narcoleptics who experience only sleep attacks very rarely exhibit sleep-onset REM periods.[‡] Instead, their attacks resemble normal NREM sleep periods. Furthermore, the nocturnal sleep of these patients appears to be essentially normal both quantitatively and qualitatively.[31,316]

[*] See references 30, 31, 89, 187, 312, 315–317, 355, 356, and 399.

[†] See references 31, 61, 88, 89, 184, 187, 189, 312, 313, 316, 317, 341, 355, 356, 399, and 402.

[‡] See references 30, 89, 187, 315, 316, 355, and 356.

These observations originally suggested[89,][334] that only patients exhibiting auxiliary symptoms should be classified as narcoleptics, since the NREM sleep attacks of independent narcoleptics could not be distinguished from the NREM sleep periods of normals. However, it has been consistently observed that narcoleptics with auxiliary symptoms may at least occasionally exhibit NREM sleep attacks and nocturnal sleep onset, that some of these patients never exhibit sleep-onset REM periods, and that NREM sleep frequently follows the sleep-onset REM period in an attack. Furthermore, imipramine, which is effective in alleviating the auxiliary symptoms of narcolepsy, but ineffective in relieving the sleep attacks,[186] has been shown to suppress REM sleep in narcoleptics.[357] On the other hand, amphetamine, phenmetrazine and methylphenidate, which are effective against sleep attacks but not against the auxiliary symptoms, have less drastic effects on REM sleep and also appear to decrease NREM sleep to a certain degree.[357] These observations have led to more recent suggestions that there is a NREM sleep disturbance in many, if not all, narcoleptics, but that REM sleep disturbances are also important in narcoleptics with auxiliary symptoms.[335,355,356]

Although the narcoleptic who exhibits sleep-onset REM periods displays an abnormal propensity to enter REM sleep, it has generally been argued that this does not reflect an excessive need to spend large amounts of time in REM sleep.[88,334,341] This conclusion is based on observations that various degrees of REM-sleep deprivation in normal subjects, with the resulting, presumed build-up of a "need" for REM sleep, only rarely produce sleep-onset REM periods during the recovery period. Furthermore, the narcoleptic's typically normal amount of nocturnal REM sleep contrasts with the rebound of REM sleep during recovery from REM deprivation in normals.

As an alternative to this explanation, Rechtschaffen and Dement[334] proposed that the REM disturbance reflects a failure of wakefulness and NREM sleep to inhibit the appearance of REM sleep. Passouant[312] and his colleagues[315] have made a similar suggestion. However, as Rechtschaffen and Dement[335] have commented more recently, the admission of an important NREM-sleep disturbance would necessitate the postulation of a failure of wakefulness to inhibit NREM as well as REM sleep.

To summarize, narcolepsy and the narcoleptic tetrad of symptoms probably affect less than 1 percent of the population, but the bothersome and sometimes dangerous nature of the attacks makes them serious public-health problems. It is generally agreed that hypothyroidism, hypoglycemia, and epilepsy are not significant etiological factors. Although the narcoleptic may develop emotional disturbance as a result of the problems caused by the disorder, there is little empirical evidence that psychological factors play a major role in the etiology of this disorder. On the other hand, disturbances of both REM and NREM sleep would seem, in some as yet unknown fashion, to be basic to the disorder. There is substantial evidence suggesting that narcoleptics who experience only sleep attacks suffer primarily from a NREM sleep disturbance. In patients who also experience the other symptoms of the narcoleptic tetrad, both the REM and NREM systems appear to be disturbed, and cataplexy, sleep paralysis, and hypnogogic hallucinations probably represent dissociated forms of REM sleep. It has been suggested that the narcoleptic's attacks reflect a failure of wakefulness to suppress REM and/or NREM sleep.

Chronic Hypersomnia

As its name implies, hypersomnia is characterized by excessive sleep. Although this disturbance may also characterize narcoleptics and patients suffering from the Pickwickian syndrome, and is a periodic manifestation in the Kleine-Levin syndrome, in chronic hypersomnia the excessive sleep is the primary chronic symptom. According to Roth[352] there are two categories of chronic hypersomnia. In the first, there is good evidence that the excessive sleep or sleepiness is associated with or precipitated by some central-nervous-system

(CNS) disorder such as skull trauma, brain tumor, encephalitis, or cerebrovascular accident, and for this reason Roth called it "symptomatic hypersomnia." Functional hypersomnia has no demonstrable organic basis. In patients with either disorder there is a notable increase in daily sleep time, and this increase may result from an excessively long nocturnal sleep period and/or frequent or long daytime sleep periods. Rechtshaffen and Roth[339] noted that these patients rarely complain of disturbed nocturnal sleep, in contrast to narcoleptics. However, they often experience extreme difficulty in awakening and postdormital confusion, or "sleep drunkenness," once they do awaken.[339,359] Daytime sleep attacks lack the compelling and irresistible nature of the narcoleptic's sleep attacks and may last for several hours or days.[339] In their latest report, Roth et al.[359] concluded that there is a complete form of hypersomnia, consisting of postdormital confusion, very deep and prolonged sleep, diurnal hypersomnia, and rapid onset of nocturnal sleep. There is also an incomplete form, which consists only of postdormital confusion and deep and prolonged sleep.

Data on the incidence of this disorder are virtually nonexistent, both because of an as yet unclear distinction between *natural long sleepers*[423] and hypersomniacs, and because of the relatively recent recognition of chronic hypersomnia as a distinct clinical entity.[352] Roth et al.[359] reported that 161 cases of hypersomnia, with and without sleep drunkenness, were seen in their clinic in Prague over the last twenty years, with 71 percent being classified as idiopathic cases. These investigators noted that incidence figures cannot be reliably based on numbers of self-selected clinic patients. They believe that many patients with hypersomnia do not seek medical help for their problem, and that the ratio of idiopathic to symptomatic cases may be higher in the general population since symptomatic cases are more likely to be seen in a clinic because of additional symptoms and more sudden changes in sleep patterns.

From the meager evidence concerning this disorder[339,359] it appears that in idiopathic cases the age of onset may range from childhood through the third or fourth decade. In symptomatic cases, the age of onset would of course depend on the age at which the CNS disorder occurred, but in one study of hypersomniacs with sleep drunkenness[359] age of onset was generally later than in idiopathic cases. In both types the disorder usually continued throughout life, with only minor periodic increases or decreases in symptomatology. From the samples of patients studied[339, 359] there is a suggestion that hypersomnia occurs about equally in the two sexes. In idiopathic cases there is frequently a family history of the disorder.[339,359]

In their study of these patients Rechtschaffen and Roth[339] described the polygraphic nocturnal sleep patterns of a rather heterogeneous group of hypersomniacs. Ages ranged from twenty to fifty-three years, and some patients were essentially normal psychologically while others showed greater or lesser degrees of psychopathology; various constellations of the hypersomnia symptom complex were present. Although there was a relative decrease in symptoms during the laboratory sleep nights, Rechtschaffen and Roth felt confident in concluding that there were no deviations from normal patterning or percentages of sleep stages in these patients. None of the patients exhibited the sleep-onset REM periods characteristic of narcoleptics. Sleep averaged 8.8 hours in length, excluding one subject who typically slept over twenty hours in the laboratory. The sleep period beyond the normal seven or eight hours was a continuation of the typical alternation of sleep stages. Although the patients often complained of difficulty in awakening, there was no evidence of abnormal amounts of slow-wave sleep, in which auditory awakening thresholds are elevated in normals.[337] In two instances of postdormital confusion the EEG showed an alternation of wakefulness and stage-1 sleep.

In a second report Roth et al.[359] described the daytime sleep patterns of hypersomniacs who experienced postdormital confusion and daytime hypersomnia. Sleep consisted primarily of alternations between stages-1 and -2 sleep, and was interrupted by frequent awakenings. Stages-3 and -4 sleep were rare, although this may have been due to the fact that most of the recordings were made in the early afternoon, when these stages are less prevalent in normals.[267] REM sleep was also absent, but the authors noted that this may have resulted from the brevity of the recording period.

Among the most suggestive results in this series of studies was the fact that hypersomniacs exhibited faster heart and respiratory rates than "good sleepers," "poor sleepers," and "deep sleepers," both before and during nocturnal sleep.[339] There was some evidence that severity of hypersomnia might be related to the degree of elevation of these rates.

Although Rechtschaffen and Roth cautioned against speculating extensively on the basis of these findings until and unless they are replicated, these investigators have suggested that the heightened activation manifested by hypersomniacs may reflect activation of neural mechanisms controlling heart and respiratory function as well as sleep, or release from centers which inhibit these functions. It may also be that the activation reflected by heart and respiratory rates produces an increased need for sleep in the hypersomniac. These are intriguing possibilities, but there remain many questions which must be answered before this disorder is fully understood. For example, Roth et al.[359] have drawn attention to the fact that there seems to be more than a chance relationship between narcolepsy and the hypersomniac symptom of sleep drunkenness, even though hypersomnia and narcolepsy are typically clearly distinguishable from each other. On the other hand, the difference between the hypersomniac and the normal "long sleeper" described by Webb and Agnew[423] is unclear, especially since postdormital confusion can occur in normals following excessive sleep.[152]

Thus we have seen that there is a distinct clinical entity of chronic hypersomnia which may be symptomatic or functional. Rapid sleep onset, deep and prolonged nocturnal sleep, postdormital confusion, and diurnal hypersomnia characterize the complete form of this disorder, while deep and prolonged sleep and postdormital confusion character-

ize the incomplete form. The few studies exploring this disorder have failed to reveal any abnormalities in the sleep patterns of hypersomniacs, although these patients appear to exhibit higher heart and respiratory rates than normals and certain other types of individuals. Neither the mechanism of this disorder nor the manner in which hypersomniacs differ from natural long sleepers and other patients who exhibit sleep attacks or excessive sleep has yet been elucidated.

The Kleine-Levin Syndrome

In 1942 Critchley and Hoffman[74] called attention to the syndrome described by Kleine[235] and Levin[245,246] and characterized by periodic hypersomnia and morbid hunger. Critchley and Hoffman proposed that this syndrome be called the Kleine-Levin syndrome and described two additional cases. In 1962 Critchley[73] reviewed the thirty-one cases reported up to that time, and emphasized several characteristics of the symptom picture. Among these were a preponderant or unique occurrence in males, a typical onset in adolescence, a spontaneous disappearance, compulsive eating rather than excessive appetite, and behavioral abnormalities. Critchley concluded that only twenty-six of the reported cases, including eleven described by him, could be considered genuine examples of this syndrome. Sours[390] confirmed the rare incidence of the disorder. He reviewed the histories of 115 patients seen at Columbia Presbyterian Medical Center in New York for various complaints of excessive sleepiness from 1932 to 1961, and did not find a single case of Kleine-Levin syndrome. Since Critchley's review in 1962 a number of new cases have been described,* but in the process Critchley's original diagnostic criteria have been somewhat broadened and modified. For example, several female cases have been described.[98,100,150] The case presented by Thacore et al.[407] began displaying symptoms at age eight and did not exhibit excessive eating, while Berti Ceroni's[29] case evolved into narcolepsy. Such differences,

* See references 24, 29, 39, 98, 100, 105, 142, 150, 157, 190, 265, and 407.

as well as others to be discussed below, led Oswald[307] and Thacore et al.[407] to conclude that the existence of a distinct nosological entity characterized by periodic hypersomnia and excessive eating has yet to be proven, and that placement of a case in this category is largely a matter of preference. Pai[310] had earlier concluded that the Kleine-Levin syndrome is not a definite clinical entity.

With this controversy in mind, we will nevertheless review some of the major findings from the reported cases. One of the two primary characteristics of Kleine-Levin patients is what has been termed periodic hypersomnolence. Oswald[307] has noted, however, that it has yet to be established that these patients in fact sleep excessively. For this to be done would require systematic monitoring of various physiological parameters, including brain waves, during the periods of so-called sleep. Although numerous investigators have reported EEG findings, the lack of precise descriptions of the patient's status (during or between exacerbations, asleep or awake) or of the examination situation (patient sitting or lying down, day or night recording, length of recording) makes it very difficult to derive a clear picture of the EEG characteristics of these patients. Furthermore, even the results which are clearly interpretable are contradictory. For example, Rosenkötter and Wende[351] reported that sleep EEG activity during sleep attacks corresponded to that of natural sleep. Barontini and Zappoli[24] found afternoon sleep during an attack to be light and unstable, but concluded that there was "no evidence of significant abnormality of the cortical biorhythms . . ." Barontini and Zappoli's patient was a twenty-nine-year-old male and the recorded sleep period lasted from 4:30 to 8:00 P.M. We have reported[224] that normal males between the ages of twenty-one and twenty-eight obtained 14 percent stage-4 sleep and 19 percent REM sleep during naps between 4 and 6 P.M. Barontini and Zappoli's patient obtained no stage-4 or REM sleep and only moderate amounts of stage-3 sleep. Thus, there did appear to be a significant lightening of this patient's sleep pattern during this hypersomnolent episode. On the other hand, other investigators[157,407] failed to detect any spindles during "sleep" attacks. Since the presence of spindles is a criterion for the existence of EEG sleep, these data indicate that true sleep may not appropriately characterize the daytime state of the Kleine-Levin patient. Garland et al.[142] reached a similar conclusion when they described their patient as withdrawn rather than somnolent during the exacerbation.

One recording made of the night sleep of a Kleine-Levin patient[24] revealed that sleep was generally light and unstable, although stage-3 sleep was moderately present. Stage-4 sleep occurred several times but never for long intervals. Only two very short REM periods occurred during the seven-hour recording period. A similar recording made following the exacerbation revealed more normal amounts of deep sleep, but REM periods were still quite short. Markman[265] confirmed this last result.

If these sleep-EEG data prove to be accurate when more subjects have been studied, it may well be argued that both the night and daytime sleep of Kleine-Levin patients is disturbed, especially in comparison to age-matched normals. From the sparse data available it would appear that these patients obtain significantly less REM and deep-stage-4 sleep at night. Their daytime sleep is either unusually light or not really sleep at all. Furthermore, even between attacks these patients seem to obtain abnormally low amounts of REM sleep at night. This last fact might indicate that this disorder is not truly periodic, as has been claimed, but that these patients suffer from persistent sleep abnormalities which are periodically exaggerated.

The second primary characteristic of this disorder is excessive eating. Although Critchley[73] considered it to be a necessary component of the clinical syndrome, subsequent cases[157,407] have not always exhibited this behavior. Critchley[73] suggested that this characteristic consisted of compulsive eating rather than bulimia, but Gilbert[150] has contested this view. Garland et al.[142] have criticized Critchley's use of various terms for overeating and Pai[310] noted that often there have been no quantitative data to support reports of overeating.

Among the other characteristics reported more or less frequently during excerbations in Kleine-Levin patients are sexual excitement or disinhibition; particular preference for sweets; irritability, especially when aroused from sleep; full or partial amnesia either during or following the attack; and depression and insomnia following the attack. Weight gains during the attacks and euphoria following them have also been reported for some patients. There have been no consistent abnormalities discovered by radiological or laboratory studies.

Critchley[73] found a psychiatric explanation of this disorder to be unsatisfactory, particularly since most of his patients appeared to be normal before the onset of symptoms. However Oswald[307] noted that many of Critchley's cases showed apparent schizophreniform abnormalities during attacks. Pai[310] concluded that the hypersomnolence and excessive eating characteristic of this disorder occur together coincidentally, and that both are hysterical in nature.

Levin[246] proposed the first organic theory of the etiology of the syndrome bearing his name. He suggested that the symptoms result from excessive inhibition or exhaustion of frontal-lobe centers controlling these behaviors. Gallinek[139] subsequently suggested that the frontal lobes and/or the hypothalamus are implicated on the basis of studies of lesions or tumors in these areas. Most authors* have agreed that dysfunction of hypothalamic or diencephalic areas is involved, in view of the disturbances in sleeping, alimentary, and sometimes sexual behavior. Several investigators have proposed that this disorder is related to narcolepsy[29,139,140,311] or to convulsive disorders.[105,311]

Interactions between psychological and organic factors have received attention from some investigators. Thus Gilbert[150] proposed that psychodynamically the Kleine-Levin exacerbation might represent an escape from a threatening environment by an individual who can sense its demands but who is unable to cope with them. According to Gilbert these psychological factors would determine the temporal occurrence of the syndrome, but an underlying diencephlic dysfunction would determine the specific manifestations of the syndrome. Earle[100] suggested that this condition is a psychosomatic disorder which emerges when individuals with psychopathology in the oral sphere also experience some pathology on the organic level, and possibly at the level of the hypothalamus. Bonkalo[39] has also proposed an interactive interpretation of the etiology of the Kleine-Levin syndrome and of other hypersomnia syndromes.

As we have seen, there is considerable debate about the exact nature of the characteristics defining the Kleine-Levin syndrome. There is suggestive evidence that patients suffering from this disorder may not in fact be truly asleep during their periodic attacks of daytime hypersomnolence; their nocturnal sleep patterns are abnormally light. In addition, two patients have shown persistent REM-sleep abnormalities following clinical improvement. Excessive eating has not been an entirely consistent finding in these patients, and there have been few quantitative descriptions of this symptom. A variety of abnormal behaviors, including sexual disinhibition, irritability, and depression, have been reported to occur during or following the attacks. Most authors agree that some dysfunction at the diencephalic or hypothalamic level is the basis for this syndrome, although several have proposed exclusively psychological or combined psychological and organic explanations. At this point, the paucity of data concerning this disorder allows only speculation as to the etiology or localization of the dysfunction. The debate about the reality of the Kleine-Levin syndrome as a distinct clinical entity may contribute to the difficulty in more fully illuminating this rather interesting set of symptoms.

The Pickwickian Syndrome

Readers of Charles Dickens's *The Posthumous Papers of the Pickwick Club* will

* See references 24, 74, 98, 105, 140, 142, 157, 190, 311, and 351.

remember the description of the rotund lad, Joe, who could not manage to stay awake. Recalling this description in 1956, Burwell and his associates[60] coined the apt term "Pickwickian syndrome" to refer to a condition characterized by marked obesity, somnolence, twitching, cyanosis, periodic respiration, secondary polycythemia, right ventricular failure, hypoxia, and hypercapnea. The syndrome had previously been described[19,233,381] under less spectacular names. Subsequent study of this condition has often failed to reveal all of the symptoms listed by Burwell et al., and obesity, hypersomnia and periodic respiration are now considered to be primary diagnostic criteria.[185,330,376] Escande et al.[106] have proposed that there are two subcategories of this syndrome, a "Burwell type," which is the most advanced form and is characterized by obesity, hypersomnolence, and alveolar hypoventilation and its concomitants, and a "Joe type," which consists only of obesity and hypersomnia.

Polygraphic studies have begun to provide some interesting information on the relationships between two of the primary symptoms of this disorder, hypersomnolence and periodic respiration. Drachman and Gumnit[97] were the first to describe the cyclical changes in EEG and respiration patterns during the sleep of these patients, and their observations have been confirmed and elaborated by others.[147,186,211,376] Very shortly after the Pickwickian patient enters sleep, apneic intervals lasting from five to sixty seconds begin to appear. During the periods of apnea typical sleep patterns occur, and the length of these intervals depends on the depth of sleep during which they occur, with deeper stages being characterized by longer, and possibly less frequent, periods of apnea. Just prior to the return of respiration there is an EEG arousal response consisting of alpha activity or a K-complex. The EEG may not necessarily show waking patterns, but only lightening of sleep. Concurrently the patient takes several deep breaths, and then the whole cycle begins again. During successive cycles the sleep stage during the apneic periods may progressively deepen. At the end of several cycles, the arousal terminating the apnea may be particularly intense and accompanied by a body movement. Eventually one of these more intense arousals becomes a more complete awakening, after which begins a new series of deepening sleep episodes terminated by arousal.

This pattern of EEG and respiratory changes has been observed during both diurnal and nocturnal sleep in Pickwickian patients. As a result, it is not surprising that a cardinal feature of their sleep, whatever the time of day, is its discontinuity. Although these patients have been reported to obtain over ten hours of sleep per twenty-four hours, this represents the sum of many short sleep periods rather than one extended sleep period.[69,145,147] The discontinuity is accompanied by further sleep abnormalities. In many cases REM and deep slow-wave sleep are absent or rare.* In other patients, REM-sleep periods may still be present but are somewhat shorter than normal.[69,211] Some investigators have reported a lessening of the apneic disturbances during REM sleep,[56,185,211] while others have found the disturbance to persist and interact with the respiratory irregularities normally characteristic of REM sleep.[376]

Since the systematic study of Pickwickian patients is relatively new, there are, understandably, insufficient data to allow full agreement on the mechanisms and etiology of this disorder. As Escande and his colleagues[106] have suggested, the parallel but virtually independent work performed by internists and electroencephalographers has also contributed to some of the debates about these matters. One widely discussed topic is the pulmonary function status of Pickwickian patients. Some investigators[97,185,330] believe that chronic hypercapnea and hypoxia, secondary to chronic alveolar hypoventilation, characterize the Pickwickian, possibly as a result of the increased work required to breathe in the extremely obese. Others[145,147] maintain that in the "pure" Pickwickian waking pulmonary function is normal enough to allow adequate

---

* See references 69, 147, 185, 211, 330, and 406.

blood-gas exchange to occur. As noted earlier, Escande et al.[106] have proposed that there may be two forms of the Pickwickian syndrome, one characterized by primary alveolar hypoventilation and the other not.

A second area of controversy is the nature of the apneic mechanism in these patients. Gastaut et al.[147] found that 80 percent of one patient's apneic episodes were peripheral or obstructive in nature, while 15 percent were of central origin and 5 percent were of mixed type. Coccagna et al.[69] also observed both central and obstructive types of apnea, but concluded that central mechanisms control the apnea, with the obstructive phenomena sometimes occurring as a result of hypotonia and thus prolonging the existent central apnea. Hishikawa et al.[185] found that apnea was obstructive in nature in their two patients, but suggested that centrally determined apnea may eventually appear as a result of the development of a permanent hyposensitivity of the respiratory centers to CO_2 retention. This would occur following the rather chronic nocturnal hypercapnea accompanying the initial obstructive apnea.

Several authors[211,376,406] have stressed the fact that the periodic respiration of Pickwickian patients is an exaggeration of respiratory changes occurring during normal sleep. In normal individuals, the onset of sleep is characterized by decreased ventilation, increased CO_2 tension, and decreased arterial oxygen saturation, and the conclusion has been that respiratory centers are less sensitive to CO_2 during sleep.[33,34,58,59] Bülow[57] has reported that CO_2 sensitivity is lower during the deeper stages of sleep than during the lighter stages. Furthermore, some normal individuals may exhibit short apneic episodes during sleep.[57,358] These observations have led to the suggestion that the nocturnal respiratory disturbances of the Pickwickian are a function of a coordinated disturbance of respiratory rhythm and sleep-waking regulation in the brain stem.[211] However, the fact that disturbed nocturnal respiration may persist even after improvement of other clinical symptoms (hypersomnolence, pulmonary ventilation) following loss of weight,[97,211,406]

suggests that these patients retain a tendency to CO_2 hyposensitivity.[211]

The postulation of an intimate relationship between disturbances in respiration and sleep-waking mechanisms naturally introduces the question of the etiology of the hypersomnolence in these patients. Jung and Kuhlo,[211] as well as others,[97] have suggested that chronic CO_2 hyposensitivity, with the resulting hypoventilation and hypercapnea, disposes the Pickwickian to diurnal sleep attacks in the absence of arousing stimuli. Another view[147,185] is that diurnal sleepiness and sleep are the result of poor and disturbed nocturnal sleep. Still another view is that a primary disturbance of the sleep-waking mechanism, analogous to that of narcoleptics, produces the daytime sleep attacks.[147] It should be noted, however, that most investigators[145,211,240,406] have clearly distinguished Pickwickians from narcoleptics, primarily on the basis of the facts that Pickwickians do not exhibit cataplexy, sleep paralysis, hypnogogic hallucinations, or the sleep-onset REM periods characteristic of many narcoleptic sleep attacks, while narcoleptics do not exhibit marked periodic respiration during sleep.

From this discussion it is clear that the Pickwickian syndrome, although relatively rare, has engendered lively interest on the part of sleep researchers. It has been confirmed that Pickwickians suffer from distinct disturbances in the maintenance and quality of sleep. These disturbances appear to be intimately related to these patients' respiratory disturbances, but the exact nature of this relationship, as well as the relationship of the sleep and respiratory disturbances to other clinical symptoms such as obesity, has yet to be fully determined.

Sleep Paralysis

Sleep paralysis, as described in the recent literature,[269,354,373] occurs during the transition between the waking and sleeping states. The individual is aware of his surroundings but is unable to move voluntarily. Respiration is not usually impaired to a significant degree. In most cases the sufferer is unable to talk, although he may manage to moan and thus attract the attention of others. Anxiety and hypnogogic hallucinations are frequent concomitants of the paralysis. In some cases the anxiety subsides as the individual becomes accustomed to the benign nature of the attacks, but in others[247] the attacks are always accompanied by anxiety. The individual experiencing hypnogogic hallucinations is generally aware of the unreal nature of his perceptions. Most sleep paralysis attacks last a maximum of several minutes, but often the time sense of the sufferer is quite distorted. The frequency of attacks is highly variable both between and within individuals. In most instances any external stimulus, and particularly a touch, will terminate the attack, although in some cases a stronger stimulus is required. If the attack is not terminated by external means, it eventually ends spontaneously. In some cases the individual must get up and move around in order to prevent a series of attacks.

This disturbance has been most frequently described as one of the constituents of the narcolepsy syndrome. Thus 34.4 percent[354] and 28 percent[439] of two samples of narcoleptic patients displayed this symptom. There are also occasional reports[251] of sleep paralysis accompanying psychosis. However, sleep paralysis as an isolated symptom has been described more and more frequently.* Although Rushton[363] and Schneck[369–371] had expressed the belief that isolated sleep paralysis is much more common than case reports would indicate, it remained for Goode[154] to support this belief with a systematic incidence study. He found that fifteen of 231 medical students, none of fifty-three nursing students, and two of seventy-five hospital inpatients reported isolated sleep paralysis. Subsequently Everett[110] reported that 15.4 percent of fifty-two medical students claimed to have experienced sleep-paralysis attacks and none had experienced either narcoleptic sleep attacks or cataplexy. In Goode's study the age of onset of sleep-paralysis attacks ranged from eight to fifty years, and among Everett's medical stu-

* See references 40, 67, 154, 247, 250, 363, 369–373, and 412.

dents the onset age ranged from childhood to the college years in those individuals who responded to this question. Of Goode's subjects, three experienced both pre- and postdormital attacks, two experienced predormital attacks only, and twelve experienced postdormital attacks only. Several of Everett's subjects reported a greater likelihood of having attacks during naps than at night. Histories of parasomnias, such as sleep hallucinations, sleepwalking and sleeptalking, were also reported by some of Goode's subjects.

There are contradictory data on the sex distribution of sleep paralysis. Approximately 80 percent of Goode's[154] subjects who reported sleep paralysis were males. However, in his survey sample over two-thirds of the respondents were males, and this may have contributed to the unequal sex distribution among the sleep-paralysis sufferers. In a study of two families with isolated sleep paralysis Roth et al.[354] found a conspicuous predominance of women with the disturbance. This study indicated that sleep paralysis is a genetically determined disturbance which is invariably transmitted by the mother. Roth et al. concluded that dominant heredity bound to the X-chromosome is the method of transmission. Other authors[154,363] have described cases with family histories of sleep paralysis.

Sleep paralysis is particularly difficult to study, both because of its variable frequency of occurrence, and because the stimulation involved in examining the patient during an attack usually terminates the paralysis. In addition, aside from the reports[354,363] that individuals suffering from isolated sleep-paralysis attacks exhibit essentially normal waking EEGs, there are no systematic descriptions of the clinical characteristics of these individuals.

As is the case with many of the sleep disorders, etiological theories of sleep paralysis tend to stress either psychological or organic factors. Langworthy and Betz[243] offered a psychological interpretation in which sleep paralysis is viewed as a neurotic defense against primary anxieties associated with realistic adjustments in interpersonal relationships. Others have suggested that the disorder is related to a state of confusion as to emotion and intention,[412] fear of destructive impulses,[40] or anxiety reflecting the individual's own specific conflicts.[251] Schneck, who has written extensively on the topic, has modified his earlier assertion that sleep paralysis is an expression of homosexual conflict,[369] and suggested more recently that general conflicts between passive and aggressive personality trends are involved.[370,371,373]

The notion of dissociation or asynchrony between various aspects of the sleep mechanism has been invoked by some as a more organic explanation of this disorder.[50,247,250] Other authors[77,436] have considered sleep paralysis to be a variant of cataplexy. However, Chodoff[67] and Goode[154] have enumerated several differences between these two phenomena, suggesting that they are not identical disorders. Still others[107,293] have proposed that sleep paralysis is a form of epilepsy. As Goode[154] notes, however, EEG recordings made during sleep-paralysis episodes offer little support for this hypothesis.[76,187,326,355]

In 1953 Aird et al.[3] advanced the hypothesis that either blockage of the reticular facilitatory system and the resultant predominance of the reticular inhibitory system, or primary stimulation of the inhibitory system, may be sufficient to produce sleep paralysis. Although it has not yet been determined whether isolated sleep-paralysis attacks are identical to narcoleptic sleep-paralysis attacks, recent polygraphic studies of narcoleptics have led to a revival of the dissociation hypothesis, in a more specific form, as the explanation of narcolepsy and of its concomitant symptoms. It has been amply demonstrated* that narcoleptics who exhibit sleep attacks and one or more of the other narcolepsy symptoms frequently experience REM periods at or soon after sleep onset. This contrasts with the normal pattern, in which the first REM period typically occurs approximately ninety minutes after sleep onset. Although earlier descriptions of EEG activity during sleep-paralysis attacks in narcoleptics[76,326] mentioned only patterns of drowsiness during the episode, more recent

---

* See references 89, 187, 188, 341, and 355.

studies[187,355] in which eye movements were monitored have indicated that the attacks are accompanied by REM sleep. Moreover, there is a loss of spinal reflexes during REM sleep in both normal subjects[191] and narcoleptics,[189] and early parts of the narcoleptic's sleep-onset REM period seem to be composed of lighter sleep than either the drowsy state, the later part of the sleep-onset REM period, or later REM periods.[185] These data suggest that the mechanism of sleep paralysis in narcoleptics involves a dissociation of REM sleep.[355] This dissociation refers to the occurrence of certain REM phenomena, such as muscular inhibition and dreamlike state, against a background of relative awareness. Roth et al.[354,355] believe that independent sleep paralysis is also due to such a disturbance in the REM system. Whether or not this is the case must be explored in future work, along with a determination of whether there is an analogous explanation for postdormital sleep-paralysis attacks.

Frightening Dreams

Polygraphic investigations have provided evidence that there are two types of unpleasant nocturnal "dream" attacks, i.e., night terrors and dream anxiety attacks. The former, also called "pavor nocturnus" in children and "incubus attacks" in adults, are characterized by a sudden scream and arousal. Intense anxiety, hypermotility, increased heart and respiration rates, confusion, unresponsiveness, hallucinations, choking sensations, and feelings of impending doom accompany the arousal. The sufferer is usually unable to remember the attack the next morning.[54,126] The dream anxiety attack is generally less intense than, and lacks the quality of panic associated with the night terror. It may, however, precipitate an arousal, and dream reports are typically more complete than after arousal from night terrors.[124] Although these two types of nightmares are usually easily differentiated on the basis of sleep EEG data, Mack[259] has pointed out that this may not be the case when only clinical reports are available.

These sleep attacks have been described in people of all ages and cultures, and are not confined to the mentally ill.[259] The incidence of night terrors appears to be much lower than that of dream anxiety attacks.[176] Fisher et al.[124] cite a report by Kurth et al.[242] according to which night terrors were described by 2.9 percent of 991 children between the ages of one and fourteen years. Hersen[183] studied 352 inpatients who were primarily diagnosed as having psychotic disorders and found that 32 percent reported having frightening dreams leading to awakening at least once a month. Among college undergraduates the analogous figure was 5 percent.[120] Whether the respondents in these two studies were reporting night terrors or anxiety attacks, or both, is not clear. After reviewing the literature on the incidence of unpleasant dreams in children, Mack[259] concluded that such dreams predominate in preschool children and that the incidence decreases after six years of age.

Sleep EEG studies[124,144] of the two types of dreams have shown that the night terror is a NREM, slow-wave sleep phenomenon, while the anxiety dream occurs during REM sleep. Most NREM sleep dreams occur during the first half of the night. During the first or second NREM period a K-complex or a burst of delta waves presages the onset of the attack. Alpha activity and investigative eye movements quickly follow, and are accompanied by sharp increases in heart and respiration rates, and by body movement and muscle contractions. With the end of the attack all measures gradually return to normal. Although Broughton[53] reported that relative tachycardia characterized the slow-wave sleep of night-terror sufferers, Fisher et al.[124] found heart and respiration rates to be normal, or even reduced, in the interval prior to the abrupt onset of the attack. They also noted that the length of the stage-4 interval preceding the attack and the quantity of delta activity during the interval were positively related to the intensity of the attack. Gastaut and Broughton[144] were able to elicit only minimal dream content from subjects following arousal from NREM attacks, but several of Fisher's[124] subjects provided lengthy reports. The content was of two types. The first consisted of a single vivid scene which appeared to occur at the same time as or just before the arousal scream. The second type was more elaborate and seemed to be related to the autonomic activity following the scream.

Autonomic activation may or may not occur before and during the arousal terminating a REM-sleep dream-anxiety attack. Fisher et al.[124] studied twenty such attacks in eleven subjects. They found that in twelve attacks which were characterized as producing mild to marked anxiety, there was no change from control levels of heart and respiratory rates. In five other attacks, less than maximal degrees of activation were present, and in the remaining three there were clear-cut increases in the heart and respiratory rates. Content elicited after REM attacks is much more elaborate than that elicited after NREM attacks, and one individual appears not to suffer from both types of attacks.[124]

There are, of course, numerous psychological interpretations of these sleep attacks,[168, 205,259] but there have been relatively few systematic studies of the variables involved. One exception is the series of studies carried out by Hersen. In the first[120] there was a significant relationship between conscious concern with death and frequency of nightmares in a college-student sample. In the second study[183] similar results were obtained with psychotic inpatients. In addition, the degree of manifest anxiety and the number of other sleep disturbances were positively related to frequency of bad dreams, while ego strength was negatively related.

Among sleep researchers there is agreement that these attacks are most probably psychological in origin. Broughton[53] suggested that NREM night terrors are disorders of arousal, similar to enuresis and somnambulism, and that the sufferers are physiologically predisposed, possibly as exhibited by their relative tachycardia during slow-wave sleep and their hyperactive heart rate during the arousal response, to experience night terrors during otherwise normal slow-wave sleep arousals. The exact precipitator of the attacks on any particular night may be the expression of repressed conflicts by mental activity released when protective barriers are lowered during the deepest stages of sleep. Or it may be that the attacks arise out of a "psychological void" and that the subjective experience of terror on arousal derives mainly from the perception of the accompanying physiological changes. In another formulation, Broughton[54] elaborated on the first explanation and proposed that unresolved conflicts alter the arousal mechanism of the night-terror sufferer, producing a psychosomatic arousal disorder.

Fisher et al.[124] believe that more immediate psychological factors precipitate both REM and NREM attacks. Specifically, increasing ego regression accompanying the progressive deepening of stage-4 sleep is suggested as the precipitator of NREM terrors, although the fact that attacks can be produced by sounding a buzzer during stage-4 sleep suggests that external stimulation may also play a precipitating role. On the other hand, the REM dream is hypothesized to have a modulating influence on anxiety, and by reducing or eliminating the physiological concomitants of anxiety it serves to guard REM sleep. This would explain the desomatization of the anxiety accompanying a majority of the REM attacks these investigators have described. When the desomatization mechanism breaks down, however, autonomic activation is seen to accompany the anxiety dream. It is the view of Fisher and his colleagues that the stage-4 nightmare represents a failure of the ego to control anxiety, and, rather than being a dream, it is a relatively rare pathological formation of NREM sleep. By contrast, the REM anxiety dream is a normal phenomenon throughout life and deals with controlled anxiety.

⟨ Secondary Sleep Disorders

Schizophrenia

Throughout the history of modern medicine, clinicians and researchers have been intrigued by the possibility of a relationship between sleep disturbances and psycho-

pathology. The apparent similarity between dreams and hallucinations has led a number of authorities to speculate upon the etiological role of disturbances in the dreaming process in the development of schizophrenia.[37,133,197,210]

The discovery of REM sleep[18] and initial reports that REM deprivation in normal subjects resulted in various psychological disturbances[82,86,364] seemed to provide tentative support for this speculation. Although later studies[83,84,215] have raised questions about the consistency and severity of these psychological effects, the earlier studies and the theories accompanying them served as compelling stimuli for polygraphic examination of the sleep of schizophrenics.

One hypothesis which attracted investigators was that the hallucinations and delusions of the schizophrenic represent eruptions of REM "pressure" into the waking state.[123] As Vogel[415] discusses, this notion, which is essentially hydraulic in nature, implies that some condition such as chronic REM deprivation exists in schizophrenics prior to the psychotic episode. In addition Vogel and Traub[416] pointed out that it has never been clear whether the intrusion of REM sleep into wakefulness represents a continuation of the build-up of REM pressure or a discharge of that pressure, and thus predictions of how REM should behave during the course of the disease are often confusing and contradictory.

In any case, persistent efforts to find evidence of REM phenomena during wakefulness and of REM abnormalities during sleep in schizophrenics have produced far from conclusive results. In examining five actively ill patients, newly admitted to the hospital, Rechtschaffen et al.[340] were unable to detect any consistent patterns of EEG, EOG, and EMG activity which indicated the presence of REM sleep during wakefulness. Chronic adult schizophrenics[62,81] and children exhibiting schizophrenia or autism[297,300,301] have shown no severe abnormalities of REM sleep, although adults at or near remission have been found to exhibit increased amounts of REM, decreased latencies to REM onset, and incomplete EMG suppression during REM sleep.[164] "Actively ill" or acute patients have not shown significant changes in REM time,[119,238,393] although changes in REM latencies have been observed in some.[117,393] Feinberg et al.[119] did observe lower REM times in short-term as compared to long-term patients. In addition, hallucinating patients have exhibited greater eye-movement densities than nonhallucinating patients.[118] Feinberg and his colleagues[118,119] have consistently failed to find any REM abnormalities in several remitted patients.

The general conclusion would seem to be that schizophrenics do not exhibit striking changes in REM sleep or evidence of REM phenomena during wakefulness. The occasional changes observed, however, may to some extent reflect drug effects, for in these studies varying degrees of control have been exercised over the drug status or length of time since drug withdrawal. In addition, the exact type and point of evolution of the patient's disease may be a significant factor. For example, Struve and Becka[398] found that "B-mitten" EEG discharges occur in a significantly greater proportion of reactive schizophrenics than process schizophrenics. Furthermore, Snyder[386] and Kupfer et al.[241] observed several patients longitudinally through the course of an acute psychotic episode and described distinct changes in various sleep parameters, including those of REM sleep, associated with both the waxing and waning phases of the episode.

Although the evidence of changes in the conventional measures of REM sleep of schizophrenics is at best inconclusive, there is suggestive evidence that the schizophrenic's response to experimental manipulation of REM sleep depends on the phase of the disease, and this may indicate that the underlying neurophysiological and biochemical mechanisms of the REM state operate differently in these patients. For example, actively ill patients exhibit little or no compensatory increase in REM sleep following several nights of REM deprivation,[442,443] but remitted patients exhibit normal[416] or even exaggerated[442,443] REM rebounds following such procedures. Zarcone and Dement[442] have updated the REM-intrusion hypothesis of

schizophrenic symptoms by suggesting that it is the behavior of pontine-geniculate-occipital (PGO) spikes which accounts for these differential effects of REM deprivation, and possibly for the psychotic symptoms. In animals, these PGO spikes are normally confined to REM-sleep periods,[52,283] and it is suspected that deprivation and rebound of these spikes, rather than of other aspects of REM sleep, produce the REM rebounds following REM-sleep deprivation.[121] When animals are administered p-chlorophenylalanine, an inhibitor of serotonin synthesis, the PGO spikes can be dissociated from REM sleep and may be discharged during the waking state.[80] With this waking discharge of PGO spikes the animals may exhibit what appear to be hallucinations accompanying the PGO spike bursts, restlessness, insomnia, and decreases in REM time.[85] Zarcone and Dement have noted that the last three symptoms are very similar to those described by Snyder[386] and Kupfer et al.[241] for patients at the onset of an acute psychotic episode. Furthermore, REM deprivation in animals exhibiting PGO spikes during the waking state does not result in a compensatory rebound of REM.[85] Zarcone and Dement have speculated that REM deprivation is ineffective because the PGO spikes are no longer confined to the REM periods. Since extended REM deprivation is not sufficient to produce a dissociation of the PGO spikes and other REM phenomena, they suggested that some abnormality of the neurochemical regulators of PGO spikes, which appear to include serotonin, must account for this dissociation of PGO spikes. Zarcone and Dement believe that such an abnormality of PGO function could determine many of the symptoms of the schizophrenic psychosis. It must be understood, however, that the existence of PGO spikes, or functionally equivalent events, in humans has yet to be demonstrated.

The early emphasis on the REM-sleep characteristics of schizophrenics resulted in a comparative neglect of the other aspects of EEG sleep. However, deficits in the stage-4 sleep of schizophrenics are well-documented,[62,117] and appear to be much more prevalent than abnormalities of REM sleep. Although some authors[435] have hesitated to attribute any specific importance to these deficits since similar types of disturbance are observed in various other disease or natural conditions, Feinberg[116] noted that the same could be said of the sporadically observed REM-sleep abnormalities. Furthermore, since sleep deprivation is ineffective in producing increased levels of stage-4 sleep in schizophrenics,[255] there is evidence equivalent to that for REM sleep that basic disturbances of the sleep mechanisms themselves are important characteristics of schizophrenia.

In conclusion, although sleep researchers have found a REM-intrusion hypothesis to be particularly attractive as an explanation of the schizophrenic's psychotic symptoms, there is little consistent evidence that the more traditional measures of REM sleep are significantly changed in many schizophrenics. However, more attention to the specific types of schizophrenics, to the changes occurring during the evolutionary course of the disease, and to the phasic events of REM sleep, may reveal specific disturbances in the basic mechanism of REM sleep. This is particularly suggested by the failure of acute schizophrenics to exhibit a compensatory REM rebound following REM-sleep deprivation. On the other hand, schizophrenics also appear to suffer from important disturbances of slow-wave sleep. It seems certain that these sleep disturbances will be found to be intimately linked to biochemical abnormalities associated with schizophrenia.[434]

Depression

Sleep disturbance is one of the more common and important features of the depressive illnesses, and it has long been thought that certain types of sleep disturbance discriminate reliably among the various subtypes of depression. Thus, delayed sleep onset has been thought to characterize reactive depression, while early awakening supposedly occurs more in endogenous depression.

The objective description of the polygraphic sleep patterns of depressed patients was initiated by Diaz-Guerrero et al. in 1946,[93] before the discovery of REM sleep. These pioneers observed that in comparison to normals, manic-depressive patients in the depressive phase of their illness exhibited difficulty falling asleep, early and frequent awakenings, greater proportions of light sleep, and greater numbers of shifts from one sleep stage to another.

Since this early study, much information has accumulated on the EEG sleep patterns of depressed patients, and many more refined descriptions have appeared. Although certain characteristics of EEG sleep have been consistently noted in these studies, other characteristics are still disputed. It has generally been observed* that depressed patients take longer to fall asleep, obtain less sleep, awaken more often, and awaken earlier than normals. In a vast majority of cases slow-wave or stage-4 sleep is moderately to markedly suppressed. Increased frequencies of stage shifts have also been noted occasionally.

These consistent observations can be contrasted with the results pertaining to REM sleep.† Many investigators have reported decreases in REM-sleep time in depressed patients, but several have also commented upon the high variability among patients with respect to REM time. Others have described normal or elevated REM times. Latency to REM onset has generally been found to be shorter than average, and sleep-onset REM periods have been observed in some cases. Measures of the density of eye movements during REM, when made, have usually been high.

Clinical improvement, whether occurring spontaneously or with the aid of pharmacological or electroconvulsive therapy, is generally accompanied by a normalization of the disturbed sleep parameters. However, slow-wave sleep may not return to normal levels even with clinical improvement.‡

Vogel et al.[417] found that experimental REM deprivation in these patients has varying effects. Some patients show evidence of REM

---

* See references 93, 158, 160, 179–181, 254, 272, 273, 308, 385, 386, and 446.
  † See references 158, 160, 174, 175, 177–181, 254, 272, 273, 308, and 385–387.
  ‡ See references 158, 160, 180, 181, 272, and 274.

"pressure" (decreased latency to REM onset, increased number of awakenings required to effect the deprivation) during deprivation and exhibit REM rebounds following the deprivation period. The REM sleep of others seems to be unaffected by the procedure. When deprivation is accompanied by the buildup of REM pressure there is a concomitant improvement in the clinical picture. A similar improvement accompanies the REM deprivation associated with administration of monoamine oxidase inhibitors.[433]

One of the most striking characteristics of the patients in these studies, and probably one of the determinants of the inconsistent results with respect to REM sleep, is the high degree of variability among patients, even within the same study. Hawkins and Mendels[179,272,273] have repeatedly emphasized this point, and have suggested that differences in severity of illness may determine much of this variability. Although these investigators[275] were unable to detect any statistically significant differences between patients rated as severely depressed and those rated mildly to moderately depressed, there was a tendency for the severely depressed patients to exhibit greater sleep disturbance. Furthermore, patients over fifty years of age tended to have more disturbed sleep than younger patients.

It appears that an even more important contributor to the variability in the EEG sleep patterns of depressed patients are differences in the diagnostic subtypes of the patients. Although there has been no consistent evidence that endogenous depressives are characterized by early awakening while reactive depressives have difficulty falling asleep, Mendels and Hawkins[275] found that psychotic depressives show significantly greater sleep disturbance than neurotic depressives. In addition, Hartmann[174,175] found that manic depressives exhibit sleep abnormalities somewhat different from those reported for groups of mixed psychotic depressives. He also observed that sleep disturbances during the depressed phase are different from those in the manic phase. However, Mendels and Hawkins[276] have reported that the sleep patterns of one hypomanic patient were generally similar to those of pa-

tients with psychotic depressive illness. Finally, Detre et al.[92] have recently described distinct differences in reported sleep patterns between bipolar and unipolar depressives, as well as evidence of hypersomnia in many patients, and particularly in bipolar depressives.

As with interpretations of the sleep disturbances characteristic of schizophrenia, some researchers have sought to relate the depressive's clinical symptoms to abnormalities in REM sleep. On the basis of his data Snyder[386] concluded that psychotic depression is accompanied and perhaps exacerbated, by the effects of REM deprivation (REM pressure). The fragmented and short sleep of these patients would gradually produce this deprivation, and therefore the degree of REM pressure should reflect the duration of earlier unrelieved sleep disturbance. Hartmann[175] also believes that REM pressure is an important aspect of depression, but he suggests that it may be intrinsic to depression rather than the result of earlier deprivation. Furthermore, according to Hartmann this REM pressure is associated with low levels of available functional norepinephrine. On the other hand, in discussing their study of experimental REM deprivation in depressives Vogel et al.[417] suggested that REM pressure produces an accumulation of catecholamines which alleviates depression.

Other researchers have taken a more global view of the depressive's sleep disturbances. Mendels and Hawkins[273] have interpreted the short, light and fragmented sleep patterns and the reductions in REM and stage-4 sleep as indicating increased activity of CNS arousal mechanisms. Presumably the heightened arousal characteristic of depression would tend to prevent these two sleep stages from occurring. More recently Whybrow and Mendels[430] reviewed neurophysiological, electromyographical, waking and sleep EEG, and chemotherapeutic evidence suggesting that in depression, and possibly mania, there is a state of CNS hyperexcitability.

Iskander and Kaelbling[195] concluded that changes in delta or stage-4 sleep are probably of greater significance in the etiology of depression than changes in REM sleep. In their opinion, the deficits in REM sleep are secondary to the deficits in slow-wave sleep since REM sleep typically occurs only after a "primer" period of delta sleep. Therefore if slow-wave sleep failed to occur, or occurred only minimally, there would be less likelihood that REM sleep would occur. Iskander and Kaelbling also suggested that the residual disturbance of delta-sleep patterns exhibited by clinically improved depressives lends further support to their conclusion.

In summary, arousal disturbances of EEG sleep (short sleep time, long sleep latency, high number of awakenings, etc.) have consistently been found to characterize depressed patients. The reduction or absence of delta sleep is also a reliable characteristic. Many patients obtain less REM sleep, but this has been less consistently observed than the above disturbances. Depressed patients appear to be rather variable in their EEG sleep patterns. Differences in severity of illness, age, and diagnostic subtype may contribute to this variability. Attempts have been made to implicate both REM- and NREM-sleep disturbances in the etiology and maintenance of depression, but, as with many clinical disorders, there is as yet no completely satisfactory explanation of this relationship.

Alcohol and Chronic Alcoholism

The effect of alcohol on human sleep patterns has received attention from researchers for several reasons. First, alcohol, caffeine and nicotine are probably the most widely used drugs in the general population, and, for this reason, all are potential contaminators of polygraphic sleep studies. Second, it is suspected that alcohol may play some role in either the precipitation or the maintenance of some types of sleep disturbance. Finally, sleep disturbance has long been observed to be one of the symptoms of various phases of the chronic alcoholic's disease process.

Administration of one g./kg. of body weight of 95 percent ethonol to normal subjects on one night resulted in a significant decrease in REM sleep.[161] Continued administration of identical amounts of alcohol either immedi-

ately before retiring,[440] or four hours before retiring,[441] for several consecutive nights, had a similar effect on REM sleep during the first one or two nights. However on subsequent nights of alcohol administration, REM returned to normal levels or above. On early recovery nights, REM remained at high levels or even increased more, but it returned to control levels by the third or fourth recovery night. When alcohol was given immediately before retiring[440] stage-2 sleep varied inversely with REM sleep, while stages 3 and 4 tended to fluctuate around control levels. There were no consistent changes in the time awake, the number of stage shifts, body movements, or latency of the first REM period. When alcohol was consumed four hours before retiring[441] the changes in REM and NREM sleep were less consistent. In a long-term study of one normal subject drinking somewhat lower doses of alcohol,[237] there was evidence of a dose-response effect in the suppression of REM, as well as an indication that increasing the dose during subsequent nights resulted in a continued suppression of REM below control levels.

From these studies of normal individuals it would appear that alcohol has an initial suppressing effect on REM sleep, that this effect decreases with continued constant doses of alcohol, that increasing doses of alcohol may sustain the effect, and that following several consecutive nightly doses of alcohol there may be a rebound of REM sleep on nonalcohol nights. Although the data are still meager, it appears that NREM sleep and certain variables reflecting wakefulness are unchanged by acute alcohol consumption.

There are no data specifically related to the use of alcohol by insomniacs. Nevertheless, it is well known by clinicians that some insomniacs use alcohol at bedtime as a hypnotic. The fact that alcohol has a stimulating effect at low doses, and must be taken in large amounts for depressant effects to appear[270,277] undoubtedly results in the insomniac's having to ingest rather large quantities to obtain the desired effect. Moreover, the demonstrated sleep-disturbing effects of alcohol may well prompt the patient to discontinue his self-treatment. Withdrawal effects on sleep patterns may then lead him to resume his use of alcohol, or perhaps some other hypnotic. In this manner he may become trapped in a vicious circle of alcohol consumption and withdrawal, both of which are accompanied by the sleep disturbance he is trying to prevent.

The nature of the sleep disturbances in the alcoholic psychoses is somewhat clearer. It appears that both delta sleep and REM sleep are disturbed throughout the various stages of this disorder. During inebriation in chronic alcoholics REM sleep is moderately to severely suppressed, at least initially.[159,162,204] Continued suppression of REM may depend on increasing dosages of alcohol.[159] However, there are nights on which "REM escape" or abnormally high amounts of REM may occur.[159,162] There is some disagreement about the exact nature of the delta-sleep disturbance during this phase. In two patients undergoing chronic alcoholization, Gross and Goodenough[162] observed an initial increase in delta sleep, followed by a decrease to normal or subnormal levels. On the other hand, Johnson et al.[204] found thirteen of fourteen patients undergoing acute alcoholization to be completely without stage-4 sleep and eight were without stage-3 sleep. They also noted that, compared to withdrawal nights, there were a greater number of stage shifts and awakenings, greater amounts of wakefulness, and fewer K-complexes during this phase. Although Gross and Goodenough[162] described disturbances in spindle activity during acute intoxication, Johnson et al. failed to find such changes in their patients. In a non-EEG study Mello and Mendelson[271] observed that chronic inebriation resulted in an increased amount of daily sleep, although sleep became more fragmented.

During the chronic alcoholic's withdrawal from alcohol ingestion, there are consistent reports of increased REM sleep on initial recovery nights, with a gradual return to normal levels on later recovery nights.[159,162,204] Johnson et al.[204] have also described decreased REM-onset times and increased numbers of REM periods in these patients. They found that the increased REM time reflected shorter intervals between REM periods rather than longer REM periods. In addition, the patients appeared to have difficulty maintaining REM sleep, as evidenced by the noticeable fragmentation of this sleep stage. There appears to be a strong relationship between this increased REM sleep during alcohol withdrawal and both the delirium and the hallucinations which are frequent signs of withdrawal. Greenberg and Pearlman[159] found that patients who exhibited delirium had more nights with increased REM sleep and showed greater increases in REM than patients who did not exhibit this symptom. Gross and Goodenough[162] observed that one patient began experiencing hallucinations on the first day of withdrawal and following a night without REM or stage-4 sleep. Another withdrawing patient with 100 percent REM sleep also exhibited hallucinations, while a third with 44 percent REM sleep did not. These authors interpreted this as evidence that the rebound of REM above a certain threshold following alcohol-induced REM suppression is the basis for the hallucinations. Gross and Goodenough[162] believe that REM rebound is also related to seizures during withdrawal.

It has also been reported[162,204] that stage 4 is absent during the withdrawal phase. Gross and Goodenough[162] have suggested that the complaints of sleep disturbance in these patients are related to this decrease in stage 4, and that "sudden and massive" return of stage 4 is signalled by the terminal sleep often observed in the recovering patient. But Johnson et al.[204] have suggested that lack of stage 4 is a characteristic of chronic alcoholics in general, and that the return of stage 4 is not a necessary condition for clinical improvement.

Insomnia is commonly accepted as one of the clinical symptoms of withdrawal. Many of the patients described by Gross and Goodenough[162] were sleepless on some nights during recovery, and these authors suggested that complete insomnia is related to a more advanced state of withdrawal. Johnson et al.[204] reported a significant improvement in various measures of restless and disturbed sleep during the withdrawal phase, as compared to the alcoholization period, but noted that their patients still appeared disturbed by normal standards. Mello and Mendelson[271] found that fragmented sleep was a frequent, but not invariable, concomitant of withdrawal. In addition, abrupt withdrawal was not necessarily accompanied by insomnia.

In summary, alcoholization in chronic alcoholics is accompanied by significant changes in REM sleep and delta sleep, as well as by fragmented or disturbed sleep. Total sleep time per day may increase, however. During withdrawal there is a rebound of REM sleep, which may be related to the appearance of both hallucinations and seizures. Delta sleep remains depressed in many cases, although a rebound of this type of sleep may accompany the terminal sleep observed in some patients. Insomnia or other complaints of sleep disturbance may occur, but they are not invariable symptoms of withdrawal. Although there is an improvement in the quality of sleep during withdrawal, these patients continue to exhibit noticeable sleep disturbances as compared to normals.

Chronic Renal Insufficiency, Hemodialysis, and Renal Transplantation

Clinical reports[296,374] have indicated that the uremic syndrome, in addition to its characteristics of lethargy, depression, restlessness, and muscular twitching, is frequently characterized by a paradoxical state of daytime drowsiness and nighttime insomnia. This disturbance has been reported to persist when the patients are maintained on hemodialysis, although Shea et al.[379] noted that the dialysis procedure may have some immediately beneficial effects on sleep. One report[278] indicated that dialyzed patients suffer predominantly from difficulty in falling asleep, and several investigators[153,278] found these patients to be particularly refractory to pharmacological treatment of the sleep disturbances.

Only two polygraphic studies of uremic patients have been reported. In 1970 Passouant et al.[314] described the sleep patterns of eighteen patients, some of whom were undergoing regular dialysis and some of whom were treated principally by dietary means. They studied five patients both before and after dialysis. Although this report is rather unclear as to the observations contributing to the data presented, the authors concluded that in the uremic syndrome sleep is characterized by decreased sleep time; increased awake time, primarily in the middle of the night; decreased slow-wave sleep; irregularity of sleep cycles; and frequent body movements. The sleep of patients regularly maintained on dialysis was not significantly disturbed, although there were some differences in sleep patterns before and after dialysis. Before dialysis, the alternations between NREM and REM were normal, but there were frequent awakenings and reductions in slow-wave and REM sleep. After dialysis, the number of awakenings decreased and slow-wave and REM sleep increased. In the patients who were dialyzed only when other means of management were temporarily ineffective, sleep problems were constant during periods of stabilization, i.e., there were frequent awakenings and decreases in slow-wave and REM sleep. The number of sleep cycles was normal and the lengths of the cycles were regular. During exacerbations the existing sleep problems were magnified, sleep cycling became very irregular, and the number of body movements increased. Dialyzing these patients, either peritoneally or by artificial kidney, resulted in increases in slow-wave and REM sleep and stabilization of REM sleep. The number of body movements remained high until several dialyses had been performed. In three patients who underwent peritoneal dialysis REM sleep appeared within ten minutes after sleep onset. Correlations among sleep and other physiological variables indicated that an increase in blood urea nitrogen was significantly correlated with decreases in slow-wave and REM sleep and increases in the number of awakenings.

In a recent study,[223] we have systematically examined the EEG sleep patterns of ten uremic patients on the night immediately preceding and the night following regular hemodialysis sessions, and have compared these patterns to those of age- and sex-matched healthy controls. In comparison to the controls, before dialysis the patients exhibited significantly shorter total sleep times, increased numbers and lengths of awakenings and percentages of awake time, decreased time from sleep onset to the first awakening, decreased ratios of total sleep time to time in bed (sleep efficiency), decreased percentages of REM and stage-2 sleep, and increased percentages of stage-3 sleep. In comparison to controls, patients after dialysis exhibited significantly lower sleep efficiency, greater percentages of awake time, longer awakenings, and lower percentages of stage-2 sleep. Direct comparisons of the patients before and after dialysis revealed no significant differences in the quantitative measures of sleep, although the fewer number of significant differences from control values in the patients after dialysis suggested that some improvement in sleep patterns had occurred as a result of the dialysis. This was further evidenced when we examined the sequence in which the various sleep stages first appeared during the first cycle. In the controls, this sequence (stage 1, 2, 3, 4, REM, 0) was identical to that usually observed in healthy subjects. Before dialysis, the sequence (1, 2, 3, 0, 4, REM) was interrupted by the early appearance of the first awakening. After dialysis, the sequence (1, 2, 4, 3, REM, 0) approached that of the controls, indicating that dialysis resulted in a more normal sleep organization during the first sleep cycle.

In a second study we examined the sleep patterns of nine uremic patients who had received kidney transplants from three months to four years before the study. Compared to age- and sex-matched controls, these patients exhibited significantly greater percentages of awake time and lengths of awakenings, greater numbers of REM periods, shorter latencies to REM sleep, and lower percentages of stage-4 sleep. The sequence of stages during the first sleep cycle was perfectly normal.

In addition to these findings, we noted that both dialysis and transplant patients showed certain qualitative changes in their sleep EEGs. Some patients exhibited an intermingling of alpha activity with delta activity.

Decreased numbers, durations, and quality of spindles were common. The K-complexes were poorly formed and had unusually low voltages. Some patients showed an increase in theta activity. Abnormally low-voltage delta activity was characteristic of many patients, both young and old. Dialysis and kidney transplantation appeared to have no significant effect on these EEG changes.

Although both dialysis and renal transplantation appear to produce some improvement in uremic patients' sleep patterns, there is never a complete normalization of sleep following these procedures. This fact suggests that chronic renal insufficiency may produce irreversible, fundamental changes in the CNS. These changes are undeniably seen at the functional level, and may even exist at the cellular level.

Pregnancy and Postpartum Emotional Disturbance

Disturbances in the sleep system have long been considered important symptoms of postpartum emotional disturbances.* Although there have been no systematic polygraphic studies of these concomitant sleep disturbances, indirect evidence from studies of other psychiatric disorders, such as depression and schizophrenia, and from studies of certain hormonal disorders would suggest that disturbed EEG sleep patterns might be an important concomitant of the postpartum emotional disturbances. More recent studies of sleep patterns during normal pregnancy and the postpartum period have provided further evidence of this. During the early stage of normal pregnancy[229] there is a noticeable increase in time spent asleep. Sleep time normalizes during the second trimester, decreases to below normal during the third, and remains low for some time following delivery. During the second trimester several additional changes begin to appear, i.e., awakenings become more frequent and the number of REM periods may temporarily increase.[228] Of even greater significance, however, is the fact that

* See references 78, 137, 171, 201, 202, 206, 258, 367, and 432.

stage-4 sleep begins to decline during this period.[228,318] Although decreased levels of stage 4 are the most striking characteristic of groups of pregnant women in their last trimester of pregnancy,[226,228,318] individual women may exhibit various degrees of variability in this pattern.[228] In some women REM sleep may decline slightly during the second trimester, only to increase sharply during the third and begin to decrease as delivery approaches.[48,318] In others, the decline in REM sleep may persist through the last trimester.[228] During the last trimester there are also increased sleep latencies, increased amounts of awake time and numbers of awakenings, and increased percentages of stage-2 sleep.[226,228]

Petre-Quadens et al.[318] observed that sleep patterns during the two weeks following delivery were similar to those of late pregnancy in their subjects (high REM, decreased or absent stage 4), and that by the third postpartum week REM and stage-4 sleep had begun to move toward normal levels. In our studies[226,228] we looked closely at the two or three nights immediately following delivery. On the first night there was a sharp increase in awake time and a sharp decrease in REM sleep. Stage-4 sleep was slightly increased above late prepartum levels. During the second and third postdelivery nights these parameters showed gradual movement toward normal levels. Nevertheless, the immediate postpartum period as a whole was still significantly disturbed in several respects. Compared to nonpregnant control subjects the new mothers exhibited longer sleep latencies, greater amounts of awake time and numbers of awakenings, decreased REM time, and decreased stage-2 sleep.[226,228] Even with the return of the menses, sleep patterns had still not completely normalized in the new mothers.[228] Although sleep latency had become more normal, there were still significantly high amounts of wakefulness and numbers of awakenings. REM sleep had essentially reached normal levels, but stage-2 sleep was somewhat depressed. The amount of stage-4 sleep was often greater than in nonpregnant controls.

These data from normal women would seem to indicate that rather profound alterations in sleep patterns are natural concomitants of the pregnancy and postpartum periods. Although sleep patterns generally normalize during the first several postpartum weeks, at the onset of the first menses following delivery there is still sufficient disturbance to suggest that this event does not represent the full attainment of the prepregnant state. The striking changes in total sleep time, and particularly in stage-4 sleep, during late pregnancy seem to be especially important since significant decreases in stage-4 sleep are concomitants of various types of psychopathology.* We may speculate that a mother's failure to recover this type of sleep following delivery is a prodromal sign of, or perhaps even an etiological factor in, postpartum emotional disturbance. This must remain a speculation, however, until more direct studies of postpartum emotional disturbances can be undertaken.

Perusal of any medical textbook and clinical experience will uncover numerous other conditions which produce or are accompanied by disordered sleep. Various CNS disorders, including infections and other toxic states, and certain nutritional and endocrine disorders, are known to be accompanied by changes in EEG sleep patterns. Many more remain to be examined by sleep researchers. From this review it should be clear that although the information produced by sleep research has raised more questions than it has answered, the sleep EEG provides a unique tool for the exploration of the neurophysiological bases of many medical and psychiatric conditions.

(Parasomnias

Sleepwalking

In sleepwalking, the individual sits up in bed, arises, and begins to move around in an uncoordinated manner. His eyes are open but

---

* See references 62, 93, 160, 179, 386, and 446.

his appearance is rather blank and dazed. Most often his movements are stereotyped and purposeless, but occasionally more complex behaviors, such as dressing or going to the bathroom, may be exhibited. The sleepwalker may mumble or emit other sounds, but rarely does he converse if spoken to. Eventually he returns to bed or is easily led there. It is very difficult to awaken the sleepwalker during his wanderings, and if he is awakened he is quite confused and disoriented. He is usually amnesic for the episode when either awakened during it or questioned about it the next morning.

The reported incidence of sleepwalking varies with the age and clinical condition of the groups sampled, and with their past or current history. From 1–33 percent of various groups have reported current histories of sleepwalking,[*] while from 3–34 percent of groups sampled have described a past history of this disturbance.[†] It is commonly stated[198] that sleepwalking occurs more often in males. However, several studies failed to reveal any significant male predominance,[299,404] and one case was remarkable for the number of female relatives of the patient who were also sleepwalkers.[101] As with this patient, many sleepwalkers show a positive family history for the disturbance.[‡]

Sleepwalking typically first appears in childhood or adolescence,[§] and in many cases disappears by the third decade.[362] However, if the disturbance persists into adulthood it often first appeared at puberty.[325] Among the various concomitants of sleepwalking in many patients are EEG evidence of epilepsy and other EEG abnormalities, CNS infection or trauma, genito-urinary complaints, and more or less severe forms of psychopathology.[¶]

Several other types of sleep disturbance are frequently observed in sleepwalkers. Pierce and Lipcon[319] found that three times as many enuretic naval recruits reported a past history of sleepwalking as did nonenuretic recruits. In a second study[321] these authors found that 47 percent of sleepwalkers reported concurrent nocturnal enuresis, whereas controls did not. Others[21,101,219] also noted the parallel occurrence of these two phenomena. Sleeptalking occurs in some sleepwalkers, as do nightmares and night terrors.[#]

Sleep-EEG studies of sleepwalking have revealed that the episodes occur during slow-wave sleep,[**] although Gastaut and Broughton[143] have reported one episode which occurred during the transition from stage-2 to REM sleep.

Gastaut and Broughton[144] described episodes whose onset consisted of intense awakening EEG reactions concomitant with or shortly preceding signs of movement. Flattening of the EEG records and then continuous ample nonreactive alpha activity followed, with the latter giving way to stage-2 or occasionally REM sleep at the end of the episode.

Jacobson et al.[200] described the episode as starting with the sudden appearance of increased EMG discharge and 1–3 cps high-voltage EEG activity. After ten to thirty seconds of this EEG pattern, lower-amplitude delta waves appeared, producing a pattern resembling slow-wave sleep. If the incidents were brief (twenty to forty seconds) this EEG pattern characterized the entire incident. If the incidents were longer, theta, alpha, and beta frequencies against a low-voltage background were characteristic. Most incidents were followed by periods of mixed spindles and slow waves, but approximately one-fourth of the incidents were followed by waking EEG activity.

Visual investigation of the environment, stereotyped movements, nonreactivity, amnesia for the event, and lack of dream recall characterized the sleepwalkers in both studies.[144,200] Further investigations showed that sleepwalkers up to sixteen years of age exhibited many more episodes of sudden rhythmical bursts of high-voltage delta activity in slow-wave sleep than did normals.[217] These

   * See references 11, 138, 309, 362, and 380.
   † See references 79, 138, 299, 319, and 404.
   ‡ See references 10, 21, 79, 219, 321, and 365.
   § See references 11, 138, 219, 325, and 391.
   ¶ See references 5, 10, 11, 115, 192, 196, 198, 212, 219, 252, 299, 309, 319–321, 365, 391, 400, 405, and 421.

   # See references 101, 198, 212, 217, 219, and 320.
   ** See references 53, 144, 198, 200, 216, and 217.

events occurred both with sleepwalking incidents and at other times, principally with some body movement. Sleepwalking has been induced in sleepwalkers[53,217] and sometimes in normals[53] by standing the subject up during slow-wave sleep. Sleepwalkers may exhibit more complex gestural movements than normals during slow-wave sleep, and appear to be more confused following forced awakenings from slow-wave sleep.[53]

The etiology postulated for sleepwalking has often depended upon the theoretical persuasion of the writer or on his particular research orientation. Thus the psychologically inclined* have considered sleepwalking to be a neurotic symptom, an immature habit pattern, a form of personality dissociation, or the acting out of a dream. In one case, sleepwalking was a prelude to an acute schizophrenic episode.[196]

On another level, several investigators† have suggested that sleepwalking is a manifestation of epilepsy. There is evidence of a genetic predisposition for the disturbance.[21] Broughton[53] suggested that sleepwalkers are physiologically predisposed to sleepwalk during slow-wave sleep arousals, whereas some other individuals are predisposed to exhibit nocturnal enuresis or night terrors. However, the nature of the specific precipitator of the sleepwalking episode remains unclear. Jacobson and Kales[198] suggested that both psychological and organic factors are involved in the disturbance. In their view the abnormal high-voltage delta-activity bursts observed in sleepwalking children may represent an organic immaturity factor, and psychological factors may be necessary to precipitate incidents in predisposed individuals.

Sleeptalking

Sleeptalking has long been of interest to physicians and laymen alike because of its supposed reflection of mental activity during sleep.[285] The nocturnal utterances may be simple, mumbled monosyllables, or close approximations of waking, conversational speech,[63] and there are many reports of sleeptalkers responding to a waking individual's questions, commands, or comments.[14,66,252,285]

The incidence of sleeptalking has been little studied. One difficulty in deriving realistic figures is that the sleeptalker is frequently unaware of this nocturnal behavior. In an early study, Child[66] found that 40 percent of a college sample between the ages of twenty and thirty years reported ever having talked in their sleep. In Gahagan's[138] later study of 559 university students, 61.5 percent reported a past history of sleeptalking and 51.2 percent reported that sleeptalking still persisted. Goode[154] found 53.1 percent of one group of medical students, 58.5 percent of a second group, 72.2 percent of student nurses, and 69.2 percent of hospital inpatients reporting histories of the phenomenon. Among fifty-five enuretic marine recruits, twenty-six had talked in their sleep during the past three months, while only fourteen of 135 nonenuretic recruits reported having done so.[28] Since these incidence figures are, in all likelihood, conservative, it would appear that at least a majority of the population has experienced sleeptalking at one time or another.

In an extensive review of the literature, Arkin[13] noted that sleepwalking may occur in the absence of any noticeable disorder,[285,418] or in conjunction with various types of physical or psychological pathology.‡ Based on his clinical experience and research, however, Arkin[13] concluded that sleeptalking "is usually benign but may reflect deeper disturbance."

The discovery of REM sleep[18] and of its relationship to dreaming[87] engendered new interest in the psychophysiological aspects of sleeptalking. Kamiya[220] was among the first to perform a polygraphic investigation of sleeptalking. He reported that 88 percent of ninety-eight sleeptalking episodes occurred during NREM sleep, and that 71 percent of the episodes were accompanied by body movements. Subsequent investigations[15,144,336] usually confirmed the predominance of sleeptalk-

---

* See references 5, 212, 252, 295, 299, 309, 320, 325, 365, 380, 391, and 405.
† See references 10, 115, 192, 319, and 320.

‡ See references 28, 163, 309, 322, 391, 405, and 418.

ing during NREM sleep, although Arkin et al.[15] and Tani et al.[403] described subjects who talked predominantly or exclusively during REM sleep. Several reports[220,336] indicate that NREM-sleep speeches are more likely to be accompanied by muscle-tension artifact than are REM-sleep speeches, making it difficult to determine the quality of the EEG activity during the episode. Nevertheless, Rechtschaffen et al.[336] reported that in NREM-sleep speeches a period of stage-2, -3, or -4 sleep would suddenly be interrupted by muscle-tension artifact accompanied by sleep speech. Occasionally a burst of high-voltage slow waves or K-complexes preceded the muscle tension by several seconds. When EEG activity was discernible through the artifact, it was usually in the 7–10 cps range and appeared to be alpha activity. The muscle-tension artifact persisted for ten to twenty seconds beyond the end of the sleep speech. The typical postepisode EEG pattern was that of stage-2 sleep. Cohen et al.[71] described one case of stage-4 sleep speech in which there was no muscle artifact. Analysis of the EEG during the speech suggested that the subject passed briefly into stage 1 during the episode. Schwartz[375] described an episode which occurred during a period of EEG wakefulness which interrupted stage-4 sleep. The subject did not recall the event when questioned about it later.

The nature of the relationship between sleeptalking and mentation during sleep has been of interest both for theoretical and for practical reasons. If it could be shown that sleeptalking is reliably related to sleep mentation, then content of sleep speeches might prove to be more "pure" than content elicited after involuntary awakenings, and might thus provide a better method of monitoring sleep mentation. After studying a small sample of sleep speeches, Rechtschaffen et al.[336] tentatively concluded that REM-sleep speeches are characterized by affect in the voice and little relationship to the experimental situation. By contrast, NREM speeches are usually flat and unemotional, tend to concern the experimental situation, and are only infrequently followed by reports of mental content with involuntary

awakening. In a more elaborate study of the degree of concordance between the content of sleep speeches and recalled mentation, Arkin et al.[16] found that 79.2 percent of REM speeches showed some degree of concordance with mentation, while 45.8 percent of stage-2 speeches, 21.1 percent of stage-3 and -4 speeches and 80 percent of stage-1-NREM speeches exhibited some degree of concordance. Whether the differences in degree of concordance in REM and NREM speeches reflect differences in recall of sleep mentation, in the mechanism of sleep speech, in types of concordance (manifest vs. latent content), or real differences in the amount of sleep mentation in the two types of sleep, remains to be determined.

Nocturnal Enuresis

Nocturnal enuresis refers to bed-wetting in individuals old enough to have acquired voluntary control of micturition. Although most writers consider a child to be enuretic if he wets his bed after three years of age, several studies[97,234,289] have shown wide individual differences, as well as possible sex differences, in the age of acquisition of urinary control, suggesting that the child who acquires control somewhat later than three years should not necessarily be considered enuretic.

The incidence of enuresis has been reported to range from 4 percent for six-year-old Child-Welfare-Clinic patients[234] to 87 percent of idiots.[409] Other incidence figures between these extremes have been reported* for groups of various ages and clinical conditions. Many authors have noted at least a slight predominance of the disorder in males,† although Frary[132] found no evidence that enuresis is a sex-linked character. There are numerous observations of a high family history for the disturbance.[132,169] Frary[132] concluded that it is determined by a single recessive gene substitution, while Hallgren[169] suggested that in "genetic cases" the mode of inheritance may be either by a dominant major gene or by the

---

* See references 8, 38, 55, 91, 167, 207, 234, 244, 280, 281, and 409.
† See references 38, 91, 132, 169, 281, and 392.

interaction of polygenes and the environment.

A wide variety of physical anomalies has been observed in enuretics, and quite frequently these anomalies have been assigned etiological roles in the disturbance. Various neuromuscular and anatomical abnormalities of the urogenital system have been described.[*] Of particular interest are the observations that the enuretic's bladder capacity may be lower than normal,[168,289,419] that some enuretics may have less concentrated urine at night,[134] and that enuretics excrete a larger amount of urine at night than normals.[327] However, Vulliamy[419] found no differences in nocturnal urine output among enuretics when diet and fluid intake were strictly controlled. Numerous other more or less relevant afflictions have received attention in the literature,[151] including epilepsy. Although high incidences of EEG epileptiform features,[411] and frequent personal and family histories of epilepsy[319] have been reported for enuretics, Poussaint et al.[328] failed to find any clinical evidence of seizure activity in what they considered to be a more representative sample of enuretics.

The psychological characteristics of enuretics have received equal attention.[†] These individuals exhibit a variety of associated behavioral problems, including nailbiting, stealing, and truancy, criminal and especially aggressive offenses, thumbsucking, speech impediments, temper tantrums, and sleepwalking. They have been characterized as being temperamental, timid, and sensitive, disturbed in the sexual realm, of loose personality organization, fearful of the opposite sex, lacking inhibitory control, emotionally immature, and passive. In one study[280] it was found that five traits—enuresis, thumbsucking, nailbiting, speech impediments, and temper tantrums—occurred more often in combination than in isolation in a sample of children. On the other hand, Lapouse and Monk[244] found no statistically significant relationship between a number of fears and worries and enuresis in a large random sample of children. Werry and Cohrssen[427] concluded that enuretic children seen by physicians tend to exhibit more psychiatric symptoms than nonenuretics, but they emphasized that more than half of their enuretic subjects were emotionally healthy. This is especially meaningful since they also suggested that children with several behavioral and somatic symptoms are more likely to be brought to a physician and thus load nonrandom samples with disturbed subjects.

Clinical EEG studies of enuretics have generally revealed a high percentage of abnormal or immature EEGs.[‡] In addition, Gunnarson and Melin[165] found more EEG abnormalities in enuretics who had never been dry than in those who had experienced a dry period. Contradictory evidence was presented by Ditman and Blinn,[94] who noted no clinical abnormalities in their patients. In a sample of sixty-eight subjects five to sixteen years old, only 10 percent of the EEGs were read as abnormal.[328] Some of these discrepancies may arise from differences in characterizing normal records for a given age.[411]

Deep sleep has been reported as a characteristic of and/or an etiological factor in enuresis,[§] principally on the basis of parents' reports and observations on the difficulty in arousing enuretics after micturition. Sleep EEG studies have revealed that enuresis can occur in all stages of sleep and during periods of nocturnal wakefulness.[¶]

Pierce et al.[324] observed an increase in restlessness and a gradual reduction of heart rate to a stable low level during the thirty minutes preceding micturition. Light sleep or waking patterns accompanied the restlessness until a final body movement signaled a change to deep-sleep patterns. Enuresis followed the body movement and slow-wave EEG activity continued throughout micturition.

Gastaut and Broughton's[144] patients typically exhibited a gradual increase in primary spontaneous bladder contractions as they

---

[*] See references 47, 51, 53, 70, 128, 130, 269, 327, and 394.

[†] See references 8, 26, 91, 149, 167, 169, 182, 248, 280, 319, 392, and 445.

[‡] See references 165, 282, 322, 377, and 411.

[§] See references 9, 44, 47, 169, 350, and 396.

[¶] See references 27, 94, 122, 144, 324, 346, 368, and 424.

passed from wakefulness to deep sleep during the early part of the night. The "enuretic episode" began with a series of bladder contractions during slow-wave sleep. There followed a series of K-complexes or a burst of rhythmic delta activity in the EEG, and then a body movement. Sleep patterns began to lighten and micturition occurred at some point following the body movement. Micturition could occur at any point along a continuum of increasing vigilance from deep to light sleep or wakefulness. Broughton[53] suggested that this finding may help reconcile some of the earlier, apparently discrepant, observations that micturition can occur in all stages of sleep and wakefulness, although differences in apparatus for signaling the onset of micturition probably contributed to some of the variability in the observations.

There is little evidence that nocturnal enuresis is related in any special way to REM sleep. Only occasional episodes have been observed during this sleep stage,[144,324,346] and, if awakened following micturition, most patients fail to recall dreams.[144,368] On the other hand, awakenings from REM periods following micturition are more likely to yield reports of dreams of micturition if the bedclothes have been left unchanged,[144] suggesting that dreams of micturition result from incorporation of external stimuli.

Etiological theories of nocturnal enuresis are varied and plentiful,[*] and the classification scheme used by Werry and Cohrssen[427] is helpful in considering them. Genetic theories are based on the high familial incidence of the disorder. Maturational theories derive from observations of physical or psychological immaturity in enuretics. Data concerning physical or psychological abnormalities in enuretics give rise to the pathological theories, while the numerous and varied observations of psychological disturbances in enuretics have produced psychogenic theories. Poor habit training has been ascribed an etiological role by some authors. As Werry and Cohrssen[427]

noted, these categories are not mutually exclusive and several writers† have emphasized the multiple etiologies of nocturnal enuresis.

Sleep EEG studies have given rise to several explanations of this disorder. Ditman and Blinn[94] and Bental[27] stressed the discrepancy between behavioral reactivity and EEG sleep before and during the enuretic event. Ditman and Blinn[94] suggested that enuretics are in a dissociative state, while Bental[27] hypothesized that the enuretic child develops a "will" to remain awake in order to avoid wetting the bed. This will is reflected in the waking EEG activity accompanying behavioral sleep. Pierce et al.[324] and Schiff[368] considered the enuretic event to be a dream equivalent or variant. On the basis of their data, Ritvo et al.[346] concluded that there are three types of enuretic events: (1) awake enuresis occurs during EEG wakefulness; (2) nonarousal enuresis occurs during stages 2, 3, or 4 and is not preceded by arousal phenomena; and (3) arousal enuresis occurs during stages 2, 3, and 4 and is preceded by arousal phenomena. According to Ritvo et al., all patients appear to have a pathophysiological substrate for enuresis, but psychological factors are probably very important in the maintenance of enuresis in patients exhibiting predominantly awake and arousal enuresis.

Broughton[53] suggested that enuresis is a slow-wave-sleep arousal phenomenon, similar to sleepwalking night terrors. In Broughton's opinion, slow-wave-sleep arousals occur in all individuals but enuretics are physiologically predisposed to enuretic attacks during the arousals. Finley[122] has also viewed enuresis as an arousal defect within the CNS.

Bruxism

Bruxism, or teethgrinding, is of interest to the physician primarily because of the damage it may cause to the teeth and related structures,[291,345] but it causes an unknown amount of annoyance to the sufferer's close associates. Although most writers consider diurnal and nocturnal bruxism to be a single entity, Red-

---

* See references 9, 20, 26, 42, 43, 47, 70, 91, 94, 113, 122, 132, 144, 149, 165, 167, 169, 170, 248, 249, 279, 280, 288, 289, 322, 324, 327, 350, 368, 377, 392, 394, 396, 409, 419, 427, and 445.

† See references 51, 149, 169, 346, and 394.

ing et al.[344] suggested that they are separate phenomena. Nocturnal bruxism is typically characterized by rhythmic patterns of masseter EMG activity which is frequently accompanied by sounds of teethgrinding,[345] while diurnal bruxism is idiosyncratic and silent, except in individuals with organic brain lesions.[264] Reding et al.[344] noted that the two phenomena occur during different states of consciousness, and that if nocturnal bruxists are awakened they appear to have no awareness of their teethgrinding. In one sample of forty-five nocturnal bruxists, none gave evidence of diurnal bruxism.[344]

Among periodontal patients 78 percent have been described as bruxists.[46] In studies of somewhat more representative samples, Reding and his associates have reported the following incidence figures: 5.1 percent of 2290 undergraduate and graduate students between the ages of sixteen and thirty-six years reported current bruxism;[343] 5.5 percent of 1157 laboratory school students ages three to seventeen years reported to be current bruxists by parents, and 15.1 percent reported to have either current or past histories;[343] and 8 percent of 2168 undergraduate and graduate students reported current or past histories.[344] Bruxism appears to affect people of all ages,[342] but seems to decline in incidence with increasing age.[343] There is some evidence that bruxism is a familial disorder.[1,343]

A primary difficulty in studying bruxism has been the reliable and artifactfree monitoring of teethgrinding. In early work[329,342] it was concluded that bruxism is temporally related to REM sleep. This conclusion has been revised with the use of stricter criteria for the detection of bruxism episodes. The latest evidence[345,366,401,403] indicates that bruxism occurs predominantly during stage-2 sleep. There is no change in the nature of sleep or in the relative proportions of sleep stages when bruxists are compared to controls. The bruxism episode, which lasts an average of nine seconds, is often preceded by a K-complex or a K-complex wave without a spindle. During the episode, trains of alpha or a temporary change toward lower-voltage, fast, random activity, without K-waves or spindles, may

occur. Heart rate may increase just before or during the episode, and subcutaneous blood vessels are constricted. Pulse rate and respiration may also change. Forearm and palm electrodermal potentials have been observed during a number of episodes. Sound stimuli during the various stages of sleep have provoked teethgrinding in some subjects. There is evidence that teethgrinding is not associated with any specific manifest content during stage-2 sleep.

Diurnal and nocturnal bruxism have been attributed to a variety of causes, including genetically determined behavior patterns,[111,112] local or intraoral factors,[137,331] lesions of the CNS,[264] and psychological factors.* Several authors have suggested that psychological disturbance is a necessary condition for the disorder and that dental problems are precipitating factors.[137,331]

The oral expression of aggression has been one of the most common psychological interpretations of bruxism. However, in a study of bruxists, presumably of both the diurnal and the nocturnal type, Frisch et al.[135] failed to find a significant relationship between degree of dental evidence of bruxism and mode of expressing aggression as determined by the Rosenzweig Picture-Frustration Study, an instrument designed to measure responses to frustration. Reding et al.[344] concluded that nocturnal bruxists and their controls do not show any statistically significant personality differences as measured by the MMPI and the Cornell Medical Index.

On the basis of their sleep EEG[345] and psychological[344] studies of nocturnal bruxists, Reding and his associates concluded[345] that none of the factors listed above plays the primary etiological role in bruxism. They proposed instead that nocturnal bruxism is a partial arousal phenomenon similar to the slow-wave-sleep arousal phenomena (sleepwalking, enuresis, and night terrors) described by Broughton.[53] Satoh and Harada[366] extended this explanation by proposing that bruxism often occurs if the dopaminergic nigrostriatal system excessively drives the areas controlling

* See references 131, 136, 173, 290, 378, 397, 408, 413, and 420.

jaw movements during the transition from sleep to wakefulness. This hypothesis is indirectly supported by a report that administration of dihydroxyphenylalanine, the precursor of dopamine, to an individual suffering from Parkinson's disease provoked bruxism.[260]

Jactatio Capitis Nocturna

Jactatio capitis nocturna, or sleep rocking, is a motor-behavior pattern consisting of rhythmical movements of the head or body prior to or during sleep. Evans,[108] who extensively reviewed the literature concerning this rather rare disorder, concluded that the movements may be regular or intermittent bursts of activity and that they may appear to be voluntary, even though the individual is usually unable to recall the episode the next morning. Mental retardation and daytime tics, and rocking movements may characterize some sufferers, but more commonly they exhibit symptoms of behavioral disorders. Most patients have rocked from the second six months of life, and the disturbance may persist into adulthood.

Only a few cases of sleep rocking have been studied in the sleep laboratory. Gastaut and Broughton[144] found that the onset of rocking associated with going to sleep is typically signaled by several slow nystagmoid eye movements. The episodes usually appear during stage-1 sleep and produce no significant EEG, cardiac, or respiratory changes. Baldy-Moulinier et al.[22] observed one case where rocking movements seemed to facilitate the return to sleep after periods of wakefulness.

Rocking movements during sleep have been observed in all phases of sleep. Slow-wave sleep episodes begin rather abruptly,[305] and seem not to produce noticeable changes in heart rate or respiration.[144,305] Although Gastaut and Broughton[144] observed no important modifications in the EEG during the episodes, Oswald[305] found that periods of slow waves and spindles were interspersed with periods of low-voltage activity as the episode ran its course.

Episodes of REM-sleep rocking also occur.[22,144,305] In one of his cases, Oswald[305] found that rocking episodes were most fre-

quent and violent during this stage. As with episodes occurring during other stages, there were no significant EEG or heart-rate changes during these REM-sleep episodes.

Evans[108] noted that both organic and psychological etiologies have been proposed for this disturbance. Evans himself suggested that the rocking movements relieve anxiety associated with sleep, and produce sleep through autohypnosis, much as the rhythmic stimulation employed by Oswald[302,303] produced sleep in an experimental situation. Oswald[305] also considers sleep rocking to be motivated, and suggested that it may reflect the use of a previously learned mechanism to relieve unhappy thoughts during sleep. Gastaut and Broughton[144] have categorized the disorder as an unconscious, semipurposeful automatism which is liberated with the depression of cortical and subcortical systems during falling asleep and during sleep.

([Sleep-Modified Disorders

In sleep there are many physiological changes which might account for modifications of various medical complaints. The changes may or may not be sleep dependent, i.e., they may be circadian. During REM sleep, pulse rate, respiration rate, and blood pressure increase and show greater variability,[208,220,388,389] penile erections occur,[126,225] and there are increases in plasma and urinary levels of 17-hydroxycorticosteroids,[263,426] brain temperature,[231,333] oxygen consumption,[49] unit neuronal discharge rates,[12,109,193] antidiuretic hormone activity,[262] and urinary 3-methoxy-4-hydroxymandelic acid.[261] Many other physiological changes occur during sleep, but this list should make the point sufficiently clear.

Several cardiovascular and respiratory disorders are exacerbated during sleep. There is great variability in the EEG sleep patterns of angina patients,[230] and nocturnal angina attacks, evidenced by ST-segment depression on the electrocardiogram, appear to occur predominantly during REM sleep.[294] Clinically it has been noted that myocardial infarctions occur with a high frequency during sleep. In our laboratory preliminary evidence suggests that myocardial infarct patients maintained on an intensive-care ward are sleep-deprived, either because of discomfort or because of disturbances produced when therapeutic procedures are carried out. We have also noted that these patients often show increases in premature ventricular contractions during REM sleep.

Paroxysmal nocturnal hemoglobinuria[75] is a rare disease affecting both sexes. It is most common between the ages of twenty and fifty and is usually fatal. Hemolysis is increased during the sleep of victims.[266]

Left ventricular failure is commonly associated with pulmonary edema at night and results in episodes of paroxysmal nocturnal dyspnea. The mechanism appears to involve an increase in plasma volume[236,422] and a shift of blood from the lower extremities to the pulmonary circulation[384] on assumption of the supine position. The resultant increase in pulmonary blood promotes pulmonary congestion and produces pulmonary edema.

Paroxysmal nocturnal headaches[23,64] are also called cluster headaches because they tend to occur in series. The patient usually awakens during the night with a severe, throbbing, unilateral headache, which may be accompanied by vomiting, watering and redness of the eyes, and stuffiness of the nose. The disorder appears to result from a periodic dilatation of the extracranial vessels in the territory of the external carotid artery.

Emphysema patients, who exhibit increased alveolar CO_2 tension and decreased arterial oxygen saturation during the waking state, suffer their most difficult periods soon after awakening. The fact that these patients show abnormal increases in alveolar CO_2 tension[349] and decreases in arterial oxygen saturation[410] while asleep may explain these postawakening exacerbations.

Sleep EEG studies of asthmatic children[218] have shown that these patients have decreased stage-4 sleep, frequent awakenings, and decreased total sleep time. Asthmatic episodes are confined to the last two-thirds of the night. In asthmatic adults[213] episodes occur throughout the night, with no relation to any specific sleep stage. The patients have shorter total sleep times and less stage 4 than controls. Johns et al.[203] found that patients experiencing dyspnea as a result of bronchial asthma reported frequent night awakenings without significant loss of sleep, and more daytime sleep than average.

Snoring is the nocturnal emission of various grunts, snorts, wheezes, buzzes, and gurgles. The immediate cause of these noises is vibration of the soft structures in the nose and throat accompanying mouth breathing during sleep. It has been estimated that one in eight persons snores most of the night.[7] In 1961 over 300 antisnore devices were recorded in the U.S. Patent Office.[114] Diverse etiologies have been suggested,[7,45] including structural abnormalities of the upper respiratory tract, sleeping position, allergies, overheated or overventilated rooms, and psychological factors. There are no known polygraphic studies of snoring. Since the etiology of this extremely common disorder is apparently mixed, such a study might help to differentiate the various types of snorers, as well as determine whether or not snoring is confined to any particular sleep stage.

Various neuromuscular conditions are exacerbated during sleep. In acroparasthesia,[141] or carpal tunnel syndrome, the patient awakens in the later part of the night with pain, tingling, and numbness in the first three or four digits of one or both hands. Attacks last for thirty minutes or more and are more frequent in women than men. This disorder appears to result from compression of the median nerves in the carpal tunnel at the wrist.

Night cramps,[382] usually of the calf, occur increasingly with age, and also during pregnancy. They are thought to result from a serum calcium deficiency in pregnant women, but the etiology in the elderly is unclear.

Tired-arm syndrome[129] affects middle-aged women, who awaken with pain in the forearm and may detect a weakness in the hand. Excessive muscular exertion has been attributed a causative role.

The elderly are primary sufferers of nocturnal pseudohemiplegia.[382] This disorder is characterized by numbness and immobility of one arm or one side of the body upon awakening at night or in the morning. It is of short duration and is possibly some form of pressure palsy.

Familial periodic paralysis[4,444] is characterized by episodes of muscular weakness and eventual flaccid paralysis. Onset is usually at night, and the attacks can last as long as several days. The apparent cause of the paralysis is an exaggeration of the normal loss of plasma potassium to the muscles, and the resulting decrease in muscle membrane excitability.

The restless-legs syndrome was first described by Wittmaack[431] as anxietas tibiarum, which is defined in *Dorland's Illustrated Medical Dictionary*[95] as "a painful condition of unrest leading to a continual change of position of limbs, and due to an increase of the muscular sense." This disorder has been briefly described by several authors,[6,32,298] but Ekbom[102,103] has presented the most detailed discussion. He coined the term "restless legs" for this syndrome and differentiated two clinical forms, asthenia crurum parasthetica and asthenia crurum dolorosa. The disorder is frequently familial in nature[41,102,257] and sleep disturbance is an almost constant concomitant.[68] Our recent study of a patient confirmed the findings of Lugaresi et al.[256] that the motor disturbances occur every twenty to thirty seconds. We also noted that the EEG burst activity signaling the limb movements became progressively stronger over a period of five to ten minutes until the patient awoke. During REM sleep the myoclonic jerks subsided, but movements of the toes continued to occur periodically. It has been proposed that restless legs is a somatic form of anxiety[298,431] or a manifestation of disturbed lower-limb circulation.[6] Several authors have attributed the disorder to disturbances in the reticular formation.[25,41,256]

Several additional medical conditions have been shown to occur or be exacerbated during sleep. Microfilaria of Wuchereria bancrofti can be found in the blood most frequently between midnight and 2 A.M.[348] Patients suffering from diabetes mellitus show a fairly wide variation in blood-sugar concentrations during sleep, whereas in normal individuals there are only small variations in blood-sugar levels.[348]

A sleep EEG study of patients with duodenal ulcers[17] revealed that the high nocturnal secretion rate of gastric acid by ulcer patients is particularly exaggerated during REM sleep. The authors suggested that content of dreams may determine the magnitude of the secretion rate.

Hypnalgia, or psychogenic pain during sleep in children, is attributed to underlying emotional disturbance.[172]

Painful nocturnal penile erections[127,222] may awaken men at night and induce a special type of sleep disturbance. They appear to be REM-related phenomena.

Nocturnal proctalgia, or proctalgia fugax,[96,382] is an early morning pain seeming to arise from the rectum. It is more common in men than in women, is reported most frequently by people twenty to fifty years old, and is often a familial disorder. It has been attributed to segmental cramp of the puboccocygeus muscle.

From this very brief review of some sleep-modified disorders it is clear that many sleep-related phenomena have yet to be studied by sleep researchers. With further study it may become necessary to reclassify some of these disorders as secondary sleep disorders. In any case, there can be no doubt that sleep research has contributed in many ways to a better understanding of numerous clinical conditions, and there is every reason to expect a similar contribution in the area of the sleep-modified disorders.

(Bibliography

1. ABE, K. and M. SHIMAKAWA. "Genetic and Developmental Aspects of Sleeptalking and Teeth-Grinding," *Acta Paedopsychiatr.* (Basel), 33 (1966), 339–344.

2. ADIE, W. J. "Idiopathic Narcolepsy: A Disease 'Sui Generis'; with Remarks on the Mechanism of Sleep," *Brain*, 49 (1926), 257–306.

3. AIRD, R. B., N. S. GORDON, and H. C.

GREGG. "Use of Phenacemide (Phenurone) in Treatment of Narcolepsy and Cataplexy. A Preliminary Report," *Arch. Neurol. Psychiatry*, 70 (1953), 510–515.

4. AITKEN, R. S., E. N. ALLOTT, L. I. M. CASTLEDEN et al. "Observations on a Case of Familial Periodic Paralysis," *Clin. Sci.*, 3 (1937), 47–57.

5. ALLEN, I. M. "Somnambulism and Dissociation of Personality," *Br. J. Med. Psychol.*, 11 (1931), 319–331.

6. ALLISON, F. G. "Obscure Pains in Chest, Back or Limbs," *Can. Med. Assoc. J.*, 48 (1943), 36–38.

7. ALTSHULER, K. Z. "Snoring: Unavoidable Nuisance or Psychological Symptom," *Psychoanal. Q.*, 33 (1964), 552–560.

8. ANDERSON, F. N. "The Psychiatric Aspects of Enuresis," *Am. J. Dis. Child.*, 40 (1930), 591–618.

9. ———. "The Psychiatric Aspects of Enuresis," *Am. J. Dis. Child.*, 40 (1930), 818–850.

10. ANDRÉ-BALISAUX, G. and R. GONSETTE. "L'Electroencéphalographie dans le somnambulisme et sa valeur pour l'établissement d'un diagnostic étiologique," *Acta Neurol. Psychiatr. Belgica*, 56 (1956), 270–281.

11. ANTHONY, J. "An Experimental Approach to the Psychopathology of Childhood: Sleep Disturbances," *Br. J. Med. Psychol.*, 32 (1959), 19–37.

12. ARDUINI, A., G. BERLUCCHI, and P. STRATA. "Pyramidal Activity during Sleep and Wakefulness," *Arch. Ital. Biol.*, 101 (1963), 530–544.

13. ARKIN, A. M. "Sleep-Talking: A Review," *J. Nerv. Ment. Dis.*, 143 (1966), 101–122.

14. ARKIN, A. M., J. M. HASTEY, and M. F. REISER. "Dialogue between Sleep-Talkers and the Experimenter." Paper presented at the Ann. Meet. of the Assoc. for the Psychophysiological Study of Sleep, Gainesville, Florida, March, 1966.

15. ARKIN, A. M., M. F. TOTH, J. BAKER et al. "The Frequency of Sleep Talking in the Laboratory among Chronic Sleep Talkers and Good Dream Recallers," *J. Nerv. Ment. Dis.*, 151 (1970), 369–374.

16. ———. "The Degree of Concordance between the Content of Sleep Talking and Mentation Recalled in Wakefulness," *J. Nerv. Ment. Dis.*, 151 (1970), 375–393.

17. ARMSTRONG, R. H., D. BURNAP, A. JACOB-SON et al. "Dreams and Gastric Secretions in Duodenal Ulcer Patients," *New Physician*, 14 (1965), 241–243.

18. ASERINSKY, E. and N. KLEITMAN. "Regularly Occurring Periods of Eye Motility, and Concomitant Phenomena, during Sleep," *Science*, 118 (1953), 273–274.

19. AUCHINCLOSS, J. H., E. COOK, and A. D. RENZETTI. "Clinical and Physiological Aspects of a Case of Obesity, Polycythemia and Alveolar Hypoventilation," *J. Clin. Invest.*, 34 (1955), 1537–1545.

20. BAKWIN, H. "Enuresis in Children," *J. Pediatr.*, 58 (1961), 806–819.

21. ———. "Sleep-Walking in Twins," *Lancet*, 2 (1970), 446–447.

22. BALDY-MOULINIER, M., M. LEVY, and P. PASSOUANT. "A Study of Jactatio Capitis during Night Sleep," *Electroencephalogr. Clin. Neurophysiol.*, 28 (1970), 87.

23. BALLA, J. I. and J. N. WALTON. "Periodic Migrainous Neuralgia," *Br. Med. J.*, 1 (1964), 219–221.

24. BARONTINI, F. and R. ZAPPOLI. "A Case of Kleine-Levin Syndrome. Clinical and Polygraphic Study," in H. Gastaut, E. Lugaresi, G. Berti Ceroni et al., eds., *The Abnormalities of Sleep in Man.* Proc. 15th Europ. Meet. Electroencephalogr., Bologna, 1967, pp. 239–245. Bologna: Aulo Gaggi, 1968.

25. BEHRMAN, S. "Disturbed Relaxation of Limbs," *Br. Med. J.*, 1 (1958), 1454–1457.

26. BENOWITZ, H. H. "The Enuretic Soldier in an AAF Basic Training Center. (A Study of 172 Cases)," *J. Nerv. Ment. Dis.*, 104 (1946), 66–79.

27. BENTAL, E. "Dissociation of Behavioural and Electroencephalographic Sleep in Two Brothers with Enuresis Nocturna," *J. Psychosom. Res.*, 5 (1961), 116–119.

28. BERDIE, R. F. and R. WALLEN. "Some Psychological Aspects of Enuresis in Adult Males," *Am. J. Orthopsychiatry*, 15 (1945), 153–159.

29. BERTI CERONI, G. "An Episode of Hypersomnia and Megaphagia and Its Evolution to a Narcoleptic Syndrome," in H. Gastaut, E. Lugaresi, G. Berti Ceroni et al., eds., *The Abnormalities of Sleep in Man.* Proc. 15th Europ. Meet. Electroencephalogr., Bologna, 1967, pp. 247–249. Bologna: Aulo Gaggi, 1968.

30. BERTI CERONI, G., G. COCCAGNA, D. GAMBI et al. "Considerazioni Clinico-Poligrafiche

sulla Narcolessia Essenziale 'A Sonno Lento'," *Sist. Nerv.*, 19 (1967), 81–89.

31. BERTI CERONI, G., G. COCCAGNA, and E. LUGARESI. "Twenty-Four Hour Polygraphic Recordings in Narcoleptics," in H. Gastaut, E. Lugaresi, G. Berti Ceroni et al., eds., *The Abnormalities of Sleep in Man.* Proc. 15th Europ. Meet. Electroencephalogr., Bologna, 1967, pp. 235–238. Bologna: Aulo Gaggi, 1968.

32. BING, R. *Lehrbuch der Nervenkrankheiten*, p. 522. Berlin: Karger, 1913.

33. BIRCHFIELD, R. I., H. O. SIEKER, and A. HEYMAN. "Alterations in Blood Gases during Natural Sleep and Narcolepsy. A Correlation with the Electroencephalographic Stages of Sleep," *Neurology (Minneap.)*, 8 (1958), 107–112.

34. ——. "Alterations in Respiratory Function during Natural Sleep," *J. Lab. Clin. Med.*, 54 (1959), 216–222.

35. BJERK, E. M. and J. J. HORNISHER. "Narcolepsy: A Case Report and a Rebuttal," *Electroencephalogr. Clin. Neurophysiol.*, 10 (1958), 550–552.

36. BLAKE, H., R. W. GERARD, and N. KLEITMAN. "Factors Influencing Brain Potentials during Sleep," *J. Neurophysiol.*, 2 (1939), 48–60.

37. BLEULER, E. (1908) *Dementia Praecox or the Group of Schizophrenias*, pp. 439–441. Translated by Z. Zinkin. New York: International Universities Press, 1950.

38. BLOMFIELD, J. M. and J. W. B. DOUGLAS. "Bedwetting, Prevalence among Children Aged 4–7 Years," *Lancet*, 1 (1956), 850–852.

39. BONKALO, A. "Hypersomnia. A Discussion of Psychiatric Implications Based on Three Cases," *Br. J. Psychiatry*, 114 (1968), 69–75.

40. BONSTEDT, T. "Emotional Aspects of the Narcolepsies. (With Report of a Case of Sleep Paralysis)," *Dis. Nerv. Syst.*, 15 (1954), 291–297.

41. BORNSTEIN, B. "Restless Legs," *Psychiatr. Neurol.*, 141 (1961), 165–201.

42. BOSTOCK, J. "Exterior Gestation, Primitive Sleep, Enuresis and Asthma: A Study in Aetiology. Part 1," *Med. J. Aust.*, 2 (1958), 149–153.

43. ——. "Exterior Gestation, Primitive Sleep, Enuresis and Asthma: A Study in Aetiology. Part 2," *Med. J. Aust.*, 2 (1958), 185–188.

44. ——. "The Deep Sleep-Enuresis Syndrome," *Med. J. Aust.*, 1 (1962), 240–243.

45. BOULWARE, M. H. "Coping with Snoring Problems of Children," *Rehabilit. Lit.*, 27 (1966), 141–142.

46. BOYENS, P. J. "Value of Autosuggestion in the Therapy of 'Bruxism' and other Biting Habits," *J. Am. Dent. Assoc.*, 27 (1940), 1773–1777.

47. BRAITHWAITE, J. V. "Enuresis in Childhood," *Practitioner*, 165 (1950), 273–281.

48. BRANCHEY, M. and O. PETRE-QUADENS. "A Comparative Study of Sleep Parameters during Pregnancy," *Acta Neurol. Belg.*, 68 (1968), 453–459.

49. BREBBIA, D. R. and K. Z. ALTSHULER. "Oxygen Consumption Rate and Electroencephalographic Stage of Sleep," *Science*, 150 (1965), 1621–1623.

50. BROCK, S. and B. WIESEL. "The Narcoleptic-Cataplectic Syndrome—an Excessive and Dissociated Reaction of the Sleep Mechanism—and Its Accompanying Mental States," *J. Nerv. Ment. Dis.*, 94 (1941), 700–712.

51. BRODNY, M. L. and S. A. ROBINS. "Enuresis. The Use of Cystourethrography in Diagnosis," *JAMA*, 126 (1944), 1000–1006.

52. BROOKS, D. C. and E. BIZZI. "Brain Stem Electrical Activity during Deep Sleep," *Arch. Ital. Biol.*, 101 (1963), 648–665.

53. BROUGHTON, R. J. "Sleep Disorders: Disorders of Arousal?" *Science*, 159 (1968), 1070–1078.

54. ——. "The Incubus Attack," *Int. Psychiatry Clin.*, 7 (1970), 188–192.

55. BROWNE, R. C. and A. FORD-SMITH. "Enuresis in Adolescents," *Br. Med. J.*, 2 (1941), 803–805.

56. BRUHOVA, S., O. NEVSIMAL, and A. OUREDNIK. "Polygraphic Study in the So Called Pickwickian Syndrome," in H. Gastaut, E. Lugaresi, G. Berti Ceroni et al., eds., *The Abnormalities of Sleep in Man.* Proc. 15th Europ. Meet. Electroencephalogr., Bologna, 1967, pp. 223–229. Bologna: Aulo Gaggi, 1968.

57. BÜLOW, K. "Respiration and Wakefulness in Man," *Acta Physiol. Scand. (Suppl.)*, 209 (1963), 1–110.

58. BÜLOW, K. and D. H. INGVAR. "Respiration and State of Wakefulness in Normals, Studied by Spirography, Capnography and EEG. A Preliminary Report," *Acta Physiol. Scand.*, 51 (1961), 230–238.

59. ———. "Respiration and Electroencephalography in Narcolepsy," *Neurology (Minneap.)*, 13 (1963), 321–326.

60. BURWELL, C. S., E. D. ROBIN, R. D. WHALEY et al. "Extreme Obesity Associated with Alveolar Hypoventilation—a Pickwickian Syndrome," *Am. J. Med.*, 21 (1956), 811–818.

61. CADILHAC, J., M. BALDY-MOULINIER, M. DELANGE et al. "Diurnal and Nocturnal Sleep in Narcolepsy," *Electroencephalogr. Clin. Neurophysiol.*, 20 (1966), 531.

62. CALDWELL, D. F. and E. F. DOMINO. "Electroencephalographic and Eye Movement Patterns during Sleep in Chronic Schizophrenic Patients," *Electroencephalogr. Clin. Neurophysiol.*, 22 (1967), 414–420.

63. CAMERON, W. B. "Some Observations and a Hypothesis Concerning Sleep-Talking," *Psychiatry*, 15 (1952), 95–96.

64. CARROLL, J. D. "Migraine: Its Variants, Differential Diagnosis and Treatment," *Res. Clin. Stud. Headache*, 1 (1967), 46–61.

65. CHEE, P. H. Y. "Ocular Manifestations of Narcolepsy," *Br. J. Ophthalmol.*, 52 (1968), 54–56.

66. CHILD, C. M. "Statistics of 'Unconscious Cerebration'," *Am. J. Psychol.*, 5 (1892), 453–463.

67. CHODOFF, P. "Sleep Paralysis. With Report of Two Cases," *J. Nerv. Ment. Dis.*, 100 (1944), 278–281.

68. COCCAGNA, G. and E. LUGARESI. "Insomnia in the Restless Legs Syndrome," in H. Gastaut, E. Lugaresi, G. Berti Ceroni et al., eds., *The Abnormalities of Sleep in Man*. Proc. 15th Europ. Meet. Electroencephalogr., Bologna, 1967, pp. 139–144. Bologna: Aulo Gaggi, 1968.

69. COCCAGNA, G., A. PETRELLA, G. BERTI CERONI et al. "Polygraphic Contribution to Hypersomnia and Respiratory Troubles in the Pickwickian Syndrome," in H. Gastaut, E. Lugaresi, G. Berti Ceroni et al., eds., *The Abnormalities of Sleep in Man*. Proc. 15th Europ. Meet. Electroencephalogr., Bologna, 1967, pp. 215–221. Bologna: Aulo Gaggi, 1968.

70. COHEN, D. L. "Nocturnal Enuresis in the Adult Male: A Urological Study," *J. Urol.*, 57 (1947), 331–337.

71. COHEN, H. D., A. SHAPIRO, D. R. GOODENOUGH et al. "The EEG during Stage 4 Sleep-Talking," Paper presented at the Ann. Meet. of the Assoc. for the Psychophysiological Study of Sleep, Washington, March, 1965.

72. COHN, R. and B. A. CRUVANT. "Relation of Narcolepsy to the Epilepsies," *Arch. Neurol. Psychiatry*, 51 (1944), 163–170.

73. CRITCHLEY, M. "Periodic Hypersomnia and Megaphagia in Adolescent Males," *Brain*, 85 (1962), 627–657.

74. CRITCHLEY, M. and H. L. HOFFMAN. "The Syndrome of Periodic Somnolence and Morbid Hunger (Kleine-Levin Syndrome)," *Br. Med. J.*, 1 (1942), 137–139.

75. DACIE, J. V. *The Haemolytic Anaemias, Congenital and Acquired*, Part 4, 2nd ed., pp. 1128–1260. New York: Grune & Stratton, 1967.

76. DALY, D. D. and R. E. YOSS. "Electroencephalogram in Narcolepsy," *Electroencephalogr. Clin. Neurophysiol.*, 9 (1957), 109–120.

77. DANIELS, L. E. "Narcolepsy," *Medicine (Baltimore)*, 13 (1934), 1–122.

78. DAVIDSON, G. M. "Concerning Schizophrenia and Manic-Depressive Psychosis Associated with Pregnancy and Childbirth," *Am. J. Psychiatry*, 92 (1936), 1331–1346.

79. DAVIS, E., M. HAYES, and B. H. KERMAN. "Somnambulism," *Lancet*, 1 (1942), 186.

80. DELORME, F., J. L. FROMENT, and M. JOUVET. "Suppression du sommeil par la *p.* chlorométhamphétamine et la *p.* chlorophénylalanine," *Compt. Rend. Soc. Biol. Filial.*, 160 (1966), 2347–2351.

81. DEMENT, W. C. "Dream Recall and Eye Movements during Sleep in Schizophrenics and Normals," *J. Nerv. Ment. Dis.*, 122 (1955), 263–269.

82. ———. "The Effect of Dream Deprivation," *Science*, 131 (1960), 1705–1707.

83. ———. "Experimental Dream Studies," in J. H. Masserman, ed., Science and Psychoanalysis. Vol. 7, *Development and Research*, pp. 129–184. Academy of Psychoanalysis. New York: Grune & Stratton, 1964.

84. ———. "Psychophysiology of Sleep and Dreams," in S. Arieti, ed., *American Handbook of Psychiatry*, 1st ed., Vol. 3, pp. 290–332. New York: Basic Books, 1966.

85. ———. "The Biological Role of REM Sleep (Circa 1968)," in A. Kales, ed., *Sleep. Physiology and Pathology. A Symposium*, pp. 245–265. Philadelphia: Lippincott, 1969.

86. DEMENT, W. C. and C. FISHER. "Experimental Interference with the Sleep Cycle," *Can. Psychiatr. Assoc. J.*, 8 (1963), 400–405.

87. DEMENT, W. C. and N. KLEITMAN. "The Relation of Eye Movements during Sleep to Dream Activity: An Objective Method for the Study of Dreaming," *J. Exp. Psychol.*, 53 (1957), 339–346.

88. DEMENT, W. C. and A. RECHTSCHAFFEN. "Narcolepsy: Polygraphic Aspects, Experimental and Theoretical Considerations," in H. Gastaut, E. Lugaresi, G. Berti Ceroni et al., eds., *The Abnormalities of Sleep in Man.* Proc. 15th Europ. Meet. Electroencephalogr., Bologna, 1967, pp. 147–164. Bologna: Aulo Gaggi, 1968.

89. DEMENT, W. C., A. RECHTSCHAFFEN, and G. GULEVICH. "The Nature of the Narcoleptic Sleep Attack," *Neurology (Minneap.)*, 16 (1966), 18–33.

90. DEPARTMENT OF HEALTH, EDUCATION AND WELFARE. *A Report to the President on Medical Care Prices.* Washington: U.S. Govt. Print. Off., 1967.

91. DESPERT, J. L. "Urinary Control and Enuresis," *Psychosom. Med.*, 6 (1944), 294–307.

92. DETRE, T., J. HIMMELHOCH, M. SWARTZBURG et al. "Hypersomnia and Manic-Depressive Disease," *Am. J. Psychiatry*, 128 (1972), 1303–1305.

93. DIAZ-GUERRERO, R., J. S. GOTTLIEB, and J. R. KNOTT. "The Sleep of Patients with Manic-Depressive Psychosis, Depressive Type. An Electroencephalographic Study," *Psychosom. Med.*, 8 (1946), 399–404.

94. DITMAN, K. S. and K. A. BLINN. "Sleep Levels in Enuresis," *Am. J. Psychiatry*, 111 (1955), 913–920.

95. DORLAND'S ILLUSTRATED MEDICAL DICTIONARY, 24th ed., p. 113. Philadelphia: Saunders, 1965.

96. DOUTHWAITE, A. H. "Proctalgia Fugax," *Br. Med. J.*, 2 (1962), 164–165.

97. DRACHMAN, D. B. and R. J. GUMNIT. "Periodic Alteration of Consciousness in the 'Pickwickian' Syndrome," *Arch. Neurol.*, 6 (1962), 471–477.

98. DUFFY, J. P. and K. DAVISON. "A Female Case of the Kleine-Levin Syndrome," *Br. J. Psychiatry*, 114 (1968), 77–84.

99. DYNES, J. B. and K. H. FINLEY. "The Electroencephalograph as an Aid in the Study of Narcolepsy," *Arch. Neurol. Psychiatry*, 46 (1941), 598–612.

100. EARLE, B. V. "Periodic Hypersomnia and Megaphagia (The Kleine-Levin Syndrome)," *Psychiatr. Q.*, 39 (1965), 79–83.

101. EDMONDS, C. "Severe Somnambulism: A Case Study," *J. Clin. Psychol.*, 23 (1967), 237–239.

102. EKBOM, K. A. "Restless Legs," *Acta Med. Scand.*, (Suppl.), 158 (1945), 1–123.

103. ———. "Restless Legs Syndrome," *Neurology (Minneap.)*, 10 (1960), 868–873.

104. ELENEWSKI, J. J. "A Study of Insomnia: The Relationship of Psychopathology to Sleep Disturbance," Ph.D. dissertation, University of Miami, 1971.

105. ELIAN, M. and B. BORNSTEIN. "The Kleine-Levin Syndrome with Intermittent Abnormality in the EEG," *Electroencephalogr. Clin. Neurophysiol.*, 27 (1969), 601–604.

106. ESCANDE, J. P., B. A. SCHWARTZ, M. GENTILINI et al. "Le Syndrome Pickwickien," *Presse Med.*, 75 (1967), 1607–1610.

107. ETHELBERG, S. "Sleep-Paralysis or Postdormitial Chalastic Fits in Cortical Lesion of the Frontal Pole," *Acta Psychiatr. Neurol. Scand.*, (Suppl.), 108 (1956), 121–130.

108. EVANS, J. "Rocking at Night," *J. Child Psychol. Psychiatry*, 2 (1961), 71–85.

109. EVARTS, E. V. "Activity of Neurons in Visual Cortex of the Cat during Sleep with Low Voltage Fast EEG Activity," *J. Neurophysiol.*, 25 (1962), 812–816.

110. EVERETT, H. C. "Sleep Paralysis in Medical Students," *J. Nerv. Ment. Dis.*, 136 (1963), 283–287.

111. EVERY, R. G. "The Significance of Extreme Mandibular Movements," *Lancet*, 2 (1960), 37–39.

112. ———. "The Teeth as Weapons. Their Influence on Behaviour," *Lancet*, 1 (1965), 685–688.

113. EYSENCK, H. J. "Learning Theory and Behaviour Therapy," *J. Ment. Sci.*, 105 (1959), 61–75.

114. FABRICANT, N. D. "Snoring," *Practitioner*, 187 (1961), 378–380.

115. FAURÉ, J., C. MARTIN, J. D'AULNAY et al. "Enurésie et somnambulisme, formes larvées de la comitialité chez l'enfant," *Arch. Fr. Pediatr.*, 8 (1951), 678–679.

116. FEINBERG, I. "Commentary on Sleep and Schizophrenia," *Schizophr. Bull.*, 4 (1971), 70–71.

117. FEINBERG, I., M. BRAUN, R. L. KORESKO et al. "Stage 4 Sleep in Schizophrenia," *Arch. Gen. Psychiatry*, 21 (1969), 262–266.

118. FEINBERG, I., R. L. KORESKO, and F. GOTTLIEB. "Further Observations on Electrophysiological Sleep Patterns in Schizophrenia," *Compr. Psychiatry*, 6 (1965), 21–24.

119. FEINBERG, I., R. L. KORESKO, F. GOTTLIEB et al. "Sleep Electroencephalographic and Eye-Movement Patterns in Schizophrenic Patients," *Compr. Psychiatry*, 5 (1964), 44–53.

120. FELDMAN, M. J. and M. HERSEN. "Attitudes towards Death in Nightmare Subjects," *J. Abnorm. Psychol.*, 72 (1967), 421–425.

121. FERGUSON, J., S. HENRIKSEN, K. MCGARR et al. "Phasic Event Deprivation in the Cat," *Psychophysiology*, 5 (1968), 238–239.

122. FINLEY, W. W. "An EEG Study of the Sleep of Enuretics at Three Age Levels," *Clin. Electroencephalogr.*, 2 (1971), 35–39.

123. FISHER, C. "Psychoanalytic Implications of Recent Research on Sleep and Dreaming. Part I: Empirical Findings," *J. Am. Psychoanal. Assoc.*, 13 (1965), 197–270.

124. FISHER, C., J. BYRNE, A. EDWARDS et al. "A Psychophysiological Study of Nightmares," *J. Am. Psychoanal. Assoc.*, 18 (1970), 747–782.

125. ———. "REM and NREM Nightmares," *Int. Psychiatry Clin.*, 7 (1970), 183–187.

126. FISHER, C., J. GROSS, and J. ZUCH. "Cycle of Penile Erection Synchronous with Dreaming (REM) Sleep. Preliminary Report," *Arch. Gen. Psychiatry*, 12 (1965), 29–45.

127. FISHER, C., E. KAHN, A. EDWARDS et al. "Total Suppression of REM Sleep with the MAO Inhibitor Nardil in a Subject with Painful Nocturnal REMP Erection," *Psychophysiology*, 9 (1972), 91.

128. FISHER, O. D. and W. I. FORSYTHE. "Micturating Cysto-Urethrography in the Investigation of Enuresis," *Arch. Dis. Child.*, 29 (1954), 460–471.

129. FORD, F. R. "The Tired Arm Syndrome," *Johns Hopkins Med. J.*, 98 (1956), 464–466.

130. FORSYTHE, W. E. and S. C. KARLAN. "Enuresis in Young Male Adults," *J. Urology*, 54 (1945), 22–38.

131. FRANKS, A. S. T. "Masticatory Muscle Hyperactivity and Temporomandibular Joint Dysfunction," *J. Prosthet. Dent.*, 15 (1965), 1122–1131.

132. FRARY, L. G. "Enuresis. A Genetic Study," *Am. J. Dis. Child.*, 49 (1935), 557–578.

133. FREUD, S. (1932–33) *New Introductory Lectures on Psycho-analysis*, in J. Strachey, ed., *Standard Edition*, Vol. 22, pp. 15–16, 221, 244–245. London: Hogarth, 1964.

134. FRIEDELL, A. "A Reversal of the Normal Concentration of the Urine in Children Having Enuresis," *Am. J. Dis. Child.*, 33 (1927), 717–721.

135. FRISCH, J., L. KATZ, and A. J. FERREIRA. "A Study on the Relationship between Bruxism and Aggression," *J. Periodontol.*, 31 (1960), 409–412.

136. FROHMAN, B. S. "Occlusal Neuroses. The Application of Psychotherapy to Dental Problems," *Psychoanal. Rev.*, 19 (1932), 297–309.

137. FÜRSTNER, C. "Ueber Schwangerschafts und Puerperalpsychosen," *Arch. Psychiatr. Nervenkr.*, 5 (1875), 505–543.

138. GAHAGAN, L. "Sex Differences in Recall of Stereotyped Dreams, Sleep-Talking, and Sleep-Walking," *J. Genet. Psychol.*, 48 (1936), 227–236.

139. GALLINEK, A. "Syndrome of Episodes of Hypersomnia, Bulimia, and Abnormal Mental States," *JAMA*, 154 (1954), 1081–1083.

140. ———. "The Kleine-Levin Syndrome: Hypersomnia, Bulimia, and Abnormal Mental States," *World Neurol.*, 3 (1962), 235–241.

141. GARLAND, H., J. P. P. BRADSHAW, and J. M. P. CLARK. "Compression of Median Nerve in Carpal Tunnel and Its Relation to Acroparaesthesiae," *Br. Med. J.*, 1 (1957), 730–734.

142. GARLAND, H., D. SUMNER, and P. FOURMAN. "The Kleine-Levin Syndrome. Some Further Observations," *Neurology*, 15 (1965), 1161–1167.

143. GASTAUT, H. and R. BROUGHTON. "Paroxysmal Psychological Events and Certain Phases of Sleep," *Percept. Mot. Skills*, 17 (1963), 362.

144. ———. "A Clinical and Polygraphic Study of Episodic Phenomena during Sleep," *Re-*

cent Adv. Biol. Psychiatry, 7 (1964), 197–221.

145. GASTAUT, H., B. DURON, J.-J. PAPY et al. "Etude polygraphique comparative du cycle nycthémérique chez les narcoleptiques, les Pickwickiens, les obèses et les insuffisants respiratoires," *Rev. Neurol. (Paris)*, 115 (1966), 456–462.

146. GASTAUT, H. and B. ROTH. "A propos des Manifestations électroencéphalographiques de 150 cas de narcolepsie avec ou sans cataplexie," *Rev. Neurol. (Paris)*, 97 (1957), 388–393.

147. GASTAUT, H., C. A. TASSINARI, and B. DURON. "Polygraphic Study of the Episodic Diurnal and Nocturnal (Hypnic and Respiratory) Manifestations of the Pickwick Syndrome," *Brain Res.*, 2 (1966), 167–186.

148. GÉLINEAU, J. B. "De la Narcolepsie," *Gaz. Hopit.*, 53 (1880), 626–628, 635–637.

149. GERARD, M. W. "Enuresis. A Study in Etiology," *Am. J. Orthopsychiatry*, 9 (1939), 48–58.

150. GILBERT, G. J. "Periodic Hypersomnia and Bulimia. The Kleine-Levin Syndrome," *Neurology (Minneap.)*, 14 (1964), 844–850.

151. GLICKLICH, L. B. "An Historical Account of Enuresis," *Pediatrics*, 8 (1951), 859–876.

152. GLOBUS, G. G. "A Syndrome Associated with Sleeping Late," *Psychosom. Med.*, 31 (1969), 528–535.

153. GONZALEZ, F. M., R. C. PABICO, H. W. BROWN et al. "Further Experience with the Use of Routine Intermittent Hemodialysis in Chronic Renal Failure," *Trans. Am. Soc. Artif. Intern. Organs*, 9 (1963), 11–17.

154. GOODE, G. B. "Sleep Paralysis," *Arch. Neurol.*, 6 (1962), 228–234.

155. GOODWIN, D. W., F. FREEMON, B. M. IANZITO et al. "Alcohol and Narcolepsy," *Br. J. Psychiatry*, 117 (1970), 705–706.

156. GRABFIELD, G. P. "The Treatment of Insomnia," *Med. Clin. North Am.*, 19 (1936), 1597–1601.

157. GREEN, L. N. and R. Q. CRACCO. "Kleine-Levin Syndrome. A Case with EEG Evidence of Periodic Brain Dysfunction," *Arch. Neurol.*, 22 (1970), 166–175.

158. GREEN, W. J. and P. P. STAJDUHAR. "The Effect of ECT on the Sleep-Dream Cycle in a Psychotic Depression," *J. Nerv. Ment. Dis.*, 143 (1966), 123–134.

159. GREENBERG, R. and C. PEARLMAN. "Delirium Tremens and Dreaming," *Am. J. Psychiatry*, 124 (1967), 133–142.

160. GRESHAM, S. C., H. W. AGNEW, JR., and R. L. WILLIAMS. "The Sleep of Depressed Patients. An EEG and Eye Movement Study," *Arch. Gen. Psychiatry*, 13 (1965), 503–507.

161. GRESHAM, S. C., W. B. WEBB, and R. L. WILLIAMS. "Alcohol and Caffeine: Effect on Inferred Visual Dreaming," *Science*, 140 (1963), 1226–1227.

162. GROSS, M. M. and D. R. GOODENOUGH. "Sleep Disturbances in the Acute Alcoholic Psychoses," *Psychiatr. Res. Rep. Am. Psychiatr. Assoc.*, 24 (1968), 132–147.

163. GROSS, M. M., D. R. GOODENOUGH, M. TOBIN et al. "Sleep Disturbances and Hallucinations in the Acute Alcoholic Psychoses," *J. Nerv. Ment. Dis.*, 142 (1966), 493–514.

164. GULEVICH, G. D., W. C. DEMENT, and V. P. ZARCONE. "All-Night Sleep Recordings of Chronic Schizophrenics in Remission," *Compr. Psychiatry*, 8 (1967), 141–149.

165. GUNNARSON, S. and K.-A. MELIN. "The Electroencephalogram in Enuresis," *Acta Paediatr. Scand.*, 40 (1951), 496–501.

166. GUNNE, L. M. and H. F. LIDVALL. "The Urinary Output of Catecholamines in Narcolepsy under Resting Conditions and following Administration of Dopamine, DOPA, and DOPS," *Scand. J. Clin. Lab. Invest.*, 18 (1966), 425–430.

167. HADER, M. "Persistent Enuresis," *Arch. Gen. Psychiatry*, 13 (1965), 296–298.

168. HADFIELD, J. A. *Dreams and Nightmares.* London: Penguin Books, 1954.

169. HALLGREN, B. "Enuresis. A Clinical and Genetic Study," *Acta Psychiatr. Neurol. Scand., (Suppl.)*, 114 (1957), 1–159.

170. HALLMAN, N. "On the Ability of Enuretic Children to Hold Urine," *Acta Paediatr. Scand.*, 39 (1950), 87–93.

171. HAMILTON, J. A. *Postpartum Psychiatric Problems.* St. Louis: Mosby, 1962.

172. HANRETTA, A. G. "Sleep in Signs, Symptoms, and Syndromes," *Dis. Nerv. Syst.*, 24 (1963), 81–94.

173. HART, H. H. "Practical Psychiatric Problems in Dentistry," *J. Dent. Med.*, 3 (1948), 83–94.

174. HARTMANN, E. "Longitudinal Studies of Sleep and Dream Patterns in Manic-De-

pressive Patients," *Arch. Gen. Psychiatry*, 19 (1968), 312–329.

175. ———. "Mania, Depression, and Sleep," in A. Kales, ed., *Sleep. Physiology and Pathology. A Symposium*, pp. 183–191. Philadelphia: Lippincott, 1969.

176. ———. "A Note on the Nightmare," *Int. Psychiatry Clin.*, 7 (1970), 192–197.

177. HARTMANN, E., P. VERDONE, and F. SNYDER. "Longitudinal Studies of Sleep and Dreaming Patterns in Psychiatric Patients," *J. Nerv. Ment. Dis.*, 142 (1966), 117–126.

178. HAURI, P. and D. R. HAWKINS. "Phasic REM, Depression, and the Relationship between Sleeping and Waking," *Arch. Gen. Psychiatry*, 25 (1971), 56–63.

179. HAWKINS, D. R. and J. MENDELS. "Sleep Disturbance in Depressive Syndromes," *Am. J. Psychiatry*, 123 (1966), 682–690.

180. ———. "The Psychophysiologic Investigation of Sleep in Patients with Depression," *Excerpta Medica Int. Congr. Ser.*, 150 (1966), 1893–1897.

181. HAWKINS, D. R., J. MENDELS, J. SCOTT et al. "The Psychophysiology of Sleep in Psychotic Depression: A Longitudinal Study," *Psychosom. Med.*, 29 (1967), 329–344.

182. HERRMAN, C. "The Treatment of Enuresis by Re-education," *Arch. Pediatr.*, 27 (1910), 600–601.

183. HERSEN, M. "Personality Characteristics of Nightmare Sufferers," *J. Nerv. Ment. Dis.*, 153 (1971), 27–31.

184. HISHIKAWA, Y. "Neurophysiological Nature of Narcoleptic Symptoms," in H. Gastaut, E. Lugaresi, G. Berti Ceroni et al., eds., *The Abnormalities of Sleep in Man*. Proc. 15th Europ. Meet. Electroencephalogr., Bologna, 1967, pp. 165–175. Bologna: Aulo Gaggi, 1968.

185. HISHIKAWA, Y., E. FURUYA, and H. WAKAMATSU. "Hypersomnia and Periodic Respiration—Presentation of Two Cases and Comment on the Physiopathogenesis of the Pickwickian Syndrome," *Folia Psychiatr. Neurol. Jap.*, 24 (1970), 163–173.

186. HISHIKAWA, Y., H. IDA, K. NAKAI et al. "Treatment of Narcolepsy with Imipramine (Tofranil) and Desmethylimipramine (Pertofran)," *J. Neurol. Sci.*, 3 (1966), 453–461.

187. HISHIKAWA, Y. and Z. KANEKO. "Electroencephalographic Study on Narcolepsy," *Electroencephalogr. Clin. Neurophysiol.*, 18 (1965), 249–259.

188. HISHIKAWA, Y., H. NAN'NO, M. TACHIBANA et al. "The Nature of Sleep Attack and Other Symptoms of Narcolepsy," *Electroencephalogr. Clin. Neurophysiol.*, 24 (1968), 1–10.

189. HISHIKAWA, Y., N. SUMITSUJI, K. MATSUMOTO et al. "H-Reflex and EMG of the Mental and Hyoid Muscles during Sleep, with Special Reference to Narcolepsy," *Electroencephalogr. Clin. Neurophysiol.*, 18 (1965), 487–492.

190. HNAYAL, A. and F. REGLI. "Contribution a l'étude clinique des anomalies du sommeil. Trois cas de 'somnolence périodique' (Kleine-Levin)," *Encephale*, 56 (1967), 33–44.

191. HODES, R. and W. C. DEMENT. "Depression of Electrically Induced Reflexes ('H-Reflexes') in Man during Low Voltage EEG 'Sleep'," *Electroencephalogr. Clin. Neurophysiol.*, 17 (1964), 617–629.

192. HUBER, Z. "EEG Investigation in 200 Somnambulic Patients," *Electroencephalogr. Clin. Neurophysiol.*, 14 (1962), 577.

193. HUTTENLOCHER, P. R. "Evoked and Spontaneous Activity in Single Units of Medial Brain Stem during Natural Sleep and Waking," *J. Neurophysiol.*, 24 (1961), 451–468.

194. IMLAH, N. "Narcolepsy in Identical Twins," *J. Neurol. Neurosurg. Psychiatry*, 24 (1961), 158–160.

195. ISKANDER, T. N. and R. KAELBLING. "Catecholamines, a Dream Sleep Model, and Depression," *Am. J. Psychiatry*, 127 (1970), 43–50.

196. JACKSON, D. D. "An Episode of Sleepwalking," *J. Am. Psychoanal. Assoc.*, 2 (1954), 503–508.

197. JACKSON, J. H. "The Factors of Insanities," in J. Taylor, G. Holmes, and F. Walshe, eds., *Selected Writings of John Hughlings Jackson*, Vol. 2, pp. 411–421. New York: Basic Books, 1958.

198. JACOBSON, A. and A. KALES. "Somnambulism: All-Night EEG and Related Studies," *Res. Publ. Assoc. Res. Nerv. Ment. Dis.*, 45 (1967), 424–448.

199. JACOBSON, A., A. KALES, D. LEHMANN et al. "Muscle Tonus in Human Subjects during Sleep and Dreaming," *Exp. Neurol.*, 10 (1964), 418–424.

200. JACOBSON, A., A. KALES, D. LEHMANN et al.

"Somnambulism: All-Night Electroencephalographic Studies," *Science*, 148 (1965),
975–977.

201. JANSSON, B. "Psychic Insufficiencies Associated with Childbearing," *Acta Psychiatr.
Scand. (Suppl.)*, 172 (1963), 1–168.

202. JELLY, A. C. "Puerperal Insanity," *Boston
Med. Surg. J.*, 144 (1901), 271–275.

203. JOHNS, M. W., P. EGAN, T. J. A. GAY et al.
"Sleep Habits and Symptoms in Male
Medical and Surgical Patients," *Br. Med.
J.*, 2 (1970), 509–512.

204. JOHNSON, L. C., J. A. BURDICK, and J. SMITH.
"Sleep during Alcohol Intake and With-
drawal in the Chronic Alcoholic," *Arch.
Gen. Psychiatry*, 22 (1970), 406–418.

205. JONES, E. *On the Nightmare*. London: Hogarth, 1949.

206. JONES, R. "Puerperal Insanity," *Br. Med. J.*,
1 (1902), 579–585.

207. JOURNAL OF THE AMERICAN MEDICAL
ASSOCIATION. Editorial. "Nocturnal Enuresis," 154 (1954), 509.

208. JOUVET, M. "Telencephalic and Rhomben-
cephalic Sleep in the Cat," in G. E. W.
Wolstenholme and M. O'Connor, eds.,
*Ciba Foundation Symposium on the Na-
ture of Sleep*, pp. 188–208. Boston: Little,
Brown, 1960.

209. ———. "Biogenic Amines and the States of
Sleep," *Science*, 163 (1969), 32–41.

210. JUNG, C. G. "The Practical Use of Dream-
Analysis," in R. F. C. Hull, transl., *The
Practice of Psychotherapy*, Vol. 16, pp.
139–143. New York: Pantheon Books,
1954.

211. JUNG, R. and W. KUHLO. "Neurophysiological Studies of Abnormal Night Sleep and
the Pickwickian Syndrome," *Prog. Brain
Res.*, 18 (1965), 140–159.

212. KAHN, B. I. and R. L. JORDAN. "Paternal
Domination as a Cause of Somnambulism,"
Calif. Med., 80 (1954), 23–25.

213. KALES, A., G. N. BEALL, G. F. BAJOR et al.
"Sleep Studies in Asthmatic Adults: Relationship of Attacks to Sleep Stage and
Time of Night," *J. Allergy*, 41 (1968),
164–173.

214. KALES, A. and G. CARY. "Treating Insomnia," in E. Robins, ed., *Psychiatry, 1971*,
pp. 55–56. New York: Medical World
News, 1971.

215. KALES, A., F. S. HOEDEMAKER, A. JACOB-
SON et al. "Dream Deprivation: An Experi-

mental Reappraisal," *Nature*, 204 (1964),
1337–1338.

216. KALES, A., A. JACOBSON, T. KUN et al.
"Somnambulism: Further All-Night EEG
Studies," *Electroencephalogr. Clin. Neu-
rophysiol.*, 21 (1966), 410.

217. KALES, A., A. JACOBSON, M. J. PAULSON et
al. "Somnambulism: Psychophysiological
Correlates. I. All-Night EEG Studies,"
Arch. Gen. Psychiatry, 14 (1966), 586–
594.

218. KALES, A., J. D. KALES, R. M. SLY
et al. "Sleep Patterns of Asthmatic Children: All-Night Electroencephalographic
Studies," *J. Allergy*, 46 (1970), 300–308.

219. KALES, A., M. J. PAULSON, A. JACOBSON
et al. "Somnambulism: Psychophysiological
Correlates. II. Psychiatric Interviews, Psychological Testing, and Discussion," *Arch.
Gen. Psychiatry*, 14 (1966), 595–604.

220. KAMIYA, J. "Behavioral, Subjective, and
Physiological Aspects of Drowsiness and
Sleep," in D. W. Fiske and S. R. Maddi,
eds., *Functions of Varied Experience*, pp.
145–174. Homewood, Ill.: Dorsey, 1961.

221. KARACAN, I. "Insomnia: All Nights Are Not
the Same," Paper presented at the Fifth
World Congress of Psychiatry, Mexico
City, November, 1971.

222. ———. "Painful Nocturnal Penile Erections," *JAMA*, 215 (1971), 1831.

223. KARACAN, I., J. BOSE, R. L. WILLIAMS et al.
"Insomnia in Hemodialytic Patients," Paper
presented at the First International Congress of the Association for the Psychophysiological Study of Sleep, Bruges,
Belgium, June, 1971.

224. KARACAN, I., W. W. FINLEY, R. L. WIL-
LIAMS et al. "Changes in Stage 1-REM
and Stage 4 Sleep during Naps," *Biol. Psychiatry*, 2 (1970), 261–265.

225. KARACAN, I., D. R. GOODENOUGH, A. SHA-
PIRO et al. "Erection Cycle during Sleep in
Relation to Dream Anxiety," *Arch. Gen.
Psychiatry*, 15 (1966), 183–189.

226. KARACAN, I., W. HEINE, H. W. AGNEW, JR.
et al. "Characteristics of Sleep Patterns
during Late Pregnancy and the Postpartum Periods," *Am. J. Obstet. Gynecol.*, 101
(1968), 579–586.

227. KARACAN, I. and R. L. WILLIAMS. "Insomnia: Old Wine in a New Bottle," *Psychiatr.
Q.*, 45 (1971), 1–15.

228. KARACAN, I., R. L. WILLIAMS, C. J. HURSCH

et al. "Some Implications of the Sleep Patterns of Pregnancy for Postpartum Emotional Disturbances," *Br. J. Psychiatry*, 115 (1969), 929–935.

229. KARACAN, I., R. L. WILLIAMS, P. J. SALIS et al. "New Approaches to the Evaluation and Treatment of Insomnia (Preliminary Results)," *Psychosomatics*, 12 (1971), 81–88.

230. KARACAN, I., R. L. WILLIAMS, and W. J. TAYLOR. "Sleep Characteristics of Patients with Angina Pectoris," *Psychosomatics*, 10 (1969), 280–284.

231. KAWAMURA, H. and C. H. SAWYER. "Elevation in Brain Temperature during Paradoxical Sleep," *Science*, 150 (1965), 912–913.

232. KEEFE, W. P., R. E. YOSS, T. G. MARTENS et al. "Ocular Manifestations of Narcolepsy," *Am. J. Ophthalmology*, 49 (1960), 953–958.

233. KERR, W. J., and J. B. LAGEN. "The Postural Syndrome Related to Obesity Leading to Postural Emphysema and Cardiorespiratory Failure," *Ann. Intern. Med.*, 10 (1936), 569–595.

234. KLACKENBERG, G. "Primary Enuresis. When Is a Child Dry at Night?" *Acta Paediatr. Scand.*, 44 (1955), 513–518.

235. KLEINE, W. "Periodische Schlafsucht," *Monatsschr. Psychiatr. Neurol.*, 57 (1925), 285–320.

236. KLEITMAN, N. *Sleep and Wakefulness*, pp. 37–39. Chicago: University of Chicago Press, 1963.

237. KNOWLES, J. B., S. G. LAVERTY, and H. A. KUECHLER. "Effects of Alcohol on REM Sleep," *Q. J. Stud. Alcohol*, 29 (1968), 342–349.

238. KORESKO, R. L., F. SNYDER, and I. FEINBERG. " 'Dream Time' in Hallucinating and Non-hallucinating Schizophrenic Patients," *Nature*, 199 (1963), 1118–1119.

239. KRABBE, E. and G. MAGNUSSEN. "On Narcolepsy. I. Familial Narcolepsy," *Acta Psychiatr. Neurol.*, 17 (1942), 149–173.

240. KUHLO, W. "Sleep Attacks with Apnea," in H. Gastaut, E. Lugaresi, G. Berti Ceroni et al., eds., *The Abnormalities of Sleep in Man*. Proc. 15th Europ. Meet. Electroencephalogr., Bologna, 1967, pp. 205–207. Bologna: Aulo Gaggi, 1968.

241. KUPFER, D. J., R. J. WYATT, J. SCOTT et al. "Sleep Disturbance in Acute Schizophrenic Patients," *Am. J. Psychiatry*, 126 (1970), 1213–1223.

242. KURTH, V. E., I. GÖHLER, and H. H. KNAAPE. "Untersuchungen über den Pavor Nocturnus bei Kindern," *Psychiatr. Neurol. Med. Psychol. (Leipz.)*, 17 (1968), 1–7.

243. LANGWORTHY, O. R. and B. J. BETZ. "Narcolepsy as a Type of Response to Emotional Conflicts," *Psychosom. Med.*, 6 (1944), 211–226.

244. LAPOUSE, R. and M. A. MONK. "Fears and Worries in a Representative Sample of Children," *Am. J. Orthopsychiatry*, 29 (1959), 803–818.

245. LEVIN, M. "Narcolepsy (Gélineau's Syndrome) and other Varieties of Morbid Somnolence," *Arch. Neurol. Psychiatry*, 22 (1929), 1172–1200.

246. ———. "Periodic Somnolence and Morbid Hunger: A New Syndrome," *Brain*, 59 (1936), 494–504.

247. ———. "Premature Waking and Post-dormitial Paralysis," *J. Nerv. Ment. Dis.*, 125 (1957), 140–141.

248. LEVINE, A. "Enuresis in the Navy," *Am. J. Psychiatry*, 100 (1943), 320–325.

249. LEVY, D. "Discussion of Michaels and Goodman," *Am. J. Orthopsychiatry*, 4 (1934), 103–106.

250. LICHTENSTEIN, B. W. and A. H. ROSENBLUM. "Sleep Paralysis," *J. Nerv. Ment. Dis.*, 95 (1942), 153–155.

251. LIDDON, S. C. "Sleep Paralysis, Psychosis, and Death," *Am. J. Psychiatry*, 126 (1970), 1027–1031.

252. LINDNER, R. M. "Hypnoanalysis in a Case of Hysterical Somnambulism," *Psychoanal. Rev.*, 32 (1945), 325–339.

253. LOEWENFELD, L. "Ueber Narkolepsie," *Munch. Med. Wochenschr.*, 49 (1902), 1041–1045.

254. LOWY, F. H., J. M. CLEGHORN, and D. J. McCLURE. "Sleep Patterns in Depression," *J. Nerv. Ment. Dis.*, 153 (1971), 10–26.

255. LUBY, E. D. and D. F. CALDWELL. "Sleep Deprivation and EEG Slow Wave Activity in Chronic Schizophrenia," *Arch. Gen. Psychiatry*, 17 (1967), 361–364.

256. LUGARESI, E., G. COCCAGNA, G. BERTI CERONI et al. "Restless Legs Syndrome and Nocturnal Myoclonus," in H. Gastaut, E. Lugaresi, G. Berti Ceroni et al., eds., *The Abnormalities of Sleep in Man*. Proc. 15th Europ. Meet. Electroencephalogr., Bo-

logna, 1967, pp. 285–294. Bologna: Aulo Gaggi, 1968.

257. LUGARESI, E., C. A. TASSINARI, G. COCCAGNA et al. "Particularités cliniques et polygraphiques du syndrome d'impatience des membres inférieurs," *Rev. Neurol. (Paris)*, 113 (1965), 545–555.

258. MACDONALD, J. "Puerperal Insanity," *Am. J. Insanity*, 4 (1847), 113–163.

259. MACK, J. E. *Nightmares and Human Conflict.* Boston: Little, Brown, 1970.

260. MAGEE, K. R. "Bruxism Related to Levodopa Therapy," *JAMA*, 214 (1970), 147.

261. MANDELL, A. J., P. L. BRILL, M. P. MANDELL. et al "Urinary Excretion of 3-Methoxy-4-Hydroxymandelic Acid during Dreaming Sleep in Man," *Life Sci. I*, 5 (1966), 169–173.

262. MANDELL, A. J., B. CHAFFEY, P. BRILL et al. "Dreaming Sleep in Man: Changes in Urine Volume and Osmolality," *Science*, 151 (1966), 1558–1560.

263. MANDELL, M. P., A. J. MANDELL, R. T. RUBIN et al. "Activation of the Pituitary-Adrenal Axis during Rapid Eye Movement Sleep in Man," *Life Sci. I*, 5 (1966), 583–587.

264. MARIE, P. and PIETKIEWICZ. "La Bruxomanie," *Rev. Stomatol.*, 14 (1907), 107–116.

265. MARKMAN, R. A. "Kleine-Levin Syndrome: Report of a Case," *Am. J. Psychiatry*, 123 1967), 1025–1026.

266. MARKS, J. "The Marchiafava Micheli Syndrome (Paroxysmal Nocturnal Haemoglobinuria)," *Q. J. Med.*, 18 (1949), 105–121.

267. MARON, L., A. RECHTSCHAFFEN, and E. A. WOLPERT. "The Sleep Cycle during Napping," *Arch. Gen. Psychiatry*, 11 (1964), 503–508.

268. MCCRARY, J. A. and J. L. SMITH. "Cortical Dyschromatopsia in Narcolepsy," *Am. J. Ophthalmol.*, 64 (1967), 153–155.

269. MCFADDEN, G. D. F. "Enuresis," *Br. Med. J.*, 1 (1964), 632.

270. MELLO, N. K. "Some Aspects of the Behavioral Pharmacology of Alcohol," in D. H. Efron, ed., *Psychopharmacology. A Review of Progress, 1957–1967.* Proc. 6th Annu. Meet. Am. Coll. Neuropsychopharmacol., San Juan, Puerto Rico, December, 1967, pp. 787–809. PHS publication no. 1836. Washington: U.S. Govt. Print. Off., 1968.

271. MELLO, N. K. and J. H. MENDELSON. "Behavioral Studies of Sleep Patterns in Alcoholics during Intoxication and Withdrawal," *J. Pharmcol. Exp. Thera.*, 175 (1970), 94–112.

272. MENDELS, J. and D. R. HAWKINS. "The Psychophysiology of Sleep in Depression," *Ment. Hyg.*, 51 (1967), 501–511.

273. ———. "Sleep and Depression. A Controlled EEG Study," *Arch. Gen. Psychiatry*, 16 (1967), 334–354.

274. ———. "Sleep and Depression. A Follow-up Study," *Arch. Gen. Psychiatry*, 16 (1967), 536–542.

275. ———. "Sleep and Depression—Further Considerations," *Arch. Gen. Psychiatry*, 19 (1968), 445–452.

276. ———. "Longitudinal Sleep Study in Hypomania," *Arch. Gen. Psychiatry*, 25 (1971), 274–277.

277. MENDELSON, J. "Biochemical Pharmocology of Alcohol," in D. H. Efron, ed., *Psychopharmacology. A Review of Progress, 1957–1967.* Proc. 6th Annu. Meet. Am. Coll. Neuropsychopharmacol., San Juan, Puerto Rico, December, 1967, pp. 769–785. PHS publication no. 1836. Washington: U.S. Govt. Print. Off., 1968.

278. MENZIES, I. C. and W. K. STEWART. "Psychiatric Observations on Patients Receiving Regular Dialysis Treatment," *Br. Med. J.*, 1 (1968), 544–547.

279. MICHAELS, J. J. "Enuresis in Murderous Aggressive Children and Adolescents," *Arch. Gen. Psychiatry*, 5 (1961), 94–97.

280. MICHAELS, J. J. and S. E. GOODMAN. "Incidence and Intercorrelations of Enuresis and Other Neuropathic Traits in So-called Normal Children," *Am. J. Orthopsychiatry*, 4 (1934), 79–102.

281. ———. "The Incidence of Enuresis and Age of Cessation in One Thousand Neuropsychiatric Patients: With a Discussion of the Relationship between Enuresis and Delinquency," *Am. J. Orthopsychiatry*, 9 (1939), 59–71.

282. MICHAELS, J. J. and L. SECUNDA. "The Relationship of Neurotic Traits to the Electroencephalogram in Children with Behavior Disorders," *Am. J. Psychiatry*, 101 (1944), 407–409.

283. MICHEL, F., M. JEANNEROD, J. MOURET et al. "Sur les Mécanismes de l'activité de pointes au niveau du système visuel au cours de la phase paradoxale du sommeil," *Compt.*

Rend. Soc. Biol. Filial., 158 (1964), 103–106.

284. MITCHELL, S. A., W. C. DEMENT, and G. D. GULEVICH. "The So-called 'Idiopathic' Narcolepsy Syndrome." Paper presented at the Ann. Meet. of the Assoc. for the Psychophysiological Study of Sleep, Gainesville, Florida, March, 1966.

285. MOLL, A. (1889) *The Study of Hypnosis*, pp. 127, 200–201. New York: Julian Press, 1958.

286. MONEYSWORTH. "Dollars and Sense," 1, no. 13, April 5, (1971), 1.

287. MONROE, L. J. "Psychological and Physiological Differences between Good and Poor Sleepers," *J. Abnorm. Psychol.*, 72 (1967), 255–264.

288. MOWRER, O. H. and W. M. MOWRER. "Enuresis—A Method for Its Study and Treatment," *Am. J. Orthopsychiatry*, 8 (1938), 436–459.

289. MUELLNER, S. R. "Development of Urinary Control in Children. Some Aspects of the Cause and Treatment of Primary Enuresis," *JAMA*, 172 (1960), 1256–1261.

290. NADLER, S. C. "Bruxism, a Classification: Critical Review," *J. Am. Dent. Assoc.*, 54 (1957), 615–622.

291. ———. "The Effects of Bruxism," *J. Periodontol.*, 37 (1966), 311–319.

292. NAN'NO, H., Y. HISHIKAWA, H. KOIDA et al. "A Neurophysiological Study of Sleep Paralysis in Narcoleptic Patients," *Electroencephalogr. Clin. Neurophysiol.*, 28 (1970), 382–390.

293. NOTKIN, J. and S. E. JELLIFFE. "The Narcolepsies. Cryptogenic and Symptomatic Types," *Arch. Neurol. Psychiatry*, 31 (1934), 615–634.

294. NOWLIN, J. B., W. G. TROYER, JR., W. S. COLLINS et al. "The Association of Nocturnal Angina Pectoris with Dreaming," *Ann. Intern. Med.*, 63 (1965), 1040–1046.

295. NOYES, A. P. and L. C. KOLB. *Modern Clinical Psychiatry*, 5th ed., pp. 62–63. Philadelphia: Saunders, 1958.

296. OLSEN, S. "The Brain in Uremia," *Acta Psychiatr. Neurol. Scand.* (Suppl.), 156 (1961), 11–20, 119–122.

297. ONHEIBER, P., P. T. WHITE, M. K. DE MYER et al. "Sleep and Dream Patterns of Child Schizophrenics," *Arch. Gen. Psychiatry*, 12 (1965), 568–571.

298. OPPENHEIM, H. *Lehrbuch der Nervenkrankheiten*, 7th ed., p. 1774. Berlin: Karger, 1923.

299. ORME, J. E. "The Incidence of Sleepwalking in Various Groups," *Acta Psychiatr. Scand.*, 43 (1967), 279–281.

300. ORNITZ, E. M., E. R. RITVO, and R. D. WALTER. "Dreaming Sleep in Autistic and Schizophrenic Children," *Am. J. Psychiatry*, 122 (1965), 419–424.

301. ———. "Dreaming Sleep in Autistic Twins," *Arch. Gen. Psychiatry*, 12 (1965), 77–79.

302. OSWALD, I. "Experimental Studies of Rhythm, Anxiety and Cerebral Vigilance," *J. Ment. Sci.*, 105 (1959), 269–294.

303. ———. "Falling Asleep Open-eyed during Intense Rhythmic Stimulation," *Br. Med. J.*, 1 (1960), 1450–1455.

304. ———. *Sleeping and Waking. Physiology and Psychology*, pp. 110, 196–200. Amsterdam: Elsevier, 1962.

305. ———. "Rocking at Night," *Electroencephalogr. Clin. Neurophysiol.*, 16 (1964), 312–313.

306. ———. "Some Psychophysiological Features of Human Sleep," *Prog. Brain Res.*, 18 (1965), 160–168.

307. ———. "Sleep and Its Disorders," in P. J. Vinken and G. W. Bruyn, eds., *Handbook of Clinical Neurology*, Vol. 3, pp. 80–111. Amsterdam: North-Holland Publishing, 1969.

308. OSWALD, I., R. J. BERGER, R. A. JARAMILLO et al. "Melancholia and Barbiturates: A Controlled EEG, Body and Eye Movement Study of Sleep," *Br. J. Psychiatry*, 109 (1963), 66–78.

309. PAI, M. N. "Sleep-Walking and Sleep Activities," *J. Ment. Sci.*, 92 (1946), 756–765.

310. ———. "Hypersomnia Syndromes," *Br. Med. J.*, 1 (1950), 522–524.

311. PALMER, H. "The Klein[e]-Levin Syndrome, Narcolepsy and Akinetic Epilepsy as Related Disorders of the Hypothalamus," *N. Z. Med. J.*, 49 (1950), 28–37.

312. PASSOUANT, P. "Problèmes physiopathologiques de la narcolepsie et périodicité du 'sommeil rapide' au cours du nycthémère," in H. Gastaut, E. Lugaresi, G. Berti Ceroni et al., eds., *The Abnormalities of Sleep in Man*. Proc. 15th Europ. Meet. Electroencephalogr., Bologna, 1967, pp. 177–189. Bologna: Aulo Gaggi, 1968.

313. PASSOUANT, P., J. CADILHAC, and M. BALDY-MOULINIER. "Physiopathologie des hyper-

somnies," *Rev. Neurol. (Paris)*, 116 (1967), 585–629.

314. Passouant, P., J. Cadilhac, M. Baldy-Moulinier et al. "Etude du sommeil nocturne chez des urémiques chroniques soumis à une épuration extrarénale," *Electroencephalogr. Clin. Neurophysiol.*, 29 (1970), 441–449.

315. Passouant, P., F. Halberg, R. Genicot et al. "La Périodicité des accès narcoleptiques et le rythme ultradien du sommeil rapide," *Rev. Neurol. (Paris)*, 121 (1969), 155–164.

316. Passouant, P., L. Popoviciu, G. Velok et al. "Étude polygraphique des narcolepsies au cours du nycthémère," *Rev. Neurol. (Paris)*, 118 (1968), 431–441.

317. Passouant, P., R.-S. Schwab, J. Cadilhac et al. "Narcolepsie-Cataplexie. Etude du sommeil de nuit et du sommeil de jour. Traitement par une amphétamine lévogyre," *Rev. Neurol. (Paris)*, 111 (1964), 415–426.

318. Petre-Quadens, O., A. M. De Barsy, J. Devos et al. "Sleep in Pregnancy: Evidence of Foetal-Sleep Characteristics," *J. Neurol. Sci.*, 4 (1967), 600–605.

319. Pierce, C. M., and H. H. Lipcon. "Clinical Relationship of Enuresis to Sleepwalking and Epilepsy," *Arch. Neurol. Psychiatry*, 76 (1956), 310–316.

320. ———. "Somnambulism: Psychiatric Interview Studies," *U.S. Armed Forces Med. J.*, 7 (1956), 1143–1153.

321. ———. "Somnambulism. Electroencephalographic Studies and Related Findings," *U.S. Armed Forces Med. J.*, 7 (1956), 1419–1426.

322. Pierce, C. M., H. H. Lipcon, J. H. McLary et al. "Enuresis: Clinical, Laboratory, and Electroencephalographic Studies," *U.S. Armed Forces Med. J.*, 7 (1956), 208–219.

323. Pierce, C. M., J. L. Mathis, and J. T. Jabbour. "Dream Patterns in Narcoleptic and Hydranencephalic Patients," *Am. J. Psychiatry*, 122 (1965), 402–404.

324. Pierce, C. M., R. M. Whitman, J. W. Maas et al., "Enuresis and Dreaming. Experimental Studies," *Arch. Gen. Psychiatry*, 4 (1961), 166–170.

325. Podolsky, E. "Somnambulistic Homicide," *Dis. Nerv. Syst.*, 20 (1959), 534–536.

326. Pond, D. A. "Narcolepsy: A Brief Critical Review and Study of Eight Cases," *J. Ment. Sci.*, 98 (1952), 595–604.

327. Poulton, E. M. and E. Hinden. "The Classification of Enuresis," *Arch. Dis. Child.*, 28 (1953), 392–397.

328. Poussaint, A. F., R. R. Koegler, and J.-L. R. Riehl. "Enuresis, Epilepsy, and the Electroencephalogram," *Am. J. Psychiatry*, 123 (1967), 1294–1295.

329. Powell, R. N. "Tooth Contact during Sleep: Association with Other Events," *J. Dent. Res.*, 44 (1965), 959–967.

330. Radonic, M., D. Dimov-Butkovic, and F. Hajnsek. "The Pickwickian Syndrome," *Lijec. Vjesn.*, 92 (1970), 465–474.

331. Ramfjord, S. P. "Bruxism, a Clinical and Electromyographic Study," *J. Am. Dent. Assoc.*, 62 (1961), 21–44.

332. Rechtschaffen, A. "Polygraphic Aspects of Insomnia," in H. Gastaut, E. Lugaresi, G. Berti Ceroni et al., eds., *The Abnormalities of Sleep in Man*. Proc. 15th Europ. Meet. Electroencephalogr., Bologna, 1967, pp. 109–125. Bologna: Aulo Gaggi, 1968.

333. Rechtschaffen, A., P. Cornwall, W. Zimmerman et al. "Brain Temperature Variations with Paradoxical Sleep: Implications for Relationships among EEG, Cerebral Metabolism, Sleep and Consciousness," Paper presented at the Symposium on Sleep and Consciousness, Lyon, France, 1965.

334. Rechtschaffen, A. and W. C. Dement. "Studies on the Relation of Narcolepsy, Cataplexy and Sleep with Low Voltage Random EEG Activity," *Res. Publ. Assoc. Res. Nerv. Ment. Dis.*, 45 (1967), 488–498.

335. ———. "Narcolepsy and Hypersomnia," in A. Kales, ed., *Sleep. Physiology and Pathology. A Symposium*, pp. 119–130. Philadelphia: Lippincott, 1969.

336. Rechtschaffen, A., D. R. Goodenough, and A. Shapiro. "Patterns of Sleep Talking," *Arch. Gen. Psychiatry*, 7 (1962), 418–426.

337. Rechtschaffen, A., P. Hauri, and M. Zeitlin. "Auditory Awakening Thresholds in REM and NREM Sleep Stages," *Percept. Mot. Skills*, 22 (1966), 927–942.

338. Rechtschaffen, A. and L. J. Monroe. "Laboratory Studies of Insomnia," in A. Kales, ed., *Sleep. Physiology and Pathology. A Symposium*, pp. 158–169. Philadelphia: Lippincott, 1969.

339. Rechtschaffen, A. and B. Roth. "Nocturnal Sleep of Hypersomniacs," *Activ.*

Nerv. Superior, 11 (1969), 229–233.

340. RECHTSCHAFFEN, A., F. SCHULSINGER, and S. A. MEDNICK. "Schizophrenia and Physiological Indices of Dreaming," *Arch. Gen. Psychiatry*, 10 (1964), 89–93.

341. RECHTSCHAFFEN, A., E. A. WOLPERT, W. C. DEMENT et al. "Nocturnal Sleep of Narcoleptics," *Electroencephalogr. Clin. Neurophysiol.*, 15 (1963), 599–609.

342. REDING, G. R., W. C. RUBRIGHT, A. RECHTSCHAFFEN et al. "Sleep Pattern of Tooth-Grinding: Its Relationship to Dreaming," *Science*, 145 (1964), 725–726.

343. REDING, G. R., W. C. RUBRIGHT, and S. O. ZIMMERMAN. "Incidence of Bruxism," *J. Dent. Res.*, 45 (1966), 1198–1204.

344. REDING, G. R., H. ZEPELIN, and L. J. MONROE. "Personality Study of Nocturnal Teeth-Grinders," *Percept. Mot. Skills*, 26 (1968), 523–531.

345. REDING, G. R., H. ZEPELIN, J. E. ROBINSON, JR. et al. "Nocturnal Teeth-Grinding: All-night Psychophysiologic Studies," *J. Dent. Res.*, 47 (1968), 786–797.

346. RITVO, E. R., E. M. ORNITZ, F. GOTTLIEB et al. "Arousal and Nonarousal Enuretic Events," *Am. J. Psychiatry*, 126 (1969), 77–84.

347. ROBERTS, H. J. "Obesity due to the Syndrome of Narcolepsy and Diabetogenic Hyperinsulinism: Clinical and Therapeutic Observations on 252 Patients," *J. Am. Geriatr. Soc.*, 15 (1967), 721–743.

348. ROBIN, E. D. "Some Interrelations between Sleep and Disease," *Arch. Int. Med.*, 102 (1958), 669–675.

349. ROBIN, E. D., R. D. WHALEY, C. H. CRUMP et al. "The Nature of the Respiratory Acidosis of Sleep and of the Respiratory Alkalosis of Hepatic Coma," *J. Clin. Invest.*, 36 (1957), 924.

350. ROLAND, S. I. "Essential Nocturnal Enuresis Treated with D-Amphetamine Sulphate," *J. Urol.*, 71 (1954), 216–218.

351. ROSENKÖTTER, L. and S. WENDE. "EEG-Befunde beim Kleine-Levin-Syndrom," *Monatsschr. Psychiatr. Neurol.*, 130 (1955), 107–122.

352. ROTH, B. *Narkolepsie und Hypersomnie.* Berlin: Verlag Volk und Gesundheit, 1962.

353. ROTH, B. and S. BRUHOVA. "Dreams in Narcolepsy, Hypersomnia and Dissociated Sleep Disorders," *Exp. Med. Surg.*, 27 (1969), 187–209.

354. ROTH, B., S. BRUHOVA, and L. BERKOVA.

"Familial Sleep Paralysis," *Arch. Suiss. Neurol. Neurochir. Psychiatr.*, 102 (1968), 321–330.

355. ROTH, B., S. BRUHOVA, and M. LEHOVSKY. "On the Problem of Pathophysiological Mechanisms of Narcolepsy, Hypersomnia and Dissociated Sleep Disturbances," in H. Gastaut, E. Lugaresi, G. Berti Ceroni et al., eds., *The Abnormalities of Sleep in Man.* Proc. 15th Europ. Meet. Electroencephalogr., Bologna, 1967, pp. 191–203. Bologna: Aulo Gaggi, 1968.

356. ———. "REM Sleep and NREM Sleep in Narcolepsy and Hypersomnia," *Electroencephalogr. Clin. Neurophysiol.*, 26 (1969), 176–182.

357. ROTH, B., J. FABER, S. NEVSIMALOVA et al. "The Influence of Imipramine, Dexphenmetrazine and Amphetaminsulphate upon the Clinical and Polygraphic Picture of Narcolepsy-Cataplexy," *Arch. Suiss. Neurol. Neurochir. Psychiatr.*, 108 (1971), 251–260.

358. ROTH, B., S. FIGAR, and O. SIMONOVA. "Respiration in Narcolepsy and Hypersomnia," *Electroencephalogr. Clin. Neurophysiol.*, 20 (1966), 283.

359. ROTH, B., S. NEVSIMALOVA, and A. RECHTSCHAFFEN. "Hypersomnia with 'Sleep Drunkenness'," *Arch. Gen. Psychiatry*, 26 (1972), 456–462.

360. ROTH, N. "Some Problems in Narcolepsy: With a Case Report," *Bull. Menninger Clin.*, 10 (1946), 160–170.

361. ROTHENBERG, S. "Psychoanalytic Insight into Insomnia," *Psychoanal. Rev.*, 34 (1947), 141–168.

362. ROTTERSMAN, W. "The Selectee and His Complaints," *Am. J. Psychiatry*, 103 (1946), 79–86.

363. RUSHTON, J. G. "Sleep Paralysis: Report of Two Cases," *Proc. Staff Meet. Mayo Clin.*, 19 (1944), 51–54.

364. SAMPSON, H. "Psychological Effects of Deprivation of Dreaming Sleep," *J. Nerv. Ment. Dis.*, 143 (1966), 305–317.

365. SANDLER, S. A. "Somnambulism in the Armed Forces," *Ment. Hyg.*, 29 (1945), 236–247.

366. SATOH, T. and Y. HARADA. "Tooth-Grinding during Sleep as an Arousal Reaction," *Experientia*, 27 (1971), 785–786.

367. SAVAGE, G. H. "Prevention and Treatment of Insanity of Pregnancy and the Puerperal Period," *Lancet*, 1 (1896), 164–165.

368. SCHIFF, S. K. "The EEG, Eye Movements and Dreaming in Adult Enuresis," *J. Nerv. Ment. Dis.*, 140 (1965), 397–404.

369. SCHNECK, J. M. "Sleep Paralysis: Psychodynamics," *Psychiatr. Q.*, 22 (1948), 462–469.

370. ———. "Sleep Paralysis," *Am. J. Psychiatry*, 108 (1952), 921–923.

371. ———. "Sleep Paralysis, a New Evaluation," *Dis. Nerv. Syst.*, 18 (1957), 144–146.

372. ———. "Sleep Paralysis without Narcolepsy or Cataplexy. Report of a Case," *JAMA*, 173 (1960), 1129–1130.

373. ———. "Personality Components in Patients with Sleep Paralysis," *Psychiatr. Q.*, 43 (1969), 343–348.

374. SCHREINER, G. E. "Mental and Personality Changes in the Uremic Syndrome," *Med. Ann. D.C.*, 28 (1959), 316–323, 362.

375. SCHWARTZ, B. A. "Discussion of N. Kleitman's Paper, 'The Nature of Dreaming'," in G. E. W. Wolstenholme and M. O'Connor, eds., *Ciba Foundation Symposium on the Nature of Sleep*, p. 366. Boston: Little, Brown, 1960.

376. SCHWARTZ, B. A., M. SEGUY, and J.-P. ESCANDE. "Corrélations E.E.G., respiratoires, oculaires et myographiques dans le 'syndrome Pickwickien' et autres affections paraissant apparentées: proposition d'une hypothèse," *Rev. Neurol. (Paris)*, 117 (1967), 145–152.

377. SECUNDA, L. and K. H. FINLEY. "Electroencephalographic Studies in Children Presenting Behavior Disorders," *N. Engl. J. Med.*, 226 (1942), 850–854.

378. SHAPIRO, S. and J. SHANON. "Bruxism as an Emotional Reactive Disturbance," *Psychosomatics*, 6 (1965), 427–430.

379. SHEA, E. J., D. F. BOGDAN, R. B. FREEMAN et al. "Hemodialysis for Chronic Renal Failure. IV. Psychological Considerations," *Ann. Intern. Med.*, 62 (1965), 558–563.

380. SHIRLEY, H. F. and J. P. KAHN. "Sleep Disturbances in Children," *Pediatr. Clin. North Am.*, 5 (1958), 629–643.

381. SIEKER, H. O., E. H. ESTES, JR., G. A. KELSER et al. "A Cardiopulmonary Syndrome Associated with Extreme Obesity," *J. Clin. Invest.*, 34 (1955), 916.

382. SIMPSON, R. G. "Nocturnal Disorders of Medical Interest," *Practitioner*, 202 (1969), 259–268.

383. SJAASTAD, O., E. HULTIN, and N. NORMAN. "Narcolepsy: Increased Urinary Excretion of Estriol. A Preliminary Report," *Acta Neurol. Scand.*, 46 (1970), 111–118.

384. SJOSTRAND, T. "Volume and Distribution of Blood and Their Significance in Regulating the Circulation," *Physiol. Rev.*, 33 (1953), 202–228.

385. SNYDER, F. "Electrographic Studies of Sleep in Depression," in N. S. Kline and E. Laska, eds., *Computers and Electronic Devices in Psychiatry*, pp. 272–303. New York: Grune & Stratton, 1968.

386. ———. "Sleep Disturbance in Relation to Acute Psychosis," in A. Kales, ed., *Sleep. Physiology and Pathology. A Symposium*, pp. 170–182. Philadelphia: Lippincott, 1969.

387. SNYDER, F., D. ANDERSON, W. BUNNEY, JR. et al. "Longitudinal Variation in the Sleep of Severely Depressed and Acutely Schizophrenic Patients with Changing Clinical Status," *Psychophysiology*, 5 (1968), 235.

388. SNYDER, F., J. A. HOBSON, and F. GOLDFRANK. "Blood Pressure Changes during Human Sleep," *Science*, 142 (1963), 1313–1314.

389. SNYDER, F., J. A. HOBSON, D. F. MORRISON et al. "Changes in Respiration, Heart Rate, and Systolic Blood Pressure in Human Sleep," *J. Appl. Physiol.*, 19 (1964), 417–422.

390. SOURS, J. A. "Narcolepsy and other Disturbances in the Sleep-Waking Rhythm: A Study of 115 Cases with a Review of the Literature," *J. Nerv. Ment. Dis.*, 137 (1963), 525–542.

391. SOURS, J. A., P. FRUMKIN, and R. R. INDERMILL. "Somnambulism. Its Clinical Significance and Dynamic Meaning in Late Adolescence and Adulthood," *Arch. Gen. Psychiatry*, 9 (1963), 400–413.

392. STALKER, H. and D. BAND. "Persistent Enuresis: A Psychosomatic Study," *J. Ment. Sci.*, 92 (1946), 324–342.

393. STERN, M., D. H. FRAM, R. WYATT et al. "All-Night Sleep Studies of Acute Schizophrenics," *Arch. Gen. Psychiatry*, 20 (1969), 470–477.

394. STOCKWELL, L. and C. K. SMITH. "Enuresis. A Study of Causes, Types and Therapeutic Results," *Am. J. Dis. Child.*, 59 (1940), 1013–1033.

395. STOUPEL, M. N. "Etude électroencéphalographique de sept cas de narcolepsiecataplexie," *Rev. Neurol. (Paris)*, 83 (1950), 563–570.

396. STROM-OLSEN, R. "Enuresis in Adults and Abnormality of Sleep," *Lancet*, 2 (1950), 133–135.

397. STROTHER, E. W. and G. E. MITCHELL. "Bruxism: A Review and a Case Report," *J. Dent. Med.*, 9 (1954), 189–201.

398. STRUVE, F. A. and D. R. BECKA. "The Relative Incidence of the B-Mitten EEG Pattern in Process and Reactive Schizophrenia," *Electroencephalogr. Clin. Neurophysiol.*, 24 (1968), 80–82.

399. SUZUKI, J. "Narcoleptic Syndrome and Paradoxical Sleep," *Folia Psychiatr. Neurol. Jap.*, 20 (1966), 123–149.

400. SZABÓ, L., O. CORFARIU, and C. CSIKY. "Electro-Clinical Aspects of Nocturnal Ambulatory Automatism (Somnambulism)," *Electroencephalogr. Clin. Neurophysiol.*, 21 (1966), 98.

401. TAKAHAMA, Y. "Bruxism," *J. Dent. Res.*, 40 (1961), 227.

402. TAKAHASHI, Y. and M. JIMBO. "Polygraphic Study of Narcoleptic Syndrome, with Special Reference to Hypnagogic Hallucination and Cataplexy," *Folia Psychiatr. Neurol. Jap. (Suppl.)*, 7 (1964), 343–347.

403. TANI, K., N. YOSHII, I. YOSHINO et al. "Electroencephalographic Study of Parasomnia: Sleep-Talking, Enuresis and Bruxism," *Physiol. Behav.*, 1 (1966), 241–243.

404. TAPIA, F., J. WERBOFF, and G. WINOKUR. "Recall of Some Phenomena of Sleep. A Comparative Study of Dreams, Somnambulism, Orgasm and Enuresis in a Control and Neurotic Population," *J. Nerv. Ment. Dis.*, 127 (1958), 119–123.

405. TEPLITZ, Z. "The Ego and Motility in Sleepwalking," *J. Am. Psychoanal. Assoc.*, 6 (1958), 95–110.

406. TERZIAN, H. "Syndrome de Pickwick et narcolepsie," *Rev. Neurol. (Paris)*, 115 (1966), 184–188.

407. THACORE, V. R., M. AHMED, and I. OSWALD. "The EEG in a Case of Periodic Hypersomnia," *Electroencephalogr. Clin. Neurophysiol.*, 27 (1969), 605–606.

408. THALLER, J. L., G. ROSEN, and S. SALTZMAN. "Study of the Relationship of Frustration and Anxiety to Bruxism," *J. Periodontol.*, 38 (1967), 193–197.

409. THORNE, F. C. "The Incidence of Nocturnal Enuresis after Age Five," *Am. J. Psychiatry*, 100 (1944), 686–689.

410. TRASK, C. H. and E. M. CREE. "Oximeter Studies on Patients with Chronic Obstructive Emphysema, Awake and during Sleep," *N. Engl. J. Med.*, 266 (1962), 639–642.

411. TURTON, E. C. and A. B. SPEAR. "E.E.G. Findings in 100 Cases of Severe Enuresis," *Arch. Dis. Child.*, 28 (1953), 316–320.

412. VAN DER HEIDE, C. and J. WEINBERG. "Sleep Paralysis and Combat Fatigue," *Psychosom. Med.*, 7 (1945), 330–334.

413. VERNALLIS, F. F. "Teeth-Grinding: Some Relationships to Anxiety, Hostility, and Hyperactivity," *J. Clin. Psychol.*, 11 (1955), 389–391.

414. VIZIOLI, R. and A. GIANCOTTI. "EEG Findings in a Case of Narcolepsy," *Electroencephalogr. Clin. Neurophysiol.*, 6 (1954), 307–309.

415. VOGEL, G. W. "REM Deprivation. III. Dreaming and Psychosis," *Arch. Gen. Psychiatry*, 18 (1968), 312–329.

416. VOGEL, G. W. and A. C. TRAUB. "REM Deprivation. I. The Effect on Schizophrenic Patients," *Arch. Gen. Psychiatry*, 18 (1968), 287–300.

417. VOGEL, G. W., A. C. TRAUB, P. BEN-HORIN et al. "REM Deprivation. II. The Effects on Depressed Patients," *Arch. Gen. Psychiatry*, 18 (1968), 301–311.

418. VOGL, M. "Sleep Disturbances of Neurotic Children," *Int. Ser. Monogr. Child Psychiatry*, 2 (1964), 123–134.

419. VULLIAMY, D. "The Day and Night Output of Urine in Enuresis," *Arch. Dis. Child.*, 31 (1956), 439–443.

420. WALSH, J. P. "The Psychogenesis of Bruxism," *J. Periodontol.*, 36 (1965), 417–420.

421. WALTON, D. "The Application of Learning Theory to the Treatment of a Case of Somnambulism," *J. Clin. Psychol.*, 17 (1961), 96–99.

422. WATERFIELD, R. L. "The Effects of Posture on the Circulating Blood Volume," *J. Physiology*, 72 (1931), 110–120.

423. WEBB, W. B. and H. W. AGNEW, JR. "Sleep Stage Characteristics of Long and Short Sleepers," *Science*, 168 (1970), 146–147.

424. WEINMANN, H. M. "Telemetric Recording of Sleep Rhythms in Enuretic Children," *Electroencephalogr. Clin. Neurophysiol.*, 24 (1968), 391.

425. WEISS, H. R., B. H. KASINOFF, and M. A. BAILEY. "An Exploration of Reported Sleep Disturbance," *J. Nerv. Ment. Dis.*, 134 (1962), 528–534.

426. WEITZMAN, E. D., H. SCHAUMBURG, and W.

FISHBEIN. "Plasma 17-Hydroxycorticoster-oid Levels during Sleep in Man," *J. Clin. Endocrinol. Metab.*, 26 (1966), 121–127.

427. WERRY, J. S. and J. COHRSSEN. "Enuresis—an Etiologic and Therapeutic Study," *J. Pediatr.*, 67 (1965), 423–431.

428. WESTPHAL, C. "Eigenthümliche mit Ein-schlafen verbundene Anfälle," *Arch. Psy-chiatr.*, 7 (1877), 631–635.

429. WEXBERG, L. E. "Insomnia as Related to Anxiety and Ambition," *J. Clin. Psycho-pathol.*, 10 (1949), 373–375.

430. WHYBROW, P. C. and J. MENDELS. "Toward a Biology of Depression: Some Suggestions from Neurophysiology," *Am. J. Psychiatry*, 125 (1969), 1491–1500.

431. WITTMAACK, T. *Pathologie und Therapie der Sensibilität-Neurosen*, pp. 458–460. Leipzig: Ernst Schafer, 1861.

432. WOLFF, H. G. and D. CURRAN. "Nature of Delirium and Allied States. The Dyser-gastic Reaction," *Arch. Neurol. Psychiatry*, 33 (1935), 1175–1215.

433. WYATT, R. J., D. H. FRAM, D. J. KUPFER et al. "Total Prolonged Drug-Induced REM Sleep Suppression in Anxious-Depressed Patients," *Arch. Gen. Psychiatry*, 24 (1971), 145–155.

434. WYATT, R. J., B. A. TERMINI, and J. DAVIS. "Biochemical and Sleep Studies of Schizo-phrenia: A Review of the Literature, 1960–1970. Part I. Biochemical Studies," *Schizo-phr. Bull.*, 4 (1971), 10–44.

435. ———. "Biochemical and Sleep Studies of Schizophrenia: A Review of the Literature, 1960–1970. Part II. Sleep Studies," *Schizo-phr. Bull.*, 4 (1971), 45–66.

436. YOSS, R. E. and D. D. DALY. "Criteria for Diagnosis of the Narcoleptic Syndrome," *Proc. Staff Meet. Mayo Clin.*, 32 (1957), 320–328.

437. ———. "Hereditary Aspects of Narcolepsy," *Trans. Am. Neurol. Assoc.*, 85 (1960), 239–240.

438. ———. "Narcolepsy," *Arch. Intern. Med.*, 106 (1960), 168–171.

439. ———. "Narcolepsy," *Med. Clin. North Am.*, 44 (1960), 953–968.

440. YULES, R. B., D. X. FREEDMAN, and K. A. CHANDLER. "The Effect of Ethyl Alcohol on Man's Electroencephalographic Sleep Cycle," *Electroencephalogr. Clin. Neuro-physiol.*, 20 (1966), 109–111.

441. YULES, R. B., M. E. LIPPMAN, and D. X. FREEDMAN. "Alcohol Administration Prior to Sleep," *Arch. Gen. Psychiatry*, 16 (1967), 94–97.

442. ZARCONE, V. and W. C. DEMENT. "Sleep Disturbances in Schizophrenia," in A. Kales, ed., *Sleep. Physiology and Pathol-ogy. A Symposium*, pp. 192–199. Philadel-phia: Lippincott, 1969.

443. ZARCONE, V., G. GULEVICH, T. PIVIK, and W. C. DEMENT. "Partial REM Phase De-privation and Schizophrenia," *Arch. Gen. Psychiatry*, 18 (1968), 194–202.

444. ZIERLER, K. L. "Diseases of Muscle," in R. H. S. Thomson and E. J. King, eds., *Biochemical Disorders in Human Disease*, pp. 598–656. New York: Academic, 1964.

445. ZUFALL, R. B. "Adult Male Enuresis: A Study of 200 Cases," *J. Urol.*, 70 (1953), 894–897.

446. ZUNG, W. W. K., W. P. WILSON, and W. E. DODSON. "Effect of Depressive Disorders on Sleep EEG Responses," *Arch. Gen. Psychiatry*, 10 (1964), 439–445.

CHAPTER 36

THE TEACHING OF PSYCHOSOMATIC MEDICINE: CONSULTATION-LIAISON PSYCHIATRY

F. Patrick McKegney

IN THIS VOLUME of the *Handbook*, the content of the field of "psychosomatic medicine" is impressively portrayed. It should be apparent that the brain and all other biological components of the human organism influence, and can be influenced by the psychological phenomena encompassed by the terms "mind," "personality," "interpersonal relationships," etc. It should also be apparent that the psychosomatic field can be discussed in terms of specific clinical disorders, normal basic mechanisms of psychosocial-physiological interactions, or specific known precipitating or causal factors. Amidst all of these approaches, one may lose sight of the fact that psychosomatic medicine also implies a broad statement of a philosophical position which directly relates to the practice of medicine. Meyer cited[30] the principle of the American Psychosomatic Society formulated more than thirty years ago:

. . . psychosomatic medicine is a way of approaching problems of health and disease. It is an approach which attempts to apply the best and most modern psychodynamic understanding of human personality function in all phases of medical practice, diagnosis, therapy and research . . . It is emphasized that psychosomatic medicine is not a specialty in medicine but rather an elaboration of medical theory and practice which takes into account the role of psychological processes in the form and functions of the body in health and disease.

As we learn more about the "role of psychological processes in . . . health and disease," we must also concern ourselves with the application of this knowledge to the improvement of health-care delivery to the sick and to the maintenance of health. Therefore, this chapter is intended as a transitional one, from the "What?" of psychosomatic medicine to the "Now What?" How can we ensure that the accumulating body of knowledge about psychosomatic medicine will be available to those who care for the disabled? How can the principles of psychosomatic medicine be finally expressed in the skills and attitudes of the "helping professions?"

Thus, this chapter will emphasize the pedagogy of psychosomatic medicine, particularly through the activity which has, somewhat ambiguously, become known as "consultation-liaison psychiatry." After presenting the need for such education, the aims and the objects of the effort will be discussed. Traditional teaching methods, their opportunities and apparent obstacles, will be contrasted with alternative educational approaches. The issues of evaluation of educational effectiveness, a frequently neglected subject, will be presented in a tentative fashion. In fact, many of the proposals in this chapter are tentative and speculative—reflecting the general neglect by psychosomatic medicine and the rest of education, to assess and improve its educational impact.

❨ The Educational Need

From the time of Hippocrates, there has been little controversy about the need for a physician to recognize the intimate relationship between the *mind* and *body*. Even the surgeon, John Hunter (1728–1793) remarked, "He who chooses to anger me holds my life in his hands." Neurologists such as John Hughlings Jackson and Sigmund Freud pursued the "concomitant phenomena" of "brain" and "mind" and emphasized the need to take both into account in clinical practice. More recently, a wide range of laboratory and clinical

researchers have identified a myriad of interactions between the biological and psychological aspects of the human organism and some of the clinical ramifications of such interactions.

Problem Incidence

Estimates of the prevalence of psychiatric illness in general or "medical populations" range from 15 to 85 percent. In a beautifully designed study by Zabarenko and co-workers,[48] psychiatrists observed physicians in their actual office practices. They found that only 6 percent of these general-practice patients had a *primary* diagnosis of "mental disorder," if very strictly defined according to the International Classification of Diseases. However, they found that there was a need for intervention in psychological problems in more than 60 percent of these patients. In another study by Cross and Bjorn of their problem-oriented general practice in Maine,[4] the five most common problems of the patient population served were: (1) depression; (2) conversion reaction; (3) obesity; (4) acute bronchitis; and (5) anxiety. These problems were more frequent than infectious diseases, arteriosclerotic cardiovascular disease, diabetes mellitus, or any other physical or social problem.

In response to the educational needs highlighted by such incidence studies, there has been a revolution in the recognition of the role of psychiatry in medicine. Medical schools rarely had departments of psychiatry before 1945. All now have full-time departments with a major segment of the students' curriculum time being devoted to psychiatry. Courses in behavioral sciences and psychopathology are now offered in almost all medical schools,[44] and considerable time is devoted to clinical clerkships on psychiatric services. Psychiatric units in general hospitals, postgraduate education courses in psychiatry for physicians, and the availability of special funding for residency training in consultation-liaison psychiatry have all become much more common since the early 1950s. It must be added that the teaching of the psychiatric aspects of medical illness has increased slightly but significantly in psychiatry departments. Werner Mendel[28] has been quoted, referring to the teaching of psychiatric consultation in medical care: "It is like motherhood—everyone is for it."

Clinical Competence

With all of this increased emphasis on psychiatry in general and also in the psychiatric teaching about our general health-care problems, is there still a need for improvement of education? The study of Zabarenko et al.,[48] cited above, found that the general physician detected and responded to only a small fraction of the 60 percent of patients needing attention for psychological problems. Peterson's study demonstrated that few physicians in general practice were able to do something about the psychiatric problems of their patients, even when recognized.[37] Mendel, who cited the general acceptance of psychiatric consultation in medical care, went on to say that "very little is being done" about the actual teaching of the psychiatric aspects of medical patients.[28] In 1966, his nationwide survey found that only 25 percent of psychiatric training programs conducted formal lectures or seminars on the consultation process.[27] The experience of consultation-liaison psychiatrists around the country would indicate that its acceptance or efficacy, as it has been traditionally pursued, still leaves much to be desired in terms of educational impact and influence on the change of medical care practice. Consultation and liaison psychiatry remains only a small component of general psychiatric training programs and represents a minor involvement in the actual practice of psychiatrists and other mental-health personnel in general. For example, the community mental-health-center movement was designed separately from general-health-care systems and is only now belatedly being considered in relationship to the growing movement toward centralized and coordinated health-care programs.

New Technology

New developments in medical care have been accompanied by new psychological problems, creating a greater need for psychiatric consultation and teaching input into medical care. Some of these problems arise from the increased survival of chronically ill patients with major disabilities and complex rehabilitative needs. Other needs result from the newly developed treatment approaches themselves, such as intensive coronary care units, chronic dialysis, and organ transplantation. In the latter two situations, the needs of the family, as well as of the patient, and the complexities of the socioeconomic aspects demand new collaborative approaches between psychiatrists and the health team. Unfortunately, the new technology also hampers the effectiveness of the psychiatrist's teaching of psychosomatic issues. By demanding careful attention to mechanical or biological details, the new medical machines and techniques tend to distract the medical team, and even the psychiatrist, from attending to the patient and his world.[31]

Therefore, the indications for the need for more education concerning psychological and psychosocial problems of general medical populations would seem obvious, based upon both the high incidence of such problems, the continuing low involvement of psychiatry in general-health-care systems and the low level of expertise of health-care professionals in those fields. But what should be the specific educational objectives of consultation-liaison psychiatry?

《 Educational Objectives

The teaching of psychosomatic medicine can be considered in terms of the three traditional pedagogical objectives: transmitting factual knowledge, developing skills, and influencing attitudes.

Consultation-liaison psychiatry, as a clinically based activity, concerns itself primarily with the last two objectives. However, many psychosomatic psychiatrists find themselves increasingly involved in teaching "content-oriented" behavioral science or psychopathology courses to first- and second-year medical students under the pressure to increase the "clinical relevance" of preclinical medical education. Thus, this chapter must touch upon the role of the consultation and liaison psychiatrist in all phases of medical- and health-care professional education.

Psychosomatic Knowledge

In terms of factual knowledge, the theory of psychosomatic medicine and its mechanismic base can be conveyed by assigned readings in the growing literature, lectures, and seminars. Yet, greater interest in and acquisition of such knowledge seems to accrue from a combination of clinical involvement of students and the transmittal of related facts. Such an approach can be used with students not involved in clinical responsibilities but it poses problems of finding appropriate patients, scheduling them and, finally, not diverting the students from the psychobiological knowledge they are being asked to acquire.

Psychosomatic Skills

Because of these difficulties, most of the teaching of psychosomatic medicine has been traditionally based in the clinical phases of medical education, and combined with the objectives of developing psychosomatic skills. The usual mode of achieving these objectives is through exercises in medical interviewing or history-taking and the clinical practice of psychiatric consultation and liaison with non-psychiatric patients. In this context the objectives can be simply stated but much more difficultly achieved or measured. They are:

1. The student should be able to *gather*, reliably, thoroughly and efficiently, the *observational* and *historical data base* about the patient *sufficient* to *understand* the patient and his problems and to *plan*, with a "sound ana-

lytical sense,"[45] the treatment approaches appropriate to these problems.

2. The student should be able to *develop a relationship* with the patient which will *enhance* objective 1. and *provide the basis* for a *collaboration* between the *physician* and the *patient* in the ongoing treatment program.[18]

3. The student should demonstrate the *abilities to synthesize the clinical data* which he gathers, independent of current theories; *to critically examine the syntheses of others*; and *to hypothesize original explanations* for the data which he observes.[8] These skills obviously have much interrelationship with student attitudes toward patients, disease, and their own roles.

Psychosomatic Attitudes

When one attempts to explicitly *teach* attitudes, the effect is frequently as if the action word were *preach*. Therefore, attitudes are usually conveyed implicitly by creating an example in the clinical situation. It is important, however, for a teacher to recognize that he has *two* roles in which modelling takes place: vis-à-vis the patient and vis-à-vis the student. The latter has been characterized as the "learning alliance" by Lazerson.[20] In both roles, the teacher can influence the students' attitudes toward the following objectives:

1. The student (and teacher) should demonstrate an appreciation and respect for the patient (and student) as a person and for the relevance of the principles of psychosomatic medicine.

2. The student (and teacher) should demonstrate a dedication to completeness, which implies that a description, if not diagnosis, of a patient's personality and adaptational capacity is necessary in *every* case.

3. The student (and teacher) should demonstrate a capacity for empathy, by which the student can communicate emotionally with the patient and convey the presence of this capacity to the patient. This objective critically interdigitates with the following one.

4. The student (and teacher) should demonstrate an ability to develop, and act accord-

ing to professional standards, to achieve a "detached concern" or an "optimal distance," to act in accordance with the needs of the patient and not in response to one's own personal needs.

Though cast in operational terms, these objectives need subdefinitions in terms of actual behaviors which are ideally quantifiable.[25] When this difficult and so far unaccomplished task is approached, the teacher must recognize there are different groups of potential learners of psychosomatic medicine, each with a distinctive background, professional role, and task-specific needs.

(Types of Learners and Learning Problems

Student Physicians

Traditionally, the primary focus of educational efforts in psychosomatic medicine has been upon the medical students, interns, and residents in University teaching hospitals, usually on the nonpsychiatric services. These consumers of the *psychosomatic educational product* are a very heterogenous lot, yet are rather strikingly uniformly negative in their regard of psychiatry,[5] the specialty with which psychosomatic medicine is usually associated. Data by Funkenstein[10] indicate that the most recent freshmen medical student groups are changing rapidly in the direction of showing greater social concern. However, whether this will be accompanied by a greater receptivity to the learning of psychosomatic medicine remains to be seen.

Given these predisposed student attitudes, the consultation-liaison psychiatrist working in the nonpsychiatric setting meets another obstacle in the nonpsychiatric teaching staff—either the full-time faculty or practicing physicians.

Full-time Faculty Staff

The full-time clinical faculty of medical schools are usually chosen for an in-depth research competence in the biological mechanisms of disease. Often, they see no patients. At most, and reluctantly, they may see a few outpatients and serve as "ward attending" six or eight weeks a year. The presence of a liaison psychiatrist or even the act of a psychiatric consultation complicates their teaching role, by asking them to look beyond the narrow field of their scholarly expertise in their role as physician in charge. Resistance to such involvement with the patient is reflected in the very small amounts of time Payson et al., found were spent discussing the "psychosomatic" aspects of patient care on teaching rounds,[34] or in patient contact.[35] This preselected or preconditioned characteristic of academic clinicians is a powerful obstacle to their and their students' learning, since these full-time faculty members are usually more powerful models for their students than their colleagues, the practicing physicians.

Practicing Physicians

Privately practicing physicians (or local medical doctors, LMD's) on the attending staffs of teaching hospitals spend much less time with the student physicians than do the full-time academic physicians. Furthermore, what exposure occurs is frequently in the context of the LMD's brief morning or evening visits with his patients, which conflict with the teaching schedule of the ward and prevent the students from participating in his visit. The student physician rarely has a meaningful involvement in the physician's daily practice of office visits, house calls, and phone contacts with his patients. Finally, most University hospital staff members are specialists or even superspecialists, and hence tend to have a narrower perspective than the psychosomatic concept implies.

The practicing physician also presents problems as a *learner* of psychosomatic medicine. His small involvement within the University hospital reduces his potential contact with the psychosomatic psychiatrist. Only rarely, and then usually for research purposes,[48] do psychiatrists spend significant time in physicians' practices. This has been one factor in the experience that continuing-education programs in psychiatry are not particularly successful.[3,7,43] Other factors relate to economics, psychiatric capability, and the availability of manpower (see below), and the probably limited flexibility of practitioners with ten to thirty years of their own style of doing things.[37,48]

Nurses and Other Health Professionals

Increasing attention to the *health team*[22] in a variety of medical-care situations has led to increased involvement by the psychosomatic teacher with nurses, physical therapists, social workers, and others delivering patient care. Since they usually spend much more time with hospital patients than do physicians or student physicians, these health professionals have many immediate and pressing problems which relate to the psychosomatic sphere. When able to ask a psychiatrist for help, they pose many pertinent and important questions about their particular role and activity in caring for and relating to the patient. Yet, this interest creates many problems for the psychosomatic teacher.

In order to convey accurate and useful opinions, the psychiatrist needs a modicum of data about the patient. The medical record is usually inadequate,[45] and the data from the individual nurse, for example, are narrow in perspective. If not requested to do so by the patient's physician, the psychiatrist cannot easily gather that data himself from the patient. Furthermore, the concern about a given patient may come independently from several sources, since the usual hospital administrative structure separates nursing, social service, physical therapy, etc., and the physician staff. The psychiatrist frequently finds himself repeating his opinions four or five times, to different professional groups, about one patient situation. Finally, any recommendation, and the learning which might accrue to the health professionals, depends in effectiveness upon the degree to which the health professionals are a *team* which *must* involve the patient's physician. The *subculture* of patient care, which operates independently of the physician, may have short-term value but has little long-range, postdischarge impact on patient and staff learning. Working solely with this subculture may be a waste of psychiatrists' teaching efforts. This nonteam aspect of health care is a major frustration for the psychiatrist or psychiatric resident in the consultation-liaison field.

The Psychiatric Resident

The psychiatrist in training is, on occasion, both a consumer of education in psychosomatic medicine and a teacher of such. Perhaps most significant is the fact that the future career teachers and practitioners of consultation-liaison psychiatry will come from the pool of psychiatric residents. Although nurses and social workers can develop many psychosomatic teaching skills and functions, the psychosomatically oriented physician should still be the main resource for the diagnostic and therapeutic planning, and management functions.[4]

The traditional role of the psychiatric resident in consultation-liaison psychiatry and its many learning opportunities will be discussed in a later section. Even after more than thirty years' experience, consultation-liaison psychiatry is not well represented in most residency training programs. Mendel's nationwide survey in 1966 showed that only 25 percent of programs offer even formal lectures or seminars on the subject.[27] Training residents to teach psychosomatic medicine above and beyond psychiatric consultations, is even less common. Some liaison services do not regularly involve psychiatric residents but rather train residents with primarily internal medicine backgrounds. This low emphasis is, at least in part, related to the characteristics of psychiatric residents. Kardener et al.,[16] for example, found that nonpsychiatric patients seen for psychiatric consultation are very low in psychiatric residents' preferences.

What are the learner characteristics which limit participation in furthering psychosomatic education? Many residents are attracted to psychiatry as a specialty for reasons which have little to do with the practice of medicine.

These may include (1) a history of personal or family emotional problems; (2) a major interest in people which may not be satisfied in other medical specialties; (3) strong social concerns which seem to be best served in psychiatry; (4) a reaction-formation to anxiety about physical disease; and (5) a wish to avoid the apparent competitiveness, pace, or responsibilities of other types of medical practice. Any of these reasons may make it more difficult for a psychiatric resident to function in the medical setting, to work with dirty, smelly, or seriously sick persons, or to identify with nonpsychiatric physicians.

As *elective* programs comprise a larger segment of medical school curricula, a student disposed toward psychiatry for such reasons can more and more avoid "medical experience." The elimination, by the National Board of Psychiatry and Neurology, of the requirements of an internship can result in a loss of valuable training for the future consultation and liaison resident.[40] Finally, the psychiatric resident in his training is increasingly exposed to the continuing departure from the *medical model* in psychiatry,[33] which may divert him from the psychosomatic context, despite some exposure to consultation and liaison training.

([Traditional Educational Techniques of Consultation–Liaison Psychiatry

The most common current model of consultation-liaison teaching dates back at least forty years to the goals of Franklin Ebaugh's Colorado program, described by Billings:[2]

1. To sensitize the physicians and students to the opportunities offered them by every patient, no matter what complaint or ailment was present, for the utilization of a common sense psychiatric approach for the betterment of the patient's condition, and for making that patient better fitted to handle his problems, somatic or personality-determined or both.
2. To establish psychobiology as an integral working part of the professional thinking of physicians and students of all branches of medicine.

3. To instill in the minds of physicians and students the need the patient-public has for tangible and practical conceptions of personality and sociological functioning.

The general strategies of a hospital consultation-liaison service fall into three categories. The following is an adaptation of Kaufman and Margolin's outline written in 1948.[17] While these authors emphasize the primary professional needs of the institution, the goals are equally applicable to any health-care setting:

1. *Psychiatric services*, i.e., the diagnosis and treatment of the hospital population (*consultation*).
2. *Teaching* involving the training of the psychiatric staff and the indoctrination and teaching of every member of the hospital staff in the principles of psychosomatic medicine (*liaison*).
3. *Research* in the field of psychosomatic medicine *and* in the process of both the consultation and liaison functions.

Margolin and Kaufman went on to add the important guiding concept that,[17] "these three functions should be regarded as *separate, chronological phases* in the development of a psychiatric service in a general hospital" (emphasis added).

In terms of specific educational tactics, a staff consultation-liaison psychiatrist is given a major assignment to one or more specific nonpsychiatric services. He usually attends the work and teaching rounds of that service and may hold special psychosomatic conferences. He sees patients upon request, and may generate the referral himself on the basis of the patient's history or his own observation of the patient on rounds. Every consultation is followed by often extensive communication with those caring for the patient in which he includes relevant concepts of psychosomatic medicine. In certain cases, the psychiatrist may assume major responsibility for the direction of patient management and aftercare, but usually he collaborates with the other health professionals, who retain their primary roles in the continuing care of the patient.

Traditional Psychiatric Resident Role

Of course, almost all training programs in psychiatry have residents assigned to see patients in the general hospital who are referred for psychiatric consultation, usually on an emergency basis. In a minority of psychiatric training programs, a few residents have consultation-liaison duties, with the additional tasks of establishing collaborative relationships, teaching, and research, as defined by Kaufman and Margolin.[17] Not all residents in a given program may have this rotation, it being either completely elective, or required for only a certain number of residents. As in the original Colorado program,[2] the psychiatric resident usually becomes involved at first as an *assistant* to the liaison staff psychiatrist, on a *part-time* basis and for brief rotations of three to six months. This resident may participate in the nonpsychiatric service's work rounds, may generate consultations, and initially evaluate all patients for whom consultation is requested. The psychiatric resident may also lead, or participate in, conferences about comprehensive patient care which are, incidentally, frequently called "social service rounds"—implying nonmedical and dispositional, as well as comprehensive-care purposes. The psychiatric resident may also hold regular or ad hoc conferences for nurses about patient care.

Certain psychiatric residents may elect longer and more advanced levels of training in consultation-liaison work. This seems to be an only occasionally exercised option; exact figures are not available. An advanced resident usually functions in a semisupervisory role, performing many of the tasks of the staff psychiatrist. He may organize and coordinate the seminars or lectures in psychosomatic medicine offered in some programs, and may also have the opportunity to pursue research activities.

Appropriately, residents with either a minor or major time commitment to consultation-liaison work usually reserve a certain amount of time for seeing outpatients. This arrangement serves two functions: it ensures the resident's being able to continue seeing psychotherapy patients for an extensive period of time throughout his residency, and it also allows him the flexibility of being able to follow certain patients initially seen in consultation. However rational, this follow-up capability frequently causes difficulty, in terms of discontinuity and/or contradiction in the resident's supervision. Should this patient be considered an "outpatient" or a "consultation patient," for administrative and supervisory purposes? Most departments have separate organizational divisions for these outpatient populations. Some programs, such as that at Johns Hopkins in the 1960s, avoided this area of potential conflict by establishing a separate outpatient service under the aegis of the psychosomatic service. Others, such as that at the University of Rochester from 1959 to 1962, considered outpatient care as crossing all departmental divisional lines and the resident continued to be supervised by the liaison staff for those outpatients originally seen in consultation. However, this scheme does add to the supervisory time per resident.

In such psychiatric residency training experiences, there are many unique learning opportunities. By being required to communicate with nonpsychiatric personnel, the resident can sharpen his psychological concepts and recognize their limitations, as he goes through the necessary process of adapting his psychiatric observations and opinions to everyday English from the jargon used so loosely among psychiatrists. However, the resident can become aware of the fact that a clear transmittal of his ideas, in and of itself, does not constitute their validation. For example, our scientific forebearers used deductive logic to precisely and irrefutably describe a large number of nonexistent creatures, such as the unicorn.[47]

Another opportunity for the psychiatric resident may present itself when he may be obliged to utilize Adolf Meyer's "life chart" concept, taking into account the biological, social, economic, and situational influences on behavior, as well as the interpersonal and intrapsychic factors emphasized in traditional psychiatric training. He may be called upon to deal with the interface between the behavioral and the somatic, and—quoting Meyerowitz— "to approach problems as a physician, but a physician who is simultaneously a behavioral expert."[31] Meyerowitz goes on to point out another learning task for the resident. "The resident as consultant frequently experiences an uncomfortable sense of time pressure, crisis and distance from his own familiar setting. He has to make practical decisions based upon relatively inadequate data and without indulgence in careful longitudinal observation. The increasing capacity to act effectively under these circumstances is a measure of his further development as a psychiatric physician."[31]

In consultation-liaison work, the resident has an opportunity to see a much larger number of patients with neurological syndromes than he would in traditional psychiatric settings. Kligerman and McKegney found in a four-year survey of 2835 inpatients seen in consultation, 14.2 percent had an acute brain syndrome, 16.8 percent a chronic brain syndrome, and 10.8 percent other neurological diseases.[19] By examining a large number of physically ill patients, the resident becomes atuned to the subtle manifestations of biological disease which, in his future patients, may initially present as a psychiatric syndrome.

Another important benefit of a consultation-liaison experience for a psychiatric resident is the opportunity of developing a sense of humility. As a consultant, the resident is considered an "expert" and is expected to contribute something of value to the medical staff and, usually, to also solve the clinical problem to everyone's satisfaction. However, frequently the psychiatric resident neither can add anything of significance, nor can he substantially affect the problem. In these situations, any consultant is liable to the temptation of trying to live up to the "expert" label, by theorizing or focussing on the minutiae of the clinical problems, usually at considerable length. As a result, the consultant bores and aggravates his busy consultees, making it less likely he will be called upon again, and may actually interfere with optimal patient care.

The psychiatric resident must learn to say in situations, in which pressing questions about complex problems are beyond his own or anyone else's expertise, "I don't know, but I will try to find out," or "I agree with what you have done and can add nothing." He must do this regardless of criticism from others and without a sense of inadequacy. As McKegney stated:[23] "The real world of the sick does not afford completely satisfactory solutions. For example, a major problem in consultation-liaison work involves the dying patient and the reactions of the medical staff. This situation highlights the relative helplessness of the psychiatrist and that of the medical staff in many other medical situations. The psychiatrist must learn, and convey the attitude to the others, that possible goals may fall far short of the optimal ones, and that all of our medical interventions may have limited efficacy."

Finally, the consultation-liaison psychiatric resident has an opportunity to learn about the *ethos* and social systems of a foreign "turf." This experience can clearly aid him in many other areas of psychiatric involvement, such as community, forensic, and military psychiatry. In contact with such conflicting value systems, the psychiatrist can learn a great deal about "countertransference" problems,[29] complementing the learning about them in individual psychotherapy.

Although this training in psychosomatic medicine has been effective for the few psychiatric residents so exposed, it hardly effects the vast potential learner population of student physicians and other health professionals. Toward this end, another major teaching effort of consultation and liaison psychiatry has been in the curricular time devoted to *interviewing* or *history taking*.

Teaching Medical Interviewing

As Kimball[18] has stated, "interviewing may be considered the basic science of clinical medicine. It is the vehicle through which all data and evaluations regarding the patient's condition are obtained, whether these be for the purpose of research or therapy." This classical position of the psychosomatic physician has never been refuted, but is rarely recognized or implemented in medical school curricula or medical practice.[6] Consultation-liaison psychiatrists are usually highly involved in teaching medical interviewing to medical students. Yet, their small numbers, the small amount of curriculum time so assigned, and the large classes of 100–200 medical students seem to preclude any significant impact of such interview teaching. Interns and residents are rarely, if ever, supervised by anyone in their contact with patients, and thus have little further opportunity for corrective feedback about their interviewing.

In a school which puts a large emphasis on teaching interviewing and clinical observation, Engel,[8] at the University of Rochester, found that 88 percent of its graduates felt better prepared than their colleagues in the ". . . overall clinical approach to the patient: . . . . This included the ability to make accurate observations and to elicit information; greater comfort in dealing with difficult patients; the capability to consider the patient as a whole and to identify, define, and respond to the patient's problems; more understanding of the implications of the psychological and social dimensions of the illness; greater skill in working with the family; and better appreciation of the viscissitudes of the doctor–patient relationship." These data indicate that such educational goals can be approached, but only by a very strong commitment to both the preclinical teaching of interviewing-observation, coupled with the clinical teaching of psychosomatic medicine via a medicine-psychiatry liaison service. Yet, very few medical schools currently make such a strong commitment to preclinical teaching. Furthermore, the shortening of the undergraduate medical curriculum may well truncate the time spent toward achieving these goals.[8,40] In that case, more attention may need to be directed to the student physicians, particularly those medical students and house officers in training on nonpsychiatric clinical services.

Student Physician Education

The teaching of psychosomatic medicine to student physicians in *nonpsychiatric* settings *seems* to have several strategic advantages toward achieving the goals cited by Billings[2]

and Engel.[8] These advantages are proposed as hypotheses, without documentation as being educationally valid. Medical education has met the tasks of goal setting and evaluation no better than other educational fields, though it has recently begun to change.[11,15]

The advantages of teaching psychosomatic medicine to student physicians in nonpsychiatric settings derive from at least four factors:

1. The student's role on the nonpsychiatric service is different from his position on a psychiatric service. On the latter, residents, clinical directors, nursing personnel, in fact everyone is concentrating on the psychological factors and understanding them more completely than the student because of an early level of sophistication and training. As a result of his "bottom-rung" role on a psychiatric service, the student often retreats from competition with the others, and neglects observing and understanding the psychological factors operating in his patients. On a nonpsychiatric service, however, and with medical or surgical patients, the student often finds he can assume an unique role among the clinical staff and achieve recognition, by emphasizing the same psychological factors he ignored or deprecated in the patient in the psychiatric setting. This "backing into" dealing with such psychological factors and concepts seems nonetheless to be an effective learning approach to these problems for the student on the nonpsychiatric service.

2. A major determinant in the student's reluctance to recognize, accept, or understand psychological factors in his patient is, of course, his own anxiety about himself. Experience suggests that such anxiety is less prominent and more readily dealt with on the nonpsychiatric service than on a psychiatric service. On the nonpsychiatric service, the primary focus of attention is on the anatomic-physiological aspects of the patients' illnesses. These aspects are less threatening and anxiety-provoking than the psychological ones and permit the student to recognize some of his own neurotic involvements, acting-out or "blind spots," without becoming overwhelmed by the additive effects of both sources of anx-

iety. If such recognition is a major element in the physician's educative process, both to increase his personal efficiency and to enable him to recognize and deal with similar psychological factors in his patients, such learning may be enhanced on a nonpsychiatric service.

3. The student has an opportunity to see, in a nonpsychiatric setting, patients in whom the organic factors have been "ruled out," in whom there is no conceivable physiological explanation for symptoms, or in whom the symptoms contrast clearly with those he finds in other patients due to organic disease. Because of this contrast, the impact on the student of the presence and importance of these psychological factors is greater than it may be in a psychiatric setting, where psychopathology is more common and, therefore, less outstanding by contrast. The *surprise value* of this contrast lends another advantage to the teaching of certain principles of psychological medicine in a medical setting rather than a psychiatric one.

4. The *relevance* of the nonpsychiatric setting and patient population to the future career goals of the student physician heighten his acceptance and learning of psychosomatic medicine. Most student physicians will not be psychiatrists. Students constantly contrast their learning experiences with their sophisticated or unsophisticated expectations of their future challenges as medical specialists or generalists. Therefore, on a nonpsychiatric service, most student physicians rightly feel *these* are the patient problems he will face as a surgeon, obstetrician, pediatrician, etc. As we broaden the clinical settings of medical student education to other than acute hospitals, the *relevance* of psychosomatic factors in medical care should become even more apparent, as the students recognize the psychosomatic nature of all patient problems and the knowledge and skills demanded for their care. However, the teaching of these student physicians on nonpsychiatric services implies a commitment of educational resources not very common in psychiatric education.

Though perhaps not because of these advantages, many of the new schools of medicine are shifting their basic teaching of psychiatry to nonpsychiatric services. For example, McMaster University's basic medical curriculum does not include the free-standing *clerkship* on a psychiatric service.[1] The core of clinical teaching of psychiatry is done in a three-month combined family practice–psychiatry clerkship using the students' experience with *nonpsychiatric* patients as a means of teaching psychiatry.

Such a shift can have serious implications for the traditional education of psychiatrists. If students do not work with psychiatrists and psychiatric patients in psychiatric settings, they will have a limited opportunity to gain experience with psychiatry as a specialty. As a result, their career choices may be made in comparative ignorance about psychiatry. The specialty field might then attract fewer and less qualified students than in the past, with a consequent detrimental impact on the large number of clearly psychiatric patients who need specialized care. This is only one of the problems related to consultation-liaison psychiatric teaching.

⟮ Obstacles to Psychosomatic Teaching

Among the obstacles to consultation-liaison teaching, the career motivation factors of psychiatric residents and psychiatrists have already been cited. Psychiatry has for some time been "riding madly in all directions," resulting in a major diffusion of psychiatry into areas outside of medicine or even of health-care systems. Indeed, "psychiatric consultation" today can refer to a psychiatrist's meeting with a group of teachers, police, or industrial managers. This departure from the "medical model" of psychiatry[33] imposes serious limitations upon student physicians' and psychiatric residents' receptiveness to traditional consultation-liaison practice.

Economic factors also limit the practice of consultation-liaison psychiatry. Since the bulk of the liaison-staff psychiatrist's activity is spent in teaching, it is not compensated by patient-care fees on an hourly basis, as in office psychotherapy. The amount of time necessary for a staff psychiatrist to perform an adequate teaching role on one nonpsychiatric inpatient unit seems to approximate ten hours per week.[23] At the current average hourly rate for psychotherapy, $50, this primary educational service could cost at least $15,000–$20,000 per year per inpatient unit, if it were not for either the academic pressures forcing the voluntary contribution of clinical faculty time, or the lower salaries paid full-time faculty. Federal funding, however munificent in the past, has never approached this figure in supporting consultation-liaison psychiatry, nor can most medical institutions underwrite such expensive teaching programs. Governmental funding of psychosomatic education of nonpsychiatrists is, paradoxically, being phased out in the face of the data increasingly substantiating the psychological needs of the general medical patient population.[4,18,37,48]

Even most national legislation concerning national health-insurance plans or health-maintenance organizations (HMO) specifically excludes payment for treatment of psychological or psychosomatic disorders. Thus, any efforts of academic institutions to maintain or expand the *teaching* of psychosomatic medicine will meet the obstacles of combined learner-consumer resistance,[5,32] patient nonacceptance, scarcity of teachers, and economic constraints. These defined obstacles would seem to indicate a need for new and different approaches to the strategies and tactics of teaching psychosomatic medicine. The areas for potential modification will be discussed in terms of curricular change and administrative-organizational change.

(Educational Approaches— Curricular Change

The Definition of Minimum Objectives

The emphasis on defining objectives of educational programs[11,15,25] has some very practical implications for the future teaching of psychosomatic medicine. Traditional approaches have involved spending approxi-mately the same amount of teaching time with *every* student, attempting to teach the *broad* range of psychosomatic medicine, without consideration of essential *core* material/abilities or differing individual student capabilities. Faculty time and curriculum hours are very precious commodities. If the *minimum* psychosomatic knowledge, skills, and attitudes needed for *all* physicians could be defined, and found acceptable even within one medical school, substantial savings could accrue in both faculty effort and student-exposure time.

Once the bare essentials for *all physicians* are defined, knowledge, skills, and attitudinal goals would be more narrowly defined for *all students* than heretofore. For example, not all medical students might need to hear a lecture or read (or more operationally, to know specific facts) about the possible psychophysiological mechanisms involving the hypothalamic-pituitary axis, however important such material may be for our future understanding of the human organism. In essence, we would not spend the faculty's and students' precious time in attempting to teach a bit about *everything* in psychosomatic medicine.

The second type of saving from goal setting would accrue from measuring *individual* student abilities for comparison with the criteria for *minimum* objectives *for all students*. It has long been recognized that students vary tremendously in their abilities and motivations to learn different things and in different amounts of time.[41] Once *minimum* objectives are set, certain students may be able to achieve these in a very short time, if they have not already done so. These students would then be freed to pursue other sets of core objectives or to select more advanced objectives in any field. These fast learners would not be required to spend their time, nor would they continue to take up faculty effort, once they had achieved the minimum psychosomatic educational goals.

The Definition of Differential Objectives

As there is clear evidence that students vary in their abilities to learn, there is evidence that different tasks in medicine require different professional aptitudes. In the case of the physician, most of the technical skills required of the cardiac surgeon are qualitatively different from those of the family physician, who may assume overall medical responsibility for a three-generation family over forty years. Given the fact of increasing specialization within medicine, the teachers of psychosomatic medicine must attempt to differentiate the educational goals in their field for the wide range of health professional roles. This setting of different objectives obviously must consider the different role-models and practice of all types of health professionals, most of which have not well defined themselves, especially vis à vis other types.

In this process of defining professional roles, many hard questions are raised, some of which confront the mythologies gradually developed through the history of medicine. For example, are all physicians expected to completely observe, define, and plan for the complete range of patient problems?[4,45] Clearly, medical practice has been specialized to the point where the answer to this question is unequivocally negative.[48] Dermatologists, anesthesiologists, surgeons, psychiatrists, neurologists, or obstetricians rarely gather a complete data base or assume primary medical managerial responsibility for the patient and his life situation. However, to explicitly remove this expertise from the responsibility of the physician-specialist is to painfully confront the mystique of the physician modeled upon Hippocrates and Osler.

Nonetheless, the teachers of psychosomatic medicine must, for efficacy and therefore maximal effectiveness, work with other medical-curriculum planners in determining the role requirements for psychosomatic education in each type of health-care practice. For example, the diagnostic role of the primary physician may require a great deal more teaching emphasis on basic psychological-physiological mechanisms than does the role of the cardiac surgeon or family psychotherapist. The emergency-room nurse needs knowledge, attitudes, and skills quite different from the rehabilitation-unit nurse[22] since their patient-responsi-

bility roles are so different. The teacher of psychosomatic medicine must be able to define and to teach, according to the different task requirements of the different health professionals. In fact, the psychosomatic psychiatrist may be a most appropriate source of educational expertise for the different health professionals in their distinguishing their own roles and educational needs.

The Problem-Oriented Approach to Care

Alvan Feinstein's conceptual approach to clinical problems[9] and Lawrence Weed's problem-oriented approach to medical records and the management of patient care[45] are among the most innovative and radical contributions to medical care in this century. Each complements the other in demanding precise definitions of diagnoses, treatments, and follow-up. The concepts of Weed and Feinstein have vast implications for all medical teaching, including psychosomatic medicine. Global diagnoses such as *rheumatic fever* or *depression* are no longer acceptable. The patient's problems must be defined according to the specific clinical phenomena of the patient, the laboratory data, and his environment. The treatment plan must include the specific approaches to the patient's behaviors, including *patient education*.[45] Each element of the patient's situation must be isolated and defined, together with its appropriate treatment.

If these approaches to medical care are valid, then psychosomatic teaching must work in accord with such principles. Grant has begun adapting the problem-oriented approach to psychiatric services,[12] but the actual psychosomatic input to the problem-oriented approach needs to be further developed. This input is needed in the screening process, the data analysis, the patient-management decision-making process—especially in the involvement of the patient and his family at each stage of care—and the evaluation of the outcome of treatment.

If such a *patient-problem oriented approach* is in operation in medical centers, the teacher of psychosomatic medicine has a clear responsibility. He must assist the staff to be efficient, reliable, thorough, and soundly analytical in the (1) collection of the data base; (2) construction of an appropriate problem list; (3) decision about a relevant treatment plan; and (4) implementation of an *appropriate follow-through* treatment and evaluation program.[45] In the problem-oriented system, the teacher of psychosomatic medicine can help the staff to develop a clear set of objectives. He can assist in the assignment of appropriate patient care and learning responsibilities to the various members of the health-care team.[22] This teaching function can be extended to students, irrespective of a specific health-care discipline, to the degree that the student is actually involved in the *useful work* of patient care.

The mechanisms of such psychosomatic teaching could be varied. The most efficient would seem to be in the *audit* of the problem-oriented patient-care medical record.[45] The thorough, reliable, efficient, and analytical problem solving of the student, house officer, or attending physician can be maintained by *peer review*, according to consensually developed criteria, with the input of the psychosomatic teacher. This educational role necessarily involves the psychosomatic teacher in the actual patient-care situation, as a participant auditor and source of feedback, especially regarding the data base, rather than as a theoretical critic or second-hand reviewer. This teaching role of the psychosomaticist requires that he be a responsible member of the patient-care team, a patient advocate, and a self-critical commentator about the treatment process. This complex, *triple-agent* role has been described by McKegney in the hemodialysis unit[24] and is not substantively different from many traditional consultation-liaison roles. The *problem-oriented approach*, however, does change the context of the psychiatrist's participation and makes new demands on him, as well as upon all other members of the health-care team.

Specific Learning Techniques

Several recently developed educational techniques can well be used by the teacher of psychosomatic medicine. The *patient-management-problem approach* developed by McGuire et al.,[21] has shown considerable promise in teaching clinical care and in the evaluation of its learning. Methodological problems have arisen because clinicians frequently do not agree on criteria for optimal result of care, or even for appropriate sequences of diagnostic and therapeutic procedures.[42] Other problems derive from the mechanics of the patient-management-problem learning-evaluation process. An random access-and-retrieval computer program is needed for best results which is frequently not readily available.

Another rather similar learning technique concerns *critical incidents*. In this approach, specific decision-making points of clinical care are presented. The student is asked to choose from among alternative courses of action and his decisions are compared to the criteria established by a panel of expert clinicians. This approach suffers from the same consensus difficulty as does the patient-management-problem technique.[42] In addition, many clinical problems, especially those involving the psychosocial sphere, are not readily presented in either the critical-incident or patient-management-problem format. Some of these difficulties arise from the admitted complexities of human behavior but others may eventually yield an improved definition of patients' problems by the psychiatrist.[12]

(Administrative-Organizational Approaches

Overall Curriculum Planning

The psychiatrist should be considered as a behavioral scientist resource to general curriculum planning,[13] although other health professionals may also be able to have such a function.[36] A psychiatrist may be important in general curriculum planning because he is more aware of behaviorally defined characteristics of different students and health practitioners. In addition, he may be able to help curriculum planners to recognize the interpersonal phenomena which distract, or at least distort, their pursuit of well-defined objectives. This role of the psychiatrist in admissions committees has already been recognized.[14] A national NIMH-sponsored conference was held in October, 1972, to examine this role. The eventual impact of this conference, entitled "The Psychiatrist as a Teacher," is still to be realized but its thrust emphasized the potential central role of the *behavioral clinician* in medical education.

Planning for New Patterns of Health-Care Delivery

Health is coming to be recognized as a "right," rather than a privilege, of every citizen. As a result, those responsible for health care are under increasing pressure to improve the effectiveness of the prevention and treatment of illness in every geographic and economic segment of the population. At the same time, the expense of medical care as currently practiced is giving rise to demands for improved efficiency in health-care delivery. Most approaches to these problems generally suggest greater coordination among the traditionally independent professional disciplines, as *teams* or groups. Furthermore, these approaches imply a more *comprehensive* approach to the patient and his problems than heretofore present in medical practice.

The psychosomatic concept and the thrust of consultation-liaison psychiatry have long advocated these goals of comprehensive and coordinated care, now being mandated by economic, social, and political forces. Psychosomatic psychiatrists may possess a unique expertise by having an overview of medical practice and an interest in the broadest definition of patient problems. They have usually become more familiar with the ranges of health-care settings, types of patient problems, medical-care practices, and abilities of different health-care professionals than any other group of physicians. As a result, psychosomatic clinicians may be able to make a unique contribution to the current demands for a revolution of medical care and health education.

Despite this historical emphasis and long clinical experience, however, psychosomatic medicine should not pretend to have answers to these complex problems. Yet, it may be able to lead in their elucidation. For example, one particular patient need, long recognized and taught in psychosomatic medicine, is that of a therapeutic relationship between the patient and physician. The traditional focus of consultation-liaison teaching about relationships has been on the student or practicing physician, since medical tradition has placed the primary patient care upon the physician.

Yet, general medical care in the future is almost surely to be delivered by a multi-professional team, each member of which will assume responsibility for certain components of the patient-care plan. For efficiency, not all team members will do the same thing or their "own thing." The responsibility for the primary, ongoing, and general therapeutic relationship will usually be given to one member of the team. Will this person be the physician member? Present time-cost considerations would indicate not. While cost-effectiveness must also be considered, effectiveness should be a function of goal-directed education. The intensively trained general physician, with his broad biological knowledge, and expertise in the diagnosis of pathology and disease, may well come to function primarily as the initial diagnostician and long-term patient-care-plan manager. As such, he will need to know a great deal about psychophysiological and psychological manifestations of disease in the general population,[18,37,46] a clear educational role for consultation-liaison psychiatry. If this role of the physician emerges, the task of developing the primary relationship with the patient may become the responsibility of the nurse or social worker, or the *physician assistant* on the team. In this case, the teaching efforts concerning the development and use of psychotherapeutic relationships in a general health-care program should be directed at nurses, social workers, or physician assistants, both as students and practitioners.

If these health professionals, other than physicians, assume major responsibilities for tasks in the health-care plan currently assumed, rightly or wrongly, to be the physicians,' who will prepare them for these tasks? Health-profession schools have regrettably ignored other professions in many ways. Faculty composition and student teaching are almost always homogeneous to the profession. Specifically, the importance of the psychotherapeutic aspects of patient care is neglected in the curricula of most professional schools, such as nursing, social work, psychology, physical therapy, etc., as it is in medicine. In the future, the same efficiency considerations forcing changes in health-care-delivery patterns should also break down these traditional educational walls. The consultation-liaison psychiatrist should be asked, or perhaps invite himself, to participate centrally in the education of other health professionals, who need to learn the knowledge, skills, and attitudes of psychosomatic medicine. Similarly, medical education should be forced to assign certain educational roles to nonphysicians. For example, many coronary-care nurses are better able to administer emergency cardiac measures than most physicians. They should teach these skills to those health-care students who need those skills—irrespective of "profession of designation." The extent to which we are in a "crisis of health care delivery," we are also in a crisis of health-care education, in which the broad concepts and concerns of psychosomatic medicine should be essential.

Determining Medical School Priorities

The changes in the political, economic, and social climate are challenging the traditional priorities of all education. A specific question is raised for psychiatry departments vis-à-vis medical school priorities. Should all schools continue to try to teach all things in medicine? If not, some schools might concentrate, for example, on developing research in basic biological mechanisms. Psychiatry departments in those schools would, consistently, need to set their highest priorities on gathering faculty with complementary expertise in basic psychobiological relationships.

Other schools may decide to put their highest priorities on teaching the physicians to be involved in the general practice of health care and not many narrow and highly trained specialist physicians, such as surgeons or psychiatrists. In such schools, the departments of psychiatry might attempt to assume a *departmental task* of consultation-liaison, in which all members make a significant contribution by participating as teacher-clinicians in non-psychiatric health-care settings. These departments could assume a primary role of collectively learning and teaching those attitudes, skills, and facts which will enable *all* health professionals to observe, understand, and respond appropriately to the behavior of the human beings for whom they have professional responsibility.[24]

These reorganizations of medical schools and departments of psychiatry will take place, if at all, over many years. In the near future, changes can be made in the organization of academic departments of psychiatry in such a way as to reduce the subspecialization connotations of consultation and liaison psychiatry. The traditional designation of a separate psychosomatically oriented "service" or "division" gave teaching responsibilities to a few select members. This designation often diminishes the departmental effectiveness in psychosomatic teaching by isolating the task from the rest of the psychiatry department. Traditionally, consultation-liaison services seem to float somewhere between departments of psychiatry and, for instance, departments of medicine, leading to a diffusion of roles only heightened by joint appointments, which are usually only titular ties between departments in two different worlds.

Many departments of psychiatry could move to broadening the teaching of psychosomatic medicine to medical students, house officers, and other health professions by increasing the commitment of most, if not all, faculty members to that educational task. New faculty members would be recruited on the basis of their interest, among other interests, in consultation-liaison work. Departmental composition would have to remain sufficiently diverse in interests and skills to provide a solid-core psychiatric-residency program. Senior psychiatric residents would go elsewhere for subspecialty areas of psychiatry not represented in depth by the particular department's faculty. Others who wished to gain more experience in the consultation-liaison field could, of course, remain. This definition of narrowed focus at advanced levels of training would presumably have a preselection effect on resident applicants and might actually reduce the identity crises found in most psychiatric residency programs.

Some very large medical school psychiatry departments may feel they are able to accept greater responsibilities for psychosomatic education of all health professionals and maintain an in-depth expertise in the many fields within psychiatry. However, with increasing limitations on growth, all departments will have to reexamine their priorities and cut back some programs to allow for expansion in others. The teaching of psychosomatic medicine has not been a high priority of psychiatry in the past. As a group of leading psychiatric educators emphasized,[26,38,39,46] it must be in the future.

❨ Bibliography

1. ADSETT, A. "Psychiatric Education in New Medical Schools—Undergraduate Programs." Paper presented at Conference on Psychiatric Education in New Medical Schools, Airlee House, Warrenton, Virginia, February 21–23, 1972.
2. BILLINGS, E. G. "The Psychiatric Liaison Department of the University of Colorado Medical Schools and Hospitals," *Am. J. Psychiatry*, 122 (1966), 28–33.
3. BRANCH, C. H. "Psychiatric Education of Physicians: What Are Our Goals?" *Am. J. Psychiatry*, 125 (1968), 237–241.
4. BJORN, J. and H. CROSS. *The Problem Oriented Private Practice of Medicine.* Chicago: Modern Hospital Press, 1970.
5. BRUHN, J. G. and O. A. PARSONS. "Attitudes toward Medical Specialties: Two Follow-up Studies," *J. Med. Educ.*, 40 (1965), 273–280.
6. DOBBS, H. I. and D. L. CAREK. "The Conceptualization and Teaching of Medical Interviewing," *J. Med. Educ.*, 47 (1972), 272–276.
7. ENELOW, A. J. and V. H. MYERS. "Postgraduate Psychiatric Education: The Ethnography of a Failure," *Am. J. Psychiatry*, 125 (1968), 627–631.
8. ENGEL, G. L. "The Education of the Physician for Clinical Observation, the Role of the Psychosomatic (Liaison) Teacher," *J. Nerv. Ment. Dis.*, 154 (1972), 159–164.
9. FEINSTEIN, A. R. *Clinical Judgement.* Baltimore: Williams & Wilkins, 1967.
10. FUNKENSTEIN, D. H. "Medical Students, Medical Schools, and Society during Three Eras," in R. H. Coombs and C. E. Vincent, eds., *Psychosocial Aspects of Medical Training,* pp. 229–281. Springfield: Charles C. Thomas, 1971.
11. GRAHAM, J. R. "Measuring Psychiatric Competence and Curriculum in Undergraduate Medical Education," *Am. J. Psychiatry*, 126 (1969), 213–219.
12. GRANT, R. and B. M. MALETZKY. "Application of the Weed System to Psychiatric Records," *Psychiatry Med.*, 3 (1972), 119–129.
13. HAMBURG, D. A., ed. *Psychiatry as a Behavioral Science.* Engelwood Cliffs, N.J.: Prentice-Hall, 1970.
14. HOFFMAN, F. H. "The Psychiatrist on the Medical School Admissions Committee," Paper presented at 123rd Meeting Am. Psychiatr. Assoc., Detroit, May 8–12, 1967.
15. JASON, H. "Defining Objectives and Setting Priorities For Instruction in Psychiatry," Paper presented at Conference on Psychiatric Education in New Medical Schools, Airlee House, Warrenton, Virginia, February 21–23, 1972.
16. KARDENER, S. H., M. FULLER, I. MENSH et al. "The Trainees' Viewpoint of Psychiatric Residency," *Am. J. Psychiatry*, 126 (1970), 1132–1143.
17. KAUFMAN, M. R. and S. G. MARGOLIN. "Theory and Practice of Psychosomatic Medicine in a General Hospital," *Med. Clin. North Am.*, 32 (1948), 611–616.
18. KIMBALL, C. P. "Techniques of Interviewing: I. Interviewing and the Meaning of the Symptom," *Ann. Intern. Med.*, 71 (1969), 147–153.
19. KLIGERMAN, M. J. and F. P. MCKEGNEY. "Patterns of Psychiatric Consultation in Two General Hospitals," *Psychiatry Med.*, 2 (1971), 126–132.
20. LAZERSON, A. M. "The Learning Alliance

and Its Relation to Psychiatric Teaching," *Psychiatry Med.*, 3 (1972), 81–91.

21. McGUIRE, C. H. and D. BABBOTT. "Simulation Technique in the Measurement of Problem Solving Skills," *J. Educ., Measur.*, 4 (1967), 1–10.

22. McKEGNEY, F. P. "Emotional and Interpersonal Aspects of Rehabilitation," in S. Licht, ed., *Rehabilitation and Medicine*, pp. 229–251. New Haven: Elizabeth Licht, 1968.

23. ———. "Consultation-Liaison Teaching of Psychosomatic Medicine: Opportunities and Obstacles," *J. Nerv. Ment. Dis.*, 154 (1972), 198–205.

24. McKEGNEY, F. P. and P. F. LANGE. "The Decision To No Longer Live on Hemodialysis," *Am. J. Psychiatry*, 128 (1971), 267–274.

25. MAGER, R. F. *Preparing Instructional Objectives*. Palo Alto: Fearon, 1962.

26. MANDELL, A. J. "Western Humanism, Liberal Politics and Psychiatric Training: Relatives, Friends or Enemies?" Paper presented 128th Annu. Meet. Am. Psychiatr. Assoc., Dallas, May 1–5, 1972.

27. MENDEL, W. M. "Psychiatric Consultation Education—1966." *Am. J. Psychiatry*, 123 (1966), 150–155.

28. ———. "A Prescription for Improving the Psychiatric Consultation," *Roche Rep.*, 4 (1967), 1–11.

29. MENDELSON, M. and E. MEYER. "Countertransference Problems of the Liaison Psychiatrist," *Psychosom. Med.*, 23 (1961), 115–122.

30. MEYER, E. M. "The Psychosomatic Concept, Use and Abuse," *J. Chronic Dis.*, 9 (1959), 298–314.

31. MEYEROWITZ, S. "Consultation," Paper presented at Conference on Psychiatric Education, Rochester, New York, March 31, 1971.

32. MOWBRAY, R. M. and B. DAVIES. "Personality Factors in Choice of Medical Specialty," *Br. J. Med. Educ.*, 5 (1971), 110–117.

33. OSMOND, H. "The Medical Model in Psychiatry," *Hosp. Community Psychiatry*, 21 (1970), 275–281.

34. PAYSON, H. E. and J. D. BARCHAS. "A Time Study of Medical Teaching Rounds," *N. Engl. J. Med.*, 273 (1965), 1468–1471.

35. PAYSON, H. E., E. C. GAENSLEN, and F. L. STARGARDTER. "Time Study of Internship on University Medical Service," *N. Engl. J. Med.*, 264 (1961), 439–443.

36. PELLEGRINO, E. D. "Research in Medical Education: The Views of a Friendly Philistine," *J. Med. Educ.*, 46 (1971), 750–756.

37. PETERSON, O. L., L. P. ANDREWS, R. SPAIN et al. "An Analytical Study of North Carolina General Practice, 1953–54," *J. Med. Educ.*, 31 (1956), 1–165.

38. REISER, M. F. "Psychiatry in the Undergraduate Medical Curriculum," Paper presented 128th Annu. Meet. Am. Psychiatr. Assoc., Dallas, May 1–5, 1972.

39. ROMANO, J. "The Teaching of Psychiatry to Medical Students: Past, Present, and Future," *Am. J. Psychiatry*, 126 (1970), 1115–1126.

40. ———. "The Elimination of the Internship— An Act of Regression," *Am. J. Psychiatry*, 126 (1970), 1565–1576.

41. SCHUMACHER, C. F. "Interest and Personality Factors as Related to Choice of Medical Career," *J. Med. Educ.*, 38 (1963), 932–942.

42. SEDLACEK, W. E. and L. W. NATRESS. "A Technique for Determining the Validity of Patient Management Problems," *J. Med. Educ.*, 47 (1972), 263–266.

43. STRATAS, N. E. "Training of Non-Psychiatric Physicians," *Am. J. Psychiatry*, 125 (1969), 1110–1111.

44. WEBSTER, T. "The Behavioral Sciences in Medical Education and Practice," in R. Coombs and C. E. Vincent, eds., *Psychosocial Aspects of Medical Training*, pp. 285–348. Springfield: Charles C. Thomas, 1971.

45. WEED, L. *Medical Records, Medical Education, and Patient Care*. Cleveland: Press of Case Western Reserve University, 1970.

46. WEST, L. J. "The Future of Psychiatric Education," *Am. J. Psychiatry*, 130 (1973), 521–528.

47. WHITE, T. H. *The Bestiary*. New York: Capricorn Books, 1954.

48. ZABARENKO, L., R. A. PITTENGER, and R. N. ZABARENKO. *Primary Medical Practice, A Psychiatric Evaluation*. St. Louis: Warren H. Green, 1968.

NAME INDEX

Note: Boldface figures indicate chapter pages.

SUBJECT INDEX

Abandonment feelings, and organ transplants, 715

Abdomen: bloating in, as conversion reaction, 657, 661; penicillin allergy and, 146; pregnancy fantasies and, 13; reaction to injury to, 10

Aberdeen, Scotland, 446

Abiotrophy, in Pick's disease, 127

Abkhasia region, 68

Aboriginal societies, and illness, 586, 587

Abortion, 303

Absence status, in epilepsy, 320, 321, 333, 339

Abscess: akinetic mutism and, 212; aphasia and, 296; epilepsy and, 337; focal pathology in, 210; psychiatric symptomatology from, 236

Abstract thinking: aphasia and, 192–193, 249–250, 253, 260; brain damage and, 185–189, 193, 205–206, 249–250; catastrophic conditions and, 195; degrees of, 187; delirium and, 45; frontal lobes and, 173; modes of behavior in, 186; schizophrenia and, 200; testing of, 205–206, 285

Acalculia, 233, 234

Acceptability rating of diseases, 601

Acceptance: chronic illness and, 30; terminal illness and, 32, 33

Accidents: alcohol and, 374, 378–379; head trauma from, 166; post-traumatic syndrome and, 172; proneness for, 593; temporal-lobe pathology and, 231

Acculturation, and hypertension, 625

Acetazolamide, 342

Acetazoleamide, 346

Acetylcholine: adrenergic transmission and, 508; autonomic nervous system and, 507; L-Dopa and, 365; encephalitis lethargica and, 157; neurotransmission with, 503,

506; physiological effects of, 507

N-acetylserotonin, 522

N-acetyltransferase, 522

Achalasia, 657, 660, 668, 686–687

Achievement: coronary artery disease and, 602; gout and, 755, 756, 757; response to disease and, 15

Achondroplasia, 469–470

Acid-base balance: epilepsy and, 338; ethanol and, 372

Acidosis: bronchial asthma and, 695; Lowe syndrome and, 468

Acid phophatases (AcP), 425, 428, 429, 430, 431

Acoustic-amnestic aphasia, 251

Acrocephalosyndactylia, 470

Acroparasthesia, 887

ACTH, see Adrenocorticotropic hormone (ACTH)

Acting out, and duodenal ulcer, 672–673

Activation theory of muscle tension, 731–732

Activity: concrete attitude and, 186; doctor-patient relationship and, 18–19; nursing homes and, 86

Activity Drive Scale, 77, 612

Activity theory of aging, 70

Actualized emotions, 191

Acute, use of term, 77

Acute brain syndrome, and delirium, 45

Acute demyelinating encephalomyelitis, 163

Acute intermittent porphyria, 408–409

Acute schizophrenia: amphetamine reaction compared with, 360; cortisol in, 302; methylphenidate and, 361; sleep in, 871, 873

Acute sclerosing panencephalitis (SSPE), 163

Acute illness, 27–28

Adams-Stokes syndrome, 318

Adaptation mechanisms: alcohol and, 380; body-image disturbances and, 828–831; congestive

heart failure and, 623; diabetes and, 307; disease and, 5, 9, 564, 585; habituation differentiated from, 542; headache as, 846; hypertension and, 632; mental retardation and, 438–440, 448–449, 456–457, 458–459, 460; rheumatoid arthritis and, 749, 750; stress and, 6

Adaptive Behavior Scales, 440

Adaptive intervention, in hospitalization, 28

Addiction, see Alcoholism; Drug addiction

Addison's disease, 301, 302–303

Adenosine 3,5 cyclic monophosphate (cyclic AMP): autonomic nervous system and, 521; bronchial asthma and, 696; immune mechanisms and, 719; norepinephrine and, 509

Adenovirus respiratory illness, 575

Adenylcyclase, 509

ADH (antidiuretic hormone), 521, 619

Ad Hoc Committee on Classification of Headache, 842

Adipose tissue, 769–770

Administration of nursing homes, 84–85, 87

Adolescence: adrenogenital syndrome and, 303; alcohol use in, 374, 393; autonomic nervous system in, 547; congestive heart failure in, 624; diabetes in, 307; functional amenorrhea in, 309; gastrointestinal disorders in, 667; head trauma in, 178; heart rate in, 531; Huntington's chorea in, 413; Klinefelter's syndrome and, 303; mental retardation in, 446; outpatient psychiatric clinics and, 73; phantom phenomena in, 830, 831; reaction to disease in, 8; sexual behavior in, 592

Adrenal: arousal and, 555; autonomic nervous system and, 504,

ease and, 123; reading, writing, and praxis disorders and, 253; parkinsonism and, 753; separation of, 216–217

Corpus striatum, and Huntington's chorea, 418, 419

Corpus subthalamicum: Huntington's chorea and, 418, 424; postencephalitic states and, 162

Cortex: abstract attitudes and, 185, 187; alcohol and, 378; Alzheimer's disease and, 113; autonomic nervous system and, 512; body image and, 816, 817; cardiovascular mechanisms and, 513; delirium and, 49; encephalitis lethargica and, 155; granular atrophy of, 97; Huntington's chorea and, 418, 419, 424, 425; integration, 271–272; migraines and, 843; neurosyphilitic conditions and, 136, 142–143, 146; nonspecific thalamo-cortical projection system and, 211; organismic approach to lesions in, 187, 188; phantom phenomena and, 849; Pick's disease and, 121–123; senile plaques in, 109; senile psychosis and, 105, 111; vasomotor control and, 515–516; Wilson's disease and, 408

Corticosteroids: Addison's disease and, 303; Cushing's syndrome and, 300, 301–302; hospitalization and, 27

Corticosterone, 619

Corticotrophin hormone, 521

Corticone-releasing hormone (CRH), 556

Cortisol: Addison's disease and, 302–303; adrenogenital syndrome and, 303; brain influences on, 556; bronchial asthma and, 701; Cushing's syndrome and, 300, 301, 302; diabetes and, 306; endocrine system and, 309, 577; lipid metabolism and, 573; stimulation and, 716

Cortisone, 301

Costs: alcoholism and, 374; reaction to disease by poor and, 11

Counseling: coronary artery disease and, 615; dying process and, 34; mental retardation and, 454, 458, 459

Countertransference, 19

County mental hospitals, 73, 74

Coxsackie B virus, 711

Cramp, occupational, 740–741

Craniofacial dystosis, 470

Craniopharyngioma, 236

Craving, drug, 382, 395

Cremasteric reflexes, in neurosyphilitic conditions, 141

Cretinism, 305, 463

Creutzfeldt-Jakob's disease, 79; Huntington's chorea differen-

tiated from, 415; myoclonic seizures in, 321

Cri-du-chat syndrome, 405, 464

Criminality, and frontal-lobe pathology, 226

Crohn's disease, 668, 683

Cross-linked theory of aging, 69

Cross tolerance in drug use, 380

Crouzon's disease, 470

Crowding: disease susceptibility and, 491–492, 592, 594, 599; immune response and, 716; psychoendocrine studies of, 556; 558, 571, 594

Crying: anarthric aphasia and, 266; pain response and, 14; pseudobulbar states and, 229

Cueing, in mental retardation, 458

Culture: alcoholism and, 375, 383; body image and, 817–821; coronary artery disease and, 609; death and dying and, 32; distribution of illnesses and, 585; doctor-patient relationship and, 19; feeding behavior and, 666; hypertension and, 628; mental retardation and, 447; pain and, 841–842; phantom phenomena and, 850; psychometric tests and, 445; psychosomatic medicine and, 492; venereal disease and, 592

Cushing's syndrome, 300–302, 303

Cyanosis, and epilepsy, 319

Cybernetic theory of aging, 70

Cyclic AMP, see Adenosine 3,5 cyclic monophosphate (cyclic AMP)

Cyclothymic personality: coronary artery disease and, 609, 612; epilepsy and, 329; neurosyphilitic conditions and, 139, 146

Cycrimine HCl, 161

Cysts, supracellar, 236

Cytochrome oxidase, 406

Cytomegalovirus infection, 163, 470–471

Cytoplasmic inclusions of Alzheimer, 123

Cystothionine, 465

Cystothionine synthetase, 465

Dalldorf mental hospital, Berlin, 136

Dancing mania, 600

Danger, and ego reaction, 485

Dawson's inclusion body encephalitis, 163

Day-care programs: mental retardation and, 454, 455; older people and, 73–74

Deafness: delirium and, 56, 59; juvenile general paralysis and, 148; paranoia and, 224–225; pure word, see Pure word deafness; testing for, 283

Death: alcohol and, 377, 393; atti-

tudes toward, 32, 33; burn patients and, 62; cardiovascular surgery and, 637, 638; delirium and, 44; diabetes and, 306; dive reflex and, 535; Edwards syndrome and, 464; fear of, 8, 32; head trauma and, 166; hyperinsulinism and, 307; hyperthyroidism and, 304; intensive care units and, 62, 634, 635; meanings of, 33; older people's attitude toward, 75; response to disease and, 18; Tay-Sachs disease and, 466; terminal illness and, 31; see also Dying process

Death anxiety, 32

Death rates: arteriosclerosis and senile psychosis and, 103; bereavement and, 75, 488

Decision-making: frontal-lobe pathology in, 226; illness and, 25–26

Dedifferentiation, in psychosomatic diseases, 485

Defense mechanisms: autonomic nervous system and, 513, 533; brain damage and, 197; cardiovascular surgery and, 637, 638; congestive heart failure and, 623, 624; coronary artery disease and, 614, 615; delirium and, 47, 57; disease and, 9, 17, 21, 31, 482; endocrine system reciprocity and, 489–490; gastrointestinal disorders and, 664, 665–666; hypertension and, 628, 630, 631, 632; hypothalamus and, 520; LSD use and, 361; muscle tension and, 729–730, 731, 733; pacemakers and, 634; parkinsonism and, 751; psychoendocrine reflections of, 561–565, 567–568, 569; psychosomatic diseases and, 485, 488, 494–495; rheumatism and, 738, 739; rheumatoid arthritis and, 744, 745; schizophrenia and, 201; ulcerative colitis and, 675

Degenerescence grumeuse, 112

Déjà entendu, and epilepsy, 326

Déjà pensée, and epilepsy, 326

Déjà-vu: epilepsy and, 326, 327; posttraumatic epilepsy and, 176; temporal-lobe pathology and, 230, 231

DeLange syndrome, 471

Delinquency, and alcohol use, 374

Deliriant drugs, and psychotic reactions, 359

Delirium, 43–66, 153; Addison's disease and, 302; alcohol-withdrawal syndrome and, 383; belladonna and, 359; brain pathophysiology and, 48–49; bromide, 358; burn patients and, 62; cardiac surgery and, 57–58; classification of, 45–46; course of, 46–47; differential diagnosis for,

Delirium (continued)
47–48; drug use and, 356, 357, 358, 359; electroencephalographic findings in, 49, 520; epilepsy and, 337; examination for, 47; eye surgery and, 56; general surgery and, 59; hallucinations in, 53–56; hepatic coma and, 61–62; herpes simplex encephalitis and, 210; history of, 44–45; hyperthyroidism and, 304; incidence of, 48; intensive care units and, 62, 636; metabolic disturbances in, 48–53; organic features of, 49–51; postcardiotomy, 636–637, 640; prevention of, 63; renal disease and, 59–61; respirator delirium in, 56–57; retarded, 47; somatic delusions in, 24; special syndromes and, 56–62; treatment of, 62–63; tricyclic antidepressants and, 365, 366

Delirium tremens: alcohol-withdrawal syndrome and, 384–385, 386, 391; death from, 393; hepatic coma and, 61; sedative withdrawal and, 358; visual hallucinations in, 234

Delivery of health care: psychosomatic medicine teaching and, 919–920; response to disease and, 13

Delta-aminolevulinic acid, 408

Delta waves, and aging process, 83

Delusions: Addison's disease and, 302; alcohol-withdrawal syndromes and, 385; aphasia and, 256, 274; cerebral arteriosclerosis and, 101; delirium and, 60; encephalitis lethargica and, 158; epilepsy and, 335; gastrointestinal disorders and, 657; headaches and, 842, 843, 845–846; hypothyroidism and, 305; intensive care units and, 636, 637; lobotomy and, 227; LSD use and, 364; neurosyphilitic conditions and, 137–138, 146; old age and, 75; parkinsonism and, 751; postcardiotomy, 57, 636; of pregnancy, 661; pruritus ani in, 661; psychoendocrine studies of, 567; rabies and, 210; somatic, 24, 659; use of term, 300; Wilson's disease and, 406

Dementia: anomia in, 262; brain weight in, 104; cerebral arteriosclerosis and, 82; definition of, 78; delirium differentiated from, 47; echolalia in, 267, 268; epilepsy and, 318, 332; Huntington's chorea and, 228, 414; limbic system and, 213; myoclonic seizures and, 321; neurosyphilitic conditions and, 136–138, 227; older people and, 75–76, 78–79; organic mental syndrome and, 174;

Pick's disease and, 118; senile, see Senile dementia; slow virus and, 79; temporal-lobe pathology and, 232; tests for, 236; Wilson's disease and, 406; word-finding difficulties in, 260

Dementia paralytica, 134

Demographic patterns: alcohol use and, 373; psychosomatic diseases and, 587–591

Demyelination, and delirium, 53

Dendrites, and head trauma, 178

Denial: alcoholism and, 394; blindness and, 219; brain damage and, 196, 197; bronchial asthma and, 701; cancer and, 715; cardiovascular surgery and, 637, 638; chronic illness and, 30, 31; congestive heart failure and, 623; coronary artery disease and, 614–615; disease and, 8, 17, 21–22, 24, 25, 32; hallucinations and, 53; hemiplegia and, 219; Huntington's chorea and, 414; intensive care units and, 634–635; mania and, 569; older people and, 77; pacemakers and, 634; phantom phenomena and, 828–829; 849–850; preoperative fear and, 59; psychological source of, 220; right hemisphere and, 218–220; semantic paraphasia and, 258; types of, 272

Denmark, 135, 347

Density, population, see Crowding

Dentate nucleus: Huntington's chorea and, 419, 421; senile psychosis and, 106

Denver Developmental Screening Tests, 455

Deoxyribonucleic acid, see DNA (deoxyribonucleic acid)

Dependency: alcohol and, 375, 379, 380–383; amenorrhea and, 309; bronchial asthma and, 702, 703; congestive heart failure and, 623; coronary artery disease and, 611, 616; delirium and, 53; dialysis and, 60; disease and, 8, 9, 16, 22, 27, 28, 30; doctor-patient relationship and, 19; duodenal ulcer and, 483–484, 669, 672, 673, 674; hypertension and, 630; intensive care units and, 634; older people and, 85; oral, 654, 655; parkinsonism and, 752; rheumatoid arthritis and, 745, 746, 749; ulcerative colitis and, 676, 677

Depersonalization: body-image disturbances in, 24; Cushing's syndrome and, 301; epilepsy and, 334

Depression, 593; Addison's disease and, 302; aging and, 72, 73, 74–76, 78; alcoholism and, 381, 383; anorexia nervosa and, 794, 797, 798, 802; aphasia and, 225; atten-

tion and, 212; bereavement and, 489; body-image disturbances in, 24; Broca's aphasia and, 273; bronchial asthma and, 703; cancer and, 715, 716; cardiac catheterization and, 633; cardiovascular surgery and, 638; cerebral arteriosclerosis and, 82; congestive heart failure and, 621, 622; coronary artery disease and, 612, 615, 616; cortical blindness and, 272; Cushing's syndrome and, 300, 301, 302; delirium and, 47, 57, 59; as description, 209; diabetes and, 306, 307; disease and, 9, 13, 18, 21, 25, 28, 29, 31, 33; electroconvulsive therapy and, 220; encephalitis lethargica and, 156, 158; endocrine disorders and, 309; epilepsy and, 319, 326, 329, 330, 334, 348; focal brain lesions and, 208; gastrointestinal disorders and, 664, 667; Huntington's chorea and, 405, 413, 414, 415, 416, 417; hyperparathyroidism and, 305; hypertension and, 627, 630, 632; hypothyroidism and, 305; intensive care units and, 634, 636; irritable bowel syndrome and, 686; juvenile meningovascular neurosyphilis and, 149; life changes and, 598; limbic system and, 213; muscle-contraction headaches and, 844, 845; muscle tension and, 730, 732, 733, 734–735, 736; neurosyphilitic conditions and, 136, 138, 139, 228; occult disorders and, 665; organic brain syndrome and, 78, 174; organ transplants and, 714; pacemakers and, 634; pain and, 842; parkinsonism and, 751; phantom phenomena and, 857; porphyria and, 408; premenstrual tension and, 307, 308; psychoendocrine studies of, 559, 567, 569–570; psychomotor epilepsy and, 230, 231; psychosomatic illness and, 588; psychotic reactions to drugs used in treatment of, 365–366; rabies and, 210; respiration and, 518; respirator delirium and, 57; rheumatism and, 737; rheumatoid arthritis and, 742, 745, 746, 748; sleep and, 873–875; somatic delusions in, 24; as symptom, 24; ulcerative colitis and, 677, 682; uremic syndrome and, 60; Wilson's disease and, 407; young adults and, 74

Deprivation, 482; circadian rhythms and, 531; delirium and, 43, 45, 46, 53, 56, 57; food seeking behavior and, 381, 770, 773; nursing homes and, 87

Dermatan sulfate, 467

Dermatomyositis, 713

and, 71, 72; *see also* Socioeconomic factors

ECT, *see* Electro-convulsive therapy (ECT)

Edema, cerebral: congestive heart failure and, 619; focal pathology of, 211; defense reactions and, 665; head trauma and, 172, 177; organic brain syndrome and, 174

Education: concerning alcoholism, 395; alcohol use correlated with, 383, 389; childhood head trauma and, 179; coronary artery disease and, 601, 610, 613; epilepsy and, 331; gout and, 755, 756; mental retardation and, 448, 453, 454, 457, 458, 460; neurosyphilitic conditions and, 137; rheumatoid arthritis and, 744

Edwards syndrome, 464

EEG, *see* Electroencephalography (EEG)

Efferent motor aphasia, 251, 265, 291

Efficiency, and response to disease, 15

Ego: abstract attitude and, 186; aging process and, 70; danger and, 485; delirium and, 63; disease and strength of, 28; hereditary disturbances and, 405; rheumatoid arthritis and, 746, 748, 749; young adult depression and, 74

Egocentricity: hypertension and, 632; response to disease and, 12

Egypt, ancient, 372

Eighteenth Amendment, 372

Eighteenth century, 383

Einheitsbestrebungen in der Medizin, 184

EKG, *see* Electrotrocardiography (EKG)

Elastic membrane: cerebral arteriosclerosis and, 99, 101; senile psychosis and, 111, 112

Elation: anarthric aphasia and, 266; Cushing's syndrome and, 300, 301; epilpsy and, 319; monoamine oxidase inhibitors and, 365; as response to disease, 13

Elderly, *see* Older people

Electric stimulation studies: avoidance behavior in, 545; infectious diseases and, 711; psychoendocrine studies with, 556

Electrocardiography (EKG), 62; congestive heart failure and, 621; coronary artery disease and, 613; delirium in, 59, 62

Electro-convulsive therapy (ECT): aphasia and, 225; body-image disturbances and, 832; bronchial asthma and, 703; hemispheric dominance and, 220, 269; Huntington's chorea and, 417; memory in, 214; muscle tension in, 735;

neurosyphilitic conditions and, 146; phantom phenomena and, 851; pseudobulbar states and, 229

Electroencephalography (EEG): aging process and, 82–83; alcohol and, 384, 391; autonomic nervous system and, 502, 503, 520–521, 532; brain tumors and, 236; bronchial asthma and, 700; bruxism and, 885; childhood head trauma and, 178, 179; Cushing's syndrome and, 301; delirium and, 44, 47, 48, 49, 56, 60, 61; depression in sleep and, 873, 874; endocrine disorders and, 309; enuresis and, 883, 884, 885; epilepsy and, 315, 317, 319, 320–321, 331, 334, 335, 336, 338–340, 341, 344, 345, 346, 347, 349; Huntington's chorea and, 415; narcolepsy and, 859, 861; neurosyphilitic conditions and, 140, 142; older people and, 75; Pick's disease and, 121; Pickwickian syndrome and, 866; post-traumatic epilepsy and, 176; pregnancy and, 878; psychomotor seizures and, 232; senile psychosis and, 112–113; sleep paralysis and, 868, 869; sleep studies with, 210, 391, 854, 855, 871, 877, 886, 888; sleeptalking and, 882; sleepwalking and, 880; temporal-lobe pathology and, 231

Electrolytes: Addison's disease and, 302; alcohol-withdrawal syndrome and, 385; autonomic nervous system and, 529, 530, 547; bronchial asthma and, 703; congestive heart failure and, 618, 619, 621; cortisol and, 300, 301; delirium and, 48, 60; endocrine disease and, 299; epilepsy and, 338, 344; learning and, 545; organ transplants and, 715

Electromyography (EMG), 502, 506; autonomic nervous system and, 520, 521; Huntington's chorea and, 415; muscle tension and, 727–728, 730, 734; occupational cramp in, 740; performance and, 540; rheumatism and, 738, 739, 740; rheumatoid arthritis and, 749, 750; sleep and, 855, 860, 871, 885

Electro-oculography (EOG): Huntington's chorea and, 415; sleep and, 855, 871

Electrophysiological studies: delirium and, 49; head trauma and, 170–171; psychoendocrinology and, 556; psychosomatic medicine and, 478–479

Eleven Item Behavioral Rating Scale, 639

Elimination: mother-child relationship and, 654, 656–657; psycho-

pathological disorders of, 662–664

Emergency services, and cardiovascular disease, 634

EMG, *see* Electromyography (EMG)

Emotionality, and alcohol use, 378

Emotions: abstract attitude impairment and, 189; actualized, 191; automatisms and, 191–192; autonomic nervous system and, 537–539; brain damage and, 183, 190–193; collective, 601; congestive heart failure and, 621; contagion effect with, 571; disease and, 13; hypertension and, 630–631; isolation and, 192; limbic system focal pathology and, 212–213; muscle tension and, 731–733; obesity and, 777, 783; pain and, 941; parkinsonism and, 753; pseudobulbar states and, 229; psychoendocrine studies of, 559–561; right hemisphere and, 219–220

Emphysema, 887

Empty speech of anomia, 260

Encephalitis: akinetic mutism in, 212; aphasia and, 294; brainstem and, 211; chronic epidemic, 116; classification and nomenclature in, 153–154; epilepsy and, 316, 318, 325, 337; hemorrhagic, 162; herpes simplex and, 210; interseizure state in, 329; mental retardation and, 471; myoclonic seizures in, 321; parkinsonism and, 751; postinfectious, 163; states after, *see* Post-encephalitic states; visual hallucinations in, 234

Encephalitis lethargica: conduct disorders in, 157–158; differential diagnosis in, 160; epidemiology of, 154–155; etiology and pathogenesis of, 155–157; eye findings in, 159; history of, 154; hypochondriasis in, 158–159; neurological and vegetative symptoms in, 159–160; pathology of, 155; psychiatric symptoms in, 157–158; schizophrenia-like reactions in, 158; work capacity in, 159

Encephalography, *see* Air encephalography

Encephalomyelitis, 152, 153

Encephalomyocarditis virus, 711

Encephalopathy: alcoholism and, 387; aphasia in, 223; boxing, 176–177; Cushing's syndrome and, 301; diphenylhydantoin and, 345; epilepsy and, 330, 338; metabolic, 223, 338; normal pressure hydrocephalus and, 228; portal-systemic, and delirium, 61–62; spongiform, 79

Encopresis, 657, 663–664

Hospitalization (*continued*)
55, 56–62, 63; epilepsy and, 348; nursing-home care versus, 87; patient's response to, 27–28; premenstrual tension and, 308; psychoendocrine studies of, 558, 559, 571, 578; psychotic drug reactions and, 366

Hospitals: delirium and conditions in, 54–55, 56–62, 63; lower socioeconomic groups and, 11; psychosocial factors in, 478; reaction to disease and environment of, 11

Hostels, for mental retardation, 455

Hostility: alcoholism and, 383, 390; arm tension and, 739; body-image and, 819, 820; cancer and, 716; chronic illness and, 30; coronary artery disease and, 612, 615; disease and, 31; doctor-patient relationship and, 19; gastrointestinal vessels and, 513; Huntington's chorea and, 414; hypertension and, 626, 627, 630, 632; hypochondriasis and, 76; intensive care units and, 636; irritable bowel syndrome and, 686; lobotomy and, 227; muscle-contraction headaches and, 845; oral, 655; parkinsonism and, 751, 753; phantom phenomena and, 850, 851; premenstrual tension and, 307; rheumatoid arthritis and, 742, 743, 744, 745, 746, 748, 749; terminal illness and, 32; ulcerative colitis and, 676, 677, 679

Host-resistance: alcoholism and, 376; early experience and, 492; endocrine system and, 494–495; environment and, 717; emotions and, 710; psychoendocrine studies of, 575; stress and, 489

Human Gastric Function (Wolff and Wolf), 481

Humoral antibody response, 710

Hungarian immigrants, and illness, 585

Hunger: anorexia nervosa and, 792, 793, 802; habituation of, 542; Kleine-Levin syndrome and, 863, 864; obesity and, 776, 777; seizures and, 326

Hunter syndrome, 467

Huntington's chorea: clinical aspects of, 412–417; diagnosis of, 415; frontal-lobe pathology in, 228; incidence of, 405, 422; management of, 415–417; nature of, 413–415; neuropathology of, 418–433; prevalence of, 413, 414; psychoses in, 404, 405, 409; treatment of, 417

Hurler syndrome, 467

Husbands, and response to disease, 17–18

Hutchinson's teeth, in juvenile general paralysis, 148

Hyalinization: Alzheimer's disease and, 117–118; Alzheimer's neurofibrillar disease and, 108; cerebral arteriosclerosis and, 92, 93–94, 99; Pick's disease and, 126; senile changes of small blood vessels and, 103–104; senile psychoses and, 111, 112

Hydantoins, and epilepsy, 342

Hydrocephalus: brain tumors and, 215; communicating, 175–176; head trauma and, 173, 177; Huntington's chorea and, 420; normal pressure (NPH), 228

Hydrochloric acid, in duodenal ulcer, 668, 674

Hydrocortisone, 28, 619

Hydrogen peroxide, in aging process, 69

17-hydroxycorticosteroids (17-OHCS): arousal and, 555; avoidance conditioning in cardiovascular disease and, 641; conditioned emotional disturbances and, 557–558; depression reactions and, 569–570; developmental studies with, 570; leukemia stress reactions and, 561–564, 566; psychotic processes and, 567–569; response to disease and, 17; response to hospitalization and, 27; sleep and, 886; social interaction studies with, 571; stress and, 557, 559–560

5-hydroxyindoleacetic acid, and LSD, 364

Hydroxyindole-O-methyltransferase (HIOMT), and light, 522, 523

5-hydroxytryptamine, and LSD, 364

Hyoscyamine, 161

Hyperactivity: alcohol and, 377, 378; brain damage and, 78; childhood head trauma and, 179; monoamine oxidase inhibitors and, 365; muscle tension and, 728; treatment of, 366

Hyperadrenalcorticism, 301

Hyperadrenalism, 340

Hyperbaric therapy, 81–82, 637

Hypercalcemia: parathyroid gland and, 305; Williams-Beuren syndrome and, 472

Hypercholesterolemia: cerebral arteriosclerosis and, 102, 103; coronary artery disease and, 613; hypertension and, 626

Hyperemia, 666

Hyperexcitability, and alcoholism, 381

Hyperglycemia: Cushing's syndrome and, 300; norepinephrine and, 509

Hyperinsulinism, 307

Hyperkinesis: epilepsy and, 330;

hyperthyroidism and, 304; predisposition to, 492; viral infections and, 153

Hyperlipidemia, 386

Hyperlipoproteinemia, 572

Hypermetamorphosia, 213

Hypermotility, 478

Hyperparathyroidism, 305

Hyperperistalsis, 665

Hyperphagia, and limbic system, 213

Hyperpituitism, 340

Hyperplasia, adrenocortical, 300

Hyperponsesis, 734

Hyperprexia, 304

Hypersalivation, 160, 482

Hypersensitivity: delirium and, 45; immune mechanisms and, 710, 712

Hypersexuality: epilepsy and, 335; limbic system and, 213, 214

Hypersomnia, chronic, 855, 861–863

Hypertension, 480; aging process and, 83; arteriosclerosis and, 102, 103; autonomic nervous system and, 514–515; biological factors in, 626–627; bronchial asthma and, 703; class and, 589; conditioning and, 503, 545; coronary artery disease and, 488, 613; Cushing's syndrome and, 300, 301; definition of, 624; delirium and, 60; early experience and, 492; emotion and, 539, 630–631; environmental factors in, 631–632; epidemiological factors in, 625; epilepsy and, 318, 340; frequency of, 586; genetic factors in, 541; hyaline degeneration and, 93–94; longitudinal studies of, 625–626; morbid sympathy and, 600; obesity and, 777, 778; parkinsonism and, 751; personality and, 631; population density and, 594; psychiatric relationships with, 627; psychobiological variables in, 625; psychological factors in, 608, 624–633; psychophysiological relationships in, 627–630; psychosomatic factors in, 484; racial differences in, 590; sex differences in, 588; stress and, 491; therapy for, 632–633, 640

Hyperthermia, 56

Hyperthyroidism, 304

Hypertriglyceridemia, 386

Hyperuricemia: gout and, 488, 755, 756; mental retardation and, 468

Hyperventilation: alcoholism and, 381, 385; epilepsy and, 339; morbid sympathy and, 600; respiration and, 518

Hypervitaminosis D, 102

Hypnalgia, 888

Hypnogogic hallucinations, in narcolepsy, 858, 859, 861

Hypnoidal state of consciousness, 490, 496

Hypnosis: body-image disturbances and, 832; bronchial asthma and, 704; cardiovascular disease and, 640; meditation changes similar to, 537; rheumatism and, 739; tuberculin reaction and, 711

Hypnotic drugs, and cross tolerances, 380

Hypoactivity, and muscle tension, 728

Hypoadrenalism: chronic schizophrenia and, 567; epilepsy and, 340

Hypocalcemia, and seizures, 316, 319, 341

Hypochloremia, 59

Hypochondriasis: abdominal bloating in, 661; aging and, 72–73; bodily preoccupations in, 810; conversion reactions in, 658, 659; coronary artery disease and, 612; encephalitis lethargica and, 158–159; focal pathology and, 210; gastrointestinal disorders and, 657; neurosyphilitic conditions and, 278; occult disorders and, 665; older people and, 75, 76–77; pain in, 842, 847–848; recovery from disease and, 29; rheumatoid arthritis and, 745; symptoms and, 24; use of medical facilities in, 25

Hypoglycemia: Addison's disease and, 302; Beckwith-Wiederman syndrome and, 472; delirium and, 49; epilepsy and, 337–338, 339, 340, 341; failure-to-grow syndrome and, 309; insulin and, 307; narcolepsy and, 859, 861; seizures and, 316, 319

Hypokalemia, 59

Hypokinesia, in Huntington's chorea, 422

Hypomagnecemia, 385

Hypomania: encephalitis lethargica and, 158; neurosyphilitic conditions and, 138

Hyponatremia: delirium and, 59; epilepsy and, 340

Hypoparathyroidism, 305–306

Hypophagia, 659

Hypopituitarism, 340

Hypoplastic degenerative cerebral arteriosclerosis, 99, 101

Hypotension: Addison's disease and, 302; operative, 58; phenothiazines and, 63

Hypothalamus, 212; asthma and, 695; autonomic afferent activity and, 511; body temperature control and, 518, 519; body weight and, 770–771, 772, 775, 776; cardiovascular mechanisms and,

513, 518; central nervous system and, 489; coronary artery disease and, 616; Cushing's syndrome and, 302; duodenal ulcer and, 668; encephalitis lethargica and, 155; endocrine system and, 555–556; failure-to-grow syndrome and, 309; focal pathology in, 213; frontal-lobe pathology and, 226; gastric secretion and, 519–520; Huntington's chorea and, 421; hypertension and, 626, 628, 630; immune responses and, 717–718, 719, 720; Korsakoff's psychosis and, 215; mutism and, 212; nonspecific thalamo-cortical projection system and, 211; norepinephrine and, 512; parkinsonism and, 753; peduncular hallucinosis and, 235; pituitary trophic hormone control and, 521; rabies and, 210; respiration and, 517, 518; sexual behavior and, 520; skeletal muscles and, 517; vasomotor control and, 515, 516; Wernicke-Korsakoff syndrome and, 389

Hyperthyroidism, 304–305; arteriosclerosis and, 102; narcolepsy and, 859, 861

Hypoventilation, 24

Hypoxia: bronchial asthma and, 695; epilepsy and, 317, 318, 324, 325, 330, 340; head trauma and, 173; posttraumatic epilepsy and, 176

Hysterectomy, 20

Hysteria, 595; abdominal bloating in, 661; anorexia nervosa and, 788, 789, 790; conversion reactions in, 658, 659; epidemic, 594, 600–601; epilepsy and, 24, 340; muscle tension in, 733; occupational cramp and, 740; reaction to disease and, 9; rheumatism and, 737; rheumatoid arthritis and, 745; tarantism and, 600

Hystero-epilepsy, 340

Id, and delirium, 47

Ideas of reference: amphetamines and, 359; cannabis and, 364; LSD use and, 363; rabies and, 210

Ideation, in eating and elimination disorders, 657, 662, 664

Identical twin studies, see Monozygotic twin studies

Identification: congestive heart failure and, 622; duodenal ulcer and, 672; response to disease and, 16, 24; rheumatoid arthritis and, 742, 744, 748

Identity: body-image and, 10; disease response and, 9, 22; psychosomatic diseases in, 595, 597; sex, see Sex identity

Identity crisis, and disease, 489

Ideomotor aprazia, 296

Ideopathic epilepsy, 317–318

Ileostomy, 682–683, 827

Illness, see Disease

Illusion: amphetamine and, 360; epilepsy and, 326, 327; psychomotor epilepsy and, 230

Ilosone, 146

Images theory of brain damage, 183, 184

Imidazole pyruvic acid, 466

Imipramine: Huntington's chorea and, 417; migraine and, 844; narcolepsy and, 861; painful phantoms and, 857

Imitation: response to disease and, 16; tarantism and, 600

Immune mechanisms: allergic disorders and, 712–713; ataxia telangiectasia and, 468; autoimmune diseases and, 713–714; bronchial asthma and, 695, 697; cancer and, 715–716; cell-mediated immune response and, 710–711; central nervous system and, 717–720; disorders of, 710–725; encephalitis lethargica and, 154; humoral antibody response in, 710; hypothalamus and, 520; infectious diseases and, 711–712; neurosyphilitic conditions and, 143; postinfectious encephalitis and, 163; organ transplants and, 714–715; psychosocial factors in, 716–717; rheumatoid arthritis and, 488; ulcerative colitis and, 675

Immunoglobulins, 710

Immunologic theory of aging, 69–70

Impotence: alcohol and, 379; Klinefelter's syndrome and, 303; limbic system and, 214; response to, 20; Scythian life and, 584

Impulsive behavior: brain damage and, 78; encephalitis lethargica and, 157; epilepsy and, 334, 335; hypertension and, 632; juvenile meningovascular neurosyphilis and, 149; limbic system and, 213; mental retardation and, 449; muscle tension and, 729; neurosyphilitic conditions and, 141; reaction to disease and, 9; temporal-lobe pathology and, 232

Inactivity, and seizures, 323

Inattention, and schizophrenia, 274

Inclusion body encephalitis, 153, 163

Incubus attacks, 861

Independence: dialysis and, 60; duodenal ulcers and, 483, 669, 671–672, 673, 674; hospitalization and, 27; hypertension and, 630; parkinsonism and, 751, 752; reaction to disease and, 8, 9; ulcerative colitis and, 682

with, 136, 137, 141, 144, 145, 146

Malignant neoplasms, adolescent, 8

Malnutrition: amenorrhea and, 309; Cockayne syndrome and, 468; delirium and, 44; Korsakoff's psychosis and, 215

Malpractice suits, 29

Mammillary bodies: memory and, 215, 216; Wernicke-Korsakoff syndrome and, 389

Management of patients, 4

Mandala formulation, 813

Manganese poisoning, 160

Mania: biogenic amines and, 573; Cushing's syndrome and, 300; dancing, 600; L-Dopa and, 365; hypertension and, 627; limbic system and, 213; monoamine oxidase inhibitors and, 365; neurosyphilitic conditions and, 136, 137, 139, 228; organic mental syndrome and, 174; psychoendocrine studies of, 569; uremic syndrome and, 60; semantic jargon and, 262; temporal-lobe pathology and, 231; uremic syndrome and, 60

Manic-depressive psychoses: euphoria in neurosyphilitic conditions differentiated from, 137; sleep and, 873, 874

Marchiafava-Bignami disease, and alcoholism, 386

Mannitol, and intracranial pressure, 172

Manual of Psychophysiological Methods (Venables and Martin), 525

Manual on Terminology and Classification in Mental Retardation (American Association on Mental Deficiency), 438, 439, 440

Man-Woman-Child Test, 822

Maple syrup urine disease, 404, 465

Maracaibo, Venezuela, 413

March of Dimes, 416

Marfan's disease, 470

Marginality, and psychosomatic disease, 591

Marijuana, and psychotic reactions, 364

Marriage: alcoholism and, 392; cardiovascular surgery and, 638; disease and, 9, 16, 17–18; epilepsy and, 347; Huntington's chorea and, 416; longevity and, 68; mental retardation and, 455, 458, 460; rheumatoid arthritis and, 744; ulcerative colitis and, 678

Masculinization, and patient's response, 20

Masochism: bronchial asthma and, 703; rheumatoid arthritis and, 746

Mass hysteria, 600–601

Mastectomy: body-image and, 829; convalescence from, 28–29; patient's response to, 20

Masturbation: anal, 661; mental retardation and, 449, 459

Maudsley Personality Inventory, 715

Mayo Clinic, 59, 858

Maze-learning, and parietal-lobe pathology, 234

Meaning: of death, 33; of illness, 20–22

Measles, 153, 155, 163, 337, 471

Mebaral, 342

Mecholyl, 698

Medial forebrain bundle, and norepinephrine, 506, 522

Medicaid, and nursing homes, 74

Medical education, and psychosomatic medicine, 905–922

Medical History of the (First) Great War, 586

Medical students: congestive heart failure in, 619; coronary artery disease in, 609; endocrine studies in, 557; hypertension in, 625–626

Medicare, and nursing homes, 74, 78

Medicine: alcoholism and, 376; alcohol use in, 373; ecologic, 584; holistic approach to, 184; psychosocial and epidemiological concepts in, 583–607; psychosocial foundations of, 3–42; socioeconomic class and knowledge of, 11

Medieval society, 68

Meditation, and autonomic nervous system, 537, 641

Medulla: cardiovascular mechanisms and, 513; Huntington's chorea and, 421, 422; nonspecific thalamo-cortical projection system and, 211; respiration and, 517; skeletal muscles and, 517; vasomotor activity and, 514, 515, 516

Megacolon disorders, 663

Megalosplanchnic type, and arteriosclerosis, 103

Megasigmoid, 663–664

Melancholia: hypertension and, 627; psychoendocrine studies of, 569; tarantism and, 600

Melanin, 106

Melatonin, 504, 522

Melody recognition, and right hemisphere, 218

Memory: alcoholism and, 387, 389–391; Alzheimer's disease and, 80; aphasia and, 193; brain damage and, 183, 201; delirium and, 45, 47, 60; denial and, 219, 273; drug use and, 357; epilepsy and,

317, 328, 330, 332–336; figure-ground organization in, 190; focal pathology in, 208; frontal lobe and, 226; herpes simplex encephalitis and, 210; Huntington's chorea and, 414; hyperparathyroidism and, 305; hypothyroidism and, 305; intensive care units and, 637; limbic system and, 215–216; neurosyphilitic conditions and, 137, 138, 227; organic brain syndrome and, 78, 174; pain and, 838, 839; reticular substance and, 211; right hemisphere and, 216; semantic aphasia and, 257; temporal-lobe pathology in, 229, 231, 233

Men: aging process in, 70, 77; alcohol use in, 373–374, 379, 388; anorexia nervosa in, 790, 792, 799–803, 805; bronchial asthma in, 700; cerebral arteriosclerosis in, 82; congestive heart failure in, 623; coronary heart disease in, 589; depression in, 75; dialysis in, 61; differences between women and, *see* Sex differences; duodenal ulcer in, 671, 744; enuresis in, 882; epilepsy in, 316; fainting in, 593; as fathers, *see* Father-child relationship; gerocomy in, 68; gout in, 754, 755–756; Hunter syndrome in, 467; Huntington's chorea in, 414; 17-hydroxycorticosteroids (17-OHCS) in, 571; hypertension in, 625, 632; individual differences in autonomic functioning in, 541; insomnia in, 857, 858; Kleine-Levin syndrome in, 863, 864; Klinefelter's syndrome in, 303; life expectancy for, 68; Lowe syndrome and, 468; mental hospital admission in old age for, 73; muscle tension in, 735; myocardial infarction in, 610; neurosyphilitic conditions in, 136; obesity in, 767, 768, 769, 774–775; personality changes in, 209; pregnancy fantasies in, 660; pruritus ani in, 661; psychosomatic diseases in, 588–589; reactions to disease in, 8–9; recovery from disease by, 28; response to disease by, 17–18, 20; rheumatoid arthritis in, 741, 744, 745, 747, 749, 750; Scythian, 584; self-assessment in older age by, 77; sexual activity in, 535; sick role in, 18; ulcerative colitis in, 677, 678

Meninges of brain: meningovascular neurosyphilis and, 147; neurosyphilitic conditions and, 134, 142, 144

Meningiomas: brain tumors and, 236; epilepsy and, 318

Micropsia: encephalitis lethargica and, 159; epilepsy and, 318, 326; temporal-lobe pathology and, 230–231

Midbrain: cardiovascular mechanisms and, 513; endocrine system and, 556; focal pathology and, 210–211; hypertension and, 515; immune mechanisms and, 717; respiration and, 517; skeletal muscles and, 517

Middle-aged people: bronchial asthma in, 700; congestive heart failure in, 623; coronary artery disease in, 612; divorces in, 592; reaction to disease in, 8; rheumatoid arthritis in, 741; syphilis in, 227

Middle Ages, 315, 584, 600, 601

Middle class: alcoholism in, 375, 388; oversocialization in, 595; psychosomatic diseases in, 591

Midline encephalitis, 214

Midtown Manhattan Study, 586, 587, 588, 589, 597

Migraine headaches, 843; clinical features of, 843; psychological features of, 843–844; treatment of, 844

Migrant laborers, and health, 590

Migration: bronchial asthma and, 700; coronary artery disease and, 602; disease and, 592; mental illness and, 592–593

Miliary sclerosis, in senile psychosis, 109

Milieu therapy, in bronchial asthma, 704

Military life: hysteria in, 595; psychoendocrine studies of, 558, 570, 575; psychiatry in, 477; rheumatism in, 736–738

Mill Hill test, 332

Milontin, 342

Mind-body dichotomy: health and, 3; psychophysiology and, 525; psychosomatic medicine and, 479–480

Minimal brain dysfunction (MBD), and viral infections, 153, 164

Minimal cerebral dysfunction syndrome, in childhood head trauma, 179

Minimization, as response to illness, 12

Minnesota Multiphasic Personality Inventory (MMPI): bruxism on, 885; coronary artery disease and, 612; epilepsy and, 330; hypertension and, 631; insomnia and, 856; muscle tension and, 733; psychomotor seizures and, 232; rheumatic arthritis and, 745–746, 748

Minority groups, and mental retardation, 439, 458

Minute memory, 214

Mitochondria, in Huntington's chorea, 429–430

MMPI, see Minnesota Multiphasic Personality Test (MMPI)

Mobility: coronary artery disease and, 610, 616; disease and, 592; gout and, 755; heart disease and, 601, 602

Modeling experiences, in mental retardation, 458

Moderation, in coronary artery disease, 616

Moneysworth (newsletter), 855

Mongolism, see Down's syndrome

Monitoring equipment, and delirium, 58

Monkeys: blood pressure in, 515; coma in, 170; Creutzfeldt-Jakob's disease and, 79; emotion and autonomic responses in, 538; fetal androgenitization in, 303; limbic system studies in, 213; psychoendocrine studies in, 556, 560, 574, 575; virus studies in, 711

Monoamine oxidase: adrenergic transmission and, 508, 509; hyperthyroidism and, 304; premenstrual tension and, 308

Monoamine oxidase inhibitors (MAOI): hypertension and, 627; psychotic reactions to, 365–366

Mononucleosis, infectious, 28, 711

Monotony: delirium and, 53, 54, 62, 63; hospital environment and, 11

Monozygotic twin studies: arteriosclerosis in, 103; autonomic functioning in, 541; bronchial asthma in, 695; coronary artery disease in, 613; dementia in, 79; duodenal ulcer in, 668, 670; epilepsy in, 318; rheumatoid arthritis in, 747; risk in psychosomatic diseases and, 488; see also Twin studies

Mood: focal pathology in, 210; menstrual cycle in, 573; premenstrual tension and, 307; temporal-lobe pathology and, 231, 232

Moray Firth, Scotland, 413

Morbidity: cardiovascular surgery and, 637, 639; chronic illness and, 30; psychosomatic disease and, 586; recent bereavement and, 9, 488–489

Morphine, 839

Mortality: cardiac catheterization and, 633; cardiac surgery and, 637, 638; early experience and, 546; infant, 595, 596; obesity and, 777–778; population density and, 594; psychosomatic disease and, 587; recent bereavement and, 9, 488–489

Mother-child relationship: body-image and, 814, 819–821; bronchial asthma and, 693, 699, 700–

701, 702, 703, 705; celiac sprue and, 684, 685; coronary artery disease and, 611; dialysis and, 60–61; disease and, 485, 494; Down's syndrome and, 463, 464; duodenal ulcer and, 487, 674, 668–670; elimination and, 654, 656–657; feeding behavior in, 654, 655; handling and adrenocortical activity in later life and, 546; heart rate in infant and, 631; hypertension and, 630, 632; illness of mother in, 16; mental retardation and, 446; personality development and, 70; rheumatoid arthritis and, 744, 745, 746, 748; stress reactions to leukemia and, 561–564, 566; ulcerative colitis and, 676, 677–678, 681

Mother-daughter relationship: amenorrhea and, 309; bronchial asthma in, 702

Motilitin, 674

Motion pictures, see Films

Motivation: alcoholism and, 381, 382, 383, 390, 392; aphasia testing and, 282; cardiovascular conditioning and, 641; conversion reactions and, 659; encephalitis lethargica and, 157; gout and, 755, 756; muscle tension and, 731; recovery from disease and, 29; rheumatoid arthritis and, 745, 747

Motor aphasia: afferent, 251, 265, 291; description of, 266; early work on, 246, 248; efferent, 251, 265, 291; posterior inferior frontal gyrus lesion in, 252

Motor behavior: alcohol and, 377, 378, 386; Alzheimer's disease and, 80; brain tumors and, 236; childhood head trauma and, 178; defense reactions and, 665; delirium and, 45, 53; emotional language and, 191; encephalitis lethargica and, 159–160; epilepsy and, 319, 320; figure and ground in, 189; focal pathology and, 208, 212; Huntington's chorea in, 414; left hemisphere in, 217; mental retardation and, 447; musculoskeletal disorders and, 727; neurosyphilitic conditions and, 138; organic mental syndrome and, 174; parkinsonism and, 753–754; pseudobulbar states in, 229; psychomotor epilepsy and, 230; seizures and, 316, 323

Mourning: mortality and morbidity and, 9, 75, 488–489; phantom phenomena and, 828, 829, 851; psychoendocrine studies of, 569; response to disease and, 21

Mouth, in neonatal behavior, 813, 814